A Practical Approach to Emergency Medicine

A Practical Approach to Emergency Medicine

Edited by

Robert J. Stine, M.D.

Associate Professor of Medicine,
University of Massachusetts Medical
School; Chief, Department of
Emergency Medicine, Worcester City
Hospital, Worcester, Massachusetts

Robert H. Marcus, M.D.

Clinical Instructor in Medicine,
New York Medical College,
Valhalla, New York; Director,
Emergency Department, Northern
Westchester Hospital Center,
Mt. Kisco, New York

Little, Brown and Company
Boston / Toronto

To Nancy for her love, understanding,
support and encouragement, and our
children, Nancy Lynn, Robert, and
Melissa, who deserve more of my
attention.   R.J.S.

To the housestaff at Barnes Hospital
for their tireless dedication to the
excellence of patient care.
                    R.H.M., R.J.S.

Contents

Contributing Authors

Marc K. Allen, M.D.

Clinical Instructor in Medicine, Case Western Reserve University School of Medicine; Research Director, Department of Emergency Medical Services, Mt. Sinai Medical Center, Cleveland, Ohio
Intracompartment Tissue Pressure Measurement

Charles B. Anderson, M.D.

Professor of Surgery and Chief, Division of General Surgery, Washington University School of Medicine; General Surgeon-in-Chief, Barnes Hospital, St. Louis, Missouri
Abdominal Emergencies

Vilray P. Blair III, M.D.

Assistant Professor of Orthopedic Surgery, Washington University School of Medicine; Assistant Surgeon of Orthopedic Surgery; Barnes Hospital and St. Louis Children's Hospital, St. Louis, Missouri
Orthopedic Emergencies

John A. Boerner, M.D.

Clinical Instructor and Cardiologist, Department of Family Medicine, University of Colorado School of Medicine, Pueblo, Colorado
Cardiac Arrhythmias; Temporary Ventricular Pacemaker Insertion

Michael E. Cain, M.D.

Assistant Professor of Medicine, Washington University School of Medicine; Director, Clinical Electrophysiology Laboratory, and Assistant Cardiologist, Barnes Hospital, St. Louis, Missouri
Cardiac Arrhythmias; Temporary Ventricular Pacemaker Insertion

J. William Campbell, M.D.

Clinical Instructor in Medicine, Washington University School of Medicine; Assistant Physician, Barnes Hospital, St. Louis, Missouri
Infectious Diseases; Microbiologic Stains

Octavio de Marchena, M.D.

Assistant Professor of Clinical Neurology, Washington University School of Medicine; Assistant Neurologist, Barnes Hospital and The Jewish Hospital of St. Louis, St. Louis, Missouri
Neurologic Emergencies; Lumbar Puncture

Paul R. Eisenberg, M.D., M.P.H.	Assistant Professor of Medicine, Washington University School of Medicine; Assistant Director, Cardiac Care Unit, Barnes Hospital, St. Louis, Missouri *Shock*
Michael B. Freeman, M.D.	Instructor in Surgery, Washington University School of Medicine; Assistant Surgeon, Barnes Hospital, St. Louis, Missouri *Abdominal Emergencies*
Robert D. Fry, M.D.	Assistant Professor of Surgery, Washington University School of Medicine; Program Director, Division of Colon and Rectal Surgery, The Jewish Hospital of St. Louis, St. Louis, Missouri *Acute Anorectal Disorders*
Lawrence A. Gans, M.D.	Assistant Professor of Ophthalmology, Washington University School of Medicine; Assistant Ophthalmologist, Barnes Hospital, St. Louis, Missouri *Ocular Emergencies; Tonometry*
Leonard D. Gaum, M.D.	Assistant Professor of Urology, Washington University School of Medicine; Assistant Surgeon, Division of Urology, The Jewish Hospital of St. Louis, St. Louis, Missouri *Urologic Emergencies; Percutaneous Suprapubic Cystostomy*
Joseph G. Gibbons, M.D.	Assistant Professor of Clinical Pediatrics, Washington University School of Medicine; Attending Pediatrician, Emergency Unit, St. Louis Children's Hospital, St. Louis, Missouri *Pediatric Emergencies*
J. Blake Goslen, M.D.	Assistant Professor of Medicine, Washington University School of Medicine; Assistant Dermatologist, Barnes Hospital, St. Louis, Missouri *Dermatology*
L. Lee Hamm III, M.D.	Assistant Professor of Medicine, Washington University School of Medicine; Assistant Physician, Barnes Hospital, St. Louis, Missouri *Acid-Base, Fluid, and Electrolyte Disturbances; Renal Disorders*
Barbel Holtmann, M.D.	Associate Professor of Surgery (Plastic and Reconstructive), Washington University School of Medicine; Plastic Surgeon, Barnes Hospital and St. Louis Children's Hospital, St. Louis, Missouri *Soft-Tissue Disorders; Regional Anesthesia; Wound-Closure Techniques*

Allan S. Jaffe, M.D.

Associate Professor of Medicine, Washington University School of Medicine; Director, Cardiac Care Unit, and Cardiologist, Barnes Hospital, St. Louis, Missouri
Myocardial, Pericardial, and Valvular Disorders; Pericardiocentesis

Arthur B. Jenny, M.D.

Assistant Professor of Neurological Surgery, Washington University School of Medicine; Assistant Surgeon, Department of Neurological Surgery, Washington University Medical Center, St. Louis, Missouri
Neurosurgical Emergencies

Jeffrey L. Kaine, M.D.

Instructor in Medicine, Washington University School of Medicine; Assistant Physician, Division of Rheumatology, Barnes Hospital and The Jewish Hospital of St. Louis, St. Louis, Missouri
Rheumatologic Disorders; Arthrocentesis and Intraarticular Injection

Robert M. Kennedy, M.D.

Instructor in Pediatrics, Washington University School of Medicine; Attending Pediatrician, Emergency Unit, St. Louis Children's Hospital, St. Louis, Missouri
Pediatric Emergencies

Ira J. Kodner, M.D.

Associate Professor of Surgery, Washington University School of Medicine; Director, Division of Colon and Rectal Surgery, The Jewish Hospital of St. Louis, St. Louis, Missouri
Acute Anorectal Disorders

Richard E. Larson, M.D.

Instructor in Medicine, University of Massachusetts Medical School; Associate Director and Attending Physician, Department of Emergency Medicine, Worcester City Hospital, Worcester, Massachusetts
Autotransfusion

Bruce D. Lindsay, M.D.

Instructor in Medicine, Washington University School of Medicine; Assistant Cardiologist, Barnes Hospital, St. Louis, Missouri
Myocardial, Pericardial, and Valvular Disorders; Pericardiocentesis

Alan P. Lyss, M.D.

Assistant Professor of Medicine, Washington University School of Medicine; Director of Clinical Oncology, Division of Hematology and Oncology, The Jewish Hospital of St. Louis, St. Louis, Missouri
Hematologic and Oncologic Emergencies

Robert H. Marcus, M.D.	Clinical Instructor in Medicine, New York Medical College, Valhalla, New York; Director and Attending Physician, Emergency Department, Northern Westchester Hospital Center, Mt. Kisco, New York *Emergency Medical Services Systems; Cardiopulmonary Resuscitation; Toxicologic Emergencies; Cricothyrotomy; Percutaneous Central Venous Catheterization; Venous Cutdowns*
J.E. Martin, Jr., M.D.	Resident, Thoracic and Cardiovascular Surgery, University of Kansas School of Medicine and Medical Center, Kansas City, Kansas *Cardiothoracic Emergencies*
Victor N. Meltzer, M.D.	Medical Director, Mid-Cities Dialysis Center; Grand Prairie, Texas *Hypertension*
Diane F. Merritt, M.D.	Instructor in Obstetrics and Gynecology, Washington University School of Medicine; Director, Pediatric and Adolescent Gynecology, St. Louis Children's Hospital; Assistant Obstetrician and Gynecologist, Washington University Medical Center, St. Louis, Missouri *Obstetric and Gynecologic Emergencies; Culdocentesis*
William W. Monafo, Jr., M.D.	Professor of Surgery, Washington University School of Medicine; Director, Burn Center and Emergency Department, Barnes Hospital; Surgeon, Barnes Hospital and St. Louis Children's Hospital, St. Louis, Missouri *Thermal Injuries*
Jon F. Moran, M.D.	Associate Professor, Thoracic and Cardiovascular Surgery, University of Kansas School of Medicine and Medical Center; Chairman, Department of Thoracic and Cardiovascular Surgery, University of Kansas Medical Center, Kansas City, Kansas *Cardiothoracic Emergencies; Tube Thoracostomy; Emergency Thoracotomy*
Harlan R. Muntz, M.D.	Assistant Professor of Otolaryngology, Washington University School of Medicine; Assistant Otolaryngologist, Barnes Hospital and St. Louis Children's Hospital, St. Louis, Missouri *Maxillofacial and Neck Trauma; Otolaryngologic Emergencies; Nasal Packing*
Matthew J. Orland, M.D.	Instructor in Medicine, Washington University School of Medicine; Assistant Director of Medical Service and Assistant Physician, Barnes Hospital, St. Louis, Missouri *Endocrine and Metabolic Emergencies*

William G. Powderly, M.B., B.Ch.	Fellow in Infectious Diseases, Washington University School of Medicine; Fellow in Medicine, Barnes Hospital, St. Louis, Missouri *Infectious Diseases; Microbiologic Stains*
Fredric G. Regenstein, M.D.	Assistant Professor of Medicine, Washington University School of Medicine; Staff Physician, Gastroenterology Section, St. Louis Veterans Administration Medical Center; Assistant Physician, Barnes Hospital, St. Louis, Missouri *Gastrointestinal Disorders*
Daniel P. Schuster, M.D.	Assistant Professor of Medicine, Washington University School of Medicine; Director, Respiratory Intensive Care Unit and Medical Intensive Care Unit, and Assistant Physician, Barnes Hospital, St. Louis, Missouri *Pulmonary Emergencies; Thoracentesis*
Allen Sclaroff, D.D.S.	Associate Professor of Oral and Maxillofacial Surgery, Washington University School of Dental Medicine; Oral and Maxillofacial Surgeon, Barnes Hospital and St. Louis Children's Hospital, St. Louis, Missouri *Oral Surgical Disorders*
Timothy I. Shoen, M.D.	Instructor in Medicine, University of Massachusetts Medical School; Attending Physician, Department of Emergency Medicine, Worcester City Hospital, Worcester, Massachusetts *Vascular Disorders*
Gregorio A. Sicard, M.D.	Associate Professor of Surgery, Washington University School of Medicine; Director, Vascular Service, and Surgeon, Barnes Hospital and St. Louis Children's Hospital, St. Louis, Missouri *Vascular Disorders*
Robert J. Stine, M.D.	Associate Professor of Medicine, University of Massachusetts Medical School; Chief and Attending Physician, Department of Emergency Medicine, Worcester City Hospital, Worcester, Massachusetts *Environmental Emergencies; Toxicologic Emergencies; Trauma; Endotracheal Intubation; MAST Suit; Percutaneous Transtracheal Ventilation; Peritoneal Lavage*
William B. Strecker, M.D.	Assistant Professor of Orthopedic Surgery, Washington University School of Medicine; Assistant Surgeon of Orthopedic Surgery, Barnes Hospital and St. Louis Children's Hospital, St. Louis, Missouri *Orthopedic Emergencies; Regional Anesthesia*

Russell E. Tackett, M.D.

Resident, Department of Surgery, Division of Urology, Washington University School of Medicine and Medical Center, St. Louis, Missouri
Urologic Emergencies; Percutaneous Suprapubic Cystostomy

John C. Vander Woude, M.D.

Resident, Cardiovascular Surgery, Texas Heart Institute, University of Texas Medical School at Houston, Houston, Texas
Vascular Disorders

Howard G. Welgus, M.D.

Assistant Professor of Medicine, Washington University School of Medicine; Director, Division of Dermatology, The Jewish Hospital of St. Louis, St. Louis, Missouri
Dermatology

Kathryn Kottemann Wire, J.D., M.B.A.

Risk Manager, Barnes Hospital, St. Louis, Missouri
Medicolegal Issues

V. Leroy Young, M.D.

Associate Professor of Surgery (Plastic and Reconstructive), Washington University School of Medicine; Plastic Surgeon, Barnes Hospital and St. Louis Children's Hospital, St. Louis, Missouri
Hand Injuries and Infections; Regional Anesthesia

Mark S. Zoccolillo, M.D.

Assistant Professor of Psychiatry, Texas Tech University Health Science Center School of Medicine, Lubbock, Texas; Texas Tech Regional Academic Health Center, Amarillo, Texas
Psychiatric Emergencies

Preface

Although in recent years several excellent books on emergency medicine have appeared, we perceived a need for a book that would be particularly useful to the practicing emergency physician in his or her day-to-day care of patients. The primary intent of this book is, as its title states, to offer a practical approach to emergency medicine. It is designed primarily for the practicing emergency physician and the emergency physician-in-training but should also be useful to medical students and other physicians who care for the acutely ill and injured.

The text is divided into five sections: Life Support, Medical Emergencies, Surgical Emergencies, Specialty Emergencies, and Issues and Procedures. It attempts to cover the scope of problems encountered in emergency medicine, ranging from truly life-threatening disorders to less serious problems commonly seen in ambulatory patients. The vast majority of the text pertains to adult emergency medicine. Pertinent pediatric emergencies, however, are included and are consolidated in Chapter 36. The last section includes a discussion of medicolegal issues as they relate to emergency medicine and a variety of procedures pertinent to the practice of emergency medicine.

The clinical sections largely take a disease or problem approach to emergency medicine rather than a symptoms approach. However, a discussion of major symptoms, including their differential diagnoses, is included. In approaching specific clinical problems, an attempt was made to include a discussion, as appropriate, of pertinent pathophysiology, etiologies, clinical features, work-up, diagnostic criteria, treatment, and disposition of the patient from the emergency department. In order to avoid a "cookbook," we have attempted, where appropriate, to provide the rationale for therapeutic modalities. In addition, to provide for continuity of care, pertinent inpatient and outpatient therapy is presented as appropriate.

This book originated at Washington University in St. Louis, Missouri. With only a few exceptions, the contributing authors either hold or held a faculty position at Washington University. They present diagnostic and therapeutic approaches to clinical problems that have worked well for them and are recommended to the reader. We realize, however, that there are other acceptable approaches that may work as well, and the reader may choose to select such alternative methods.

Every effort was made to make *A Practical Approach to Emergency Medicine* as up to date as possible and to include the most current recommendations regarding diagnostic approaches and therapeutic modalities. We realize, however, that emergency medicine is a dynamic field and that new recommendations will likely appear by the time this book is in print. The reader is urged to supplement the material presented in this book with recent advances in emergency medicine.

The editors are deeply indebted to the following people who were responsible for making this book a reality: the individual authors for their tireless effort in the preparation and revisions of their manuscripts; Ms. Jeannie Barenkamp for her typographical assistance; Spectrum Emergency Care, Inc. (particularly Ms. Sandi Eggelston and Ms. Sheila Broeker) for technical assistance in preparation of the manuscript; Doctors Demos Agiomavritis, Marc Allen, Richard Larson and Timothy Shoen of Worcester City Hospital and Timothy Haydock of Northern Westchester Medical Center for review of the manuscript; Ms. Vicki Friedman and Ms. Marcy Hartstein of Washington University for the artwork; and Mr. James Krosschell, Mr. Robert

Davis, and the editorial staff of Little,
Brown and Company for their guidance
and helpful suggestions. A special
thanks goes to Mrs. Carol Bloom for her
dedication, perseverance, and excellent
administrative and typographical assistance in the preparation of this book.

R.J.S.
R.H.M.

Life Support

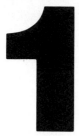

Emergency Medical Services Systems

Robert H. Marcus

Emergency medical services (EMS) systems are community-wide, coordinated means of responding to sudden illness or injury. They concern themselves with the management of various emergencies (including cardiac, trauma, burn, poison, behavioral, spinal cord, and neonatal) and disasters.

Emergency Medical Services (EMS) Components

The EMS system consists of distinct components that together form a system for providing emergency care.

I. **Care provided by an EMS system**
   A. **Prehospital care**
      1. **Entry**
         a. **Discovery** is the recognition of an emergency.
         b. **Access.** A simple, standard, and well-publicized telephone number makes access to the system easiest. The "911" number meets these criteria but is not universally operational. When gaining access to the EMS system, specifics such as the nature and location of the emergency must be given to the EMS operator.
      2. **Rescue**
         a. **The first responder** is one trained in basic life support, which includes prevention of circulatory and respiratory arrest through prompt recognition and intervention and the capability of performing cardiopulmonary resuscitation (CPR). A model EMS system is capable of providing basic life support within 4 minutes. This can be accomplished with large-scale community training of lay persons in basic life support.
         b. **The second responder** is one trained in advanced life support, which includes basic life support plus the use of adjunctive procedures such as endotracheal intubation, intravenous (IV) lifeline placement, drug administration, cardiac monitoring, and defibrillation. A model EMS system provides advanced life support within 8 minutes. This may be accomplished through a rapid response system and well-trained paramedic personnel.
      3. **Transport.** EMS transportation units are capable of providing basic or advanced life support depending on the training of the attendants.
         a. **Ground transportation.** Ambulance design standards are established by the Department of Transportation. Ambulances should be large enough to hold all equipment necessary to deliver advanced life support and provide adequate room for rescue personnel to function. Essential equipment for ambulances is outlined by the American College of Surgeons [8]. Land vehicles are most effective for a range of up to 30–50 miles, depending on the terrain.
         b. **Air ambulances.** Operational guidelines for air ambulances are provided by the American College of Surgeons [5].
            (1) The success of **helicopter transport** was demonstrated during the Vietnam war and subsequently in the civilian experience. Its effectiveness in reducing morbidity and mortality in the critically ill or injured patient is due to the rapid delivery of health care to patients in the field and rapid transport to a definitive care facility. Helicopter use is particularly effective in inaccessible areas or rural areas where sophisticated medical care is unavailable. However, **problems** with the use of helicopters include the following:
               (a) Unavailability of landing sites at the scene and possibly at the destination.

Table 1-1. JCAH categorization of emergency services

Level I	A hospital that provides comprehensive emergency care 24 hours a day with at least one physician experienced in emergency care on duty in the emergency department. Inhospital physician coverage (or a suitable equivalent) shall be provided by at least the medical, surgical, orthopedic, obstetric/gynecologic, pediatric, and anesthesiology services. Other specialty consultations shall be available within 30 minutes. Inhospital capabilities shall provide for management of physical and related emotional problems on a definitive basis.
Level II	A hospital that provides emergency care 24 hours a day with at least one physician experienced in emergency care on duty in the emergency department. Inhospital capabilities shall provide for managing physical and related emotional problems with provision for patient transfers to another facility when needed. Specialty consultation shall be available within 30 minutes.
Level III	A hospital that provides emergency care 24 hours a day with at least one physician available to the emergency care area within 30 minutes. Specialty consultation shall be available by the attending medical staff or by transfer to a designated hospital where definitive care can be provided.
Level IV	A hospital that has the capability of determining whether an emergency exists, rendering lifesaving first aid, and making appropriate referral to a facility capable of providing needed services. Provisions for physician coverage shall be defined by the medical staff.

Source: Adapted from *Accreditation Manual for Hospitals AMH/87.* Chicago: Joint Commission on Accreditation of Hospitals, 1986.

- **(b)** Difficulty in providing advanced life support during transport (patients should be stabilized as much as possible prior to transport).
- **(c)** A decrease in atmospheric oxygen with an increase in altitude, necessitating supplemental oxygen for most patients.
- **(d)** Worsening of conditions in which there is trapped air subject to changes in atmospheric pressure, such as a bowel obstruction (nasogastric suction should be instituted prior to transport), pneumothorax (a chest tube generally should be inserted prior to transport), and use of air splints (pressure should be monitored during transport).
- **(2) Fixed wing aircraft** should be used for the rapid transport of patients for distances greater than 100 miles. Land or helicopter transport must be available at each end of the flight.
- B. **Emergency department care** should include assessment of ill or injured patients and delivery of definitive or stabilizing care, depending on the capabilities of the hospital. Specific guidelines for provision of emergency department care have been developed by the American College of Emergency Physicians [2]. The Joint Commission on Accreditation of Hospitals (JCAH) has classified hospitals according to their capabilities in providing emergency medical services to the community (Table 1-1). This scheme, however, does not include categorization or designation of specialty (e.g., trauma, burn, spinal cord, neonatal) referral centers.
- C. **Inhospital care** may be provided by general hospitals or specialty hospitals (e.g., trauma centers, burn centers, spinal cord centers, rehabilitation institutes).
- II. **Organizational considerations**
  - A. **Medical control** is the entity accountable for the medical competence of an EMS system. The basic functions of medical control include the assurance that field personnel have available immediate expert direction for emergency care, assurance of a continued high quality of performance, and provisions for ongoing review of community EMS activities.
    - 1. The **medical director** is a designated physician responsible for the direction of medical care by all personnel involved in an EMS system.
    - 2. The **resource (base) hospital** is the medical control institution, whereas other hospitals in the system are referred to as associate hospitals. The resource hospital coordinates the many complex elements in the system, including provision of medical direction in the field, referral of victims to appropriate hospitals, and notification of receiving hospitals regarding the arrival of patients and the care provided to the patients in the field.

3. **Immediate medical control** may be accomplished by two mechanisms:
   a. **Protocol systems,** where EMS units operate on standing protocols.
   b. **Nonprotocol systems,** where EMS units operate on direct contact with the resource hospital.
B. The **communication center** is where most components of the EMS system are set into action and coordinated. It allows access to the system, dispatches rescue and public safety units, maintains voice and electrocardiogram (ECG) telemetry contact between the rescuer at the scene and the resource hospital, and coordinates hospital emergency facilities, especially during disasters.
C. **EMS units** include the teams of personnel (and their vehicles and equipment) who assess the status of patients on the scene, provide emergency care, and transport patients to appropriate facilities when necessary. The capabilities of EMS units can be divided into three categories depending on the training of their personnel.
   1. **EMT-1s (EMT-As, EMT-Basics)** are trained to recognize life-threatening conditions and render advanced first aid and basic life support, which includes the ability to perform CPR, immobilize the spine, extricate victims, maintain an airway through noninvasive techniques, administer oxygen, and apply splints and dressings. Requirements are a minimum of 81 hours of instruction with variable clinical experience.
   2. **EMT-Ps (paramedics)** are trained in advanced life support (see sec. **I.A.2.b**) and communication skills. Requirements include completion of a standard course of 15 modules developed by the Department of Transportation.
   3. **Intermediate EMTs** are trained in basic life support plus designated aspects of advanced life support (e.g., EMT-Trauma, EMT-Cardiac).
D. **Public education** involves informing the public about EMS systems, particularly the means to gain access to the system and the location of hospital emergency facilities. It also involves educating the public regarding the prevention of diseases and accidents and training them in bystander response.

Field Stabilization and Disposition

The amount of time spent in field stabilization depends on several factors, including the distance to the nearest appropriate hospital, the nature of the illness or injury, and the ability to provide definitive care in the field. For seriously ill or injured patients, the first 40 minutes after insult is critical, with survival directly related to the time to definitive care (survival rates drop 10% for each 10 minutes that definitive care is delayed in some situations) [11]. Although stabilizing measures may be of value in buying time for seriously ill or injured patients, these measures should be initiated expeditiously and, moreover, abandoned if not technically feasible within strict time constraints. Every effort should be made to avoid undue delays in all phases of operations. Generally, time in the field should not exceed 30 minutes if definitive care cannot be provided there. The disposition of patients should take into account the abilities of facilities to care for particular illnesses or injuries. A major cause of inadequate patient care is the delivery of patients to the nearest hospital rather than to other hospitals more capable of appropriately caring for the patients. **Specific guidelines for field stabilization and disposition are dictated by local EMS authorities, and decisions regarding the care of ill or injured patients in the field should be in accordance with local policy.** The following, however, is intended as a general approach to field stabilization and disposition.
I. **Emergency cardiac care (ECC)** is a subdivision of the EMS system that specifically deals with the recognition of early warning signs of a myocardial infarction, efforts to prevent complications, prompt availability of basic and advanced cardiac life support, and transfer to an appropriate facility. The importance of ECC is shown by the fact that of the approximately 1.5 million people in the United States who sustain a myocardial infarction yearly, over 40% of them will die, and over half of these deaths will occur outside the hospital with most occurring within the first 2 hours after the onset of symptoms [17]. The ability to save victims of cardiac arrest out of the hospital can be inferred from various studies documenting a 60–80% successful resuscitation rate in selected subgroups of patients suffering cardiac arrest [9]. More than 40% of patients with ventricular fibrillation (responsible for the majority of early deaths from coronary artery disease) have been successfully resuscitated when CPR was performed within 4 minutes and definitive care was provided within 8 minutes [15].
   A. **Symptomatic ischemic heart disease.** It is important to attempt to stabilize conscious cardiac victims at the scene, since it is difficult to initiate basic or advanced

cardiac life support in a moving ambulance. In addition, stabilization in the field may obviate the need for high-speed transport requiring the use of sirens, which themselves may increase the incidence of arrhythmias, and measures to stabilize patients in the field may avert life-threatening complications in transit. Stabilization of cardiac patients in the field has resulted in as much as a fivefold reduction in the incidence of cardiac arrest in transit [17].

1. The **first responder** (see **EMS Components**, sec. **I.A.2.a**) should identify symptoms characteristic of ischemic heart disease, advise the victim to stop activity and sit or lie down, attempt to calm the victim through reassurance, and monitor the victim's pulse. The EMS system should be activated if the patient has no known angina pectoris and symptoms persist for more than 2 minutes or if the patient has known angina pectoris and three nitroglycerin tablets are used within 10 minutes without complete resolution of symptoms.

2. The **second responder** (see **EMS Components**, sec. **I.A.2.b**) should assure adequate oxygenation, preferably by administering supplemental oxygen; establish an IV line for delivery of cardiac drugs and fluids as needed; monitor the patient's ECG, blood pressure, and respiration; initiate treatment of arrhythmias that are symptomatic or precursors of cardiac decompensation; attempt to relieve pain as indicated; and establish communications with the resource hospital for consultation and notification of transport of the patient.

3. **Disposition**

   a. Patients with potentially life-threatening cardiac conditions (e.g., chest pain of suspected cardiac origin, potentially life-threatening arrhythmias) should be transported to a hospital by an ambulance capable of providing advanced cardiac life support, since their status may decompensate at any time without warning.

   b. Patients with potentially life-threatening cardiac conditions should be treated in a facility where close monitoring in a coronary care unit or its equivalent is available.

   c. Patients who develop cardiac complications that may be amenable to emergent surgical care (e.g., ruptured interventricular septum or papillary muscle) should be transferred to an institution where these conditions can be treated.

B. **Cardiac arrest.** Successful treatment of cardiac arrest is directly related to the rapidity with which an effective circulation can be restored. Restoring adequate spontaneous circulation at the scene is more likely to result in the victim's survival than use of basic life support measures en route; thus, every effort should be made to stabilize the victim at the scene within a reasonable time period.

1. **Basic cardiac life support** (see Chap. 2). Immediate initiation of basic life support is vital. In the absence of prompt initiation of bystander CPR, resuscitation of prehospital cardiac arrest victims is less than half as successful, despite the availability of a well-trained paramedic team with a rapid response time [17].

2. **Advanced cardiac life support** (see Chap. 2) is essential. CPR is only a holding action that will maintain viability of patients for only a brief period of time [17]. Thus, definitive measures (e.g., defibrillation, drug administration) must be instituted promptly if an effective circulation is to be restored and the victim saved.

3. **Transport**

   a. Patients should be transported immediately to the nearest appropriate emergency facility if the rescuer cannot deliver advanced cardiac life support at the scene or the victim does not respond to advanced cardiac life support.

   b. If needed, CPR should be continued during loading and transportation and should not be interrupted for more than 30 seconds. In addition, the patient should not be moved to a more convenient site until the patient is stabilized and is ready for transport or arrangements have been made for CPR during movement [9].

II. **Trauma.** The improved survival rate of trauma victims during the Vietnam conflict can be attributed to the presence of well-trained paramedics in the field; rapid transportation by helicopters, which bypassed local aid stations and delivered the victims to facilities equipped to handle the injuries; and technical advances in emergency care. In the civilian experience, it has been demonstrated that overall mortality of trauma victims can be reduced significantly by appropriate prehospital care and rapid transport to a facility capable of treating the severely traumatized patient [10, 18, 19].

A. Field stabilization. Severely traumatized patients often require emergency care (e.g., blood transfusions, operative intervention) that cannot be provided in the field. Thus, every effort should be directed toward providing **rapid transportation to a facility equipped to treat the injured**, with minimal time spent attempting to stabilize the victims in the field. Time is a critical factor; morbidity and mortality are reduced significantly if definitive care can be instituted within 2 hours after the insult, preferably within 1 hour (the golden hour) [19]. The following are general guidelines for field stabilization of trauma victims.

1. **Victims must be extricated carefully** to avoid inflicting further injury (e.g., to the spinal cord).
2. **Basic life support** should be instituted as needed.
3. The **cervical spine must be immobilized** if there is suspected injury (e.g., diving accidents; significant injuries to the face, head, or neck; traumatized patients with altered mental status). The head, neck, and chest should be aligned when moving these patients, and a semirigid cervical collar should be used when available. After extrication, patients should be immobilized on a backboard.
4. **External bleeding usually can be controlled by direct pressure** and, when appropriate, elevation of the affected extremity (rarely are tourniquets indicated).
5. In general, **supplemental oxygen should be administered** to trauma victims.
6. The **Military Anti-Shock Trousers (MAST)** suit is a valuable asset in treating the seriously injured trauma victim by splinting pelvic and lower extremity fractures, tamponading bleeding sites under the trousers, and raising the blood pressure. The MAST suit is indicated in hypotensive patients and should be applied prior to attempting placement of an IV line, since it will raise the blood pressure and thus increase the likelihood of successful IV cannulation.
7. If a peripheral vein is readily accessible, then a **large-bore catheter** (i.e., 14- or 16-gauge in adults) should be placed and **Ringer's lactate solution** infused at a rate capable of maintaining the systolic blood pressure greater than 90 mm Hg. Note: It may be difficult to obtain venous access in these patients; however, **valuable time must not be lost in the field with multiple attempts at IV placement.**
8. In a patient with a suspected **tension pneumothorax** and significant hemodynamic compromise, a catheter with a flutter valve [12] should be placed through the chest wall at the second intercostal space in the midclavicular line.
9. In a patient with a **sucking chest wound,** the wound should be covered with an airtight sterile dressing. If the patient develops signs of tension pneumothorax, the seal should be broken, allowing air to escape.
10. Patients with a **flail chest** may be managed by applying constant firm pressure or sandbags over the flailed area.
11. In patients with **eviscerated organs,** the organs should be covered with a moist sterile dressing; placing the organs back into the peritoneal cavity should not be attempted unless there is circulatory compromise.
12. **Impaled objects** should be stabilized in place with a sterile dressing without an attempt at removal.
13. Obvious **fractures should be splinted,** if time allows, by immobilizing the joint above and below the fracture. Severely angulated fractures should be aligned, but no attempt should be made to reduce open fractures below the skin.
14. **The blood pressure, respirations, mental status, and ECG must be monitored continuously.** Agitation in a trauma patient may indicate intoxication, head injury, shock, hypoxia, or a distended bladder.

B. Disposition. In the handling of trauma victims, trauma systems have significantly decreased morbidity and mortality [10, 19]. **Trauma systems function by transporting victims to facilities capable of handling specific injuries,** often bypassing closer facilities. Trauma systems require categorization of facilities according to their capabilities, good prehospital triage with immediate identification of seriously injured patients, and rapid transport of victims to appropriate facilities.

1. Various **triage methods** have been developed for the purpose of identifying the seriously traumatized patient. These methods include the trauma score (Table 1-2) [14], the CRAMS scale [16], and the American College of Surgeons method [6]. However, **local EMS authorities should be consulted for specific local guidelines concerning field categorization of trauma victims.**
2. **Trauma centers.** Trauma statistics show that 85% of trauma victims can be

Table 1-2. Trauma score

Respiratory rate	10–24/min		4
	25–35/min		3
	>35/min		2
	<10/min		1
	None		0
Respiratory effort	Normal		1
	Shallow or retractive		0
Systolic blood pressure	>90 mm Hg		4
	70–90 mm Hg		3
	50–69 mm Hg		2
	<50 mm Hg		1
	No pulse		0
Capillary refill	Normal (<2 sec)		2
	Delayed (>2 sec)		1
	None		0
Glasgow coma scale (GCS)			
Eye opening	Spontaneous	4	
	To voice	3	
	To pain	2	
	None	1	
Verbal response	Oriented	5	
	Confused	4	
	Inappropriate words	3	
	Incomprehensible words	2	
	None	1	
Motor response	Obeys command	6	
	Purposeful movement (to pain)	5	
	Withdrawal (to pain)	4	
	Flexion (to pain)	3	
	Extension (to pain)	2	
	None	1	
	Total GCS Points		
		14–15	5
		11–13	4
		8–10	3
		5–7	2
		3–4	1
Total trauma score[a,b]			1–16

[a]The trauma score is a physiologic measure of severity of injury. The score is obtained by summing the numbers assigned to each parameter. The score correlates inversely with injury severity and directly with the probability of survival.
[b]Patients with a trauma score of 12 or less likely will benefit from care delivered at a trauma center.
Source: Adapted from H. R. Champion et al., Trauma score. *Crit. Care Med.* 9:672, 1981. Copyright Williams & Wilkins, 1981. With permission.

managed at a local level, 10% need further care in a standard intensive care unit (ICU) setting, and 5% need special care that is available only at a designated trauma center [10]. These statistics are reversed for spinal cord and burn injuries, with 85% requiring a specialized center [10]. Regional categorization of trauma centers should follow the American College of Surgeons guidelines [3, 4].

    a. Level I centers are comprehensive hospitals that have made a substantial commitment to the care of the seriously injured. These institutions have the resources and ready availability of staff specialists to manage definitively the critically injured multiple trauma victims. In addition, a commitment to research and a quality assurance program are integral components of these centers.

      b. Level II centers have a serious commitment to trauma care but may not have the availability of staff specialists at all times. This level institution may handle the largest volume of trauma in a geographic area.

      c. Level III centers have a commitment to providing initial trauma care; they should use established protocols.

III. Guidelines for prehospital care of other emergencies (e.g., hypoglycemia, burns, drownings, anaphylaxis, seizures, drug overdosage, behavioral disturbances, obstetric complications, neonatal problems) should be provided by local EMS authorities.

Disaster Planning

A disaster is the occurrence of an incident that produces casualties in numbers too great and at too fast a rate for a community service to handle. Disasters can be classified as either natural (e.g., floods, earthquakes, storms) or man-made (e.g., transportation accidents, fires, explosions, riots, wars).

I. Disaster planning establishes a system that ensures optimal utilization of personnel and facilities during a disaster.

  A. All **communities** should have a written disaster plan that is rehearsed periodically to familiarize involved individuals with operations during a disaster.

  B. All **hospitals** should have a written disaster plan that is rehearsed at least twice per year as required by the Joint Commission on Accreditation of Hospitals [1].

II. Prehospital phase

  A. A disaster is identified, and the **disaster plan is activated** according to the preestablished plan.

  B. A **disaster control center** is established with centralization of authority to coordinate management efforts.

  C. A **communications network** is established between the disaster control center, the rescue site, medical facilities, and other participating agencies.

  D. A **command post** is established at the disaster site and acts as a casualty collection area and site for ambulance arrivals and departures. This site should be manned by supervisory personnel responsible for communications and direction of rescue efforts.

  E. Triage is essential for optimal efficiency in caring for large numbers of casualties. Triage is an ongoing process that begins at the scene; it involves rapid categorization of victims (according to injury severity) and treatment (e.g., airway management, control of external bleeding) directed only at correcting immediately life-threatening conditions. Triaged victims should be identified with colored tags or bands that specify management priorities and disposition. Priorities can be divided into four categories.

    1. First priority victims are severely injured but have a good chance of survival with prompt care.

    2. Second priority victims are seriously injured, but their care can be delayed temporarily without undue threat to life or limb.

    3. Third priority victims are not seriously injured, and treatment can be delayed for prolonged periods.

    4. Fourth priority victims are deemed unsalvageable due to their extensive injuries or are dead.

  F. The **police** and **fire departments** are important components in disaster management; they are instrumental in controlling crowds and traffic, assuring the safety of victims and bystanders, putting out fires, and carrying out rescue operations.

  G. Victims should be transported to appropriate facilities (e.g., hospitals, shelter areas, morgues) as soon as possible.

III. Hospital phase

  A. On notification of a disaster situation, the **hospital disaster plan is activated** by a designated individual.

  B. A **control center with an individual in charge** (e.g., the chief of surgery) is established within the hospital to centralize medical authority. This control center is responsible for continual review of the hospital's resources and capabilities; identification of those hospitalized patients who may be discharged or transferred; establishment of a communications network between the disaster control center and key areas both within and outside the hospital; assignment of personnel; and overall coordination of hospital activities.

  C. Security arrangements are necessary to minimize the presence of unauthorized individuals and vehicles in or near the hospital complex.

D. Specific care areas that are properly staffed should be available for the initial handling of victims. These include a triage area, a resuscitation area, a minimal care area, a holding area (for those deemed unsalvageable and those seriously injured victims for whom delayed care will not be detrimental), a decontamination area (if necessary), a psychiatric area, and a morgue. In addition, the operating suite must be made readily available for those victims requiring immediate surgery.

E. Incoming **victims are triaged** to the appropriate areas according to the nature and severity of their injuries. They are assigned **disaster tags** for identification purposes, as well as for recording pertinent information regarding their injuries. Laboratory results and x-rays should remain with the victims to their final destinations; however, judicious use of x-rays and laboratory tests is necessary to reduce overburdening those departments.

Bibliography

1. *Accreditation Manual for Hospitals AMH/87.* Chicago: Joint Commission on Accreditation of Hospitals, 1986.
2. American College of Emergency Physicians. Emergency care guidelines. *Ann. Emerg. Med.* 11:222, 1982.
3. American College of Surgeons Committee on Trauma. Hospital resources for the optimal care of the injured patient. *Bull. Am. Coll. Surg.* 64(8):43, 1979.
4. American College of Surgeons Committee on Trauma. Qualifications of trauma care personnel. *Bull. Am. Coll. Surg.* 65(2):10, 1980.
5. American College of Surgeons Committee on Trauma. Air ambulance operations. *Bull. Am. Coll. Surg.* 65(2):16, 1980.
6. American College of Surgeons Committee on Trauma. Field categorization of trauma patients and hospital trauma index. *Bull. Am. Coll. Surg.* 65(2):28, 1980.
7. American College of Surgeons Committee on Trauma. Treatment protocol for prehospital management of the trauma patient. *Bull. Am. Coll. Surg.* 65(2):23, 1980.
8. American College of Surgeons Committee on Trauma. Essential equipment for ambulances. *Bull. Am. Coll. Surg.* 66(6):17, 1981.
9. American Heart Association. Standards and guidelines for cardiopulmonary resuscitation (CPR) and emergency cardiac care (ECC). *J.A.M.A.* 255:2905, 1986.
10. Boyd, D. R. Trauma—a controllable disease in the 1980s (Fourth Annual Stone Lecture, American Trauma Society). *J. Trauma* 20:14, 1980.
11. Brill, J. C., and Geiderman, J. M. A rationale for scoop-and-run: Identifying a subset of time-critical patients. *Top. Emerg. Med.* 3:37, 1981.
12. Caroline, N. L. *Emergency Care in the Streets* (2nd ed.). Boston: Little, Brown, 1983.
13. Carveth, S. W., et al. (eds.). *A Manual for Instructors of Basic Cardiac Life Support.* Dallas: American Heart Association, 1977.
14. Champion, H. R., et al. Trauma score. *Crit. Care Med.* 9:672, 1981.
15. Eisenberg, M. S., et al. Cardiac resuscitation in the community: Importance of rapid provision and implications for program planning. *J.A.M.A.* 241:1905, 1979.
16. Gormicon, S. P. CRAMS scale: Field triage of trauma victims. *Ann. Emerg. Med.* 11:132, 1982.
17. McIntyre, K. M., and Lewis, A. J. (eds.). *Textbook of Advanced Cardiac Life Support.* Dallas: American Heart Association, 1983.
18. Trunkey, D. D. Regionalization of trauma care. *Top. Emerg. Med.* 3:91, 1981.
19. Trunkey, D. D. The value of trauma centers. *Bull. Am. Coll. Surg.* 67(10):5, 1982.

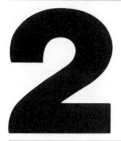

Cardiopulmonary Resuscitation

Robert H. Marcus

Cardiac arrest is the cessation of breathing and circulation. It is recognized by apnea and pulselessness in an unconscious victim. Management of the cardiac arrest victim should follow the current recommendations of the American Heart Association [1, 12, 16, 17]. However, these recommendations are subject to change as a result of the widespread research being performed in this field.

I. **Initiation of cardiopulmonary resuscitation (CPR)**. In the emergency department, it is often necessary to make a decision whether to initiate CPR on patients with only a minimal history. The current standard of care dictates that the decision to withhold CPR should not be made arbitrarily, and full resuscitative measures should be instituted when there is any doubt concerning this issue. If indicated, the decision to limit or terminate care may be made at a later time when more information is available. Specifically, CPR should be initiated when there is a possibility of brain viability and there is no legal or medical reason to withhold resuscitative measures. However, **withholding CPR** may be acceptable in the following situations:

   A. There is reliable evidence of death (e.g., decapitation, rigor mortis, evidence of tissue decomposition, extreme dependent lividity).

   B. The decision to withhold CPR was made (on justifiable grounds) prior to the patient's arrival in the emergency department.

   C. The patient is known to be in the terminal stages of an incurable disease.

   D. The patient was pulseless and apneic for a prolonged period of time (i.e., > 10 minutes) prior to initiation of resuscitative measures (this must take into account the reliability of the observer and the presence of factors that may favorably affect outcome, such as the patient being a child or the presence of hypothermia or drug overdosage).

II. **Immediate response** entails establishing unresponsiveness, calling for help, and placing the victim in a supine position on a hard surface (taking care when there is possible spinal injury).

III. **Airway management.** In the unconscious victim, the tongue is the most common cause of airway obstruction, since the muscles supporting the mandible relax, allowing the tongue to fall posteriorly. Other causes of upper airway obstruction include infection, foreign body, tumor, trauma, laryngeal edema, and laryngospasm. It is essential to establish and maintain an open airway, since this measure alone may restore breathing and prevent cardiac arrest or anoxic brain damage. Furthermore, a patent airway is essential to ventilate anoxic or hypoxic patients.

   A. Airway maneuvers

   1. The **head tilt–chin lift** is the most effective airway maneuver. This method is performed by tilting the victim's head backward by applying firm pressure to the forehead, while the fingers of the other hand are placed under the chin bringing the mandible anteriorly; the operator's thumb may be used to retract the lower lip to keep the mouth open. An alternative airway maneuver is the **jaw thrust** with or without head tilt (see **2**).

   2. For **suspected cervical spine–injured** victims, the **jaw thrust without head tilt** maneuver is recommended. This method is performed by grasping the angles of the mandibles and displacing the mandible anteriorly without moving the head or neck.

   B. Adjuncts to airway management

   1. **Suction devices** are useful adjuncts in clearing oropharyngeal secretions and/or gastric contents from the upper airway, as well as clearing secretions from the lower respiratory tract in the intubated patient. Flexible suction catheters may be inserted orally, nasally, or through an endotracheal tube or tracheos-

tomy site. The rigid pharyngeal suction tips must be inserted orally and are most useful in removing thick secretions or food particles.

2. **The oro- and nasopharyngeal airways** hold the tongue away from the posterior wall of the pharynx and obviate obstruction from the lips and teeth; in addition, the oropharyngeal airway provides access for oropharyngeal suctioning and prevents bite injuries to the tongue and orotracheal tube. The oropharyngeal airway should be used only in unconscious victims, since otherwise it may stimulate vomiting or laryngospasm. Nasopharyngeal airways are better tolerated in responsive patients and are preferred if the mouth cannot be opened.

3. **The esophageal obturator airway (EOA)** is a device that utilizes a face mask attached to a blind tube with a distal 35-cc balloon. The tube is inserted blindly into the esophagus, the mask is fitted tightly over the face, and the balloon is inflated, occluding the esophagus. Oxygen is delivered through the proximal end of the tube and exits through side holes adjacent to the pharynx, thus entering the lungs. The EOA should be used only in comatose patients over 16 years old. Contraindications include known or suspected esophageal disease or injury. Since removal of the EOA may be followed by regurgitation of stomach contents, a suction device should be available and, in the comatose patient, an endotracheal tube inserted and the cuff inflated prior to removal of the EOA. Complications associated with use of the EOA include tracheal compression if the balloon is inflated above the carina, esophageal injury, and inadvertent endotracheal intubation. Presently there is controversy regarding the efficacy of the EOA, with some studies indicating poor ventilation, problems maintaining an airway, and difficulty with EOA insertion [23]. Thus, the EOA should be used only if endotracheal intubation cannot be performed.

4. **Oro- or nasotracheal intubation** (see Chap. 38) is the preferred method of establishing an airway in the cardiac arrest victim, since it ensures patency of the upper airway, isolates the airway for suctioning and ventilation, and decreases the likelihood of pulmonary aspiration. Oxygenation with the bag-valve-mask or mouth-to-mouth technique always should be performed prior to attempts at tracheal intubation, and CPR should not be interrupted for more than 30 seconds during attempts at tracheal intubation. The nasal route is preferred in patients in whom there is difficulty gaining oral access or suspected cervical spine injury. Blind nasotracheal intubation, however, is not recommended in nonbreathing patients or patients with laryngeal edema.

5. **Surgical procedures.** When an airway cannot be established by any of the above methods, transtracheal catheter ventilation (see Chap. 38), cricothyrotomy (see Chap. 38), or, rarely, tracheostomy should be performed, preferably by personnel well trained in the technique.

C. **In foreign-body upper airway obstruction** (see Chap. 28 for non-foreign-body upper airway obstruction), there is usually a preceding history of eating or aspiration of foreign material. In the awake patient, agitation, dyspnea, stridor, weak cough, inability to speak, and/or cyanosis may be present. In the unconscious victim, this condition may be recognized by an inability to ventilate the patient using the bag-valve-mask or mouth-to-mouth technique.

1. **In upper airway obstruction with adequate ventilation**, the victim usually is capable of breathing, speaking, and coughing. In these patients, no emergency procedures are immediately necessary. Appropriate diagnostic tests, such as soft-tissue neck x-rays, and specialty consultation are indicated.

2. **Upper airway obstruction with inadequate ventilation**
   a. In the **conscious victim**, manual thrusts should be performed immediately. Manual thrust consists of an inward thrust with the operator's fist or heel of the hand applied to the victim's upper abdomen (abdominal thrust or Heimlich maneuver) or chest (chest thrust); the chest thrust is indicated only for markedly obese patients or patients in advanced pregnancy. Manual thrusts should be repeated until the foreign body is dislodged or the victim becomes unconscious.
   b. In the **unconscious victim**, an attempt to open the airway (see sec. III.A) and ventilate the patient should be undertaken. If unsuccessful, 6–10 manual thrusts should be delivered. If still unsuccessful, manual removal should be attempted immediately. If proper equipment is readily available, removal of the obstructing foreign body with a clamp or forceps under direct visualization with a laryngoscope should be attempted. In the absence of

appropriate equipment, manual removal should be attempted by grasping the tongue and lower jaw between the thumb and fingers and lifting the mandible (tongue-jaw lift), followed by sweeping the index finger of the other hand across the posterior pharynx (this maneuver should be used only in the unconscious victim). If these attempts fail, an airway must be established without delay distal to the site of obstruction by percutaneous transtracheal ventilation (see Chap. 38), cricothyrotomy (see Chap. 38), or rarely, tracheostomy.

IV. Rescue **breathing** should be initiated with two breaths of 1–1.5 seconds each if adequate respiratory exchange does not occur once the airway is open. In victims with a pulse (for no pulse, see sec. **V**) but inadequate respiratory exchange, one ventilation every 5 seconds should be delivered. Methods of rescue breathing are as follows:

   A. Mouth-to-mouth breathing, which is effective, requires no equipment but only delivers an FiO_2 of 16–17%. Alternative methods include mouth-to-nose (if the victim cannot be ventilated by the mouth-to-mouth method) and mouth-to-stoma.

   B. The **bag-valve-mask device** should be used only by experienced personnel due to the difficulties encountered with its usage, and an oro- or nasopharyngeal airway generally is required with this device to maintain an open airway. The bag-valve-mask device usually provides lower tidal volumes than the mouth-to-mouth technique due to problems in providing a leak-proof seal with the mask while maintaining a patent airway and compressing the bag [17]. Gastric distention is a problem with the bag-valve-mask device, as well as with the mouth-to-mouth method.

   C. Other adjuncts to rescue breathing include use of the EOA and ventilation through an endotracheal tube, transtracheal catheter, cricothyrotomy, or tracheostomy (see Chap. 38).

V. Circulation

   A. External chest compressions are initiated if no pulse is palpable. This technique consists of rhythmically compressing with the heels of the operator's hands the lower half of the patient's sternum 4–5 cm using a 50% compression and 50% relaxation cycle. For a single rescuer, a compression-ventilation ratio of 15:2 with a compression rate of 80–100/minute is recommended. For two rescuers, a compression-ventilation ratio of 5:1 with a compression rate of 80–100/minute is indicated. Even under optimal conditions, external cardiac compressions usually provide a cardiac output of less than one-third of normal; thus, it is important that compressions be performed on a hard surface in a supine victim to maximize carotid blood flow and venous return to the heart.

   It is important to remember that CPR alone may not prevent deterioration of cardiac arrest victims; clinical studies indicate that if definitive care (e.g., defibrillation, intubation, drug administration) is not provided within 8 minutes, overall survival rates fall dramatically [7]. Furthermore, it is essential not to stop CPR for more than 7 seconds except under special circumstances, such as endotracheal intubation, and then cessation should not exceed 30 seconds. Complications encountered with external chest compressions include fractured ribs, a fractured sternum, costochondral separation, pneumothorax, hemothorax, lung contusion, myocardial contusion, laceration of the liver, and fat embolism.

   B. Internal cardiac massage has been shown to produce a cardiac and stroke index about twice that of external cardiac compressions, as well as producing a mean circulation time within the normal physiologic range [5]. Despite the superior hemodynamics achieved with internal cardiac massage, technical difficulties and significant complication have limited this procedure to qualified physicians in the setting of cardiac arrest associated with penetrating chest trauma, cardiac tamponade, crushed chest injuries when the chest cannot be stabilized laterally, anatomic deformities of the chest that preclude adequate closed chest compressions, operative cases in which the chest is already open, and rarely, failure of adequately applied closed chest compressions.

   C. New methods for improving cardiac output generated during CPR include a 60% compression duration during external cardiac massage [25], use of the Military Anti-Shock Trousers (MAST) suit [15], and use of interposed abdominal compressions (IAC-CPR) [26]. However, the ability of these procedures to improve survival significantly has not been proved conclusively.

VI. Intravenous (IV) therapy and other routes for drug administration

   A. A **large-bore IV line** is essential. Initially, upper-extremity peripheral access is preferred, if readily available. Intravenous catheter placement below the diaphragm is not recommended, since there is evidence supporting preferential blood flow to the upper body during CPR [8]. Later, a central venous catheter placed above the diaphragm will be useful to deliver drugs directly into the central circulation, resulting in higher cardiac drug concentrations and a faster delivery time to the heart, compared to the peripheral route [14]. Ideally, CPR should not be interrupted for central venous cannulation.

B. The **endotracheal route** is an alternative method for drug administration in patients with an endotracheal tube in place when IV access is delayed or cannot be obtained. Drugs that have been shown to be well absorbed by this route include epinephrine, atropine, lidocaine, naloxone, and diazepam [8].

C. Intracardiac injections generally are not recommended due to the significant complications (e.g., pneumothorax, hemothorax, cardiac tamponade, myocardial or coronary laceration, and intramyocardial injection) encountered with this route.

VII. Drug therapy

A. Supplemental **oxygen** at 100% concentration should be delivered as soon as possible.

B. **Epinephrine**, an alpha- and beta-adrenergic agonist, stimulates spontaneous cardiac contractions, elevates perfusion pressure during CPR, improves the myocardial contractile state, and may convert a fine ventricular fibrillation to a coarse pattern that is more amenable to electrical defibrillation. It is useful in asystole, electromechanical dissociation, and ventricular fibrillation. The recommended dosage is 0.5–1.0 mg (5–10 ml of a 1:10,000 solution) IV q5 minutes as needed. An epinephrine drip may be prepared by adding 1 mg of epinephrine to 250 ml of 5% D/W and titrating to the desired effect.

C. **Sodium bicarbonate** is indicated for correction of significant metabolic acidosis, which may depress normal electrical activity, lower the ventricular fibrillation threshold, and inhibit the action of catecholamines. However, there is little data indicating that bicarbonate therapy improves outcome of cardiac arrest victims [1]. Furthermore, bicarbonate has not improved the ability to defibrillate or improved survival rates in experimental animals [1]. Presently, there is evidence that bicarbonate administration during cardiac arrest may (1) induce hyperosmolarity, hypernatremia, and extracellular alkalosis; (2) inhibit the release of oxygen from hemoglobin by shifting the oxyhemoglobin dissociation curve; and (3) produce a paradoxical acidosis by generating carbon dioxide, which is freely diffusable into myocardial and cerebral cells, depressing their function [1].

Currently, sodium bicarbonate administration during cardiac arrest is recommended only after ensuring adequate alveolar ventilation and following the use of other standard modalities, such as defibrillation and pharmacologic therapies (e.g., epinephrine, antiarrhythmic agents). Generally, sodium bicarbonate therapy will not be necessary until after 10 minutes of resuscitative efforts. Indications for early use of sodium bicarbonate during cardiac arrest include (1) a documented significant metabolic acidosis after the patient has been hyperventilated, (2) a preexisting acidosis, and (3) hyperkalemia. Ideally, bicarbonate therapy should be guided by arterial blood gas (ABG) determinations. However, if ABG results are unavailable, an initial bolus of 1 mEq/kg can be given IV, if deemed necessary, and followed by half that dose q10-15 minutes as needed. Calcium salts and catecholamines should not be administered along with sodium bicarbonate, since calcium precipitates and catecholamines are inactivated in this solution.

D. **Atropine**, a vagolytic drug, enhances the rate of discharge of the sinoatrial node and improves atrioventricular conduction. It is useful in treating bradyarrhythmias with associated hemodynamic compromise or ventricular premature depolarizations. Atropine may also be effective in restoring electrical activity in asystole. The recommended dosage is 0.5 mg (1.0 mg in asystole) IV, repeated q5 minutes as needed to a total dose of 2.0 mg.

E. **Isoproterenol** is a pure beta-agonist with potent inotropic and chronotropic properties (at the expense of increasing myocardial oxygen demands). It is indicated for hemodynamically significant, atropine-resistant bradyarrhythmias as a temporary measure pending pacemaker placement. An infusion is made by adding 1 or 2 mg of isoproterenol to 500 ml of 5% D/W (2 or 4 µg/ml) and titrating (usually 2–20 µg/minute) to the desired heart rate. The American Heart Association no longer recommends isoproterenol as adjunctive therapy in asystole and electromechanical dissociation since there is evidence that isoproterenol may be detrimental in cardiac arrest by decreasing peripheral vascular resistance and thus decreasing coronary artery perfusion pressure during CPR [11].

F. Calcium ions play an important role in myocardial excitation-contraction coupling. Calcium increases myocardial contractility and may enhance ventricular automaticity (but it also suppresses sinus impulse formation). However, studies have not demonstrated benefit from the use of calcium in cardiac arrest victims [1]. Furthermore, there is evidence suggesting that toxic levels result from administration of previously recommended dosages [6], that the drug is of questionable effectiveness in treating asystole and electro-mechanical dissociation [24], and that there are detrimental effects on post-hypoxic cerebral ischemia [27] and possibly myocardial ischemia. Thus, current recommendations for the use of calcium include hyperkalemia, hypocalcemia (e.g., after multiple blood transfusions), and toxicity from calcium channel blocking agents. The dosage is 2 ml (2–4 mg/kg) of a 10% calcium chloride solution IV, repeated at 10 minutes intervals as needed. Calcium glucectate, 5–7 ml, and calcium gluconate, 5–8 ml, are equivalent calcium preparations; however, calcium chloride is the preferred salt due to the increased availability of active ionized calcium. In the beating heart, calcium should be given slowly, since otherwise it may produce severe ventricular or bradyarrhythmias. Since calcium potentiates the effects of digitalis, it should be given cautiously to patients taking a digitalis preparation.

G. Lidocaine suppresses discharges from ventricular ectopic foci, increases the myocardial fibrillation threshold, and may terminate reentrant ventricular arrhythmias. Lidocaine is the drug of choice for treatment of ventricular tachycardia and as adjunctive therapy in the management of ventricular fibrillation. It should also be used prophylactically following conversion of these arrhythmias to a supraventricular rhythm. The dosage is 1.0 mg/kg IV initially, followed by 0.5 mg/kg q8–10 minutes as needed, to a maximum of 3 mg/kg. On termination of the ventricular arrhythmia, an infusion of 2–4 mg/minute should be started. With the exception of the initial dose in patients with ventricular fibrillation, loading (bolus) and maintenance doses should be reduced 50% in the presence of liver dysfunction or decreased hepatic blood flow (e.g., secondary to congestive heart failure, shock) and in patients over 70 years old. Toxicity is manifested by central nervous system signs and symptoms (e.g., slurred speech, altered mental status, seizures).

H. Bretylium tosylate produces an initial catecholamine release, followed by adrenergic blockade. Bretylium may terminate ventricular reentrant arrhythmias, increase the ventricular fibrillation threshold, and facilitate electrical defibrillation; in addition, it may have direct defibrillatory activity. Despite these properties, it is not considered a first-line drug in the treatment of ventricular arrhythmias. It is recommended for the treatment of resistant ventricular fibrillation or tachycardia, that is, (1) ventricular fibrillation or pulseless ventricular tachycardia refractory to defibrillation and lidocaine (2) ventricular tachycardia with a pulse not controlled by lidocaine, procainamide, and cardioversion as appropriate (see Fig. 2-2) [1]. In refractory ventricular fibrillation or pulseless ventricular tachycardia, the initial dose is 5 mg/kg by rapid IV injection, followed by repeat doses of 10 mg/kg at 15–30-minute intervals as needed to a total dosage of 30 mg/kg. In refractory ventricular tachycardia associated with a pulse, the initial dose is 5–10 mg/kg (diluted to 50 ml with 5% D/W), given by slow IV infusion over 8–10 minutes. For continued arrhythmia suppression, a continuous infusion of 1–2 mg/minute may be used. Complications include nausea, vomiting, and initial hypertension and increased frequency of arrhythmias, followed by hypotension (especially orthostatic hypotension). Caution should be used in administering bretylium to patients with possible digitalis toxicity, since the initial catecholamine release may aggravate digitalis-toxic arrhythmias.

I. Procainamide suppresses ventricular ectopic activity and may terminate reentrant arrhythmias. It is recommended as a second-line antiarrhythmic agent (after lidocaine) for treatment of ventricular tachycardia and suppression of ventricular ectopy. Procainamide is administered IV at a rate of 20 mg/minute (10 mg/minute in stable patients) until the arrhythmia is suppressed, 1 gm has been given, the QRS widens by 50% of its original width, or hypotension occurs. A maintenance infusion of 1–4 mg/minute may be used for continuous arrhythmia suppression. The dosage should be reduced in the presence of renal impairment or severe cardiac dysfunction.

J. Dopamine is an alpha-, beta-, and dopaminergic-receptor stimulator. It differs from other vasopressors in its selective dose-related response. Dopamine is indicated for hemodynamically significant hypotension not secondary to hypovolemia and possibly as adjunctive therapy during cardiac arrest [20]. An infusion is made by adding 400 or 800 mg of dopamine to 500 ml of 5% D/W (800 or 1600 μg/ml) and titrating (usually 2–50 μg/kg/minute) to the desired effect.

K. Norepinephrine has alpha- and beta-adrenergic properties and is useful in nonhypovolemic hypotension. Because of its potent vasoconstricting activity, norepinephrine may increase coronary perfusion during CPR and thus may be a beneficial adjunct in treating cardiac arrest [28]. An infusion is prepared by adding 4 mg of norepinephrine (levarterenol) base to 500 ml of 5% D/W (8 μg/ml of base) and infused at an initial rate of 16–24 μg/minute, titrating to the desired blood pressure.

VIII. Defibrillation, electrical cardioversion, and precordial thump

A. Electrical defibrillation with an unsynchronized direct current (DC) shock is the treatment of choice for ventricular fibrillation. This electric current depolarizes a critical mass of the heart, ideally allowing for uniform repolarization followed by an organized rhythm. Ventricular fibrillation should always be confirmed clinically (e.g., a pulseless, unconscious victim) prior to attempted defibrillation, and CPR should be continued until provisions for defibrillation are ready. The quick-look paddles allow for rapid evaluation of the cardiac rhythm and subsequent defibrillation, if necessary.

1. Factors influencing electrical defibrillation

   a. Since the **time to first shock** is inversely proportional to success [13], time-consuming procedures (e.g., endotracheal intubation, IV placement) should be avoided initially and immediate defibrillation attempted. The rapidity of defibrillation is the major determinant of survival in cardiac arrest from ventricular fibrillation [1].

   b. Correct paddle placement is important to depolarize a critical mass of the heart. Electrical defibrillation or cardioversion is performed by placing one paddle to the right of the upper sternum and the other paddle to left of the apex, or one paddle over the precordium and the other paddle posteriorly behind the heart.

   c. Reducing the transthoracic resistance will increase the delivered energy. This is accomplished by reducing the skin resistance through the use of conductive materials, applying firm pressure to the paddles over the chest wall, using optimal size (10 cm in diameter) paddles, and delivering shortly spaced repetitive shocks at end expiration.

   d. Factors that decrease the success rate of attempted defibrillation include hypoxia, acidosis, hypothermia, electrolyte imbalance, drug toxicity, and the presence of underlying pathology (e.g., congestive heart failure, acute myocardial infarction). To optimize the chance for successful defibrillation, these factors must be corrected, if possible.

Fig. 2-1. Ventricular fibrillation (and pulseless ventricular tachycardia). This sequence was developed to treat a broad range of patients with ventricular fibrillation (VF) or pulseless ventricular tachycardia (VT). Some patients may require care not specified herein. This algorithm should not be construed as prohibiting such flexibility. Flow of algorithm presumes that VF is continuing. CPR indicates cardiopulmonary resuscitation.

[a] Pulseless VT should be treated identically to VF.

[b] Check pulse and rhythm after each shock. If VF recurs after transiently converting (rather than persists without ever converting), use whatever energy level has previously been successful for defibrillation.

[c] Epinephrine should be repeated every five minutes.

[d] Intubation is preferable. If it can be accomplished simultaneously with other techniques, then the earlier the better. However, defibrillation and epinephrine are more important initially if the patient can be ventilated without intubation.

[e] Some may prefer repeated doses of lidocaine, which may be given in 0.5-mg/kg boluses every eight minutes to a total dose of 3 mg/kg.

[f] Value of sodium bicarbonate is questionable during cardiac arrest, and it is not recommended for routine cardiac arrest sequence. Consideration of its use in a dose of 1 mEq/kg is appropriate at this point. Half of original dose may be repeated every ten minutes if it is used.

Source: From American Heart Association, Standards and guidelines for cardiopulmonary resuscitation (CPR) and emergency cardiac care (ECC). *J.A.M.A.* 255:2905, 1986. With permission. Copyright 1986, American Medical Association.

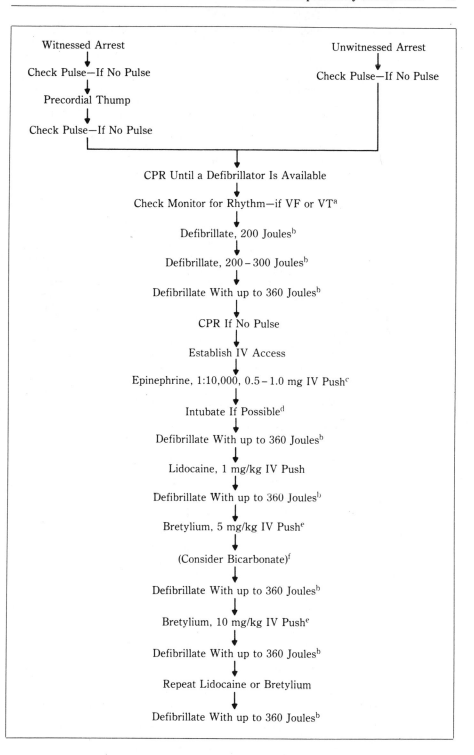

Witnessed Arrest

Check Pulse—If No Pulse

Precordial Thump

Check Pulse—If No Pulse

Unwitnessed Arrest

Check Pulse—If No Pulse

CPR Until a Defibrillator Is Available

Check Monitor for Rhythm—if VF or VT[a]

Defibrillate, 200 Joules[b]

Defibrillate, 200 – 300 Joules[b]

Defibrillate With up to 360 Joules[b]

CPR If No Pulse

Establish IV Access

Epinephrine, 1:10,000, 0.5 – 1.0 mg IV Push[c]

Intubate If Possible[d]

Defibrillate With up to 360 Joules[b]

Lidocaine, 1 mg/kg IV Push

Defibrillate With up to 360 Joules[b]

Bretylium, 5 mg/kg IV Push[e]

(Consider Bicarbonate)[f]

Defibrillate With up to 360 Joules[b]

Bretylium, 10 mg/kg IV Push[e]

Defibrillate With up to 360 Joules[b]

Repeat Lidocaine or Bretylium

Defibrillate With up to 360 Joules[b]

    2. Blind defibrillation is indicated in cardiac arrest when a defibrillator is readily available and a monitor is not. Immediate defibrillation in this setting may be lifesaving since the majority of sudden cardiac deaths are due to ventricular fibrillation. Also, this shock may convert ventricular tachycardia and will not be harmful in the presence of asystole.

    3. Energy requirements. Although there is a relationship between body size and the energy needed for defibrillation (with infants and children requiring less energy than adults), size does not appear to be a clinically important variable in determining the energy requirements for defibrillation over the range of weights in most adults [1]. Thus, current guidelines call for the initiation of defibrillation in adults with three consecutive shocks, with the initial energy level at 200 joules; second and third shocks, if needed, should be at 200–300 joules and up to 360 joules, respectively [1]. If these are unsuccessful, further shocks of up to 360 joules should be delived following adjunctive therapy.

    4. Myocardial necrosis can occur with cumulative delivered energies of more than 425 joules. Use of small-diameter paddles and short intervals (i.e., < 3 minutes) between shocks also increase the likelihood of myocardial damage [8].

  B. Electrical cardioversion (see Chap. 4, **Treatment,** sec. **VII**) is the termination of arrhythmias other than ventricular fibrillation, preferably by a synchronized DC shock (if time permits) to reduce the potential for induction of ventricular fibrillation. Emergency cardioversion is indicated for rapid ventricular or supraventricular rhythms (amenable to electrical therapy) in which immediate arrhythmia termination is essential to prevent clinical deterioration. Generally, the need for emergent cardioversion should be based on the patient's clinical status rather than the specific rhythm disturbance. There are no absolute contraindications to emergent cardioversion when this therapy is necessary. However, in certain circumstances (e.g., digitalis toxicity) where complications from electrical therapy may be significant, emergent cardioversion should be done with great caution; this generally demands administering an antiarrhythmic agent prior to cardioversion and using the lowest effective energy level. In these high-risk instances, the use of other therapies (e.g., antiarrhythmic drugs, cardiac pacing), when appropriate, should be strongly considered.

  C. The **precordial thump** is accomplished by delivering a sharp blow to the midsternum with the ulnar aspect of the rescuer's fist from 20–30 cm above the sternum. This produces a small electric stimulus of about 4 joules that may convert ventricular tachycardia or ventricular fibrillation of recent onset or generate a beat in ventricular asystole secondary to complete heart block. Since rapid defibrillation is a major determinant of successful resuscitation, one precordial thump is recommended in patients with monitored ventricular fibrillation and in witnessed cardiac arrest if a defibrillator is not available. When a precordial thump is used in patients with ventricular tachycardia who have a pulse, a monitor-defibrillator should be available since a thump can induce ventricular fibrillation [1]. Controversially, there is evidence that the precordial thump is ineffective in converting ventricular fibrillation and, furthermore, may precipitate deterioration of other cardiac rhythms [18].

IX. Emergent cardiac pacing

  A. Transvenous or **transthoracic pacemakers** are indicated in hemodynamically significant, medically refractory bradyarrhythmias and possibly asystole. During CPR, the subxiphoid transthoracic approach may be preferable, since it enables direct electrode placement without interrupting CPR.

  B. The **external cardiac pacemaker** is safe and effective; it can be applied rapidly and requires little training to use. Thus, its application in the emergency setting for selected cases appears quite promising [9].

X. Arrhythmia management. Successful management of arrhythmias requires adequate coronary perfusion; correction of acidosis, hypoxia, and electrolyte disorders; and correct drug usage. See Figs. 2-1 through 2-7 for arrhythmia management algorithms.

XI. Continuous monitoring of cardiac arrest victims is essential to ensure adequate therapy. This includes cardiac monitoring, periodic arterial blood gas determinations to evaluate oxygenation and acid-base status, and monitoring of arterial pulsations to check the adequacy of chest compressions.

XII. Termination of CPR. Indications for termination of CPR in the acute setting include the following:

  A. The rescuer is exhausted and unable to continue CPR.

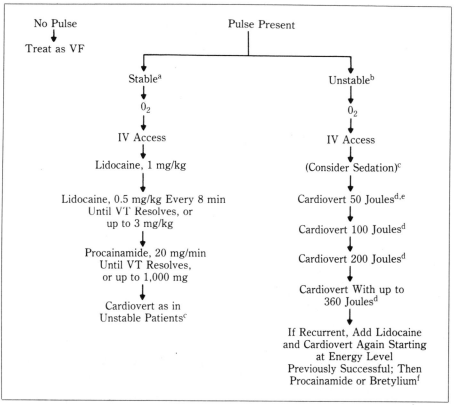

Fig. 2-2. Sustained ventricular tachycardia (VT). This sequence was developed to treat a broad range of patients with sustained VT. Some patients may require care not specified herein. This algorithm should not be construed as prohibiting such flexibility. Flow of algorithm presumes that VT is continuing. VF indicates ventricular fibrillation.
[a] If patient becomes unstable (see footnote b for definition) at any time, move to "Unstable" arm of algorithm.
[b] Unstable indicates symptoms (e.g., chest pain or dyspnea), hypotension (systolic blood pressure < 90 mm Hg), congestive heart failure, ischemia, or infarction.
[c] Sedation should be considered for all patients, including those defined in footnote b as unstable, except those who are hemodynamically unstable (e.g., hypotensive, in pulmonary edema, or unconscious).
[d] If hypotension, pulmonary edema, or unconsciousness is present, unsynchronized cardioversion should be done to avoid delay associated with synchronization.
[e] In the absence of hypotension, pulmonary edema, or unconsciousness, a precordial thump may be employed prior to cardioversion.
[f] Once VT has resolved, begin intravenous (IV) infusion of antiarrhythmic agent that has aided resolution of VT. If hypotension, pulmonary edema, or unconsciousness is present, use lidocaine if cardioversion alone is unsuccessful, followed by bretylium. In all other patients, recommended order of therapy is lidocaine, procainamide, and then bretylium.
Source: From American Heart Association, Standards and guidelines for cardiopulmonary resuscitation (CPR) and emergency cardiac care (ECC). *J.A.M.A.* 255:2905, 1986. Copyright 1986, American Medical Association. With permission.

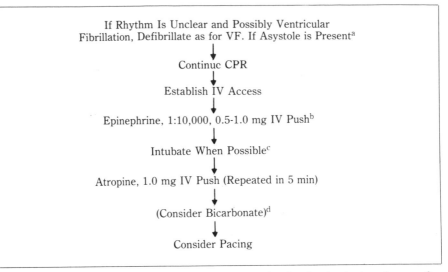

If Rhythm Is Unclear and Possibly Ventricular
Fibrillation, Defibrillate as for VF. If Asystole is Present[a]
↓
Continue CPR
↓
Establish IV Access
↓
Epinephrine, 1:10,000, 0.5-1.0 mg IV Push[b]
↓
Intubate When Possible[c]
↓
Atropine, 1.0 mg IV Push (Repeated in 5 min)
↓
(Consider Bicarbonate)[d]
↓
Consider Pacing

Fig. 2-3. Asystole (cardiac standstill). This sequence was developed to treat a broad range of patients with asystole. Some patients may require care not specified herein. This algorithm should not be construed to prohibit such flexibility. Flow of algorithm presumes asystole is continuing. VF indicates ventricular fibrillation; IV, intravenous.
[a] Asystole should be confirmed in two leads.
[b] Epinephrine should be repeated every five minutes.
[c] Intubation is preferable; if it can be accomplished simultaneously with other techniques, then the earlier the better. However, cardiopulmonary resuscitation (CPR) and use of epinephrine are more important initially if patient can be ventilated without intubation. (Endotracheal epinephrine may be used.)
[d] Value of sodium bicarbonate is questionable during cardiac arrest, and it is not recommended for the routine cardiac arrest sequence. Consideration of its use in a dose of 1 mEq/kg is appropriate at this point. Half of original dose may be repeated every ten minutes if it is used.
Source: From American Heart Association, Standards and guidelines for cardiopulmonary resuscitation (CPR) and emergency cardiac care (ECC). *J.A.M.A.* 255:2905, 1986. Copyright 1986, American Medical Association. With permission.

B. **The responsibility has been transferred to others** who are capable of continuing resuscitative efforts.
C. **The patient is deemed unresuscitatable.** This decision should be made on the basis of **cardiovascular unresponsiveness,** that is, the inability to restore cardiovascular functioning after an adequate trial of standard resuscitative therapy. CPR should not be terminated on the basis of suspected brain death, since in the acute setting signs of brain death may be unreliable and in the brain-dead victim premature termination of CPR will hamper potential salvage of organs for transplantation. Signs of brain death are particularly unreliable in the presence of hypothermia, hypovolemia, and drug intoxication and in children. Thus, in these settings, a prolonged resuscitative effort is indicated.
D. **The patient is successfully resuscitated.** Postresuscitation care includes the following:
   1. **Transfer to an intensive care unit.** Initially, continuous monitoring is essential, since the postresuscitative period is a high-risk period for recurrent cardiac arrest.
   2. **Cerebral resuscitation.** Presently, methods of ameliorating anoxic brain damage incurred during cardiac arrest include measures to reduce intracranial pressure (i.e., hyperventilation, administration of loop and osmotic diuretics, elevation of the head of the bed 30 degrees, and fluid restriction). The use of steroids, calcium channel blockers, barbiturate coma, and induced hypothermia, however, are of unproved efficacy at this time [17, 27].

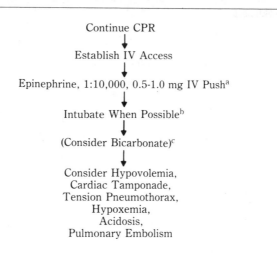

Fig. 2-4. Electromechanical dissociation. This sequence was developed to treat a broad range of patients with electromechanical dissociation. Some patients may require care not specified herein. This algorithm should not be construed to prohibit such flexibility. Flow of algorithm presumes that electromechanical dissociation is continuing. CPR indicates cardiopulmonary resuscitation; IV, intravenous.

[a] Epinephrine should be repeated every five minutes.

[b] Intubation is preferable. If it can be accomplished simultaneously with other techniques, then the earlier the better. However, epinephrine is more important initially if the patient can be ventilated without intubation.

[d] Value of sodium bicarbonate is questionable during cardiac arrest, and it is not recommended for routine cardiac arrest sequence. Consideration of its use in a dose of 1 mEq/kg is appropriate at this point. Half of original dose may be repeated every ten minutes if it is used.

Source: From American Heart Association, Standards and guidelines for cardiopulmonary resuscitation (CPR) and emergency cardiac care (ECC). *J.A.M.A.* 255:2905, 1986. Copyright 1986, American Medical Association. With permission.

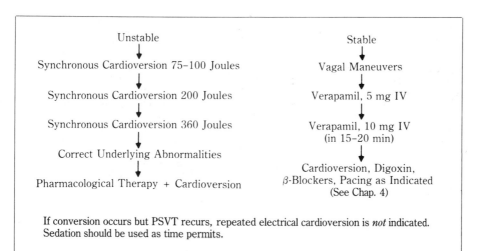

Fig. 2-5. Paroxysmal supraventricular tachycardia (PSVT). This sequence was developed to treat a broad range of patients with sustained PSVT. Some patients may require care not specified herein. This algorithm should not be construed as prohibiting such flexibility. Flow of algorithm presumes PSVT is continuing. (Source: From American Heart Association, Standards and guidelines for cardiopulmonary resuscitation (CPR) and emergency cardiac care (ECC). *J.A.M.A.* 255:2905, 1986. Copyright 1986, American Medical Association. With permission.)

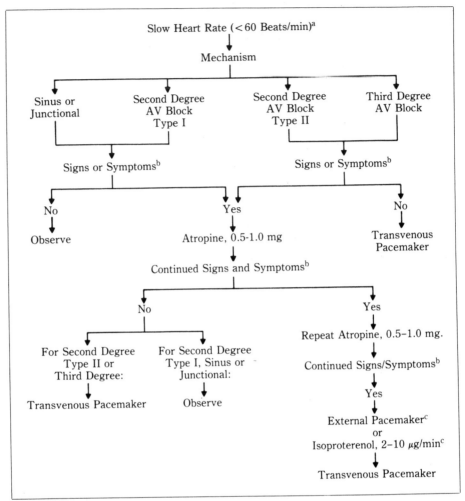

Fig. 2-6. Bradycardia. This sequence was developed to treat a broad range of patients with bradycardia. Some patients may require care not specified herein. This algorithm should not be construed to prohibit such flexibility. AV indicates atrioventricular.
[a] A solitary chest thump or cough may stimulate cardiac electrical activity and result in improved cardiac output and may be used at this point.
[b] Hypotension (blood pressure < 90 mm Hg), premature ventricular contractions, altered mental status or symptoms (e.g., chest pain or dyspnea), ischemia, or infarction.
[c] Temporizing therapy
Source: From American Heart Association, Standards and guidelines for cardiopulmonary resuscitation (CPR) and emergency cardiac care (ECC). *J.A.M.A.* 255:2905, 1986. Copyright 1986, American Medical Association. With permission.

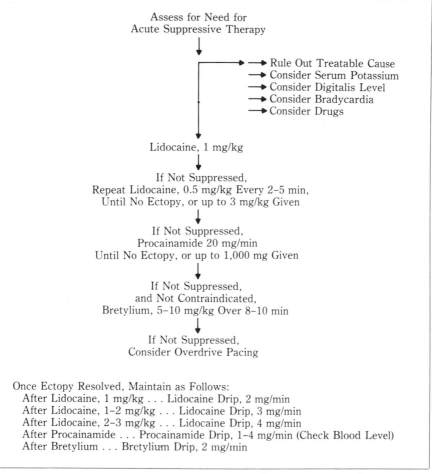

Assess for Need for
Acute Suppressive Therapy

→ Rule Out Treatable Cause
→ Consider Serum Potassium
→ Consider Digitalis Level
→ Consider Bradycardia
→ Consider Drugs

Lidocaine, 1 mg/kg

If Not Suppressed,
Repeat Lidocaine, 0.5 mg/kg Every 2–5 min,
Until No Ectopy, or up to 3 mg/kg Given

If Not Suppressed,
Procainamide 20 mg/min
Until No Ectopy, or up to 1,000 mg Given

If Not Suppressed,
and Not Contraindicated,
Bretylium, 5–10 mg/kg Over 8–10 min

If Not Suppressed,
Consider Overdrive Pacing

Once Ectopy Resolved, Maintain as Follows:
After Lidocaine, 1 mg/kg . . . Lidocaine Drip, 2 mg/min
After Lidocaine, 1–2 mg/kg . . . Lidocaine Drip, 3 mg/min
After Lidocaine, 2–3 mg/kg . . . Lidocaine Drip, 4 mg/min
After Procainamide . . . Procainamide Drip, 1–4 mg/min (Check Blood Level)
After Bretylium . . . Bretylium Drip, 2 mg/min

Fig. 2-7. Ventricular ectopy: acute suppressive therapy. This sequence was developed to treat a broad range of patients with ventricular ectopy. Some patients may require therapy not specified herein. This algorithm should not be construed as prohibiting such flexibility. Source: From American Heart Association, Standards and guidelines for cardiopulmonary resuscitation (CPR) and emergency cardiac care (ECC). *J.A.M.A.* 255:2905, 1986. Copyright 1986, American Medical Association. With permission.

Bibliography

1. American Heart Association. Standards and guidelines for cardiopulmonary resuscitation (CPR) and emergency cardiac care (ECC). *J.A.M.A.* 255:2905, 1986
2. Babbs, C. F. New versus old theories of blood flow during CPR. *Crit. Care Med.* 8:191, 1980.
3. Bishop, R. L., and Weisfeldt, M. L. Sodium bicarbonate administration during cardiac arrest. *J.A.M.A.* 235:506, 1976.
4. Chipman, C., et al. Criteria for cessation of CPR in the emergency department. *Ann. Emerg. Med.* 10:11, 1981.
5. Del Guerico, D., et al. Comparison of blood flow during external and internal cardiac massage in man. *Circulation* 31(Suppl.):171, 1965.
6. Dembo, D. H. Calcium in advanced life support. *Crit. Care Med.* 9:358, 1981.
7. Eisenberg, M. S., et al., Cardiac resuscitation in the community: Importance of rapid provision and implications for program planning. *J.A.M.A.* 241:1905, 1979.
8. Ewy, G. A. Recent advances in cardiopulmonary resuscitation and defibrillation. *Curr. Probl. Cardiol.*, Vol. VIII, April 1983.

9. Falk, R. H., et al. Safety and efficacy of noninvasive cardiac pacing. *N. Engl. J. Med.* 309:1166, 1983.

10. Gascho, J. A., et al. Determinants of ventricular defibrillation in adults. *Circulation* 60:231, 1979.

11. Holmes, H. R., et al. Influence of adrenergic drugs upon vital organ perfusion during CPR. *Crit. Care Med.* 8:137, 1980.

12. Kaye, W., and Paraskos, J. A. (eds.). *Instructors Manual for Advanced Cardiac Life Support.* Dallas: American Heart Association, 1982.

13. Kerber, R. E., and Sarnat, W. Factors influencing the success of ventricular defibrillation in man. *Circulation* 60:226, 1979.

14. Kuhn, G. J., et al. Peripheral vs. central circulation times during CPR: A pilot study. *Ann. Emerg. Med.* 10:417, 1981.

15. Lee, H. R., et al. MAST augmentation of external cardiac compression: Role of changing intrapleural pressure. *Ann. Emerg. Med.* 10:560, 1981.

16. Lewis, A. J., et al. *A Manual for Instructors of Basic Cardiac Life Support.* Dallas: American Heart Association, 1981.

17. McIntyre, K. M., and Lewis, A. J. (eds.). *Textbook of Advanced Cardiac Life Support.* Dallas: American Heart Association, 1983.

18. Miller, J., et al. The precordial thumb—useful or detrimental? (abstract). *Ann. Emerg. Med.* 12:246, 1983.

19. Niemann, J. T. Coronary perfusion pressure during experimental cardiopulmonary resuscitation. *Ann. Emerg. Med.* 11:127, 1982.

20. Otto, C. W., et al. Comparison of dopamine, dobutamine, and epinephrine in CPR. *Crit. Care Med.* 9:640, 1981.

21. Report of the Medical Consultants on the Diagnosis of Death to the Presidents Commission for the Study of Ethical Problems in Medicine and Biomedical and Behavioral Research. Guidelines for the determination of death. *J.A.M.A.* 246:2184, 1981.

22. Reznekov, L. Calcium antagonist drugs: Myocardial preservation and reduced vulnerability to ventricular fibrillation during CPR. *Crit. Care Med.* 9:360, 1981.

23. Smith, J. P., et al. The esophageal obturator airway: A review. *J.A.M.A.* 250:1081, 1983.

24. Stevins, J. P., et al. Use of calcium in prehospital cardiac arrest. *Ann. Emerg. Med.* 12:136, 1983.

25. Taylor, G. J., et al. Importance of prolonged compression during cardiopulmonary resuscitation in man. *N. Engl. J. Med.* 296:1515, 1977.

26. Voorhees, W. D., et al. Improved oxygen delivery during cardiopulmonary resuscitation with interposed abdominal compression. *Ann. Emerg. Med.* 12:128, 1983.

27. White, B. C., et al. Effect of flunarizine on canine cerebral cortical blood flow and vascular resistance post cardiac arrest. *Ann. Emerg. Med.* 11:119, 1982.

28. Yakaitis, R. W., et al. Relative importance of alpha and beta adrenergic receptors during resuscitation. *Crit. Care Med.* 7:293, 1979.

3

Shock

Paul R. Eisenberg

General Principles

Shock is a syndrome of tissue hypoperfusion leading to impaired cellular metabolism and ultimately organ failure.

I. **Classification.** The pathophysiology of shock remains controversial. However, all shock syndromes are characterized by tissue hypoperfusion. Perfusion failure may be due to decreased cardiac output, maldistribution of blood flow, or both. A classification that recognizes these pathophysiologic differences is presented in Table 3-1.

II. **Pathophysiology**

A. **Cellular hypoxia.** All shock syndromes lead to inadequate substrate delivery to cells. The consequent cellular hypoxia leads to anaerobic metabolism, resulting in increased lactate production (i.e., acidosis) and reduced adenosine triphosphate (ATP) production. Depletion of ATP reduces substrate for energy-dependent metabolic processes and results in cell membrane dysfunction. Release of lysosomal enzymes may also contribute to membrane disruption and proteolysis. In addition, direct damage to cell membranes may occur with such agents as endotoxin. Ultimately, if not reversed, these processes lead to cell death.

B. **Reflex responses.** Increased sympathetic activity occurs in response to hypotension and is mediated by carotid and aortic baroreceptors. Catecholamine secretion causes vasoconstriction, tachycardia, and increased cardiac output (in the absence of overriding limiting factors). Stretch receptors in the atria and vena cavae may also be important in some types of shock; decreased atrial pressure, as during hypovolemia, results in decreased stimulation and thus decreased efferent activity of these receptors. This leads to ADH secretion, renal vasoconstriction, and ultimately renin and angiotensin secretion. Thus sodium and water retention generally occurs.

C. **Cardiac function.** Altered cardiac function is characteristic of shock. In most forms of shock, cardiac output is depressed as a result of a decreased venous return (preload), primary cardiac dysfunction, or in some cases mechanical factors extrinsic to the heart (see Table 3-1). In addition, various factors may interact to further compromise cardiac function (see Fig. 3-1). As a result, it is not unusual in prolonged shock states for irreversible left ventricular dysfunction to develop.

Catecholamine secretion may increase cardiac output early in the course of shock (if decreased preload or impaired contractility is not a limiting factor). Thus in some shock states (e.g., sepsis), cardiac output may be elevated initially.

D. **Pulmonary function.** Alterations in pulmonary function are common in shock and range from compensatory changes in response to metabolic acidosis to frank respiratory failure. The latter is most often due to the adult respiratory distress syndrome (noncardiogenic pulmonary edema).

1. **Respiratory alkalosis** is common in the early stages of shock as a result of sympathetic stimulation. However, metabolic acidosis usually predominates as tissue hypoperfusion progresses, resulting in acidemia.

2. **Impaired oxygenation** due to complicating factors, such as increased left ventricular filling pressures, increased pulmonary capillary permeability, aspiration, infection, pulmonary embolism, or injury, is often present.

3. **Respiratory acidosis** or alveolar hypoventilation may occur secondary to depressed central nervous system (CNS) function.

4. **The adult respiratory distress syndrome (ARDS)** (see Chap. 7) is the most serious pulmonary complication of shock, with a case fatality rate of greater than 50%. This syndrome is characterized by the accumulation of extravascular

Table 3-1. Classification of shock syndromes

I. Distributive (maldistribution of blood flow)
   A. Septic
   B. Neurogenic
   C. Anaphylactic
   D. Toxic shock syndrome
   E. Metabolic
II. Hypovolemic (decreased cardiac output secondary to loss of intravascular volume)
   A. Hemorrhagic
   B. Nonhemorrhagic
      1. Gastrointestinal fluid loss (e.g., vomiting, diarrhea)
      2. Renal loss (e.g., diabetes insipidus, osmotic diuresis)
      3. Severe dehydration
      4. Severe burns
      5. Third-space loss (e.g., peritonitis, pancreatitis)
III. Cardiogenic (decreased cardiac output due to cardiac factors)
   A. Impaired left ventricular contractility (e.g., ischemia, infarction, congestive myopathy)
   B. Impaired right ventricular contractility (e.g., right ventricular infarction)
   C. Acute regurgitant lesions (e.g., mitral or aortic regurgitation, intraventricular septal rupture)
   D. Obstructive cardiac lesions (e.g., aortic stenosis, subaortic stenosis)
   E. Bradyarrhythmias or tachyarrhythmias
IV. Obstructive (decreased cardiac output due to factors extrinsic to the heart)
   A. Pericardial tamponade
   B. Pneumothorax
   C. Pulmonary embolism
   D. Severe pulmonary hypertension

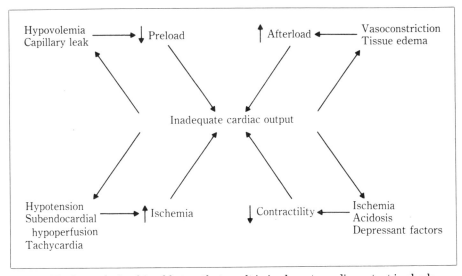

Fig. 3-1. The interrelationship of factors that result in inadequate cardiac output in shock. (From K. I. Shine et al., Aspects of the management of shock. *Ann. Intern. Med.* 93:723, 1980. With permission.)

lung water due to increased alveolocapillary permeability. The mechanisms responsible are complex and incompletely understood. However, several risk factors for the development of this syndrome have been identified, including sepsis, multiple fractures, multiple transfusions, disseminated intravascular coagulation, and aspiration. In one series, the presence of more than one risk factor was associated with an increased incidence of ARDS [8].

E. **Renal function.** Oliguria is the most common manifestation of renal involvement in shock.

   1. **Oliguria** occurs early in most shock syndromes due primarily to profound renal vasoconstriction and a decrease in renal blood flow. The increased vascular tone is mediated by increased sympathetic activity and the renin-angiotension system. Renal cortical perfusion is decreased, while medullary perfusion is increased. These alterations result in a decreased glomerular filtration rate that may be further compromised by endothelial cell swelling. A concentrated urine due to increased sodium resorption and free-water retention results. With prompt improvement of hypovolemia and increased renal perfusion, this state is often reversible. However, prolonged hypoperfusion commonly results in acute renal failure.

   2. **Acute renal failure** in shock is most often a result of acute vasomotor nephropathy. The pathogenesis of acute vasomotor nephropathy is primarily hypoxic cellular injury due to prolonged renal hypoperfusion. Other factors likely are important; however, they are not completely elucidated. Furthermore, renal injury may be exacerbated by vasopressors, antibiotics (e.g., aminoglycosides), myoglobin, sepsis, or disseminated intravascular coagulation. Often renal failure in this setting is reversible.

F. **Cerebral** ischemia is infrequent in shock when mean arterial pressure is above 60 mm Hg, the range in which autoregulation is effective. With marked and prolonged hypotension, however, global ischemia occurs, often resulting in brain death.

G. **Liver** function is frequently impaired with prolonged hypotension. Metabolic dysfunction and hepatocellular necrosis may result. Although hepatic dysfunction usually does not contribute to the acute manifestations of shock, decreased hepatic clearance of drugs and their metabolites may lead to toxicity (e.g., decreased lidocaine clearance).

H. **Bowel** ischemia and hemorrhagic necrosis may occur if hypotension is prolonged. Depending on the severity of the hypotension, intestinal submucosal hemorrhage, ileus, and rarely bowel perforation may occur.

I. **Metabolic effects.** Elevation of the blood glucose is common in shock, primarily from sympathetic stimulated glycogenolysis. Lipolysis also occurs; however, decreased perfusion of adipose tissue and possibly impaired metabolism may limit the use of free fatty acids as an energy source.

J. **Other factors,** such as vasoactive hormones, endorphins, enkephalins, and prostaglandins, have been implicated in the pathophysiology of shock in a variety of experimental models. However, the precise role of these mediators remains undetermined.

III. **Management**
   A. **General measures**
      1. **Initial assessment** of the hypotensive patient must be rapid yet thorough, with particular attention directed at evidence of **organ hypoperfusion.** In patients with profound hypotension (e.g., systolic blood pressure < 60 mm Hg), tissue hypoxia is almost invariably present. However, shock (i.e., tissue hypoperfusion) may be present with higher systolic blood pressures. In some instances, hypotension may only be apparent if the patient sits or stands up (orthostasis). Typically, the patient in shock will have cool clammy extremities; a thready, rapid pulse; and impaired consciousness. However, some patients with septic shock initially have warm extremities and borderline hypotension. Correct diagnosis of the latter group is essential if early aggressive treatment is to be initiated.

      2. **Adequate ventilation** must be assured. Both patency of the airway and the presence of bilateral breath sounds should be confirmed. If necessary, endotracheal intubation (see Chap. 38) should be performed promptly; most patients with severe shock will require intubation. Supplemental oxygen should be administered by nasal cannula, face mask, or endotracheal tube, initially at a concentration of 100% and later adjusted to maintain an arterial $PO_2 > 60$ mm Hg.

3. **Venous access** is the second priority in the immediate management of the patient with shock. Initially, one or more large-bore (18-gauge or larger) peripheral intravenous catheters should be inserted. The number of intravenous lines needed is dictated by the etiology and severity of the hypotension. If adequate peripheral access is not available, central venous catheterization (e.g., subclavian, internal jugular, or femoral vein catheterization) or a peripheral vein (e.g., saphenous vein) cutdown should be performed. Placement of central venous lines should always be performed using the best possible sterile procedure without sacrificing rapidity. Once the patient is stabilized, replacement of these lines using more optimal sterile technique should be routine practice.

4. **Further assessment**
   a. The **pulmonary** examination should assess for pulmonary edema, infiltrates, consolidation, and pneumothorax.
   b. The **cardiovascular** examination should be directed at detecting cardiogenic or obstructive shock. A dyskinetic cardiac impulse with an S3 gallop suggests cardiogenic shock. Elevation of the jugular venous pulse may indicate pericardial effusion or biventricular or right ventricular failure (see Chap. 5). Asymmetry or absence of peripheral pulses should be assessed, as these findings may be the only indication of an aortic dissection. Perfusion of the extremities should be noted; although poor perfusion may be a sign of shock, it is both nonspecific and insensitive in assessing the severity of shock.
   c. **Central nervous system** hypoxia is associated with confusion, agitation, or impairment of consciousness. Focal neurologic deficits, however, are infrequent and usually indicate a complicating primary neurologic event.
   d. The **abdominal** examination is important in the early evaluation of shock to assess for evidence of intraabdominal infection or blood loss (e.g., secondary to ruptured ectopic pregnancy, aortic aneurysm, or trauma). A rectal examination and assessment of the stool for blood are essential. If upper gastrointestinal bleeding is suspected, a nasogastric tube should be placed (with appropriate protection of the airway as indicated) to diagnose the presence of blood and judge the rate of blood loss. A pelvic examination should be performed, particularly when septic shock, toxic shock, or an ectopic pregnancy is considered.
   e. Careful examination of the **skin** may be of help in the differential diagnosis. A diffuse erythroderma in a menstruating female is consistent with toxic shock; hyperpigmentation may indicate adrenocortical insufficiency; urticaria may signify anaphylactic shock; and petechiae or ecchymoses may indicate a coagulopathy or meningococcemia.
   f. **Renal** hypoperfusion usually results in oliguria, which should be monitored by placement of an indwelling urethral catheter. A urine flow of less than 30–50 ml/hour is usually observed during hypoperfusion and improves with successful circulatory resuscitation.

5. **Initial laboratory** investigations should include serum electrolytes, creatinine, and blood urea nitrogen; a complete blood count and differential; a platelet count, prothrombin time, and activated partial thromboplastin time; and arterial blood gases. In all females of childbearing age, a pregnancy test is mandatory. An electrocardiogram and chest x-ray are indicated as well. Other studies (e.g., cultures, additional radiographic studies) will depend on the circumstances and likely diagnosis.

6. **Monitoring** of the patient in shock initially includes noninvasive determination of the blood pressure, heart rate, respiratory rate, cardiac rhythm, fluid status, and urinary output. When hypotension is profound and/or unresponsive to initial resuscitative measures, invasive hemodynamic monitoring is indicated. If invasive monitoring is not immediately available, the urinary output and signs of congestive heart failure (i.e., S3 gallop or pulmonary crackles) may be followed as an indication of adequate or excessive fluid resuscitation, respectively.
   a. **Arterial catheterization** is utilized to assess the central arterial pressure, since auscultated blood pressures may be inaccurate in the persistently hypotensive patient and in the presence of vasopressors. The femoral, axillary, or radial artery is usually chosen for catheterization; however, when profound vasoconstriction is present, radial artery pressures may not reflect central aortic pressures. It is essential that catheterization be performed under optimal sterile conditions. Since the mean arterial pressure is less prone to measurement variation than the systolic blood pressure, therapy

should be titrated using a mean arterial pressure of greater than 70 mm Hg as an end point. When pressure monitoring equipment is not available, **Doppler** aided blood pressure measurements are fairly accurate [3].

b. **The central venous pressure** (CVP), although not accurate in monitoring volume resuscitation, can be followed and kept less than 10–15 cm of H_2O. In addition, an initially low CVP (i.e., < 5 cm of H_2O) may be useful in determining the presence of hypovolemia.

c. **Pulmonary artery catheterization** is helpful in the management of shock not readily responding to initial therapy. Determinations of the pulmonary artery wedge pressure (normal 10–14 mm Hg) and cardiac index (normal > 2.4 liter/minute/m^2) may be used to guide fluid and pressor therapy. Accurate determination of these values is useful, since hemodynamic patterns vary considerably in shock and the clinical assessment is often inaccurate [4, 6]. In addition, determination of right heart and other pulmonary pressures, as well as the characteristics of the waveforms, may be diagnostically useful (e.g., pulmonary hypertension, cardiac tamponade). Pulmonary artery catheterization also allows for determination of mixed venous oxygenation. When the mixed venous oxygen tension is less than 30 mm Hg (or O_2 saturation is less than 60%), inadequate tissue oxygen delivery or, less often, increased oxygen consumption is likely. However, a normal or high (i.e., > 35 mm Hg) value in patients with shock may occur in the presence of arteriovenous shunting and septic shock.

B. Treatment of the shock state

1. **Fluid resuscitation** remains one of the most controversial areas in the management of shock. Although it is clear that adequate volume resuscitation is one of the most important early interventions in shock, there remains considerable debate as to the choice of fluids used and the criteria for adequacy [14, 15, 16].

   a. **Crystalloids** (e.g., usually normal saline or Ringer's lactate solution) are the most commonly administered forms of fluid therapy for volume replacement. Despite variability in personal preference, there is no proved difference between normal saline and Ringer's lactate as agents for volume resuscitation. Since crystalloids diffuse freely between the extravascular and intravascular compartments, large amounts of crystalloid resuscitation often lead to interstitial edema and may contribute to dilution of plasma proteins. Some investigators believe that this dilution leads to a decreased colloid oncotic pressure and may exacerbate noncardiogenic pulmonary edema; however, other studies do not support this view.

   Crystalloid solutions are inexpensive and usually immediately available. They should be considered definitive therapy for water and electrolyte volume loss (e.g., vomiting, diarrhea). In addition, crystalloids can be used as primary therapy for all forms of hypovolemic and distributive shock, even if colloids are added.

   b. **Colloids** are solutions containing nondiffusible high-molecular-weight molecules, usually either albumin or synthetic macromolecules. Since colloid solutions do not diffuse rapidly from the intravascular compartment, they are more effective acutely for intravascular volume expansion than an equivalent volume of crystalloid. Some physicians prefer colloid resuscitation, reasoning that less edema and interstitial fluid accumulation should result. However, consistent evidence that colloid resuscitation either reduces or exacerbates noncardiogenic pulmonary edema is not available.

   Presently available colloid solutions are expensive and have several drawbacks. Plasma protein fraction (plasmanate) has been associated with hypotensive reactions, presumably due to the presence of bradykinin or other impurities. High-molecular-weight dextran interferes with platelet function and thus may increase bleeding. Newer agents such as hetastarch may have less adverse effects and may be preferable.

   c. **Whole blood** is an effective volume expander; however its use should be limited to severe hemorrhage. Packed red blood cells (including type-specific or O-negative blood) are useful for increasing the oxygen carrying capacity [5, 22]. In hemorrhagic shock, transfusion of blood is indicated in the presence of persistent hypotension following the infusion of 2 liters of crystalloid. (See Chap. 17 for further discussion of blood products.)

   d. The "**crystalloid versus colloid**" debate continues; however, sufficient evidence is not available to recommend one approach of therapy in preference to the other. Generally, if the systolic blood pressure is greater than 60 mm Hg or there is no evidence of symptomatic cardiac or cerebral hypoperfusion, initial therapy with crystalloids should be adequate. An initial fluid challenge of 300–500 ml of crystalloid over 15 minutes or less is recommended. If after 2 liters of fluid the blood pressure has not improved and further fluids are indicated, a colloid solution or blood (packed red blood cells) may be added. When marked hypotension and cardiac or cerebral dysfunction are present, initial therapy using rapid crystalloid infusion and, if desired, colloids is indicated; a vasopressor may need to be added and hopefully can be tapered as volume resuscitation is successful. The amount of fluids administered should be based on the occurrence of a physiologic response rather than an arbitrary volume. Following the initial volume challenge, fluid administration of up to 2–3 liters/hour may be necessary. Initially the best response to follow is improvement in the blood pressure. Subsequently, whenever possible, the best indication of adequate volume resuscitation is a pulmonary artery wedge pressure or pulmonary artery diastolic pressure of 15–18 mm Hg.

2. The **Military Anti-Shock Trousers (MAST) suit** is an important device in the early management of shock (see Chap. 38). This device is an inflatable trouser and an abdominal binder that provides circumferential external pressure of up to 104 mm Hg (generally 10–40 mm Hg inflation is used). Once inflated, the blood pressure is increased by the MAST suit, effecting an increase in peripheral resistance and a modest (100–400 ml) "autotransfusion" of blood from the capacitance vessels to the central circulation, allowing for preferential perfusion of the vital organs (i.e., the heart and brain). In addition, the MAST suit tamponades bleeding from sites beneath the device and stabilizes pelvic and femur fractures. The device is useful in treating those forms of shock in which an increase in afterload would not be detrimental.

3. **Pharmacologic** support of the circulation is accomplished by the use of sympathomimetic drugs. These agents should be used whenever initial volume replacement does not promptly improve the blood pressure. Several agents are available; selection of a particular agent should be based on the hemodynamic action required.

   a. **Norepinephrine (Levophed)** is both an alpha- and beta-agonist. The primary effect is vasoconstriction (alpha-receptors) with resultant increased total peripheral resistance. This results in increased cardiac and cerebral perfusion, while other organs may be hypoperfused. Stimulation of cardiac receptors (beta-1) results in a tachycardia, but the cardiac output may not change or may decrease due to an increased afterload.

      Norepinephrine should be prepared as an 8–16 mg/liter solution (8–16 µg/ml) using either 5% dextrose or 5% dextrose and saline and initially infused at a rate (usually 2–8 µg/minute) to maintain a systolic blood pressure of greater than 90 mm Hg.

   b. **Dopamine** has become the most frequently used sympathomimetic agent for shock because of its ability to maintain splanchnic and renal blood flow in addition to alpha- and beta-agonist activity. The hemodynamic effects depend on the dose administered. At a dosage of 1–5 µg/kg/minute, total peripheral resistance may decrease while splanchnic and renal blood flow increase. At 5–8 µg/kg/minute, cardiac (beta-1) stimulation predominates, and thus the cardiac output (positive inotropy) and blood pressure usually increase. At dosages above 10 µg/kg/minute, alpha-adrenergic stimulation occurs, resulting in generalized vasoconstriction and splanchnic and renal blood flow decrease. Dopamine is usually prepared as an 800 mg/liter solution (8 µg/ml) using either 5% dextrose or 5% dextrose and saline.

   c. **Methoxamine and phenylephrine** are pure alpha-agonists. Total peripheral resistance increases, and cardiac output usually decreases. These agents are used when hypotension is due to decreased sympathetic tone (e.g., spinal shock, postanesthetic hypotension, certain drug overdosages). Methoxamine is generally administered IV as a 3- to 5-mg bolus, which will increase the blood pressure for 20–40 minutes. Phenylephrine is administered slowly IV in a dosage of 0.1–0.5 mg or as an infusion of 10 mg in 500 ml of either 5% dextrose or 0.9% saline, titrated to physiologic response.

   d. **Isoproterenol** is a pure beta-agonist with both cardiac (beta-1) and vascular (beta-2) effects. Cardiac output increases, while peripheral resistance falls.

The blood pressure decreases or is unchanged depending on the increase in cardiac output. Because of its positive chronotropic effects, it is useful in treating atropine-resistant bradyarrhythmias (see Chap. 2).

e. **Dobutamine** is a beta- and alpha-agonist; however, beta-1 stimulation predominates. Cardiac output and heart rate increase, and total peripheral resistance falls. The utility of dobutamine is based on its positive inotropic properties. When used for this purpose, the initial dosage is 1–2 µg/kg/minute, and the dosage is titrated to a maximum of 10–15 µg/kg/minute to achieve the desired increase in cardiac output (see Chap. 5).

f. **Metaraminol** is metabolized to norepinephrine and thus is an indirect alpha- and beta-agonist. Metaraminol is adminstered as an infusion of 15–100 mg in 500 ml of either 5% dextrose or 0.9% saline. An intravenous bolus of 0.5–5.0 mg may be used when a rapid effect is desired in severe shock.

4. **Sodium bicarbonate** is of benefit in treating the metabolic acidosis (secondary to lactate production) common to most shock states. It should be administered when the pH is less than 7.2. Usually 1 mEq/kg is administered initially; further administration should be guided by arterial blood gas results. Respiratory acidosis should be treated by endotracheal intubation and increased alveolar ventilation.

IV. **Disposition.** Patients with shock require hospitalization, usually in an intensive care unit.

Specific Shock States

I. **Hemorrhagic shock** occurs with rapid loss of more than 30–40% of the blood volume.

A. **Common etiologies** include trauma, gastrointestinal bleeding, ruptured abdominal aortic aneurysm, and ruptured ectopic pregnancy.

B. The **hemodynamic** alterations are due to hypovolemia with decreased venous return and thus reduced ventricular filling pressures (preload). Stroke volume falls, and hypotension ensues. Compensatory marked sympathetic stimulation and oliguria occur.

C. **Initial examination** usually reveals a patient who is pale, tachycardiac, tachypneic, and hypotensive. Gross hemorrhage or signs of intraabdominal or intrathoracic bleeding are usually but not always present.

D. **Specific laboratory studies** should include a complete blood count, platelet count, coagulation studies, serum electrolytes, arterial blood gas, pregnancy test, and serum calcium. A spun hematocrit should be obtained in the emergency department; however, it is not an accurate indicator of the degree of blood loss until after hemodilution has occurred (3–4 hours).

E. **Immediate management**

1. The **airway** should be assured. Oxygen should be administered by face mask or endotracheal tube at a concentration of 100% unless carbon dioxide retention is a known problem. In severe anemia, the contribution of dissolved oxygen to total oxygen delivery may be significant.

2. **Peripheral venous access** should be established with two to three large-bore catheters (14- to 16-gauge). If necessary, jugular, subclavian, femoral, or saphenous vein access may be used, although usually only the latter accommodates a large-bore tube for rapid fluid administration.

3. **Volume infusion.** A crystalloid fluid challenge of 300–500 ml should be given whenever there is clinical evidence of shock and the blood pressure is less than 70–80 mm Hg. If the blood pressure does not improve, an additional 1–2 liters are then administered by rapid infusion. Transfusion of whole blood or packed red blood cells is indicated if the systolic blood pressure does not increase to greater than 90 mm Hg after 2 liters of fluid administration. In trauma patients with intrathoracic hemorrhage, autotransfusion may be used (see Chap. 38). Generally, the hematocrit should be maintained above 30%.

When shock is more severe and the initial systolic blood pressure is less than 60–70 mm Hg or when cardiac or cerebral dysfunction is present, more aggressive volume therapy including blood products (O-negative packed cells), colloids, and pressors may be necessary. Colloid therapy has been suggested as initial therapy for this degree of hypotension.

When **massive blood transfusion** is necessary, several complications may occur. Dilution of clotting factors and platelets in some patients may result in inadequate hemostasis. Fresh frozen plasma and platelets should be administered when this occurs. Hypocalcemia may occur with rapid administration of stored blood due to citrate binding of ionized calcium. Administration of calcium chloride, 14.5 mEq, is indicated should there be bradycardia, arrhythmias, hypotension, or other evidence of hypocalcemia. Hypothermia may also occur with massive transfusion of cold banked red blood cells but can be prevented by using a blood warming device [5].

4. The **MAST suit** is useful in hemorrhagic shock and should be used as part of the initial resuscitative effort to improve cardiac and cerebral perfusion.

5. **Pressors** may be needed to support cerebral and cardiac perfusion. Dopamine is preferred and is started at a high dosage (5–10 μg/kg/minute) and tapered rapidly to maintain the systolic blood pressure at a minimum of 90 mm Hg. The general rule of both pressor and volume therapy is to ensure vital organ function while restoring intravascular volume. As aggressive volume resuscitation is successful, the dosage of pressor is decreased as rapidly as consistent with vital organ perfusion.

6. The narcotic antagonist **naloxone hydrochloride** has improved survival in animal models of hemorrhagic shock. However, this agent has not been used in human studies and remains investigative [9].

7. **Monitoring** of the vital signs, cardiac rhythm, volume infused, pressor dosage, and urine output is essential. When persistent hypotension or cardiac dysfunction occurs, invasive hemodynamic monitoring is indicated.

II. **Hypovolemic shock** not due to hemorrhage is a consequence of either fluid and electrolyte loss or "third-space" sequestration. Examples of the former are severe vomiting and diarrhea, salt-wasting nephropathy, diabetes mellitus, diabetes insipidus, and extensive burns. Third-space losses occur with severe pancreatitis, bowel obstruction or ischemia, peritonitis, and some types of trauma.

A. The **hemodynamics** are similar to hemorrhagic shock, with intense sympathetic stimulation due to hypovolemia.

B. **Initial presentation** of the patient is similar to that of hemorrhagic shock, with tachycardia, tachypnea, and hypotension. Abdominal evaluation may be helpful in establishing the presence of ascites or an infectious process.

C. **Laboratory studies.** Measurement of serum electrolytes frequently is important in determining fluid and electrolyte replacement. The hematocrit may be increased due to hemoconcentration. Serum calcium and magnesium may be decreased in some disorders (e.g., pancreatitis, salt-wasting nephropathy).

D. **Immediate management**

1. The **airway** should be stabilized and oxygen administered at a sufficient concentration to keep the arterial oxygen tension greater than 60 mm Hg.

2. **Volume resuscitation** with crystalloid generally is definitive therapy for most nonhemorrhagic hypovolemic shock. However, if hypotension is severe, colloids may be added. Aggressive therapy directed at obtaining a systolic blood pressure greater than 90 mm Hg is essential. When anemia is present, packed red blood cells should be added to maintain the hematocrit about 30%. The MAST suit may be used initially while volume therapy is being initiated.

3. The indications for **pressor therapy** (see sec. I.E.5) are similar to those for all types of shock and include persistent hypotension after initial volume resuscitation and significant cardiac or cerebral hypoperfusion.

4. **Monitoring** of the vital signs and fluid input and output is essential. When hypotension is persistent or requires pressor therapy, or when cardiac dysfunction is suggested by the history or physical examination, consideration should be given to invasive hemodynamic monitoring.

III. Although **septic shock** is hemodynamically heterogenous, the physiology is often characterized by maldistribution of blood flow rather than by true hypovolemia.

A. The most common **etiologic agents** are gram-negative bacteria; however, gram-positive bacteria, rickettsiae, fungi, viruses, and protozoa have been reported to cause a similar syndrome.

B. **Pathophysiology.** Most experimental models of septic shock have employed administration of gram-negative bacteria or endotoxin to initiate shock. Endotoxin, the large lipopolysaccharide associated with gram-negative bacterial cell walls, is the essential factor, and antibodies directed against this molecule prevent the development of shock. The pathogenesis of shock due to endotoxin involves many factors including complement activation, kinin system activation, release of mediators from leukocytes, impaired coagulation (including disseminated intravascular coagulation), and direct damage of cell membranes by endotoxin. The pathophysiology of shock due to organisms without endotoxin has not been well studied; however, presumably similar events occur.

C. The **hemodynamic** alterations of septic shock may antedate clinically apparent shock. Both the more typical "cold shock" (characterized by vasoconstriction and a decreased cardiac output) and "warm shock" may occur. The latter is characterized by a hemodynamic pattern of decreased total peripheral resistance, cutaneous vasodilatation, and an increased cardiac output. Tissue hypoxia and lactic acidosis occur despite a normal mixed venous oxygen tension. This pattern is thought to be due to maldistribution of blood flow and possibly arteriovenous shunting.

D. The **clinical presentation** is variable. Some patients present with hypotension, hypothermia, tachycardia, tachypnea, and oliguria. Others may have warm skin and mild hypotension, with evidence of organ hypoperfusion in the form of confusion or oliguria. When septic shock is suspected, a source of infection should be sought.

E. **Laboratory studies.** A urinalysis is essential. Cultures of blood, urine, cerebrospinal fluid, or other sources of infection should be obtained prior to antibiotic administration. The leukocyte count may be either elevated or depressed; the latter suggests a poor prognosis. Thrombocytopenia and coagulation abnormalities are common.

F. **Immediate management**

1. Assurance of **airway** patency and adequate ventilation is always the first priority. Supplemental oxygen usually is indicated.

2. **Volume resuscitation** is generally started with a 300- to 500-ml crystalloid fluid challenge. The MAST device may also be used to improve vital organ perfusion. When large amounts of crystalloid (i.e., > 2–3 liters) appear necessary, colloid may be of benefit. Red blood cells should be administered if the hematocrit is less than 30%. When cardiac or cerebral dysfunction is present, pressors should be initiated while volume is being administered.

3. Empiric **antibiotic** therapy is indicated whenever septic shock is suspected (after cultures of all possible sources of infection are obtained). Since gram-negative bacilli are the most common etiologic agents, an aminoglycoside is administered; gentamycin or tobramycin should be given as an initial intravenous bolus of 2 mg/kg, with subsequent dosing based on the patient's renal function. Amikacin may be used if resistance to the other aminoglycosides is suspected. The choice of a second antibiotic depends on the suspected source of infection, for example ticarcillin for *Pseudomonas*, clindamycin for abdominal anaerobes, oxacillin or nafcillin for penicillinase-producing gram-positive organisms, and ampicillin for enteric gram-negative bacilli (see Chap. 12).

4. **Surgical incision and drainage** and/or debridement should be performed promptly when indicated.

5. The use of **corticosteroids** in the initial treatment of septic shock has been advocated based on both experimental and clinical data. Improved survival when steroids are administered prior to or very early after the administration of endotoxins has been shown in animal models [11]. One clinical study found a decreased mortality in patients with septic shock given steroids early [17]. However, a recent prospective randomized trial found that despite early improvement in patients with septic shock treated with steroids the in-hospital mortality was the same as in patients not treated with steroids [19]. Thus, the data is inconclusive, and the benefit of steroids is not uniformly accepted. If steroids are used, either methylprednisolone, 30 mg/kg, or dexamethasone, 3 mg/kg, should be administered early in the course and may be repeated once 4–8 hours later.

6. **Antiserum** to a mutant *Escherichia coli* recently has been found to decrease mortality in patients with septic shock [24]. However this therapy is not yet available for clinical use.

7. **Naloxone hydrochloride** has been shown to improve survival in experimental models of septic shock and improve hypotension in patients with septic shock [7, 13]. However, there have been no controlled studies using this agent, and there is no consensus as to the proper dosage. More important, there is no evidence in humans that naloxone alters the course of septic shock. Therefore, at the present time its use should be considered investigational.

8. **Other agents,** most notably indomethacin, have been shown to improve survival in experimental models. However, none has been shown to be applicable to human use.

IV. The **toxic shock syndrome** is thought to be due to a toxin produced by some strains of *Staphylococcus aureus*. Most often, it has been associated with tampon use in menstruating females; however, cases due to other sites of staphylococcal infection have been reported, including cutaneous lesions, surgical wound infections, postpartum infections, and abscesses.

   A. The **hemodynamics** are best characterized as a distributive type of shock and are similar to those described for septic shock.

   B. The **clinical diagnosis** of toxic shock is based on the presence of each of the following: a temperature greater than 38.9°C; skin erythroderma or desquamation, hypotension or orthostatic syncope, and mucosal (conjunctival, pharyngeal, or vaginal) hyperemia; however, mucosal hyperemia is not an essential criterion. In addition to the major criteria, there should be evidence of involvement of at least three organ systems. Common clinical manifestations include confusion, headache, myalgias, nausea, vomiting, diarrhea, and respiratory failure. Toxic shock should always be considered in the differential diagnosis of shock in menstruating women, particularly when an erythroderma is present.

   C. Common **laboratory** findings associated with toxic shock include a leukocytosis with increased band forms, thrombocytopenia, prolonged clotting studies, an elevated blood urea nitrogen, an elevated creatine phosphokinase, low serum proteins, elevated liver function tests, hypocalcemia, hypomagnesemia, and a sterile pyuria. Cultures of blood, wounds, and vaginal or cervical exudates should always be obtained to look for *S. aureus*.

   D. **Immediate management** of toxic shock follows the same guidelines as for septic shock, except for the choice of antibiotics. Since the diagnosis is likely to be equivocal on presentation, both an aminoglycoside and an antistaphylococcal agent generally are chosen initially. Most isolates associated with toxic shock have been sensitive to oxacillin or nafcillin. Resistant strains are treated with vancomycin (see Chap. 12).
   Electrolyte abnormalities, such as hypocalcemia, are common with toxic shock and should be treated with intravenous replacement.

   E. **Complications** of toxic shock, as with all types of shock, include disseminated intravascular coagulation, acute vasomotor nephropathy, and the adult respiratory distress syndrome.

V. **Anaphylactic shock** is an acute, distributive form of shock that occurs in response to antigen exposure in a sensitized individual. The reaction is mediated by IgE antibodies and involves the release of multiple mediators from mast cells and basophils. These mediators include histamine, leukotrienes, prostaglandins, kinins, catecholamines, and chemotactic factors.

   A. **Etiologic agents.** Substances that may cause anaphylaxis include insect stings, drugs, foreign serum, radiographic contrast agents, pollen, and food products.

   B. The **hemodynamic** pattern is an acute decrease in total peripheral resistance, venous return, and cardiac output. Intravascular volume depletion may also occur due to increased capillary permeability.

   C. **Clinical features.** Hypotension is prominent. Ventilatory compromise may occur due to bronchospasm, laryngospasm, and/or laryngeal edema. Rarely, noncardiogenic pulmonary edema may be the only manifestation. Often urticaria, angioedema, or diffuse erythema is present. There may or may not be a history of known allergy.

   D. **Immediate management**
      1. To assure **adequate ventilation,** endotracheal intubation is often required and should not be delayed. Intubation may be difficult due to laryngeal edema, and in some instances cricothyrotomy may be required. Administration of 100% oxygen is indicated.
      2. **Epinephrine** is the drug of choice for the initial therapy of anaphylactic reactions. The dose is 0.5 mg SQ (0.5 ml of 1:1000 solution) or, in severe cases (i.e., respiratory distress, shock), IV (5 ml of 1:10,000 solution); in the latter situation, sublingual or endotracheal administration is effective when intravenous access is delayed. The subcutaneous dose may be repeated every 20–30 minutes (for up to 3 doses) and the intravenous dose every 5–10 minutes as needed.
      3. **Bronchospasm** that persists after initial therapy should be treated with intravenous aminophylline (6 mg/kg loading dose over 30 minutes, followed by a maintenance infusion of 0.5 mg/kg/hour).
      4. **Volume resuscitation** with crystalloids is often necessary, even when epinephrine is effective, and requirements may be large.
      5. **Pressors** are administered when hypotension persists or vital organ perfusion is compromised (see sec. **I.E.5**). The MAST suit may also be used to treat persistent hypotension.

6. **Corticosteroids** are of value in preventing recurrence of anaphylaxis but not in treating the initial episode. Generally, hydrocortisone, 500 mg IV q6h, or its equivalent is administered.

7. **Antihistamines,** such as diphenhydramine (50–100 mg IV), may be of some benefit by preventing histamine binding to target tissues. This may prevent relapses.

VI. In **neurogenic shock,** there is loss of sympathetic tone at the level of the CNS. In the emergency setting, cervical spinal cord trauma is the most common etiology. A similar syndrome is also seen with high spinal anesthesia, marked elevations of the cerebrospinal fluid pressure, and some instances of profound toxic depression of the CNS. However, neurogenic shock is generally not a sequela of cerebrovascular accidents, focal CNS lesions, or cerebral trauma.

A. The **hemodynamic** consequences of loss of sympathetic tone are vasodilatation resulting in a decreased preload and cardiac output and thus hypotension. Frequently, a bradycardia is noted.

B. The **clinical presentation** most often is that of hypotension in association with cervical trauma. The hypotension in some cases may be well tolerated by the patient.

C. Immediate management

1. A secure **airway** must be established as needed without aggravating any spinal cord injury (see Chap. 17). Administration of supplemental oxygen is indicated.

2. **Volume resuscitation** should be cautious. Unless there is associated blood loss, administration of large amounts of fluid, with the attendant risk of CNS and pulmonary edema, may not be required. Achieving and maintaining a systolic blood pressure of 80–90 mm Hg generally is acceptable and well tolerated by the patient.

3. The **MAST suit** is a useful adjunct in the management of these patients.

4. A **pressor** may be needed in conjunction with volume resuscitation. In this setting, an agent with predominant alpha-adrenergic activity (e.g., methoxamine, phenylephrine) is often used.

VII. Cardiogenic shock. See Chap. 5.

Bibliography

1. Abraham, E., et al. Sequential cardiorespiratory patterns in septic shock. *Crit. Care Med.* 11:799, 1983.

2. Altura, B. M., Lefer, A. M., and Shumer, W. *Handbook of Shock and Trauma. Volume I: Basic Science.* New York: Raven, 1984.

3. Buggs, H., et al. Comparison of systolic arterial blood pressure by transcutaneous Doppler probe and conventional methods in hypotensive patients. *Anesth. Analg.* (Cleve.) 52:776, 1973.

4. Connors, A. F., McCafree, D. R., and Gray, B. A. Evaluation of right heart catheterization in the critically ill patient without myocardial infarction. *N. Engl. J. Med.* 308:263, 1983.

5. Cowley, R. A., and Dunham, C. M. *Shock Trauma/Critical Care Manual.* Initial Assessment and Management. Baltimore: University Park Press, 1982. Pp. 35–42.

6. Eisenberg, P. R., Jaffe A. S., and Schuster, D. P. Clinical evaluation compared to pulmonary artery catheterization in the hemodynamic assessment of critically ill patients. *Crit. Care Med.* 12:549, 1984.

7. Faden, A. I., and Holaday, J. W. Experimental endotoxin shock: The pathophysiologic function of endorphins and treatment with opiate antagonists. *J. Infect. Dis.* 142:229, 1980.

8. Fowler, A. A., et al. Adult respiratory distress syndrome: Risk with common predispositions. *Ann. Intern. Med.* 99:293, 1983.

9. Gurll, N. J., et al. Opiate receptors and endorphins in the pathophysiology of hemorrhagic shock. *Surgery* 89:364, 1981.

10. Hess, M. L., Hastillo, A., and Greenfield L. J. Spectrum of cardiovascular function during gram negative sepsis. *Prog. Cardiovasc. Dis.* 23:279, 1981.

11. Hinshaw, L. B., Beller-Todd, B. K., and Archer, L. T. Current management of the septic shock patient: Experimental basis for treatment. *Circ. Shock* 9:543, 1982.

12. Pelligra, R., and Sandberg, E. C. Control of intractable abdominal bleeding by external counterpressure. *J.A.M.A.* 24:708, 1979.

13. Peters, W. P., et al. Pressor effect of naloxone in septic shock. *Lancet* 1:529, 1981.

14. Rackow, E. C., et al. Fluid resuscitation in circulatory shock: A comparison of the

cardiorespiratory effects of albumin, hetastarch, and saline solutions in patients with hypovolemic and septic shock. *Crit. Care Med.* 11:839, 1983.

15. Shine, K. I., et al. Aspects of the management of shock. *Ann. Intern. Med.* 93:723, 1980.
16. Shoemaker, W. C., and Hauser, C. J. Critique of crystalloid versus colloid in shock and shock lung. *Crit. Care Med.* 7:117, 1979.
17. Shumer, W. Steroids in the treatment of clinical septic shock. *Ann. Surg.* 184:333, 1976.
18. Sobel, B. E. Cardiac and Noncardiac Forms of Acute Circulatory Failure. In E. Braunwald (ed.), *Heart Disease* (2nd ed.). Philadelphia: Saunders, 1984.
19. Sprung, C. L., et al. The effects of high-dose corticosteroids in patients with septic shock: A prospective, controlled study. *N. Engl. J. Med.* 311:1137, 1984.
20. Tarazi, R. C. Sympathomimetic agents in the treatment of shock. *Ann. Intern. Med.* 81:364, 1974.
21. The toxic shock syndrome (conference). *Ann. Intern. Med.* 96:831, 1982.
22. Walt, A. J. (ed.). *Early Care of the Injured Patient* (3rd ed.). Philadelphia: Saunders, 1982.
23. Wayne, M. A., and Macdonald, S. C. Clinical evaluation of the antishock trouser: Retrospective analysis of five years' experience. *Ann. Emerg. Med.* 12:342, 1980.
24. Ziegler, E. J., et al. Treatment of gram negative bacteremia and shock with human antiserum to a mutant *Escherichia coli*. *N. Engl. J. Med.* 307:1225, 1982.

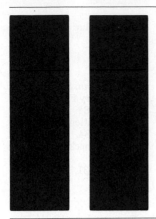

Medical Emergencies

4

Cardiac Arrhythmias

John A. Boerner and
Michael E. Cain

Assessment

Cardiac arrhythmias are common and frequently serious problems in emergency medicine. Proper management requires prompt and accurate assessment.

I. **History.** The duration of the present episode and the presence of associated symptoms should be determined. In addition, the frequency of previous episodes and the modes of initiation and termination should be noted. Having the patient reproduce the rate and rhythm of the palpitations by finger tapping provides an important diagnostic clue. The presence of any underlying disease and precipitating events should be elicited. Furthermore, a careful drug history is imperative.

II. **Physical examination** (Table 4-1). Examination of the jugular venous pulse during an arrhythmia, especially the timing of the *a* and *v* waves and the presence or absence of cannon *a* waves, provides information about the pattern of atrioventricular (AV) conduction. The intensity of the first heart sound (S1) (loud or soft, constant or variable) also reflects the degree of AV synchrony. The response to carotid sinus massage has diagnostic and therapeutic value. Evidence of cardiomegaly, congestive heart failure (CHF), or hypotension provides information regarding the etiology and hemodynamic consequence of the arrhythmia. In addition, the general examination provides clues to other relevant disorders, such as hyper- or hypothyroidism.

III. **Evaluation of the electrocardiogram (ECG).** The pattern and relationship of atrial and ventricular activity is important (Table 4-1). Assessment of atrial activity may be facilitated by the following.

   A. Multiple lead **rhythm strips.** Leads aVF and V_1, recorded at a paper speed of 50 mm/second, are particularly useful for identifying atrial activity.

   B. Bipolar "Lewis" lead. The left arm lead (lead I) is placed posteriorly or over the left ventricular apex and the right arm lead is used to explore the precordium.

   C. **Carotid sinus massage** and other vagotonic maneuvers often alter the ventricular response, facilitating identification of atrial activity. The patient should be supine, with an intravenous (IV) line in place and the ECG monitored. The carotid arteries should be auscultated initially, since a bruit is a relative contraindication to this maneuver. If there are no contraindications, the right carotid sinus is massaged firmly for no more than 10 seconds. If there is no response, the left carotid sinus is then massaged. **Both carotid sinuses, however, should not be massaged simultaneously.** The Valsalva maneuver may be tried in conjunction with carotid sinus massage.

   D. **Esophageal lead.** If a conventional esophageal lead is not available, one can be made by passing a pacemaker wire through a nasogastric (NG) tube. The pacemaker wire, however, should not extend beyond the distal part of the tube during passage into the esophagus. After the NG tube and pacemaker wire are placed approximately 50 cm into the esophagus, the pacing wire is connected to an exploring (V lead) electrode. The pacemaker wire is then extended through the distal end of the NG tube, and a search is made for electrical activity. If atrial activity is not evident, the NG tube and pacemaker wire should be withdrawn slowly in 1-cm increments until P waves and QRS complexes are identified. Having the patient hold his or her breath during midinspiration reduces respiratory interference.

   E. **Intraatrial electrogram.** This procedure must be done under sterile conditions with a well-grounded ECG machine or special amplifier.

IV. **Laboratory studies.** Important precipitating factors may be identified by obtaining a chest x-ray, arterial blood gas, serum electrolytes (including calcium and magnesium), serum creatinine, serum creatine kinase (CK) and MB-CK, thyroid function tests, and drug levels (especially of antiarrhythmic agents) as indicated; decisions regarding selec-

Table 4-1. Cardiac arrhythmias: physical examination and electrocardiographic characteristics

Arrhythmia	Intensity of S_1	Jugular venous pulse	Ventricular response to carotid sinus massage[a]	P waves			QRS complexes		
				Rate	Rhythm	Morphology	Rate	Rhythm	Morphology
Sinus tachycardia	Constant	Normal	Gradual slowing and return to former rate	100–180	Regular	May be peaked	100–180[b]	Regular	Normal
Sinus bradycardia	Constant	Normal	Gradual slowing and return to former rate	< 60	Regular	Normal	< 60[b]	Regular	Normal
Atrial premature depolarizations (APDs)	May be soft with very premature beats	Constant	Gradual slowing of underlying rhythm and return to former rate; variable effect on frequency of APDs	Variable	Irregular	Variable	Variable[b]	Irregular	Normal
Atrial flutter	Constant; variable if AV block variable	Flutter a waves	Abrupt slowing and return to former rate; atrial flutter remains	250–350	Regular	Sawtooth	75–175	Regular in absence of drugs or disease	Normal
Atrial fibrillation	Variable	No a waves	Gradual slowing; gross irregularity remains	400–600	Grossly irregular	Baseline undulation without clear p waves	100–180	Grossly irregular	Normal
Paroxysmal supraventricular tachycardia (PSVT)	Constant, usually decreased	Constant, usually with cannon a waves	Abrupt slowing due to either termination of arrhythmia or increase in AV block with atrial tachycardia remaining	120–250	Regular	Dependent on mechanism[c]	120–250[b]	Regular	Normal

Arrhythmia	First heart sound	Venous pulse	Response to carotid sinus massage[a]	Atrial rate	Atrial rhythm	AV conduction	Ventricular rate	Ventricular rhythm	QRS complex
Atrial tachycardia with block	Constant; variable if AV block variable	More a waves than v waves	Abrupt slowing and return to former rate; atrial tachycardia remains	150–250	Regular	Abnormal	75–200	Regular in absence of drugs or disease	Normal
Multifocal atrial tachycardia	Variable	Variable relation of a to v waves	No response or gradual slowing with atrial irregularity continuing	100–150	Grossly irregular	Variable	100–150[b]	Grossly irregular	Normal
Nonparoxysmal AV junctional tachycardia	Variable[d]	Intermittent cannon a waves[d]	None (slight slowing may occur)	60–100[e]	Regular	Normal	70–130	Regular	Normal; may be abnormal but < 0.12 sec
Ventricular premature depolarizations (VPDs)	Variable	Intermittent cannon a waves	Gradual slowing of underlying rhythm and return to former rate; variable effect on VPDs	60–100[e]	Regular	Normal	60–100	Irregular	Normal except for VPDs
Accelerated idioventricular rhythm	Variable[d]	Intermittent cannon a waves[d]	None	60–100[e]	Regular	Normal	50–110	Fairly regular	Abnormal, > 0.12 sec
Ventricular tachycardia	Variable[d]	Intermittent cannon a waves[d]	None	60–100[e]	Regular	Normal	110–250	Regular	Abnormal, > 0.12 sec
Ventricular flutter	Soft or absent	Cannon a waves	None	60–100[e]	Regular	Normal	250–300	Regular	Sine wave
Ventricular fibrillation	Soft or absent	Usually absent	None	60–100[e]	Regular	Normal	400–600	Grossly irregular	Baseline undulation; no QRS complexes

[a] Lack of a response to carotid sinus massage may occur with any arrhythmia.
[b] Ventricular rate equals atrial rate in absence of AV block.
[c] See Table 4-2.
[d] Any independent atrial arrhythmia may exist, or the atria may be captured retrogradely.
[e] Constant if atria are captured retrogradely.
Source: Adapted from D. P. Zipes, Specific Arrhythmias: Diagnosis and Treatment. In E. Braunwald (ed.), *Heart Disease: A Textbook for Cardiovascular Medicine* (2nd ed.). Philadelphia: Saunders Company, 1984.

tion of these laboratory tests are based on the historical and physical findings. Echocardiography, radionuclide ventriculography, and cardiac catheterization are more definitive procedures available for evaluating electively the extent of underlying cardiac disease. Invasive electrophysiology testing may be required for adequate management.

Treatment

The armamentaria for treating cardiac arrhythmias include an increasing number of pharmacologic agents, as well as electrical cardioversion and cardiac pacing.

I. **Class Ia drugs. Quinidine, procainamide, and disopyramide** are direct membrane depressants that decrease conduction velocity, prolong refractoriness, decrease automaticity, and reduce the heterogeneity in repolarization in the ventricular conduction system. These agents are used for treating a variety of **atrial** and **ventricular arrhythmias.** Quinidine, procainamide, and disopyramide share similar cardiac **toxicities.** The QRS and QT intervals widen as serum concentrations increase. Toxic doses may precipitate ventricular arrhythmias including torsade de pointes and ventricular fibrillation (VF). At high concentrations, sinoatrial block, sinus arrest, high-grade AV block, or asystole may occur. These agents slow intraatrial conduction and have an indirect vagolytic effect on AV node conduction. As a result, when used as single agents for the treatment of atrial fibrillation or flutter, the atrial rate may slow, more atrial impulses may penetrate the AV node, and the ventricular rate may paradoxically increase. In addition, these agents produce **myocardial depression** and **vasodilatation.**

A. **Quinidine**
   1. **Absorption and excretion.** After oral administration, quinidine is virtually completely absorbed, with peak serum levels achieved in 90 minutes (quinidine sulfate) to 3 hours (quinidine gluconate). Intramuscular (IM) administration is associated with incomplete absorption and tissue necrosis and is rarely indicated. Quinidine may be given IV but must be infused cautiously to avoid severe hypotension. Quinidine is metabolized primarily by the liver, and the parent drug and metabolites are excreted in the urine. The serum half-life is 5–10 hours in normal subjects but shows marked interpatient variability. Drug clearance is reduced in the presence of hepatic dysfunction, CHF, and renal insufficiency. **Serum levels** from 1.3–5.0 μg/ml correlate with clinical efficacy.

   2. **Clinical indications**
      a. Suppression of symptomatic **atrial** and **ventricular premature depolarizations** (APDs and VPDs).
      b. **Conversion of atrial fibrillation and flutter** to sinus rhythm. Successful conversion occurs in 10–20% of patients during treatment with quinidine, especially if atrial fibrillation or flutter is of recent onset and the atria are not enlarged. Following successful conversion, quinidine is effective in maintaining sinus rhythm for up to 6 months. However, long-term prevention has not been demonstrated conclusively.
      c. Termination and prevention of **automatic and reentrant supraventricular tachycardias** (SVTs).
      d. Termination of **ventricular tachycardia** (VT).
      e. **Prevention** of recurrent **VT** and **VF.**

   3. **Toxicity and precautions**
      a. Since **quinidine may enhance AV conduction,** it should not be administered to patients with atrial flutter or fibrillation unless the ventricular rate has been controlled adequately (e.g., with digitalis or propranolol).
      b. Quinidine should not be administered to patients with preexisting second- or third-degree **AV block** without a temporary or permanent pacemaker in place and should be used with caution in patients with sick sinus syndrome or **bundle branch block.** Quinidine should be discontinued if the QRS duration increases by more than 50% (or 25% in patients with an underlying intraventricular conduction delay).
      c. Quinidine should not be administered to patients with **QT$_c$ prolongation** (normal upper limit of QT$_c$ is 0.46 for men and 0.47 for women) and should be discontinued if the QT$_c$ interval [QT$_c$ = QT (sec) ÷ $\sqrt{\text{RR interval(sec)}}$] increases by more than 25%. On rare occasions, syncope and sudden death have occurred without substantial QT$_c$ prolongation.
      d. Quinidine may exacerbate CHF and should not be used in patients with severe **CHF** or **shock.**

   e. Gastrointestinal side effects include diarrhea, nausea, vomiting, and anorexia.
   f. Central nervous system toxicity includes tinnitus, hearing loss, vertigo, visual disturbances, headache, confusion, delirium, and psychosis.
   g. Hypotension (especially with parenteral administration) may occur due to vasodilatation and myocardial depression.
   h. Other reactions include rash, fever, thrombocytopenia, hemolytic anemia, hepatitis, proteinuria, and angioedema.
4. **Drug interactions**
   a. Serum digoxin levels increase twofold with quinidine administration.
   b. The effects of coumadin are potentiated by quinidine.
   c. Antacids delay quinidine absorption.
   d. Phenobarbital and phenytoin shorten the serum half-life of quinidine.
5. **Preparations and dosages**
   a. Quinidine sulfate. The usual oral dosage is 200–600 mg q6h. Extentabs (Quinidex, 300 mg) are administered as 600 mg q8–12h.
   b. Quinidine polygalacturonate (Cardioquin) may cause less gastric irritation. Each tablet contains a dose equivalent to 200 mg of quinidine sulfate. The recommended dosage is 1–3 tablets q8–12h.
   c. Quinidine gluconate (Quinaglute, Duraquin). Each tablet of this sustained-release preparation is equivalent to 250 mg of quinidine sulfate. The recommended dosage is 1–2 tablets q8h. A **parenteral formulation** is available; it should be diluted (i.e., 800 mg in 50 ml of 5% D/W) and infused at a rate of 1 ml/minute to a dosage 6–10 mg/kg, with careful monitoring of the blood pressure and ECG.
B. **Procainamide**
   1. **Absorption and excretion.** Procainamide is absorbed well with an oral bio-availability of 80%. Initial effects are seen within 20 minutes, and the peak plasma concentration occurs 1 hour after oral ingestion. Initial effects are seen 5–10 minutes after IM injection and immediately following IV administration. Normally, 70–90% of the drug is eliminated by renal excretion; the remainder is metablized by the liver, chiefly to N-acetylprocainamide (NAPA), which is then excreted by the kidneys. The serum half-life of procainamide is 3 hours in normal individuals but may be prolonged to 6–12 hours by CHF and renal insufficiency. A newer sustained-release formulation extends the duration of action to 6 hours, but bioavailability is lower than that of the standard capsules. Since NAPA may accumulate to toxic levels in the presence of renal dysfunction, it is important to monitor serum levels of both procainamide and NAPA. **Serum levels** of procainamide from 4–12 µg/ml correlate with clinical efficacy.
   2. **Clinical indications**
      a. Suppression of symptomatic **APDs and VPDs.**
      b. Conversion and prevention of **atrial fibrillation and flutter.** The efficacy of procainamide is comparable to quinidine.
      c. Termination and prevention of **automatic and reentrant SVTs.**
      d. Termination of **VT.**
      e. Prevention of recurrent **VT** and **VF.**
   3. **Toxicity and precautions**
      a. Same as in sec. **I.A.3.a** and **b**.
      b. Prolongation of the QT_c interval occurs less frequently with procainamide than with quinidine or disopyramide. Nonetheless, the drug should not be administered to patients with QT_c prolongation and should be discontinued if the QT_c interval increases by more than 25% during therapy.
      c. Procainamide may exacerbate CHF and should be used with caution in patients with severe **myocardial dysfunction.**
      d. Hypotension, especially with IV administration, may occur due to vasodilatation and myocardial depression.
      e. A **lupuslike syndrome** develops in up to 30% of patients treated chronically. Manifestations include fever, arthritis, pleuropericarditis, and hepatomegaly. The brain and kidneys are generally not involved, and the syndrome is reversible when the drug is stopped. Up to 70% of patients develop a positive antinuclear antibody (ANA), which in the absence of symptoms is not an indication to stop treatment.
      f. Other reactions include diaphoresis, fever, skin rash, myalgias, digital vas-

culitis, Raynaud's phenomenon, gastrointestinal disturbances, depression, psychosis, and agranulocytosis.

4. Drug interactions. Procainamide does not interact with coumadin or digoxin.

5. Preparation and dosages

    a. Oral. For ventricular arrhythmias, a loading dose of 750–1000 mg may be given, followed by a maintenance dosage of 250–1000 mg q3h up to a total daily dose of 6 gm. For atrial arrhythmias, an initial dose of 1250 mg may be followed in 1 hour by 750 mg if there have been no ECG changes. A dosage of 500–1000 mg q2h may then be given until the arrhythmia is interrupted or side effects occur. The sustained-release preparation (Procan-SR) is administered at a dosage of 500–1500 mg q6h.

    b. Intramuscular. The IM dosage is 500–1000 mg q6h.

    c. Intravenous. The drug should be diluted in 5% D/W and administered (by direct IV injection or preferably continuous infusion) at a rate not to exceed 50 mg/minute until the arrhythmia is terminated or a total dose of 1 gm is reached. A maintenance infusion of 2–6 mg/minute (e.g., 2 gm of procainamide in 500 ml of 5% D/W at 0.5–1.5 ml/minute) may then be administered.

C. Disopyramide

1. Absorption and excretion. Disopyramide has an 80–90% oral bioavailability. The peak plasma concentration is reached in 2 hours. Following administration, 40–60% of the drug is excreted unchanged in the urine; the remainder is metabolized by the liver, with some metabolites excreted by the kidneys. The serum half-life ranges from 4–10 hours in normal individuals. Renal, hepatic, and cardiac insufficiency prolong the half-life and require careful adjustment of dosage. **Serum levels** of 2.8–7.5 µg/ml correlate with clinical efficacy.

2. Clinical indications

    a. Suppression of symptomatic **APDs and VPDs.**

    b. Conversion and prevention of **atrial fibrillation and flutter** (although not approved by the FDA for this use). Disopyramide is comparable to quinidine and procainamide in converting atrial fibrillation and flutter to sinus rhythm.

    c. Termination and prevention of **automatic and reentrant SVTs** (although not approved by the FDA for this use).

    d. Prevention of recurrent **VT** and **VF.**

3. Toxicity and precautions

    a. Same as in sec. I.A.3.a, b, and c.

    b. Disopyramide depresses myocardial function to a greater extent than quinidine or procainamide and thus should not be used in patients with CHF or a left ventricular ejection fraction of less than 30%.

    c. Disopyramide has marked **parasympatholytic properties** and thus may cause blurred vision, dry mouth, urinary retention, constipation, and exacerbation of glaucoma and myasthenia gravis.

4. Drug interactions

    a. Phenytoin and phenobarbital may decrease the serum half-life of disopyramide.

    b. Disopyramide does not alter serum digoxin levels.

5. Preparation and dosages. Disopyramide is available only for oral administration. The usual oral dosage is 100–300 mg q6h. A loading dose of 300 mg may be given initially. In patients with moderate renal insufficiency (i.e., creatinine clearance > 40 ml/minute), hepatic insufficiency, or CHF, the recommended dosage is 100 mg q6h, with or without a loading dose of 200 mg. In patients with marked renal insufficiency, the recommended dosage (with or without a loading dose of 150 mg) is 100 mg q8h, q12h, and q24h for creatinine clearances of 30–40, 15–30, and < 15 ml/minute, respectively.

II. Class Ib drugs. Lidocaine, mexiletine, tocainide, and phenytoin are effective against both automatic and reentrant ventricular arrhythmias but not supraventricular arrhythmias. Lidocaine and phenytoin are also effective in treating tachyarrhythmias complicating digitalis toxicity. Alterations in electrophysiologic parameters induced by these drugs vary with the tissue studied and the extracellular potassium concentration. In tissues partially depolarized, especially due to ischemia, these agents markedly slow conduction velocity. However, at therapeutic concentrations they have little effect on sinus, atrial, or AV nodal tissues.

A. Lidocaine

1. Absorption and excretion. Oral administration of lidocaine is not practical due to extensive first-pass hepatic metabolism. Following IM injection, effective serum levels occur in 15 minutes. The duration of action is usually 90 minutes. Following IV administration, the onset of action is immediate, with an initial distribution half-life of 8–17 minutes. About 90% of the drug is metabolized by the liver, with less than 10% excreted unchanged in the urine. After attainment of steady-state kinetics, the elimination half-life is 1–2 hours in normal subjects, 4 hours in patients with uncomplicated myocardial infarction (MI), and over 10 hours in patients with CHF, hepatic dysfunction, shock, or age greater than 70 years. Therapeutic **serum levels** are 2–6 µg/ml.

  2. **Clinical indications**
    a. Lidocaine is the drug of choice for the emergent treatment of **VPDs** and **VT** and for prevention of recurrent **VF.** Many authorities recommend lidocaine prophylactically for patients with an acute MI.
    b. Lidocaine should be used **prophylactically if ventricular arrhythmias are anticipated during electrical cardioversion.**
  3. **Toxicities and precautions**
    a. Dose-related **central nervous system toxicity** is the most common side effect and includes dizziness, paresthesia, confusion, delirium, stupor, coma, seizures, and rarely respiratory arrest.
    b. **Myocardial depression,** especially in patients with severe CHF, may occur.
    c. Patients with sinus node dysfunction, His-Purkinje disease, or junctional escape rhythms may develop **depressed cardiac automaticity or conduction** (e.g., sinus arrest, AV block).
    d. Augmentation of anterograde AV conduction through an accessory pathway in some patients with the Wolff-Parkinson-White (WPW) syndrome and atrial fibrillation or flutter may result in an accelerated ventricular rate.
  4. **Drug interactions**
    a. **Decreased metabolism** of lidocaine occurs with concomitant administration of isoniazid, chloramphenicol, propranolol, and norepinephrine.
    b. **Increased metabolism** occurs with phenobarbital and isoproterenol.
    c. Large doses of lidocaine may enhance the muscle-relaxant properties of succinylcholine.
  5. **Preparations and dosages.** Lidocaine is supplied at 1% and 2% solutions; it is available in ampules of 50 or 100 mg for IV bolus therapy and in single-use vials of 1–2 gm for preparing IV infusions.
    a. **Initial IV therapy** should begin with a 1 mg/kg bolus. At the same time, a continuous infusion of 2–4 mg/minute should be started. Second and third boluses of 0.5 mg/kg each should be given at 5-minute intervals to prevent subtherapeutic serum levels as a result of the rapid distribution of lidocaine to the tissue compartment.
    b. **Maintenance therapy** consists of a continuous IV infusion of 1–4 mg/minute (e.g., 2 gm of lidocaine in 500 ml of 5% D/W at 0.25–1.0 ml/minute). The initial bolus and maintenance dosages should be reduced by 50% in patients with CHF, shock, or hepatic dysfunction and in patients over 70 years of age.
    c. **IM administration** should be used only when IV administration is not possible; the dosage is 4–5 mg/kg.
B. **Mexiletine** is a new antiarrhythmic drug recently approved by the FDA. Mexiletine is similar to lidocaine in its chemical structure, electrophysiologic properties, clinical spectrum of antiarrhythmic activity, and toxicities.
  1. **Absorption and excretion.** Approximately 88% of mexiletine is absorbed following ingestion, with peak plasma concentrations observed within 2–4 hours; however, absorption may be delayed and less complete in patients during acute MI. Approximately 70% of mexiletine in serum is protein-bound. It is eliminated primarily by the liver, but 3–15% may be excreted by the kidneys. Renal excretion increases with acidification of the urine and decreases with alkalinization of the urine. The half-life in normal patients is 8–10 hours, but a variable increase may be observed in patients during acute MI, in whom the half-life may exceed 20 hours. Hepatic congestion and liver disease may be expected to delay clearance of mexiletine. The margin between **therapeutic** (0.75–2.0 µg/ml) and **toxic** (> 2.0 µg/ml) concentrations is narrow.
  2. **Clinical indications.** Mexiletine is effective in reducing the frequency of VPDs, and it may be useful in the prophylactic control of ventricular tachyarrhythmias. Further study is required to determine if mexiletine reduces the incidence of sudden death. It may have a role in the treatment of long QT interval

syndromes (torsade de pointes). On the basis of its electrophysiologic properties it is unlikely to have a role in the treatment of supraventricular arrhythmias.

3. **Toxicity and precautions.** Side effects of long-term oral therapy are dose-dependent. The frequency and severity of adverse effects are markedly increased with plasma concentrations above 2.0 μg/ml.

   a. **Nausea or vomiting** is common.

   b. **Central nervous system toxicity** includes fine tremor, dizziness, and blurred vision. Higher levels of mexiletine may result in dysarthria, diplopia, nystagmus, and an impaired level of consciousness.

   c. **Cardiovascular.** A depressant effect on sinus node function may be observed in patients with sick sinus syndrome. It should be used with caution in patients having intraventricular conduction disease. Mexiletine has minimal myocardial depressant effects; however, it should be used cautiously in patients with advanced heart failure. Hypotension may occur with higher dosages.

4. **Drug interactions.** Cumulative toxicity may be observed with concomitant use of mexiletine and lidocaine. The electrophysiologic effects of mexiletine are additive with those of other antiarrhythmic agents.

5. **Preparations and dosages.** Mexiletine is available in 50-, 100-, and 200-mg tablets. A loading dose is not indicated for chronic prophylaxis of ventricular arrhythmias. The usual maintenance dosage is 200 mg q8h. Some patients may require up to 1200 mg/day, but toxicity is dose-dependent.

C. **Tocainide**

1. **Absorption and excretion.** Approximately 95% of tocainide is absorbed, with peak plasma concentrations occurring within 2 hours. Absorption is complete but delayed if tocainide is given with meals. Approximately 30% of an administered dose is eliminated in the urine, and much of the remainder undergoes hepatic metabolism. Renal clearance is reduced by alkalinization of the urine. The half-life ranges from 10–14 hours and appears to be prolonged in patients during acute MI. **Therapeutic serum levels** are 3–10 μg/ml. Increased toxicity is observed with levels exceeding 10 μg/ml.

2. **Clinical indications.** Tocainide reduces the frequency of VPDs in patients with acute MI and appears to be effective in reducing ventricular ectopy with chronic oral use. Its efficacy in reducing the incidence of sudden death or VT requires further study.

3. **Toxicity and precautions**

   a. **Neurologic symptoms** such as dizziness, tremor, paresthesia, and confusion are the most common reported adverse reactions.

   b. **Nausea or vomiting** is relatively common.

   c. **A lupuslike illness** has been reported as a rare complication. Rash, pneumonitis, and lymphopenia have been described.

   d. **Cardiovascular.** Tocainide has little effect on sinus node automaticity or intracardiac conduction, but it should be used with caution in patients having sinus node dysfunction. Although hemodynamic effects are minor, tocainide should be used cautiously in patients with advanced heart failure.

4. **Drug interactions.** The electrophysiologic effects of tocainide are additive with other antiarrhythmic agents, particularly lidocaine. Asystole has been reported with concurrent tocainide and metoprolol therapy.

5. **Preparations and dosages.** Tocainide is available in 400- and 600-mg tablets. The usual daily dosage of tocainide is 1200–1800 mg PO in divided doses q8–12h. Some patients may have fewer side effects if tocainide is taken with food.

D. **Phenytoin**

1. **Absorption and excretion.** Absorption following oral administration is incomplete and delayed and varies with the commercial preparation. The peak plasma concentration occurs 8–12 hours after IM injection; however, IM administration causes pain, muscle necrosis, and sterile abscesses and is associated with variable absorption due to the insolubility of phenytoin at physiologic pH. Following IV administration, the onset of action is prompt. The drug is metabolized by the liver and has a mean half-life of 24 hours. However, the rate of metabolism is variable and affected by a variety of medications. It is essential to monitor plasma concentrations of phenytoin when changing dosages or altering other medications. **Serum levels** of 10–20 μg/ml correlate with clinical efficacy.

2. **Clinical indications**
   a. **Digitalis-induced arrhythmias** (supraventricular and ventricular).
   b. Phenytoin may be useful in combination with other antiarrhythmic agents (e.g., quinidine, procainamide, or disopyramide) in the treatment of non-digitalis-induced ventricular arrhythmias, particularly when prolongation in the QT_c interval has occurred.
3. **Toxicity and precautions**
   a. Common adverse reactions are dose related and include nystagmus, ataxia, drowsiness, stupor, and coma.
   b. **Hypotension, sinus bradycardia, and respiratory depression** may follow rapid IV administration. These effects may be mediated by the IV vehicle (propylene glycol) and can be minimized by slow ($\leq$ 50 mg/minute) administration.
   c. Other toxic effects include nausea, epigastric pain, anorexia, skin rash, gingival hyperplasia, megaloblastic anemia, lymphadenopathy, agranulocytosis, a lupuslike syndrome, hyperglycemia, and osteomalacia.
   d. Due to the acidity of the parenteral drug, sterile abscesses (following IM injection) and thrombophlebitis (following IV infusion) may occur.
4. **Drug interactions**
   a. **Increased metabolism** of phenytoin resulting in a shortened half-life can occur with administration of any drug that induces hepatic enzymes (e.g., phenobarbital).
   b. **Decreased metabolism** and increased serum levels can occur with concomitant use of phenylbutazone, coumadin, isoniazid, chloramphenicol, tolbutamide, diazepam, phenothiazines, and many other medications.
   c. Phenytoin decreases the efficacy of corticosteroids, coumadin, oral contraceptives, quinidine, and vitamin D.
5. **Preparations and dosages**
   a. **Oral.** A loading dose of 1000 mg is followed by 500 mg/day on days 2 and 3 and then a maintenance dosage of 300–400 mg/day. The drug may be given once or twice daily depending on the commercial preparation. Serum levels should be monitored.
   b. **Intramuscular** administration is associated with erratic absorption and results in sterile abscesses; it is not recommended.
   c. **Intravenous.** Phenytoin should be given by **slow** IV push at a rate not to exceed 50 mg/minute until the arrhythmia is controlled, adverse effects result, or a total dose of 1000 mg is given. Frequent monitoring of the ECG and blood pressure is required. Subsequent doses may be given as 150–200 mg bid (again, at rates not to exceed 50 mg/minute) until oral therapy is possible.

III. **Class Ic drugs**
   A. **Flecainide** is a new drug recently approved by the FDA. Flecainide profoundly depresses the maximum rate of rise of phase O of the action potential and markedly slows conduction. It has little effect on the resting potential, action potential duration, or effective refractory period (ERP). This agent appears to have profound effects on conduction in the His-Purkinje system and ventricular myocardium. It also slows conduction in the AV node. Automaticity is decreased in the sinus node, Purkinje fibers, and ventricular tissue. Flecainide has minor effects on slow channel-mediated potentials. The ECG characteristically shows a widening of the QRS and lengthening of the QT_c interval, but the ST segment is not significantly changed.
   1. **Absorption and excretion.** Flecainide is a benzamide derivative that is almost completely absorbed following oral ingestion. Absorption is not effected by food. Peak plasma levels are observed in about 3 hours. Less than 40% of flecainide is bound to plasma proteins. The mean plasma elimination half-life in patients is 20 hours (range 12–27 hours). Renal excretion accounts for 86% of elimination as flecainide or its metabolites. Metabolites have little or no intrinsic electrophysiologic activity. Urinary excretion decreases with alkalinization of the urine. Approximately 5% of flecainide is excreted in the bile.
   2. **Clinical indications**
      a. **Suppression of VPDs and VT.** Flecainide produces marked suppression of ventricular arrhythmias. It appears to be more potent in suppressing VPDs than conventional antiarrhythmic agents. Its efficacy in preventing ventric-

ular arrhythmias induced by programmed electrical stimulation requires further study.

  b. **Supraventricular tachycardia.** The efficacy of flecainide in the treatment of SVT is unknown. It has been reported to terminate AV node reentry and orthodromic SVT in patients with accessory pathways.

3. **Toxicity and precautions**

  a. Flecainide has **marked effects on cardiac conduction** and should be used with caution in patients with AV conduction delay. A 20% increase in the PR and QRS intervals is commonly observed and is not cause for concern. Patients having an increase of more than 50% in the PR and QRS intervals should be closely monitored. If bifascicular block or second- or third-degree AV block occurs, the dosage should be reduced or the drug discontinued.

  b. Flecainide may **increase pacing thresholds** of the atria and ventricles by 200%. It should be used with caution in pacemaker-dependent patients. Chronic use of flecainide may require adjustment in pacemaker parameters.

  c. **Exacerbation of ventricular arrhythmias** has been reported in 4–12% of patients. Serum levels above 1000 ng/ml appear to be associated with a higher risk of sustained ventricular arrhythmias, which may be refractory to conventional resuscitative measures.

  d. Other common side effects include blurred vision, dizziness, nausea, and headache.

4. **Preparations and dosages.** Flecainide is available in 100-mg scored tablets. It may take 5–7 days to reach steady-state plasma levels. The initial dosage is 100 mg bid. The dosage may be increased cautiously by 50 mg bid every fourth day until clinical efficacy is obtained or a total daily dose of 400 mg (200 mg bid) is reached. Dosages exceeding 400 mg/day should be avoided in patients with heart failure or renal failure, and plasma levels should be followed. **Therapeutic serum levels** range from 400–900 ng/ml. It is recommended that the dosage not exceed 600 mg/day. Some patients may require a q8h dosage interval.

IV. **Class II drugs: beta-blockers.** Although many beta-blockers are available for use in the United States, only propranolol and timolol are approved for use as antiarrhythmic agents to prevent sudden death following MI. Other beta-blockers most likely have similar effects and in some instances offer advantages in selected patients. Propranolol will be discussed as the prototype drug.

Although propranolol in high doses has direct membrane-depressant effects, its major antiarrhythmic action is due to the competitive blockade of cardiac beta-receptors. Propranolol slows the sinus rate and helps decrease myocardial oxygen demand in the setting of myocardial ischemia. Propranolol prolongs the conduction and refractory properties of the AV node, thus decreasing the ventricular rate during atrial fibrillation and flutter and in many cases abolishing automatic and reentrant arrhythmias involving the AV node. However, propranolol has little direct effect on conduction and refractoriness of His-Purkinje tissue and ventricular muscle.

Beta-blockade also accounts for propranolol's **toxicity,** including sinus bradycardia, AV node block, myocardial depression, bronchoconstriction, and vasoconstriction.

A. **Absorption and excretion.** Following oral ingestion, propranolol is rapidly and completely absorbed, but substantial first-pass hepatic metabolism reduces bioavailability to 10–30%, with significant interpatient variability. The peak effect occurs in 1.0–1.5 hours. Beta-blockade occurs almost immediately following IV administration. A dose of 1 mg IV is comparable to 10 mg PO. The serum half-life varies from 2–6 hours, but there is no simple correlation between the dosage or plasma level and therapeutic effect. Effective beta-blockade may persist for prolonged periods, and the dosage should be titrated according to the clinical response (e.g., changes in the resting heart rate or prevention of exercise-induced tachycardia). The half-life of propranolol is prolonged in patients with hepatic dysfunction and CHF.

B. **Clinical indications**

  1. **Atrial fibrillation and flutter.** Propranolol may be used alone or in conjunction with digitalis or verapamil to decrease the ventricular rate during atrial fibrillation or flutter.

  2. **Reentrant SVTs** involving the sinus or AV nodes may be terminated or prevented. The ventricular response during other forms of SVT (e.g., automatic or intraatrial reentry) may be slowed.

  3. **Digitalis-induced arrhythmias** (both atrial and ventricular) may respond to

propranolol. However, if significant AV block is present, lidocaine or phenytoin is preferable.

4. **Ventricular arrhythmias** are generally unresponsive, except those occurring in the setting of acute ischemia (e.g., during exercise) or high catecholamines (e.g., with pheochromocytoma or emotion, thyrotoxicosis, or general anesthesia).

5. **Sinus tachycardia** usually is a secondary state and does not by itself need treatment. However, when sinus tachycardia complicates ongoing myocardial ischemia or thyrotoxicosis, treatment with a beta-blocker may be beneficial.

6. **Post–myocardial infarction.** Patients recovering from a MI appear to have reduced sudden and overall mortality when treated with a beta-blocker.

C. **Toxicity and precautions**

1. In patients with **CHF** or **shock**, propranolol should be used only if the clinical state is directly due to a tachyarrhythmia. Concomitant digitalis administration, however, may permit the use of small doses of propranolol. The **myocardial-depressant effects** of propranolol may be reversed with inotropic agents, including dopamine and dobutamine.

2. **Bradycardia** due to sinus node dysfunction or AV node block may occur.

3. **Bronchoconstriction** may precipitate respiratory failure in patients with asthma or chronic obstructive pulmonary disease (COPD).

4. **Sudden withdrawal of propranolol may precipitate arrhythmias or angina** in patients receiving chronic therapy. Thus, beta-blockers should be tapered over several days before being discontinued.

5. Since the premonitory signs and symptoms of acute hypoglycemia may be prevented, beta-blockers should be used cautiously in patients receiving hypoglycemic agents.

6. Other toxic effects include mental depression, Raynaud's phenomenon, claudication, epigastric distress, and sexual dysfunction.

D. **Drug interactions.** Propranolol may accentuate the **negative chronotropic effects** of digitalis and verapamil and the **negative inotropic effects** of other antiarrhythmic agents.

E. **Preparations and dosages**

1. **Oral.** The dosage required to achieve a salutary effect varies considerably among patients. The dosage must be titrated according to the clinical effect. Dosages of 20–80 mg q6h are usually adequate for an antiarrhythmic effect.

2. **Intravenous.** Propranolol is administered IV when immediate beta-blockade is required. The rate of administration should not exceed 1 mg/minute or a total dosage of 0.15 mg/kg. A dosage of 1–3 mg is often sufficient.

V. **Class III drugs. Amiodarone and bretylium** are powerful drugs that markedly prolong action potential duration and repolarization to a greater extent than they depress conduction velocity. As a consequence, refractoriness is prolonged and the ability of the membrane to undergo spontaneous diastolic depolarization is delayed. These drugs appear to suppress arrhythmias mediated by reentry as well as those due to disturbances in automaticity.

A. **Amiodarone** is a new antiarrhythmic drug recently approved by the FDA. Amiodarone is a benzofuran derivative with a chemical structure similar to thyroxine (T_4). Amiodarone prolongs action potential duration, repolarization, and refractoriness in atrial and ventricular tissue. It slows the sinus node discharge rate and recovery time and prolongs AV node conduction. Amiodarone blocks the peripheral conversion of T_4 to triiodothyronine (T_3). It is a noncompetitive alpha- and beta-adrenergic antagonist and inhibits release of neurotransmitter from presynaptic adrenergic neurons. Systemic vascular resistance and mean arterial blood pressure are reduced without a significant change in left ventricular function; however, hemodynamic deterioration has been reported in patients with severe underlying left ventricular failure.

1. **Absorption and excretion.** Approximately 50% of an oral dose is absorbed and a peak plasma concentration occurs 3–8 hours after ingestion. Amiodarone undergoes a complex distribution and equilibration. It is highly lipophilic and is detected in many organs and tissues. A loading period of 10 days or longer is required to achieve steady-state kinetics. The slow uptake and release from reservoir tissues contributes to its long half-life. It has a biphasic elimination pattern suggesting discordant rates of release from different tissue compartments. The exact process of elimination is unknown, but renal elimination of amiodarone and its metabolite is negligible. The terminal half-life of amiodarone has a range of 18–40 days. There is substantial overlap between

therapeutic (1.5–3.0 µg/ml) and toxic serum levels. Measurement of serum concentrations of amiodarone are of only limited value in monitoring a maintenance dosage.

2. **Clinical indications.** Amiodarone is a powerful antiarrhythmic agent with significant toxicity. This agent should only be used in patients with documented sustained arrhythmias that are refractory to more conventional agents or in patients in whom conventional agents produce intolerable side effects.

   a. **Supraventricular arrhythmias.** Amiodarone has been reported to prevent recurrences of atrial fibrillation and atrial flutter and can result in chemical conversion of atrial fibrillation to sinus rhythm. It effectively slows the ventricular rate in patients having chronic atrial fibrillation, but the onset of this effect is slow in comparison to conventional agents. Amiodarone is effective in the chronic treatment of AV nodal reentrant SVT.

   b. **Wolff-Parkinson-White (WPW) syndrome.** Amiodarone prolongs the ERP of the atrium, AV node, and accessory pathways and is effective in preventing recurrence of sustained orthodromic SVT and atrial fibrillation.

   c. **Sustained VT or VF.** Amiodarone prevents the recurrence of sustained spontaneous VT or VF (not associated with acute MI) in up to 60% of patients. A therapeutic latency of 5–15 days exists before beneficial antiarrhythmic effects are observed, and full suppression of arrhythmias may not be obtained for a month or more after initiating therapy.

3. **Toxicity and precautions.**

   a. **Corneal microdeposits,** detectable on slit-lamp examination, develop in virtually all patients. Their occurrence is dose-dependent and is reversible with discontinuation of the drug. These deposits rarely interfere with vision, although occasional patients may notice halos around lights at night.

   b. **Photosensitivity** is a common adverse reaction, and some patients develop a violaceous facial discoloration.

   c. **Hypothyroidism** and **hyperthyroidism** have been reported with an incidence of approximately 3%. Thyroid function should be monitored routinely. Amiodarone blocks peripheral conversion of T_4 to T_3; thus, most euthyroid patients treated with amiodarone demonstrate mild elevations of T_4 and a decrease in T_3 levels. The diagnosis of **hyperthyroidism** may be obscured by elevation of T_4 observed routinely during chronic amiodarone therapy but is confirmed by high free T_3 levels or failure of thryoid-stimulating hormone (TSH) to respond to administration of thyrotropin-releasing hormone. **Hypothyroidism** is diagnosed by the clinical features, low T_3 and T_4 levels, and a markedly increased TSH level.

   d. **Pulmonary fibrosis** has been reported with an incidence of 5–15%. It may occur early or late in the course of therapy at a wide range of dosages. Patients characteristically present with dry cough and dyspnea associated with pulmonary infiltrates and rales. The process appears to be reversible if detected early. Serial chest x-rays should be obtained every 4–6 months to detect interstitial changes. Results of pulmonary function tests do not appear to be predictive of amiodarone pulmonary toxicity.

   e. **Cardiovascular.** Asymptomatic sinus bradycardia and prolonged AV node conduction are frequently observed; however, in rare instances a permanent pacemaker may be required to treat severe bradycardia or high-grade AV block. Exacerbation of ventricular arrhythmias has been reported but occurs less commonly than observed with class I agents. Severe hypotension may occur with a rapid IV injection of amiodarone. The ECG effects of amiodarone are a lengthened PR interval, QRS duration, and QT interval. Torsade de pointes has been reported with the use of amiodarone as a rare complication.

   f. **Miscellaneous.** Nausea, anorexia, and constipation may occur. Chemical hepatitis is a rare complication. Tremor, ataxia, and peripheral neuropathy have been reported with an increasing incidence.

   g. **Drug interactions.** Amiodarone has been reported to markedly potentiate the effects of **coumadin** and to increase **digoxin** levels. Maintenance dosages of digoxin and coumadin should be routinely reduced by one-half when amiodarone is started.

4. **Preparations and dosages.**

   a. **Oral.** Amiodarone is available in 200-mg scored tablets. The initial loading schedules are empiric and vary from 800–1600 mg daily for 1–2 weeks. The usual daily maintenance dosage is 200–600 mg (5–10 mg/kg).

   b. Intravenous. An IV solution is available in 3-ml vials containing 150 mg of amiodarone. The solution is irritating and should be administered through a central venous line. The usual initial dosage is 5 mg/kg injected over 2–3 minutes. Onset of action is 5–10 minutes after IV injection. The major problems with IV injection are abrupt hypotension and AV block. Maintenance therapy consists of 10 mg/kg/day divided into 3 equal solutions with each infused over 8 hours.

B. Bretylium has direct electrophysiologic effects as well as important interactions with the autonomic nervous system. In Purkinje fibers, bretylium has no direct effect on normal phase 4 depolarization. However, automaticity transiently increases after drug exposure because of the initial release of norepinephrine from adrenergic nerve terminals. Bretylium markedly prolongs action potential duration and ERP in Purkinje fibers and ventricular muscle. These effects appear to be more prominent in normal than ischemic tissue. This differential effect reduces the disparity in ERP between normal and infarcted zones. Bretylium has no consistent effect on resting membrane potential, rate of phase 0 depolarization, membrane responsiveness, or conduction velocity. Efficacy in terminating reentrant arrhythmias is probably related to marked alterations in refractoriness or stabilization of sympathetic tone.

The **toxicity** of this agent is primarily due to its interaction with the autonomic nervous system. Bretylium accumulates in peripheral adrenergic nerve terminals, resulting in an initial release of norepinephrine, producing a sympathomimetic effect. Subsequently, bretylium inhibits the release of norepinephrine by producing adrenergic neuronal blockade and may cause hypotension.

   1. Absorption and excretion. The onset of action is prompt with IV administration, **although maximum efficacy may require 15–20 minutes.** When given IM, the drug requires 30 minutes to reach therapeutic levels. The serum half-life varies from 4–17 hours. Myocardial binding is intense, and serum levels may not reflect pharmacologic efficacy. After 24 hours, 70–80% of bretylium is excreted unchanged in the urine.

   2. Clinical indications
   a. Refractory ventricular arrhythmias, including VT and VF, constitute the primary indication for the use of this drug. It may be effective during cardiac arrest, even if VF has been present for long periods and is refractory to conventional maneuvers including lidocaine and defibrillation.
   b. Ventricular arrhythmias associated with digitalis intoxication may respond to bretylium, but conventional agents (i.e., potassium, phenytoin) should be tried first.

   3. Toxicity and precautions
   a. Supine and orthostatic **hypotension.**
   b. Initial elaboration of catecholamines may exacerbate arrhythmias including those caused by toxicity to digitalis.
   c. Other side effects include nausea, vomiting, parotid pain and swelling, lightheadedness, rash, emotional lability, and renal dysfunction.

   4. Drug interactions
   a. Bretylium's effectiveness may be reduced when used with other antiarrhythmic drugs.
   b. Bretylium may heighten the response to infused catecholamines.
   c. The hypotensive effects of diuretics or vasodilator drugs may be augmented during bretylium administration.

   5. Preparation and dosages. Parenteral bretylium is available in 500-mg ampules.
   a. Ventricular fibrillation. An initial IV bolus of 5–10 mg/kg is followed by a continuous maintenance infusion of 1–2 mg/minute or repetitive IM or IV dosages of 5–10 mg/kg q6–8h.
   b. Ventricular tachycardia. Dilute 500 mg of bretylium in 40 ml of 5% D/W (10 mg/ml). An initial IV bolus of 5–10 mg/kg should be given over an 8- to 10-minute period, followed by a maintenance infusion of 1–2 mg/minute or repetitive boluses of 5–10 mg/kg IV q6–8h. IM administration is less reliable and may be associated with local tissue necrosis unless the dose is divided and injection sites rotated.

VI. Class IV drugs: calcium antagonists (channel blockers)

A. Verapamil blocks the slow inward calcium current responsible for sinus and AV node depolarizations. Verapamil directly slows the sinus rate and prolongs conduction and refractoriness in the AV node. Some of these direct effects, however, are attenuated by a reflex increase in sympathetic tone secondary to verapamil-induced vasodilatation. Verapamil has little direct electrophysiologic effects on atrial muscle, His-Purkinje tissue, and ventricular muscle. In addition, verapamil does not directly affect the electrical properties of accessory pathways associated with the WPW syndrome; however, reflex sympathetic stimulation may enhance anterograde conduction through the bypass tract and result in further acceleration of the ventricular rate during atrial fibrillation or flutter.

Since the predominant electrophysiologic effect of verapamil is on the AV node, verapamil is particularly useful in the treatment of supraventricular arrhythmias. However, verapamil may reduce abnormal ventricular automaticity in some settings, including ischemia and digitalis toxicity. Concomitant administration of a beta-blocker enhances the effects of verapamil but may aggravate toxic manifestations.

Calcium channel blockade impairs cardiac and vascular excitation-contraction coupling, resulting in myocardial depression and vasodilatation.

Diltiazem has electrophysiologic properties similar to verapamil but at present does not have FDA approval for the treatment of arrhythmias.

1. **Absorption and excretion.** Following **oral** administration, verapamil is 90% absorbed but undergoes extensive first-pass hepatic metabolism, resulting in a bioavailability of only 20–35%. The peak plasma concentration occurs in 1–2 hours. The onset of action following **IV** administration occurs within 2 minutes, with a peak effect at 10–15 minutes. Verapamil is metabolized by the liver, and the metabolites are excreted by the kidneys. The serum half-life ranges from 2–5 hours in normal individuals but is prolonged in patients with hepatic dysfunction. The electrophysiologic effects persist up to 6 hours following a single dose, whereas the hemodynamic effects dissipate in 10–20 minutes.

2. **Clinical indications**
   a. **Rapid conversion to sinus rhythm of SVTs** utilizing the sinus or AV nodes as part of a reentrant circuit (e.g., sinus node and AV nodal reentry, reentry utilizing a manifest or concealed bypass tract).
   b. **Control of the ventricular rate** during atrial fibrillation, atrial flutter, intra-atrial reentry, and automatic atrial tachycardias. Verapamil can be used in conjunction with digitalis or propranolol, although such combinations must be used cautiously.
   c. Verapamil is generally not effective in treating ventricular arrhythmias.

3. **Toxicity and precautions**
   a. **Bradycardia, high-degree AV block,** and **asystole** have been reported. Verapamil should not be administered to patients with preexisting second- or third-degree AV block or to patients with sinus node dysfunction unless a temporary or permanent pacemaker is present. In addition, concomitant use of a beta-blocker can aggravate these adverse effects by attenuating reflex sympathetic stimulation.
   b. **Patients with WPW having atrial fibrillation or flutter** may experience a dangerous acceleration in the ventricular rate due to the reflex sympathetic stimulation associated with administration of verapamil; degeneration to VF can result.
   c. Marked **hypotension** due to vasodilatation and cardiac depression is observed in up to 10% of patients receiving verapamil IV. Treatment with fluids and vasopressors may be required.
   d. **Myocardial depression** (often counterbalanced by the reduction in afterload resulting from verapamil-induced vasodilatation) may aggravate or precipitate CHF. Thus, verapamil is contraindicated in the presence of severe CHF or shock.
   e. **Transient ventricular ectopy** may follow conversion of supraventricular arrhythmias to sinus rhythm but is generally benign and requires no treatment.
   f. Other adverse reactions include dizziness, headache, nausea, abdominal discomfort, and constipation.

4. **Drug interactions**
   a. **The negative inotropic and chronotropic effects** of verapamil are additive

with beta-blockers, quinidine, procainamide, and disopyramide. Combined therapy must be used with caution; in particular, combined treatment of verapamil and disopyramide should be avoided.

b. Verapamil causes a 50–70% increase in serum digoxin levels and can result in digitalis toxicity, including profound AV block.

c. Verapamil may augment the effects of antihypertensive agents.

5. Preparations and dosages

a. Intravenous. Verapamil is administered IV as a 5- to 10-mg bolus over 2–3 minutes. A repeat dose of 10 mg may be given after 15–30 minutes if the initial response is not adequate.

b. Oral. The oral dose of verapamil is 80–120 mg tid–qid.

VII. Direct-current (DC) cardioversion is achieved most commonly with an external unit synchronized to the QRS complex to avoid discharge during the vulnerable period of the ventricle. Electrical cardioversion can effectively terminate reentrant arrhythmias but is unlikely to terminate automatic arrhythmias (i.e., some forms of atrial tachycardias with or without block, nonparoxysmal AV junctional tachycardia, and accelerated idioventricular rhythms). Cardioversion should be performed using the lowest possible energy to reduce the incidence of complication and the degree of discomfort. The incidence of major complications is small if attention is paid to proper patient selection and avoidance of digitalis toxicity. Successful cardioversion does not obviate the need for antiarrhythmic therapy.

A. Clinical indications

1. Atrial fibrillation. Emergent cardioversion can be used as the initial treatment of atrial fibrillation or when atrial fibrillation precipitates angina or hemodynamic compromise. Elective cardioversion is indicated when initial medical therapy has been unsuccessful in restoring sinus rhythm. Cardioversion is especially successful when atrial fibrillation is of recent onset. On the other hand, sinus rhythm is rarely maintained long-term if the left atrial size measured echocardiographically exceeds 4.5 cm.

2. Atrial flutter is difficult to control medically, and cardioversion is frequently the initial treatment of choice. Low energies (i.e., <50 joules) are usually effective. Cardioversion should be performed emergently if angina or hemodynamic compromise is present.

3. Reentrant supraventricular tachycardias (involving the SA node, AV node, atrium, or a manifest or concealed bypass tract) respond readily to cardioversion, usually with 25–100 joules. Emergent cardioversion should be performed if angina, CHF, or hypotension is present. Elective cardioversion may be used in stable patients if other measures are not effective.

4. Ventricular tachycardia. Cardioversion is the treatment of choice for sustained VT accompanied by angina, CHF, or hypotension. Cardioversion often can be accomplished with 50 joules. However, pulseless patients should receive 200 joules initially, followed by 200–300 joules and then 360 joules if not effective.

5. Ventricular flutter and fibrillation. Immediate cardioversion/defibrillation is essential to survival (see Chap. 2).

B. Relative contraindications

1. Digitalis toxicity. Therapeutic levels of digoxin are not a contraindication to cardioversion; however, refractory ventricular arrhythmias may develop if toxic levels of digoxin are present. If cardioversion cannot be delayed and high serum levels of digoxin are suspected, lidocaine should be administered and the lowest possible energy setting used. The energy level should be increased progressively until reversion is achieved or evidence of increased ventricular instability occurs.

2. Automatic tachycardia (including some forms of SVT with and without block, multifocal atrial tachycardia, nonparoxysmal junctional tachycardia, and accelerated idioventricular rhythm) are not responsive to cardioversion. Many digitalis-induced arrhythmias fall into this category.

3. Repetitive, nonsustained tachycardias.

4. Sinus node dysfunction or conduction system disease, including a slow ventricular rate during atrial fibrillation (particularly in the absence of medications). Marked sinus bradycardia, sinus pause or arrest, history of the bradycardia-tachycardia syndrome (especially with a history of syncope), and complete AV block are contraindications unless a temporary or permanent pacemaker has been inserted.

5. Presence of underlying diseases, including hyperthyroidism, marked left atrial enlargement, pericarditis, and marked metabolic derangements that make it unlikely that sinus rhythm will be maintained. Whenever possible, the underlying pathology should be corrected prior to cardioversion. If hemodynamic compromise is present, immediate cardioversion may be necessary as a temporizing measure.

6. **Recurrent supraventricular arrhythmias previously converted to sinus rhythm** should not be treated by repeated cardioversion unless the patient has not received adequate antiarrhythmic therapy. Rapid atrial pacing is often a better approach for patients with recurrent reentrant SVT or atrial flutter, allowing repeated conversions over a short period while the efficacy of different antiarrhythmic medications are evaluated; however, rapid atrial pacing is not effective for atrial fibrillation or automatic SVTs.

C. **Technique of cardioversion**

1. When cardioversion is performed electively, the patient should be fasting for 6–8 hours prior to the procedure, and serum electrolytes and drug levels (especially digitalis) should be normal. An anticoagulant and antiarrhythmic agent (e.g., procainamide or quinidine) should be administered prior to the procedure in most cases of atrial fibrillation and flutter.

2. A 12-lead ECG should be obtained prior to and following cardioversion. The rhythm should be monitored continuously throughout the procedure.

3. The patient should be supine, with the paddles coated with electrode gel and in firm contact with the chest. Two paddle positions are acceptable:

   a. A posterior paddle is positioned in the left interscapular region, with the anterior paddle over the sternum in the third interspace.

   b. One paddle is placed to the right of the sternum at the level of the second interspace and the other in the left midaxillary line at the fourth or fifth interspace.

4. Sedation and amnesia should be induced with IV diazepam and/or a short-acting barbiturate. An IV line should be in place, and personnel skilled in endotracheal intubation should be in attendance.

5. **The synchronization artifact** should be clearly evident on the monitor. A synchronized shock (delivered during the QRS complex) should be used for all cardioversions except for ventricular flutter and fibrillation.

6. **Initial energy settings** should be **25–50 joules for atrial flutter and SVT, 100–200 joules for atrial fibrillation, 25–200 joules** (50 joules if hemodynamically compromised, 200 joules if pulseless) **for VT, and 200 joules for VF.** Stepwise increases in energy settings should be used if termination of the arrhythmia is not successful. However, if sinus rhythm is achieved only transiently, higher energy settings are of no value. If ventricular arrhythmias occur, a 50- to 100-mg bolus of lidocaine should be administered if the procedure is to be continued. If symptomatic bradycardia occurs, 0.5–1.0 mg of atropine should be administered IV. A temporary pacemaker may be required occasionally.

7. After sinus rhythm is restored, appropriate antiarrhythmic therapy should be initiated or continued.

D. **Complications.** Serious ventricular arrhythmias are rare if proper QRS synchronization is maintained and digitalis toxicity avoided. Transient atrial and ventricular arrhythmias may be precipitated by the autonomic discharge accompanying cardioversion but usually do not require treatment. Bradycardia or cardiac standstill may occur in predisposed patients. Skin irritation and muscle soreness are common. Elevation of total CK and lactic dehydrogenase (LDH) may occur due to muscle trauma, but MB-CK generally remains normal unless cumulative energies greater than 425 joules are used. Transient ST elevation may be noted without other evidence of myocardial injury. Embolic phenomena may occur following successful cardioversion, especially in patients cardioverted from atrial fibrillation; prophylactic anticoagulation may, however, reduce the risk of this complication.

VIII. **Cardiac pacing** may be required in patients with symptomatic brady- or tachyarrhythmias. Temporary pacemakers are usually right ventricular endocardial electrodes placed percutaneously or through a cutdown. During cardiac arrest, a transthoracic pacemaker may be necessary. Permanent pacemakers use endocardial electrodes placed transvenously or epicardial electrodes placed during cardiac surgery. A variety of programmable sensing and pacing modes are available, allowing considerable flexibility in pacemaker function. Patients with temporary or permanent pacemakers require close monitoring.

A. Indications for temporary pacing
  1. Bradyarrhythmias
   a. Symptomatic sinus bradycardia or second- or third-degree heart block due to transient drug intoxication or electrolyte imbalance.
   b. Complete heart block, Mobitz II AV block, or during an acute MI the development of new bundle branch block patterns including right bundle branch block (RBBB) with left axis deviation (LAD), RBBB with right axis deviation (RAD), alternating RBBB and LBBB, and LBBB with PR prolongation. However, most patients with complete heart block complicating an acute inferior MI have an escape rhythm manifesting a narrow QRS complex at a rate of 45–60 beats/minute that may be adequate to maintain an acceptable blood pressure; insertion of a pacemaker may be deferred in these patients. Marked sinus bradycardia due to an acute inferior MI is usually responsive to atropine; however, refractory cases may require pacing.
   c. Symptomatic sinus bradycardia, atrial fibrillation with a slow ventricular rate, or other manifestations of **conduction system disease** may require temporary pacing until a permanent pacemaker can be inserted.
   d. Asystole or marked bradycardia during cardiac arrest that is unresponsive to medications (see Chap. 2).
  2. Tachyarrhythmias are best managed by medications or DC cardioversion. If these measures are not effective or contraindicated or if the arrhythmias recur frequently while therapy is being optimized, temporary pacing may be useful.
   a. Atrial flutter can be terminated successfully in nearly all cases (except atypical flutter having atrial rates over 400 beats/minute). This technique may be particularly useful in patients with atrial flutter who have received substantial doses of digitalis in an unsuccessful attempt to decrease the ventricular rate or in whom signs of digitalis intoxication make cardioversion relatively contraindicated. Atrial fibrillation, however, cannot be terminated with atrial pacing.
   b. Reentrant SVTs (e.g., sinus or AV node reentry, or reentry using a manifest or concealed bypass tract).
   c. Automatic or digitalis-induced SVTs cannot be terminated by pacing; however, atrial pacing at a rate greater than the intrinsic atrial rate can be used to increase the degree of AV block and thereby slow the ventricular response (e.g., changing an SVT with an atrial rate of 140 beats/minute having a 1:1 ventricular response to an atrial paced rate of 180 beats/minute with 2:1 AV block, resulting in a ventricular rate of 90 beats/minute).
   d. Recurrent sustained VT can be terminated in many instances by overdrive ventricular pacing. Underdrive ventricular pacing is effective occasionally when the rate of the VT is less than 150 beats/minute. Cardiac pacing during VT, however, should be performed only by experienced physicians, since degeneration to VF may occur.
   e. Bradycardia-dependent VT or VT/VF complicating intrinsic or drug-induced QT prolongation (torsade de pointes) can often be prevented by pacing at a rate faster than the intrinsic sinus rate.
B. Indications for permanent pacing
  1. Bradyarrhythmias
   a. Symptomatic bradycardia or prolonged symptomatic pauses following termination of atrial tachyarrhythmias (e.g., sick sinus syndrome, carotid sinus hypersensitivity).
   b. Second- or third-degree block that is symptomatic or due to His-Purkinje disease (intra-His or infra-His block).
   c. Transient complete heart block in the setting of acute anterior MI, even if the conduction disturbance resolves, since a high incidence of recurrent complete heart block occurs in this population. Transient complete heart block complicating an inferior MI, however, does not usually require prophylactic permanent pacing.
   d. Marked first-degree block in the His-Purkinje system (i.e., HV $\geq$ 100 msec, or 60–99 msec if symptoms present).
   e. Congenital complete heart block if the heart rate fails to accelerate with exercise or other stress.
  2. Tachyarrhythmias. Patient-activated radio-frequency underdrive and overdrive pacemakers are available for medically refractory reentrant SVTs. Simi-

larly, underdrive patient-activated pacemakers are available for patients with refractory VT, and overdrive burst pacing units for VT are under development. Patients considered for pacemaker therapy should first undergo extensive electrophysiologic testing to determine the mechanism of the arrhythmia and document a favorable response to the proposed pacing method.

C. Complications of permanent pacing
1. **Battery failure** is the most common cause of pacemaker failure.
2. **Loss of capture** due to development of local fibrosis or electrode dislodgement.
3. **Perforation of the myocardium** with loss of ventricular capture or stimulation of the diaphragm or chest wall.
4. **Stimulation of chest wall muscles or the diaphragm,** even in the absence of cardiac perforation.
5. **Sensing dysfunction,** particularly with bipolar pacing units. Conversion to a unipolar mode may correct the problem.
6. **Mechanically induced ventricular ectopy.**
7. **Electrode fracture** resulting in intermittent as well as persistent failure.
8. **"Endless loop" tachycardias** (with AV sequential pacemakers in DDD mode only).
9. Rarely, a pacemaker wire may induce significant tricuspid insufficiency.
10. Loss of atrial contribution to ventricular filling during ventricular pacing can result in hypotension and pulmonary congestion in patients with "stiff" or hypertrophied ventricles or mitral stenosis. AV sequential pacing may be helpful in this setting.
11. **Infection** at the site of electrode insertion or pacemaker pocket. However, bacteremia from other sites is not in itself an indication for pacemaker removal.

Management of Specific Arrhythmias

Optimal management of cardiac arrhythmias requires a thorough understanding of the various mechanisms underlying them and the therapeutic methods available.

I. Sinus tachycardia is a normal physiologic response to a variety of stresses, or it may be secondary to a number of drugs, including catecholamines, theophylline, and caffeine.
  A. ECG recognition. The atrial rate is 100–180 beats/minute; the P waves have a normal morphology, and each P wave is followed by a QRS complex at a constant PR interval (unless concomitant AV block is present). The onset and termination of sinus tachycardia are gradual. Carotid sinus massage results in a gradual slowing, with return to the initial rate after release; however, marked sinus tachycardia may not respond to vagal maneuvers.
  B. Therapy
    1. When sinus tachycardia is an appropriate physiologic response (e.g., fever), specific treatment is generally not required. **Therapy should be directed at the underlying cause.**
    2. In circumstances such as thyrotoxicosis, toxicity to sympathomimetic drugs, or severe mitral stenosis with pulmonary edema or ongoing ischemia, specific therapy may be required. **Propranolol** may be given IV in 1.0-mg increments q1–5 minutes (with the total dosage not to exceed 0.15 mg/kg) to control the heart rate; alternatively, oral therapy may be given in dosages of 10–80 mg q6h as needed to control the heart rate. Digitalis is not helpful unless CHF is responsible for the sinus tachycardia. Administration of verapamil IV is frequently associated with a sinus tachycardia due to reflex sympathetic stimulation; oral administration of verapamil, however, often produces a slowing in sinus rate.
  C. Disposition depends on the underlying abnormality responsible for the tachycardia and the patient's hemodynamic status. Patients having cardiovascular symptoms as a direct consequence of sinus tachycardia should be hospitalized. Use of IV propranolol requires a monitored bed and close supervision.
II. Sinus bradycardia is a normal physiologic response to decreased sympathetic or increased parasympathetic tone as occurs in well-trained athletes, during sleep, or in response to such stimuli as vomiting, pain, or increased intracranial pressure. Sinus bradycardia may also occur with hypothyroidism, with hypothermia, or in response to certain drugs including propranolol and verapamil. In addition, sinus bradycardia may be due to primary sinus node dysfunction and result in hemodynamic compromise.
  A. ECG recognition. The atrial rate is less than 60 beats/minute. P waves have a

normal contour and occur before each QRS complex with a constant PR interval exceeding 0.12 seconds (unless concomitant AV block is present). Sinus arrhythmia often coexists.

B. Therapy

1. **Asymptomatic patients require no specific therapy** other than correction of any underlying pathology.

2. If cardiac output is inadequate or ventricular arrhythmias complicate the slow rate, **atropine** (0.5–1.0 mg IV, repeated as necessary) or, in the absence of myocardial ischemia, **isoproterenol** (1–10 μg/minute by continuous infusion) will augment the heart rate. Cardiac pacing may be required for acute and chronic management.

C. Disposition

1. Patients with asymptomatic sinus bradycardia detected incidentally should be referred for outpatient evaluation directed at determining whether the bradycardia is physiologic or a result of sinus node dysfunction.

2. Patients having symptomatic sinus bradycardia require hospitalization and ECG monitoring.

III. Sinus pause or sinus arrest is due to failure of sinus node automaticity and results in atrial and ventricular asystole unless a subsidiary pacemaker discharges. Sinus node dysfunction may be secondary to a primary degenerative process (as in sick sinus syndrome), acute ischemia, excess vagal tone, or toxic effects of most antiarrhythmic drugs. The clinical consequences depend on the rate of discharge of subsidiary pacemakers and the underlying state of the patient.

A. ECG recognition. Sinus pause or arrest is manifest as a sudden pause in sinus rhythm. The PP interval delimiting the pause is not a multiple of the basic PP interval prior to the pause. The pause may last for several seconds, and the beat ending the pause may be sinus, junctional, or ventricular in origin.

B. Therapy

1. **Asymptomatic individuals do not require specific therapy** other than correction of any underlying abnormality.

2. Symptomatic patients may be managed acutely with **atropine, isoproterenol, or temporary pacing** as described for the treatment of sinus bradycardia (see sec. **II.B.2**). A permanent pacemaker may be required for long-term management.

C. Disposition

1. Patients without symptoms should be referred for outpatient evaluation directed at determining the severity of sinus node dysfunction.

2. Symptomatic patients require hospitalization.

IV. Sinoatrial exit block. In sinoatrial (SA) exit block, the sinus node discharges normally, but conduction block occurs in the perinodal tissue. As a result, atrial and ventricular asystole ensue unless a subsidiary pacemaker discharges. SA exit block may be due to excessive vagal stimulation, acute myocarditis or infarction, atrial fibrosis, or toxic effects of antiarrhythmic agents. Clinical consequences depend on the duration of the ensuing pause. It is important to identify and correct any underlying abnormality.

A. ECG recognition. SA exit block is diagnosed electrocardiographically by a sudden absence of P waves. In contrast to a sinus pause, the PP interval delimiting the subsequent pause is a multiple of the basic PP interval. SA exit block results in a PP interval approximately two, three, or four times the normal PP interval. SA exit block may manifest a Wenckebach periodicity with progressive shortening in the PP intervals prior to the pause.

B. Therapy

1. **Asymptomatic individuals do not require specific therapy.** Precipitating abnormalities should be searched for and treated, if present.

2. Symptomatic patients may be treated acutely with **atropine, isoproterenol, or temporary pacing** as described for the treatment of sinus bradycardia (see sec. **II.B.2**).

C. Disposition

1. Patients without symptoms should be referred for outpatient evaluation directed at determining the severity of sinus node dysfunction.

2. Symptomatic patients require hospitalization.

V. Wandering atrial pacemaker is due to a shift in the site of the dominant pacemaker focus from the sinus node to other atrial sites or AV junctional tissue. It occurs when the rate of sinus node discharge is less than that of latent pacemakers. A wandering atrial pacemaker may be observed normally, expecially in athletes, presumably due to enhanced vagal tone, but more commonly indicates intrinsic sinus node dysfunction or other underlying heart disease.

A. ECG recognition. The atrial rate is 45–100 beats/minute. The P-wave morphology and PP interval are variable. Each P wave is followed by a QRS complex (in the absence of concomitant AV block), but the PR interval may vary as the site of atrial depolarization shifts in relation to the AV node. The change in pacemaker focus is usually gradual, occurring over several beats.

B. Therapy

    1. Patients are usually asymptomatic, and no therapy is required acutely.

    2. If **symptoms are present** (due to severe bradycardia), treatment should be initiated as outlined for sinus bradycardia (see sec. **II.B.2**).

C. Disposition

    1. Patients without symptoms should be referred for outpatient evaluation.

    2. Symptomatic patients require hospitalization.

VI. Atrial premature depolarizations (APDs) represent premature atrial depolarizations that occur earlier than the normal sinus interval. They are normal phenomenon at all ages but frequently reflect the presence of underlying heart disease. APDs may be exacerbated by myocardial or pericardial inflammation, myocardial ischemia, emotional stress, or a variety of medications or drugs including caffeine, tobacco, and alcohol. The clinical consequences depend on the frequency of APDs and their role in initiating other atrial or ventricular tachyarrhythmias (most commonly atrial fibrillation/flutter and SVT).

A. ECG recognition. APDs are manifest as premature P waves with morphologies that usually differ from sinus P waves. Examination of multiple leads may be necessary to identify P waves properly, especially when they are superimposed on the preceding T wave. AV conduction following an APD depends on the inherent function of the AV conduction system. In general, the PR interval of an APD varies inversely with its prematurity. Late-coupled APDs may be conducted normally, but early APDs are associated with a prolonged PR interval or aberrant conduction (simulating VPDs if the P wave is not identified correctly). Very early APDs may block in the AV node or His-bundle and result in a pause simulating a sinus pause or exit block.

B. Therapy

    1. Asymptomatic individuals without evidence for sustained atrial tachyarrhythmias, including atrial fibrillation/flutter or SVT, require **no specific therapy** acutely other than the elimination of any underlying or precipitating disorders.

    2. Patients with **symptomatic** APDs may be treated electively (generally as outpatients) with **quinidine, procainamide, or disopyramide.** Patients with a history of atrial fibrillation or flutter, however, should not receive these drugs without concomitant therapy with AV nodal depressant drugs (i.e., digitalis, propranolol, or verapamil) to control the ventricular rate (see sec. **VIII.B.2**). Patients with catecholamine-related APDs may be treated effectively with propranolol alone.

    3. Patients with APDs that initiate **atrial fibrillation or flutter** should be treated with a combination of drugs directed at suppressing the APDs (i.e., quinidine, procainamide, or dysopyramide) and at slowing the ventricular response (i.e., digitalis, propranolol, or verapamil).

    4. Patients with APDs initiating **recurrent SVT** should be treated as outlined in sec. **IX.B.3**.

C. Disposition

    1. Patients with asymptomatic or symptomatic APDs should be referred for outpatient evaluation directed at determining whether organic heart disease is present.

    2. Initiating therapy in patients experiencing atrial fibrillation/flutter or SVT generally requires hospital admission, preferably to a monitored bed.

VII. Atrial flutter may be paroxysmal or persistent and frequently degenerates to atrial fibrillation. Atrial flutter may complicate any cardiac disease causing atrial dilatation or develop as a consequence of pericarditis, thyrotoxicosis, alcohol ingestion, or pulmonary embolism. Since the atria contract during atrial flutter, the incidence of embolism is less than with atrial fibrillation.

A. ECG recognition. The atrial rate is 250–350 beats/minute with regular sawtooth flutter waves seen best in leads II, III, aVF, and V_1. The ventricular rate is most often half the atrial rate because of 2:1 AV block. In children and patients with preexcitation syndromes, thyrotoxicosis, or conditions of catecholamine excess, 1:1

conduction may occur. Quinidine, procainamide, or disopyramide when administered alone may slow the atrial rate, resulting in 1:1 AV conduction and acceleration of the ventricular rate. Digitalis, beta-blockers, and verapamil slow AV conduction. The QRS complex is narrow unless aberrant conduction is present. During vagal maneuvers such as carotid sinus massage, a stepwise decrease in ventricular rate due to increased AV block may occur; the atrial rate, however, is not affected by such maneuvers.

B. Therapy

1. If the patient is **hemodynamically unstable,** cardioversion should be performed immediately. Frequently, low energies (i.e., 25–50 joules) are successful. If cardioversion results in atrial fibrillation, a second shock at a higher energy (i.e., 50–200 joules) may restore sinus rhythm; alternatively, if atrial fibrillation is tolerated better, the patient can be treated medically (see sec. VIII.B.2).

2. If the patient is **hemodynamically stable** and atrial flutter is of new onset or paroxysmal, DC cardioversion may be performed electively (as described under **Treatment,** sec. VII.C). Alternatively, medical management or rapid atrial pacing can be utilized, depending on physician and patient preference and the presence of associated diseases. If atrial flutter is chronic and detected incidentally, no specific treatment is required acutely.

   a. If **medical therapy** is elected, the ventricular rate should be controlled first with AV nodal depressant drugs (i.e., digitalis, propranolol, or verapamil) used alone or in combination. Pharmacologic conversion to sinus rhythm can then be attempted with quinidine, procainamide, or disopyramide. If successful, the patient should continue to receive both the AV nodal depressant drug and the membrane depressant drug that achieved conversion. If pharmacologic therapy is not effective, DC cardioversion or rapid atrial pacing should be performed.

   b. If **rapid atrial pacing** is elected, a temporary atrial pacemaker is inserted and positioned in the high right atrium. Successful termination is critically dependent on the rate and duration of pacing. The optimal pacing rate is 125% of the atrial flutter rate. Pacing should be continued until a change in the flutter wave morphology, typically from negative to positive, is observed in the inferior leads. Rapid atrial pacing is particularly useful for patients receiving large doses of digitalis. Pacing may result in degeneration to atrial fibrillation, most often accompanied by a slower ventricular rate and clinical improvement.

3. **Prevention** depends on the correction of underlying abnormalities and the use of quinidine, procainamide, or disopyramide in conjunction with an AV nodal depressant drug (i.e., digitalis, beta-blocker, or verapamil).

C. Disposition

1. Patients with atrial flutter associated with hemodynamic instability require hospitalization and monitoring.

2. Patients with hemodynamically stable atrial flutter of new onset should be admitted for pharmacologic or electrical cardioversion. Cardiovascular evaluation should be directed at determining the presence and extent of underlying heart disease.

VIII. Atrial fibrillation, like atrial flutter, may be paroxysmal or chronic. Atrial fibrillation may complicate any condition causing atrial dilatation or irritation, including coronary artery disease, hypertension, mitral or tricuspid valve disease, cardiomyopathy, pericarditis, and pulmonary embolism. Moreover, it may accompany hyperthyroidism or alcohol ingestion, and on occasion, it occurs in otherwise normal individuals. During atrial fibrillation, the atria do not contract effectively, resulting in the loss of the atrial contribution to ventricular filling and a proclivity to systemic embolism. The ability to restore and maintain sinus rhythm is inversely related to the atrial size and duration of atrial fibrillation.

A. ECG recognition. Atrial depolarization is chaotic and is manifested electrocardiographically as small, irregular baseline undulations of variable amplitude and morphology. Discrete P waves are not seen. The ventricular rhythm, in the absence of drugs, generally is "irregularly irregular" at a rate of 100–200 beats/minute. Carotid sinus massage transiently slows the ventricular rate.

1. Atrial fibrillation with a **regular ventricular response** should raise suspicion of digitalis toxicity, as it may represent AV dissociation with an accelerated junctional pacemaker.

2. Atrial fibrillation with a **slow ventricular response** in the untreated patient

implies underlying AV node disease. These patients often have concomitant sinus node disease, and attempted conversion to sinus rhythm may result in prolonged asystole.

3. Atrial fibrillation in some patients with preexcitation syndromes may be associated with an extremely rapid ventricular response that may result in syncope or degenerate to VF. Electrocardiographically, a **rapid irregular wide-complex tachycardia** is observed. Digitalis or verapamil may worsen the situation and should not be used in such situations.

B. Therapy

1. **Hemodynamically unstable** patients require emergent cardioversion; energies of 100–200 joules are usually effective. If cardioversion is not successful, the ventricular rate may be slowed acutely with IV administration of digitalis, verapamil, or propranolol; a combination of these drugs may occasionally be necessary. Once the ventricular rate has been controlled acutely, maintenance dosages should be started (PO or IV, depending on the clinical situation) and the patient managed as outlined in sec. **VIII.B.2**

2. **Hemodynamically stable patients**

   a. **Control of ventricular rate.** Patients hemodynamically stable with new onset or paroxysmal atrial fibrillation associated with a moderate or rapid ventricular response (i.e., >100 beats/minute) should be treated acutely with **digitalis, propranolol, or verapamil** (IV or PO, depending on the clinical situation) to control the ventricular rate. Propranolol may be used in patients with pulmonary edema if it is a consequence of diseases inhibiting ventricular filling (e.g., mitral stenosis, idiopathic hypertrophic subaortic stenosis). Maintenance therapy is usually required, and the dosage should be titrated to maintain the ventricular rate between 60 and 90 beats/minute. Serum digoxin levels considered toxic in other circumstances may be required to control the ventricular rate adequately. In addition, a combination of digitalis and propranolol or verapamil may be beneficial.

   b. **Elective restoration** to sinus rhythm can then be attempted pharmacologically. Administration of **procainamide, quinidine, or disopyramide** for 2–3 days restores sinus rhythm in up to 30% of patients. However, if atrial fibrillation persists, cardioversion can be attempted electrically. Synchronized energies of 100–200 joules are generally effective. If sinus rhythm is restored, maintenance dosages of both the AV node depressant agent and membrane depressant agent should be continued. If sinus rhythm cannot be restored, the AV node depressant drug that controlled the ventricular rate best should be continued and the membrane depressant agent discontinued.

3. Patients manifesting a **wide-complex irregular tachycardia** may have atrial fibrillation with ventricular preexcitation (e.g., WPW syndrome). Digitalis or verapamil should not be administered to slow the ventricular response, since paradoxical acceleration of the ventricular rate and degeneration to VF may occur. If cardioversion is not successful, the ventricular rate may be controlled acutely with IV procainamide, which slows conduction through the bypass tract.

4. **Anticoagulation** should be considered for patients with atrial fibrillation, especially those with paroxysmal atrial fibrillation or mitral valve disease.

   a. Patients requiring **emergent cardioversion** should receive heparin prior to cardioversion if time permits. If not contraindicated, anticoagulant therapy should be continued for 2–3 weeks if cardioversion is succesful.

   b. Patients **cardioverted electively** (with drugs or electrically) should receive anticoagulant therapy for 2–3 weeks prior to cardioversion and for 2–3 weeks following successful restoration of sinus rhythm.

5. If atrial fibrillation is chronic and the ventricular response well controlled, no acute treatment is required.

C. Disposition

1. All patients presenting with atrial fibrillation complicated by hemodynamic decompensation require hospitalization and monitoring.

2. Patients hemodynamically stable with new onset or paroxysmal atrial fibrillation should be admitted for acute and chronic therapy, as well as evaluation directed at determining whether heart disease is present.

3. The patient with chronic atrial fibrillation and a controlled ventricular response should be referred for outpatient evaluation directed at determining whether underlying heart disease is present.

IX. Paroxysmal supraventricular tachycardia (PSVT) may occur in patients of all ages,

Table 4-2. ECG diagnosis of PSVT subtype: P–QRS relationship

Type	ECG
AV node reentry	Retrograde P wave is buried in QRS or immediately follows QRS (RP < 50% RR).
AV reentry utilizing a bypass tract (orthodromic SVT)	P wave immediately follows the QRS (RP < 50% RR) and is usually negative in lead I.
Sinus node reentry	P-wave morphology is identical to sinus rhythm, with PR related to PSVT rate (RP > 50% RR).
Intraatrial reentry	P-wave morphology depends on site of intraatrial circuit, with PR related to PSVT rate (RP > 50% RR).
Automatic atrial tachycardia	P-wave morphology depends on site of ectopic focus, with PR related to PSVT rate (RP > 50% RR); first and subsequent P waves have same morphology.

with or without underlying heart disease. PSVT may be due to disturbances in automaticity or reentrant circuits involving the sinus or AV node, a bypass tract, or atrial muscle. The response to therapy depends on the mechanism involved. In general, automatic atrial tachycardias are not terminated by cardioversion, vagal maneuvers, or drugs directed at the AV node; however, quinidine, procainamide, or disopyramide may be effective. Reentrant rhythms are generally terminated successfully by cardioversion; in addition, reentrant rhythms involving the sinus or AV node (i.e., sinus node or AV node reentry, reentry utilizing a bypass tract) are often terminated successfully by vagal maneuvers or pharmacologically with verapamil, digitalis, or propranolol. Careful scrutiny of the 12-lead ECG during PSVT, as well as the effects of certain drugs and maneuvers, provides valuable information relating to the mechanism responsible for the PSVT. In some instances, invasive electrophysiologic studies are required; for a complete discussion, see Josephson and Seides (1979).

A. ECG recognition (Table 4-2). The rate ranges from 120–250 beats/minute. The QRS complex is narrow in the absence of aberration or preexisting bundle branch block.

1. **AV node reentry** is the most common cause of PSVT, accounting for 60% of cases. The reentrant circuit is localized to the AV node and is due to the longitudinal dissociation of the AV node into two functionally distinct pathways. During PSVT, anterograde conduction occurs over one pathway and retrograde conduction over the other, resulting in near simultaneous ventricular and atrial activation. As a result, **retrograde P waves (negative in leads II, III, and aVF) are buried within the QRS complexes and are not visible on the surface ECG or appear immediately following the QRS complex** (with the RP interval < 50% of RR interval). AV node reentry cannot exist in the presence of AV node block but can persist if AV block is intra- or infra-His. Since intra-His and infra-His blocks are uncommon, especially in young patients, the presence of AV block during PSVT reduces markedly the chance that AV node reentry is the responsible mechanism.

2. **PSVT complicating the WPW syndrome** is the second most common form and accounts for 25% of cases. The reentrant circuit is large and involves the atria, AV node, His-Purkinje system, ventricular muscle, and a bypass tract. Bypass tracts may be manifest or concealed. In patients with manifest WPW, the bypass tract can conduct anterograde and retrograde, and characteristic delta waves are observed in the ECG recorded during sinus rhythm. Concealed bypass tracts (CBTs) only conduct retrograde, and ventricular preexcitation is not present during sinus rhythm. Patients with manifest or concealed bypass tracts are predisposed to develop orthodromic PSVT. Patients with manifest WPW are also susceptible to other supraventricular arrhythmias.

   a. **PSVT associated with a CBT.** During orthodromic PSVT, anterograde conduction occurs through the normal AV node to the ventricles and then returns retrograde through the bypass tract to excite the atria; thus, **P waves are seen immediately following the QRS complex**, reflecting the sequential ventricular to atrial activation sequence. Since in most patients with CBTs, the bypass tract is left-sided, retrograde atrial activation proceeds left to right during SVT and consequently **the P waves generally are**

negative in lead I. Since orthodromic PSVT due to a bypass tract cannot occur in the presence of AV block, if AV block is present during the PSVT, the PSVT is not due to a bypass tract.

b. **Supraventricular arrhythmias in patients with manifest WPW.** See sec. XVI.

3. **Sinus node reentry** accounts for 5% of cases of PSVT. The reentrant circuit is localized to the sinus node and perinodal tissue. As a result, the **P-wave morphology during PSVT is identical or very similar to that during normal sinus rhythm.** Since the AV node is not an integral part of the reentry circuit, the PR interval or presence of AV block during sinus node reentry depends solely on the intrinsic properties of the AV node.

4. During **intraatrial reentry,** which accounts for 5% of cases of PSVT, the reentrant circuit involves atrial muscle. The **P-wave morphology depends on the site of the circuit within the atria.** The AV node is not part of the reentrant circuit, and AV conduction during intraatrial reentry depends on the intrinsic properties of the AV node.

5. **Automatic atrial foci** account for 5% of cases of PSVT. During PSVT, the **P-wave morphology depends on the location of the ectopic pacemaker.** Importantly, in automatic PSVT, the P-wave morphology of the first beat initiating the PSVT is identical to that of subsequent P waves. In contrast, in reentrant forms of PSVT, the P-wave morphology of the APD triggering the reentrant circuit differs from the P-wave morphology during PSVT. In automatic PSVT, as in PSVT due to sinus node or intraatrial reentry, the AV node is not an integral part of the underlying mechanism; thus, the PR interval or presence of AV block depends on the inherent function of the AV conduction system.

B. **Therapy**

1. If the patient is **hemodynamically compromised** or experiencing **angina,** immediate electrical cardioversion is indicated. Energies of 25–50 joules are usually successful.

2. If the patient is **stable,** the choice of therapy should be guided by the mechanism responsible for the PSVT. If the mechanism cannot be determined, the following guidelines are helpful.

a. **Vagal stimulation,** including the **Valsalva maneuver** and **carotid sinus massage,** alters the electrical properties of the sinus and AV nodes and should be performed first. Vagal stimulation may terminate PSVT due to sinus or AV node reentry or orthodromic PSVT using a CBT. Vagal maneuvers, however, do not terminate intraatrial or automatic PSVTs but may increase AV block and slow the ventricular rate.

(1) **Diving reflex.** More intense vagal stimulation can be achieved with the diving reflex by placing the patient's forehead, cheeks, and temples into ice water. However, this maneuver can cause ventricular ectopy or asystole and should not be performed in older patients or those with a history of ventricular ectopy or conduction system disease.

(2) **Drugs.** Vagal stimulation can also be augmented by the administration of the following drugs; however, this approach is now considered **secondline** behind the use of verapamil.

(a) **Edrophonium** should be given as a 1.0-mg test dose and then as 10 mg IV push over 30 seconds. Carotid sinus massage should then be repeated. Edrophonium, however, should not be used in hypotensive patients.

(b) **Methoxamine, phenylephrine,** or **metaraminol** may be given IV over 2–3 minutes in a dosage of 3–5 mg for methoxamine, 0.1–0.5 mg for phenylephrine, and 0.5–1.0 mg for metaraminol. These agents enhance blood pressure and reflexively increase vagal tone. They should not be used in hypertensive patients.

b. **Verapamil** (see **Treatment,** sec. **VI**), generally as an IV bolus of 5–10 mg over 2–3 minutes (repeated once in a dosage of 10 mg if necessary), is the **drug of choice** for terminating PSVT due to sinus or AV node reentry or that utilizing a CBT. By increasing AV block, verapamil may also slow the ventricular rate during automatic or intraatrial reentrant PSVT. Caution regarding its use must be exercised in hypotensive patients.

c. **Propranolol** given IV or PO (see **Treatment,** sec. **IV**) may terminate PSVT due to reentrant circuits involving the sinus or AV nodes or a CBT and slow AV conduction in automatic or intraatrial reentrant SVT.

d. Digoxin slows AV node conduction and may terminate PSVT due to AV node reentry or reentry using a CBT. Like verapamil and propranolol, digoxin may increase AV block and slow the ventricular response to other forms of PSVT. Digoxin should be given in a dose of 0.5–0.75 mg IV or PO initially, followed by aliquots of 0.25 mg q2h as needed. The total dose in the first 24 hours, however, should not exceed 1.5 mg. If ouabain is used, the initial dose is 0.2–0.3 mg IV, followed by 0.1 mg q30–60 minutes for 2–4 doses. Carotid sinus massage should be repeated after each dose of these digitalis preparations.

e. Quinidine or procainamide in conventional dosages may be helpful in terminating PSVT utilizing a CBT, intraatrial reentry, or automatic PSVT.

f. Electrical cardioversion or **rapid atrial pacing** can be used if the above methods are unsuccessful. The reentrant forms of PSVT are almost always responsive, but automatic PSVT generally continues unabated. In such a circumstance, the ventricular response should be controlled with propranolol, verapamil, digitalis, or rapid atrial pacing.

3. Prophylaxis against recurrence is often more difficult than termination of the acute episode. Decisions regarding prophylactic therapy should be based on the PSVT mechanism, frequency of episodes, nature of underlying heart disease (if any), and symptoms. In general, PSVT is recurrent. Patients with infrequent episodes that are not associated with disabling symptoms may prefer intermittent acute treatment (e.g., single PO or IV administration of an effective antiarrhythmic drug) to chronic therapy. On the other hand, patients with frequent episodes or episodes associated with disabling symptoms should be treated chronically. Invasive electrophysiologic study may be necessary to determine the mechanism and optimal treatment.

a. Although PSVT due to **AV node reentry** is the most common form, it is one of the most difficult to control, in part due to the profound autonomic influences on the AV node. In 70% of cases, AV node depressant agents, including digitalis, beta-blockers, and verapamil, are effective and exert their beneficial actions primarily on the anterograde limb of the microreentrant circuit. In 30% of cases, procainamide, quinidine, and disopyramide are effective as single agents by affecting retrograde conduction primarily. Rarely, a combination of both types of agents is effective, but generally such combinations offset the salutary effects of each drug.

b. Reentry using a CBT is prevented best by procainamide, quinidine, or disopyramide, since these agents affect directly the electrical properties of the accessory pathway. AV node depressant drugs, when used alone, are also effective. The combination of an AV node depressant agent and a type I membrane depressant drug is generally not more effective than a single drug from either group alone.

c. Sinus node reentry is generally prevented with beta-blockers.

d. Intraatrial reentry and **automatic PSVT** are prevented best with quinidine or procainamide. Concomitant treatment with an AV node depressant drug is recommended for intraatrial reentrant and automatic PSVTs if the ventricular rate is rapid.

C. Disposition. All patients hemodynamically unstable or having ischemic chest pain and most patients with new onset PSVT require admission to a monitored hospital bed for observation, evaluation, and therapy. Patients with well-tolerated PSVT, especially those having a clear precipitating event, can often have their PSVT terminated in the emergency department and be referred for outpatient evaluation directed at determining whether underlying heart disease is present.

X. Atrial tachycardia with block (PAT with block) is due in 50–75% of cases to **digitalis toxicity.** Other causes include coronary artery disease, with or without infarction, and cor pulmonale. This arrhythmia probably represents increased automaticity of an ectopic atrial pacemaker, making it a form of automatic SVT. The symptoms and prognosis are related to the etiology and underlying cardiac status.

A. ECG recognition. The atrial rate is usually 150–200 beats/minute. The P-wave morphology depends on the location of the ectopic atrial pacemaker. By definition, some degree of AV block is present, resulting in a ventricular rate that is slower than the atrial rate. Frequently, other manifestations of digitalis toxicity, including ventricular ectopy, are present.

B. Therapy

1. If the patient is receiving digitalis, it must be assumed that digitalis toxicity is responsible and the drug stopped immediately. If the serum potassium concentration is low, potassium should be administered cautiously to yield a high normal level of 4.5–5.0 mmol/liter. The patient must be monitored closely, since increased AV block can occur during potassium replacement. Phenytoin or propranolol may occasionally terminate the arrhythmia. **Often, withholding digitalis and careful monitoring are all that are necessary. Electrical cardioversion is contraindicated.**

   2. If the patient has not been receiving digitalis, digitalis or propranolol may be given carefully, if necessary, to further increase the AV block and slow the ventricular rate. Procainamide, quinidine, or disopyramide may then terminate the arrhythmia in some patients. Electrical cardioversion is unlikely to be effective.

  C. Disposition. As these patients nearly all have digitalis toxicity or severe underlying heart disease, they should be hospitalized in a monitored bed.

XI. Multifocal (chaotic) atrial tachycardia (MAT) occurs most commonly in patients with severe pulmonary disease, often during treatment with theophylline and/or catecholamines. It occurs occasionally in diabetics, patients with acute CHF, and children and rarely as a consequence of digitalis toxicity. The prognosis depends primarily on the underlying condition responsible for the arrhythmia rather than the ill effects of the arrhythmia itself. MAT may degenerate to atrial fibrillation.

  A. ECG recognition. The atrial rate is 100–250 beats/minute with multiple (at least three) P-wave morphologies and varying PP and PR intervals. Unlike atrial fibrillation, an isoelectric baseline exists between P waves. The ventricular rate depends on the inherent conduction properties of the AV node. Frequently, blocked APDs may be present. The QRS complex is narrow in the absence of aberrancy.

  B. Therapy. Effective therapy depends primarily on **correction of the underlying condition.** Specific antiarrhythmic therapy is usually not effective and often ill advised. It is important to distinguish this rhythm from atrial fibrillation, since digitalis is often not effective in slowing the ventricular rate and excess digitalis in the face of underlying hypoxia or catecholamine administration may lead to a fatal ventricular arrhythmia. Rarely, patients may respond to propranolol, but such therapy is contraindicated in the presence of severe lung disease. Verapamil may help slow the ventricular rate in some patients, although little experience with this therapy is available.

  C. Disposition. Admission to a monitored hospital bed is indicated for all symptomatic patients.

XII. Nonparoxysmal AV junctional tachycardia is probably caused by derangements in automaticity in or near the AV node. It may be due to digitalis toxicity, inferior infarction, or myocarditis; follow open-heart surgery; or occur rarely in otherwise healthy individuals. The consequences and therapy depend on the underlying cause. It is important to suspect digitalis toxicity.

  A. ECG recognition. Nonparoxysmal AV junctional tachycardia is characterized by a fairly regular ventricular rate of 65–130 beats/minute. The QRS complex has a normal supraventricular configuration (in the absence of preexisting bundle branch block). Retrograde atrial activation (with a negative P wave in leads II, III, and aVF occurring just before or just after each QRS complex) may be present, or the atria may be controlled by an entirely independent means (e.g., atrial fibrillation). Atrial fibrillation with a regular ventricular rate, however, suggests digitalis toxicity. Further administration of digitalis in an attempt to slow the ventricular response will aggravate the situation and may result in a fatal arrhythmia. Carotid sinus massage may transiently slow the ventricular rate. Occasionally, the ventricular rate may reveal a Wenckebach periodicity due to exit block from the AV junctional focus.

  B. Therapy

   1. If the patient is being treated with digitalis, digitalis toxicity must be assumed to be responsible and the drug stopped. If necessary, potassium, lidocaine, phenytoin, or propranolol may be administered as described in the management of digitalis-induced arrhythmias (see sec. **XVII.A**).

   2. If the patient has not been on digitalis and the rate is rapid and causing hemodynamic compromise, digitalis should be given to slow the ventricular response. Cardioversion may be attempted but is unlikely to be successful. Usually, careful monitoring and attention to the underlying heart disease will suffice, and the arrhythmia will abate spontaneously.

Table 4-3. Wide-complex tachycardia: supraventricular versus ventricular

Supports supraventricular origin with aberrancy
1. QRS width of 0.12 sec
2. Initial QRS deflection identical to baseline QRS complexes
3. RBBB configuration at a rate > 170 beats/min
4. Triphasic rsR configuration in lead V_1, especially with Q waves in leads I and V_6
5. Onset with a premature P wave
6. P and QRS rate and rhythm linked, suggesting that ventricular activation depends on atrial discharge (e.g., 2:1 AV block)
7. Slowing or termination by increased vagal tone
8. Long-short cycle sequence

Supports ventricular origin
1. QRS width > 0.14 sec
2. Left-axis deviation, often marked
3. RBBB complexes with monophasic (R), biphasic (qR, RS), or Rsr configuration in lead V_1; and R, rS, QS, or QR configuration in lead V_6
4. LBBB complexes with a qR or QS configuration in lead V_6
5. A concordant precordial pattern (QRS complexes positive or negative in all precordial leads)
6. Fusion or capture beats
7. AV dissociation
8. P and QRS rate and rhythm linked, suggesting that atrial activation depends on ventricular discharge (e.g., 2:1 VA block)
9. "Compensatory" pause

Source: Adapted from H. J. Wellens, F. W. Bar, and K. I. Lie, The value of the electrocardiogram in the differential diagnosis of a tachycardia with a widened QRS complex. *Am. J. Med.* 64:27, 1978.

   C. **Disposition.** In general, most patients should be hospitalized to determine the precipitating factor and assess the extent of underlying heart disease.
XIII. **Ventricular premature depolarizations (VPDs)** are due to intraventricular reentry or disturbances in automaticity and occur in normal subjects and patients with underlying heart disease. Although some patients experience discomfort or disturbances in circulatory function from VPDs themselves, their general importance lies in their possible role as harbingers of VT or VF. However, in the absence of underlying heart disease, VPDs are not generally associated with an increased risk of sudden death. In the presence of heart disease, particularly coronary artery disease and various forms of cardiomyopathy, VPDs may be more ominous.
   A. **ECG recognition.** VPDs are premature QRS complexes, generally bizarre in morphology, and greater than 0.12 seconds in duration. The T wave is usually large and opposite in direction to the major deflection of the QRS. The QRS is not preceded by a premature P wave, although a sinus P wave occurring at its usual time may be present. A retrograde P wave may follow the QRS complex, or the P wave may be obscured by the QRS and not be visible on the surface ECG. Although differentiation of a VPD from a supraventricular beat conducted aberrantly is not always possible, presence of a compensatory pause, fusion beats, initial QRS forces different in direction from normal sinus beats, or certain morphologic characteristics as described in Table 4-3 favor a ventricular origin. **Ventricular parasystole** is characterized by monomorphic VPDs occurring at varying coupling intervals and having RR intervals related mathematically (i.e., each RR interval is a multiple of an underlying RR interval). The parasystolic rate may range from 20–400 beats/minute but is usually 30–60 beats/minute.
   B. **Therapy.** Theoretic indications for treating patients with VPDs include reducing symptoms accompanying an irregular heart rhythm and preventing sustained VT/VF.
      1. Patients with **symptomatic VPDs** can be treated empirically, with alleviation of symptoms serving as an objective therapeutic endpoint.
      2. The issue of treating patients with asymptomatic VPDs to reduce the risk of sudden cardiac death remains controversial. Decisions to treat patients with **asymptomatic VPDs** should be made only after considering the benefit-to-risk ratio of administering antiarrhythmic agents to asymptomatic patients. Ap-

proximately 30% of patients receiving quinidine, procainamide, or disopyramide develop adverse reactions necessitating discontinuation of these agents. Moreover, antiarrhythmic agents have been shown to aggravate ventricular arrhythmias in up to 15% of patients. Since VPDs in the absence of organic heart disease are not generally associated with an increased risk of sudden death, most investigators do not recommend specific treatment in the absence of symptoms. VPDs in the presence of organic heart disease may be more ominous, but there are no definitive data demonstrating that their presence specifically identifies patients at increased risk for sudden death or that empiric treatment reduces the incidence of sudden death. Nevertheless, many investigators recommend that patients with severe left ventricular dysfunction (i.e., ejection fraction < 30%) manifesting complex VPDs (i.e., R-on-T phenomenon, multiform VPDs, > 5 VPDs/minute, a bigeminal pattern, or couplets or salvos of 3 or more) merit treatment.

   a. VPDs may be suppressed **acutely** with IV lidocaine or procainamide.

   b. VPDs may be suppressed **chronically** with oral quinidine, procainamide, disopyramide, or rarely propranolol. Newer agents including tocainide, mexiletine, and flecainide appear to be as efficacious as the more conventional drugs in suppressing VPDs.

   c. Some patients with **bradycardia-dependent ventricular ectopy** can be managed with cardiac pacing, with or without concomitant use of antiarrhythmic agents.

C. Disposition

   1. Patients with symptomatic VPDs require hospital admission, as do patients in whom acute suppression is indicated.

   2. Patients with asymptomatic VPDs detected incidentally should be referred for outpatient evaluation directed at determining whether underlying heart disease is present.

XIV. Ventricular tachycardia (VT) occurs most often in the setting of ischemic heart disease, including classic or variant angina or an acute MI, and following recovery from MI, particularly those complicated by development of a ventricular aneurysm. Other common causes include a cardiomyopathy, prolonged QT syndrome, mitral valve prolapse, drug toxicity, and metabolic disorders. In addition, VT may occur occasionally in otherwise healthy individuals. In most patients, VT is due to a reentrant mechanism, although in some instances disturbances in automaticity may be responsible. An **accelerated idioventricular rhythm** and **torsade de pointes** are particular forms of VT and are discussed separately.

A. ECG recognition. VT is defined as a series of three or more wide QRS complexes (with a duration > 0.12 seconds) of abnormal morphology, occurring at a rate of 100–250 beats/minute and accompanied by ST and T-wave changes in a direction opposite to the major QRS deflection. VT is often classified as nonsustained or sustained. Although arbitrary, sustained VT is defined as VT lasting longer than 30 seconds or associated with immediate hemodynamic collapse. The QRS contours may be uniform, multiform, or vary in a more or less repetitive manner (i.e., torsade de pointes, bidirectional VT). Retrograde atrial activation may be apparent, or the atria may be independent and exhibit AV and VA dissociation. Differentiation of VT from SVT with aberrancy based on analysis of the surface ECG can be difficult and at times impossible. Major features differentiating these arrhythmias are described in Table 4-3. Intracardiac recordings are required occasionally.

B. Therapy

   1. Acute therapy

      a. If sustained VT is associated with **hemodynamic compromise** or **angina,** immediate cardioversion is indicated. If the patient is without a pulse, countershock with 200 joules should be performed, followed by countershock with 200–300 joules and then with 360 joules if VT continues. In less dire circumstances, cardioversion should be attempted with a synchronized discharge of 50 joules, followed by progressively higher energies if initial attempts are not successful. Administration of IV lidocaine (or procainamide or bretylium when appropriate) should be done concomitantly.

      b. If the patient is **hemodynamically stable,** lidocaine may be used as initial therapy. If lidocaine is not effective, procainamide or bretylium may be administered IV. If conversion to sinus rhythm does not occur promptly or the patient's condition deteriorates, immediate electrical cardioversion is indicated. Underdrive or overdrive ventricular pacing may be used occasionally to terminate VT but should be performed only by experienced personnel.

2. Chronic therapy

a. Quinidine, procainamide, or **disopyramide,** often in a relatively high dosage, is the drug of choice for prevention of recurrent VT. Unfortunately, empiric trials with these drugs have at best a 35% chance of success. Furthermore, patients refractory to one of these drugs are unlikely to respond to another drug. Invasive electrophysiologic testing utilizing programmed ventricular stimulation appears to predict accurately the clinical efficacy of these drugs and is often indicated when dealing with sustained VT not associated with an acute MI.

b. Phenytoin may be used alone or in combination with one of the above drugs but is generally not efficacious outside the setting of digitalis toxicity or VT associated with the long QT syndrome.

c. Propranolol is generally not effective except for catecholamine- or ischemia-induced VT.

d. Overdrive pacing may be helpful in preventing bradycardia-dependent VT but is generally not effective if the intrinsic heart rate is over 60 beats/minute.

e. Underdrive pacing is occasionally effective in terminating recurrent episodes of medically refractory VT but should be utilized only by experienced personnel following invasive electrophysiologic testing.

f. Newly approved drugs including amiodarone, flecainide, mexiletine, and tocainide offer promise in cases refractory to conventional therapy. These newer agents appear to be effective in preventing a recurrence of VT in 25–50% of cases.

g. Various **surgical procedures** have been used effectively in patients with medically refractory VT, especially those with ventricular aneurysms.

C. Variants of VT

1. Accelerated idioventricular rhythm most likely represents enhanced automaticity of an infrajunctional pacemaker (i.e., His-Purkinje system, ventricular myocardium) and occurs usually in the setting of an acute MI or digitalis toxicity. The ventricular rate is generally 60–110 beats/minute. Episodes are generally transient and well tolerated. Degeneration of acclerated idioventricular rhythm to rapid VT or VF is uncommon. **Treatment is not necessary in most cases.** If necessary, the rhythm may be suppressed by increasing the atrial rate with atropine or atrial pacing or by administration of lidocaine, procainamide, quinidine, disopyramide, or bretylium.

2. Torsade de pointes refers to a form of VT characterized by QRS complexes of changing amplitude and morphology that appear to twist around the isoelectric line. It is associated with prolongation of the QT interval, most commonly due to toxic levels of quinidine, disopyramide, or procainamide. Some cases may be congenital or due to hypokalemia or phenothiazine toxicity. **Treatment** consists of stopping the offending agent and, if necessary, overdrive suppression by atrial or ventricular pacing at a rate of 100–120 beats/minute. Isoproterenol can be used cautiously until pacing is initiated. Lidocaine or phenytoin may also be helpful. Quinidine, procainamide, and disopyramide are specifically contraindicated.

D. Disposition. All patients presenting with sustained VT require immediate medical attention and admission to a monitored hospital bed.

XV. Ventricular flutter and fibrillation occur most commonly in patients with severe underlying heart disease but may occasionally be due to drug toxicity, electric shock, or other causes. They are rapidly fatal and account for most cases of sudden death. The mechanism appears to be reentry, which in the case of VF becomes totally disorganized.

A. ECG recognition. Ventricular flutter appears as a continuous sine wave at a rate of 250–300 beats/minute. VF appears as a disorganized irregular oscillation of the baseline without clear QRS complexes. P waves, ST segments, and T waves are generally not distinguishable.

B. Therapy

1. Acute therapy. See Chap. 2.

2. Chronic therapy is similar to that for VT (see sec. **XIV.B.2**).

XVI. Heart block refers to a transient or permanent disturbance in impulse conduction. This discussion will be limited to conduction disturbances in the AV node and His-Purkinje system. Heart block may be due to idiopathic degeneration of the conduction system, encroachment by perivalvular calcification, replacement by granuloma in sarcoidosis, MI, drug toxicity, or a variety of other causes. Acute and chronic therapy is dictated by the clinical state of the patient and the underlying pathology.

A. ECG recognition

1. **First-degree AV block** is characterized by 1:1 AV conduction (with each P wave followed by a QRS complex) with a prolonged PR interval exceeding 0.2 seconds.

2. **Mobitz I (Wenckebach) second-degree AV block** is characterized by progressive PR prolongation until a P wave fails to conduct to the ventricles. Additional ECG findings include the following:

    a. The PR interval of the complex following the pause is shorter than the PR interval of the beat preceding the pause.

    b. The pause is less than twice the RR interval preceding the pause.

    c. Regular group beating occurs if the sinus rhythm is regular.

3. **Mobitz II second-degree AV block** is intermittent sudden failure of conduction, whereby a P wave is not followed by a QRS complex. The PR intervals of conducted beats preceding and following the nonconducted P wave are constant.

4. **Third-degree AV block** is complete failure of AV conduction with no atrial activity transmitted to the ventricle.

B. Therapy and disposition

1. **First-degree AV block** rarely requires treatment acutely. Patients presenting with a history of syncope, presyncope, or intermittent symptoms of diminished cardiac output in whom first-degree AV block is the only abnormality detected should be admitted to a monitored bed, since this abnormality may be associated with more severe disturbances in conduction. Patients without symptoms in whom first-degree AV block is detected incidentally do not require any immediate attention but should be referred for outpatient evaluation directed at determining if significant conduction system disease is present.

2. **Mobitz I (Wenckebach) AV block** rarely requires emergent treatment. Patients with symptoms, however, require hospitalization. On the other hand, patients without symptoms or an obvious precipitating event in whom Mobitz I AV block is discovered incidentally do not require immediate attention and should be referred for outpatient evaluation directed at determining if significant conduction system disease is present.

3. Patients with **Mobitz II AV block** or **third-degree AV block** require hospitalization and monitoring. If these high-grade AV blocks are accompanied by hemodynamic decompensation, atropine or isoproterenol may be useful acutely. Temporary and permanent cardiac pacing are generally required.

XVII. Wolff-Parkinson-White (WPW) syndrome is the most common form of ventricular preexcitation and is due to a bypass tract (Kent bundle) connecting the atria and ventricles. Kent bundles, however, do not demonstrate decremental conduction (i.e., progressive slowing of conduction during faster heart rates) characteristic of normal AV nodal tissue. Patients with the WPW syndrome are susceptible to two types of arrhythmias. First, atrial-ventricular reentrant SVT may occur with anterograde conduction through the normal AV pathway (orthodromic SVT) and retrograde conduction through the Kent bundle; rarely, this reentrant circuit involves anterograde conduction through the Kent bundle with retrograde conduction through the normal AV pathway (antidromic SVT). Second, atrial fibrillation may be associated with a rapid ventricular rate resulting from anterograde conduction through the Kent bundle, with loss of the protective decremental conduction properties of the AV node. In patients with Kent bundles having short refractory periods, ventricular response rates exceeding 300 beats/minute may occur and result in hemodynamic collapse with degeneration to VF. **The concept of concealed Kent bundles is discussed in sec. IX.**

A. ECG recognition

1. During **sinus rhythm** in patients in whom the WPW syndrome is manifest, the surface ECG reflects ventricular fusion resulting from anterograde conduction through the normal AV conduction pathway and the Kent bundle. Each P wave is followed by a QRS complex with a short (i.e., < 0.12 seconds) PR interval. The QRS complex is wide, with a slurred onset known as a delta wave. Secondary ST–T wave changes are present in a direction generally opposite to the major delta and QRS vectors. These patterns may mimic bundle branch block, MI, or ventricular hypertrophy.

2. During **orthodromic SVT,** the QRS complexes are usually normal (unless aber-

rancy or preexisting bundle branch block is present), since anterograde conduction is exclusively through the normal AV conduction system. Each QRS complex is followed by a P wave with a short RP interval, exactly as in patients with SVT due to a CBT (see sec. **IX.A.2.a).** Rarely, patients may have an antidromic SVT, with anterograde conduction through the bypass tract during SVT causing a wide-complex regular tachycardia, with P waves again following the QRS complexes with a short RP interval.

3. **Atrial fibrillation** with anterograde conduction through the bypass tract predominantly appears as a **rapid, irregular wide-complex tachycardia** simulating VT.

B. Therapy

1. **Asymptomatic patients** without SVT in general do not require treatment. However, those patients having an accessory pathway with a short anterograde refractory property are at risk for sudden death due to a rapid ventricular rate during atrial fibrillation and should be managed medically or surgically as described in sec. **XVII.B.3–5.** Assessment of the refractory properties of a Kent bundle usually requires invasive electrophysiologic study.

2. Patients with **recurrent orthodromic SVT** may be treated with drugs that alter AV node conduction (i.e., digitalis, propranolol, or verapamil) or conduction through the Kent bundle (i.e., quinidine, procainamide, disopyramide, or lidocaine). In general, membrane depressant agents are more effective than AV node depressant agents. **AV node depressant agents, however, should not be used empirically** in patients with WPW unless the results of electrophysiologic testing demonstrate that the Kent bundle has a long refractory period.

3. Patients with **atrial fibrillation** and a short anterograde refractory period of their Kent bundle are at risk for a rapid ventricular rate that may degenerate to VF. Digitalis and verapamil may enhance conduction further and should not be used as single agents in patients with WPW unless prior electrophysiologic study has demonstrated a long refractory period for the bypass tract. Procainamide, quinidine, and disopyramide can be used to slow conduction through the accessory pathway.

4. **If a sustained tachyarrhythmia is refractory to drug therapy or if the patient is compromised hemodynamically, cardioversion should be performed.** Some epidoses of SVT refractory to medical management can be managed by underdrive or overdrive pacing.

5. Surgical ablation is an effective therapy that is available at a few centers.

C. Disposition

1. Patients without symptoms in whom WPW is detected incidentally should be referred for outpatient evaluation.

2. Patients with orthodromic SVT should be admitted to the hospital to facilitate optimal medical management.

3. Patients with WPW and a rapid ventricular response to atrial fibrillation require hospitalization.

XVIII. Digitalis-induced arrhythmias can take the form of nearly all known rhythm disturbances, including tachyarrhythmias (generally due to disturbances in automaticity) and bradyarrhythmias (due to heart block). Common forms include sinus exit block and arrest, PAT with block, Mobitz I second-degree AV block, complete heart block, nonparoxysmal junctional tachycardia, and complex ventricular ectopy including VT and VF. Since there are no specific ECG features that are unique to digitalis toxicity, a high index of suspicion must be maintained to allow prompt recognition and therapy.

A. Therapy

1. **Digitalis must be stopped promptly.** Further therapy depends on the clinical state of the patient and the specific arrhythmia.

2. **Supraventricular arrhythmias,** including PAT with block and junctional tachycardia, are usually stable and generally require only **observation. Potassium** supplementation is indicated if serum levels are low and second- or third-degree AV block is not present. When drug therapy is necessary, **phenytoin** is the drug of choice. Lidocaine, verapamil, and cardioversion generally are not effective.

3. **Complex ventricular ectopy** frequently requires therapy.

a. In the absence of AV block, **potassium** should be administered to maintain the serum level in the high normal range.

b. **Lidocaine** is the drug of choice if additional therapy is required.

c. **Phenytoin** may also be effective.

d. **Procainamide** (either IV or PO) can be used if the above agents fail, but AV block may be exacerbated. Disopyramide may also be used, but quinidine causes increased digoxin levels and is relatively contraindicated.

    e. Propranolol is an alternative second-line agent but should not be used if second- or third-degree block is present unless an electronic ventricular pacemaker is in place.

    f. Temporary overdrive suppression is effective occasionally for medically refractory cases. However, there is an increased risk of mechanically induced VT during catheter manipulation in this clinical setting.

    g. For refractory life-threatening cases, **Fab antibody fragment** can be used; this has been associated with excellent results.

    h. Certain measures are relatively contraindicated. As mentioned, **quinidine** will increase serum digoxin levels. **Bretylium** causes an initial release of catecholamines that can be deleterious. **Cardioversion** can precipitate fatal ventricular arrhythmias. Hypokalemia can aggravate digitalis-induced arrhythmias.

  4. Heart block, whether sinoatrial or atrioventricular, requires close observation in a monitored setting. **Atropine,** 0.5–1.0 mg IV, may be used initially if the patient's hemodynamic status is compromised. A **temporary transvenous pacemaker** is indicated if the response to atropine is incomplete or if high-grade (i.e., Mobitz type II or third-degree) AV block is present. **Contraindicated** are potassium (which aggravates AV block) and isoproterenol (which aggravates ventricular ectopy).

  B. Disposition. All patients with digitalis-induced arrhythmias require admission to a monitored hospital bed.

XIX. Sick sinus syndrome (SSS) refers to a spectrum of disorders due to sinus and AV node dysfunction. Patients with SSS manifest bradycardia, a slow ventricular rate during atrial fibrillation, sinus arrest or exit block, or varying degrees of AV nodal block. In addition, some patients have recurrent supraventricular tachyarrhythmias (the tachycardia-bradycardia syndrome) that terminate with long pauses before resumption of sinus rhythm.

  A. Symptoms and signs include palpitations, fatigue, presyncope or syncope, CHF, angina, and pulmonary edema.

  B. The **diagnosis** may be made by ECG or electrophysiologic testing, but prolonged monitoring (either as an inpatient or outpatient) is especially useful not only to document the rhythm disorder but also to correlate symptoms.

  C. Therapy. In general, chronic drug or pacemaker therapy should be instituted only after careful evaluation; failure to do so will often meet with disappointing results.

    1. Asymptomatic patients do not require therapy. The incidence of sudden death as the first manifestation of SSS is extremely low.

    2. Symptoms clearly documented to be due to excessive **bradycardia or prolonged pauses** require implantation of a permanent pacemaker. Acute management, if necessary, consists of administration of atropine or isoproterenol or temporary pacing.

    3. Patients with the **tachycardia-bradycardia** syndrome may require pacemaker placement prior to drug therapy directed at controlling the tachyarrhythmia (which would otherwise aggravate the bradycardia). In general, all antiarrhythmic agents, including digitalis, must be used with extreme caution in patients with the SSS.

  D. Disposition

    1. Patients without symptoms in whom evidence of SSS is observed incidentally should be referred for outpatient evaluation.

    2. Patients with symptomatic SSS require hospitalization, preferably in a monitored bed.

    3. Patients with asymptomatic SSS who require antiarrhythmic drugs for other reasons should be admitted, since such agents may aggravate this disorder.

XX. Carotid sinus hypersensitivity (CSH) is a syndrome of enhanced responsiveness to carotid sinus stimulation. Two subtypes are observed clinically: (1) *cardioinhibitory* hypersensitivity, which is defined as ventricular asystole exceeding 3 seconds in duration during carotid sinus stimulation; and (2) *vasodepressor* hypersensitivity, which is defined as a decrease in systolic blood pressure of at least 50 mm Hg (due to vasodilatation) without associated cardiac slowing, or a decrease in systolic blood pressure exceeding 30 mm Hg associated with reproduction of the patient's clinical symptoms. Some patients have a combination of the two forms. Either subtype may result in presyncope or syncope during such maneuvers as head turning or neck extension or during direct carotid sinus massage. Since many elderly patients satisfy the criteria for CSH but do not have associated symptoms, it is essential to reproduce the clinical symptoms during testing (i.e., carotid sinus massage) prior to initiation of therapy.

A. Therapy

1. **Asymptomatic** patients do not require therapy.
2. Patients with **infrequent and mild symptoms** can often be managed by avoidance of tight collars and rapid neck movements.
3. Therapy for patients with **severe symptoms** depends on the subtype. **Cardioinhibitory CSH** requires implantation of a permanent ventricular pacemaker. **Vasodepressor CSH** is much more difficult to treat, and severe cases may require radiation therapy or surgical denervation of the carotid sinus. Atropine will abolish acutely the bradycardia response but not prevent vasodilatation.
4. Drugs including digitalis, propranolol, alpha methyldopa, and clonidine may enhance CSH and be responsible for symptoms in some patients; these drugs should be avoided if possible.

B. Disposition. Symptomatic patients require hospitalization.

XXI. Pacemaker failure can take the form of an altered paced rate, failure to pace (due to failure to deliver a stimulus or failure to capture), or failure to sense intrinsic activity. The result can be pacemaker-induced tachycardia or more commonly bradycardia. The most common cause of failure to sense or capture is lead dislodgement or myocardial perforation; but a variety of other causes may be at fault, including lead fracture, pulse generator component failure, increased stimulation threshold due to fibrosis or electrolyte imbalance, or inappropriate programming in parameters of sensitivity or stimulus strength. The most common cause of slowing of the pacemaker rate is battery failure, although oversensing of T waves or extracardiac potentials may be responsible. The diagnosis and management of pacemaker malfunction requires an intimate knowledge of the individual pacemaker model and programmable functions.

A. Evaluation of apparent pacemaker failure should include a check of the pacemaker rate, with or without conversion to the fixed-rate nonsensing (V00) mode by application of a magnet to the pulse generator; evaluation of the ECG for an altered QRS axis or morphology (compared to a prior tracing), which might indicate lead dislodgement or failure to sense and capture appropriately; and careful inspection of a chest x-ray to look for lead fracture, dislodgement, or myocardial perforation. The pacemaker can be interrogated noninvasively or reprogrammed to check the sensitivity and stimulus specifications using special equipment. Experienced personnel are often required for final analysis and therapeutic recommendations.

B. The disposition will depend on both the apparent problem and the underlying disease that initially dictated pacemaker placement. If pacemaker malfunction is suspected or, when identified, cannot be rectified easily by reprogramming, the patient should be admitted to a monitored hospital bed.

Bibliography

1. Chou, T. C. *Electrocardiography in Clinical Practice.* New York: Grune & Stratton, 1979.
2. Chung, E. K. Appraisal of multifocal atrial tachycardia. *Br. Heart J.* 33:500, 1971.
3. Josephson, M. E., and Seides, S. F. *Clinical Cardiac Electrophysiology: Techniques and Interpretations.* Philadelphia: Lea & Febiger, 1979.
4. Mancini, G. B., and Goldberger, A. T. Cardioversion of atrial fibrillation: Consideration of embolization, anticoagulation, prophylactic pacemaker, and long-term success. *Am. Heart J.* 104:617, 1982.
5. Smith, W. M., and Gallagher, J. J. "Les Torsade de Pointes": An unusual ventricular arrhythmia. *Ann. Intern. Med.* 93:578, 1980.
6. Wellens, H. J., Bar, F. W., and Lie, K. I. The value of the electrocardiogram in the differential diagnosis of a tachycardia with a widened QRS complex. *Am. J. Med.* 64:27, 1978.
7. Zipes, D. P. Management of Cardiac Arrhythmias: Pharmacological, Electrical, and Surgical Techniques, and Specific Arrhythmias: Diagnosis and Treatment. In E. Braunwald (ed.), *Heart Disease* (2nd ed.). Philadelphia: Saunders, 1984.

Myocardial, Pericardial, and Valvular Disorders

Bruce D. Lindsay and
Allan S. Jaffe

Chest Pain

I. **Evaluation.** A brief history, physical examination, and electrocardiogram provide the basis for managing patients who present with chest pain. Medical records may improve diagnostic accuracy, but the evaluation, treatment, and disposition should not be delayed if they are not readily available.
   A. **History.** A concise history is most important. Assessment of chest pain should characterize its quality, location, pattern of radiation, duration, precipitating factors, and the means by which relief is obtained. It is important also to establish whether the pain has occurred previously and if its frequency or severity has changed. Risk factors for heart disease should be identified.
   B. **Physical examination.** A brief but careful physical examination should be performed promptly, since findings associated with myocardial ischemia may be transient. The general appearance of the patient provides a useful gauge of the severity of the illness. An ashen complexion, diaphoresis, dyspnea, agitation, or impaired mentation may be associated with a variety of serious causes of chest pain. Vital signs are the most immediate objective indication of the patient's condition. Careful examination of the lungs, heart, abdomen, and peripheral pulses is also mandatory.
   C. **Diagnostic studies**
      1. **Electrocardiogram (ECG).** An ECG should be performed in any patient having an arrhythmia, heart failure, or symptoms suggestive of angina, myocardial infarction, or pericarditis. It should be repeated to look for changes as soon as the chest pain resolves.
      2. **Radiographic studies.** A chest x-ray is most useful in the diagnosis of pulmonary diseases; it is also helpful in assessing the presence and severity of heart failure. However, the disposition of a critically ill patient should not be delayed to obtain a chest x-ray in the emergency department. Patients with musculoskeletal pain may require x-rays of the area in question.
      3. **Arterial blood gas (ABG).** An ABG should be obtained in patients who manifest respiratory distress or are suspected of having a pulmonary embolus or myocardial ischemia (i.e., chest pain or ECG changes) unless the administration of thrombolytic therapy is anticipated. Endotracheal intubation should not be delayed to await the results of an ABG in the presence of overt respiratory failure.
II. **Differential diagnosis of chest pain.** Part of the difficulty in evaluating patients with chest discomfort is due to the overlapping distribution of visceral pain fibers in the cervical spinal cord. Thus, myocardial pain may be perceived as radiating to the neck or inner aspects of the arms. Other visceral pains may do the same and mimic the pain of myocardial ischemia. Table 5-1 lists the major differential diagnoses of episodic chest pain. In most instances, a brief but careful history, physical examination, and ECG will provide the data needed for appropriate management.
   A. **Angina** (see **Myocardial Disorders,** sec. I). Many patients with angina deny pain and refer to chest discomfort as a substernal heaviness or squeezing sensation precipitated by exertion. It may radiate over the precordium, to the inner aspects of either arm, or to the shoulders, neck, or jaw. Angina typically lasts 2–10 minutes and frequently is accompanied by nausea, diaphoresis, or dyspnea. An S4 gallop is usually appreciated. The systolic murmur of papillary muscle dysfunction may occur concomitantly. Associated findings also may include arrhythmias, congestive heart failure (CHF), and hypotension or hypertension. An appropriately timed ECG usually demonstrates transient ST-segment or T-wave abnormalities.
   B. **Myocardial infarction** (see **Myocardial Disorders,** sec. II). The characteristic discomfort of myocardial infarction (MI) is similar to that of angina but tends to be

Table 5-1. Differential diagnosis of chest pain—typical features

Etiology	Duration	Quality	Location/radiation	Factors that provoke	Relief of pain
Angina	2–15 min	Pressure	Precordium, neck, shoulders, arms	Exertion, stress, cold	Rest, TNG
Variant angina	2–15 min	Pressure	Precordium, neck, shoulders, arms	Sleep, cold	Rest, TNG, calcium blockers
Myocardial infarction	>20 min	Pressure	Precordium, neck, shoulders, arms	Exertion, stress; however, may occur at rest	Morphine
Aortic dissection	Constant	Severe, aching, tearing	Precordium, neck, back	Hypertension, exertion	Morphine and treatment of dissection
Pericarditis	Minutes to hours	Aching, pleuritic	Precordium, trapezium	Inspiration, supine position	Upright position, aspirin
Pleuritis	Minutes to hours	Sharp	Localized chest	Inspiration, coughing	Analgesics, aspirin
Pulmonary embolism	Minutes to hours	Aching, pleuritic	Localized chest	Inspiration, coughing	Analgesics
Esophageal	Minutes to hours	Aching, burning	Precordium, throat	Eating, bending	Antacids, TNG, sitting-up
Musculoskeletal	Variable	Aching, sharp	Focal	Movement or pressure	Rest, analgesics
Anxiety	Variable	Dull ache, sharp	Anterior chest below left breast	Stress	Sedation, time, reassurance
Mitral valve prolapse	Variable	Aching, sharp	Anterior chest	None	Time, reassurance

Key: TNG = sublingual nitroglycerin.

more severe. It most often begins at rest and lasts more than 20 minutes; however, more severe and longer episodes do not distinguish infarction from unstable angina in all instances. The physical findings associated with angina (see sec. **II.A**) tend to be more pronounced with infarction. Hypotension, tachycardia, and CHF are adverse prognostic signs. The initial ECG may demonstrate characteristic ST-segment elevation; however, the ST-segment and T-wave changes of small MIs may be nonspecific, or the ECG may be normal.

C. **Aortic dissection** (see **Aortic Dissection**). Patients with dissection of the aorta present with pain that is severe, is sudden in onset, and frequently radiates to the back (especially to the left scapular area). Patients may be agitated, since the pain frequently has a tearing quality and may radiate widely, mimicking other chest pain syndromes. Nausea, diaphoresis, and light-headedness are common. Hypertension usually is present, as it is an important cause of dissection. Hypotension suggests rupture or cardiac tamponade. Other physical findings characteristically are transient and include pulse deficits, aortic regurgitation, and nervous system dysfunction (central or peripheral). The chest x-ray may show widening of mediastinum but is often nondiagnostic. The definitive diagnostic study is aortic angiography.

D. **Pericarditis** (see **Pericardial Disease**, sec. **I**). The pain associated with pericarditis generally is retrosternal and may radiate to the left precordium, neck, or trapezius ridge. It may be dull or sharp and may be worse with deep inspiration or recumbency. Relief is obtained at times by sitting up and leaning forward. Pericardial friction rubs are often evanescent. Rubs have a scratchy quality and classically have three components: one during atrial contraction (present in about 70% of cases), one during ventricular systole (always present), and one during early diastole due to rapid ventricular filling (difficult to hear). Rubs generally are heard best along the left sternal border with the patient leaning forward during held expiration or inspiration. Pericardial rubs can mimic the auscultatory finding of many other disease entities.

E. **Pleuritis** is an inflammation of the pleura and is manifested as a sharp stabbing pain. It is generally localized and aggravated by deep inspirations, coughing, or a change of position. It may be associated with pericarditis, viral infection, pneumonia, or pulmonary emboli. Pneumonia may present with few physical findings; however, rales, rhonchi, diminished breath sounds, or bronchial breathing suggests consolidation. In some instances, a pleural effusion or empyema may develop. A spontaneous pneumothorax also may cause pleuritic chest pain. The pain characteristically is sudden in onset, and the physical examination may reveal ipsilateral loss of breath sounds and hyperresonance to percussion.

F. **Pulmonary embolism** (see Chap. 7) is a difficult bedside diagnosis. The most common symptoms are dyspnea and pleuritic chest pain. Anxiety, cough, hemoptysis, or syncope may occur. Tachypnea, tachycardia, rales, and less frequently an increased pulmonic component to S2 may be observed. In the absence of pulmonary infarction, the chest x-ray may show oligemia distal to the affected vessel, enlargement of a pulmonary artery, right ventricular enlargement, or loss of lung volume. Signs of parenchymal consolidation are associated with pulmonary infarction. A variety of ECG abnormalities may occur, including nonspecific ST-segment and T-wave changes and arrhythmias.

G. **Musculoskeletal disease.** Musculoskeletal pain generally has a sharp or aching quality. Usually, point tenderness is present, and movement evokes or exacerbates the pain. The thoracic outlet syndrome (see Chap. 25) may present with chest, shoulder, or arm pain. Compression of the nerves to the arm and upper chest by cervical ribs, the scalenus anticus muscle, or anomalous ligaments may cause aching and paresthesis along the inner aspect of the arm to the hand in response to specific arm positions. Peripheral sensory or motor deficits may not occur unless nerve compression is of long duration. The pain of cervical spine disease (see Chap. 25) may radiate to the shoulders, arms, or upper chest and is typically exacerbated by movement of the neck.

H. **Esophageal disease** (see Chap. 10). Reflux esophagitis has a burning quality, often referred to as heartburn. The discomfort may be epigastric or substernal, worse after a large meal, or aggravated by bending or lying. The reflux of acid may cause a sour taste. Food or antacids may provide relief. The diagnosis is clinical but can be confirmed by esophagoscopy or an upper gastrointestinal (GI) series. Esophageal spasm is typically precipitated by swallowing and aggravated by hot or cold liquids. Although esophageal spasm is not caused by exertion, the quality of the pain may mimic angina and respond to nitroglycerin. Changes in blood pressure, heart rate, and ST segments or T waves can occur. If the symptoms are suggestive of angina, it is best to assume the cause is coronary artery disease until a definitive diagnosis is reached.

I. **Anxiety.** Anxious patients may complain of sharp or vague dull precordial chest discomfort that is of variable duration. Frequently the discomfort is localized beneath the left breast. Associated symptoms are common, especially paresthesias due to hyperventilation. Tension is a common exacerbant, but the discomfort is uncommon during exertion.

J. **Mitral valve prolapse.** Although the cause is unknown, mitral valve prolapse is frequently associated with chest pain. The pain may resemble angina or be atypical. Mitral valve prolapse may be used to explain atypical pain in young patients; however, in older patients, ischemic heart disease and mitral valve prolapse may coexist. In general, the presence or absence of mitral valve prolapse should not affect the disposition.

III. **Disposition.** Patients who are critically ill should be transported expeditiously to an intensive care unit. Such patients include those with a high likelihood of acute MI, unstable angina, aortic dissection, or pulmonary embolus. Complications associated with these conditions (e.g., CHF, hypotension, or rhythm disturbances) need not be present. New-onset angina does not mandate hospitalization unless it is precipitated by mild exertion or has an unstable pattern.

When chest pain is atypical for angina, serial physical examinations and ECGs are helpful. A new S4 or S3 gallop or labile ST-segment or T-wave abnormalities suggest ischemia. The presence of multiple risk factors for coronary artery disease is evidence in favor of ischemic chest discomfort. If it appears that the pain is of cardiac origin, then admission for diagnosis is generally warranted; however, for some patients who are stable, an outpatient evaluation can be arranged.

Myocardial Disorders

I. **Angina**

A. **Pathophysiology**

1. **Ischemia** (the most frequent manifestation of which is angina) results when there are **imbalances between myocardial oxygen demand and oxygen delivery** (i.e., coronary blood flow).

   a. **Coronary blood flow** is determined by coronary artery perfusion pressure, heart rate, coronary artery size, wall stress, and metabolic and autonomic regulatory factors. In normal people, coronary flow is maintained as long as the mean blood pressure (BP) ([systolic BP + (2 × diastolic BP)] ÷ 3) is 70 mm Hg. An increase in heart rate shortens diastole, reducing coronary blood flow while increasing oxygen demand. High wall stress inhibits flow to the subendocardium. A reduction in the cross-sectional area of the coronary artery makes autoregulation more difficult, in which case coronary flow can only be maintained at rest by dilation of the distal coronary vessels.

   Patients with ischemia may have both a limitation to flow due to atherosclerotic obstruction and dynamic changes in coronary tone that limit increase in oxygen delivery. A small number (approximately 4%) of patients have coronary artery spasm in the absence of fixed obstructive disease.

   b. **Myocardial oxygen consumption** depends on heart rate, wall tension, volume work, and inotropic state. Clinically, these factors are related to heart rate, blood pressure, and stroke volume. Hypertension, tachycardia, and circumstances that demand a high cardiac output (e.g., exercise) increase oxygen consumption.

2. **Ischemia may impair systolic and diastolic ventricular function,** leading to reduced cardiac output and pulmonary venous congestion. The attendant reduction in oxygenation and increase in wall stress further exacerbate ischemia. Ischemia may also predispose to supraventricular or ventricular arrhythmias with further compromise of ventricular performance and worsening of ischemia.

B. **Clinical features**

1. **History**

   a. **Characteristic features.** Myocardial ischemia commonly results in substernal heaviness, pressure, or a squeezing sensation; less often, it may cause epigastric burning or a gaseous feeling. It may radiate across the chest to the shoulders, neck, jaw, or inner aspect of either arm. Typically angina lasts 2–10 minutes, abating with rest or in response to nitroglycerin. Longer episodes may represent infarction. Pain lasting only a few seconds generally is not angina. Angina frequently is accompanied by nausea, diaphoresis, and dyspnea. Arrhythmias may be induced by ischemia or may be a precipitant. The patient should be asked about changes in the frequency, severity, and duration of anginal episodes. The number of sublingual nitroglycerin required to relieve angina acutely and the number of nitroglycerin consumed weekly should be determined.

  b. **Precipitating factors.** Angina pectoris usually is precipitated by physical exertion (e.g., walking up an incline or upper extremity exercise) or emotional stress. Angina also may occur with less exertion following a meal or exposure to cold weather. The physician should inquire about the patient's life-style and the events leading to the emergency department visit to identify possible exacerbants of discomfort.

  c. The presence of **risk factors** for coronary artery disease reinforce the suspicion of angina in a patient with atypical chest pain. Major risk factors include hypertension, diabetes mellitus, hyperlipidemia, a family history of coronary artery disease before age 55, and smoking. Patients with a history of hypertension or diabetes may present with less typical symptoms.

  2. **Physical examination**

    a. **General appearance.** Patients with severe angina or infarction tend to be ashen, diaphoretic, and dyspneic and may hold a clenched fist over the precordium. They usually are relatively still in contrast to patients with a dissecting aortic aneurysm, who frequently are agitated.

    b. The **vital signs** are the most immediate indications of a patient's condition. They must be obtained and recorded promptly, as they are prone to sudden change. Tachycardia may be due to discomfort, an arrhythmia, CHF, hypoxia, or any combination of these. Transient bradycardia may occur with angina or infarction and usually is vagally mediated. Hypotension may be associated with brady- or tachyarrhythmias or excessive use of antianginal agents. Hypertension may precipitate ischemia, or it may be a concomitant. The respiratory rate may be elevated by anxiety, but in general, tachypnea suggests serious cardiopulmonary compromise.

    c. **A properly timed cardiac examination** should reveal signs compatible with ischemia. An S4 gallop reflects the need for an augmented atrial contraction to fill a stiff ventricle and is a very common finding. Transient systolic murmurs may be indicative of papillary muscle dysfunction. The murmurs of aortic valvular disease or hypertrophic cardiomyopathy may provide clues to alternative etiologies for ischemia (i.e., other than coronary artery disease). It is important to evalulate the patient closely for signs of CHF (e.g., an S3 gallop, internal jugular vein distention, and rales).

    d. **Examination of the peripheral and retinal blood vessels** provides indirect information about disease affecting the coronary arteries. Atherosclerotic and hypertensive retinal changes frequently coexist and include narrowing of the arteriolar lumen, tortuosity of vessels, and arteriolar venous compression. Diseased peripheral arteries result in diminished or absent pulses.

C. Classification. Angina may be categorized as chronic stable angina, new-onset angina, unstable angina, or variant angina. Patients with chronic stable angina have little change in the frequency or severity of their angina or in their exercise tolerance. New-onset angina generally indicates the onset of symptoms within about 4 weeks of evaluation. Patients with unstable angina are those having angina of increased severity or duration, a recent decrease in exercise tolerance, angina at rest, or new-onset angina precipitated by minimal exertion.

D. Diagnostic studies

  1. **Electrocardiograms** must be performed promptly because the changes of ischemia are transient. In the absence of a previous ECG, all abnormalities should be considered acute. Characteristic changes indicative of ischemia are ST-segment depression and T-wave flattening or inversion. ST-segment elevation suggests transmural injury, as observed with coronary vasospasm or infarction. Ischemic abnormalities tend to resolve, whereas those associated with infarction persist. Thus, it is helpful to compare the tracing during pain with one obtained after relief of pain. Patients with prolonged ongoing chest pain are more likely to have distinct ECG abnormalities; however, a normal ECG does not exclude coronary artery disease.

  2. **Exercise testing** is useful for the diagnosis of coronary artery disease and

Table 5-2. Mechanisms by which antianginal agents prevent ischemia

Drug	Coronary vasodilation	Oxygen demand		
		Heart rate	Left ventricular volume	Impedance
Nitrates	↑	↑	↓ ↓ ↓	↓
β-adrenergic blockers	—	↓ ↓ ↓	↑	— or ↑
Nifedipine	↑ ↑ ↑	↑	↓ ↓	↓ ↓ ↓
Verapamil	↑ ↑	↓	↑	↓ ↓
Diltiazem	↑ ↑ ↑	↓ ↓	—	↓

Key: — = no effect, ↑ = increase, ↓ = decrease; magnitude of effect (i.e., mild, moderate, marked) is given by the number of arrows.

assessment of exercise capacity. The standard treadmill test is used most commonly. Exercise testing in combination with radionuclide imaging techniques may improve sensitivity and specificity but at a substantial increase in cost. Contraindications to exercise testing are unstable angina, CHF, aortic stenosis, hypertrophic cardiomyopathy, uncontrolled hypertension, uncontrolled arrhythmias, second- or third-degree AV block, and any major systemic illness that interferes with exercise. Radionuclide studies are particularly useful in evaluating patients with baseline ECG abnormalities (e.g., left bundle branch block) that preclude interpretation of ST-segment changes with exercise. It is preferable that digoxin be discontinued days prior to exercise testing, because it can induce ST-segment abnormalities and interfere with interpretation of the test. The referring physician should discontinue antianginal agents 24 hours prior to the test if possible because they may cause false-negative results.

3. **Cardiac catheterization** may be indicated to evaluate atypical chest pain, to define the severity of coronary artery disease, or to identify acquired or congenital lesions that may be corrected surgically.

E. **Pharmacologic therapy of angina.** Pharmacologic agents for the treatment of angina attempt to improve oxygen delivery or reduce oxygen demand (Table 5-2). If angina does not respond to maximal doses of a single agent, a second drug should be added; however, it is best to avoid combining agents with similar pharmacologic actions or shared adverse effects.

1. **Nitrates** relieve ischemia primarily by inducing venous pooling with a resultant reduction in ventricular volume and thus wall stress. A minor reduction in peripheral impedance and coronary vasodilating effects also play a role. Nitrates are the drugs of first choice for the treatment of ischemia.

a. **Sublingual nitroglycerin** (TNG) may be taken prophylactically or used for relief acutely; the available dosages are 0.3, 0.4, and 0.6 mg. The onset of action is 2 minutes with sustained benefit for 15–30 minutes. The recommended dosage is 0.4 mg every 5 minutes while pain lasts. If there is no relief after 3 tablets, the patient should be taken to an emergency facility. Adverse effects are headache, flushing, hypotension, and reflex tachycardia. Patients should sit when taking TNG to avoid these effects. An initial test dose should be administered under supervision to assess tolerance. If stored in airtight amber bottles, TNG has a shelf life of 6 months.

b. **Long-acting nitrates** undergo variable GI absorption and rapid hepatic metabolism. Nonetheless, prolonged hemodynamic and antianginal effects occur. Topical preparations avoid first-pass hepatic metabolism, but absorption through the skin is variable. The use of long-acting nitrates is prophylactic.

2. **Beta-adrenergic blocking agents** reduce oxygen demand predominantly by slowing the heart rate; they also reduce myocardial contractility. Their effects are most pronounced during periods of exercise when adrenergic tone is greatest. Beta-1 "selective" agents (e.g., metaprolol) at low dosages reduce the propensity to bronchospasm, peripheral vasoconstriction, and hypoglycemia. Agents with intrinsic sympathomimetic activity (e.g., pindolol) preserve resting heart rate and dilate rather than constrict peripheral vessels at rest; otherwise, they have similar effects to other beta-adrenergic blockers. Beta-adrenergic blockers should be gradually titrated to attain a resting heart rate of 50–60

Table 5-3. In vivo effects of calcium channel blockers

Drug	Net ventricular performance	Sinus rate	AV node conduction	Peripheral vasodilation	Coronary vasodilation
Nifedipine	↑	↑		↑ ↑ ↑	↑ ↑ ↑
Verapamil	↓	↓	↓ ↓	↑ ↑	↑ ↑
Diltiazem	—	↓ ↓	↓	↑	↑ ↑ ↑

Key: — = no effect, ↑ = increase, ↓ = decrease; magnitude of effect (i.e., mild, moderate, marked) is given by the number of arrows.

beats/minute with an increase of less than 30 beats/minute with exertion. Acutely, intravenous (IV) agents can be used to treat selected supraventricular tachycardias, relieve ischemic chest pain, or limit infarct size. The dosage of IV propranolol is 1 mg given over 1 minute and repeated q5 minutes to a maximum dosage of 0.15 mg/kg. Alternatively, 5 mg of metoprolol may be given IV and the dose repeated q5 minutes to a maximum dosage of 15 mg. Adverse effects include bronchospasm, heart failure, fatigue, peripheral vasoconstriction, diarrhea, and hypoglycemia in insulin-dependent diabetics.

3. **Calcium channel blockers** (Table 5-3) exert their effects through complex cellular interactions, some of which involve calcium. All are vasodilators and are effective in the treatment of angina, especially variant angina.

   a. **Nifedipine** is a potent peripheral and coronary vasodilator. It reduces impedance, improving ventricular performance, and dilates the coronary bed, improving coronary blood flow. A starting dosage of 10 mg PO tid is titrated according to blood pressure and clinical response. In acute situations, the drug can be given sublingually. Adverse effects include headache, dizziness, flushing, and peripheral edema. In addition, nifedipine may exacerbate angina if reflex tachycardia or blood pressure reduction is marked. It is especially effective in combination with beta-adrenergic blockers.

   b. **Verapamil** also is a potent vasodilator. It slows the heart rate and atrioventricular (AV) node conduction and reduces myocardial contractility. It is contraindicated in patients with marked sinus bradycardia, sick sinus syndrome, or AV conduction delay, and it may exacerbate CHF in some patients. Since the hemodynamic and electrophysiologic effects of verapamil are similar to those of beta-adrenergic blockers, it should be used cautiously in concert with these agents. The dosage of verapamil is 80–160 mg PO tid. It can cause constipation, especially at high dosages in older patients.

   c. **Diltiazem** is a potent coronary dilator but has less peripheral vasodilating effects. It slows the heart rate but produces little depression of myocardial contractility. It should be avoided in patients with sinus bradycardia, sick sinus syndrome, or impaired AV node conduction. The dosage of diltiazem is 30–90 mg qid. Since it has similar effects, diltiazem manifests less therapeutic synergism with beta-adrenergic blockers than with other agents. It can be substituted in appropriate patients as first-line therapy. Adverse effects are less frequent with this agent than with other calcium channel blockers.

F. **Initial management**
   1. **Chronic stable angina**
      a. **Diagnostic studies.** Exercise testing is generally performed to assess the patient's exercise capacity and to confirm the diagnosis. Hypotension or marked ST-segment depression early in the course of exercise is indicative of severe coronary disease.
      b. **Management.** Chronic stable angina that occurs infrequently may be treated adequately with sublingual nitroglycerin as needed. Prophylactic agents are useful in the treatment of stable angina that occurs more frequently with mild to moderate exertion; nitrates, beta-adrenergic blockers, or calcium blockers can be used as first-line agents. Outpatient management is appropriate.
   2. **New-onset angina**
      a. **Diagnostic studies.** New-onset angina that only occurs with moderate to heavy exertion may be assessed with exercise testing. If angina occurs at rest or with mild exertion, exercise testing is contraindicated, and cardiac catheterization should be considered.

b. Management. New-onset angina that occurs at rest or with mild exertion is treated as unstable angina (see sec. **I.F.3.b**). Angina that occurs only with moderate to heavy exertion may be treated the same as stable angina (see sec. **I.F.1.b**). The patient should be admitted for observation if the pattern of angina is not clear.

3. **Unstable angina**
   a. **Diagnostic studies.** Exercise testing is contraindicated. Cardiac catheterization is recommended if the patient is a surgical candidate.
   b. **Management.** Admission to an intensive care unit is warranted. A combination of at least two antianginal agents should be used. Beta-adrenergic blockade is the mainstay of therapy. Intravenous nitroglycerin may be particularly useful for the acute management of frequent severe angina episodes. Coronary artery bypass grafting should be considered in all such patients, since many have severe disease, including left main coronary involvement in up to 20%.

4. **Variant angina**
   a. **Diagnostic studies.** The diagnosis is confirmed by an ECG demonstrating ST-segment elevation during pain. Holter monitoring may be helpful in documenting ST-segment elevation, since asymptomatic episodes of ST-segment elevation are common. Exercise testing is characteristically normal. In the absence of concomitant severe obstructive coronary artery disease, ergonovine may be administered during cardiac catheterization to promote coronary artery spasm. Ergonovine testing is potentially dangerous and should not be performed in the emergency department.
   b. **Management.** Admission to the hospital generally is advised. Nitrates and calcium channel blockers, used alone or in combination, are the agents of choice. Coronary artery bypass grafting is not of benefit in the absence of significant fixed obstructive coronary disease.

II. **Acute myocardial infarction (AMI)**
   A. **Pathophysiology.** Most acute transmural infarctions occur when thrombosis is superimposed on an obstructing coronary atheroma. The events leading to thrombosis are incompletely defined but appear to involve intimal defects, mediators of coagulation, and perhaps vasospasm. The incidence and course of spontaneous clot lysis is unknown. Some "nontransmural" infarctions occur in the absence of total coronary occlusion, presumably due to an imbalance between oxygen supply and demand. The immediate consequences of MI result in changes in cellular electrophysiology, ventricular compliance, and contractility.
   1. **Alterations in the electrical properties of cells** in the ischemic region may lead to electrophysiologic inhomogeneity, providing a substrate for ventricular tachycardia and fibrillation, which occur most frequently during the first 20–30 minutes of infarction. Reperfusion may transiently accentuate electrophysiologic abnormalities and exacerbate ventricular arrhythmias.
   2. **The mechanical effects of ischemia** are increased ventricular stiffness and loss of myocardial fiber shortening, followed by passive systolic lengthening and an increased end-diastolic fiber length. The contractile abnormalities progress sequentially from dyssynchrony to hypokinesis to akinesis and frequently to dyskinesis in the completed infarction. Changes in global left ventricular function are dependent on the site and extent of the damaged area. CHF is due to shifts in the left ventricular end-diastolic pressure-volume curve (increased stiffness) and the loss of myocardial cells. This usually becomes clinically apparent after 20% of the left ventricle is infarcted, and cardiogenic shock ensues when more than 40% of the left ventricle is irreversibly compromised. Scar formation begins during the first week after infarction but requires 2–3 months to be completed. Rupture of the free wall of the left ventricle occurs in about 10% of patients who die in the hospital and generally involves the anterior or lateral wall. Such patients usually are older, hypertensive, and female and have infarction as the initial manifestation of ischemic heart disease. The formation of an aneurysm may occur with stretching of akinetic infarcted tissue. This complication develops in 12–15% of infarctions and most commonly involves the apex of the left ventricle. Left ventricular aneurysms rarely rupture, but enlargement and paradoxical systolic bulging may reduce cardiac output and precipitate heart failure. In addition, the margins of an aneurysm frequently provide the substrate for arrhythmias.
   3. **Myocardial salvage.** The survival and prognosis of patients who reach the

Table 5-4. Drug dosages for acute relief of pain during angina

Drug	Route	Dosage	Comment
Nitroglycerin	SL	0.3–0.4 mg	Repeat q5min prn.
	IV	Start infusion at 10 μg/min	Increase infusion 5–10 μg/min q5min to desired effect. Monitor BP
Nifedipine	SL	10 mg	Chew capsule, or extract contents with a syringe and swish in mouth or place under tongue. Monitor BP.
Propranolol	IV	1 mg over 1 min; repeat q5 min to a maximum dosage of 0.15 mg/kg	Titrate to heart rate of 60 beats/min or systolic pressure of 110 mm Hg.
Metoprolol	IV	1 mg/min; maximum cumulative dose of 15 mg	Titrate to heart rate of 60 beats/min or systolic pressure of 110 mm Hg.
Morphine	IV	2–4 mg q10min prn	Repeat until pain is controlled. Monitor respirations and BP.
Meperidine	IV	25–50 mg q10min prn	Repeat until pain is controlled. Monitor respirations and BP.

hospital is determined primarily by the amount of myocardium that is damaged. This is a function of myocardial oxygen demand and the extent and magnitude of the reduction in coronary flow. In some patients, thrombosis may impair flow to a large area of myocardium, whereas in others, either a smaller area may be compromised or the area may be maintained by collateral reperfusion. Either spontaneous or pharmacologic reperfusion may salvage ischemic tissue. Experimental data indicate that early reperfusion salvages more tissue. In the clinical setting, the precise time of coronary occlusion and the extent of collaterol flow are unknown; thus, the time constraints for myocardial salvage are less accurately defined. However, it appears that attempts to limit the initial extent of infarction with beta-blockers, nitrates, or thrombolysis should be confined to patients whose infarctions are less than 4 hours from onset.

- **B. Clinical features.** The history and physical examination of patients with AMI are similar to those of angina except that the symptoms have a longer duration and the physical findings usually are more pronounced. AMI occurs most frequently when patients are at rest, and many (25% or more) do not have a history of angina. Elderly, diabetic, and hypertensive patients are apt to present atypically, for instance with CHF, weakness, nausea, or systemic symptoms rather than with typical chest discomfort. In addition, it can be difficult to distinguish acute GI illness and unstable angina from MI.
- **C. Initial management.** Prompt admission to a coronary care unit (CCU) is indicated if there is suspicion of infarction because mortality is greatest in the early hours of AMI.
  - 1. A **large IV** should be inserted to assure good venous access.
  - 2. **Electrocardiographic monitoring** should be initiated at once.
  - 3. **Supplemental oxygen** should be administered at a rate of 2–4 liters/minute through a nasal cannula.
  - 4. **Analgesia** (Table 5-4). Morphine sulfate is the agent of choice and should be administered in 2- to 4-mg doses until pain is controlled, provided signs of toxicity do not occur. Hypotension, depression of respirations, nausea, and vomiting may limit the use of morphine in an occasional patient. Intravenous beta-adrenergic blockers and nitrates are reserved for refractory patients. Thus, their use as analgesic agents is rarely necessary in the emergency department.
  - 5. **Antiarrhythmia prophylaxis.** The prophylactic use of lidocaine generally is recommended. A common regimen is a bolus of 1 mg/kg given IV over 2 minutes followed by a continuous infusion; a second bolus of 0.5 mg/kg is given 10 minutes later. A reasonable maintenance infusion rate is 50 μg/kg/minute.

This should be reduced to 20 μg/kg/minute in patients with CHF, with liver disease, or greater than 70 years of age. Many drugs (e.g., propranolol, cimetidine) delay the clearance of lidocaine; thus the use of such agents mandates cautious adjustment of the lidocaine infusion rate. Toxicity includes somnolence, seizures, tremulousness, nausea, and vomiting. When available, blood levels are helpful.

D. Diagnostic studies. In most instances, initial diagnostic studies should be limited to an ECG and blood gases. No delay should be engendered waiting for diagnostic studies.

1. **Electrocardiogram.** An ECG is performed to diagnose the presence of ischemia and to exclude rhythm and conduction abnormalities. The initial ECG is diagnostic in 50–60% of patients. Serial ECGs increase the accuracy to 85–90%. Convex ST-segment elevation is classic for acute infarction; however, this pattern may not be present initially. The ECG changes of a nontransmural infarction are ST-segment depression and T-wave inversion. These ECG criteria usually reflect the general location of the injury but do not accurately define the pathologic extent (transmural versus nontransmural) of necrosis. ST-segment elevation involving the inferior or precordial leads suggests involvement of the inferior or anterior regions of the left ventricle, respectively. ST-segment depression and an R:S ratio greater than 1.0 in V_1 and V_2 suggest posterior infarction, a frequent concomitant of inferior MI. Right ventricular involvement is suggested by ST-segment elevation in V_{4r}. Right bundle branch block (RBBB) does not alter identification of Q waves, but left bundle branch block (LBBB) does. Although Q waves in leads I, aVL, V_5, or V_6 suggest infarction in patients with LBBB, enzyme markers are required for a definitive diagnosis.

2. **Arterial blood gas.** An ABG is recommended to guide oxygen therapy unless thrombolytic therapy is anticipated. In this circumstance, the ABG should be deferred unless essential to management.

3. **Creatine kinase (CK).** In the absence of reperfusion, plasma total CK and the MB fraction rise within 6–8 hours of the onset of infarction, peak at about 24 hours, and remain elevated for 2–3 days. Elevation of the MB fraction is highly specific and sensitive for AMI. Serial levels (q6–12h) are essential since MB-CK determinations may be normal early after infarction. Thus, a normal MB-CK level cannot be used to aid initial disposition.

E. Complications of AMI

1. **Arrhythmias**

   a. **Sinus bradycardia.** Inferior AMIs often cause vagal stimulation and sinus bradycardia, junctional escape rhythms, or varying degrees of AV block, especially during the first 6 hours of infarction. Hypotension, symptoms of hypoperfusion, and increased ventricular ectopy occur more commonly when the ventricular rate is less than 50 beats/minute. Symptomatic bradycardia should be treated with an IV bolus of 0.5–1.0 mg of atropine. A paradoxical response, however, may be seen with doses lower than 0.5 mg. Atropine may be repeated at 5-minute intervals. In general, 2 mg of atropine provides total vagal blockade. Higher doses must be used cautiously, as they may cause unwanted agitation or confusion. Patients who are refractory to atropine or require repeated doses should have a temporary pacemaker inserted.

   b. **Atrioventricular block**

      (1) **First-degree AV block** does not require treatment, but a PR interval exceeding 0.24 seconds is a relative contraindication to the use of digoxin, verapamil, or beta-adrenergic blockers.

      (2) **Mobitz I second-degree AV block** is commonly seen with inferior-posterior myocardial infarctions and generally has a transient benign course. The indications for atropine or pacemaker insertion are the same as for sinus bradycardia.

      (3) **Mobitz II second-degree AV block** generally occurs with anterior infarctions and is associated with a high risk of progression to complete block. Its presence warrants insertion of a temporary pacemaker.

      (4) **Complete heart block** is an unstable periinfarctional rhythm and mandates a temporary pacemaker. If a slow wide (ventricular) escape rhythm is present, atropine may be tried first but will likely be ineffective. Low doses of isoproterenol (2–10 μg/min) may accelerate the heart rate to 40–50 beats/minute, or an external pacemaker can be used until a temporary pacemaker can be placed. Infusion rates of isoproterenol

greater than 10 μg/minute are likely to induce ventricular ectopy and ischemia. Patients who progress to complete AV block via an antecedent bundle branch block require a permanent pacemaker.

c. **Sinus tachycardia** is common with AMI and is an adverse prognostic sign. It may occur due to heart failure, hypotension, hyperthyroidism, or complications such as pulmonary embolism, fever, or anemia. When sinus tachycardia does not respond to relief of pain and the etiology is unclear, insertion of a Swan-Ganz catheter is indicated. If sinus tachycardia persists after the central hemodynamics have been optimized and no other etiologies for tachycardia are apparent, a hyperdynamic state secondary to catecholamine excess may exist. Such patients generally have an anterior MI, hypertension, and a high cardiac output; they may benefit from beta-adrenergic blockade.

d. **Atrial fibrillation, atrial flutter, and paroxysmal supraventricular tachycardia (PSVT)** are common when heart failure is present and may be refractory unless the heart failure is improved.

   (1) Patients with a **rapid ventricular response** should be cardioverted immediately, since hemodynamic compromise is likely to occur. Atrial fibrillation usually requires a synchronized discharge of 100 joules, atrial flutter 25 joules, and PSVT 100 joules.

   (2) If the **ventricular response is slow,** a temporary pacemaker is recommended before direct-current (DC) cardioversion because there is an increased risk of asystole immediately following cardioversion.

   (3) **Recurrent arrhythmias.** If atrial fibrillation, atrial flutter, or PSVT is recurrent, the goal of therapy is to slow the ventricular response to 60–100/minute. Verapamil, digoxin, or propranolol can be used depending on hemodynamic and conducting system considerations. Once the ventricular response is controlled, some patients may convert to sinus rhythm. The addition of either procainamide or quinidine may promote conversion to a sinus rhythm and prevent recurrence.

e. **Ventricular premature depolarizations (VPDs).** If not initiated prophylactically, lidocaine should be used in the treatment of VPDs that are frequent (> 6/minute), are multiform, impinge on the ascending limb of the T wave, or appear in couplets or runs (three or more VPDs at a rate > 100/minute). The loading dosage and maintenance infusion rate of lidocaine are given in sec. **II.C.5.**

f. **Accelerated idioventricular rhythm (AIVR)** is a ventricular rhythm (rate 60–100/minute) that is common during the first 48 hours after infarction. It may be a sign of reperfusion in patients receiving thrombolytic therapy. An accelerated idioventricular rhythm may be a ventricular escape rhythm, or it may be precipitated by a VPD. In most instances, AIVR is transient; thus no therapy is needed. On occasion, more sustained AIVR can cause clinical decompensation by uncoupling atrial contraction. In this situation, atropine accelerates the sinus node and may abolish AIVR. If atropine is unsuccessful, lidocaine can be used. Occasionally, overdrive ventricular pacing may be required. Patients with AIVR may develop ventricular tachycardia at twice the rate of the AIVR.

g. **Ventricular tachycardia** severely compromises left ventricular function and may deteriorate into ventricular fibrillation. It can be treated with a precordial thump or a bolus of intravenous lidocaine, but DC countershock (synchronized if possible) using 10–25 joules is usually preferred. Bretylium and procainamide (Table 5-5) are useful in the management of resistant or recurrent ventricular tachycardia.

h. **Ventricular fibrillation.** See Chap. 2.

2. **Hypotension** may result from massive infarction, arrhythmias, hypovolemia, a reflex reduction in peripheral resistance, right ventricular infarction, or cardiac rupture.

   a. **Specific entities**

      (1) **Right ventricular infarction** is a commonly overlooked cause for hypotension in patients with inferior MI. Physical manifestations of predominant right ventricular infarction include right-sided gallops, jugular venous distention, and Kussmaul's sign (i.e., jugular venous distention with inspiration). Pulmonary congestion may be present or absent. Hypotension is a result of low flow due to a reduction in right

Table 5-5. Drug dosages for ventricular arrhythmias in acute myocardial infarction

Drug	Route	Dosage	Comment
Lidocaine	IV	1 mg/kg bolus over 2 min. Repeat 0.5 mg/kg bolus in 10 min; then maintenance infusion of 2–4 mg/min.	Decrease infusion rate if patient is older than 70 years or if CHF, shock, or hepatic disease is present.
Procainamide	IV	Infuse at a maximum rate of 50 mg/min to a total dose of 1000 mg; then maintenance infusion of 2–6 mg/min.	Monitor BP.
Bretylium	IV	If emergent, give 5–10 mg/kg bolus; if nonemergent, dilute 1:8 and infuse over 8 min. Constant infusion rate is 1–2 mg/min.	Reserve for ventricular tachycardia or ventricular fibrillation. Monitor BP. Full antiarrhythmic effect may not be observed for 30 min.

ventricular stroke volume. Noninvasive tests (e.g., echocardiography or radionuclide imaging) or placement of a Swan-Ganz catheter, which may unmask a high right ventricular pressure, a characteristic right atrial pressure tracing (rapid Y descent), and a normal to low pulmonary artery occlusive pressure, can be used for diagnosis. The appropriate treatment of right ventricular infarction is administration of fluid and dobutamine.

(2) **Cardiac rupture** occurs in approximately 10% of fatal MIs and is far more common than rupture of the papillary muscle or ventricular septum. It occurs most often in hypertensive, elderly patients with otherwise uncomplicated transmural MI (i.e., without CHF or aneurysm formation). The clinical diagnosis should be suspected if chest pain occurs in such patients in the absence of ECG changes. Sinus or junctional bradycardia and signs of cardiac tamponade may follow. Rupture is most likely to occur 2–4 days after MI. Rupture of the left ventricle is usually fatal within minutes, but confinement by the pericardium may limit hemorrhage and allow time for diagnosis by aspiration of grossly hemorrhagic pericardial fluid. Most patients require an immediate operation, but a few present less acutely and can undergo angiography prior to surgery. On occasion, the extravasation of blood is limited by the pericardium and a fibrotic false aneurysm with a connection to the left ventricle. This is known as a pseudoaneurysm and frequently results in rupture and death unless it is suspected and repaired surgically.

(3) If the **peripheral resistance** is low, another disease process, such as heat stroke, sepsis, or hyperthyroidism, may be complicating infarction. The short-term use of norepinephrine may be effective in some of these patients. Patients who are markedly vasoconstricted require a central arterial catheter, since peripheral readings may underestimate the true blood pressure.

b. **Treatment** of hypotension is cause-specific. Arrhythmias and heart failure (see sec. **III**) should be treated expeditiously. In the absence of heart failure, patients should be treated with leg elevation and judicious boluses of saline. If a fluid challenge of 500 ml of saline fails to correct hypotension, dopamine should be started at 5 μg/kg/minute and titrated to maintain a systolic pressure greater than 90 mm Hg. A Swan-Ganz catheter should be placed to establish the cause of hypotension and to guide management.

3. **Hypertension** increases myocardial oxygen demand and probably increases infarct size. If hypertension (i.e., systolic pressure > 160 mm Hg or diastolic pressure > 90 mm Hg) does not abate after sedation and relief of pain, the use of parenteral agents is indicated. Propranolol, 0.1 mg/kg, or an equivalent dosage of another beta-blocker can be given over 15 minutes if there are no contraindications; it may be especially useful if a hyperdynamic circulating state is present. Intravenous nitroglycerin is particularly effective in lowering blood pres-

sure when concomitant heart failure is present. In the absence of heart failure, nitroprusside is preferred. The blood pressure should be titrated to a systolic pressure less than 140 mm Hg and a diastolic pressure less than 90 mm Hg. A tachycardia in response to nitroprusside or nitroglycerin implies an inadequate intravascular volume.

4. **Persistent chest pain** is most effectively treated with repeated doses of morphine sulfate. There is little evidence to suggest that nitrates or propranolol alleviate the pain of evolving infarction as effectively. The parenteral use of these agents may provide relief in the presence of recurrent ischemia.

III. **Heart Failure**

A. **Pathophysiology.** Heart failure is present when the cardiac output is inadequate to satisfy systemic oxygen requirements. Most commonly, the mechanism is impaired cardiac performance and inadequate output rather than excessive oxygen demand. Forward cardiac output can be reduced for a variety of reasons (e.g., inadequate filling, valvular regurgitation) but most frequently is due to cardiac muscle dysfunction. The compensatory changes of heart failure include increased peripheral resistance, plasma volume expansion, and myocardial hypertrophy and dilation, which all result in higher myocardial oxygen demand. Symptoms occur when the systolic and diastolic properties of the heart deteriorate beyond the capacity of these mechanisms to compensate.

1. **Adrenergic stimulation.** When ventricular performance deteriorates, reflex baroreceptors activate sympathetic mechanisms that augment contractility and increase the heart rate and arterial vasoconstriction.

2. **Intravascular volume expansion.** Sympathetic mechanisms also mediate venoconstriction, decreased visceral blood flow, and shunting from peripheral to central veins to increase the cardiac volume. A decreased renal perfusion pressure and a decreased renal sodium concentration stimulate the renin-angiotensin system and aldosterone secretion, leading to further arterial vasoconstriction and salt retention. Volume expansion results in an increase in myocardial fiber length and improvement in forward cardiac output at the expense of a rise in ventricular pressure. If the heart is stiff, small changes in volume result in large changes in pressure and may precipitate pulmonary congestion. In patients with myocardial infarction, pulmonary fluid extravasation tends to begin at a left ventricular end-diastolic pressure (LVEDP) of 18 mm Hg, and an LVEDP above 25 mm Hg is usually associated with pulmonary edema. Increased pulmonary congestion reduces vital capacity and pulmonary compliance, increases the work of breathing, and widens the alveolar-arterial oxygen difference. The net effect of these attempts to increase the cardiac output is an increased myocardial oxygen demand.

3. **Myocardial hypertrophy and dilation.** Hypertrophy develops in response to increased myocardial work. Pure pressure overload, such as is seen with aortic stenosis or chronic hypertension, evokes marked hypertrophy. In contrast, volume overload states such as occur with regurgitant aortic or mitral valve lesions cause ventricular dilation but less pronounced wall thickening. Dilation generally does not occur in response to pressure overload until contractile performance is diminished or a volume overload state has developed. Hypertrophy and dilation are compensations to maintain cardiac output, but these responses ultimately lead to increased wall stress and increased myocardial work.

B. **Etiologies.** The major causes of acute heart failure include myocardial ischemia, infarction, and severe acute valvular dysfunction (e.g., malfunctioning prosthesis or ruptured chordae tendinae). Exacerbants can be arrhythmias, pulmonary emboli, sepsis, or malignant hypertension. Any of the preceding etiologies predispose to a subacute presentation of heart failure developing over days or weeks preceding evaluation in the emergency department. Other causes such as thyroid disease or chronic anemia are less common. Chronic heart failure is usually a manifestation of coronary artery disease, hypertension, valvular heart disease, or cardiomyopathy.

C. **Clinical features**

1. **Symptoms**

a. **Compensatory increases in the ventricular volume-pressure relationship** lead to increased lung water, poor gas exchange, and increased airway resistance. These effects result in dyspnea on exertion and occasionally cough. Dyspnea precipitated by recumbency (i.e., **orthopnea**) reflects the inability to accept an augmented venous return; it can be avoided by elevating the head of the bed. Urgent and profound respiratory distress awakening the patient from sleep is termed **paroxysmal nocturnal dyspnea (PND).**

   b. A **reduced cardiac output** results in poor peripheral perfusion, muscle fatigue, and diminished urine output; progressive deterioration causes somnolence, cold extremities, and Cheyne-Stokes respiration. Renal blood flow improves at night, resulting in nocturia.

2. **Physical examination.** Patients with mild heart failure appear well at rest; however, dyspnea is usually apparent with exercise or more severe dysfunction. Orthopnea, paroxysmal nocturnal dyspnea (PND), and Cheyne-Stokes respiration may be observed with heart failure of greater severity. Compensatory increases in adrenergic tone cause tachycardia. Pulses alternans (i.e., alternating weak and strong peripheral pulses) is commonly present. Fluid retention and extravasation into tissue spaces (i.e., legs, abdomen, lungs, and pleural space) develop as CHF increases and implies a component of right heart failure. Rales are common, and pleural effusions may be present. An elevated venous pressure is manifested by jugular venous distention and congestive hepatomegaly; the latter can result in abdominal pain, ascites, hepatic pulsations, nausea, and vomiting. Sustained, firm compression over the liver for 1 minute may elicit persistent neck vein distention when heart failure is present (hepatojugular reflux). The apical impulse is laterally displaced and frequently enlarged. S3 gallops are low-frequency sounds heard just after the S2; they are best appreciated at the cardiac apex using the bell of the stethoscope with the patient in the 45-degree left lateral decubitus position.

D. **Disposition.** The appropriate disposition of patients with heart failure depends on its severity and abruptness of onset. Acute (i.e., onset within minutes or hours) or severe heart failure warrants admission to the intensive care unit. Heart failure that is subacute (i.e., onset within days or weeks) or of moderate severity is best treated initially in the hospital. Patients with chronic stable heart failure frequently can be managed as outpatients if the failure is mild.

E. **Therapy** is oriented toward detecting and treating the underlying cause (e.g., thyrotoxicosis, anemia, ischemia) and alleviating the failure itself. There are several approaches to therapy, which most often are combined. These include reducing preload (volume) by decreasing venous return or blood volume or reducing impedance to ventricular ejection. Both of these interventions may reduce wall stress, but pulmonary congestion is more directly treated by reduction of preload. Inotropic agents can be used to improve contractility. Oxygen supplementation should be employed if hypoxia is present.

1. **Oxygen** therapy should be started immediately if the patient is dyspneic. A rate of 4–6 liters/minute is a reasonable first approximation in patients without a propensity to carbon dioxide retention. Endotracheal intubation is indicated to reduce the work of breathing for patients with labored respirations if acute ischemia is present or progressive clinical deterioration occurs.

2. **Preload reduction** is commonly implemented with diuretics and/or nitrates. Both are effective, and the combination may be synergistic. Excessive reduction in preload, however, may cause hypotension. Thus, it is prudent to assess the response to one agent before adding a second.

   a. Diuretics, such as furosemide and ethacrynic acid, have their initial effect within 5 minutes, reducing preload by an increase in venous capacitance. Subsequently (within 20 minutes), renal effects initiate a diuresis. The initial dosage of furosemide is 20–40 mg IV and of ethacrynic acid 25–50 mg IV. Higher dosages may be necessary in patients with renal failure; however, an excessive diuresis will result in intravascular volume depletion, a reduced cardiac output, and hypotension.

   b. Nitrates dilate the venous system, thereby reducing preload. If the heart is noncompliant, changes in volume substantially reduce LVEDP and thus pulmonary congestion and wall stress. The peripheral arterial effects of sublingual and oral nitrates are minor, although coronary dilatation does occur. Sublingual TNG (0.4 mg) has a rapid onset of action (within 30 seconds), maximal effect at 8 minutes, and a duration of action of about 20 minutes. High doses of long-acting nitrates have similar effects and can be utilized for chronic therapy. Intravenous nitrate therapy can be utilized for patients with severe heart failure in whom greater peripheral arterial effects are necessary.

Table 5-6. Cardiovascular effects of inotropic agents

Drug	Heart rate	Cardiac output	LVEDP	Peripheral vascular resistance
Norepinephrine	↑ ↑	—	↑ ↑	↑ ↑ ↑
Dopamine				
Low dosage	↑	↑ ↑	— or ↑	— or ↑
High dosage	↑ ↑	↑	↑ ↑	↑ ↑ ↑
Dobutamine	↑	↑ ↑ ↑	—	—
Isoproterenol	↑ ↑ ↑ ↑	↑ ↑	—	—
Digoxin	— or ↓	↑	↓	—
Amrinone	— or ↓	↑ ↑ ↑	↓	↓

Key: — = no effect, ↑ = increase, ↓ = decrease; magnitude of effect (i.e., mild, moderate, marked) is given by the number of arrows.

3. **Impedance reduction.** Most patients with heart failure have a high peripheral resistance. Agents that reduce peripheral resistance improve cardiac output while inducing little change in heart rate or blood pressure. Agents available for this purpose include intravenous nitroglycerin and nitroprusside, which are best administered with hemodynamic monitoring. Captopril, hydralazine, prazosin, and nifedipine are all useful in the more chronic management of heart failure.

   a. **Sodium nitroprusside** is a smooth-muscle dilator with arterial and venous effects. Increased cardiac output and reduced pulmonary congestion accompany increased venous capacitance and a reduction in peripheral resistance. However, cardiac output will fall if the preload is lowered excessively, and hypotension may ensue, since arterial vasodilatation continues. In addition, there is concern that nitroprusside may exacerbate ischemia in patients with coronary artery disease. The initial infusion rate is 0.5 μg/kg/minute with increases of 0.1–0.5 μg/kg/minute every 5 minutes until the desired hemodynamic effect is reached. Thiocyanate toxicity can occur in patients with renal failure or at high dosages.

   b. **Intravenous nitrates** have effects similar to nitroprusside in patients with heart failure; however, nitrates lose most of their arterial effects when preload becomes normalized. In patients with CHF and coronary disease, nitrates are preferred to nitroprusside, since they concomitantly benefit ischemia. Parenteral agents usually necessitate invasive hemodynamic monitoring for appropriate use, especially in patients with ischemic heart disease.

   c. **Chronic agents.** Hydralazine, captopril, prazosin, and nifedipine are useful chronically. Hydralazine and nifedipine have predominant arterial effects, while captopril and prazosin have balanced effects on the arterial and venous beds. Hydralazine may exacerbate ischemia.

4. **Inotropic agents** (Table 5-6). The choice of an inotropic agent depends on its cardiac and vascular effects. Dobutamine is the preferred agent for heart failure, but dopamine is preferred in the presence of hypotension. Amrinone has been approved for intravenous use and has effects similar to dobutamine.

   a. **Dobutamine** is a potent beta-1 agonist with some beta-2 effects. It is a weak alpha-agonist but invariably results in reflex arterial vasodilatation. Thus, dobutamine increases cardiac output and decreases arterial and pulmonary venous pressure. Hemodynamic monitoring is usually necessary for titration of the hemodynamic effects, especially in patients with ischemic heart disease. The initial infusion rate is 2.5–10.0 μg/kg/minute. Excessive dosages may induce arrhythmias and potentiate ischemia.

   b. **Dopamine** is a direct beta-1 agonist with alpha-adrenergic effects at higher dosages. At a low dosage (2–5 μg/kg/minute), renal blood flow improves with little change in heart rate, peripheral resistance, or preload. At higher infusion rates (>10 μg/kg/minute), these effects are lost, and peripheral resistance and preload increase. Higher infusion rates also induce a tachycardia. Thus, higher dosages of dopamine may exacerbate heart failure,

Table 5-7. Drug dosages for acute management of pulmonary edema

Drug	Route	Dosage	Comment
Nitroglycerin	SL	0.3–0.4 mg q5min prn	Monitor BP.
	IV	Start infusion at 10 µg/min; increase infusion 5–10 µg/min q5min to desired effect	Monitor BP.
Morphine	IV	2–4 mg q10min as needed to relieve dyspnea and anxiety	Monitor BP and respirations.
Furosemide	IV	20–40 mg, repeated prn	Monitor BP.
Nitroprusside	IV	Start infusion at 0.5 µg/kg/min; increase infusion 0.1–0.5 µg/kg/min q5min to desired effect	Monitor BP.
Nifedipine	SL	10 mg	Chew capsule, or extract contents with a syringe and place under tongue or swish in mouth. Monitor BP.

arrhythmias, and ischemia. Nonetheless, in the presence of marked hypotension, dopamine remains the agent of choice.

   c. Norepinephrine is a potent inotrope and vasoconstrictor. Its hemodynamic effects are similar to those of high-dose dopamine. Some authorities believe it is the agent of choice in septic shock.

   d. Isoproteronol is a potent beta-1 agonist with both arterial and venous dilating effects. Its use of CHF is contraindicated in patients with ischemic heart disease because it may induce hypotension and exacerbate ischemia.

   e. Digoxin is a weak inotrope with substantial toxicity. Thus, it has little role in the treatment of acute severe heart failure. It may be useful in some patients with chronic CHF.

   f. Amrinone is synthetic inotropic agent with vasodilating properties recently approved for intravenous use in the short-term management of CHF. Its mechanism of action has not been fully elucidated; however, it appears to influence the myocardial levels of cyclic nucleotides. It is not a beta-adrenergic agonist, nor does it affect sodium-potassium triphosphatase activity; its metabolites are excreted primarily through the kidneys. It has a half-life of approximately 5–6 hours in patients with CHF. Its hemodynamic effects are to increase cardiac output and to decrease pulmonary wedge pressure and peripheral resistance. A mild decrease in the mean arterial pressure usually is observed, and myocardial oxygen consumption generally is unchanged. The most common adverse affect is a dose-related thrombocytopenia; arrhythmias, hypotension, nausea, hepatocellular dysfunction, and fever have also been reported. Therapy is initiated with a 0.75 mg/kg bolus given IV over 3 minutes, and a maintenance infusion of 5–10 µg/kg/minute is administered. Therapy should be guided by hemodynamic monitoring with a Swan-Ganz catheter, especially in patients with ischemic heart disease. Based on the clinical response, a second bolus may be given 30 minutes after therapy is initiated. The total daily dosage, however, should not exceed 10 mg/kg.

F. Pulmonary edema

  1. Clinical features. Pulmonary edema represents the extreme of pulmonary congestion. Patients are extremely dyspneic, ashen, cyanotic, and diaphoretic, and frothy pink sputum may be observed. Rales, rhonchi, an S3 gallop, and tachycardia are common; hypertension and wheezing occur frequently.

  2. Treatment (Table 5-7)

    a. Oxygen, 4–6 liters/minute, should be administered with the patient sitting up. Marked respiratory distress or clinical deterioration is an indication for endotracheal intubation.

    b. Morphine sulfate, 4–6 mg IV, should be given to reduce venous return and relieve anxiety.

    c. Nitroglycerin, 0.3–0.4 mg SL, may be given immediately to reduce venous return and peripheral resistance and to treat ischemia, the most common cause of pulmonary edema.

   d. Furosemide, 40 mg IV, also causes venous pooling and later induces a diuresis.

   e. Vasodilator therapy with intravenous nitroglycerin, nitroprusside, or sublingual nifedipine can be used to reduce impedance, especially when hypertension is present.

   f. Rotating tourniquets and phlebotomy are useful mechanical measures to reduce venous return.

 3. **Disposition.** The patient should be admitted to an intensive care unit. Hemodynamic monitoring usually is indicated unless rapid compensation occurs.

G. **Cardiogenic shock**

 1. **Clinical features.** Concomitant pulmonary congestion and peripheral hypoperfusion represent the terminal phase of CHF. It is essential to exclude mechanical factors (e.g., flail mitral leaflet, prosthetic valve malfunction, acute ventricular septal rupture), since these are potentially reversible lesions. In general, both preload and impedance are high, and cardiac output is low; impaired oxygenation and poor peripheral perfusion are the rule. Patients typically have a tachycardia and appear dyspneic, ashen, and diaphoretic; half have impaired mentation, and most have a systolic blood pressure less than 80 mm Hg, or a 90 mm Hg fall from previous levels.

 2. **Treatment.** Dobutamine is the preferred inotrope, but if marked hypotension is present, dopamine is preferred. Impedance reduction may be helpful but frequently exacerbates hypotension. Intraaortic balloon counterpulsation should be employed in patients with refractory hypotension when there are mechanical factors that can be surgically corrected. However, patients with cardiogenic shock without a reversible mechanical component are unlikely to benefit from intraaortic balloon counterpulsation.

IV. **Cardiomyopathy**

A. **Dilated cardiomyopathy** is characterized by primary myocardial dysfunction, a large heart, and CHF (see sec. III). The cause of dilated cardiomyopathy is usually difficult to identify. Several metabolic abnormalities, toxins, and infectious agents have been implicated. Treatment is directed at CHF.

B. **Restrictive cardiomyopathy** is characterized by impaired diastolic compliance. Cardiac contractility may be normal early in the course. Etiologies of restrictive myopathy include amyloidosis, sarcoidosis, hemochromatosis, Fabry's disease, Gaucher's disease, and Löffler's endocarditis. Treatment is supportive, but excess diuresis must be avoided. In patients with hemochromatosis, repeated phlebotomy or the use of desferrioxamine, an iron chelating agent, may improve cardiac function.

C. **Hypertrophic cardiomyopathy** is a genetically transmitted disorder characterized microscopically by myocardial fiber disarray. Patients with hypertrophic myopathy have impaired ventricular diastolic compliance similar to that of patients with restrictive cardiomyopathy; however, contractility is increased. In some patients, a reduced ventricular volume leads to dynamic outflow tract obstruction, especially when the septum is markedly hypertrophied. The diastolic abnormalities reduce the stroke volume and elevate the left atrial pressure. The atrial contribution to ventricular filling becomes critical as the ventricle becomes stiffer.

 1. **Clinical features**

   a. **Presentation and complications.** Patients with hypertrophic cardiomyopathy commonly present during the teenage and young adult years, although many patients are not recognized until much later. Dyspnea, palpitations, angina, syncope, and presyncope are common complaints. Angina may occur generally due to increased wall stress. Syncope may be caused by arrhythmias (ventricular or atrial) or occur after exercise when the cardiac output is inadequate to sustain blood pressure in the vasodilated state. Sudden death can also occur after exercise. Mitral regurgitation and atrial fibrillation are frequent complications. Atrial fibrillation may impair cardiac filling, leading to a reduced cardiac output and pulmonary congestion. Systemic emboli are common in patients with hypertrophic cardiomyopathy and atrial fibrillation.

   b. Characteristic **physical findings** are an apical impulse with two or three components (e.g., palpable atrial impulse, a late systolic bulge); an S4 gallop, and a dynamic carotid pulse. A harsh systolic murmur usually is best heard along the sternal border, although it may have a blowing quality toward the apex. The murmur may be unimpressive unless provocative maneuvers such as Valsalva, rising from a squat, or amyl nitrite are employed; however, maneuvers should not be performed in critically ill patients, as they may be detrimental and misleading. The murmur may behave atypically in hypertensive patients with hypertrophic cardiomyopathy.

2. **Diagnostic studies.** The ECG usually demonstrates ST-segment and T-wave abnormalities and criteria for left ventricular hypertrophy. Pseudoinfarction patterns occur attributable to prominent septal Q waves. Cardiomegaly may or may not be present. Echocardiography is extremely helpful in distinguishing hypertrophic cardiomyopathy from mitral or aortic valvular disease.

3. **Management**
   a. **General measures.** Agents that reduce ventricular size (e.g., nitrates, diuretics) and inotropic agents (e.g., digoxin) should be avoided if possible. Patients should be instructed to avoid strenous exercise and to taper exercise gradually.
   b. **Beta-adrenergic blockade** is the mainstay of medical therapy. Beta-adrenergic blockers improve diastolic filling and reduce outflow obstruction. Many authorities advocate very high dosages of propranolol (e.g., 640 mg/day).
   c. **Calcium channel blockers.** Verapamil promotes diastolic relaxation, which improves ventricular filling and reduces outflow obstruction. Verapamil appears as beneficial (hemodynamically) as beta-adrenergic blockers; however, in a rare patient, verapamil can precipitate hypotension with attendant syncope and even death. Nifedipine also improves ventricular relaxation but is more likely to result in hypotension.
   d. **Surgical myotomy-myectomy** should be considered for patients who are refractory to medical therapy.
   e. **Acute atrial fibrillation** leads to hemodynamic decompensation and pulmonary edema and requires immediate DC cardioversion. If atrial fibrillation recurs, control of the rate with beta-blockers or verapamil frequently is of benefit, since the abnormality is one of filling, not contractility. Patients with hypertrophic myopathy and atrial fibrillation should be anticoagulated to prevent systemic emboli.

V. **Myocarditis**
   A. **Etiology.** At present, definitive information concerning inflammatory myopathies is lacking. The underlying cause is rarely identified unless the patient has a known underlying disease state, such as systemic lupus erythmatosus, rheumatic fever, or alcohol abuse. In most patients, viral infection or an autoimmune process is suspected. Several putative viruses (e.g., Coxsackie A and B, echovirus, and influenza) have been implicated, as have abnormalities in the immune response. On rare occasions in the United States, fungal, parasitic, or rickettsial organisms cause myocarditis.
   B. **Clinical features.** In most instances, signs and symptoms of myocarditis follow a viral illness and range from mild to fulminant. Heart failure may be prominent, or arrhythmias, conduction disturbances, fever, or chest pain may dominate the clinical picture. Physical findings are nonspecific and vary with the severity of the disease process.
   C. **Diagnostic studies.** ECG changes such as nonspecific ST-segment and T-wave abnormalities are common but may be transient. Atrioventricular and intraventricular conduction abnormalities (e.g., first-degree AV block in acute rheumatic myocarditis) may be seen. The chest x-ray may show heart failure. Enzymatic markers of myocardial injury may be persistently elevated in a small subset. Gallium-67 imaging and myocardial biopsy have been advocated to improve the diagnostic accuracy and to guide management; however, the value of these procedures is speculative. Viral cultures of stool, throat, and blood, or a fourfold rise of serum antibody titers support the diagnosis of a viral etiology.
   D. **Management.** Patients with acute myocarditis should be admitted to the hospital. The management of myocarditis is supportive, including bed rest and the standard treatment of heart failure and arrhythmias. If digoxin is indicated, it should be used cautiously, because patients with acute myocarditis are easily susceptible to digoxin toxicity. Correctable etiologies (e.g., alcohol, ischemia) should be identified and treated appropriately. A subset of patients may improve with beta-blockers. The use of immunosuppressive agents is popular but unproved.

Pericardial Disease

I. Acute pericarditis

A. Etiologies. Most pericarditis is thought to be related to antecedent viral infection or myocardial infarction. Periinfarction pericarditis is common during the first 72 hours following a transmural infarction. A second type of pericarditis, Dressler's syndrome, can occur from 1 week to many months after a myocardial infarction, presumably due to antimyocardial antibodies. Uremia, chest trauma, neoplasia, tuberculosis, and bacterial infection are less common causes.

B. Clinical features.

1. **Symptoms.** The pain of pericarditis varies, but it usually arises from inflammation of the adjacent pleura and is appreciated over the left chest; true pericardial pain is referred to the trapezius ridge. The pain is often pleuritic, frequently increased with recumbency, and decreased with sitting and leaning forward. The pain may vary with respiration. Severe dyspnea raises the possibility of tamponade.

2. **Physical examination.** The characteristic sign of pericarditis is a three-component pericardial friction rub. The components correspond to ventricular systole, rapid ventricular filling, and atrial contraction. Friction rubs should be listened for at the lower left sternal border, with the patient both supine and seated and the breath held in inspiration and expiration. Pericardial friction rubs and one or more of the components are often transient. When a rub is present, the ventricular systolic component is invariably heard.

C. Diagnostic studies. The diagnosis is established on clinical grounds. The typical ECG changes of pericarditis are not invariably present. Characteristically, diffuse concave ST-segment elevation is observed without reciprocal changes. A few days later, the ST segments return to normal, and T-wave flattening is noted. Subsequently, T-wave inversion may occur and persist for weeks or months. Mild MB-CK elevations occur rarely and imply myocardial involvement. Echocardiography is a sensitive method for detecting pericardial fluid but adds little to the clinical diagnosis. The sedimentation rate is usually elevated.

D. Management. Admission to the hospital is generally advised if the diagnosis is in question or symptoms are severe. Pericarditis is usually a self-limited disorder resolving over 2–6 weeks; therefore, therapy is primarily symptomatic. Most patients obtain relief with aspirin, 650 mg qid, or indomethacin, 25–50 mg tid. Recent data suggest that indomethacin may have adverse effects in patients with ischemia or infarction. Steroids are reserved for patients with refractory symptoms, since these drugs may impair scar formation in patients with infarction and are frequently associated with recurrent symptoms upon tapering. Anticoagulants should be used with caution in patients with pericarditis because they may predispose to tamponade.

II. Pericardial tamponade

A. Pathophysiology. The pericardial sac normally contains 15–50 ml of fluid, and intrapericardial pressure is several mm Hg lower than the ventricular end-diastolic pressure. A rise in pericardial pressure elevates both the left and right ventricular end-diastolic pressures, impairs diastolic filling, and reduces stroke volume. Pericardial tamponade occurs when the pericardial pressure rises to or over the level of the ventricular end-diastolic pressure. Tamponade can be precipitated by as little as 80 ml of fluid if the accumulation is rapid or the pericardium is stiff; however, more gradual accumulation of 1–2 liters may be tolerated before tamponade occurs.

B. Etiology. Pericardial tamponade may occur with any cause of pericarditis but is more common with uremic, neoplastic, or bacterial etiologies. Anticoagulant therapy increases the risk of tamponade.

C. Clinical features. Patients with tamponade are dyspneic, have a tachycardia, and may complain of chest heaviness. Signs on physical examination include jugular venous distention with a blunted Y descent, tachypnea, and an abnormal pulsus paradoxus (i.e., a difference in blood pressure between inspiration and expiration exceeding 10 mm Hg or 25% of the pulse pressure). Pulsus paradoxus is easily appreciated by palpation of the carotid or femoral artery and may be quantitated by blood pressure measurement. Patients may have hypotension, diminished heart sounds, and/or a pericardial friction rub. Pulmonary congestion usually is absent. Kussmaul's sign, an increase in jugular venous distention with inspiration, although common in constrictive pericarditis, occurs rarely in acute pericardial tamponade.

D. **Differential diagnosis.** Other conditions causing jugular venous distention and pulsus paradoxus in the absence of pulmonary congestion include right ventricular infarction, massive pulmonary embolus, restrictive cardiomyopathy, and constrictive pericarditis.

E. **Diagnostic studies**
1. The **chest x-ray** may show a large globular heart with separation of the pericardial fat pad in a slowly accumulating large pericardial effusion, but the silhouette may appear normal when less fluid is present.
2. **Echocardiography** is most useful in demonstrating an effusion.
3. The **ECG** may show low voltage, electrical alternans, or diffuse ST-segment elevation.
4. **Swan-Ganz catheterization** can be used to confirm the diagnosis in the occasional patient in whom a clinical decision is difficult. Typical findings are equalization of the pulmonary artery occlusive pressure, right ventricular end-diastolic pressure, and right atrial pressure. The right atrial wave form characteristically has a diminished Y descent.

F. **Management.** Once the diagnosis of tamponade is made, treatment must be undertaken expeditiously.
1. The goal of **pharmacologic therapy** is to sustain the patient until more definitive therapy can be performed. A bolus of 500–1000 ml of normal saline should be administered rapidly if the patient is hypotensive. A dopamine infusion may also help sustain the blood pressure and cardiac output. Nitroprusside can be used to improve the cardiac output if the blood pressure is adequate.
2. **Pericardiotomy** is the preferred treatment. It is safe, provides greater diagnostic information, and more complete drainage than pericardiocentesis.
3. Blind **pericardiocentesis** (see Chap. 38) should only be performed during the period prior to surgical intervention in patients refractory to fluids and pharmacologic support.

Valvular Heart Disease

I. **Aortic stenosis**
A. **Clinical features.** Patients with aortic stenosis (AS) are asymptomatic until late in the course of the disease. Symptoms such as angina, syncope, and exertional dyspnea in patients with significant stenosis are an indication for surgery. Angina may occur with or without coronary artery disease; conversely, the absence of angina does not exclude coronary disease. Syncope is most often caused by exertional hypotension induced by inappropriate vasodilation but may also be attributed to arrhythmias. Heart failure usually indicates advanced disease and frequently concomitant mitral regurgitation. The atrial contribution to ventricular filling becomes essential when the ventricle is hypertrophied and stiff; thus, atrial fibrillation can be a potentially catastrophic complication. The **physical findings** of AS are a slowly rising carotid pulse, a diffuse sustained apical impulse, a soft or absent A2, a harsh systolic ejection murmur radiating to the carotid arteries, a prominent S4 gallop, and an aortic ejection click. Patients who are elderly or have a low cardiac output may have less prominent findings.
B. **Diagnostic studies.** The chest x-ray is helpful if calcification of the aortic valve is seen. ECG criteria for left ventricular hypertrophy with repolarization abnormalities is a fairly sensitive but nonspecific finding. Echocardiography and Doppler flow studies are frequently helpful in confirming severe aortic stenosis. Cardiac catheterization is necessary to exclude additional valvular or coronary abnormalities.
C. **Management.** Patients with symptomatic AS should be admitted for cardiac catheterization and surgery. Syncope, severe angina, or severe heart failure is criterion for admission to a CCU. Acutely, diuretic therapy for pulmonary congestion can be employed, but excessive diuresis can be catastrophic. Dobutamine may be used as an inotrope but with caution. Similarly, nitrates can be used for angina. Acute atrial fibrillation may severely compromise the cardiac output and should be treated with prompt cardioversion.

II. **Acute aortic regurgitation**
A. **Etiologies.** The most common causes of acute aortic regurgitation are endocarditis

and aortic dissection. Staphylococcus and enterococcus are the most common infecting organisms. Closed chest trauma and spontaneous rupture of a leaflet are other causes.

    B. Clinical features. The onset of heart failure generally is sudden and severe, since regurgitation occurs into a small, stiff left ventricle. Characteristic physical findings are tachycardia, lack of a widened pulse pressure, a dynamic but nondisplaced apical impulse, a soft S1, a systolic flow murmur, a short early diastolic murmur reflecting early equilibration of aortic and ventricular pressures, an apical middiastolic rumble (Austin Flint murmur), and an S3 gallop. In addition, patients with endocarditis may have systemic emboli and AV conduction disturbances.

    C. Diagnostic studies. The chest x-ray usually shows severe pulmonary congestion; however, cardiomegaly is present only if a component of the cardiac disease is chronic. Combined echocardiography and Doppler flow studies may demonstrate a flail leaflet or vegetation and provide a qualitative estimate of the severity of regurgitation.

    D. Management. Afterload reduction with nitroprusside is the first line of therapy. Inotropic agents are rarely useful, and intraaortic balloon counterpulsation is contraindicated. Patients with shock must undergo immediate valve replacement. If endocarditis is suspected, blood cultures should be obtained immediately, and antibiotic therapy should be initiated promptly. Such patients benefit from 7–10 days of antibiotics before valve replacement; however, surgery rarely is avoided and should not be delayed if hemodynamic compromise is severe.

III. Mitral stenosis

    A. Etiology. Almost all mitral stenosis is caused by rheumatic heart disease; thus, mitral stenosis is often accompanied by mitral regurgitation.

    B. Clinical features. The principal symptom of mitral stenosis is dyspnea due to either pulmonary congestion or poor cardiac output. Atrial fibrillation frequently leads to clinical deterioration. Thromboembolism is common, age related, and more apt to occur in patients with atrial fibrillation. Characteristic **physical findings** are a right ventricular lift, a palpable P2, an apical diastolic thrill, an accentuated S1, an opening snap, and an apical diastolic rumble with presystolic accentuation (if sinus rhythm is present).

    C. Diagnostic studies. The ECG and chest x-ray demonstrate the effects of the lesion, that is, right ventricular hypertrophy, left atrial enlargement, and pulmonary venous and pulmonary arterial hypertension. Fluoroscopy is often required to appreciate the calcification of the mitral valve. The diagnosis of mitral stenosis is easily confirmed with M-mode echocardiography, and the severity can be estimated with combined 2-D echocardiogaphy and Doppler studies.

    D. Management. Patients with severe symptoms should be admitted to the hospital and evaluated for surgery. Frequently, decompensation is precipitated by acute atrial fibrillation. The ventricular response to atrial fibrillation must be controlled with digoxin, verapamil, or a beta-adrenergic blocker. Cardioversion is mandated for patients who are hemodynamically compromised by acute atrial fibrillation. The treatment of pulmonary congestion with diuretics must be undertaken cautiously, since a high atrial pressure is needed for left ventricular filling in the presence of severe mitral stenosis. Anticoagulant therapy and antibiotic prophylaxis are routine.

IV. Acute mitral regurgitation

    A. Etiologies. Acute mitral regurgitation usually occurs due to chordal or papillary muscle rupture. MI and endocarditis are the most common causes. Most patients with acute mitral regurgitation caused by MI have an inferior or posterior infarction with damage to the posterior papillary muscle. Other causes include rheumatic chordal involvement, Marfan's syndrome, acute rheumatic fever, and trauma.

    B. Clinical features. Acute mitral regurgitation presents with an abrupt onset of symptoms, a new systolic murmur, and a normal heart size. The severity of symptoms relates in part to the nature of the pathologic lesion, that is, chordal versus papillary muscle involvement and total versus partial rupture. The characteristic murmur is an early systolic decrescendo murmur reflecting a reduced intensity in late systole due to atrial and ventricular pressure equilibration; however, no murmur may be appreciated when the cardiac output is very low. The murmur radiates to the base if the posterior apparatus is involved or to the axilla if the anterior apparatus is involved. A hyperdynamic pulse, low-amplitude carotid pulsations, S4 and S3 gallops, and a widely split S2 are characteristic.

    C. Diagnostic studies. The ECG and chest x-ray may help establish the etiology, but

Prosthesis type	Mitral prosthesis	Acoustic characteristics	Aortic prosthesis	Acoustic characteristics
Ball valves	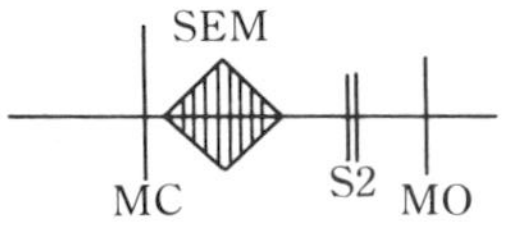	1) A2–MO interval 0.07–0.11 sec 2) MO>MC 3) II–III/VI SEM 4) No diastolic murmur	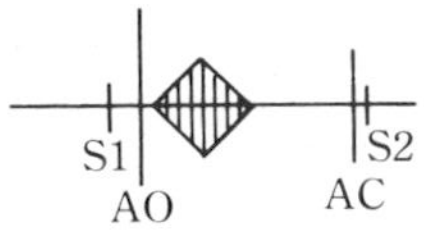	1) S1–AO interval 0.07 sec. 2) AO>AC 3) II/VI harsh SEM 4) No diastolic murmur
Disk valves	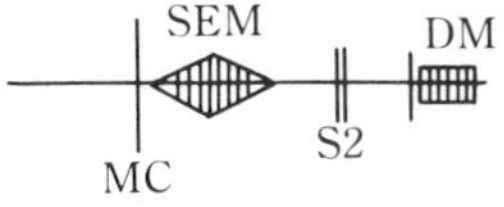	1) A2–MO interval 0.05–0.09 sec 2) MO is rarely heard 3) II/VI SEM is usually heard 4) I–II/VI diastolic rumble is usually heard	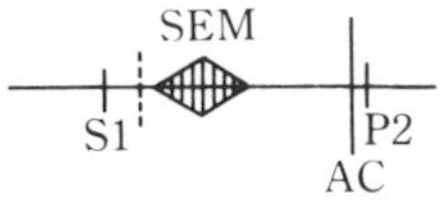	1) S1–AO interval 0.04 sec. 2) AO is uncommonly heard, AC is usually heard 3) II/VI SEM is usually heard 4) Occasional diastolic murmur
Porcine valves	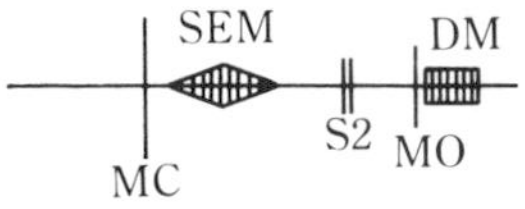	1) A2–MO interval 0.1 sec 2) MO is audible 50% 3) I–II/VI apical SEM 50% 4) Diastolic rumble ½–⅔	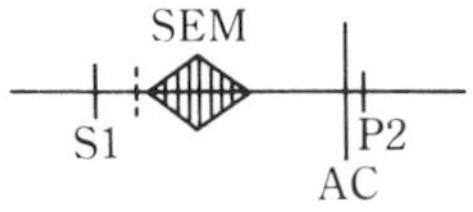	1) S1–AO interval 0.03–0.08 sec. 2) AO is uncommonly heard, AC is usually heard 3) II/VI SEM in most 4) No diastolic murmur
Bileaflet valve (St. Jude)			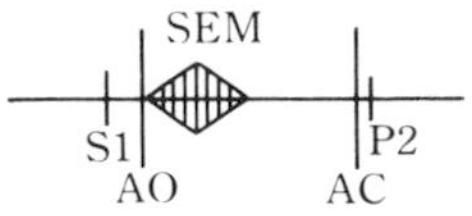	1) AO and AC commonly heard 2) A soft SEM is common

Fig. 5-1. Auscultatory characteristics of prosthetic heart valves. (Reproduced from N. D. Smith, V. Raizada, and J. Abrams, Auscultation of the normally functioning prosthetic valve. *Ann. Intern. Med.* 95:594, 1981. With permission).
Key: SEM = systolic ejection murmur; DM = diastolic murmur; AO = aortic valve opening sound; AC = aortic valve closure sound; MO = mitral valve opening sound; MC = mitral valve closure sound; S1 = first heart sound; S2 = second heart sound; A2 = aortic second sound; P2 = pulmonic second sound.

the diagnosis is a clinical one. The chest x-ray usually shows severe pulmonary congestion, but cardiomegaly is absent unless a component of chronic heart disease is present. Echocardiography and Doppler studies are helpful to assess the presence of vegetations and the stability of the mitral valve apparatus and to exclude other lesions. Cardiac catheterization definitively identifies the severity of mitral regurgitation and concomitant coronary artery disease.

D. Management. The immediate goal is to stabilize the patient in preparation for cardiac catheterization and mitral valve replacement. Impedance reduction with nitroprusside is the mainstay of therapy. Patients with shock require intraaortic balloon counterpulsation. Dobutamine may be helpful. If endocarditis is suspected, antibiotic therapy should be started after blood cultures are obtained.

V. Complications of prosthetic heart valves. A large number of prosthetic heart valves are now in use, and each has different auscultatory characteristics (Fig. 5-1). Thromboemboli, vegetations, or mechanical failure may alter these characteristics and provide a clue to the presence of prosthetic dysfunction. The complications of prosthetic heart valves include thromboembolism, hemolytic anemia, endocarditis, and mechanical failure.

A. Thromboembolism is more common with tilting disk and ball valves than with tissue valves. Thromboemboli may be clinically silent but can result in a cerebrovascular accident, MI, renal failure, retinal infarction, or obstruction of peripheral arteries. The treatment of thromboemboli is adequate anticoagulation or, if persistent, valve replacement.

B. Hemolysis frequently occurs with the caged ball and some disk valves and normally is mild; it is less common with tissue valves. Care is generally supportive (e.g., administration of folate). Severe hemolysis may be a sign of significant dysfunction of the prosthesis.

C. Paravalvular leaks may occur with any type of prosthesis, especially if the annulus is abnormal. Extensive paravalvular leaks may not result in impressive murmurs despite severe heart failure. Thus, progressive heart failure in a patient with a prosthetic valve mandates investigation. Fluoroscopy and echocardiography are helpful, but Doppler studies are likely to be of more benefit. Cardiac catheterization may be required to evaluate heart failure when noninvasive studies fail to identify the problem. Surgical repair is indicated when paravalvular leaks precipitate heart failure.

D. Endocarditis (see Chap. 12) is the most common complication of prosthetic valves. During the first 2 months after surgery, the most common pathogens are *Staphylococcus epidermidis, Staphylococcus aureus,* gram-negative organisms, and *Candida.* The most common etiologies thereafter are *Streptococcus viridans, S. epidermidis, S. aureus,* and enterococcus. Endocarditis should be considered in the differential diagnosis whenever fever, heart failure, or systemic emboli occur in a patient with a prosthetic valve. The diagnosis is established with blood cultures. When endocarditis occurs in patients with prosthetic valves, early operative intervention should be considered, since cure with antibiotics alone is unusual.

E. Mechanical failure may occur due to thrombi, endothelial encroachment on the valve, or mechanical wear. Ball valves or disk valves develop changes in shape or restricted movement, whereas tissue valves may calcify, especially in children. Thromboemboli, severe hemolysis, heart failure, or auscultatory changes may be associated with mechanical failure. The treatment is valve replacement.

Aortic Dissection

I. Classification. Proximal aortic dissections involve the ascending aorta and arch and frequently are fatal. Distal dissections (beginning beyond the left subclavian artery) have lower complication and mortality rates.

II. Etiologies. Aortic dissections occur more commonly in men than women, occur in the sixth and seventh decade, and almost invariably are associated with hypertension. Cystic medial necrosis, Marfan's syndrome, Ehlers-Danlos syndrome, aortitis, vasculitis, and pregnancy are less common causes.

III. Clinical features

A. Symptoms. The pain of aortic dissection usually is severe and sudden in onset. Patients frequently are restless because the pain is typically tearing or ripping. Proximal dissections tend to radiate to the anterior thorax, neck, and jaw, whereas distal dissections tend to radiate posteriorly to the interscapular area. Nausea, vomiting, profuse diuresis, apprehension, and faintness are common.

Table 5-8. Drug dosages for acute management of aortic dissection

Drug	Route	Dosage	Comment
Propranolol	IV	1 mg over 1 min q5min prn to a maximum total dosage of 0.15 mg/kg	Titrate to heart rate of 60 beats/minute or systolic pressure of 110 mm Hg.
Nitroprusside	IV	Start infusion at 0.5 μg/kg/min; increase infusion 0.1–0.5 μg/kg/min q5min to desired effect	Titrate to systolic pressure of 100–120 mm Hg.
Trimethaphan	IV	Start infusion at 1 mg/min, and titrate to desired effect	Elevate head to 45-degree angle. Titrate to systolic pressure of 100–120 mm Hg.

   B. Physical examination. Physical findings are characteristically transient. Hypertension is generally present. Hypotension suggests dissection into the pericardium with tamponade, aortic rupture, or acute aortic valve regurgitation. Proximal dissection can be accompanied by pulse deficits, aortic valve regurgitation, neurologic deficits, or dissection of the coronary artery with infarction. The murmur of acute aortic regurgitation is short, harsh, and early diastolic. Central neurologic deficits are more common with proximal dissection; however, neurologic impairment of the spinal cord can occur with either proximal or distal dissections. Horner's syndrome or hoarseness can occur from nerve compression.
IV. Diagnostic studies. The chest x-ray may show widening of the mediastinum or the aortic arch, but the chest x-ray is not adequate for diagnosis. Echocardiography may be helpful in the detection of a proximal dissection, pericardial tamponade, and aortic regurgitation. The definitive study, however, is aortic angiography; in addition to confirming the diagnosis, angiography defines the site and extent of the dissection. CT scanning with contrast also is useful.
V. Management
   A. Medical Therapy. Patients with either type of dissection should be admitted to an intensive care unit. Pain should be relieved with morphine sulfate. The combination of nitroprusside and a beta-adrenergic blocker (Table 5-8) is the therapy of choice to reduce the systolic pressure to 100–120 mm Hg. Propranolol should be given IV until the heart rate is 60–80 beats/minute at the desired pressure. Less desirable alternatives include trimethaphan, reserpine, or alpha methyldopa. If trimethaphan is used, it may be necessary to place the patient at a 45-degree angle to control hypertension. Hydralazine and diazoxide are contraindicated because they induce a reflex tachycardia and increase shear stresses on the aorta. Patients should undergo aortic angiography after an attempt at stabilization. Medical therapy is superior for patients with uncomplicated distal dissections and patients with stable aortic dissections presenting 2 or more weeks after onset of symptoms.
   B. Surgical therapy. Urgent surgical intervention is required for the treatment of acute proximal dissections, since severe complications commonly accompany progression of the dissection. Surgery is indicated for distal dissections when vital organ function is compromised or progression occurs despite medical therapy.

Bibliography

1. Bates, R. J., et al. Cardiac rupture—challenge in diagnosis and management. *Am. J. Cardiol.* 40:429, 1977.
2. Canedo, M. I., Frank, M. J., and Abdulla, A. M. Rhythm disturbances in hypertrophic cardiomyopathy: Prevalence, relation to symptoms, and management. *Am. J. Cardiol.* 45:848, 1980.
3. Cohen, J. N., et al. Right ventricular infarction. Clinical and hemodynamic features. *Am. J. Cardiol.* 33:209, 1974.
4. Dalen, J. E., and Alpert, J. S. *Valvular Heart Disease.* Boston: Little, Brown, 1981.
5. Debusk, R. F., and Harrison, D. C. The clinical spectrum of papillary muscle disease. *N. Engl. J. Med.* 281:1458, 1969.
6. Doroghazi, R. M., et al. Long-term survival of patients with treated aortic dissection. *J. Am. Coll. Cardiol.* 3:1026, 1984.

7. Hancock, E. W. On the elastic and rigid forms of constrictive pericarditis. *Am. Heart J.* 100:917, 1980.
8. Hillis, L. D., and Braunwald, E. Myocardial ischemia. *N. Engl. J. Med.* 296:971, 1977.
9. Hillis, L. D., and Braunwald, E. Coronary artery spasm. *N. Engl. J. Med.* 299:695, 1977.
10. Johnson, R. A., and Palacios, I. Dilated cardiomyopathies of the adult. *N. Engl. J. Med.* 307:1051, 1982.
11. Lie, K. I., et al. Lidocaine in the prevention of primary ventricular fibrillation. A double-blind, randomized study of 212 consecutive patients. *N. Engl. J. Med.* 291:1324, 1974.
12. Lorell, B., et al. Right ventricular infarction. Clinical diagnosis and differentiation from cardiac tamponade and pericardial constriction. *Am. J. Cardiol.* 43:465, 1979.
13. Luchi, R. J., Chahine, R. A., and Raizner, A. E. Coronary artery spasm. *Ann. Intern. Med.* 91:441, 1979.
14. Oliva, P. B. Unstable angina with ST segment depression. Pathophysiologic considerations and therapeutic implications. *Ann. Intern. Med.* 100:424, 1984.
15. Sampson, J. J., and Cheitlen, M. D. Pathophysiology and differential diagnosis of cardiac pain. *Prog. Cardiovasc. Dis.* 13:507, 1971.
16. Sanders, C. A., et al. Etiology and differential diagnosis of acute mitral regurgitation. *Prog. Cardiovasc. Dis.* 14:129, 1971.
17. Smith, N. D., Raizada, V., and Abrams, J. Auscultation of the normally functioning prosthetic valve. *Ann. Intern. Med.* 95:594, 1981.
18. Spodick, D. H. Acute cardiac tamponade: Pathologic physiology, diagnosis, and management. *Prog. Cardiovasc. Dis.* 10:64, 1967.
19. Spodick, D. H. Differential diagnosis of acute pericarditis. *Prog. Cardiovasc. Dis.* 14:192, 1971.
20. Spodick, D. H. Pericardial rub: Prospective, multiple observer investigation of pericardial friction in 100 patients. *Am. J. Cardiol.* 35:357, 1975.
21. Stein, L., Shubin, H., and Weil, M. H. Recognition and management of pericardial tamponade. *J.A.M.A.* 225:503, 1973.
22. Stein, P. D., et al. The electrocardiogram in acute pulmonary embolism. *Prog. Cardiovasc. Dis.* 17:247, 1975.
23. Wigle, J. R., and LaGrosse, C. J. Sudden severe, aortic insufficiency. *Circulation* 32:708, 1965.

Hypertension

Victor N. Meltzer

Hypertension, arbitrarily defined as a diastolic blood pressure (BP) exceeding 90 mm Hg or a systolic BP greater than 160 mm Hg, afflicts more than 60,000,000 persons in the United States. Consequently, hypertension is not an uncommon finding in the emergency department, either as a process responsible for the patient's acute symptoms or unrelated to the presenting complaint. This wide spectrum of clinical presentation necessitates diverse approaches in management. Thus, it is important to consider the entire clinical picture, rather than solely the sphygmomanometer reading, in order to institute appropriate management of the hypertensive patient.

Hypertensive States and Related Problems

Because hypertension is generally an asymptomatic state, patients presenting to the emergency department do so because of (1) an unrelated medical or surgical problem, (2) an impending complication of the hypertensive state (hypertensive urgency), (3) a life-threatening complication related to the hypertension (hypertensive emergency), or (4) a symptom or sign caused by antihypertensive medication. To manage such patients appropriately, the emergency physician must determine from the clinical presentation which situation exists. This demands a careful evaluation, including a thorough history (including chart review), complete physical examination, and appropriate laboratory tests (generally, serum electrolytes and creatinine, urinalysis, electrocardiogram [ECG], and perhaps a chest x-ray). Emphasis should be directed toward determining whether the patient has labile or chronic hypertension, signs of end-organ damage (e.g., retinopathy, left ventricular hypertrophy), an impending or life-threatening complication of hypertension, or problems (including noncompliance) with antihypertensive medications.

I. **Hypertension unrelated to presenting symptoms.** While some patients experience headaches, dizziness, or epistaxis when their BP is elevated, such symptoms appear as commonly in the nonhypertensive population [38]. Thus, a causal relationship between hypertension and these symptoms should not necessarily be invoked. Moreover, many nonhypertensive patients with such symptoms temporarily become hypertensive in the emergency department milieu, probably as a result of the release of catecholamines and other endogenous pressors. Thus, a prior history of hypertension and signs of end-organ damage (e.g., retinopathy, left ventricular hypertrophy, azotemia) should be sought to distinguish patients with chronic hypertension from those with labile hypertension.

A. If **hypertension has not been documented** previously and there are no signs of chronic hypertension or significant risk for near-term complications (i.e., diastolic BP < 110 mm Hg and no evidence of underlying cardiovascular disease), the patient should receive appropriate treatment for the symptomatic condition and arrangements made for follow-up BP checks on an outpatient basis, beginning within 2 weeks if the diastolic BP is 100–109 mm Hg or within 2 months if the diastolic BP is 90–99 mm Hg, to determine whether the patient has chronic hypertension. However, patients with evidence of chronic hypertension (e.g., signs of end-organ damage) and those judged to be at high risk for near-term complications (i.e., patients with diastolic BP ≥ 110 mm Hg or underlying heart disease) should be considered candidates for initiation of oral antihypertensive drug therapy prior to discharge from the emergency department. See sec. **I.F** for principles of drug therapy.

B. For patients with **confirmed chronic hypertension** presenting with unrelated symptoms, attention should be directed toward factors known to correlate with increased risk of morbidity, that is, a diastolic BP ≥ 110 mm Hg or the presence of target organ damage (e.g., retinopathy, history of ischemic heart disease, left ventricular hypertrophy on the ECG, creatinine elevation, claudication, prior stroke, or transient ischemic attack). Patients at increased risk deserve more aggressive drug therapy (see sec. I.F) with more rapid (within 1 week) control of the BP than patients with mild hypertension. BP control for patients in this latter group may be achieved over several weeks using drug or nondrug therapy [27]. Hospitalization for control of chronic, uncomplicated hypertension is not generally required, but follow-up within 2 weeks should be arranged. Counselling by the physician will often reinforce the patient's understanding of hypertension and the drug regimen prescribed, thus enhancing compliance.

C. Some consideration of the **secondary causes of hypertension** is appropriate, although a thorough evaluation is usually reserved for a follow-up appointment. Emergency physicians should take special note of hypokalemia (suggestive of hyperaldosteronism, either primary from an adenoma or hyperplasia or secondary from diuretics or unilateral renal artery stenosis). Other findings suggestive of secondary hypertension include an abdominal bruit (renal artery stenosis), hypertension with orthostatic hypotension (pheochromocytoma), recurrent hypertension after years of good control (renal artery stenosis), and hypertension that is difficult to control despite compliance with medical therapy (renal artery stenosis). Grade III or IV hypertensive retinopathy plus a diastolic BP greater than 125 mm Hg has a high correlation with hypertension of renovascular origin [10]. Secondary hypertension may also result from the ingestion of various medications, including oral contraceptive agents, estrogens, sympathomimetics, steroids, nonsteroidal antiinflammatory agents, appetite suppressants, and tricyclic antidepressants; such agents also reduce the effectiveness of some antihypertensive drugs the patient may be taking. Discontinuance of such interfering substances may allow normalization of the BP without additional therapy.

D. **Systolic hypertension** (i.e., a systolic BP > 160 mm Hg with a diastolic BP < 90 mm Hg) is not uncommon in the elderly population, nor is it confined to this age group. The risk of cardiovascular and cerebrovascular complications is well documented, but the benefits of therapy are unproved [18]. Nonetheless, treatment is generally initiated when systolic hypertension is confirmed, with the goal of reducing the systolic BP below 160 mm Hg. Treatment usually should begin at a low dosage (half of usual) of a diuretic, beta-blocker, or prazosin. Careful surveillance for adverse effects is important, particularly before dosage increments.

E. **Pseudohypertension.** Some patients, particularly the elderly, manifest spuriously elevated sphygmomanometric readings due to sclerosed peripheral arteries, while the true intraarterial BP is normal or only mildly elevated (pseudohypertension) [33]. Drug therapy in such patients may produce intraarterial hypotension, characterized by dizziness and syncope; this entity should be considered when these symptoms develop on antihypertensive therapy. Pseudohypertension should be suspected when the pulseless brachial or radial artery remains palpable during proximal occlusion of the artery by the inflated BP cuff (so-called Osler's maneuver) [25]. Pseudohypertension is diagnosed by comparing sphygmomanometric readings with those obtained by intraarterial placement of a catheter attached to a pressure transducer. Other causes of dizziness and syncope in patients on antihypertensive drug therapy (e.g., volume depletion, arrhythmia, vasomotor syncope) should also be considered.

F. **General principles of antihypertensive therapy.** The approach to antihypertensive therapy ideally should be based on the pathophysiologic mechanisms generating the increased peripheral vascular resistance. Then the mechanism of the hypertension should be determined to be "sensitive" to the prescribed drug(s). Unfortunately, such information usually is not known. Thus, drug selection is often based on such considerations as incidence of and types of side effects, secondary benefits, ease of administration, and cost.

1. One approach is called **stepped-care,** an effective, empiric method by which therapy is initiated with a diuretic. If adequate BP control is not achieved, an antiadrenergic agent (e.g., beta-blocker, methyldopa, clonidine, guanabenz, reserpine) is added. If this combination fails to control the BP, a vasodilator (e.g., hydralazine, prazosin) is added. At each of these three steps, the dosage prescribed is increased until the BP is controlled, an adverse effect is encountered, or the maximum recommended dosage is tried.

2. **Newer concepts.** More recent data have emphasized the value of nondrug therapy [3, 19] and broadened the categories of drugs acceptable for initial antihypertensive therapy. Diuretics and beta-blockers have been shown to be of

nearly equal efficacy and safety as single-drug therapy in patients with mild hypertension. In addition, studies comparing prazosin or captopril with other "first-line" agents have shown the safety and effectiveness of such drugs as initial therapy for mild to moderate hypertension. Individual cases may have specific aspects that contraindicate a certain drug or display a potential for secondary benefits from a particular antihypertensive drug. Such considerations may make one drug more attractive than another. For further information regarding the outpatient management of hypertension, the reader is referred to recent reviews [11, 17].

II. **Hypertension with impending complications** (hypertensive urgency) requires prompt BP control within several hours to 1 day to avert potential morbid events. This category includes such conditions as a diastolic BP greater than 120 mm Hg without other acute complications, perioperative hypertension, preeclampsia, and malignant hypertension. This is in contrast to hypertension plus a life-threatening complication, such as a dissecting aortic aneurysm or hypertensive encephalopathy, which constitutes a hypertensive emergency and requires immediate, aggressive BP control (see sec. III). Since a distinction may not always be clear, clinical judgment must be applied. Hypertensive urgencies usually are handled with oral agents. Depending on the clinical situation, hospitalization may not be necessary in reliable patients. Prompt follow-up (within 7 days), however, is essential. Specific information regarding drug administration is found in the section on **Antihypertensive Agents.**

   A. **Severe but uncomplicated hypertension** qualifies as a hypertensive urgency. The diastolic BP exceeds 120 mm Hg, but signs of retinopathy, encephalopathy, or other conditions requiring immediate intervention are absent. While no emergency condition exists, these patients should receive prompt care to prevent impending complications. The goal is to achieve a diastolic BP of 100–110 mm Hg within 4–6 hours. Useful agents include clonidine or sublingual nifedipine. Failure to lower the diastolic BP to 110 mm Hg is sufficient indication to warrant hospitalization. Once the BP is adequately controlled, an appropriate outpatient regimen should be prescribed and follow-up provided within 7 days.

   B. **Hypertension in the perioperative setting** is generally a hypertensive urgency. Cardiac work and tension on vascular suture lines must be minimized. Hypertensive patients who require surgery should remain on their oral antihypertensive agents as long as possible. Diuretic-induced hypokalemia should be corrected preoperatively to avoid enhanced ventricular excitability. During the peri- and intraoperative periods, intravenously administered drugs like hydralazine, methyldopate, nitroprusside, or nitroglycerin may be required for control of the BP, due to both restricted oral intake and impaired absorption of oral agents following anesthesia. Phentolamine is the parenteral agent of choice for the perioperative control of hypertension due to a pheochromocytoma (see sec. II.G). Trimethaphan may prolong the anesthetic-induced delay in return of bladder and bowel function.

   C. **Azotemic patients** (see also sec. II.F). Hypertension in patients with chronic renal failure is a risk factor for further reduction in renal function and cardiovascular and cerebrovascular complications. Severe hypertension (i.e., a diastolic BP > 115 mm Hg) should be reduced gradually over a 24-hour period. For patients with a glomerular filtration rate (GFR) less than 20 ml/minute, this requires either close outpatient follow-up or hospitalization, because the GFR may transiently fall further while control of the BP is established; however, after several days of BP control, the GFR usually returns to the pretreatment level. Patients with a GFR above 20 ml/minute can be treated safely on an outpatient basis. An effective outpatient regimen often includes a combination of a diuretic, antiadrenergic drug, and vasodilator. Loop diuretics and potent drugs, such as captopril and minoxidil, may be needed. Agents that reduce renal blood flow (RBF) (e.g., reserpine, guanethidine) should be avoided, while those that maintain it (e.g., clonidine, captopril, methyldopa, prazosin, hydralazine, minoxidil) are preferred. Beta-blockers have been demonstrated to produce variable effects on RBF but generally are thought to be safe for azotemic patients [37]. However, captopril may impair the function of a solitary kidney supplied by a stenosed renal artery [9, 15].

   D. **Hypertension in hemodialysis patients** is usually volume-dependent, that is, responsive to removal of excess extracellular fluid by ultrafiltration. However, a near-normal BP is desirable prior to heparinization for dialysis. Thus, patients with a predialysis diastolic BP greater than 120 mm Hg generally should be given a rapidly acting antihypertensive agent, preferably one with a short duration of action. Either hydralazine, 5–10 mg IV, repeated in 20–30 minutes if needed, or nifedipine, 10–20 mg sublingually, usually will reduce the BP rapidly and still allow fluid removal without drug-induced hypotension during the dialytic process. This approach may also effect temporary correction of non-volume-dependent hypertension in hemodialysis patients. Thus, the factors generating the hypertensive state need not be known prior to giving hydralazine or nifedipine. However, elective evaluation to establish the etiology of the hypertension may be indicated.

E. Preeclampsia (see Chap. 33).

    1. Clinical features. Hypertension in pregnancy is diagnosed if the BP exceeds 140/90 mm Hg, or the systolic or diastolic BP rises by more than 30 mm Hg or 15 mm Hg, respectively. The hypertension may be pregnancy-induced or chronic due to underlying essential hypertension, endocrinopathy, or renal disease [6, 12]. Preeclampia refers to the hypertensive state, which may be associated with nondependent edema and/or proteinuria. Preliminary data on the mechanism of preeclampsia implicate a decrement in plasma volume [13], perhaps due to abnormally "leaky" capillaries and glomeruli, resulting in interstitial edema formation and proteinuria, respectively. According to this scenario, hypertension follows because of hyperreactivity of the abnormal vasculature to compensatory circulating pressors. Primigravidas and women with prior hypertension are at increased risk for the development of preeclampsia. Maternal diastolic hypertension is associated with increased infant mortality [21, 29] and maternal morbidity.

    2. Management of hypertension in pregnancy is somewhat controversial. Patients with a diastolic BP of 90–100 mm Hg generally should be admitted for bed rest and observation. Those with a diastolic BP over 100 mm Hg should be admitted, placed at bed rest, and perhaps given oral antihypertensive drug therapy. Methyldopa, hydralazine, propranolol, metoprolol, and atenolol are effective agents, although their use is not universally recommended [32]. Diuretics should probably be avoided, particularly if hypovolemia and placental hypoperfusion are factors in the pathogenesis of preeclampsia. In animal studies, captopril and clonidine appear to induce fetal death and embryopathy, respectively; both should be avoided. The role of therapeutic intravascular volume expansion in preeclampsia is under investigation but cannot be recommended at present. **Magnesium sulfate** ($MgSO_4$) is given (see sec. **III.F.2.b**) if mental status abnormalities develop or diastolic BP exceeds 110 mm Hg. $MgSO_4$ inhibits labor and prevents seizures. These actions may be associated with a mild decline in BP, but $MgSO_4$ should not be considered an antihypertensive agent. Near-term patients are candidates for induction and delivery. Patients in whom the medical approach fails to achieve an adequate response (establishment of diastolic BP $\leq$ 90 mm Hg) become candidates for delivery, regardless of fetal maturity. During labor and delivery, maternal and fetal monitoring are instituted. If maternal diastolic BP exceeds 105 mm Hg, hydralazine (5-mg IV boluses) should probably be given [22]. Resistant hypertension usually responds to diazoxide (30-mg IV boluses). Nitroprusside may be associated with fetal cyanide toxicity and is best avoided.

F. Malignant hypertension

    1. Clinical features. The **diagnosis** of malignant hypertension is established by the combination of severe hypertension (generally a diastolic BP > 120 mm Hg) and fresh hemorrhages and/or papilledema on funduscopy. The vasculopathy, characterized by fibrinoid necrosis involving small arterioles, leads to renal insufficiency. Renin levels are extremely high but need not be measured. While most cases represent progression of poorly controlled essential hypertension [31], consideration must be given to potential secondary causes of malignant hypertension, such as scleroderma and other collagen-vascular diseases involving the kidneys, renovascular hypertension, pheochromocytoma, and acute or subacute glomerulonephritis.

    2. Pertinent **laboratory tests** include a complete blood count (CBC), urinalysis, serum creatinine and electrolytes, an ECG, and chest x-ray. Subsequently, tests to exclude secondary forms of hypertension may be indicated.

    3. Management

        a. Prompt BP control. The BP should be promptly reduced using an oral agent, if possible. Clonidine loading may be the best choice (see **Antihypertensive Agents**, sec. **I.A**), although captopril, labetalol, and nifedipine have been used successfully. Oral agents such as these may be used if the patient is alert and not vomiting. Alternatively, nitroprusside, diazoxide, labetalol, reserpine, or hydralazine can be given but is seldom required.

b. **Bed rest and salt restriction.** Patients should be hospitalized and placed at bed rest on a low-salt diet (i.e., 6–8 gm of NaCl daily).

c. **Potassium repletion.** The hyperreninemia of malignant hypertension generates secondary hyperaldosteronism with subsequent kaliuresis. Thus, patients frequently will require potassium supplementation. This must be given carefully in the face of chronic renal insufficiency. The serum potassium concentration should be followed until a safe level is established.

d. **Oral antihypertensive therapy.** If a parenteral antihypertensive agent is used initially, the change to oral therapy should begin as soon as the BP is brought under control and the patient can tolerate oral medication. This usually involves the combination of a diuretic (i.e., a thiazide if the GFR is > 30 ml/minute, furosemide or bumetanide if the GFR is < 30 ml/minute), an antiadrenergic drug (i.e., a beta-blocker, clonidine, or methyldopa), and a vasodilator (i.e., hydralazine, prazosin, or minoxidil). Alternatively, patients may be controlled with captopril plus a diuretic. Nifedipine has been useful in combination therapy as well.

e. Bilateral nephrectomies are rarely required for control of malignant hypertension now that highly potent antihypertensive drugs are available. That operation may be indicated for seriously hypertensive, high-renin dialysis patients who desire renal transplantation.

4. **Course.** A transient decline in GFR may follow rapid BP lowering, perhaps due to renal hypoperfusion. This generally resolves spontaneously over several days and should not deter efforts to achieve good BP control. However, other causes of renal insufficiency should also be considered, such as dehydration from overdiuresis, congestive heart failure due to cardiodepression from ischemic heart disease or beta-blockade, captopril-induced hypoperfusion of a single kidney having a stenosed renal artery [9], or interstitial nephritis secondary to allopurinol, antibiotics, or nonsteroidal anti-inflammatory agents. The retinal abnormalities of malignant hypertension usually resolve after 1–2 weeks of good BP control.

G. **Pheochromocytoma**

1. **Clinical features.** A pheochromocytoma may present with mild to severe hypertension and subtle clinical clues, such as orthostatic hypotension, nervousness, palpitations, headaches, nausea, vomiting, sweating, a tachycardia, and cool extremities. The hypertension results primarily from norepinephrine secretion and may be absent in patients with tumors secreting primarily epinephrine.

2. **Evaluation.** Measuring the urinary excretion of cathecholamines and their metabolites has been the standard diagnostic approach. However, serum catecholamine levels, particularly when drawn under rigidly controlled conditions, may be diagnostic [4]. A CT scan is useful for anatomic localization. The clonidine suppression test [5] may be useful.

3. **Management** involves control of the BP by alpha-blockade in preparation for surgical removal of the tumor.

a. **Parenteral therapy. Phentolamine** (Regitine), 5 mg IV, is the agent of choice for control of hypertensive episodes. However, orthostatic hypotension and tachyarrhythmias can result from blockade of alpha-2 receptors. Nitroprusside is also effective, but alpha-blockade is more physiologically appropriate in view of the norepinephrine-based mechanism. Beta-blockade can be accomplished with any of several agents to prevent or attenuate the tachycardia and tachyarrhythmias that may ensue from nonspecific alpha-blockade and endogenous catecholamine excess; however beta-blockade should only be given after alpha-blockade has been established to avoid unopposed alpha-induced vasoconstriction that will exacerbate the hypertension.

b. **Oral therapy. Oral phenoxybenzamine,** 10–20 mg tid–qid, is useful for alpha-blockade in patients awaiting surgical removal of pheochromocytoma and in patients with hypertension from nonresectable tumors. Prazosin, 2–5 mg bid–qid, may also be used in the preoperative management of patients with pheochromocytoma [28]. Although alpha-methyl-tyrosine is not available in the United States, it has been used successfully in other countries for control of hypertension and symptoms associated with pheochromocytoma; the drug inhibits catecholamine synthesis.

H. Clonidine withdrawal hypertension may mimic pheochromocytoma in presentation, symptoms, and blood and urine catecholamine levels. In addition, abrupt discontinuance of other antihypertensive agents may produce a similar syndrome, characterized by marked hypertension. **Management** with reinstitution of clonidine is usually sufficient for control of the blood pressure, although phentolamine or nitroprusside may also be used. Patient reeducation should be provided or another drug substituted.

I. Patients with **severe burns** or acute **quadriplegia** may develop severe hypertension, although the pathophysiologic mechanisms are uncertain. Although such patients are acutely ill from the burn or injury, the severe hypertension may also become a serious condition. Nitroprusside or diazoxide is effective in these patients. Oral clonidine loading may also be used.

III. Hypertension plus a related life-threatening complication (hypertensive emergency) requires immediate, aggressive control of the BP and appropriate treatment of the complication. Drugs selected to reduce the BP (see **Antihypertensive Agents),** however, should not interfere with the assessment or therapy of the associated problem. Hypertensive emergencies generally occur in patients with chronic hypertension. Some complications (e.g., encephalopathy) occur as a direct result of the hypertension, whereas others (e.g., acute myocardial infarction) occur in association with underlying vascular disease produced by the hypertension and other factors. Patients with hypertension plus one of these complications require hospitalization, preferably in an intensive care unit.

A. Hypertensive encephalopathy

1. **Clinical features.** Hypertensive encephalopathy usually develops in patients with underlying malignant hypertension; thus, the retinal findings of malignant hypertension usually are present. Diffuse cerebral dysfunction is prominent, as manifest by confusion, seizures, stupor, or coma. A headache is usually present, and transient focal neurologic deficits may occur. A diastolic BP greater than 130 mm Hg is typical. Pulmonary edema is not uncommon.

2. The **pathophysiology** of hypertensive encephalopathy is not completely understood but appears to involve autoregulatory failure by damaged arterioles in the brain, allowing leakage of plasma components through arterial walls with generation of cerebral edema.

3. **The differential diagnosis** includes thrombotic or hemorrhagic stroke, an intracranial mass lesion, uremic encephalopathy, and drug intoxication. The gradual onset of hypertensive encephalopathy over 24–48 hours helps distinguish it from an acute cerebrovascular event.

4. **Evaluation.** In addition to the laboratory tests recommended for malignant hypertension (see sec. **II.F**), a CT scan of the head is useful in eliminating primary neurologic disorders. A lumbar puncture usually is not required, unless neck stiffness or fever is present.

5. **Management.** Hospitalization is mandatory, as the disease can be fatal in the absence of aggressive care. Prompt reduction of the BP takes precedence over investigation into the etiology (e.g., essential hypertension, glomerulonephritis, renal artery stenosis, pheochromocytoma). **Parenteral agents must be used.** However, drugs that alter the mental status (e.g., methyldopa, reserpine) or impair left ventricular function (e.g., beta-blockers) should be avoided. Diazoxide is the simplest to administer and may obviate the need for subsequent intensive-care-unit monitoring. Alternatively, nitroprusside or trimethaphan is effective and may also be considered a drug of choice. The diastolic BP should be reduced to about 100 mm Hg within 30–60 minutes.

6. **Prognosis.** The entire clinical picture resolves following BP control, although renal function frequently remains abnormal due to underlying renal damage present prior to the encephalopathic episode. If the mental status fails to improve with BP control, the diagnosis must be questioned. A trial of dialysis may be required to exclude uremic encephalopathy in patients with a GFR less than 10 ml/minute.

B. Hypertension plus a hemorrhagic stroke (see Chap. 32).

1. **Clinical features.** This combination generally presents as a severe headache and rapid neurologic deterioration. Anatomically, the bleeding is intracerebral or subarachnoid. Intracerebral bleeds tend to originate from aneurysms of the striate arteries and occur almost exclusively in hypertensive persons. Subarachnoid bleeds occur from Berry aneurysms (sometimes associated with polycystic

kidney disease or coarctation of the aorta) or from vascular malformations (angiomas). Small bleeds may be clinically indistinguishable from thrombotic strokes. Nuchal rigidity suggests blood in the cerebrospinal fluid.

2. **Evaluation.** Laboratory studies should include a CBC, urinalysis, serum creatinine and electrolytes, coagulation profile, chest x-ray, and ECG. A CT scan of the head and spinal fluid examination are useful in confirming the diagnosis. Angiography may be required and should differentiate vascular malformations from aneurysmal bleeds.

3. **Management.** Patients with hemorrhagic strokes, either intracerebral or subarachnoid, require intensive-care monitoring, neurologic or neurosurgical consultation, and frequent neurologic examinations. Although controversial, reduction of the diastolic BP to 100–110 mm Hg generally is accepted. The drug of choice for BP control is **nitroprusside,** which can be titrated to achieve the appropriate BP level. Drugs that depress the sensorium (e.g., reserpine, methyldopate) or may cause excessive hypotension (e.g., diazoxide) should be avoided. Trimethaphan generally is not used, because patients frequently are unable to remain in the head-up position required for maximum effectiveness of ganglionic blockade. Fluid intake should be minimized in the euvolemic patient to avoid increasing the intracranial pressure. Further details regarding management can be found in Chap. 32.

C. **Pulmonary edema** (see Chap. 5) may be precipitated or exacerbated by systemic hypertension. Correction of the hypertension alone may be adequate to restore the cardiac output when left ventricular function is not seriously impaired. A reduced cardiac output associated with systemic hypertension (i.e., an elevated total peripheral resistance) responds well to afterload reduction through vasodilator therapy. However, vasodilators should be used cautiously or be avoided in patients with left ventricular outflow obstruction (e.g., aortic valvular stenosis, idiopathic hypertrophic subaortic stenosis).

1. **Acute management.** Initially, the usual measures for treating pulmonary edema should be instituted (see Chap. 5). Tests to exclude acute myocardial infarction are usually indicated. Persistent hypertension, particularly in the absence of significant clinical improvement, demands aggressive vasodilator therapy and restoration of a normal BP. The most effective antihypertensive vasodilator is **nitroprusside,** which dilates both the arterial and venous systems, thus reducing afterload and preload, respectively; the dose is titrated according to the clinical and hemodynamic response. Trimethaphan can be used if nitroprusside is contraindicated or unavailable. **Nitroglycerin** IV is a potent venodilator with a mild to moderate afterload reducing effect; it may be used in combination with nitroprusside, with careful hemodynamic monitoring, or it may be adequate as the sole antihypertensive agent. It is of special value when myocardial ischemia is also present. Phentolamine produces tachycardia and adverse gastrointestinal symptoms; it should be avoided. Since diazoxide and hydralazine cause fluid retention, an enhanced heart rate, and increased myocardial contractility, they should also be avoided. Amrinone, which possesses inotropic and mixed vasodilator properties, may find a place in the armamentarium for treating this hypertensive emergency.

   Hypertensive patients requiring **intubation** deserve very close BP monitoring. The BP may drop significantly within minutes following intubation, perhaps because the patient calms and sympathetic outflow is reduced. This may necessitate a prompt reduction in the dosage of antihypertensive agent administered to avoid drug-induced hypotension.

2. **Disposition.** Hospitalization is warranted. Hemodynamic monitoring in an intensive care unit is indicated if there is associated myocardial ischemia or infarction or if the patient has an inadequate response to the therapy instituted in the emergency department.

3. **Chronic management.** Orally administered vasodilators generally are effective in the management of pulmonary edema–prone patients on a chronic basis. Useful agents include nitrates, hydralazine, prazosin, captopril, nifedipine, and minoxidil. Labetalol and pindolol may also be useful. The addition of a diuretic is usually required, and the serum potassium should be kept within normal limits. Although nitrates are effective venodilators, they will control systemic hypertension of only the mildest degree. Arteriolar vasodilators should be avoided in patients with significant left ventricular outflow obstruction.

D. Dissecting aortic aneurysm (see Chap. 5) is a potentially lethal complication of hypertension, requiring astute diagnostic acumen and a coordinated team approach for successful management [39].

1. **Clinical features.** Patients usually have a history of hypertension unless another predisposing cause is present (e.g., Marfan's syndrome, third trimester of pregnancy, blunt chest trauma). The most prominent feature is usually severe pain in the chest, abdomen, or back. Other symptoms and signs are usually the result of impaired vascular supply to the brain, heart, abdominal viscera, and/or extremities due to the dissection. In addition, aortic valvular insufficiency may develop, producing a diastolic murmur; cardiac tamponade may occur, with resultant hypotension and dyspnea.

2. **Diagnostic evaluation.** Although chest x-ray, echocardiography, and CT scanning are useful, aortography is the definitive study to establish the diagnosis. It should be undertaken once the patient is stabilized and the BP is controlled. In addition, an acute myocardial infarction should be ruled in or out, particularly for proximal dissections (i.e., those originating proximal to the left subclavian artery).

3. **Management** requires prompt BP control prior to diagnostic maneuvers. The treatment of choice is either **trimethaphan** or the combination of **nitroprusside plus beta-blockade.** Both regimens are of approximately equal effectiveness. Morphine may be required for pain relief. Constant monitoring of the vital signs, urine output, mental status, and peripheral pulses is required. The BP should be reduced to the minimum level that allows adequate tissue perfusion (i.e., ideally a systolic BP of 100–110 mm Hg). Dissections involving the aortic root are best treated surgically, while those distal to the left subclavian artery usually can be treated medically. However, surgery is indicated for distal dissections in which the hematoma progresses despite medical therapy. Further details on management can be found in Chap. 5.

E. Angina or myocardial infarction (see Chap. 5) will be exacerbated by hypertension, as the increased afterload augments myocardial oxygen demand [34]. The precise effect of hypertension on the extent of myocardial necrosis is uncertain, but it is likely that control of the hypertension will salvage some jeopardized myocardium. Reduction of hypertension should be undertaken with an agent that can be carefully and quickly titrated. **Nitroprusside** or **trimethaphan** is the agent of choice. Intravenous nitroglycerin may also be useful, especially when congestive heart failure is present. Hydralazine should be avoided, as it tends to increase the heart rate and myocardial contractility (both of which increase the myocardial oxygen requirement). Diazoxide should be avoided for similar reasons, as well as the fact that hypotension may occur and exacerbate coronary insufficiency. Oral antihypertensive agents that may be useful after the BP has been brought under control include beta-blockers, which offer antiarrhythmic actions and appear to reduce the risk of reinfarction and sudden death, and those calcium-channel blockers that reduce the BP (e.g., nifedipine).

F. Eclampsia (see Chap. 33).

1. **Clinical features.** Eclampsia is an emergency condition characterized by hypertension in pregnancy (see sec. **II.E**) and seizures or coma. The neurologic features may represent a form of hypertensive encephalopathy. Proteinuria is present, and azotemia may develop.

2. **Management.** Obstetric consultation should be obtained.

   a. The patient is kept NPO, and **fetal monitoring** is begun.

   b. **Magnesium sulfate** ($MgSO_4$), 4 gm, is given IV and followed by a maintenance dosage of 1–3 gm/hour IV. The deep-tendon reflexes, respirations, and serum magnesium levels are assessed as measures of magnesium toxicity.

   c. **The urine output** is carefully monitored. If oliguria develops, Swan-Ganz catheter measurements may be required to assess the adequacy of the intravascular volume. Oliguria, despite both an adequate intravascular volume and cardiac output, is an indication for prompt delivery.

   d. **Hypertension** (diastolic BP > 105 mm Hg) is treated with **hydralazine** IV or IM, with monitoring of the BP q5minutes. Following a 5-mg test dose, 5–10 mg is given q20minutes until a diastolic BP of 90–100 mm Hg is reached. Failure of hydralazine to control the BP also indicates the need for prompt delivery, regardless of fetal maturity. Diazoxide given in 30-mg IV boluses is often useful in patients resistant to hydralazine.

   e. **Prompt delivery** of the fetus is essential. Following delivery, the BP gradually returns to normal; however, methyldopa or hydralazine may be useful in the interim. MgSO$_4$ should be continued as 5 gm IM q6h for 36 hours after delivery. Neurotoxic signs must still be monitored.

Antihypertensive Agents

Therapeutic agents that are useful in the emergency department setting are briefly summarized below. For more information on oral antihypertensive agents and their use in nonemergency and nonurgent BP control, the reader is referred to other sources [11, 17].

I. **Oral agents** can be used when immediate BP reduction is not critical, the patient is awake and alert, drug absorption is expected to be normal, and precise titration to a specific BP level is not critical.

    A. **Clonidine (Catapres)** is a centrally acting alpha-agonist that produces its hypotensive effect within 1 hour and its peak effect in 2–4 hours [23]. Clonidine loading has been effective in reducing the BP over 4–6 hours when given as 0.2 mg PO followed hourly by 0.1 mg until the BP is controlled (i.e., a diastolic BP of 100–110 mm Hg is obtained) or the patient has received a total dose of 0.7–0.9 mg [1, 36]. In most patients, BP control can be achieved within 4 hours. After the last dose, a further decline in the diastolic BP of 10–15 mm Hg over the ensuing 1–2 hours generally is seen and should be anticipated. The total required dose generally can be divided by three and administered q8h along with a diuretic for maintenance outpatient BP control. Patients thus treated should be seen for follow-up within 1 week, as dose titration may be required. **Side effects** include sedation, drowsiness, a dry mouth, and orthostatic hypotension. Sudden discontinuance of therapy may result in rebound hypertension, which can be marked. Patients should be warned about this.

    B. **Nifedipine (Procardia)** is a calcium-channel blocker with vasodilating effects. Although not currently approved by the FDA as an antihypertensive agent, it promptly reduces the BP in many hypertensive patients after sublingual administration [2, 24]. A 10-mg capsule is punctured and the contents emptied under the patient's tongue. The fall in BP correlates with the pretreatment BP, with higher levels responding with greater declines. The effect is seen within 5 minutes, peaks in about 30 minutes, and may last up to several hours. The oral route (10–30 mg tid–qid) is also effective, although it is slower and has a less marked hypotensive effect. As a mixed (arterial and venous) vasodilator, nifedipine may be particularly useful in the management of hypertensive heart failure, hypertension plus angina pectoris, and hypertension in patients undergoing hemodialysis. **Side effects** include flushing, dizziness, headache, rash, edema, and palpitations.

    C. **Captopril (Capoten)** is an angiotensin-converting-enzyme inhibitor that also has additional mechanisms implicated in its antihypertensive actions [41]. A prompt decline in BP usually follows a 25-mg dose in patients with renin-dependent hypertension. However, the renin dependency of hypertension is not usually known to the emergency department physician, thus limiting the usefulness of this approach. The drug should be avoided in pregnancy, based on laboratory animal studies demonstrating reduced placental perfusion and increased fetal wastage. A reduction in the GFR following institution of captopril therapy may indicate nephrotoxicity or underlying bilateral renal artery stenoses or arterial stenosis to a solitary kidney [9, 15].

II. **Parenteral agents** should be used when immediate BP lowering is required or the oral route cannot be relied on. Some agents require intensive-care-unit monitoring and thus carry substantial additional costs and personnel requirements; thus, other agents should be used when possible.

    A. **Hydralazine (Apresoline)** is a potent direct arterial vasodilator, given IM or IV. The initial dosage is 5–10 mg, which can be repeated at 20- to 30-minute intervals up to 40 mg. It is inexpensive and usually effective. **Drawbacks** include an unpredictable magnitude of the hypotensive response, a reflex tachycardia (which can be attenuated by beta-blockade), and fluid retention (which can be minimized by concomitant diuretic administration). Because of these adverse effects, hydralazine should be avoided in patients with coronary artery disease or a dissecting aortic aneurysm.

    B. **Diazoxide (Hyperstat)** is a direct arterial vasodilator.

        1. **Dosage.** Diazoxide usually is administered as a 300-mg bolus by rapid IV push. The BP is monitored at 5- to 10-minute intervals for the first 30–60 minutes and q15minutes until it stabilizes [20]. If hypertension recurs or the desired BP

is not attained, another 300-mg dose may be given after 30 minutes. Alternatively, particularly in patients with other antihypertensive agents on board, diazoxide may be given in doses of 150 mg instead of 300 mg. This may avoid drug-induced hypotension, which can aggravate or precipitate coronary or cerebral insufficiency in predisposed patients. This risk may also be reduced by continuously infusing the drug slowly IV; clinical experience with this technique is limited, and it offers little advantage over nitroprusside. Oral agents should be started when the diastolic BP is less than 110 mm Hg and the patient is stable.

  2. **Side effects.** As with hydralazine, the heart rate and cardiac output rise. However, the addition of a beta-blocker will limit these effects. In addition, a diuretic (e.g., furosemide, 20–80 mg, or bumetanide, 0.5–2.0 mg) should be given to combat fluid retention. Since the medication has a pH of 11.6, care must be taken not to allow it to extravasate. Drug-induced hyperglycemia and hyperuricemia have been reported. Because of the drug-induced tachycardia and increased cardiac output, diazoxide should not be used in patients with coronary insufficiency or a dissecting aortic aneurysm.

C. **Nitroprusside (Nipride)** is a mixed (arterial and venous) vasodilator useful in most hypertensive emergencies, particularly because of its immediate but short-lived antihypertensive effect [8, 30].

  1. **Dosage.** A solution of nitroprusside is prepared by placing 50 mg in 500 ml (100 μg/ml) or in 250 ml (200 μg/ml) of 5% D/W and shielding it from light. The initial dosage is 0.5 μg/kg/minute by infusion pump, which is essential to avoid infusion failure or bolus infusion. Since the BP must be followed continuously, intensive-care-unit monitoring is advised. The dosage may be progressively increased to a maximum of 10 μg/kg/minute, although the average dosage required is 3 μg/kg/minute. Since the BP will promptly rise upon cessation of therapy, oral agents should be initiated as soon as possible.

  2. **Toxicity.** Nitroprusside combines with sulfhydryl groups in red blood cells to release cyanide, which is metabolized in the liver to thiocyanate for subsequent renal excretion. **Thiocyanate toxicity** (manifested by tinnitus, blurred vision, and delirium) may result from prolonged (i.e., exceeding 5 days) infusion, excessive doses, or renal or hepatic insufficiency. In patients at risk, plasma thiocyanate levels should be monitored and kept under 10 mg/dl. In addition, the appearance of a metabolic acidosis may indicate the development of **cyanide toxicity** (see Chap. 16), which is not detected by thiocyanate levels. Should a metabolic acidosis appear, another drug should be instituted in lieu of nitroprusside and nitrites administered to promote formation of methemoglobin, which will free cytochrome oxidase from cyanide; sodium thiosulfate, 12.5 gm in 50 ml of 5% D/W is then given IV over 10 minutes to serve as a substrate for the conversion of cyanide to sodium thiocyanate by rhodanese in the liver.

D. **Trimethaphan (Arfonad)** is a potent ganglionic blocker with a rapid onset and short duration of action (1–2 minutes). The drug reduces the BP as well as the cardiac output and left ventricular ejection rate. Since the major antihypertensive effect is posture-dependent, patients should be treated sitting up in bed if possible. A 500-mg ampule is diluted in 500 ml of 5% D/W and infused continuously by infusion pump at an initial rate of 1 mg/minute (or 1 ml/minute). The dosage can be increased as needed to a maximum rate of 6 mg/minute. As with nitroprusside, the BP must be monitored closely. **Side effects** are those of parasympathetic blockade (e.g., paralytic ileus, urinary retention, mydriasis) and intravascular volume expansion that opposes the drug's hypotensive action. A diuretic (e.g., furosemide, 20–80 mg, or bumetanide, 0.5–2.0 mg) can be given IV to restore the hypotensive effect.

E. **Nitroglycerine** (intravenous) is a potent venodilator with mild to moderate arteriolar dilating effects. It is finding acceptance as an effective agent for controlling hypertension intra- and perioperatively and in patients with hypertension plus angina, myocardial infarction, or pulmonary edema [14, 16]. The usual dosage is 10–200 μg/minute. The onset of action is within 5 minutes. Because it is supplied in an ethanol diluent, high doses may produce alcohol intoxication [35]. **Side effects** include tachycardia, flushing, headache, and methemoglobinemia.

F. **Phentolamine (Regitine)** is a nonspecific alpha-blocker that is particularly useful in controlling the hypertension of catecholamine excess secondary to pheochromocytoma, clonidine withdrawal, or tyramine ingestion in patients on monoamine oxidase inhibitors. A 5-mg dose is given IV or IM and may be repeated q5–10 minutes as needed. The effect of a single bolus lasts only 15–20 minutes. An oral form (50-

Table 6-1. Adverse effects of oral antihypertensive drugs*

Sign or Symptom	Drug	Sign or Symptom	Drug
Anemia (hemolytic)	Methyldopa	Hypertension	See Withdrawal syndrome
Angina	Hydralazine, abrupt discontinuance of beta-blockers	Hypokalemia	Diuretics
		Hyponatremia	Diuretics
Asthma	Beta-blockers	Hypotension (postural)	Prazosin, guanethidine, methyldopa, hydralazine
AV block	Beta-blockers, verapamil plus digoxin		
		Impotence	Diuretics, guanethidine, methyldopa, clonidine, beta-blockers
Bradycardia	Beta-blockers		
Congestive heart failure	Beta-blockers		
Claudication	Beta-blockers	Lethargy	Methyldopa, clonidine
Cold extremities	Beta-blockers	Lupus	Hydralazine
		Myalgia	Diuretics, hydralazine, beta-blockers
Confusion	Clonidine		
Constipation	Clonidine	Pericardial effusion	Minoxidil
Depression	Reserpine		
Diarrhea	Methyldopa	Rash	Captopril, hydralazine
Dry mouth	Methyldopa, clonidine	Raynaud's phenomenon	Beta-blockers
Edema	Minoxidil, Nifedipine		
Fatigue (especially with exercise)	Beta-blockers	Sedation	Methyldopa, clonidine
		Sleep disturbance	Beta-blockers, especially if lipid-soluble
Fever	Methyldopa, hydralazine		
		Syncope	Prazosin (especially after first dose), any antihypertensive agent in patients with pseudo-hypertension
Gout	Diuretics		
Hepatitis	Methyldopa		
Hirsutism	Minoxidil		
Hypercalcemia	Thiazides		
Hyperglycemia	Thiazides		
Hyperkalemia	Spironolactone, triamterene, amiloride, beta-blockers, captopril	Tachycardia	Diuretics, hydralazine, minoxidil
		Withdrawal syndrome	Clonidine, methyldopa, beta-blockers, minoxidil

*This list is not meant to be all-inclusive. Additional signs and symptoms, as well as additional drugs, may be found in more detailed texts.

mg tablets) may be given 4–6 times daily. **Side effects** include tachyarrhythmias, orthostatic dizziness, flushing, and gastrointestinal distress. These limit its application to the above settings.

    G. **Methyldopate (Aldomet)**, the ethyl ester of methyldopa, is given by IV infusion. A dosage of 250–500 mg is added to 100 ml of 5% D/W, infused over 30–60 minutes, and repeated q6h. The drug requires decarboxylation in the central nervous system for activation, thus delaying the onset of action by 4–6 hours. **Adverse effects** include sedation, headache, dizziness, and an occasional paradoxical pressor response. Because it alters the mental status, methyldopate should be avoided in patients with hypertensive encephalopathy and hemorrhagic or thrombotic stroke.

    H. **Reserpine (Serpasil)**, 1–5 mg IM, is convenient and produces its effect in 2–3 hours. However, it depresses the sensorium and may obscure the neurologic evaluation.

   I. Other parenteral agents may be of value but have had little clinical testing in hypertensive emergencies. They may not be adequate when used alone but may add to the effectiveness of another agent. In the future, some may prove useful in certain clinical situations.

      1. **Verapamil (Calan, Isoptin),** a calcium-channel blocker, is useful in treating supraventricular tachyarrhythmias and has mild antihypertensive action. It may be of value in select situations, such as moderate hypertension plus angina pectoris or moderate hypertension plus a supraventricular tachyarrhythmia. Because it depresses myocardial contractility and slows atrioventricular (AV) conduction, it should be avoided in patients with left ventricular dysfunction and patients on beta-blockers or digoxin. A dosage of 5–10 mg IV over 1–2 minutes produces a hypotensive effect within 3–5 minutes, but the effect lasts only about 60 minutes.

      2. **Propranolol (Inderal)** is a nonspecific beta-blocker, useful when combined with nitroprusside in the treatment of a dissecting aortic aneurysm. It is given IV in a dosage of 1 mg over 1–2 minutes. The onset of action is within 30 minutes. It can be repeated q15minutes as needed to a maximum dosage of 0.15 mg/kg to keep the heart rate at 55–70/minute. The purpose of the drug in this situation is to reduce the cardiac output and aortic shearing force (torque). It should be avoided in patients with heart failure, AV block, obstructive lung disease, or bradycardia.

      3. **Labetalol (Normodyne, Trandate),** has alpha-1 plus nonspecific beta-adrenergic receptor blocking activity, thus functioning as a vasodilator [26]. Preliminary experience suggests that it may be useful in some hypertensive emergencies when given as a series of miniboluses (i.e., 20 mg, followed by doubling of the bolus size up to 80 mg) at 10-minute intervals until the BP is controlled or a maximum dosage of 400 mg is given [40]. The average total dose required is 200 mg. **Adverse effects** include hypotension, nausea, vomiting, paresthesias, and flushing. Patients should be supine for at least 2 hours after the last dose to avoid orthostatic hypotension.

III. Adverse effects of antihypertensive agents. Patients may present to the emergency department with a symptom or sign related to an adverse effect of an oral antihypertensive drug. Some of the more common adverse effects attributed to oral antihypertensive agents are listed in Table 6-1. When an adverse effect is suspected, the physician must decide whether a dosage reduction is indicated or a different medication should be substituted for the current agent. Traditional treatment of the symptom may also be indicated. In addition, it is important to consider that a cause other than the drug may account for the patient's symptom, despite the fact that the drug may be associated with that particular symptom. For example, many drugs are associated with impotence, but psychologic factors may be responsible for this symptom in a given patient. A causal relationship may not be clearly defined even if the symptom resolves following discontinuance of the drug. Reexposure to the drug may be indicated when the relationship between the drug and the symptom is unclear and must be determined. Under such circumstances, the risk-benefit relationship must be evaluated by the physician, and the patient must be properly informed about the reasons for recommending reexposure.

Bibliography

1. Anderson, R. J., et al. Oral clonidine loading in hypertensive urgencies. *J.A.M.A.* 246:848, 1981.
2. Bertel, O., et al. Nifedipine in hypertensive emergencies. *Br. Med. J.* 286:19, 1983.
3. Black, H. R. Nonpharmacologic therapy for hypertension. *Am. J. Med.* 66:837, 1979.
4. Bravo, E. L., and Clifford, R. W. Pheochromocytoma: Diagnosis, localization and management. *N. Engl. J. Med.* 311:1298, 1984.
5. Bravo, E. L., et al. Clonidine-suppression test. A useful aid in the diagnosis of pheochromocytoma. *N. Engl. J. Med.* 305:623, 1981.
6. Chesley, L. C. Hypertension in pregnancy: Definition, familial factor, and remote prognosis. *Kidney Int.* 18:234, 1980.
7. Cohn, J. N. Calcium, vascular smooth muscle, and calcium entry blockers in hypertension. *Ann. Intern. Med.* 98:806, 1983.
8. Cohn, J. N., and Burke, L. P. Nitroprusside. *Ann. Intern. Med.* 91:752, 1979.
9. Curtis, J. J., et al. Inhibition of angiotensin-converting enzyme in renal-transplant recipients with hypertension. *N. Engl. J. Med.* 308:377, 1983.

10. Davis, B. A., et al. Prevalence of renovascular hypertension in patients with grade III or IV hypertensive retinopathy. *N. Engl. J. Med.* 301:1273, 1979.
11. Fields, L., and Wickline, S. Hypertension. In M. J. Orland and R. J. Saltman (eds.), Manual of Medical Therapeutics (25th ed.). Boston: Little, Brown, 1986.
12. Fisher, K. A., et al. Hypertension in pregnancy: Clinical-pathological correlations and remote prognosis. *Medicine* 60:267, 1981.
13. Groenendijk, R., et al. Hemodynamic measurements in preeclampsia: Preliminary observations. *Am. J. Obstet. Gynecol.* 150:232, 1984.
14. Hill, N. S., et al. Intravenous nitroglycerin: A review of pharmacology, indications, therapeutic effects and complications. *Chest* 79:69, 1981.
15. Hricik, D. E., et al. Captopril-induced functional renal insufficiency in patients with bilateral renal-artery stenoses or renal-artery stenosis in a solitary kidney. *N. Engl. J. Med.* 308:373, 1983.
16. Jaffe, A. S., and Roberts, R. The use of intravenous nitroglycerin in cardiovascular disease. *Pharmacotherapy* 2:273, 1982.
17. Joint National Committee. 1984 report of the joint national committee on detection, evaluation, and treatment of high blood pressure. *Ann. Intern. Med.* 144:1045, 1984.
18. Kannel, W. B. Perspectives on systolic hypertension: The Framingham study. *Circulation* 61:1179, 1980.
19. Kaplan, N. M. Non-drug treatment of hypertension. *Ann. Intern. Med.* 102:359, 1985.
20. Koch-Weser, J. Diazoxide. *N. Engl. J. Med.* 294:1271, 1976.
21. Lin, C. C., et al. Fetal outcome in hypertensive disorders of pregnancy. *Am. J. Obstet. Gynecol.* 142:255, 1982.
22. Lindheimer, M. D., and Katz, A. I. Hypertension in pregnancy. *N. Engl. J. Med.* 313:675, 1985.
23. Lowenstein, J. Clonidine. *Ann. Intern. Med.* 92:74, 1980.
24. Magometschnigg, D., and Pichler, M. Effective and safe treatment of hypertensive crisis with nifedipine. *Am. J. Cardiol.* 47:469, 1981.
25. Messerli, F. H., et al. Osler's maneuver and pseudohypertension. *N. Engl. J. Med.* 312:1548, 1985.
26. Michelson, E. L., and Frishman, W. H. Labetalol: An alpha- and beta-adrenoceptor blocking drug. *Ann. Intern. Med.* 99:553, 1984.
27. Narins, R. G. Mild hypertension: A therapeutic dilemma. *Kidney Int.* 26:881, 1984.
28. Nicholson, J. P., Jr., et al. Pheochromocytoma and prazosin. *Ann. Intern. Med.* 99:477, 1983.
29. Page, E. W., and Christianson, R. The impact of mean arterial pressure in the middle trimester upon the outcome of pregnancy. *Am. J. Obstet. Gynecol.* 125:740, 1976.
30. Palmer, R. F., and Lasseter, K. C. Sodium nitroprusside. *N. Engl. J. Med.* 292:294, 1975.
31. Ramos, O. Malignant hypertension: The Brazilian experience. *Kidney Int.* 26:209, 1984.
32. Redman, C. W. G. Treatment of hypertension in pregnancy. *Kidney Int.* 18:267, 1980.
33. Rosenfeld, J. Hypertension in the elderly. *Kidney Int.* 23:540, 1983.
34. Shell, W. E., and Sobel, B. E. Protection of ischemic myocardium by reduced ventricular afterload. *N. Engl. J. Med.* 291:481, 1974.
35. Shook, T. L., et al. Ethanol intoxication complicating intravenous nitroglycerin therapy. *Ann. Intern. Med.* 101:498, 1984.
36. Spitalewitz, S., et al. Use of oral clonidine for rapid titration of blood pressure in severe hypertension. *Chest* (Suppl. 83):404, 1983.
37. Weber, M. A., and Drayer, J. I. M. Renal effects of beta-adrenoceptor blockade. *Kidney Int.* 18:686, 1980.
38. Weiss, N. S. Relation of high blood pressure to headache, epistaxis, and selected other symptoms. *N. Engl. J. Med.* 287:631, 1972.
39. Wheat, M. W., Jr. Acute dissecting aneurysms of the aorta: Diagnosis and treatment—1979. *Am. Heart J.* 99:373, 1980.
40. Wilson, D. J., et al. Intravenous labetalol in the treatment of severe hypertension and hypertensive emergencies. *Am. J. Med.* 75(4A):95, 1983.
41. Zusman, R. M. Renin- and non-renin-mediated antihypertensive actions of converting enzyme inhibitors. *Kidney Int.* 25:969, 1984.

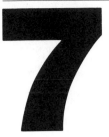

Pulmonary Emergencies

Daniel P. Schuster

The major function of the respiratory system is to maintain an adequate exchange of oxygen (O_2) and carbon dioxide (CO_2). Any acute process or disorder that interferes with this vital function can be properly considered a pulmonary emergency. Complete interruption of O_2 transfer results in life-threatening hypoxemia in 1–2 minutes; likewise, a complete lack of CO_2 elimination usually causes the arterial PCO_2 to rise 3–4 mm Hg/minute, with serious acidemia occurring in several minutes. Clearly, rapid recognition of processes that threaten an adequate respiratory gas exchange, along with timely and appropriate intervention, is of paramount importance to patient management in the emergency department.

Physiology and Pathophysiology

The major components of the respiratory system include the airways, lung parenchyma, pleural space, thoracic blood vessels, lymphatics, and the respiratory muscles with their nervous system connections. Major disruption in the normal function of any one of these components can cause serious dysfunction in one or more of the other components.

I. **Gas exchange.** Effective O_2 uptake and CO_2 elimination depend on an appropriate matching of regional ventilation to perfusion. This matching is a complex function of gravity, cardiac output, blood volume, the pattern of ventilation, and the local influence of vasomotor and bronchomotor tone.

   A. **Intrapulmonary shunting.** When the local ventilation-perfusion ($\dot{V}/\dot{Q}$) ratio in any given lung region decreases, blood that drains that region is incompletely oxygenated. Systemic hypoxemia results, because the O_2-carrying capacity of hemoglobin is limited. Normal areas of lung cannot compensate for areas of lung with low $\dot{V}/\dot{Q}$ ratios. This process of adding incompletely oxygenated blood to blood from other areas of lung with normal oxygenation is called **venous admixture. Intrapulmonary shunt** is an area of lung with a $\dot{V}/\dot{Q}$ ratio of 0; "physiologic shunt" represents venous admixture in areas of lung with a $\dot{V}/\dot{Q}$ ratio between normal (about 0.8) and that of shunt (0).

   B. **Alveolar dead space.** In contrast to shunt, CO_2 elimination progressively decreases in areas of lung that develop $\dot{V}/\dot{Q}$ ratios **greater** than 1.0. Such areas are poorly perfused relative to their ventilation. An area of lung without perfusion at all (a $\dot{V}/\dot{Q}$ ratio of infinity) eliminates no CO_2 and is known as alveolar dead space (to be distinguished from anatomic dead space [e.g., the trachea, which is not perfused by pulmonary arterial blood but does carry respiratory gases]).

   C. **Respiratory failure** results when one or more components of the respiratory system fail to achieve either effective O_2 uptake (defined as >90% saturation of the circulating mass of hemoglobin) and/or effective CO_2 elimination (as determined by the maintenance of a normal pH). Both the severity of the gas exchange abnormality and the rapidity with which it develops are relevant. **Acute respiratory failure (ARF)** may occur in patients with a previously normal respiratory system or may be superimposed on preexisting abnormalities in gas exchange. ARF is often defined as a PaO_2 less than 50 mm Hg while breathing room air ("oxygenation failure") and/or a $PaCO_2$ greater than 50 mm Hg with a pH less than 7.3 ("ventilatory failure").

II. **Lung mechanics.** Whereas the primary purpose of the lung is to exchange CO_2 and O_2 effectively, the primary purpose of the rest of the respiratory system is to move air in and out of the lung. The respiratory muscles, of which the diaphragm is the most important, are a major compensatory mechanism during acute respiratory failure (especially ventilatory failure). **Respiratory muscle weakness by itself,** as in any form of neuromuscular paralysis, can lead to ventilatory failure (hypercarbia). Likewise, because respiratory muscle effort is markedly increased in the presence of parenchymal or airway disease, **respiratory muscle fatigue** may make mechanical ventilatory support necessary. Early recognition of respiratory muscle weakness or fatigue is an important part of the emergency assessment of patients with impending ARF.

   A. **Function residual capacity (FRC).** The volume of gas within the lung at the end of each tidal volume is referred to as the FRC. At this time, the normal tendency of the lung to collapse is precisely balanced by an equal tendency of the chest wall to expand. The FRC is an important benchmark because airway resistance, pulmonary vascular resistance, and the work of breathing are minimized when the FRC is near normal predicted values. However, the FRC is not easily measured at the bedside, and therefore changes in the FRC are usually inferred. Changes in the FRC are often correlated with diseases known to change the normal pressure-volume relationship (i.e., compliance) of the respiratory system. Lung diseases that either acutely or chronically decrease lung or chest wall compliance (e.g., interstitial fibrosis, pulmonary edema, obesity, ascites) will cause the FRC to decrease. Conversely, processes that increase compliance or cause air-trapping (e.g., emphysema, asthma, flail chest) will increase the FRC.

   B. **Work of breathing.** The respiratory muscles are most efficient (and thus the work of breathing is minimized) when they begin to contract at their greatest fiber length. As hyperinflation (increased FRC) occurs, the diaphragm in particular begins to contract at less than its maximally stretched length and thus is forced to operate at a considerable mechanical disadvantage. The work of breathing can also be increased by higher-than-normal airways resistance (nonelastic work) or by diminished respiratory system compliance (elastic work). All of these factors may promote respiratory muscle fatigue and subsequent ventilatory failure (hypercarbia).

Signs and Symptoms of Pulmonary Disease

The history and physical examination are of obvious importance in the emergency evaluation of patients with pulmonary disorders, but treatment must often begin before a definitive diagnosis can be made. Therefore, the presenting signs and symptoms assume special importance in directing initial management. Further treatment often depends on the underlying cause; thus, the differential diagnosis for each complaint must be carefully considered.

   I. **Dyspnea (shortness of breath).** This subjective sensation is often described as difficulty getting air into the lungs and is sometimes termed air hunger. It is to be distinguished from other causes of breathlessness (e.g., pleuritic pain, hyperventilation syndromes including those resulting from a metabolic acidosis or certain poisonings such as salicylism). Tachypnea (rapid, shallow breathing) usually accompanies dyspnea, as does a tachycardia. Other accompanying signs depend on the etiology.

   A. **Etiology.** Dyspnea is a very nonspecific symptom that may be due to disease of any component of the respiratory system or may be of nonpulmonary origin (usually cardiac). A very acute onset should suggest pulmonary edema (cardiac or noncardiac), pulmonary embolism, a pneumothorax, foreign body aspiration, or sometimes asthma. More commonly, the dyspnea that accompanies asthma is subacute in onset, as is also true of the various pneumonias. Dyspnea may also be chronic, as with chronic obstructive pulmonary disease (COPD), any of the restrictive lung diseases, or chronic congestive heart failure. **Orthopnea** (or dyspnea with recumbency) does not reliably distinguish pulmonary from nonpulmonary causes of dyspnea. On the other hand, **paroxysmal nocturnal dyspnea** (PND) in its classic form (dyspnea occurring after several hours of recumbency) is a more reliable indicator that cardiac disease exists. Other less common causes of dyspnea include anemia, hyperthyroidism, chronic upper airway disease, obesity, and some of the psychoneuroses.

   B. **Treatment** is directed toward the specific underlying illness involved. In addition, most patients with dyspnea at rest will benefit from temporary administration of supplemental O_2.

   II. **Wheezing.** This musical sound is due to the turbulent movement of air through a constricted airway; it may occur during either inhalation or exhalation.

   A. **Etiologies.** The most common cause is bronchospasm due to either asthma or chronic lung disease with a bronchospastic component. Dyspnea, tachypnea, and tachycardia commonly accompany wheezing. Other less common causes of wheezing include congestive heart failure, endobronchial obstruction (e.g., due to tumor, granuloma, or a foreign body), and pulmonary embolism.

   B. **Evaluation.** See **Obstructive Lung Disease,** sec. I.B.

    C. Treatment is directed at the specific etiology (see **Obstructive Lung Disease**, sec. I.D).

III. Stridor is often confused with inspiratory wheezing but is due to critical upper airway obstruction. The airway may be only 2–3 mm wide. Any further obstruction may rapidly lead to asphyxiation and death. Thus, the distinction from bronchospasm is crucial.

    A. Etiologies include epiglottitis, other soft-tissue infections of the pharnyx, tumor, granuloma, vocal cord paralysis, foreign body aspiration, and trauma.

    B. Evaluation. The presence of inspiratory wheezing should always raise the possibility of stridor. If the wheezing sound is loudest over the upper airway and of less intensity over the periphery of the lung, emergency inspection of the glottic opening by a trained specialist (usually an otolaryngologist) should be obtained. Soft-tissue radiographs are also helpful in the evaluation of patients with stridor, but these should be obtained in the emergency department where close supervision of the patient is possible.

    C. Treatment. In almost all cases, either endotracheal intubation, cricothyrotomy, or tracheostomy will be required, depending on the nature of the upper airway obstruction. This is often best managed in the operating suite, if time permits.

IV. Cyanosis. This sign is present when the skin or mucous membranes appear bluish because of the presence of an abnormal amount of desaturated (reduced) hemoglobin in the blood. When cyanosis is generalized, it is referred to as "central" and is most commonly due to arterial hypoxemia. Central cyanosis implies that at least 5 gm/dl or reduced hemoglobin is present; thus, the actual PO_2 at which cyanosis occurs will vary depending on the level of hemoglobin (i.e., anemia versus polycythemia). On the other hand, "peripheral" cyanosis is the result of a stagnant circulation through peripheral vascular beds.

    A. Etiologies

        1. Central cyanosis may result from lung disease with associated arterial hypoxemia, a right-to-left cardiac shunt (e.g., congenital cyanotic heart disease), or hemoglobin abnormalities (met- or sulfhemoglobinemia).

        2. Peripheral cyanosis is most commonly seen when the cardiac output is reduced for any reason but may also result from exposure to cold (e.g., Raynaud's phenomenon) or arterial or venous obstruction.

    B. Evaluation. Regardless of the etiology, recognition of cyanosis means that an arterial blood gas must be immediately obtained to rule out significant arterial hypoxemia. Depending on the clinical circumstances, a methemoglobin determination may also be indicated.

    C. Treatment

        1. Central cyanosis is treated with supplemental inspired O_2.

        2. The treatment of **peripheral cyanosis** includes, in addition to supplemental O_2, measures to increase blood flow to compromised vascular beds.

V. Hemoptysis. Death due to asphyxiation is the major cause for concern with hemoptysis. The unpredictability of airway bleeding means that a conservative approach is necessary, and almost all patients with gross hemoptysis should be admitted if this is a new complaint.

    A. Etiologies. Hemoptysis may be due to airway or parenchymal lung infection, neoplasm, cardiovascular disease (e.g., mitral stenosis, pulmonary embolus, vascular anomalies), and coagulation disorders, as well as a variety of less common disorders (e.g., Goodpasture's syndrome, Wegener's granulomatosis, pulmonary sequestration, idiopathic pulmonary hemosiderosis). Minor amounts of hemoptysis, as in blood-streaked sputum, are most commonly due to airway inflammation (e.g., bronchitis, bronchiectasis, lung abscess, tuberculosis, fungal disease, pneumonia). It is important to distinguish hemoptysis from other sources of bleeding, especially nasopharyngeal lesions.

    B. Evaluation. Although quantitation of hemoptysis is often difficult and is of questionable clinical utility, massive hemoptysis is usually defined as greater than 500 ml of expectorated blood/24 hours. Much more important, however, is the clinical status of the patient on initial examination. The mental status, overall muscle strength (important in evaluating cough to keep the airway clear), and the presence or absence of any underlying pulmonary disorder are important factors to consider. A chest x-ray, complete blood count (CBC), hemostasis profile, and arterial blood gases are appropriate laboratory tests. Additional workup, including bronchoscopy and arteriography may be needed to establish a diagnosis and to identify the site of bleeding. If bleeding is brisk, emergency cardiothoracic consultation should be obtained.

C. Treatment

    1. Airway. Ensuring a secure, patent airway is of paramount importance. It is often useful to place the patient with the bleeding side down, if known, to avoid aspiration into the other lung. The decision to intubate the patient must be individualized and will depend on the patient's ability to handle blood in the airway. Intubation with a double-lumen endotracheal tube (e.g., a Carlen's tube) or a main-stem endobronchial intubation of the nonbleeding side is an option to consider, but these procedures require additional skill and experience and are often less important than providing routine endotracheal intubation, with humidification and suctioning.

    2. Supportive measures, such as administration of supplemental O_2 and blood tranfusions, should be initiated as appropriate. Any airway infection or inflammation should be treated with appropriate antibiotics and any coagulation abnormalities corrected. Drugs that suppress cough (e.g., codeine) are rarely useful.

    3. Definitive treatment, including possible surgery, will depend on the underlying cause.

VI. Chest pain (see Chap. 5). The differential diagnosis here most commonly includes ischemic heart disease, aortic dissection, pericarditis, pleurisy, pulmonary embolism, gastrointestinal disorders, and musculoskeletal discomfort.

VII. Cough. When cited as the sole problem, this symptom is almost always due to upper respiratory infection. However, any cause of dyspnea (see sec. I) may result in coughing, and occasionally the sole manifestation of asthma is the acute or subacute onset of coughing.

A. Evaluation

    1. Acute cough. A chest x-ray is not indicated unless other evidence of lung disease (e.g., pneumonia) is present. Depending on the clinical situation, it may be necessary to search for a foreign body (see Chap. 28).

    2. The workup of a **chronic cough** is best handled on an outpatient basis. A careful examination of the upper airway and chest x-ray are both indicated. Further workup may include laryngoscopy, bronchoscopy, or computed tomography (CT) examination.

B. Treatment generally includes use of an expectorant and/or cough suppressant such as guaifenesin and codeine, respectively. If there is evidence of bacterial infection, an antibiotic is indicated. Further treatment is directed at the underlying disease.

Clinical Assessment

I. Oxygenation. The diagnosis of ARF often requires a high index of suspicion because clinical signs such as cyanosis, although useful when clearly present, may occur only when gas exchange is markedly impaired. The most sensitive clue may be the respiratory rate, which is almost always abnormal during ARF. Ultimately, the diagnosis of ARF depends on an analysis of arterial blood gases (ABGs).

A. Arterial blood gases. Arterial oxygenation is inadequate when the hemoglobin saturation is less than 90% ($PaO_2 < 60$ mm Hg), and most patients become symptomatic when the PaO_2 falls below 40–50 mm Hg. The danger of hypoxemia (a reduced amount of O_2 in arterial blood) is that it will lead to hypoxia (decreased tissue oxygenation) with impaired vital organ function. O_2 delivery to the tissues depends on an intact respiratory system, an adequate circulating mass of hemoglobin, and an appropriate cardiac output. The quantity of O_2 in blood is dependent on the amount of hemoglobin present and its saturation with oxygen. Because of the sigmoidal shape of the oxyhemoglobin saturation curve, a PaO_2 of 60 mm Hg usually ensures a hemoglobin saturation of at least 90%.

B. Alveolar-arterial oxygen ([A-a]PO_2) gradient. To calculate the [A-a]PO_2 gradient, the inspired O_2 concentration (FIO_2) must be accurately determined since

PAO_2 = (barometric pressure − water vapor pressure) × FIO_2 − ($PaCO_2$/respiratory quotient)

This is usually not possible unless the patient is breathing room air or is intubated. Thus, at sea level,

[A-a]$PO_2 = [(713 \times FIO_2) - (PaCO_2/0.8)] - PaO_2$

Any cause of hypoxemia (except alveolar hypoventilation) will cause this gradient to widen. Thus, a normal [A-a]PO_2 difference suggests that alveolar hypoventilation (hypercarbia) must be the cause of hypoxemia, whereas a widened [A-a]PO_2 gradient (i.e., > 15 mm Hg) indicates that O_2 uptake is impaired, even if the PaO_2 seems to be normal (as sometimes occurs in the dyspneic patient with hypocarbia).

C. **Other methods for assessing oxygenation** include the calculation of the percentage of cardiac output perfusing nonventilated lung (intrapulmonary shunt), the calculation of systemic oxygen transport, and a direct measure of the mixed venous PO_2. The data required to assess oxygenation by these methods require pulmonary artery catheterization, and thus such data are rarely available in the emergency situation.

II. **Alveolar ventilation** is most directly assessed by the arterial carbon dioxide tension. The $PaCO_2$ varies directly with the amount of CO_2 produced/unit time ($\dot{V}CO_2$) and inversely with alveolar ventilation ($\dot{V}_A$). Alveolar ventilation, in turn, is equal to the minute ventilation minus the dead-space ventilation ($\dot{V}_A = \dot{V}_E - \dot{V}_D$). Because $PaCO_2$ is proportional to the ratio of $\dot{V}CO_2/\dot{V}_A$, $PaCO_2 = K(\dot{V}CO_2/[\dot{V}_E - \dot{V}_D])$, where K is a constant. Thus, the CO_2 tension may rise inappropriately (ventilation failure) when any of three conditions occur: (a) CO_2 production rises (e.g., fever, shivering, seizures) and is unmatched by a rise in alveolar ventilation, (b) total minute ventilation decreases (e.g., depressed consciousness, muscle paralysis, or, rarely, intrinsic pulmonary disease), or (c) dead-space ventilation increases and is not compensated by an increase in minute ventilation. Increases in dead space occur when areas of lung are ventilated but not perfused (e.g., pulmonary embolus) or when decreases in regional pulmonary perfusion exceed decreases in regional ventilation (e.g., emphysema, shock, mechanical ventilation). The consequences of ventilatory failure, and the subsequent rise in $PaCO_2$, are respiratory acidosis, hypoxemia, and at times, depressed ventilatory responsiveness to CO_2. An acute rise in $PaCO_2$ to 45–50 mm Hg will drop the pH below its normal lower limit of 7.35, whereas a slow rise over days or weeks will produce less of an effect on pH because of compensatory bicarbonate retention.

III. **Mechanics.** A few simple observations and tests are sufficient to assess the performance of the respiratory muscles in the emergency setting.

A. **Respiratory rate.** The work of breathing increases directly in proportion to increases in the respiratory rate. Respiratory rates greater than 30/minute are difficult to maintain for any length of time. The key to lowering the rate (if unrelated to anxiety) is to treat the underlying problem, but mechanical ventilatory assistance may be necessary first.

B. **Spirometric tests.** Measurements of the peak expiratory flow rate (PEFR), vital capacity (VC), and/or the forced expiratory volume in 1 second (FEV_1) are often useful in evaluating patients with bronchospasm or acute exacerbations of chronic obstructive lung disease, especially to judge the severity of the attack and the response to bronchodilator therapy. They are particularly useful when previous values are available for comparison (> 20–50% reduction from previous values is significant).

   1. The **FEV_1** is somewhat less dependent on patient cooperation than the PEFR. An FEV_1 less than 700–1000 ml or a PEFR less than 100 liters/minute indicates severe airway obstruction, especially when the FEV_1/FVC ratio is less than 60%.

   2. The **VC** is low in restrictive lung diseases (e.g., idiopathic pulmonary fibrosis). The VC is particularly useful when primary respiratory muscle weakness (as in neuromuscular paralysis) may be an important consideration. The VC measurement is often combined with a measure of negative inspiratory force (NIF), in which the patient inspires against a closed airway while the pressure change is measured; low values for both tests (VC < 15 ml/kg, NIF < 25 cm H_2O) indicate severe muscle weakness, usually requiring mechanical ventilatory support.

C. The **work of breathing** is difficult to assess per se. Instead, the respiratory rate, the patient's facial expression, and the presence or absence of use of accessory muscles, abdominal paradox, respiratory alternans, and diaphoresis serve as clues to whether respiratory muscle work is increased.

Management Principles of Respiratory Care

The most important principle of emergency respiratory care is to make sure that the airway is secure and that adequate ventilation is assured. Guidelines for elective intubation and initiation of mechanical ventilation are given in Table 7-1.

Table 7-1. Guidelines for elective intubation and mechanical ventilation for acute respiratory failure

Process	Usual indication(s)	Useful parameters	Comment
Acute respiratory failure without underlying respiratory disease			
Neuromuscular illness (e.g., Guillain-Barré syndrome, myasthenia gravis)	Imminent failure of respiratory pump	Inspiratory pressure < 25 cm H_2O; Vital capacity < 15 ml/kg; Respiratory rate > 30–40/min	Onset of abnormalities in gas exchange is often sudden and follows signs of weakness
Central airway obstruction	Presence of inspiratory stridor		Emergency tracheostomy may be necessary
Lung parenchymal or airway disease (e.g., ARDS, pulmonary edema, pneumonia, asthma)	Progressive refractory hypoxemia; Progressive respiratory acidosis; Excessive work of breathing	PaO_2 < 60 mm Hg, with FiO_2 > 0.6; $PaCO_2$ > 45 mm Hg; pH < 7.3; Respiratory rate > 30–40/min	Hypercapnea is often a late manifestation
Stupor or coma (e.g., drug overdose)	Airway protection	Poor gag reflex, ineffective cough	Onset of apnea may be abrupt
Circulatory failure (e.g., myocardial infarction, cardiogenic shock)	Inadequate gas exchange; Increased O_2 consumption	As above (lung parenchymal or airway disease)	Decreased work load for the severely failing or ischemic heart can be critical
Acute-on-chronic respiratory failure (e.g., acute exacerbation of COPD or chronic neuromuscular disease)	Impaired mental status; Refractory hypoxemia; Progressive respiratory acidosis	PaO_2 < 35–45 mm Hg despite controlled O_2 therapy; pH < 7.20–7.25; Respiratory rate > 30–40/min	Implies hypoxia or CO_2 narcosis; O_2 therapy resulting in progressive respiratory acidosis is an indication for mechanical ventilation

Source: E. P. Trulock III and D. P. Schuster, Acute Respiratory Failure. In M. J. Orland and R. J. Saltman (eds.), *Manual of Medical Therapeutics* (25th ed.). Boston: Little, Brown, 1986. With permission.

I. **Improving oxygenation**
   A. **Increasing the FIO_2.** Commonly used oxygen delivery systems provide a varying FIO_2 (except during mechanical ventilation) depending on the balance between the patient's minute ventilation and the gas flow of the delivery system. A high minute ventilation will result in a lower than expected FIO_2.
   1. **Nasal cannulas** (prongs) are comfortable and are effective in raising the FIO_2 in nontachypneic patients, including "mouth breathers." Oxygen flow rates of 1 and 2 liters/minute provide approximate O_2 concentrations of 24% and 28%, respectively.
   2. Light, comfortable plastic **masks** can provide 50–60% O_2 at a flow rate of 6 liters/minute. "Non-rebreathing" masks provide an even higher FIO_2 (70–90%) in nontachypneic patients.
   3. The **Ventimask** delivers a controlled maximum O_2 concentration by entraining ambient air around a jet of O_2. Concentrations available vary from 24 to 50%.
   B. **Increasing airway pressure** is required when an increase in FIO_2 alone does not adequately treat oxygenation failure (i.e., $PaO_2 < 60$ mm Hg). By maintaining positive airway pressure throughout the respiratory cycle, airways remain open, the FRC increases, and ventilation-perfusion matching improves. Endotracheal intubation (see sec. **III**) and mechanical ventilation (see sec. **IV**) are necessary for the majority of patients who require **continuous positive airway pressure (CPAP).** An alternative, which is occasionally useful, is "face-mask CPAP," in which a tight-fitting face mask is put in place and the patient exhales against a device that maintains positive airway pressure. This approach can be useful when less than 10 cm H_2O CPAP is required to improve oxygenation and when the work of breathing is not excessive. Gaseous distention of the stomach with emesis and aspiration are potential problems, and therefore face-mask CPAP should not be used in obtunded patients. The mask must be removed periodically to prevent pressure necrosis. Thus, prolonged use for many days is usually impractical.
II. **Improving alveolar ventilation**
   A. When failure to eliminate CO_2 is associated with **mild acidosis** (e.g., pH 7.30–7.35) and the patient is both alert and cooperative, temporizing measures, such as **intermittent positive-pressure breathing (IPPB),** deep breathing, and airway care, may prove beneficial. IPPB may be useful when CO_2 retention is due to any of the neuromuscular diseases or chest wall deformities (e.g., amyotrophic lateral sclerosis, severe kyphoscoliosis). IPPB is prescribed by tidal volume (10–12 ml/kg), with a pressure limit of 30–40 cm H_2O. Higher pressures may result in a pneumothorax.
   B. More **severe degrees of respiratory acidosis,** especially with mental status changes, require **endotracheal intubation** (see sec. **III**) and **mechanical ventilation** (see sec. **IV**).
III. **Artificial airways.** Endotracheal tubes with high-volume, low-pressure cuffs should be used to minimize the risk of tracheal necrosis.
   A. **Indications for endotracheal intubation** include initiation of mechanical ventilation, maintenance of continuous positive airway pressure (usually termed **positive end-expiratory pressure [PEEP]** in this context), facilitation of tracheal suctioning, prevention of aspiration, and relief of upper airway obstruction.
   B. **Site of placement.** Initially, either nasotracheal or orotracheal intubation is performed. Emergent bedside cricothyrotomy or tracheostomy is not indicated unless the patient has an upper airway obstruction that cannot be cleared for placement of an endotracheal tube. Orotracheal tubes are preferred for emergency intubation, especially in patients with underlying chronic lung disease. Nasotracheal tubes are easier to stabilize and are more comfortable, but the use of small-diameter (and thus high-resistance) tubes may lead to difficulty in weaning, particularly in the patient with chronic lung disease.
   C. **Method of placement.** See Chap. 38.
IV. **Mechanical ventilation** is a **supportive** tool. The decision to institute mechanical ventilation should take into account the reversibility of the process causing respiratory failure. The **clinical setting** should be one of the factors considered in making this decision.
   A. **Ventilator types and mode.** Almost all modern ventilators provide volume-controlled assisted ventilation. The mechanics of each are sufficiently different that physicians should be aware of the specifications of the ventilators used by their institution. Ventilators may be insensitive to a patient's effort to breathe spontaneously ("controlled ventilation"), may be set to be "triggered" by a patient's spontaneous effort ("assisted ventilation"), or may provide a dual system in which a given

number of controlled or assisted breaths are given each minute interspersed by unassisted spontaneous breathing (synchronized or unsynchronized intermittent mandatory ventilation [SIMV or IMV]). In general, use of either the assist-control mode with a "backup" rate of 10–15 breaths/minute or use of the IMV mode at the same initial rate will be satisfactory immediately after intubation. Later adjustments are made on the basis of ABGs.

B. **Initial ventilator orders.** When the patient has been intubated, the physician must select the FIO_2, minute ventilation (V_E), PEEP, and mode of mechanical ventilation.

1. **FIO_2.** Hypoxemia and hypoxia are more dangerous than brief overoxygenation. An initial FIO_2 of 0.9–1.0 alleviates hypoxemia due to all but the lowest of $\dot{V}_A/\dot{Q}$ ratios. After initial oxygenation, the FIO_2 may be changed to obtain a PaO_2 of 60–100 mm Hg.

2. **A minute ventilation ($\dot{V}_E$)** of 100 ml/kg is an appropriate starting point. This can be accomplished at a respiratory rate of 8–15 breaths/minute and tidal volume of 10–15 ml/kg. Minute ventilation should be adjusted until a normal pH is achieved. If the IMV mode is used, the total respiratory rate (including the patient's own spontaneous breaths) should be less than 20–25 breaths/minute to allow the respiratory muscles time to rest. Slower rates may be preferred in obstructive lung disease, while faster rates may be useful when pulmonary compliance is diminished (e.g., any cause of pulmonary edema).

3. **PEEP.** Many physicians use small amounts of PEEP (2–5 cm H_2O) immediately because many causes of acute respiratory failure are associated with a decreased FRC. However, such practice is probably inappropriate when respiratory failure is the result of severe bronchospasm, when the potential for serious air-trapping exists.

The **optimal level of PEEP** is controversial. A conservative approach is to choose the least amount of PEEP that provides 90% saturation of blood at an FIO_2 of less than 0.6.

V. **Complications of respiratory care**

A. **Improper placement of the endotracheal tube** in the right main stem bronchus may cause inadequate ventilation, hypoxemia, or a pneumothorax; placement in the esophagus will result in inadequate ventilation and gastric distention.

B. Cuff overinflation regularly produces late development of **tracheal stricture.**

C. **Endotracheal tube dislodgement or cuff leak** should be suspected when there is a sudden decrease in expired volume associated with a fall in airway pressure.

D. **Barotrauma.** Subcutaneous emphysema, pneumomediastinum, simple pneumothorax, and tension pneumothorax are associated with high peak airway pressures and PEEP (usually greater than 45–50 cm H_2O and 10 cm H_2O, respectively). A pneumothorax should be considered when lung compliance or blood pressure falls suddenly. Frequent palpation of the neck for crepitation and auscultation of the lung should be routine. Tube thoracostomy equipment should be readily available for mechanically ventilated patients.

E. **Oxygen toxicity** results from high concentrations of inspired oxygen. Histologic changes may occur within days when 100% O_2 is used, while a longer period (several weeks) may be necessary with concentrations near 60%. Ultimately, a syndrome indistinguishable from the adult respiratory distress syndrome (ARDS) with subsequent pulmonary fibrosis will result.

F. Rapid **acid-base shifts** can occur when sudden overventilation results in hypocapnia and respiratory alkalosis. The result may be a decreased cardiac output, cardiac arrhythmias, and central nervous system disturbances. **Altered acid-base states should be corrected at a rate proportional to their development.**

G. **Hemodynamic effects.** Positive pressure ventilation, especially in conjunction with PEEP, can result in decreased venous return, especially if associated with extracellular fluid volume depletion. This may decrease cardiac output and blood pressure. The treatment includes volume expansion and vasoactive agents if necessary.

Obstructive Lung Disease

I. **Asthma** is a chronic episodic illness, the cardinal feature of which is reversible airway obstruction. Precipitating factors include a variety of allergens and chemical irritants, infections, cold exposure, drugs, and exercise.

A. **Pathophysiology.** By incompletely understood mechanisms, constriction of bronchial smooth muscle, mucosal edema, and hypersecretion of mucus occur. The smooth-muscle hyperreactivity may respond rapidly to therapy, but the mucosal abnormalities usually abate more slowly. The increase in airway obstruction leads to a marked increase in airway resistance during both the inspiratory and expiratory phases of breathing. As a result, the work of breathing is proportionately increased. As the attack continues, the patient ultimately begins to fatigue. Eventually, effective alveolar ventilation cannot be sustained, and hypercapneic respiratory acidosis, hypoxemia, and even cardiorespiratory arrest ensue. The last is often particularly difficult to manage, because simple intubation does not relieve the airway obstruction and effective ventilation may not be possible. Thus, every effort must be made to avoid this complication.

B. Assessment. Efforts have been made to formulate scoring systems that are predictive of the need for hospitalization. None have met with uniform success. Such systems correlate reasonably well the severity of airway obstruction with the need for hospitalization but are less successful in predicting the response to therapy. The following are offerred as guidelines to the initial assessment of the asthmatic patient.

   1. The **history** should elicit at least the following information: current symptoms, duration of the current episode, history of similar episodes in past, severity of the attack in relation to previous episodes, history of recent emergency department visits, the need for prior hospitalization or intubation, current medications and compliance with same, any history of cardiac disease, and complications due to treatment.

   2. The **physical examination** should note the general appearance of the patient, vital signs, whether wheezing is localized or diffuse, the extent of air movement, whether other pulmonary findings (e.g., rales) are present, and whether or not cardiac abnormalities (e.g., murmurs or signs suggestive of heart failure) are present.

     a. Wheezing itself correlates poorly with the severity of airflow obstruction and only indicates that at least some degree of airflow obstruction is present.

     b. Cyanosis or an **abnormal mental status** in a wheezing patient is an ominous sign that indicates hypoxemia or severe hypercapnea. Such a patient often requires immediate intubation.

     c. Use of **accessory muscles of breathing** (e.g., the sternocleidomastoids), **diaphoresis,** an increased **pulsus paradoxicus** (> 15 mm Hg), and obvious and **severe dyspnea** all correlate with **severe airway obstruction** (i.e., an $FEV_1 < 700–1000$ ml). Such patients should be considered at great risk for rapid deterioration and almost all will require hospitalization.

   3. Objective evaluation

     a. Bedside **spirometry and arterial blood gases** may be used to quantitate the severity of severe airway obstruction. Patients with severe illness, who have begun to fatigue, will demonstrate progressive CO_2 retention and respiratory acidosis; this is especially common when the FEV_1 falls below 700–1000 ml or the PEFR is less than 100 liters/second.

     b. A **chest radiograph** is not necessary for a routine attack, especially in a young patient with a previous characteristic history. A chest radiograph, however, is recommended if the attack fails to respond to initial therapy or there is any evidence of an infectious process, cardiac disease, pneumothorax, or foreign body aspiration.

C. Differential diagnosis. Other illnesses that can mimic asthma because of wheezing include upper airway obstruction (e.g., due to tumor, foreign body, or edema), congestive heart failure, allergic reactions (including anaphylaxis), and bronchitis.

D. Treatment

   1. Oxygen (2–3 liters/minute by nasal prongs) should be administered to all patients with asthma, pending blood gas results or rapid clinical improvement.

   2. Bronchodilators

     a. Sympathomimetic agents are first-line drugs (unless contraindicated) in the management of asthma. Parenteral, inhaled, and oral forms are available. Agents with greater beta-2 selectivity (e.g., metaproterenol) may decrease the incidence of cardiotoxicity.

       (1) Parenteral forms include aqueous epinephrine (0.3–0.5 ml of a 1:1000 dilution q20–30minutes for 1–3 doses) and terbutaline (0.25–0.5 mg q4h); both are given SQ. The duration of action of epinephrine is short (20 minutes) compared to that of terbutaline (3–4 hours), but the onset of action of the latter drug (30–60 minutes) is delayed compared to that of epinephrine (several minutes). Despite the beta-2 selectivity of terbutaline, both drugs can cause severe tachycardia when given parenterally and therefore should be used with caution in older patients and those with cardiovascular disease.

(2) **All of the inhaled forms** are approximately equivalent in effectiveness. Commonly used agents include metaproterenol (0.2–0.3 ml in 2.5 ml of saline or 2 inhalations via a metered-dose inhaler q4–6h), albuterol (2 inhalations via a metered-dose inhaler q4–6h), or isoetharine (0.5 ml in 2.5 ml of saline q1–4h). Occasionally, the aerosol, acting as an irritant, can cause an exacerbation of bronchospasm. IPPB for the administration of aerosols is usually less effective than spontaneous breathing and provides an unnecessary risk of pneumothorax.

(3) The most commonly used **oral** agent is terbutaline (2.5–5.0 mg q8h). Tachycardia and tremulousness can occur when this agent is administered this way but are less common than when it is given parenterally. The combined use of oral terbutaline and an inhaled sympathomimetic agent is common practice during severe attacks but is often unnecessary in milder episodes. Metaproterenol and albuterol are other oral agents.

b. **Theophylline** is a standard of initial management of asthma but should not be used to replace sympathomimetics as long as the latter are not contraindicated. If the patient has not been taking an oral form of the drug, the loading dose is 6 mg/kg IV over 20–30 minutes; otherwise, the loading dose should be based on a serum level or be halved or eliminated entirely. Calculations for the loading dose are generally based on total body weight, except in cases of massive obesity, when a more conservative estimate of body weight (closer to ideal) should be used. The maintenance infusion is started at 0.5 mg/kg/hour (based on the **ideal** body weight) in most patients. A reduction in the maintenance dose should be anticipated in patients with congestive heart failure, liver disease, or advanced age and in patients receiving cimetidine or erythromycin (which slow the metabolism of theophylline); conversely, smokers and adolescents often require higher maintenance dosages (1.0 mg/kg/hour). Alterations in the maintenance dosage schedule should be made in association with early and repeated determinations of serum theophylline concentrations (therapeutic range of 10–20 μg/ml).

c. **Anticholinergic agents.** An inhalable form will be marketed in the near future. When atropine itself is used, the dosage is usually 0.025–0.05 mg/kg in 3 ml of saline. The appropriate indication for its use in the setting of acute asthma is not established. For the present, it is probably best to reserve its use for those instances in which conventional therapy has not been satisfactorily effective.

3. **Corticosteroids** should be given to any patient not responding well to bronchodilator therapy within a few hours, particularly when steroid use has been necessary previously. The mechanism of action is not understood, but their efficacy in this clinical setting is well established. The appropriate initial dosage is not established, but 0.5 mg/kg of methylprednisolone (or its equivalent) q6h is an effective regimen. Beneficial effects (with improvement in FEV_1), however, may not be apparent until 12–24 hours after initiating steroid treatment.

4. **Other measures**

a. Adequate (but not exuberant) **hydration,** either orally or parenterally, should be initiated in all cases.

b. **Antibiotics** are required only when the sputum is grossly purulent or pneumonia is present on a chest radiograph.

c. Percussion and postural drainage usually are not helpful in mobilizing secretions or mucous plugs in most asthmatics and can actually exacerbate symptoms.

d. **Sedatives are contraindicated** unless mechanical ventilation is instituted.

5. **Initial management** in the emergency department largely depends on the severity of the attack. Patients who are only mildly to moderately ill can often be managed solely with rapidly absorbable oral and inhalable forms of theophylline and sympathomimetic agents. Not all patients need subcutaneous epinephrine and intravenous aminophylline. More seriously ill patients, however, will usually benefit by initiating therapy with parenteral forms of these same agents.

6. Patients with severe and/or unresponsive respiratory acidosis require **endotracheal intubation** and **mechanically assisted ventilation.** Since the onset of

cardiorespiratory arrest is often precipitous in asthmatics, the threshold for intubation and mechanical ventilatory support should be somewhat lower than in other situations (e.g., exacerbation of COPD). After successful intubation, it is often necessary to sedate and paralyze the patient to achieve acceptable ventilation.

E. **Disposition.** This decision is based on a number of factors, the most important of which include the severity of the attack, the duration of the attack, the initial response to treatment, and the history of outcome of prior attacks. Any patient who does not have a marked salutary response to treatment (as evidenced by failure of the FEV_1 to improve and to exceed 1600 ml within 4–6 hours of presentation) should be hospitalized. However, patients who do have such a response should not be discharged automatically. Patients who have a particularly severe attack (as evidenced by an initial FEV_1 < 700–1000 ml or respiratory acidosis), have a history of a previous relapse, have recently made another emergency department visit, or have an attack exceeding 24–48 hours in duration usually should be admitted.

Patients who are discharged should be sent home on a regimen that represents an incremental increase from their standard program. Often this will mean a short (5- to 10-day) course of corticosteroids (beginning with a dosage of 40–60 mg/day of prednisone or its equivalent) and/or an increase in the dosage of theophylline preparation. Patients previously taking sympathomimetic agents should continue this medication. Early follow-up within the next 1–2 days by the primary care physician is advised.

II. **Chronic obstructive pulmonary disease (COPD)** is the rubric given to any pulmonary illness that causes an abnormal limitation in the rate of expired airflow. Asthma fits into such a category, but current usage usually limits the term *COPD* to chronic bronchitis and emphysema. Both conditions usually coexist in the same patient, although one or the other may dominate. The obstruction to airflow in the former case is due to mucous gland hyperplasia and hypersecretion. In the latter case, the pathogenesis is not as clear, although loss of the normal parenchymal supporting structure with diminished elastic recoil is considered by many to be the most important factor. Bronchial smooth muscle hyperreactivity with concomitant wheezing is often part of the spectrum of COPD as well, further complicating the clinical picture.

A. **Assessment**
   1. Typical **symptoms** include worsening shortness of breath, dyspnea on exertion, and worsening cough with sputum production.
   2. Characteristic **physical findings** include a prolonged expiratory phase, hyperexpansion of the chest, pursed-lip breathing, and cigarette stains on the fingers; milder cases, however, are usually less obvious.
   3. Classic findings on a **chest radiograph** include flattened diaphragms, an increased anteroposterior diameter, and the presence of bullae; patients with significant COPD, however, may not have any of these abnormalities.
   4. **Bedside spirometry** is very useful. Reductions in the FEV_1, FVC, and FEV_1/FVC ratio will in most cases secure the diagnosis.
   5. **Arterial blood gases** generally reveal hypoxemia. ABGs may also reveal a compensated or uncompensated respiratory acidosis, depending on the acuity of the situation.

B. Initial **treatment** is directed toward the relief of symptoms, which generally are related to abnormalities in gas exchange and increases in the work of breathing associated with worsening airflow obstruction. It is important to keep in mind that patients with severe chronic CO_2 retention (e.g., PCO_2 > 60–70 mm Hg) often have a pH near 7.3, even when stable. Under such circumstances, the patient's mental status is the best index of the acuity of the disease process. Although patients with chronic hypercapnea (and a normal pH) may have diminished CO_2 responsiveness, in most cases respiratory drive is not dependent on borderline hypoxemia. Although severe acute hypercarbia does indeed lead to "CO_2 narcosis," most patients will tolerate oxygen administration without developing this problem. In fact, often more harm is done by withholding O_2 from a hypoxemic patient than by administering O_2.
   1. **Improving oxygenation.** In most circumstances, O_2 by nasal prongs (2–3 liters/minute) or by 28–35% Ventimask will be satisfactory. Worsening CO_2 retention, with acidemia (e.g., pH < 7.25) and mental status changes, however, is an indication for intubation and assisted ventilation.

2. **Improving alveolar ventilation**
   a. **Airway care** is improved by expectoration of mucus and is possibly improved by percussion and postural drainage maneuvers.
   b. **Respiratory muscle strength** is improved with rest, administration of oxygen, nutrition, and possibly theophylline administration.
   c. In the emergency setting, the focus should be on the **relief of bronchospasm** (see sec. **I.D.2**). Many patients with COPD, even without demonstrable wheezing or response to bronchodilators by spirometry, seem to benefit from administration of a sympathomimetic agent (if not contraindicated) or a theophylline preparation and a short course of glucocorticoids (see sec. **I.D.3**).
3. **Decreasing the work of breathing.** This is accomplished primarily by relief of airway obstruction (e.g., bronchospasm, airway mucus) or by intubation and mechanical ventilation.
4. **Treating associated problems.** Patients with significant COPD have little reserve in the face of other pulmonary problems. Thus, although worsening dyspnea may be the complaint, pneumonia, congestive heart failure, a pneumothorax, or pulmonary embolus may be the precipitating cause. These problems should be considered whenever a patient with COPD deteriorates and should be appropriately treated, if present. Another common problem is acute bronchitis. Patients with grossly purulent sputum, especially if recently changed in character, or with fever should be treated with an antibiotic (e.g., ampicillin or tetracycline, 500 mg q6h). However, routine use of antibiotics is not recommended.

C. **Disposition.** Most patients with well-documented COPD who have significant worsening of symptoms will need to be hospitalized. Certainly a clear-cut deterioration in baseline blood gases or the presence of associated complications (e.g., pneumonia, pneumothorax) is a major indication for hospitalization. Even without such abnormalities, these patients often need hospitalization, because they are often elderly, the response to therapy is unpredictable, and coexisting causes of dyspnea are common. However, patients with only mild to moderate obstruction whose exacerbation is mild and whose response to therapy in the emergency department is significant (with return of symptoms and objective data to near baseline) can usually be sent home on a regimen of increased bronchodilator therapy and/or a short-course of steroids. An antibiotic should be given if there is evidence of an acute bronchitis. Arrangements should be made for early follow-up.

D. **Cor pulmonale.** Patients with cor pulmonale show evidence of right-sided heart failure (i.e., right-sided S_3 and ventricular heave, elevated jugular venous pressure, hepatojugular reflux, hepatic distention, and peripheral edema) due to chronic increases in the pulmonary vascular resistance (PVR). The increase in PVR is usually due to chronic hypoxemia and loss of pulmonary vasculature as a result of destructive emphysema. Because of the hypoxemia, these patients also are often cyanotic, plethoric, and polycythemic. Most patients will have to be hospitalized if they present with significant worsening of symptoms. The following therapeutic considerations should be kept in mind.
   1. **Relief of hypoxemia** is perhaps the single most important therapeutic maneuver, because it will improve cardiac function and will decrease the severity of pulmonary hypertension.
   2. The administration of digitalis for isolated right heart failure is probably not useful.
   3. The use of diuretics to treat peripheral edema should be cautious because of the risk of reducing preload to a heart that depends on high right-sided filling pressures.
   4. **Every effort should be made to treat reversible airway disease** (bronchospasm, mucus hypersecretion), parenchymal disease (pneumonia), and left-sided cardiac disease when present.

Adult Respiratory Distress Syndrome (ARDS)

I. **Pathophysiology.** Pulmonary edema occurs whenever the extravascular water content of the lung is increased. Increases in extravascular water result from two processes: (1) increases in hydrostatic pressure at the pulmonary capillary level (as in cardiogenic pulmonary edema) and (2) increases in alveolocapillary membrane permeability (as in all forms of noncardiogenic pulmonary edema). The former is most commonly the result of left ventricular heart failure, whereas the latter is often the initial step that results in the cascade of events known as ARDS. These two processes (i.e., cardiogenic and noncardiogenic edema) are not mutually exclusive; they may coexist in the same patient, and the diagnosis of one in no way excludes the other. (See Chap. 5 for a discussion of cardiogenic pulmonary edema.)

II. **Clinical features.** In all instances, the onset of ARDS is acute. Dyspnea, which is usually marked, generally develops after alveolar flooding has occurred. Areas of low $\dot{V}/\dot{Q}$ and shunt develop rapidly, leading to serious hypoxemia. If chronic lung disease is not present, hypercapnia is usually absent; indeed, most patients are hypocapneic. To some extent this may be due to a concurrent metabolic acidosis (due to tissue hypoxia or hypoperfusion if shock is also present). Tachypnea is uniformly present due in part to stimulation of the interstitial J-receptors and also to the diminished lung compliance that is a cardinal feature of ARDS. These factors in turn cause the work of breathing to increase, setting the stage for respiratory muscle fatigue. Once the latter occurs, rapid clinical deterioration follows, with cardiopulmonary arrest a common end point.

III. **Etiologies.** Although the causes of noncardiogenic pulmonary edema are numerous, appropriate clinical processes that are likely to be encountered in the emergency department include viral pneumonia, sepsis, severe trauma, severe head injury, gastric aspiration, near-drowning, smoke or noxious gas inhalation, and intravenous illicit-drug overdose (e.g., heroin).

IV. **Diagnosis.** ARDS should be considered if the following are present: (1) an appropriate clinical setting (see sec. III), (2) severe respiratory distress (with tachypnea and tachycardia), (3) severe hypoxemia (e.g., $PaO_2 < 60$ mm Hg with $FiO_2 > 0.6$), (4) diffuse pulmonary infiltrates on chest radiograph, (5) diminished respiratory system compliance (either inferred or measured directly during mechanical ventilation), and (6) no evidence that heart failure is the principal cause of the pulmonary infiltrates. The last criterion may require pulmonary artery catheterization in an intensive care unit. ARDS often develops hours after the initial insult and may not be clinically evident until after the patient has left the emergency department.

V. **Treatment.** Since little can be done at present to reverse noncardiogenic pulmonary edema per se, the principal goal of initial therapy is to maintain adequate tissue oxygenation by maintaining forward cardiac output, an adequate circulating mass of hemoglobin, and a PaO_2 greater than 60 mm Hg (to achieve 90% saturation of hemoglobin).

   A. Since ARDS often develops in the context of shock or trauma, **the first priority is to ensure an adequate circulation and blood pressure** with either volume infusion or use of pressors, as appropriate. The choice of fluids for volume infusion (crystalloid versus colloid) is controversial, and no one regimen has proved uniformly successful or safe. If anemia is present, blood transfusion is the ideal choice. Otherwise, crystalloid infusion is probably as effective as colloid infusion and is definitely less expensive. To minimize aggravating the extent of pulmonary edema, left-sided cardiac filling pressures (as estimated by the pulmonary artery occlusion or "wedge" pressure) should be kept as low as consistent with adequate cardiac function (often best evaluated by measurement of the mixed venous oxygen tension or saturation).

   B. If the airway is at all compromised because of trauma or because of a depressed mental status, **endotracheal intubation** (or occasionally tracheostomy) should be performed immediately.

   C. **Adequate arterial oxygenation** should be achieved as promptly as possible. Endotracheal intubation and mechanical ventilation eventually become necessary in almost all cases. If so, the initial FiO_2 should be 0.9–1.0. Although O_2 toxicity is an important concern, it is not a factor to consider during the initial management. Furthermore, even though **PEEP** has not been shown to forestall ARDS, its early use should be anticipated in any patient with developing ARDS. Sufficient PEEP to bring the PaO_2 above 60 mm Hg at an FiO_2 less than 0.6 should be instituted on a progressive basis, as required. Pulmonary artery catheterization for monitoring the cardiac output and mixed venous oxygenation are often necessary to balance the negative effect of PEEP on cardiac performance against improvements in arterial oxygenation.

   D. The use of corticosteroids during ARDS is controversial. The evidence for a beneficial effect at present is conflicting, which may reflect the diverse etiologies that cause the syndrome. Most investigators agree, however, that if steroids are to be useful, they must be given as early as possible after the initial lung injury. The dosage most commonly recommended is 30 mg/kg of methylprednisolone, and little harm can be done if one such dose is given. At some centers, the dose is repeated q6h for 48–72 hrs. This is not recommended because of a lack of evidence supporting a beneficial effect and concern that such a regimen might cause immunosuppression with subsequent nosocomial infection in a compromised host.

VI. Disposition

1. **All patients with ARDS** need to be hospitalized because of the seriousness of the underlying illness and the severity of the gas exchange abnormality. Unlike congestive heart failure, treatment of ARDS is not immediately satisfactory, and dramatic improvements in the first hours after intubation should not be anticipated.

2. Young, healthy patients who present to the emergency department without symptoms associated with ARDS but are at **risk for the subsequent development of the syndrome** (e.g., smoke or other noxious gas inhalation) may be sent home if the patient is asymptomatic at the time of discharge, the chest x-ray is clear, the ABGs are normal, close observation is available at home, and quick return to the hospital is possible should breathlessness develop. On the other hand, patients at risk for ARDS who are elderly or have a serious underlying medical illness should probably be hospitalized for overnight observation, but such cases should be handled on an individual basis.

Pulmonary Embolism

I. Assessment

A. **Clinical features.** The chief complaint is usually dyspnea and/or pleuritic pain. Some patients will also have hemoptysis. The nonspecific nature of these complaints, however, places pulmonary embolism in the differential diagnosis of a wide variety of pulmonary illnesses. Occasionally, when more than 60% of the pulmonary circulation is obstructed, the initial presentation may include syncope or shock. Tachypnea and tachycardia are generally present, and the diagnosis is suspect when they are not. Signs of right-sided cardiac pressure overload on physical examination or ECG are occasionally, but not commonly, present.

B. **Risk factors.** Since most pulmonary emboli arise from deep venous thrombosis, the risk factors for these two conditions are similar: a past history of either condition, cardiomegaly, heart failure, recent myocardial infarction, venous disease of the lower extremities, recent hip fracture, recent major surgery, malignancy, obesity, oral contraceptive use, and prolonged bed rest.

C. **Arterial blood gases.** The alveolar-arterial oxygen gradient is almost always widened; the PaO_2 is usually (approximately 90% of the time) less than 90 mm Hg; hypocarbia is usually present. The absence of any of these findings, however, should not be used to exclude the diagnosis. On the other hand, the presence of a respiratory alkalosis in a patient with COPD and chronic hypercapnia may be an important diagnostic clue to the possibility of a pulmonary embolus.

D. The **chest radiograph** is usually normal but may show a pleural effusion, a pleural-based infiltrate, platelike atelectasis, or elevation of a hemidiaphragm.

E. A **perfusion** or **ventilation-perfusion** ($\dot{V}/\dot{Q}$) lung scan is probably the first test of choice (depending on availability) in establishing or excluding the diagnosis of pulmonary embolism. The information obtained, however, depends not only on the quality and interpretation of the scan, but also on the likelihood of pulmonary emboli in the patient population being studied (the so-called prior probability). Thus, if the prior probability is extremely low, even a highly characteristic $\dot{V}/\dot{Q}$ scan would not definitely confirm the diagnosis. This kind of problem is especially important in the emergency department, where the question of pulmonary embolism is often raised because of the nonspecific complaint of pleuritic pain in otherwise young and healthy individuals. Unless a pleural effusion or evidence of deep venous thrombosis is present or a history of factors associated with veno-occlusive disease is obtained (see sec. **I.B**), the prior probability of pulmonary emboli in healthy patients under the age of 40 with the sole complaint of pleuritic pain is extremely low ($<$ 3%). Thus, further diagnostic testing (such as $\dot{V}/\dot{Q}$ scanning) in such a patient population would not be of value. On the other hand, a $\dot{V}/\dot{Q}$ scan in other patient populations at risk for pulmonary embolism can either confirm or exclude the diagnosis.

F. **Pulmonary angiography** is necessary when the data obtained above do not allow a confident conclusion either for or against the diagnosis. In some cases, however, even this test may not be definitive.

II. Treatment

A. Most patients require **supplemental oxygen.**

B. Hypotension and diminished cardiac output due to massive pulmonary emboli should be managed with a combination of volume expansion and vasoactive agents (e.g., dopamine).

Pulmonary artery catheterization can be useful in such circumstances to monitor the cardiac output and mixed venous PO_2; the wedge pressure, however, should be interpreted with caution since it is usually not possible to be certain that the vasculature between the catheter tip and left atrium is patent when pulmonary emboli are present. Elevations in the mean pulmonary artery pressure ($>$ 25 mm Hg) in patients without a prior history or reason for pulmonary hypertension may identify a group of patients at special risk for developing shock, should repeat embolization occur. Treatment of such patients is currently controversial, but some recommend prophylactic vena caval interruption, usually with an umbrella or similar device.

C. In all patients, a major goal of treatment is the **prevention of new emboli.** This is accomplished with systemic anticoagulation and/or vena caval interruption.

    1. A variety of **anticoagulation** dosing schemes with heparin have been advocated, each trying to balance the incidence of recurrence of emboli against bleeding complications. One such regimen consists of administering 10,000 units of heparin IV as a bolus, followed by a continuous infusion of 1000 units/ hour. Adjustments are subsequently made based on activated partial thromboplastin time (aPTT) determinations. The maintenance dosage necessary to achieve an increase in the aPTT to 1.5–2.0 times control values is often higher in the first 2–3 days after embolization than subsequently.

    2. If heparin cannot be administered (e.g., the patient has had recent significant upper gastrointestinal bleeding) or recurrent embolization has occurred despite adequate anticoagulation, **vena caval interruption** should be considered. If an umbrella is placed in the vena cava, heparin therapy may be continued (unless otherwise contraindicated), since heparin will prevent extension of an already existing clot. With the Greenfield filter, chronic anticoagulation is probably not necessary.

D. Thrombolytic therapy (with streptokinase or urokinase) is primarily indicated in the patient with massive pulmonary embolization ($>$ 50% of the pulmonary vasculature) and hemodynamic instability or with deep venous thrombosis extending to or beyond the iliac veins. Angiography is usually required prior to initiation of thrombolytic therapy to be certain of the diagnosis. Initiation of thrombolytic therapy more than 2–3 days after embolization has occurred often does not result in significant clot lysis.

E. Pulmonary embolectomy. With the advent of thrombolytic therapy, pulmonary embolectomy is rarely indicated in the acute setting.

F. All patients should be kept at **bed rest** to assist in the prevention of further embolization of an existing clot.

III. Disposition. All patients with proven or suspected pulmonary emboli need to be hospitalized.

Aspiration Syndromes

Any foreign material that is accidentally inhaled into the lung has been "aspirated." The consequences vary, however, depending on the nature of the aspirate. The clinical presentation is the result of airway obstruction, direct chemical injury to the airway mucosa, or secondary infection.

I. Aspiration of gastric contents usually occurs in patients with an altered mental status (e.g., during cardiopulmonary resuscitation). If the pH of the aspirate is low ($<$ 2.5), the adult respiratory distress syndrome may result. Airway obstruction with hypoxemia and atelectasis occurs when the volume of the aspirate is large. Both airway obstruction and secondary pneumonia may occur if large food particles are aspirated. Despite these risks, as many as one-third of patients improve spontaneously within 48 hours. Thus, **routine use of glucocorticoids or prophylactic antibiotics is not recommended.** Instead, patients should be hospitalized and supported as indicated by the severity of their gas exchange abnormality. Bronchoscopy should be performed to relieve airway obstruction due to aspiration of large food particles or foreign objects. A subsequent deterioration in pulmonary status after 36–48 hours (with respiratory distress and worsening hypoxemia) may indicate the emergence of a secondary pneumonia. In such cases, the most common offending organism is a gram-negative aerobe, and appropriate antibiotics should be given.

II. **Aspiration of oropharyngeal contents.** To a certain extent, all normal individuals probably aspirate small quantities of oropharyngeal secretions, especially while sleeping. However, pneumonia does not occur because of normal host defense mechanisms. In contrast, individuals with altered pulmonary defenses are more likely to develop a community-acquired pneumonia after aspiration; patients with COPD or alcohol abuse, especially those with poor oral hygiene, are at especially high risk. The pneumonia that develops depends on the resident flora in the given individual, but **anaerobic pneumonia** is particularly common. A classic clinical presentation is that of an alcoholic with complaints of breathlessness, insidious weight loss, fever, and a pulmonary infiltrate in a dependent lung segment on chest x-ray (e.g., the superior segment of either lower lobe) that may or may not be accompanied by cavitation or a pleural effusion. If the latter is present, material obtained appropriately for anaerobic culture may later prove to be diagnostic. The initial management of these patients includes hospitalization, appropriate, supportive care for any gas exchange abnormality, antibiotics (including penicillin if no contraindication exists), and postural drainage if an abscess is present.

III. **Foreign body aspiration.** See Chaps. 2 and 28.

IV. **Near-drowning.** See Chap. 15.

Pleural Effusion

A **pleural effusion** refers to fluid in the pleural space. Visualization on an upright chest x-ray implies at least 500 ml of fluid is present, whereas visualization on a lateral decubitus view is possible with less than 50 ml of fluid. Bilateral decubitus films should be obtained whenever possible to confirm the diagnosis and visualize the parenchyma of the "up" lung. A pleural effusion in association with a pneumonia is often referred to as parapneumonic, but this term does not necessarily imply that the fluid itself is infected (empyema).

I. **Etiologies** include heart failure, malignancy, pulmonary embolism, pulmonary infarction, pneumonia, trauma, collagen-vascular disease, pancreatitis, renal failure, hepatic failure with ascites, and esophageal rupture.

II. **Assessment.** A diagnostic thoracentesis (see Chap. 38) should be performed unless there is good reason to expect that the effusion is due to a noninfectious, benign cause, such as congestive heart failure or hepatic failure with ascites (i.e., that the fluid is a transudate). The fluid can be submitted for the following studies.

A. **Cell count and differential.** Gross blood is seen with pulmonary infarction, tumor, or trauma. The total white blood cell count is not of much value.

B. **Fluid pH.** A pH less than 7.3 is seen with empyema, malignancy, or collagen vascular disease. A pH less than 7.0–7.1 usually means that thoracostomy drainage will be required.

C. **Glucose.** A glucose concentration less than 40 mg/dl is associated with empyema, rheumatoid arthritis, or tuberculosis.

D. **Amylase and triglycerides.** Elevation in amylase occurs with pancreatitis, renal failure, or esophageal rupture, whereas elevation of triglycerides is seen in chylous effusions.

E. **Protein and lactic dehydrogenase (LDH) determinations.** When values are approximately twice as high as serum values, the fluid is an exudate rather than a transudate. Further diagnostic evaluation of transudates is generally unnecessary.

F. **Stains and cultures** for bacteria, mycobacteria, and fungi can be obtained.

G. **Cytology.** Several hundred milliliters of pleural fluid should be submitted, if possible.

III. **Management.** The primary therapeutic question is whether the effusion will resolve spontaneously or not. Infected pleural fluid (as evidenced by a positive stain, gross purulence, or a positive culture), fluid with a pH less than 7.0–7.1, and grossly bloody fluid generally will not resolve spontaneously and therefore will require tube thoracostomy drainage. Two other indications for this procedure include very large effusions that cause symptoms (e.g., dyspnea) and effusions that recur rapidly after initial attempts to drain them by simple needle aspiration. No more than 1 liter of fluid should be drained at a time (unless the fluid is bloody due to trauma) because of the risk of reexpansion pulmonary edema. Sclerosis or surgical ablation of the pleural space may be necessary in the case of recurrent symptomatic effusion.

IV. **Disposition.** Patients with a new pleural effusion should be hospitalized for diagnosis and treatment. In contrast, patients with chronic effusions that are relatively stable in size and do not cause significant respiratory distress may not require hospitalization; early follow-up for such patients is usually appropriate.

Bibliography

1. Dantzker, D. R. Mechanisms of Hypoxemia and Hypercapnia. In R. C. Bone (ed.), *Critical Care: A Comprehensive Approach*. Park Ridge, Ill.: American College of Chest Physicians, 1984. Pp. 1–14.
2. Dantzker, D. R. Respiratory Muscle Function and Fatigue. In R. C. Bone (ed.), *Critical Care: A Comprehensive Approach*. Park Ridge, Ill.: American College of Chest Physicians, 1984. Pp. 48–59.
3. Fanta, C. H., Rossing, T. H., and McFadden, E. R., Jr. Glucocorticoids in acute asthma: A critical control trial. *Am. J. Med.* 74:845, 1983.
4. Hopewell, P. C., and Miller, R. T. Pathophysiology and management of severe asthma. *Clin. Chest Med.* 5:623, 1984.
5. Hudson, L. D. Causes of the adult respiratory distress syndrome: Clinical recognition. *Clin. Chest Med.* 3:195, 1982.
6. Jay, S. J. Diagnostic procedures for pleural disease. *Clin. Chest Med.* 6:33, 1985.
7. Make, B. Medical management of emphysema. *Clin. Chest Med.* 4:465, 1983.
8. Nowak, R. M., et al. Spirometric evaluation of acute bronchial asthma. *J.A.C.E.P.* 8:9, 1979.
9. Nowak, R. M., et al. Comparison of peak expiratory flow and FEV_1 admission criteria for acute bronchial asthma. *Ann. Emerg. Med.* 11:64, 1982.
10. Petty, T. L. Principles of Mechanical Ventilation. In T. L. Petty (ed.), *Intensive and Rehabilitative Respiratory Care*. Philadelphia: Lea & Febiger, 1982. Pp. 88–113.
11. Polak, J. F., and McNeil, B. J. Pulmonary scintigraphy and the diagnosis of pulmonary embolism: A perspective. *Clin. Chest Med.* 5:457, 1984.
12. Rossing, T. H., et al. Emergency therapy of asthma: Comparison of the acute effects of parenteral and inhaled sympathomimetics and infused aminophylline. *Am. Rev. Respir. Dis.* 122:365, 1980.
13. Stauffer, J. L. Establishment and Care of the Airway. In T. L. Petty (ed.), *Intensive and Rehabilitative Respiratory Care*. Philadelphia: Lea & Febiger, 1982. Pp. 22–73.
14. Volgesang, G. B., and Bell, W. R. Treatment of pulmonary embolism and deep vein thrombosis with thrombolytic therapy. *Clin. Chest Med.* 5:487, 1984.

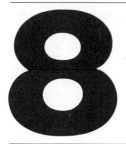

Acid-Base, Fluid, and Electrolyte Disturbances

L. Lee Hamm III

Disorders of fluid and electrolyte balance and acid-base homeostasis may be primary or secondary to other illnesses. However, since many of these disorders do not have specific symptoms or findings on physical examination, routine laboratory tests such as serum electrolytes and arterial blood gases provide invaluable information; they should be obtained wisely, but not reluctantly. The history and physical examination are extremely useful in guiding the selection of the laboratory investigation and in establishing etiologic diagnoses.

Acid-Base Disturbances

I. Physiology and general assessment

A. Acid-base homeostasis is maintained by three interrelated components: body buffers, ventilatory control of carbon dioxide (CO_2), and renal handling of bicarbonate (HCO_3^-). Changes in pH are moderated by various buffer systems, particularly blood and tissue proteins, bone, and the CO_2/HCO_3^- buffer system. The last is especially important both in diagnostic and physiologic terms, since both CO_2 and HCO_3^- can be adjusted independently by the body.

B. The **Henderson-Hasselbach equation,**

$$pH = 6.1 + \log \frac{[HCO_3^-]}{0.03 \times PCO_2},$$

defines the obligatory interrelationship of pH, HCO_3^- concentration in mEq/liter, and PCO_2 in mm Hg. This relationship is depicted graphically in Fig. 8-1 as the acid-base nomogram. On the nomogram, the intersection of any two of the three components (i.e., pH, PCO_2, $[HCO_3^-]$) should define the third. Any major deviation from this relationship suggests a laboratory error. The total CO_2 reported with the serum electrolytes is HCO_3^- plus dissolved CO_2; since the latter is small, the total CO_2 and the calculated HCO_3^- reported with the blood gases are nearly equal.

1. Primary changes

a. Metabolic disturbances. Primary changes in HCO_3^- are metabolic disturbances. A primary decrease in plasma HCO_3^- is a metabolic acidosis; this can result from large exogenous acid loads, large endogenous acid loads (e.g., ketoacids, lactic acid), gastrointestinal (GI) HCO_3^- losses, or failure of the kidneys to resorb HCO_3^- or excrete acid appropriately. A metabolic alkalosis (i.e., a primary increase in HCO_3^-) can result from large exogenous alkali loads but usually follows inappropriate loss of acid from the GI tract (usually as gastric acid) or the kidneys.

b. Respiratory disturbances. Primary changes in PCO_2 result from respiratory disturbances. A respiratory acidosis results from excess accumulation of CO_2 (i.e., a rise in PCO_2); in contrast, a respiratory alkalosis (i.e., a primary decrease in PCO_2) occurs from inappropriately high ventilation.

2. Compensation. Primary disorders of PCO_2 (respiratory disorders) should lead to compensatory changes in HCO_3^- in the same direction. This tends to normalize the HCO_3^-/PCO_2 ratio and hence the blood pH. Most of the change in HCO_3^- results from changes in the renal handling of HCO_3^-. Likewise, primary disturbances in HCO_3^- should lead to compensatory changes in PCO_2 in the same direction. Ventilatory compensation with PCO_2 (in response to metabolic disorders) usually takes hours to develop; renal compensation of HCO_3^- handling in response to respiratory disorders often takes days to develop fully. The **predicted compensatory response** is given in Table 8-1. These are also

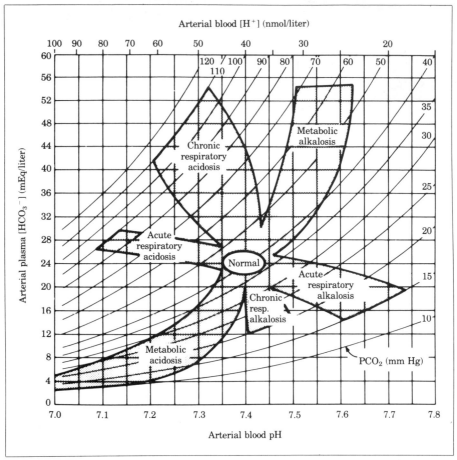

Fig. 8-1. Acid-base nomogram showing 95% confidence limits of respiratory and metabolic compensations for primary, simple acid-base disturbances. The pH, [HCO$_3^-$], and PCO$_2$ should intersect for any blood gas sample. To predict the pH change with changes in [HCO$_3^-$] or PCO$_2$, trace along the diagonal lines for changes in [HCO$_3^-$] with constant PCO$_2$ or trace along the horizontal lines for changes in PCO$_2$ with constant [HCO$_3^-$]. (Reproduced from M. G. Cogan, F. C. Rector, and D. W. Seldin, Acid-Base Disorders. In B. M. Brenner and F. C. Rector (eds.), *The Kidney.* Philadelphia: Saunders, 1981. With permission.)

incorporated in the acid-base nomogram (see Fig. 8-1). The respiratory compensation to a metabolic acid-base disorder and the metabolic compensation (i.e., renal compensation in chronic disorders) to respiratory disorders are an integral result of the primary disorder. Failure of compensation, after the hours or days required for its full development, implies an additional acid-base disorder. For example, if a metabolic acidosis produced a fall in HCO$_3^-$ (ΔHCO$_3^-$ in mEq/liter) from 25 to 15 mEq/liter, the PCO$_2$ should fall to 26–30 mm Hg from 40 mm Hg after several hours (see Predicted Response in Table 8-1); however, if the PCO$_2$ remained at 40 mm Hg, then a respiratory acidosis would be present in addition to the metabolic acidosis.

C. **Clues to the presence of an acid-base disorder** can come from the **history** (e.g., a history of vomiting should lead to the suspicion of a metabolic alkalosis), the **physical examination** (e.g., Kussmaul's respirations should suggest a metabolic acidosis), or **electrolyte abnormalities** detected on routine laboratory determinations. Of particular note regarding the last are changes in plasma HCO$_3^-$ or chloride (Cl$^-$) as presented in Table 8-1. Abnormalities of chloride should be considered in proportion to the sodium (Na$^+$) concentration. For instance, with hyponatremia (e.g., a serum

Table 8-1. Diagnosis of acid-base disorders

Primary disorder	pH	PCO_2	$[HCO_3^-]$	$[Cl^-]$	Predicted response
Metabolic acidosis	Low	Low	Low*	$\uparrow$ or $\rightarrow$	$\Delta PCO_2(\downarrow) = (1.0-1.4)\Delta\ HCO_3^-$
Respiratory acidosis	Low	High*	High	$\downarrow$	Acute: $\Delta HCO_3^-(\uparrow) = 0.1\Delta PCO_2$ Chronic: $\Delta HCO_3^-(\uparrow) = (0.25-0.55)\Delta PCO^2$
Metabolic alkalosis	High	High	High*	$\downarrow$	$\Delta PCO_2(\uparrow) = (0.4-0.9)\Delta HCO_3^-$
Respiratory alkalosis	High	Low*	Low	$\uparrow$	Acute: $\Delta HCO_3^-(\downarrow) = (0.2-0.25)\Delta PCO_2$ Chronic: $\Delta HCO_3^-(\downarrow) = (0.4-0.5)\Delta PCO_2$

*Initiating disturbance.
Key: $\rightarrow$ = no change; $\uparrow$ = increase; $\downarrow$ = decrease

Table 8-2. Important causes of an abnormal anion gap

Increased anion gap	Decreased anion gap

Metabolic acidosis
  Uremia
  Ketoacidosis
  Lactic acidosis
  Intoxications (e.g., methanol, ethyl-
  ene glycol, salicylate, paraldehyde)
Alkalosis
Hyperalbuminemia (dehydration)
Administered anions (e.g., citrate, car-
benicillin, penicillin)
	Hypoalbuminemia
	Paraprotein (myeloma)
	Falsely low measured serum Na^+ (hy-
	perviscosity, extreme hypernatremia)
	Falsely high measured Cl^- (bromism)

Na^+ of 120 mEq/liter), the chloride concentration usually will fall simultaneously (e.g., to approximately 85 mEq/liter).

1. The **anion gap** is also a useful guide in diagnosing acid-base disorders. The anion gap is usually calculated as $[Na^+] - ([HCO_3^-] + [Cl^-])$ and is normally 8–16 mEq/liter. Important causes of an abnormal anion gap are listed in Table 8-2. An anion gap greater than 30 mEq/liter is almost always associated with a metabolic acidosis; an anion gap between 20 and 30 mEq/liter is usually associated with a metabolic acidosis.

2. **Arterial blood gases** (ABGs) are the definitive guide to the diagnosis of acid-base disturbances. Simple acid-base disorders are those with only one primary disturbance (and its compensatory response); a guide to the diagnosis of these is given in Table 8-1. Mixed acid-base disorders are those with two or more primary disturbances (e.g., a metabolic acidosis and primary respiratory alkalosis); these are discussed in sec. II.E. Using Table 8-1, the predominant disorder can be diagnosed. For example, if the pH is low, a metabolic or respiratory acidosis is predominant, and these can be differentiated by the PCO_2 and HCO_3^-. If the pH and HCO_3^- are low and the PCO_2 is high, then a mixed metabolic and respiratory acidosis is present.

II. **Specific acid-base disturbances**
   A. **Respiratory acidosis**
      1. **Etiologies** of a respiratory acidosis are those of respiratory failure. Acute respiratory acidosis is often caused by sedative overdose, neuromuscular illnesses or injuries, airway obstruction, pulmonary edema, or acute illnesses or injuries involving the lungs or the thoracic cage. Chronic respiratory acidosis is usually caused by chronic obstructive pulmonary disease but may result from chronic neuromuscular illnesses or severe restrictive pulmonary disease.
      2. **Manifestations.** Acute and chronic respiratory acidoses differ in many important aspects. Clinically, acute hypercapnia and respiratory acidosis are often

marked by restlessness, dyspnea, tachypnea, and a declining mental status. Chronic hypercapnia, on the other hand, frequently is less symptomatic but may also result in an altered mental status (e.g., somnolence, confusion), asterixis, headache, and signs of increased intracranial pressure; in addition, signs of chronic pulmonary disease are often present with chronic respiratory acidosis. Hypoxia usually accompanies both acute and chronic respiratory acidoses and may be the more emergent problem.

3. **Arterial blood gases** should readily differentiate a respiratory acidosis from a metabolic acidosis (see Table 8-1). Acute hypercapnia causes a large fall in pH with a small rise in plasma HCO_3^- (see Table 8-1 and Fig. 8-1); an acute increase in PCO_2 of 20 mm Hg should cause approximately a 0.15-unit fall in arterial pH but only a 2 mEq/liter increase in HCO_3^-. In contrast, after several days of renal compensation to chronic respiratory acidosis, the HCO_3^- increases significantly and the pH rises toward normal; chronically, the same 20 mm Hg increase in PCO_2 should cause a 5–11 mEq/liter increase in HCO_3^- with a pH exceeding 7.32. Therefore, with chronic hypercapnia, acidemia is mild. Acute exacerbations of CO_2 retention in chronic pulmonary disease are frequent occurrences and result in intermediate changes in the pH and HCO_3^- for the level of PCO_2.

4. **Treatment** of respiratory acidosis usually involves the management of respiratory failure. Hence, therapy includes both improving oxygenation and increasing ventilation to lessen hypercapnia and acidemia. Use of sodium bicarbonate ($NaHCO_3$) to treat the acidemia should be avoided, since any benefits will be temporary. Instead, efforts should be directed at increasing ventilation. However, lowering the PCO_2 should be gradual in patients with chronic respiratory acidosis to avoid a posthypercapneic metabolic alkalosis. Also, although oxygen administration is usually needed in both acute and chronic respiratory acidoses, high inspired oxygen concentrations generally should be avoided initially in patients with chronic respiratory acidosis (if not on controlled mechanical ventilation) to avoid precipitously removing their hypoxic ventilatory drive; this is necessary because the normal hypercapneic ventilatory drive is impaired in these patients. During the initial therapy of both acute and chronic respiratory acidoses, ABGs should be obtained frequently to ensure adequate oxygenation and normalization of the blood pH (at least within the range of 7.25–7.50).

5. **Disposition.** In general, patients with acute respiratory acidosis, worsening of chronic respiratory acidosis, significant acidemia (i.e., pH < 7.3), or other complications (e.g., a metabolic acidosis or alkalosis, hypo- or hyperkalemia) should be hospitalized for treatment.

B. A **respiratory alkalosis** is caused by excessive ventilatory excretion of CO_2. Of course, increased ventilation (i.e., either an increased tidal volume or respiratory rate) is appropriate in the presence of hypoxia but often inappropriate for the acid-base status.

1. **Etiologies** of respiratory alkalosis include pulmonary disorders (such as hypoxia without CO_2 retention, pulmonary embolism, pulmonary edema, or pneumonia), anxiety, pain, central nervous system (CNS) lesions, sepsis, severe liver disease, salicylate overdosage, and excessive mechanical ventilation. In addition, rapid correction of plasma HCO_3^- in patients with a metabolic acidosis may produce a picture of respiratory alkalosis. Recognition of the presence of respiratory alkalosis can be the initial clue to the diagnosis of unsuspected salicylate intoxication, sepsis, pulmonary embolism, or early shock.

2. **Manifestations.** Clinically, a respiratory alkalosis frequently causes perioral and peripheral paresthesias and may lead to frank signs of neuromuscular irritability, such as hyperreflexia, tetany, and seizures. Severe alkalemia can cause refractory cardiac arrhythmias, and alkalemia can also worsen hepatic encephalopathy. In addition, hypocapnia reduces cerebral blood flow.

3. **Arterial blood gases** show a high pH and a low PCO_2 and HCO_3^- (see Table 8-1). A high HCO_3^- would also indicate a mixed respiratory and metabolic alkalosis. The PCO_2 is also low with a metabolic acidosis; however, the pH is low, not high. A mixed respiratory alkalosis and metabolic acidosis is a common mixed disturbance, which is discussed in sec. **II.E.**

4. **Treatment** of mild respiratory alkalosis consists of the therapy of the underlying illness (e.g., pneumonia, salicylate intoxication, hypoxia) in many cases. Anxiety-induced hyperventilation is treated by efforts to calm the patient and having the patient rebreathe CO_2 (into a paper bag) to lessen the symptoms of

Table 8-3. Important causes of a metabolic acidosis

High anion gap	Normal anion gap
Renal failure	GI loss of HCO_3^- (e.g., diarrhea, ureterosigmoidostomy)
Ketoacidosis (diabetic, alcoholic)	
Lactic acidosis	Renal tubular acidosis (including carbonic anhydrase inhibitors and hypoaldosteronism)
Intoxications (e.g., ethylene glycol, methanol, salicylate, paraldehyde)	
	Hyperalimentation
	"Dilution" acidosis
	Renal failure
	Ketoacidosis

alkalemia, such as paresthesias, which further produce anxiety. In patients on mechanical ventilation, the tidal volume or respiratory rate can be lowered as allowed by adequate oxygenation; increasing the dead space will also raise the PCO_2. Severe respiratory alkalosis in seriously ill patients requires specific aggressive therapy, as the associated mortality is high.

   5. **Disposition** will depend on the etiology of the respiratory alkalosis. Since respiratory alkalosis can indicate the presence of an otherwise inapparent significant illness, the etiology should be established; this may require hospitalization.

C. **Metabolic acidosis**

   1. The **etiologic categories** of a metabolic acidosis include large acid loads (exogenous or endogenous) that consume plasma HCO_3^-, loss of HCO_3^- from the GI tract or the kidneys, and failure of the kidneys to excrete acid. A useful clinical classification, based on the anion gap, is given in Table 8-3. Renal failure and ketoacidosis usually result in a high anion gap but may cause metabolic acidosis without an elevated anion gap in some cases. Simple laboratory tests (i.e., serum creatinine or blood urea nitrogen [BUN], glucose, ketones, lactate, and toxicology tests) can aid in establishing the etiology of a high anion gap metabolic acidosis.

   2. **Manifestations** of a metabolic acidosis may include hyperventilation, hyperkalemia, hypotension, pulmonary edema (particularly with volume expansion in the setting of severe acidemia), and an altered mental status; the last, however, may be a reflection of other physiologic derangements in severely ill patients with an acute metabolic acidosis. An acidosis also stimulates catecholamine release. The plasma HCO_3^- is low unless there are additional acid-base disorders, such as a chronic respiratory acidosis or metabolic alkalosis. An elevated anion gap or chloride may also be a clue to the presence of a metabolic acidosis. The blood pH and arterial PCO_2 will be low (see Table 8-1 and Fig. 8-1); if the PCO_2 is normal or high, a respiratory acidosis is superimposed. Patients presenting with a metabolic acidosis should have a urine pH measured prior to treatment to assess the ability of the kidneys to acidify the urine; patients with a hyperchloremic acidosis without diarrhea may have renal tubular acidosis (RTA), which represents a category of metabolic acidosis caused by the inability of the kidneys to adequately resorb HCO_3^- (proximal RTA) or excrete acid by acidifying the urine (distal RTA).

   3. **Treatment** of metabolic acidosis generally is unnecessary if the acidosis is mild to moderate (i.e., pH > 7.2) and the underlying cause is being corrected. Severe acute metabolic acidosis, however, should be treated with intravenous $NaHCO_3$ to raise the pH to 7.2.

      a. **Administration of bicarbonate.** Estimating HCO_3^- needs is often unnecessary and inaccurate, as HCO_3^- may be continually consumed by acid production (e.g., uncontrolled lactic acidosis) or may be produced as organic acids (e.g., lactate, ketoacids) are metabolized to HCO_3^-. One approach is to give patients with severe metabolic acidosis 2–4 ampules of $NaHCO_3$ (1 ampule = 44 mEq HCO_3^-) and remeasure the blood pH. The HCO_3^- (and pH) should be monitored frequently to estimate subsequent needs, aiming for a plasma HCO_3^- of 15 mEq/liter (or a pH of 7.2).
      Administration of $NaHCO_3$ frequently is complicated by hypernatremia and

volume overload. HCO_3^- administration may also precipitate hypokalemia in potassium-depleted patients, since the untreated acidemia can mask the potassium depletion. HCO_3^- administration can also precipitate paresthesias and tetany in hypocalcemic patients.

b. Dialysis. In very severe acidosis (particularly lactic acidosis with cardiovascular and renal compromise), continual HCO_3^- needs may exceed volume excretion; in such a situation, hemodialysis or peritoneal dialysis can sometimes be attempted to treat both the acidemia and the volume overload.

c. Ventilation. Treatment of acidemia should also include appropriate ventilation to eliminate the CO_2 formed. In addition, for example, an HCO_3^- of 10 with a metabolic acidosis should be accompanied by a PCO_2 of 20–25 mm Hg and a pH of about 7.25 (see Fig. 8-1 and Table 8-1); however, if the PCO_2 were 40 mm Hg (i.e., a concomitant respiratory acidosis), the pH would be 7.0, and correction of the "inapparent" respiratory disorder would drastically improve the arterial pH.

4. Specific forms of acidosis. Diabetic ketoacidosis and renal failure are discussed in Chaps. 9 and 13, respectively.

a. Lactic acidosis

(1) Etiologies. Lactic acidosis is usually caused by tissue hypoxia, resulting from inadequate perfusion or acute hypoxemia. The disorder often occurs in the setting of septic shock, cardiogenic shock, or hypovolemic shock. Grand mal seizures, diabetic ketoacidosis, and ethanol ingestion are also commonly accompanied by some degree of lactic acidosis. Other less frequent causes include various drugs and toxins, certain hereditary metabolic disorders, and some malignancies.

(2) The **diagnosis** of lactic acidosis is made by the finding of an elevated lactate level in the presence of a metabolic acidosis. However, the diagnosis is strongly suggested by the presence of a high anion-gap metabolic acidosis in the absence of renal failure, ketoacidosis, and the intoxications listed in Table 8-3.

(3) Treatment of lactic acidosis requires reversal of the underlying etiology, including restoration of tissue perfusion and blood pressure and maintenance of adequate oxygenation. Treatment of the acidosis per se frequently requires administration of HCO_3^- as described in sec. **II.C.3.a.** However, the HCO_3^- requirements are often large and continuous until the underlying cause is treated. Furosemide may aid in the excretion of excess volume and sodium loads associated with $NaHCO_3$ administration. However, hemodialysis or peritoneal dialysis using bicarbonate dialysate may be necessary.

b. Ketoacidosis is sometimes found in the absence of diabetic ketoacidosis (discussed in Chap. 9). The usual circumstance is a malnourished or starved patient with a history of heavy alcohol comsumption (alcoholic ketoacidosis). Vomiting is usually present. Lactic acidosis, volume depletion, and electrolyte deficiencies (particularly involving potassium, magnesium, and phosphate) often are present. Plasma glucose may be low to moderately elevated. Other acid-base disorders (e.g., a metabolic alkalosis from vomiting or a respiratory alkalosis) may be mixed with the metabolic acidosis. The usual nitroprusside test (Acetest) for ketones is insensitive because β-hydroxybutyrate exceeds acetoacetate. Treatment consists of volume repletion and administration of glucose, electrolytes, and vitamins (e.g., thiamine).

c. Intoxications. Certain poisonings (see Table 8-3) can produce a high anion-gap metabolic acidosis; the acidosis can be a clue to the diagnosis of these. Early recognition of salicylate, ethylene glycol, and methanol poisoning is important for successful treatment. Specific treatment of these poisonings is discussed in Chap. 16.

(1) Salicylate poisoning can cause metabolic acidosis, respiratory alkalosis, or a combination. Suspicion of this disorder should arise in patients with a high anion-gap acidosis or a respiratory alkalosis.

(2) Ethylene glycol, the main ingredient in antifreeze, causes CNS manifestations (i.e., inebriation leading to coma), cardiovascular collapse, a severe high anion-gap metabolic acidosis, and later renal failure.

(3) Methanol causes retinitis (leading to blindness) and a severe metabolic acidosis, appearing several hours after ingestion.

Table 8-4. Metabolic alkalosis: common causes

Associated with volume depletion: urine chloride < 10 mEq/liter
  Gastrointestinal disorders (usually vomiting or gastric drainage)
  Diuretics
Mineralocorticoid excess: urine chloride > 20 mEq/liter
Posthypercapneic syndrome
Milk-alkali syndrome

---

5. **Disposition.** Patients with metabolic acidosis should be hospitalized for evaluation and treatment unless the problem is mild and chronic and the etiology is known.

D. **Metabolic alkalosis** is characterized by a high HCO_3^- concentration, pH, and PCO_2. Under normal conditions, the kidneys have an enormous capacity to excrete HCO_3^- rapidly. Therefore, a metabolic alkalosis is usually associated with some abnormality that serves to "maintain" excess HCO_3^-.

1. **Etiologies** of a metabolic alkalosis are given in Table 8-4. The most common cause is vomiting or gastric drainage; the associated volume (NaCl) depletion serves to maintain the alkalosis by preventing the kidneys from excreting the excess HCO_3^-. Diuretics and some uncommon forms of diarrhea are also associated with a metabolic alkalosis and volume depletion. All these disorders are marked by a low urine chloride; however, diuretics may induce a metabolic alkalosis without a low urine chloride and in edematous states without volume depletion. The second major category of metabolic alkalosis is that caused by mineralocorticoid excess; this group includes primary hyperaldosteronism and Cushing's syndrome, among others, and is marked by some evidence of volume overload and a high urine chloride. Another, usually transient, form of metabolic alkalosis is posthypercapneic metabolic alkalosis; this occurs when chronic respiratory acidosis with compensatory retention of HCO_3^- is rapidly treated with improved ventilation, leaving an HCO_3^- concentration disproportionately high for the PCO_2. Alkali administration (e.g., HCO_3^-, antacids, citrate) in the presence of renal insufficiency may also cause a metabolic alkalosis. The milk-alkali syndrome is similar; combined calcium and antacid ingestion results in nephrocalcinosis and renal insufficiency, which prevents the appropriate excretion of HCO_3^-.

2. **Manifestations** of a metabolic alkalosis may include hypoventilation, hypokalemia, and occasionally problems secondary to alkalemia, such as neuromuscular irritability (e.g., tetany) and arrhythmias. The history and physical examination may provide clues to the diagnosis (e.g., a history of vomiting, signs of volume depletion). The pH, HCO_3^-, and PCO_2 will be elevated in simple metabolic alkalosis (see Table 8-1). The respiratory compensation to a metabolic alkalosis (hypoventilation) is variable and usually produces a PCO_2 less than 55 mm Hg. A metabolic alkalosis may worsen ventilation in chronic pulmonary disease and hinder weaning patients off ventilatory support. A low plasma Cl^- is another manifestation of a metabolic alkalosis in some cases.

3. **Treatment** of a metabolic alkalosis associated with volume depletion usually can be accomplished by NaCl administration. Usually there are concomitant potassium deficits that require KCl administration. Inhibition of gastric acid secretion (e.g., with cimetidine) may be helpful when continued gastric suction is necessary. Patients with mineralocorticoid excess can be aided by administration of spironolactone (a mineralocorticoid antagonist) and potassium while the source of excess mineralocorticoids is investigated and removed. Acetazolamide, a carbonic anhydrase inhibitor, can be used to induce an $NaHCO_3$ diuresis in patients with adequate renal function, volume overload, and a metabolic alkalosis (e.g., a diuretic-induced metabolic alkalosis in patients with congestive heart failure). In patients with a simultaneous respiratory alkalosis, treatment of the respiratory component (to raise the PCO_2) may rapidly lower the pH toward normal. In extreme cases of a metabolic alkalosis and alkalemia, intravenous acid (i.e., dilute HCl, NH_4Cl, arginine hydrochloride) or hemodialysis may be used.

    4. Disposition. Most patients with metabolic alkalosis should be hospitalized for evaluation and treatment.

  E. Mixed acid-base disorders are not uncommon and occur when an illness produces two or three of the "simple" acid-base disorders. An example is the patient with cardiopulmonary arrest who has both a lactic acidosis and a respiratory acidosis.

    1. Assessment. These mixed disorders require a thorough history and physical examination and careful evaluation of both the arterial blood gases and serum electrolytes.

      a. Arterial blood gases that fail to conform to one of the patterns shown on the nomogram (Fig. 8-1) represent mixed disorders, assuming sufficient time has elapsed for appropriate compensation. Likewise, the predicted responses given in Table 8-1 can be used similarly. For example, if a patient has a pH of 7.2, PCO_2 of 40 mm Hg, and HCO_3^- of 15 mEq/liter, the predominant disorder is a metabolic acidosis. However, this example falls between a respiratory acidosis and metabolic acidosis on the nomogram, and using Table 8-1, the expected $PCO_2 = 40 - [1.2 \times (25 - 15)] = 40 - 12 = 28$ mm Hg. Since the measured PCO_2 is significantly higher, the patient has a respiratory acidosis in addition to the metabolic acidosis. However, such an approach fails in some circumstances. For instance, a pH of 7.26, PCO_2 of 60, and HCO_3^- of 26 appear on the nomogram to be an acute respiratory acidosis; however, if the history were of chronic respiratory failure, these blood gas values could represent a chronic respiratory acidosis with a superimposed metabolic acidosis.

      b. The **anion gap and chloride concentration** can also be clues to the presence of mixed disorders. For instance, in the last example in sec. **a**, an elevated anion gap would readily diagnose the presence of a metabolic acidosis. Similarly, the chloride concentration, using Table 8-1, can provide a clue to the presence of an otherwise inapparent diagnosis. For example, if $Na^+ = 140$ mEq/liter, $HCO_3^- = 15$ mEq/liter, and $Cl^- = 90$ mEq/liter, the elevated anion gap (35 mEq/liter) virtually diagnoses a metabolic acidosis; however, the low Cl^- implies a simultaneous respiratory acidosis or metabolic alkalosis (see Table 8-1).

    2. The **management** of mixed acid-base disorders first requires the recognition of all of the component disorders. Treatment then depends on that defined for the individual disorders. The physician must recognize that treating only one component of a mixed acidosis and alkalosis may worsen the blood pH. For example, a diuretic-induced metabolic alkalosis is common in patients with a chronic respiratory acidosis; in these patients, rapidly lowering the PCO_2 may cause a severe alkalemia.

Fluid and Electrolyte Disturbances

This section deals with disorders of salt, water, and potassium homeostasis. Disorders of other extracellular ions (i.e., Ca^{++}, Mg^{++}, and phosphate) are discussed in Chap. 9.

I. Physiology and assessment

  A. Volume and salt homeostasis

    1. The **fluid compartments** of the body are divided into the **intracellular** and **extracellular** compartments. Water moves freely between the two compartments, keeping the osmolality equal. Potassium is the major intracellular cationic solute; sodium is the major extracellular cationic solute. Since sodium is effectively restricted to the extracellular compartment, sodium balance is the main determinant of the extracellular fluid volume. If salt (NaCl) is retained, as in congestive heart failure, the extracellular fluid volume expands; the reverse is also true. The extracellular fluid volume is about 20% of the body weight, that is, about 14 liters in a 70-kg adult.

      a. The **extracellular fluid volume and salt homeostasis** ordinarily are regulated by the kidneys. The sensors of extracellular fluid volume include both extrarenal baroreceptors and intrarenal sensors. In the kidneys, glomerular filtration and subsequent renal tubular resorption determine sodium excretion. Normally, large amounts of sodium are filtered across the glomeruli each day.

$$\text{Filtered Na}^+ = \text{glomerular filtration rate (or creatinine clearance)}$$
$$\times \text{ plasma Na}^+ = 100 \text{ ml/minute} \times 140 \text{ mEq/liter}$$
$$= 14 \text{ mEq/minute} = 20,160 \text{ mEq/day}$$

Of this, greater than 95% is normally resorbed by the renal tubules and reenters the circulation. Tubular sodium resorption is altered by numerous factors, including aldosterone and peritubular protein. Adrenal aldosterone secretion is primarily determined by the renin-angiotensin system. Normally, the entire system (i.e., the sensors and kidneys) maintains a relatively constant extracellular fluid volume despite wide variations in salt intake, as Na^+ intake is matched by Na^+ excretion. However, in certain illnesses (e.g., heart failure, cirrhosis, nephrotic syndrome), Na^+ retention continues despite an expanded extracellular fluid volume.

   b. The **extracellular fluid compartment** includes the **interstitial compartment** and the **intravascular compartment.** Blood proteins and cellular elements are relatively restricted to the intravascular space. In contrast, electrolytes, such as NaCl, diffuse freely between the vascular compartment and the larger interstitial compartment. Of course, integrity of the intravascular volume is the critical factor for an adequate circulation. Under certain conditions (e.g., severe hypoalbuminemia), the relationship between the intravascular volume and total extracellular volume becomes deranged, usually with the former decreased and the latter increased.

2. **Assessment** of the extracellular fluid volume depends predominantly on a thorough history and physical examination. Certain laboratory values are also useful in assessing the volume status. For example, a high BUN/creatinine ratio (greater than 10:1) and a low urine Na^+ concentration (less than 10 mEq/liter) are frequently found in volume-depleted patients. Of course, measurements of the central venous pressure and pulmonary capillary wedge pressure are the most accurate gauge of the right and left ventricular filling pressures, respectively. In addition, accurate weights, particularly in the hospitalized patient, are invaluable in estimating changes in the volume status.

   a. **Volume depletion** (Table 8-5) can be suggested by a history of fluid losses (e.g., vomiting, diarrhea, profuse sweating, diuretic use), third-spacing of fluid, or inadequate salt and fluid intake. The volume-depleted patient may complain of thirst, fatigue, weakness, or malaise. There usually is a decreased urine output. Signs of volume depletion on examination include orthostatic changes in the pulse and blood-pressure, tachycardia, hypotension, dry mucous membranes, decreased skin turgor, and absent axillary sweat. Laboratory data suggestive of volume depletion include an increased hematocrit, increased plasma protein, increased BUN/creatinine ratio, a urine Na^+ less than 10 mEq/liter, and fractional excretion of Na^+ less than 1% (see Chap. 13). However, the urine Na^+ and fractional excretion of Na^+ will not be low in patients with volume depletion caused by renal losses of salt (Table 8-5).

   b. The cardinal sign of **extracellular fluid volume excess** is edema. Of course, localized edema can have other causes, such as lymphatic obstruction. Edema is best found in dependent areas, such as the back of a bedridden patient or the ankles of an ambulatory person. Signs of **intravascular fluid excess** may include hypertension, an increased central venous pressure (as estimated by the jugular venous height), and signs of heart failure, such as rales and an S3 gallop.

B. **Water homeostasis**
   1. **Water balance** determines the osmolality and sodium concentration. Hyponatremia and hypernatremia usually represent disorders of water homeostasis. Sodium balance is regulated as discussed in sec **I.A.1.a.** Water balance is regulated independently of sodium balance by urine concentration and dilution. The need for urine concentration or dilution depends predominantly on the oral intake of water (regulated in part by thirst), insensible water losses, and other fluid losses (e.g., vomiting, diarrhea).

   a. **Urine dilution** requires adequate tubular fluid delivery to and intact function of the thick ascending limb of Henle, the so-called diluting segment. In this part of the kidney, NaCl is resorbed without water resorption, producing a dilute fluid. Adequate delivery to this distal segment requires intact glo-

Table 8-5. Causes of volume depletion

Extrarenal losses
  Hemorrhage (external or occult internal)
  GI fluid losses (e.g., diarrhea, vomiting)
  Skin (e.g., excessive sweating, burns)
Renal losses
  Osmotic agents: endogenous (e.g., glucose, urea), exogenous (e.g., mannitol, contrast agents)
  Diuretics
  Mineralocorticoid deficiencies
  Salt-wasting renal disease (e.g., recovering acute renal failure, postobstruction, chronic renal insufficiency with sudden decreased salt intake)
Sequestration of fluid (e.g., pancreatitis, intestinal obstruction, peritonitis, rhabdomyolysis, sepsis with vasodilation)
Inadequate salt intake

merular filtration and less than maximal proximal fluid resorption. Hence, with renal insufficiency or severe volume depletion, which induces maximal proximal resorption, the diluting capacity is diminished.

b. Urine concentration requires NaCl resorption from the thick limb plus a hypertonic renal medullary interstitium and a collecting tubule made permeable to water by antidiuretic hormone (ADH). NaCl resorption by the thick ascending limb is necessary, since this initiates formation of the hypertonic medullary interstitium. With ADH present, the collecting tubule becomes permeable to water, and water diffuses from the tubule into the hypertonic medullary interstitium. Therefore, ADH controls urine concentration.

ADH is released from the posterior pituitary when small increases in the plasma osmolality above the normal of 280–290 mOsm/kg occur. ADH then leads to water resorption in the collecting tubule, thus reducing the plasma osmolality. ADH can also be released by a variety of nonosmotic stimuli mediated through the parasympathetic system; these stimuli include pain, stress, hypoxia, liver disease, adrenal insufficiency, heart failure, and, most importantly, volume depletion. Volume depletion, however, has to be at least 10% to cause ADH release.

c. Oral intake. The same stimuli that release ADH (e.g., hypertonicity, volume depletion) cause thirst. Only rarely are derangements of oral intake severe enough to cause clinical problems in patients with normal kidney function.

2. **Assessment** of the patient with a suspected altered water balance includes a thorough history of fluid and solute intake, urine output, thirst, medications, neurologic symptoms, and symptoms of other illnesses. Patients may present with polydipsia or polyuria as the sole manifestation of disorders of urine concentration and dilution. Laboratory data that should be obtained in most cases include a serum Na^+, osmolality, and creatinine and a urine Na^+, osmolality, and creatinine.

C. Potassium homeostasis

1. **Potassium physiology.** Potassium is the major intracellular cation, and therefore the total body potassium content is large, approximately 3500 mEq. The serum or extracellular K^+ usually (although not invariably) reflects the total body K^+. Most of the normal K^+ intake (approximately 100 mEq/day) is excreted by the kidneys, which are the major regulatory organ for K^+ balance. Urinary excretion of K^+ occurs primarily in the distal tubule and is increased by mineralocorticoids (aldosterone), a high distal tubule flow and sodium delivery (diuretics), alkalosis, and a high K^+ intake. However, serum K^+ can be altered more acutely (in minutes) by nonrenal factors that affect the distribution of K^+ between the extracellular fluid and the much larger intracellular pool; acidemia acutely drives K^+ out of cells, whereas alkalemia drives K^+ into cells. As a very rough estimate, each 0.1-unit change in pH changes the serum K^+ 0.6 mEq/liter in the opposite direction. Also, insulin and, to a lesser extent,

catecholamines move K^+ into cells, a major defense mechanism in acute hyper-kalemia.

2. **Assessment** of a suspected K^+ derangement includes an immediate serum K^+ and an electrocardiogram (ECG). The history should include an assessment of K^+ intake, a medication list (especially for various diuretics and digitalis), and clues for such illnesses as diabetes mellitus and renal disease. On physical examination, cardiovascular and neuromuscular manifestations predominate in K^+ disorders. Additional laboratory assessment includes serum electrolytes and creatinine, ABGs, and urine electrolytes.

II. Disorders of fluid volume
A. Volume depletion

1. **Major causes** of volume depletion are listed in Table 8-5. This classification based on the site of lost volume is useful in defining the etiologies of volume depletion and in reminding the clinician of possible volume depletion in the listed conditions. Since the kidneys can adapt to a very low Na^+ intake, inade-quate salt intake is usually only a contributing factor in volume depletion.

2. The **manifestations** of volume depletion are given in sec. **I.A.2.a.**

3. **Treatment** of volume depletion obviously depends on the etiology and extent of volume depletion. At one extreme is hypovolemic shock, the management of which is described in Chap. 3. At the other extreme is mild volume depletion without symptoms, which can be managed with oral intake of food and water and treatment of the primary process.

   a. **Intravenous replacement fluid** in volume-depleted patients should usually be **normal saline** (0.9% NaCl). Ringer's lactate solution is comparable but also contains 4 mEq/liter of K^+ and Ca^{++}. NaCl can be given as glucose-containing solutions as well. If the patient also requires HCO_3^-, some of the Na^+ can be given as $NaHCO_3$ (e.g., 0.45% NaCl plus 1–2 ampules of $NaHCO_3$) or as Ringer's lactate in patients without severe acidosis, since the lactate is converted to HCO_3^-. If the patient is mildly volume-depleted and hypernatremic (secondary to loss of H_2O in excess of salt), 0.45% NaCl can be used. With normal renal function, however, replacement of fluid and electrolytes does not have to match exactly that lost; the kidneys will return the body to proper homeostasis when provided with sufficient electrolytes and water. Many volume-depleted patients have other associated electrolyte deficits that will require attention (e.g., potassium, magnesium). The rate of fluid administration should be commensurate with the clinical situation.

   b. **Other fluids.** Ordinarily, 5% D/W should not be viewed as a replacement fluid (or a maintenance fluid) for volume depletion, since this fluid is not retained in the extracellular compartment. In some extreme cases, particu-larly with hypoalbuminemia, colloid solutions such as albumin are useful; however, the effect is temporary, since the albumin is rapidly metabolized. Mannitol can also be used to shift fluid quickly to the intravascular compart-ment. Whole blood is an excellent volume-expanding agent that may be used not only in hemorrhage but also in other cases requiring a colloid (e.g., an edematous patient with a low intravascular volume).

4. **Disposition.** Since severe volume depletion usually results from or causes other major clinical problems, hospital admission for intravenous volume repletion is usually required. On the other hand, mild volume depletion (without orthostatic hypotension) in a patient with good kidney function may be managed in an outpatient setting if the precipitating problem has resolved and the patient is able to maintain oral intake.

B. Volume excess

1. The **causes** of volume overload are given in Table 8-6. Congestive heart failure and cirrhosis are discussed in Chaps. 5 and 10, respectively; the nephrotic syndrome and renal failure are discussed in Chap. 13. Renal insufficiency does not usually lead to large volume overloads unless the glomerular filtration rate is severely reduced (i.e., < 20 ml/minute) or salt intake is increased abruptly.

2. The cardinal **manifestation** of extracellular fluid volume overload is **edema**. However, in some circumstances, the intravascular volume and total extracellu-lar volume are disparate, that is, one is increased and the other decreased. Whereas congestive heart failure, cirrhosis, and the nephrotic syndrome are characterized by edema, the intravascular volume or "effective intravascular volume" is often low, which is at least part of the mechanism for the salt

Table 8-6. Causes of volume overload (edema)

Congestive heart failure
Cirrhosis
Hypoalbuminemia (nephrotic syndrome, malnutrition, cirrhosis)
Renal insufficiency
Miscellaneous salt-retaining states (e.g., idiopathic cyclic edema, acute glomerulonephritis, vasodilators)

retention by the kidneys. The signs of intravascular volume excess are given in sec. **I.A.2.b.**

3. **Treatment** of volume overload depends greatly on the clinical circumstance. Obviously, impaired cardiopulmonary function, as in cardiogenic pulmonary edema, demands aggressive treatment; but mild peripheral edema may be little more than a cosmetic problem justifying only conservative treatment (e.g., salt restriction). More severe peripheral edema, however, is uncomfortable, limits activity, imposes risks of skin infection and injury, and therefore justifies treatment.
   a. Appropriate **treatment of the primary disease** is of paramount importance. See the appropriate sections of this book for the treatment of the various disorders causing volume overload.
   b. **Treatment of the volume load** per se usually includes bed rest (which alone will cause a diuresis), salt restriction, and use of diuretics. Furosemide is the most widely used single agent for the treatment of volume overload; ethacrynic acid and bumetanide are similar drugs used less frequently. In emergent situations, furosemide should be given IV; otherwise it can be given PO. To initiate a diuresis, 20–40 mg or the patient's oral dose (if already on furosemide) can be given IV and repetitively doubled (up to 320 mg) until a response is obtained. Thiazide diuretics (e.g., hydrochlorothiazide) are less potent diuretics that can be used effectively in treating mild cases of volume overload and hypertension. The combination of metolazone (a thiazide diuretic) and furosemide is frequently useful in cases of volume overload refractory to furosemide alone; however, the combination can lead to severe K^+ wasting. Amiloride, spironolactone, and triamterene are mild "K^+-sparing" diuretics. Acetazolamide is a mild diuretic that may be particularly useful in treating the combination of volume overload and a metabolic alkalosis. Frequent complications of diuretics include intravascular volume depletion (when the rate of diuresis is too fast), hypokalemia, a metabolic alkalosis, and hyponatremia. Hyperkalemia can result from the K^+-sparing diuretics.

4. The **disposition** will depend on the primary disease causing the volume overload and the degree of volume overload. Generally, patients with acute onset of significant edema, severe edema, or volume overload associated with cardiopulmonary dysfunction require hospitalization. On the other hand, mild to moderate exacerbations of chronic edema (with <10 pounds of weight gain) usually can be managed outside the hospital with dietary instructions, increases in diuretic dosages, and frequent follow-up.

III. **Disorders of sodium concentration**
   A. **Hyponatremia** usually represents a disorder of water (not Na^+) homeostasis, resulting in a low plasma osmolality.
      1. The **etiologies** of hyponatremia are listed in Table 8-7.
      2. The **manifestations** of hyponatremia (with a low plasma osmolality) include confusion, lethargy, coma, and seizures. The severity of the manifestations depend not only on the magnitude of the low osmolality but also on the rate of decrease in the osmolality.
      3. **Assessment**
         a. **Hyponatremia with a normal plasma osmolality.** The assessment of the patient with hyponatremia should begin with a consideration of the disorders that cause hyponatremia with a normal measured osmolality (see Table 8-7). Measurement of the plasma osmolality is helpful but not always neces-

Table 8-7. Causes of hyponatremia

With normal plasma osmolality
    Caused by other solutes (e.g., hyperglycemia, mannitol, alcohols, ethylene glycol)
    Factitious (severe hyperproteinemia or hyperlipidemia)
With low plasma osmolality
    Volume depletion (see Table 8-5)
    Volume overload (congestive heart failure, nephrotic syndrome, cirrhosis, renal failure)
    Clinical euvolemia
        Water intoxication
        Drugs (e.g., tricyclic antidepressants, prostaglandin inhibitors, morphine, aceta-
          minophen, barbiturates, chlorpropamide, vincristine, clofibrate, cyclophosphamide,
          nicotine)
        Hypothyroidism
        Addison's disease
        Stress/pain
        Syndrome of inappropriate antidiuretic hormone (SIADH)
          Tumors (e.g., lung, pancreas, brain)
          Pulmonary disease or positive-pressure ventilation
          CNS disease (tumor, trauma, cerebrovascular accident)
          Acute intermittent porphyria

sary. Hyperglycemia is a common cause of a low sodium concentration with a normal osmolality. Glucose is an osmotically active solute, and high concentrations of glucose shift water from the intracellular to the extracellular fluid, thus lowering the sodium concentration. A useful guideline is that the plasma Na^+ is expected to fall by 1.6 mEq/liter for each 100 mg/dl increase in the blood glucose. Thus, with a glucose of 1100 mg/dl, the plasma sodium should fall 16 mEq/liter. Other solutes (see Table 8-7) occasionally can cause a similar situation. Also severe hyperlipidemia or hyperproteinemia can cause hyponatremia with a normal osmolality; lipids and proteins displace plasma water and hence electrolytes in a given volume of plasma. All of the disorders of hyponatremia with a normal osmolality (except hyperglycemia) cause the measured osmolality to differ significantly (i.e., >10 mOsm/kg) from the calculated osmolality:

$$\text{Calculated osmolality} = 2(Na^+ + K^+) + \frac{\text{glucose}}{18} + \frac{\text{BUN}}{2.8}$$

  b. Hyponatremia with a low plasma osmolality (see Table 8-7) is assessed clinically by first evaluating the volume status of the patient (see sec. **I.A.2**).

    (1) Volume depletion of any etiology (see Table 8-5) can cause hyponatremia, particularly if water is used to replace lost fluid. Common causes include vomiting and the use of diuretics. Occasionally, especially with diuretics, overt signs of volume depletion are absent.

    (2) In the **edematous disorders** with hyponatremia (i.e., congestive heart failure, cirrhosis, nephrotic syndrome), the primary illness is usually clinically apparent; in these disorders, hyponatremia results from nonosmotic stimuli to ADH release and an impaired diluting ability of the kidneys. Hyponatremia associated with renal failure usually results from water intake or administration in excess of that excreted plus insensible losses.

    (3) The **euvolemic, hyponatremic disorders** include a variety of illnesses (see Table 8-7). Water intoxication per se usually requires greater than 10 liters/day of water intake to cause hyponatremia when there is normal renal function and normal solute (protein and salt) intake. However, with severely decreased solute intake, patients can become hyponatremic with normal water ingestion even with a normal urine diluting mechanism. In all of the other causes of euvolemic hyponatremia, a disorder of urine dilution is present; the urine in these other disorders should be more concentrated than 50–100 mOsm/kg, the normal lower limit of urine dilution, despite a low plasma osmolality. A variety of drugs, hypothyroidism, and Addison's disease have to be considered in the euvolemic hyponatremic patient. The syndrome of inappropriate ADH (SIADH) is a diagnosis of exclusion, since ADH levels are not routinely available. The usual causes of SIADH are given in Table 8-7. SIADH is usually characterized by hyponatremia, a urine that is not maximally dilute (e.g., urine osmolality > 150 mOsm/kg H_2O), and no signs of volume overload or depletion. Serum uric acid is frequently low.

4. The **treatment** of hyponatremia depends on the etiology and the clinical manifestations. Identification and treatment of the primary disorder (see Table 8-7) are always necessary.

   a. The disorders with **normal osmolality** (see Table 8-7) require no specific treatment for the hyponatremia per se.

   b. The conditions with **volume depletion** generally should be treated with isotonic saline (0.9% NaCl).

   c. In contrast, water restriction is the primary mode of therapy for the **euvolemic and edematous disorders.** When water restriction is unsuccessful in treating SIADH, demeclocycline, 300–600 mg bid, is useful to allow larger water intakes; however, it should not be used in patients with liver disease.

   d. For **severe, symptomatic hyponatremia** characterized by neurologic signs, such as seizures or coma, hypertonic saline (3% NaCl) should be given to increase the plasma osmolality quickly; 300–500 ml of 3% NaCl can be given over 6–8 hours and the Na^+ concentration remeasured. However, this treatment expands the plasma volume rapidly and therefore can precipitate pulmonary edema. To lessen the volume load, furosemide can be administered simultaneously. In less extreme cases, normal saline (0.9% NaCl) can be given with furosemide; furosemide causes excretion of a hypotonic urine, while the Na^+ is replaced with the more hypertonic solution, 0.9% NaCl. The goal of these treatments is to raise the Na^+ concentration to 125 mEq/liter (not to normal) and alleviate the neurologic manifestations. (Raising serum sodium too quickly above 120–125 mEq/liter can cause additional neurologic problems.) Slower methods, using water restriction or isotonic saline as appropriate, can then be used to normalize the sodium concentration completely.

5. **Disposition.** Almost all patients with hyponatremia should be admitted to the hospital, both for diagnosis and treatment. The only exception is very mild hyponatremia (i.e., serum $Na^+ > 130$ mEq/liter) with a clear etiology (e.g., volume depletion).

B. **Hypernatremia** usually represents a disorder of water balance rather than Na^+ balance.

1. The **etiologies** of hypernatremia are listed in Table 8-8. The classification in Table 8-8 is again based on the volume status, dividing the causes into those associated with volume depletion, euvolemia, and volume overload.

2. **Manifestations.** Hypernatremia, reflecting a high plasma osmolality, has the following manifestations, which are predominantly neurologic: thirst, confusion, lethargy, ataxia, neuromuscular irritability, seizures, and coma. Focal neurologic signs may also develop from CNS hemorrhage, both parenchymal and subarachnoid.

3. Two **protective mechanisms,** that is, urine concentration (water retention) and thirst (leading to water intake), usually operate to prevent hypernatremia. Urine concentration requires an intact ADH release and kidneys able to respond to ADH appropriately. **Central diabetes insipidus (DI)** represents a lack of secretion of ADH from the posterior pituitary; **nephrogenic DI** represents a failure of urine concentration in response to ADH. However, both of these disorders frequently present only with polydipsia and polyuria, with a normal osmolality if thirst mechanisms are intact and water is available.

4. **Assessment** of the patient with hypernatremia should include a history of fluid intake and loss and medication usage; evaluation of the volume status; and determination of the plasma and urine osmolalities and serum creatinine, Ca^{++}, and K^+. The origin of H_2O loss and/or the cause of inadequate H_2O intake should be identified. In particular, clinical assessment of the volume status is useful in differentiating the various causes of hypernatremia (see Table 8-8).

Table 8-8. Causes of hypernatremia

$H_2O > NaCl$ losses (volume-depleted patients)
  Renal (osmotic diuretics)
  Nonrenal (insensible H_2O losses, sweating, GI losses)
H_2O losses (euvolemic patients)
  Extrarenal (insensible H_2O losses)
  Renal
    Central diabetes insipidus (e.g., tumor or trauma involving the pituitary gland)
    Nephrogenic diabetes insipidus
      Congenital
      Chronic renal disease
      Hypercalcemia
      Hypokalemia
      Drugs (e.g., alcohol, lithium, demeclocycline, amphotericin, vinblastine, colchicine)
      Starvation
Na^+ gain (volume-overloaded patients)
  Endogenous (hyperaldosteronism, Cushing's syndrome)
  Exogenous ($NaCl$, $NaHCO_3$, hemodialysis error)

        a. Volume-depleted patients with hypernatremia have lost both salt and water, but more of the latter. This is probably the most common setting of hypernatremia; that is, the mentally impaired or bedridden patient not receiving adequate water or adequate water and salt. Obligatory water losses (i.e., insensible water loss plus a minimal urine output) usually exceed salt losses, since the kidneys can conserve NaCl well.
        b. Euvolemic state. Patients with **pure H_2O losses** (e.g., diabetes insipidus) usually do not have any signs of volume depletion. Renal water losses (i.e., central or nephrogenic diabetes insipidus) are characterized by a less than maximally concentrated urine in the presence of a high plasma osmolality indicative of a renal concentrating defect. Inappropriate renal salt and water losses (e.g., an osmotic diuresis), however, also cause a concentrating defect. Central and nephrogenic DI are distinguished by their response to exogenous vasopressin, urine concentration occurring in central DI but not in nephrogenic DI.
        c. Volume-overloaded state. Hypernatremia caused by a **pure Na^+ gain** is unusual. Severe hypernatremia, however, may be caused by exogenous Na^+ gain (most frequently $NaHCO_3$ administration during cardiopulmonary resuscitation) but not by endogenous mechanisms.
     5. Treatment of hypernatremia depends partly on the volume status of the patient. Hypernatremia per se is treated with hypotonic fluids, that is, free water (usually 5% D/W). The calculated water deficit (in liters) should be corrected slowly, over approximately 48 hours, to avoid producing cerebral edema:

$$\text{Calculated water deficit} = \frac{[Na^+] \text{ measured} \times TBW}{[Na^+] \text{ desired}} - TBW$$

       where total body water (TBW) is usually taken as 60% of body weight (in kg). Ongoing water losses should also be taken into account.
        a. The **severely volume-depleted hypernatremic patient** usually should receive normal saline initially to restore the intravascular volume.
        b. Exogenous Na^+ excess usually should be treated not only with free water (i.e., 5% D/W) but also with a diuretic or dialysis to remove the excess Na^+.
        c. In cases of **central DI** with large ongoing water losses, vasopressin (Pitressin) may be needed.
     6. Disposition. Significant hypernatremia (i.e., serum $Na^+ > 150$ mEq/liter) should be treated in the hospital.
  IV. Disorders of potassium
    A. Hypokalemia
      1. Etiologies. Major causes of hypokalemia are listed in Table 8-9. In the absence of a severely reduced K^+ intake, K^+ loss through the kidneys or GI tract is the usual cause of hypokalemia. In the presence of a K^+ deficiency, urinary losses of K^+ should be minimal. Therefore, a urine K^+ greater than 20 mEq/liter in the

Table 8-9. Causes of hypokalemia

Cellular shift without K^+ deficiency (e.g., alkalosis, periodic paralysis)
Inadequate K^+ intake (starvation, alcohol abuse)
Excessive losses
  Gastrointestinal (e.g., vomiting, diarrhea)
  Renal
    Diuretics, including osmotic diuretics (e.g., glucose)
    Primary mineralocorticoid excess (e.g., Cushing's disease, primary aldosteronism)
    Secondary mineralocorticoid excess, hyperreninemia (e.g., edematous disorders, malignant hypertension, renovascular hypertension, volume depletion)
    Renal tubular acidosis
    Bartter's syndrome
    Antibiotics (e.g., amphotericin, gentamicin, carbenicillin)
    Acute leukemia

presence of hypokalemia usually indicates renal K^+ losses. With loss of gastric fluid (due to vomiting or nasogastric suction), the major K^+ loss is usually through the kidneys because of the simultaneous alkalosis and volume depletion leading to high renins and aldosterone.

2. **Manifestations.** Severe hypokalemia and K^+ deficiency can lead to a variety of problems: arrhythmias (including ventricular ectopy, especially in patients on digitalis), neuromuscular depression manifested by muscle weakness (leading to paralysis and respiratory depression) and intestinal ileus, and rhabdomyolysis. If K^+ depletion causes rhabdomyolysis, the serum K^+ will increase and may even become high as K^+ is released from the damaged muscles. Similarly, K^+ depletion without hypokalemia may be present in acidosis and in uremia. Other less severe or less common manifestations of hypokalemia include glucose intolerance, worsening of hepatic encephalopathy, and nephrogenic diabetes insipidus.

3. **Treatment**
   a. Management of hypokalemia requires **identification and treatment of ongoing K^+ losses** (e.g., secondary to diuretics).
   b. **Potassium administration.** Since rapid administration of K^+ can produce toxicity from hyperkalemia, most cases of hypokalemia should be treated slowly. In addition, K^+ supplements and K^+-sparing diuretics should be used with great caution in patients with renal insufficiency, low urine flow, or diabetes mellitus; such patients can rapidly become hyperkalemic.
      (1) **Mild to moderate hypokalemia** (i.e., serum $K^+ > 2.0$–2.5 mEq/liter) without severe manifestations can be treated with either oral K^+ (usually 40–80 mEq/day in divided doses) or slow intravenous K^+ (i.e., < 10 mEq/hour in a solution containing ≤ 30 mEq K^+/liter) administered peripherally. Since hypokalemia usually reflects a K^+ deficit of a few hundred milliequivalents, several days of therapy will be required to replenish deficits.
      (2) **Severe hypokalemia** with major complications (e.g., paralysis, arrhythmias) requires more aggressive treatment with intravenous K^+ in rates up to 40 mEq/hour in solutions containing up to 60 mEq/liter, administered peripherally. However, the patients should be monitored closely and the serum K^+ checked frequently, since manifestations of hyperkalemia may develop with the more rapid rates of administration. Since manifestations of hyperkalemia depend on the extracellular-to-intracellular K^+ ratio and the latter is low in potassium depletion, rapid K^+ entry into the relatively small extracellular pool can cause hyperkalemic manifestations.
   4. **Disposition.** Severe hypokalemia (i.e., serum $K^+ < 2$ mEq/liter) or hypokalemia associated with arrhythmias or neuromuscular problems should be treated in the hospital. Also, hypokalemia with ongoing losses of K^+ (e.g., caused by diuretics) may require hospitalization for successful treatment, since manipulation of dosages of K^+ and other medications is often required.
B. **Hyperkalemia**
   1. **Etiologies.** Major causes of hyperkalemia are classified in Table 8-10.

Table 8-10. Causes of hyperkalemia

Pseudohyperkalemia (prolonged tourniquet, hemolysis of drawn blood, extreme elevation of leukocytes or platelets)

Exogenous K^+ load (e.g., dietary, transfusions, potassium penicillin)

Endogenous K^+ load or shift
   Tissue damage (e.g., crush injuries, rhabdomyolysis, ischemic organ, intravascular hemolysis)
   Chemotherapy, especially involving large tumor masses
   Acidosis
   Drugs (e.g., massive digitalis overdose, arginine, succinylcholine)
   Acute hyperosmolality
   Hyperkalemic periodic paralysis

Decreased renal K^+ excretion
   Renal failure
   K^+-sparing diuretics
   Mineralocorticoid deficiency (e.g., Addison's disease, type IV RTA)
   Tubular defects in K^+ excretion

---

    a. Pseudohyperkalemia includes conditions where K^+ is normal in the circulating blood but is released during or after blood drawing. In this situation, the ECG should never reflect the changes of hyperkalemia.

    b. Exogenous K^+ loads will not usually cause hyperkalemia unless the load is massive and acute or there is impaired K^+ excretion.

    c. Endogenous K^+ loads can be massive, since the amount of intracellular K^+ is very large.

    d. Decreased renal K^+ excretion commonly contributes to hyperkalemia. With chronic moderate renal insufficiency, potassium excretion "adaptation" occurs and hyperkalemia is unusual unless a large K^+ load or another defect is suddenly imposed. With acute renal failure, oliguria worsens the propensity for hyperkalemia; thus, potassium should be restricted. Potassium-sparing diuretics (and captopril), mineralocorticoid deficiency, and certain renal tubular defects (e.g., some patients with lupus erythematosus, renal transplants, or sickle cell disease) all lead to decreased renal K^+ excretion despite otherwise normal kidney function. Type IV RTA (or hyporeninemic hypoaldosteronism) is a relatively common disorder seen in patients with mild renal insufficiency, particularly diabetics; these patients have hyperkalemia and a mild to moderate hyperchloremic metabolic acidosis. Hyperkalemia in this disorder may result from both hypoaldosterone and a tubule secretory defect for K^+.

2. Manifestations depend not only on the level of hyperkalemia but also on the rate of rise. Hyperkalemia is frequently asymptomatic until complications develop. These include hypotension, arrhythmias, and cardiac arrest (asystole). The ECG may demonstrate sequential changes: tall peaked T waves, ST depression, prolonged PR interval, loss of P waves, and widening of the QRS leading to a sine wave pattern; hypotension and cardiac arrest may occur at any point in the sequence. Another occasional manifestation of hyperkalemia is weakness leading to paralysis.

3. Contributing problems. Although diabetes mellitus per se does not cause hyperkalemia, diabetics are particularly prone to acute hyperkalemia from other causes. Normally, hyperkalemia stimulates insulin release (as well as aldosterone and catecholamine release), which drives K^+ into cells. With insulin deficiency, this protective mechanism is lost. Similarly, beta-adrenergic blockers and nonsteroidal anti-inflammatory agents have been implicated as worsening the propensity to hyperkalemia.

4. Treatment should be guided by the severity of the hyperkalemia. ECG changes demand immediate treatment. A K^+ level exceeding 6.5 mEq/liter (even without ECG changes) should also be treated promptly. With all forms of therapy, the ECG should be monitored until the hyperkalemic changes disappear, and the serum K^+ should be followed closely to ensure that therapy is effective.

    a. Calcium gluconate, 5–10 ml of a 10% solution given IV over 2 minutes and repeated in 5 minutes if necessary, immediately antagonizes the effects of hyperkalemia. However, raising the blood Ca^{++} is effective for less than 1 hour, and other therapy should be initiated simultaneously. Calcium usually should not be given to patients on digitalis.

   b. Sodium bicarbonate causes K^+ to shift into cells. One ampule (44 mEq) of $NaHCO_3$ can be injected over 2–5 minutes and repeated in 10–15 minutes. The beneficial effect starts within minutes but only lasts 1–2 hours. Bicarbonate is particularly useful in hyperkalemia associated with acidemia. Volume overload and hypernatremia are potential complications if large amounts of $NaHCO_3$ are given.

   c. Glucose and insulin administration also shifts K^+ into cells due to the effect of insulin on cellular K^+ uptake. A useful combination is 1 ampule (50 ml) of D50 (25 gm of dextrose) by IV push along with 5–10 units of regular insulin given IV over 5 minutes. Also, a combination of glucose, insulin, and $NaHCO_3$ is very effective; 1 liter of D10 with 2 ampules of $NaHCO_3$ added is given over 2–3 hours (more rapid at the start), and approximately 25 units of regular insulin is administered subcutaneously. These maneuvers, however, have a limited duration of action, since K^+ is not removed but only shifted intracellularly.

   d. Sodium polystyrene sulfonate (Kayexalate). This resin exchanges sodium for potassium; it can be given orally or rectally. Orally, 50 gm of Kayexalate mixed in 100 ml of 20% sorbitol (as an osmotic laxative) can be given every 3–4 hours. If oral administration is not possible, 50 gm of Kayexalate may be mixed in 200 ml of water with 50 gm of sorbitol added or in 200 ml of 20% dextrose and given as a retention enema (to be retained for 30–60 minutes). Although Kayexalate is slower in lowering the serum K^+ than the aforementioned methods, K^+ is actually removed from the body.

   e. Dialysis. Peritoneal dialysis removes K^+ very slowly. Hemodialysis is efficient but usually should not be the first line of therapy.

  5. Disposition. Hyperkalemia of sufficient magnitude to require immediate treatment (usually > 5.5–6.0 mEq/liter) should be treated in the hospital. Lesser degrees of hyperkalemia caused by K^+ administration, which can be managed by lowering or eliminating the amount prescribed, can be treated on an outpatient basis with early follow-up.

Bibliography

1. Berl, T., and Schrier, R. W. Disorders of Water Metabolism. In R. W. Schrier (ed.), *Renal and Electrolyte Disorders* (3rd ed.). Boston: Little, Brown, 1986.
2. Cogan, M. G., Rector, F. C., and Seldin, D. W. Acid-Base Disorders. In B. M. Brenner and F. C. Rector (eds.), *The Kidney*. Philadelphia: Saunders, 1981. Pp. 841–907.
3. DeFronzo, R. A. Hyperkalemia and hyporeninemic hypoaldosteronism. *Kidney Int.* 17:118, 1980.
4. Dirks, J. H. Mechanisms of action and clinical uses of diuretics. *Hosp. Pract.* 14:99, 1979.
5. Gennari, F. J. Serum osmolality: Uses and limitations. *N. Engl. J. Med.* 310:102, 1984.
6. Kreisberg, R. A. Lactate homeostasis and lactic acidosis. *Ann. Intern. Med.* 92:227, 1980.
7. Kunau, R. T., and Stein, J. H. Disorders of hypo- and hyperkalemia. *Clin. Nephrol.* 7:173, 1977.
8. Narins, R. G., and Emmett, M. Simple and mixed acid-base disorders: A practical approach. *Medicine* 59:161, 1980.
9. Narins, R. G., et al. Diagnostic strategies in disorders of fluid, electrolyte and acid-base homeostasis. *Am. J. Med.* 72:496, 1982.
10. Oh, M. S., and Carroll, H. J. The anion gap. *N. Engl. J. Med.* 297:814, 1977.
11. Reineck, H. J., and Stein, J. H. Regulation of Sodium Balance. In M. H. Maxwell and C. R. Kleeman (eds.), *Clinical Disorders of Fluid and Electrolyte Metabolism*. New York: McGraw-Hill, 1980.

Endocrine and Metabolic Emergencies

Matthew J. Orland

Diabetes Mellitus

I. **Physiology of glucose metabolism.** A balance of production, absorption, and clearance of glucose is affected by diet and by the actions of insulin and several counterregulatory hormones.
  A. **Hepatic glucose production** is responsible for the maintenance of plasma glucose in the fasting state.
  B. **Dietary intake,** primarily of sugar and refined carbohydrates, produces postprandial plasma glucose elevation.
  C. **Clearance of glucose** from the blood results mainly from cellular uptake. Muscle metabolism accounts for a significant fraction of glucose utilization, increasing with physical activity. Urinary glucose clearance occurs only when the plasma level exceeds the renal glucose threshold of 150–350 mg/dl.
  D. **Insulin** lowers plasma glucose by reducing hepatic glucose production and by stimulating cellular glucose uptake. Estimates suggest that a normal pancreas produces roughly 50 units (2 mg) of insulin daily. About half of normal insulin production is devoted to basal nutrient metabolism; the remainder is secreted in response to meals [14].
  E. **Glucagon, epinephrine, cortisol, and growth hormone** antagonize insulin-induced hypoglycemia and may produce hyperglycemia when insulin is deficient. Insulin-treated patients rely particularly on glucagon and epinephrine to maintain plasma glucose and avoid serious hypoglycemia [3].
II. **Pathophysiology of diabetes mellitus.** Patients with diabetes mellitus secrete insulin in quantities insufficient to meet metabolic needs. Hyperglycemia is the primary manifestation of insulin lack or resistance to insulin action. Ketogenesis results from more severe insulin deficit.
  A. **Diabetes mellitus** is divided into three subclasses.
    1. **Type I (insulin-dependent) diabetes mellitus** results from virtually total loss of insulin production. Onset of this disease is usually before age 30. Presentation may be with diabetic ketoacidosis (DKA), and patients are prone to recurrent DKA and death without insulin treatment.
    2. **Type II (non-insulin-dependent) diabetes mellitus** is due to relative insulin deficit, promoted by insulin resistance in many cases. The majority of patients with diabetes belong to this group. The onset is typically after age 40. Presentation may be with the nonketotic hyperosmolar syndrome (NKHS). Most patients are obese and can ameliorate hyperglycemia with weight loss. Although most can survive without exogenous insulin, insulin treatment is important for the management of persistent hyperglycemia. A stress, such as infection, may promote ketoacidosis in patients with type II diabetes mellitus, but this is uncommon.
    3. **Other (secondary) diabetes mellitus** refers to development of hyperglycemia resulting from another recognized cause. In patients with chronic pancreatitis, hemochromatosis, or pancreatic carcinoma, or following pancreatectomy, insulin production is deficient. In Cushing's syndrome and acromegaly, hormonally mediated insulin resistance occurs.
  B. **Impaired glucose tolerance** exists in some individuals who do not have overt diabetes, constituting a distinct diagnostic group at increased risk of developing diabetes in the future.
  C. **Gestational diabetes mellitus** refers to the onset of abnormal glucose homeostasis during pregnancy (see Chap. 33).
III. **The diagnosis of diabetes mellitus** may be suggested by symptoms or follow discovery of hyperglycemia or glycosuria in an asymptomatic patient. In either situation, it is

Table 9-1. Factors that promote hyperglycemia in patients with diabetes mellitus*

I. Increased dietary intake (particularly of carbohydrate)
II. Limitation of physical activity
III. Change in hypoglycemic therapy
IV. Limitation of insulin production
    A. Pancreatic diseases (or pancreatectomy)†
    B. Drug treatment, including
       1. Diazoxide
       2. Thiazide diuretics
       3. Phenytoin
V. Development of insulin resistance
    A. Infection
    B. Inflammation
    C. Pregnancy
    D. Trauma (including surgery)
    E. Drug treatment, including
       1. Glucocorticoids
       2. Oral contraceptives (or synthetic estrogens)
       3. Sympathomimetic agents
       4. Nicotinic acid
    F. Antibodies to insulin
    G. Antibodies to insulin receptors†

*These factors (particularly IV and V) should also be investigated in patients with diabetic keto-acidosis or nonketotic hyperosmolar syndrome.
†These factors are less important in diagnosis of acute hyperglycemic exacerbations.
Source: M. J. Orland, Diabetes Mellitus. In M. J. Orland and R. J. Saltman (eds.), *Manual of Medical Therapeutics* (25th ed.). Boston: Little, Brown, 1986. With permission.

important to consider potentially reversible factors promoting hyperglycemia (see Table 9-1) before a permanent diagnosis is established [6].
  A. Symptomatic patients. The association of polyuria, polydipsia, and weight loss with a plasma glucose exceeding 200 mg/dl is sufficient for the diagnosis of diabetes mellitus when reversible factors are not evident.
    1. Clinical manifestations of hyperglycemia may also include lethargy, nocturia, visual blurring, and morning headache. Orthostasis is frequently evident; severe volume depletion may suggest DKA or NKHS. Diabetic retinopathy or other complications may occur in patients with long-standing hyperglycemia, prompting a presumptive diagnosis of diabetes mellitus (see sec. **IV.D–J**).
    2. Laboratory evaluation should include measurement of serum electrolytes and blood urea nitrogen (BUN) to assess for DKA and NKHS (see sec. **IV.B–C**).
  B. Asymptomatic patients. Newly recognized hyperglycemia should be evaluated with respect to stress of illness and temporal association with meals. A plasma glucose of greater than 200 mg/dl suggests the need for diagnostic evaluation.
  C. Diagnostic tests. The following are appropriate for unstressed, nonpregnant individuals.
    1. Fasting plasma glucose should be determined in all patients with suspected diabetes mellitus. A fasting plasma glucose exceeding 140 mg/dl on more than one occasion is considered diagnostic.
    2. Oral glucose tolerance testing may be used for patients with a normal or equivocal fasting plasma glucose. The test is valid only when the daily carbohydrate intake is greater than 150 gm and physical activity is unrestricted. Adults are given 75 gm of glucose in the morning following an overnight fast. The plasma glucose is measured at 0, 30, 60, 90, and 120 minutes. A positive test includes a plasma glucose of greater than 200 mg/dl at 120 minutes and at one other time during the test. The test should be abnormal on more than one occasion for diagnosis.
  D. Diagnosis in pregnancy is discussed in Chap. 33.
  E. Disposition for diagnostic evaluation. Hospitalization facilitates management of insulin-dependent (type I) diabetes. Admission solely for diagnosis of type II diabetes mellitus should be discouraged.
IV. Complications of diabetes mellitus include the acute consequences of insulin insufficiency and the manifestations of long-standing disease.

A. **Hyperglycemia** should be approached with consideration of associated symptoms and chronicity. The duration of glucose elevation may be deduced from the history of symptoms or review of records. Chronic hyperglycemia implies inadequate treatment, whereas a change from a stable glucose profile indicates a precipitating stress (see Table 9-1). Dietary changes and limitation of activity should be investigated. Compliance to a therapeutic regimen should be ascertained.

1. **Clinical manifestations** of hyperglycemia are discussed in sec. **III.A.** Orthostatic pulse and blood pressure measurements should be sufficient to establish the volume status in most patients; however, postural hypotension with an absent pulse response may occur as a result of diabetic autonomic neuropathy.

2. **Laboratory evaluation** should confirm hyperglycemia and should include measurement of electrolytes and BUN to screen for a metabolic acidosis or hyperosmolarity. A hemoglobin A_{1C} determination may help to establish the severity and chronicity of hyperglycemia and evaluate the efficacy of home therapy. Urine should be screened for ketones. A complete blood count and cultures should be obtained when an infection is suspected.

3. The **disposition** depends on the condition of the patient and support available outside of the hospital. Educated patients may be able to manage hyperglycemia at home. Admission may be considered for educational purposes when outpatient resources are inadequate. Hospital care is appropriate for patients with polydipsia, polyuria, and weight loss and is strongly advised for those with significant volume deficit or mental status impairment.

4. **Therapy.** All discharged patients should have a plan for management of hyperglycemia, including a return or referral appointment. The goals and possible complications of therapy should be discussed to ensure patient safety until more detailed instruction can be provided. The discipline required for optimum care should be conveyed.

   a. **Dietary management** is important for all patients. A minimum requirement is a reduction of refined sugar in the diet. Foods with a high sugar content should be ingested only as part of a balanced meal or in the management of hypoglycemia. Obese patients with type II diabetes may improve on a regimen further emphasizing caloric reduction. Nonobese individuals generally do not require caloric limits [12].

      (1) **Patients receiving insulin or oral agents** need to maintain a regular meal schedule to aid in the management of hyperglycemia and to prevent serious hypoglycemia. In most cases, the meal plan should include breakfast, lunch, dinner, and a bedtime snack. Work schedules and physical activity must be considered when a diet is prescribed.

      (2) **Alcohol intake should be limited.** Most alcoholic beverages contain sugar and can promote hyperglycemia. Excessive alcohol intake may limit hepatic glucose production, variably augmenting the hypoglycemic effects of insulin and oral agents.

   b. **Oral hypoglycemic agents** reduce plasma glucose in many patients with non-insulin-dependent (type II) diabetes mellitus. Oral agents may be beneficial to patients usually controlled by diet alone who develop worsening hyperglycemia in association with a transient illness. The efficacy of chronic oral agent therapy may be limited in some patients, and a possibility of increased cardiovascular mortality with these drugs is recognized. Tolbutamide, 250 mg PO bid, represents an acceptable starting regimen when accompanied by appropriate dietary management. Care should be taken to avoid hypoglycemia (see sec. **V.A**). Oral hypoglycemic medications should not be used in insulin-dependent (type I) diabetes mellitus. Table 9-2 lists the oral hypoglycemic drugs [9].

   c. **Insulin therapy** may be initiated or adjusted without hospitalization in well-educated patients when the diagnosis of diabetes mellitus has been established and prompt follow-up has been arranged.

      (1) **Initial dosages of insulin** in type II diabetes mellitus are generally between 10 and 20 units of an intermediate-acting preparation daily (Table 9-3), administered SQ before breakfast. The level of hyperglycemia and extent of obesity help to determine a starting dosage within this range and also influence the rate of adjustment.

      (2) **Subcutaneous injection.** The anterior abdomen and thighs represent suitable sites for injections. Patients should be instructed to rotate injection sites. The skin should be clean, and areas of infection, dermopathy,

Table 9-2. Characteristics of oral hypoglycemic drugs (sulfonylureas)

Generic name	Dosage range* (mg/day)†	Onset of action (hours)	Duration of action (hours)†
Tolbutamide	500–3000	0.5–1.0	6–12
Tolazamide	100–1000	4–6	10–24
Glipizide	5–40	1–3	12–24
Acetohexamide	250–1500	0.5–1.0	12–24
Glyburide	2.5–20.0	0.5–1.0	24–60
Chlorpropamide	100–500	1–2	60–90

*Higher dosages should be divided.
†Activity of the sulfonylureas is prolonged in both hepatic and renal failure.
Source: M. J. Orland, Diabetes Mellitus. In M. J. Orland and R. J. Saltman (eds.), *Manual of Medical Therapeutics* (25th ed.). Boston: Little, Brown, 1986. With permission.

Table 9-3. Pharmacokinetics of subcutaneous insulin preparations

Insulin preparation	Onset of action (hours)	Peak effect (hours)	Duration of action (hours)
Rapid-acting			
Regular	0.25–1.0	2–6	4–12
Semilente	0.5–1.0	3–6	8–16
Intermediate-acting			
NPH	1.5–4.0	6–16	12–24
Lente	1–4	6–16	12–28
Long-acting			
Protamine, Zinc, & Iletin (PZI)	3–8	14–24	24–48
Ultralente	3–8	14–24	24–48

Note: Variations in pharmacokinetics (i.e., ranges) result from patient differences and insulin dosage. Large dosages may have prolonged activity. Activity is also prolonged in renal failure.
Source: M. J. Orland, Diabetes Mellitus. In M. J. Orland and R. J. Saltman (eds.), *Manual of Medical Therapeutics* (25th ed.). Boston: Little, Brown, 1986. With permission.

      scarring, or irritation should be avoided. Family members should be present when patients are instructed in the injection technique.

    (3) Purified insulin of human or porcine composition should be prescribed for patients with a history of previous insulin use who are restarting insulin therapy; this may reduce the incidence of insulin allergy [7]. Similarly, patients for whom short-term use of insulin is anticipated should use a purified, single-species insulin.

  d. Home glucose monitoring is essential for patients taking insulin, is strongly recommended for patients taking oral hypoglycemic agents, and is useful for patients managed by diet alone. Capillary blood glucose measurement is preferred. Urine monitoring represents a poor alternative to blood testing but may be used to monitor hyperglycemia greater than the renal glucose threshold. A starting regimen for insulin-treated patients includes a fasting morning measurement and a measurement either before dinner or at bedtime. Measurements should be recorded to aid subsequent therapeutic adjustments. Education is essential to ensure proper technique.

  e. Urine ketone measurements should supplement blood glucose monitoring when patients are at risk for diabetic ketoacidosis. These measurements should be performed regularly when the patient is ill or when the blood glucose is greater than 400 mg/dl.

B. Diabetic ketoacidosis (DKA). The development of DKA follows severe insulin insufficiency. A tendency toward DKA is characteristic of patients with insulin-dependent (type I) diabetes mellitus. Evaluation should reveal an interruption of insulin therapy or a precipitating stress (see Table 9-1).

  1. Clinical manifestations. The spectrum of severity of DKA ranges from asymptomatic patients to patients presenting in overt shock or coma. Typical symptoms include weight loss, polyuria, polydipsia, vomiting, and abdominal pain that is typically vague and without localizing signs. Volume depletion may produce supine or postural hypotension. Significant acidosis promotes hyperventilation and altered mental status. The patient's breath may smell of acetone. Ophthalmoscopy may reveal lipemia retinalis. **Attention should be given to the diagnosis and treatment of an underlying illness.** Specific symptoms may suggest infection or myocardial infarction. Septic shock may occur without fever or overt infection. Although diffuse abdominal pain is often present in DKA, localizing findings indicate the need for diagnostic evaluation and specific therapy (see Chap. 19).

2. **Laboratory evaluation** should begin with bedside measurement of plasma glucose and urine ketones. Definitive diagnosis requires documentation of metabolic acidosis, including (a) an arterial pH of less than 7.35, (b) a depressed serum bicarbonate, and (c) an increased anion gap. Before initiating therapy, serum ketones should be documented. Lactic acidosis may accompany DKA, reflecting sepsis or volume deficit.

   a. **Measurements of plasma glucose, sodium, potassium, and bicarbonate are important in guiding therapy.** A low plasma sodium may reflect the contribution of glucose to the total osmolarity or the presence of lipemia. Elevation of plasma potassium usually reflects acidosis, as total body stores generally are depleted; a potassium deficit is evident when the pH is corrected. Initial evaluation of hyperkalemia should include an electrocardiogram (ECG). An elevated serum creatinine may indicate renal insufficiency or volume depletion but may be spurious due to interference from serum ketones in many clinical assays.

   b. **Precipitating factors.** Cultures of blood and urine should be obtained when the underlying stress leading to DKA is not apparent because of a significant incidence of occult infection. A chest radiograph may disclose pneumonia not apparent on initial examination of the volume-depleted patient. The ECG should be evaluated for myocardial infarction, which may occur particularly in patients over age 40 or with diabetes of greater than 10 years' duration. Serum amylase is frequently elevated in diabetic ketoacidosis without discernible pancreatic or bowel pathology.

3. **Differential diagnosis.** Coexistence of ketonuria and hyperglycemia does not establish a diagnosis of DKA; urine ketones may reflect fasting in an otherwise stable patient. Hyperglycemia is usually evident in patients with DKA, but the glucose may not be strikingly elevated, particularly in insulin-treated patients. The history is the most helpful determinant in differentiating DKA from alcoholic ketoacidosis (see Chap. 8).

4. **Management.** Stabilization of patients in shock and management of coma (see Chaps. 3 and 32) take precedence over the specific therapy of DKA. Administration of 50% dextrose in an attempt to awaken a comatose patient in the field will not greatly affect subsequent management, but capillary glucose should be measured when possible to preclude excessive glucose administration. The specific therapy of DKA includes three ordered phases: correction of volume deficit, reversal of the ketogenic process, and control of plasma glucose.

   a. **The volume deficit** should be managed initially with isotonic saline or Ringer's lactate solution. In most cases, the first liter should be given within 1 hour; shock should prompt more rapid fluid administration. When roughly half of the estimated volume deficit is replaced, salt concentration in intravenous fluids should be reduced, and maintenance fluids (e.g., 0.45% saline) should be continued at 150–250 ml/hour in uncomplicated cases until the ketoacidosis is reversed and oral intake is tolerated. When volume management is complicated by renal failure, heart failure, or myocardial infarction, central venous pressure or Swan-Ganz monitoring may be indicated. Bladder catheterization should be avoided when patients can urinate without difficulty, but it may be necessary to measure the urinary output in hypotensive patients.

   b. **Electrolyte balance** should be maintained. Hourly measurement of electrolytes is appropriate during emergency department management.

      (1) **Bicarbonate administration** is recommended when DKA is accompanied by shock or coma, initial arterial pH is less than 7.1, or severe hyperkalemia is present. Bolus administration should be avoided unless judged to be a lifesaving measure. Two ampules of sodium bicarbonate

(88 mEq Na$^+$) may be added to a liter of 0.45% saline and infused as described in sec. **IV.B.4.a** until the indications for use are no longer present.

(2) Potassium administration should begin when ECG evidence of hyperkalemia has resolved. Peripheral IV infusion should contain potassium chloride to provide 20–40 mEq K$^+$/liter. When plasma potassium is less than 4.0 mEq/liter, the treatment should be more aggressive; the infusion of potassium chloride may be increased to 15 mEq/hour if needed. Urine output should be monitored, and potassium therapy must be followed with particular care in oliguric patients.

(3) Phosphate administration should be limited in the emergency department, since complicated hypophosphatemia is rare and large doses of IV phosphate may precipitate hypocalcemia and renal failure. Asymptomatic phosphate depletion may be managed with oral phosphate supplements when patients regain the ability to eat (see **Disorders of Calcium, Magnesium, and Phosphate**, sec. **III.B**).

c. **Administration of insulin.** After initiation of fluids, insulin is used to reverse the ketogenic process. Careful note should be made of any insulin administration preceding emergency department presentation, as this may affect management.

(1) Initial treatment should include 10–20 units of regular insulin, given as an IV bolus.

(2) Intravenous insulin infusion represents safe and practical therapy when an automated device is available. **Regular insulin,** 100 units, can be added to 500 ml of 0.45% sodium chloride and infused initially at 50–75 ml/hour (i.e., 10–15 units/hour). Since insulin adheres to plastic tubing, infusion sets should be flushed with 50–100 ml of the insulin solution before initiating treatment.

(3) Intramuscular insulin injections are an alternative to intravenous infusion when shock or hypotension is not present. The initial IV bolus should be followed by regular insulin, 5–10 units IM q1h. Subcutaneous regular insulin treatment should be avoided in DKA.

(4) Adjustment of insulin dosage should be guided initially by blood or plasma glucose, which can be measured frequently (i.e., at 30-minute intervals) during emergency department management. Without a dextrose infusion (see sec. **IV.B.4.d**), the glucose level should fall by roughly 50 mg/dl/hour during treatment. A slower fall in glucose indicates insulin resistance; in such a situation, the dosage of insulin should be increased by 50–100%. When the glucose level cannot be used as a therapeutic parameter, the responses of plasma bicarbonate and the anion gap should be assessed.

d. **Administration of dextrose** is usually necessary to maintain plasma glucose during continued insulin therapy of DKA. Fluids should contain 5% dextrose when plasma glucose falls to 250 mg/dl; in some cases, this recommendation implies supplementation of the initial intravenous fluid regimen.

5. **Disposition.** Patients with DKA should be hospitalized. Management of patients with severely altered mental status or shock may be facilitated in an intensive care unit.

C. **Nonketotic hyperosmolar syndrome (NKHS)** is peculiar to non-insulin-dependent (type II) diabetes mellitus. NKHS follows a period of negative free-water balance that leads to hyperosmolarity and a volume deficit. Insufficiency of insulin is not severe enough to allow ketogenesis. NKHS may be the presenting manifestation of diabetes and may occur as a sequel to stroke, infection, corticosteroid therapy, excessive carbohydrate intake or renal failure. The diagnosis of NKHS should be considered in all elderly patients who present in coma.

1. **Clinical manifestations.** Patients with NKHS typically present with an altered mental status. The history usually reveals a stress promoting insulin resistance (see Table 9-1) and a reason for a volume deficit, including poor oral intake, gastrointestinal losses, use of diuretic medications, or osmotic diuresis. Focal neurologic findings should suggest a cerebrovascular accident (CVA). Recent trauma may incapacitate a patient prone to the disorder. Pregnancy also should be considered. A history of glucocorticoid therapy should prompt investigation regarding recent treatment. Although corticosteroids may promote NKHS, they should not be withheld if adrenal insufficiency is suspected.

2. **Laboratory evaluation.** The diagnosis of NKHS is established by (a) hypergly-cemia, usually greater than 600 mg/dl, (b) absence of ketonemia, and (c) a plasma osmolarity exceeding 350 mOsm/liter, either calculated (see Chap. 16) or measured. Cultures of blood and urine and a chest radiograph should be obtained to evaluate for infection. An ECG should be examined to assess for a recent myocardial infarction. Acidosis with an elevated anion gap may suggest DKA or reveal excessive lactic acid production resulting from hypovolemia, sepsis, or necrotizing inflammation.

3. **Management.** Goals in therapy include restoration of plasma volume and osmo-larity and treatment of hyperglycemia. Considerations in the treatment of DKA apply (see sec. **IV.B.4**); management of shock and coma takes precedence over the specific therapy of NKHS.

   a. **Fluid and electrolyte therapy.** The initial choice of fluids in NKHS usually precedes the laboratory diagnosis, and it is appropriate to administer **iso-tonic sodium chloride** for volume repletion until the extent of hyperosmo-larity is documented. Fluids should be given rapidly until roughly half of the estimated volume deficit is restored. Maintenance fluids should then be infused at 150–250 ml/hour, with considerations of cardiac and renal func-tion affecting subsequent adjustment. Serial glucose and electrolyte mea-surements should guide fluid therapy.

      (1) **Correction of hyperosmolarity.** When hyperosmolarity is documented, half-normal (0.45%) saline may be given. Immediate correction of hy-perosmolarity is not indicated; 5% D/W should be reserved for patients in the hospital whose hyperosmolarity does not correct with the saline-containing fluids given in the emergency department.

      (2) **Electrolyte repletion.** A potassium deficit should be anticipated; as in DKA, the serum potassium declines during insulin therapy. Sodium bicarbonate may be added to the IV fluids of patients who demonstrate a severe metabolic acidosis (i.e., pH less than 7.1, or a measured bicarbon-ate less than 15 mEq/liter), accompanying efforts to delineate a cause. Phosphate repletion is not part of the emergency therapy of NKHS but should be considered in later management.

   b. **Administration of insulin.** Regular insulin, 20 units IV, should be given when the plasma glucose is greater than 600 mg/dl. A smaller bolus may be given when hyperglycemia is less marked. Subsequent insulin may be given IV or IM, as described for DKA (see sec. **IV.B.4.c**). The insulin dosage should be adjusted according to changes in blood glucose. Care should be taken to avoid hypoglycemia; the glucose level should be kept greater than 250 mg/dl in the emergency department.

4. **Disposition.** Patients with NKHS should be hospitalized. Shock, severe mental status impairment, or a CVA suggests the need for an intensive care facility.

D. **Visual disturbances in the diabetic patient**

1. **Etiologies.** Diabetic retinopathy, cataract formation, or glaucoma may limit vision in patients with long-standing diabetes mellitus. Acute monocular visual loss can result from intravitreous hemorrhage, preretinal hemorrhage involv-ing the macula, retinal detachment, or emboli to the retinal vasculature. Bilat-eral visual loss suggests a CVA but may also be the perceived result of a dominant monocular visual loss when vision in the nondominant eye has been insidiously impaired. Blurring of vision may reflect lens changes associated with fluctuations in the plasma glucose. Diplopia may indicate development of a cranial nerve palsy.

2. **Management. Funduscopic examination should be performed routinely in diabetic patients.** Acute visual impairment warrants prompt ophthalmologic evaluation. Recognition of proliferative diabetic retinopathy should prompt re-ferral to an ophthalmologist for photocoagulation therapy.

E. **Diabetic neuropathy** may present with sensory symptoms or deficit, motor impair-ment, or autonomic dysfunction.

1. **Pain** is often associated with hyperesthesia in the distribution of a peripheral nerve. In the distal extremities, a nerve entrapment must be considered; pro-vocative testing may be helpful in establishing a diagnosis (see Chap. 32). In the trunk, differentiation from radiculopathy may be difficult. There is no satisfac-tory therapy for painful diabetic neuropathy. Improvement in glycemic control is helpful to some patients. Treatment with opioid analgesics is indicated for incapacitating pain.

2. **A sensory deficit** has no specific treatment. Patient education is important to avoid insidious trauma, burns, and neuropathic ulcers. Painless bone or joint injury requires specialized care.
3. **A motor deficit** results from a cranial nerve palsy or peripheral neuropathy, producing distal muscular weakness and atrophy. Other causes of weakness must be excluded (see Chap. 32). Physical therapy may be beneficial.
4. **Autonomic neuropathy** may cause orthostatic hypotension, a neurogenic bladder, impotence, urinary or fecal incontinence, or loss of hypoglycemic counterregulation. Management of the complications of autonomic neuropathy is symptomatic; postural hypotension may warrant hospital admission.
F. **Renal disease** as a result of diabetes may present with nonnephrotic proteinuria, the nephrotic syndrome, or an insidious decrease in glomerular filtration rate (GFR).
   1. **Hypertension** may accelerate the renal and cardiovascular complications of diabetes. Aggressive antihypertensive therapy is usually indicated (see Chap. 6).
   2. **Urinary tract infection** should be treated (see sec. **IV.J.1**).
   3. **Hypoglycemia** may develop in patients who maintain insulin or sulfonylurea therapy despite a decreasing GFR. In the presence of a decreased GFR, dosages of these agents should be reduced (see sec. **V.A**).
G. **Vascular disease** is accelerated in diabetic patients. Complications include cardiac disease, stroke, and peripheral ischemia. Pain as a symptom of ischemic vascular disease may not be present in patients afflicted with diabetic neuropathy.
H. **Coronary heart disease and myocardial infarction** result from vascular disease. A cardiomyopathy may also occur. Heart disease must be considered when dyspnea, hyperglycemia, or acidosis occurs, even if pain is atypical or absent. A young age should not preclude the diagnosis of coronary disease. An ECG may be helpful in establishing a diagnosis.
I. **Foot ulcers** resulting from repeated trauma, arterial disease, or chronic venous stasis represent difficult management problems. **Patients with neuropathic ulcers must totally avoid local pressure to promote healing;** hospital care is often appropriate. Suspicion of an infected ulcer warrants investigation for osteomyelitis and admission for antibiotic therapy, particularly when circulatory compromise is present. Minor ulcerations or abrasions may respond to a change of shoes and meticulous avoidance of recurrent trauma. A careful debridement of necrotic tissue aids healing.
J. **Infection.** Immune compromise should be anticipated in patients with uncontrolled diabetes mellitus, predisposing them to infection. The coexistence of infection and diabetes mellitus complicates management of both.
   1. **Urinary tract infection** (UTI) occurs with high frequency in women with diabetes. Enteric gram-negative organisms are the most common pathogens; *Staphylococcus aureus* and streptococci are also associated with UTIs in diabetic patients. Single-dose antibiotic therapy for cystitis is often not sufficient (see Chap. 12). **Pyelonephritis** warrants hospitalization for intravenous antibiotic therapy. Fungal infections of the lower urinary tract may be difficult to eradicate and warrant treatment if metabolic control is compromised. Careful control of hyperglycemia aids treatment of UTI. Recurrent infections and a neurogenic bladder are indications for chronic urinary tract prophylaxis.
   2. **Cellulitis** is common in diabetic patients. Gram-positive pathogens are most commonly involved; staphylococcal infections may follow abrasions not recognized by patients with a sensory deficit. A significant incidence of gram-negative cellulitis warrants use of an aminoglycoside in initial therapy, and anaerobic bacterial infection should also be considered. Cellulitis accompanying vascular insufficiency or neuropathy should prompt hospitalization.
   3. **Vulvovaginitis** (see Chap. 33) is commonly the result of infection with *Candida albicans* and is an indication for investigation of hyperglycemic control and use of antifungal therapy.
   4. **Skin abscesses,** frequently caused by *S. aureus*, occur in patients with hyperglycemia. Management includes incision and drainage of abscesses and administration of an oral antibiotic. Control of glucose aids healing and may inhibit the recurrence of infections.
V. **Complications of the treatment of diabetes mellitus**
   A. **Hypoglycemia** complicates therapy with oral hypoglycemic agents and insulin. Management includes prompt treatment of hypoglycemia and correction of causes.

Hypoglycemia usually results from a medication overdose, a change in the content or timing of meals (including missed meals), or a change in physical activity. The duration of action of insulin or oral agent preparations (see Tables 9-2 and 9-3) affects the clinical course and should influence decisions in management.

1. **Clinical manifestations.** Many insulin-treated patients recognize the occurrence of irritability, tremulousness, diaphoresis, tachycardia, and confusion as an "insulin reaction." A similar syndrome occurs when hypoglycemia is produced by oral agents. Inadequate hypoglycemic counterregulation (which may follow treatment with beta-adrenergic antagonists) or medication overdose may lead to more serious manifestations, such as seizures, stupor, or coma. Focal neurologic findings may develop and may resolve with restoration of a normal plasma glucose.

2. **Laboratory evaluation.** Measurement of the plasma glucose should verify hypoglycemia (see **Hypoglycemia**). Use of a glucose oxidase reagent strip will give a rapid and reliable estimate of the blood glucose.

3. **Treatment** should be guided by the mental status of the patient, the cause and anticipated course of symptoms, and the degree of plasma glucose depression.

   a. **Oral glucose or sugar-containing liquids,** such as orange juice, may be sufficient for alert patients when drug overdose is not apparent and the plasma glucose is greater than 30 mg/dl. Ensuing treatment should include a meal containing carbohydrate.

   b. **Intravenous dextrose** should be administered to patients when mental function is impaired, insulin or sulfonylurea overdose is suspected, or prolonged hypoglycemia is anticipated. Patients should receive 25 gm of dextrose (50 ml of 50% D/W), preferably after a blood specimen is obtained for glucose determination. Glucose should be raised to greater than 100 mg/dl, as verified by repeated measurements. A maintenance intravenous infusion should contain 5–10% dextrose. Patients should be fed when able to eat. Plasma potassium should be measured when 50 gm or more of dextrose is given in therapy.

   c. **Glucagon,** 1 mg IM, may be given to treat hypoglycemia when intravenous access is difficult. Patients prone to develop recurrent hypoglycemia should have glucagon available for home emergency; a family member should be instructed in the preparation and injection technique.

4. **Disposition.** Hospitalization is warranted for severe or prolonged hypoglycemia or when medication overdose is evident. Patients taking an intermediate- or long-acting insulin should be admitted if recurrence of hypoglycemia is feared or if adjustment of therapy is apt to be complicated. Patients who are unable to eat or who are taking sulfonylureas should also be admitted. Intensive care is indicated when the clinical course is apt to warrant frequent monitoring. Patients discharged from the emergency department require close follow-up.

5. **Adjustment of drug therapy** may be appropriate for the prevention of recurrent hypoglycemia in patients discharged from the emergency department.

   a. **Inability to maintain dietary intake** may follow gastrointestinal illness, oral surgery, trauma, or depression. Patients with non-insulin-dependent (type II) diabetes may require cessation of oral drug therapy during this period. Insulin-treated patients should continue insulin in small doses to prevent sensitization (see sec. **V.B**). Patients with insulin-dependent (type I) diabetes may reduce their total daily insulin to 40–50% of normal, with the reduction primarily of meal-related doses (see sec. **I.D**).

   b. **Changes in physical activity** should be modulated to conform with dietary and drug therapy. Patients must be instructed to eat more or to reduce insulin dosage in conjunction with exercise (see sec. **I.C**).

   c. An **alternative to beta-adrenergic antagonist therapy** should be considered for patients taking these drugs and having a history of recurrent or severe hypoglycemia.

B. **Insulin allergy** is seen in as many as 5% of patients with insulin-treated diabetes. Usually the reaction to insulin is local, with erythema, induration, or pruritus at a recent injection site. Generalized urticaria may be seen; dyspnea and anaphylactic reactions are rare. Reactions to insulin occur typically in patients previously sensitized to an insulin preparation who, after a lapse in therapy, restart insulin treatment. Skin tests may aid diagnosis [7]. Management of local reactions or urticaria includes a change in therapy to a purified insulin of porcine or human composition. Diphenhydramine, 25 mg PO tid, or hydroxyzine hydrochloride, 25–50 mg PO qid, may limit pruritus. More serious allergic symptoms warrant hospitalization. Patients should be advised to avoid intermittent insulin treatment.

   C. Antibody-mediated insulin resistance may cause a sudden rise in the dosage of insulin necessary to manage hyperglycemia. Development of insulin antibodies may occur at any time but is more common in the first 6 months of insulin therapy. Hospitalization is warranted when antibody-mediated insulin resistance is suspected, as management may be difficult [7].

VI. Special considerations in the treatment of diabetes mellitus

   A. Surgical patients usually require revision of diabetes therapy. When postoperative oral intake is apt to be limited, patients should be given 50% of their daily insulin dosage by infusion (see sec. **IV.B.4.c.(2)**) or as an intermediate- or long-acting insulin before surgery; subcutaneous regular insulin should be avoided. Patients normally managed with diet or oral hypoglycemic therapy may be given a purified, single-species insulin preparation preoperatively if hyperglycemia (i.e., a plasma glucose greater than 200 mg/dl) suggests the need for treatment. Elective surgery should be deferred until hyperglycemia is controlled. Emergency surgery, however, may be necessary despite hyperglycemia, DKA, or NKHS; in such a situation, intensive monitoring is indicated [13].

   B. Initiation of drug therapy for other disorders

      1. Corticosteroid therapy promotes insulin resistance. Treatment with pharmacologic doses of glucocorticoids should prompt patient education and attention to home glucose monitoring. Topical, intraarticular, or inhalent therapy poses fewer problems in hyperglycemic control, but intensification of monitoring is prudent.

      2. Oral contraceptive therapy may promote insulin resistance. Patients with diabetes who anticipate oral contraceptive therapy should intensify home monitoring.

   C. Management of patients using continuous subcutaneous insulin infusion devices (insulin pumps) is similar to that of conventionally treated patients.

      1. Complications peculiar to this method of insulin administration include hyperglycemia or DKA following insidious pump failure and infection at catheter insertion sites. Hypoglycemia may be severe but is often of short duration when only regular insulin is infused.

      2. If discontinuation of pump therapy is necessary, patients can be treated with injections of insulin that emulate pump action. The daily maintenance infusion dosage should be divided into two injections of intermediate- or long-acting insulin. Meal doses can be emulated with subcutaneous injections of regular insulin.

   D. Diabetes mellitus in pregnant patients. See Chap. 33.

Hypoglycemia

  I. Evaluation of low plasma glucose. Low plasma glucose is seen in insulin-treated patients (see **Diabetes Mellitus**, sec. **V.A**) but also occurs outside of this context.

   A. Spurious hypoglycemia should be excluded. Poor technique in the use of glucose oxidase strips often leads to underestimation of glucose values. Glycolysis may lower plasma glucose in a laboratory sample, particularly when processing is delayed; this may be minimized when glycolytic inhibitors are used.

   B. Verified plasma glucose below 50 mg/dl warrants evaluation.

  II. Management of hypoglycemic disorders. Disposition is facilitated when occurrence of spontaneous hypoglycemia is associated with either a fasting or postprandial state.

   A. Fasting hypoglycemia. Normal adults can maintain a normal plasma glucose despite 72 hours of fasting; thus, the occurrence of hypoglycemia in patients subjected to a fast of shorter duration warrants a diagnostic evaluation.

      1. Etiologies. Fasting hypoglycemia is most often the result of hyperinsulinism, and in patients not using exogenous insulin or sulfonylurea drugs, it suggests an insulinoma. Fasting hypoglycemia can also result from an inability to maintain hepatic glucose production, as is seen in severe liver disease or following alcohol intoxication. Emaciated patients may not be able to produce sufficient substrate for hepatic gluconeogenesis, but this degree of cachexia is uncommon in the United States. Malnourished patients with renal failure are prone to hypoglycemia. Fasting hypoglycemia may also accompany adrenocortical insufficiency, myxedema, or growth hormone deficit [16].

2. **Clinical manifestations.** Although a plasma glucose of less than 40 mg/dl can produce an adrenergic response and impaired mental functioning, patients with long-standing hypoglycemia may be alert and remarkably asymptomatic. Fasting hypoglycemia should be considered in the evaluation of dementia, seizures, and psychiatric symptoms, particularly when they occur at night or early in the morning. Presentation may follow acute alcohol intoxication or limitation of food intake in susceptible individuals.

3. **Laboratory evaluation.** Insulin levels may be obtained for subsequent interpretation; the circumstances at the time of collection should be documented. Sulfonylurea levels may be obtained to assess for factitious hypoglycemia.

4. **Disposition.** A fasting plasma glucose of less than 50 mg/dl is a criterion for admission, but suspicion of fasting hypoglycemia may warrant hospitalization even when a low glucose level is not documented in the emergency department.

B. **Reactive hypoglycemia** occurs in the postprandial state and represents the action of insulin secreted in response to meals.

1. **Clinical manifestations.** Symptoms of irritability, agitation, tremulousness, diaphoresis, confusion or an altered sensorium, and hunger occur 1–4 hours after meals. Symptomatic relief from food is common. Serious functional disability and mental impairment may occur, particularly as a sequel to a partial gastrectomy. In most cases, however, a counterregulatory adrenergic response develops before the mental status is compromised.

2. **Laboratory evaluation.** Reactive hypoglycemia can be substantiated by home blood glucose monitoring or results of a 5-hour glucose tolerance test, performed in a fashion analogous to that of the 2-hour test (see **Diabetes Mellitus,** sec. **III.C.2**). A positive test correlates presence of symptoms with the nadir of the plasma glucose.

3. **Disposition.** Outpatient diagnostic evaluation is preferable. Admission should be considered in patients who give a history of a serious mental status aberration.

4. **Specific therapy.** Discharged patients should be managed with frequent feedings, until complete outpatient evaluation suggests more specific dietary or drug management.

III. **Treatment of hypoglycemia**

A. **Intravenous dextrose** should be given when a seizure or mental status impairment is evident. An initial bolus of 50 ml of 50% D/W IV should be followed by a 5% D/W infusion to maintain the plasma glucose greater than 100 mg/dl (see **Diabetes Mellitus,** sec. **V.A**).

B. **Oral glucose or sugar-containing liquids,** such as orange juice, may be sufficient for mild hypoglycemia (i.e., a plasma glucose of 35–50 mg/dl) associated with adrenergic symptoms.

C. **Drug therapy for recurrent hypoglycemia,** including oral diazoxide or phenytoin for fasting hypoglycemia or propantheline bromide or propranolol for reactive hypoglycemia, is best reserved until full diagnostic evaluation has been accomplished outside of the emergency department.

Thyroid Disorders

I. **Thyroid physiology.** The thyroid gland serves as a metabolic regulator. Thyroid function is reflected by manifestations in remote organs, sharing increased or decreased metabolic activity depending on the status of hormone secretion.

A. **Thyroid hormones** include thyroxine (T_4) and triiodothyronine (T_3). T_4 is most abundant. T_3 is the principal regulator of cellular response. The majority of T_3 is made from conversion of T_4 by peripheral tissue enzymes. T_4 and T_3 circulate largely bound to plasma proteins, of which thyroxine-binding globulin (TBG) is the most important. Both the peripheral production of T_3 and TBG levels are affected by nutritional status, pregnancy, and disease states. Physiologic effects of T_3 and T_4 are conferred by the free hormones, circulating in equilibrium with their protein carriers.

B. **Thyroid regulation**

1. **Thyroid-stimulating hormone** (TSH), secreted by the pituitary gland, influences the growth of thyroid tissue and the production of thyroid hormones. When pituitary function is normal, levels of TSH are regulated by the status of thyroid hormone secretion. High TSH levels are seen in primary hypothyroidism, and low levels are seen in primary hyperthyroidism.

    2. Thyrotropin releasing hormone (TRH) is a hypothalamic product that modulates TSH secretion [4].

II. Evaluation of thyroid function

  A. Clinical manifestations of functional thyroid disease are best recognized in an unstressed, otherwise healthy patient. It may be difficult to recognize abnormal thyroid function in the presence of significant nonthyroidal illness, trauma, or pregnancy. In such cases, the clinical presentation must be evaluated in terms of an appropriate metabolic status for the patient, and the clinical suspicion of thyroid disease should prompt a laboratory evaluation (see secs. **III** and **IV**).

  B. Laboratory evaluation. Chemical analysis should serve primarily to substantiate a clinical diagnosis.

    1. Initial thyroid function testing should include a total T_4 and a T_3 resin uptake (T_3RU). The T_3RU estimates thyroid hormone binding to TBG and other serum proteins. The free T_4 index (T_4I) is a calculated value based on total T_4 and the T_3RU, which gives an artificial but often clinically useful correction of the total T_4 for fluctuations in TBG.

    2. Secondary thyroid tests may be used for diagnosis of specific disease states or to aid interpretation when initial thyroid function testing does not match a clinical assessment. A TSH assay is important in the diagnosis of hypothyroidism and can be useful in the diagnosis of hyperthyroidism when low levels are measured accurately [17]. Direct measurement of a free T_4 level (not to be confused with the calculated free T_4 index) may be helpful in evaluating hypothyroidism when total T_4 is reduced in nonthyroidal illness [20]. Measurement of serum T_3 may be helpful in the diagnosis of hyperthyroidism.

    3. Drugs may interfere with thyroid testing, and a medication history should be obtained when tests are ordered. Phenytoin lowers the total T_4. Synthetic estrogens raise total T_4 and TBG [8].

III. Hypothyroidism. The spectrum of hypothyroidism ranges from asymptomatic individuals to those lapsing into myxedema coma. Occult hypothyroidism occurs frequently in elderly patients. Hypothyroidism as a result of chronic lymphocytic thyroiditis (Hashimoto's disease) is most common and is more prevalent in women. Hypothyroidism may appear in the course of patients with Graves' disease, particularly following treatment. Secondary hypothyroidism occurs with hypopituitarism and TSH deficiency.

  A. Clinical manifestations. Patients with mild hypothyroidism may present with weight gain, intolerance of cold, forgetfulness, constipation, changes in the skin, hair loss, or an altered menstrual pattern including hypermenorrhea. Severe hypothyroidism is associated with slowed mental functioning leading to stupor or coma and the development of anasarca. There may be facial edema, thickening of the tongue, and a delay in the relaxation phase of deep tendon reflexes.

    1. Edema, enlarged heart, and bradycardia may suggest congestive heart failure; however, hemodynamic compromise is unusual without an underlying primary cardiac disease. Pericardial effusion may occur, but tamponade is rare. Cardiomyopathy may accompany long-standing hypothyroidism.

    2. Goiter is a hallmark of primary thyroid disease but is not necessary to establish a diagnosis of hypothyroidism. Diffuse enlargement with a firm, rubbery texture is typical of lymphocytic thyroiditis. A nodular appearance or texture suggests multinodular goiter. A neck scar may suggest a previous thyroidectomy, supporting a presumptive diagnosis of hypothyroidism in comatose patients.

  B. Laboratory evaluation should include measurement of total T_4, T_3RU, and TSH. The combination of a low T_4, normal or low T_3RU, and elevated TSH suggests primary thyroid disease.

    1. Enlargement of the cardiac silhouette on a radiograph of the chest is common in primary hypothyroidism. A small heart shadow should raise the suspicion of coexisting adrenal insufficiency.

    2. Other abnormalities include a normocytic, normochromic anemia, hyponatremia, and hypercholesterolemia. Creatine kinase elevation is common and is mostly of muscle origin. Unless these findings are associated with symptoms, further evaluation can follow correction of the hypothyroid state.

    3. Thyroid antibody determinations may help to establish the presence of autoimmune thyroid disease.

  C. Therapy with thyroxine (T_4), 100–200 µg/day PO, should be initiated in outpatients when the diagnosis of hypothyroidism is established. Selection of the initial dosage is influenced by body weight and age; in elderly patients, smaller dosages may prove sufficient for thyroid hormone replacement. Therapy should be adjusted to ameliorate symptoms and to maintain the serum total T_4 within a normal range. Patients with severe cardiac or pulmonary disease may be prone to complications when thyroid hormone is initiated. These patients can be treated initially with T_4, 25–50 µg/day PO and their dosage can be increased to 100–200 µg PO qd over 2–3 weeks. Follow-up should address cardiorespiratory function and the occurrence of symptoms such as angina pectoris.

D. **The disposition** is based largely on the severity of hypothyroid symptoms and the nature of any underlying disease. Patients with a significant impairment of mental status should be hospitalized. Those with severe coronary artery disease or incapacitating pulmonary disease with hypoxemia may be admitted to monitor for complications of therapy. Admission for diagnostic evaluation in an ambulatory patient is not warranted. Patients not hospitalized should be referred promptly for outpatient follow-up.

E. **Complications of therapy.** Symptoms of hypothyroidism or hyperthyroidism are indications for adjustment of therapy if (1) compliance is ascertained, (2) measurement of total T_4 has been ordered to verify the abnormality, and (3) an appropriate dosage adjustment has not been made within 2 weeks of the evaluation. Occasionally, therapy may be complicated due to low-level autonomous thyroid hormone secretion. Preparations containing T_3 may cause hyperthyroidism when taken in excess, yet serum T_4 levels may be normal or low; when these are used, a serum T_3 and TSH must be measured to follow therapy.

F. **Myxedema coma.** Hypothyroidism leading to stupor represents a medical emergency requiring attention to multiple organ system dysfunction. Most often, myxedema coma results from infection, trauma, cold exposure, or central nervous system (CNS) depressant drugs in a labile hypothyroid patient. A mortality approaching 50% may be anticipated [19].

1. **Clinical manifestations.** Myxedema is recognized in the stuporous or comatose patient by the presence of edema, hypothermia, bradypnea, and bradycardia. The deep tendon reflexes should exhibit a delayed relaxation phase.

2. **Laboratory evaluation.** Before treatment with thyroid hormone, serum should be obtained for total T_4, T_3RU, and TSH. Free T_4 may be ordered for later evaluation, as nonthyroidal illness may complicate a chemical diagnosis. Arterial blood gases often reveal hypoxemia and hypercarbia. ECG abnormalities include PR prolongation, decreased QRS amplitude, and T-wave flattening. Other abnormalities peculiar to hypothyroidism also occur (see sec. **III.B**). Hyponatremia may be severe.

3. **Disposition.** All patients with myxedema coma should be admitted; most are candidates for intensive care.

4. **Management** includes maintenance of vital functions and administration of thyroid hormone.
   a. **Ventilation.** Although hypoventilation responds to correction of the hypothyroid state, endotracheal intubation and assisted ventilation should be considered, particularly in patients with primary lung disease. Macroglossia, CNS dysfunction, goiter, and edema may lead to obstruction of the airway and may complicate endotracheal intubation. Paralytic agents and CNS depressants should be avoided in emergency department therapy.
   b. **Cardiovascular therapy.** Hypothyroidism reduces the cardiac output. Thyroid hormone replacement improves the cardiovascular tone but may also increase demands for cardiac reserve, complicating management.
      (1) **Hypotension** is an indication for Swan-Ganz and ECG monitoring, as fluids may promote heart failure and pressors may cause arrhythmias.
      (2) **Pericardial effusion** rarely causes hemodynamic compromise; however, neck vein distention and pulsus paradoxus suggest the need for Swan-Ganz monitoring to assess the cardiovascular status.
   c. **Hypothermia** should be treated with rewarming (see Chap. 15), anticipating a response to thyroid hormone.
   d. **Hyponatremia** is caused by a depressed renal blood flow and inadequate water excretion. A plasma sodium of less than 120 mEq/liter is an indication for an isotonic saline infusion and free-water restriction.
   e. **Specific therapy** includes emergent treatment with thyroid hormone after the possible complication of adrenal insufficiency has been circumvented [19]. Patients may be treated on the basis of clinical suspicion as a lifesaving measure, while awaiting a laboratory confirmation of the diagnosis.

(1) **Hydrocortisone sodium succinate** (Solu-Cortef), 100 mg IV q6h, should be given. Oral and intramuscular administration should be avoided because of slow and unpredictable absorption. Steroids may be tapered when stability ensues.

(2) **Sodium levothyroxine,** 200–500 μg, should be given IV over 1 hour. The selection of a dosage is affected by the size of the patient, severity of manifestations, age, and suspicion of organic heart disease. The dosage should be relatively low in elderly patients. Patients with suspected coronary artery disease should receive ECG monitoring for arrhythmia. Lower initial dosages of levothyroxine (i.e., 200 μg) should be given when the diagnosis of myxedema is in question.

   f. **Beta-adrenergic antagonists and lithium carbonate should be withheld** until patients are well into the recovery phase of therapy, because hypothyroidism may confer markedly increased sensitivity to these agents.

G. **Surgical patients** with untreated hypothyroidism are at increased risk for developing perioperative complications, such as hypotension from a depressed cardiac output, respiratory failure, or an impairment of CNS function leading to coma. Coagulopathy may also occur, due to abnormalities of both platelets and protein factors. Elective surgery should be postponed until the hypothyroid state is corrected. If trauma or acute decompensation warrants immediate surgery, levothyroxine, 200–500 μg IV, is indicated preoperatively. ECG and Swan-Ganz monitoring facilitates perioperative management. Patients already receiving appropriate thyroid replacement pose no additional surgical risk, and emergent thyroxine treatment is not needed [18].

IV. **Hyperthyroidism.** Excessive thyroid hormone leads to increased metabolic activity. Graves' disease accounts for the majority of hyperthyroidism; this autoimmune disease is more prevalent in women. The availability of thyroid hormone and its popularity in the treatment of obesity should raise a consideration of factitious disease in diagnosis. The spectrum of affliction includes asymptomatic individuals, particularly among the elderly, and patients whose organ function is critically impaired. Severity of manifestations should guide management.

A. **Clinical manifestations.** Patients often present with fatigue, weakness, weight loss, intolerance of heat, agitation, tachycardia, and changes in menstrual pattern, including hypomenorrhea. Thin skin and fine hair may be evident. Owing to the prevalence of Graves' disease, goiter, ophthalmopathy, or dermopathy may be the presenting manifestation in a mildly hyperthyroid (or euthyroid) patient. Less commonly, patients may notice polyuria or bowel habits tending to loose or more frequent stools.

   1. **Tachycardia** is nearly universal in young patients with hyperthyroidism but is less prevalent in the elderly. An irregular pulse should suggest atrial fibrillation; both supraventricular and ventricular arrhythmias may occur. High cardiac output is a feature of hyperthyroidism and may be associated with heart failure.

   2. **Fever** is unusual; when present, it indicates underlying illness or severe hormone excess. Peripheral vasodilation is common even without fever. Flushing may be noted.

   3. **Neurologic** manifestations include seizures and psychosis. A fine tremor is usually present, which is best appreciated by palpation of the patient's extended hands.

   4. **Thyroid enlargement** is often present in hyperthyroid patients. Hyperthyroidism may accompany multinodular goiter (see sec. **VII**) or toxic adenoma.

B. **Laboratory evaluation** should include total T_4 and T_3RU. These tests are sufficient when the T_4 is elevated in patients with a clear clinical presentation. Clinical hyperthyroidism with equivocal or depressed total T_4 should be evaluated with T_3 and free T_4 determinations. TSH measurement is helpful only when levels below the normal range can be measured accurately [17]. Excessive TSH production is rare. Chemical diagnosis in equivocal cases may require the TRH stimulation test [4].

   1. **The diagnosis of Graves' disease** may be supported by the determination of thyroid-stimulating immunoglobulins, but clinical presentation often precludes the need for this test.

   2. **Radioiodine (^{131}I, RAI) uptake** by the thyroid gland may be helpful in the differential diagnosis of hyperthyroidism. This test is useful only if there has been no excessive iodine intake, as from the treatment of hyperthyroidism or contrast-dependent radiologic procedures, for 6 weeks preceding the test. A high

RAI uptake suggests Graves' disease or a toxic goiter. A very low uptake suggests thyroiditis. RAI uptake is reduced by thionamide drugs.

C. **The disposition** should be based on severity of manifestations and on any complications that might be anticipated in outpatient management. Hospitalization is warranted when cardiovascular or CNS complications are present. Arrhythmias, including digoxin-resistant atrial fibrillation, paroxysmal atrial tachycardia, and frequent ventricular premature contractions, may warrant admission to a facility providing continuous ECG monitoring.

D. **Symptomatic control.** Outpatients with symptomatic tachycardia or agitation should be treated with propranolol, initially 10–20 mg PO qid, in anticipation of specific therapy. The dosage can be titrated over a few days to achieve a symptomatic response. Patients with a contraindication to propranolol may require hospitalization or referral for specific therapy.

E. **Specific therapy** of uncomplicated hyperthyroidism, including radioiodine, antithyroid drugs, or surgery, generally should be reserved for hospitalized patients or for outpatients referred to regular care. Thionamide drugs, including propylthiouracil (PTU), 100 mg PO tid, or methimazole, 10 mg PO tid, may be started if prompt follow-up is assured.

F. **Complications of therapy** include side effects of drug treatment and fluctuations in thyroid hormone production. Both recurrence of hyperthyroidism and development of hypothyroidism commonly occur, underscoring the need for a prompt follow-up evaluation.

1. **Thionamide drug therapy** often needs adjustment. Changes in dosage should be followed by prompt referral to the prescribing physician. Intermittent symptoms of hyperthyroidism may be managed with propranolol (see sec. **IV.D**). Side effects of thionamide drug therapy, including skin rash or hematopoietic suppression, may indicate a need to discontinue these agents. Patients who develop viral or bacterial infections while taking PTU or methimazole should receive a complete blood count with differential to screen for granulocytopenia.

2. **Radioiodine therapy** may worsen hyperthyroidism within the first few weeks after treatment. Mild exacerbations may be treated with propranolol (see sec. **IV.D**); referral should follow. When hypothyroidism is evident, it usually indicates irreversible loss of thyroid function; thyroid hormone therapy is then indicated (see sec. **III.C**).

G. **Complicated hyperthyroidism and thyroid storm.** Hyperthyroidism complicated by critical organ compromise represents a medical emergency requiring prompt management. Thyroid storm is a rare disorder, most often precipitated by a nonthyroidal stress such as surgery or trauma [19].

1. **Clinical manifestations** of thyroid storm include abrupt onset of fever and worsening tachycardia in a labile, hyperthyroid patient. Presentation usually includes evidence of cardiovascular, CNS, and gastrointestinal impairment. Cardiovascular complications may include supraventricular or ventricular arrhythmias and high-output heart failure, often leading to hypotension or pulmonary edema. The CNS abnormalities may include hyperkinesis, seizures, psychosis, somnolence, stupor, or coma. Gastrointestinal manifestations may include diarrhea, abdominal pain, hepatomegaly, or jaundice.

2. **Laboratory evaluation** should include measurement of T_4 and T_3RU. ECG monitoring is also indicated.

3. **Disposition.** Patients with complicated hyperthyroidism should be hospitalized, preferably in an intensive care unit.

4. **Management** is in anticipation of hospital admission.

a. **Cardiovascular assessment** should be ongoing with attention to cardiac rhythm and function. Volume status should be estimated. Hypotension not responding to isotonic saline is an indication for hemodynamic monitoring. Dopamine may be used to support the blood pressure when any volume deficit has been replaced; the potential for arrhythmias must be recognized. Swan-Ganz catheterization should reveal a high cardiac output; fluid management should be based on maintenance of a normal pulmonary artery occlusive pressure. Cardiomyopathy may complicate management; digoxin, diuretics, and nitrates are appropriate for treatment of heart failure. Arterial blood gases should be obtained to monitor oxygenation.

b. **Hyperthermia** should be treated with a cooling blanket, aiming for near normalization of the core temperature. Acetaminophen may be given as adjunctive therapy for temperature reduction.

    c. Central nervous system manifestations require supportive care. Comatose patients should be intubated to avoid aspiration of gastric contents.

    d. Treatment of hyperthyroid manifestations may be accomplished with propranolol, 0.5–1.0 mg IV q5minutes, titrating dosage to maintain a pulse of 100/minute. Heart failure with tachycardia does not contraindicate use of propranolol, but Swan-Ganz monitoring is prudent in these cases. Treatment with reserpine (1–5 mg IM, followed by 1–2 mg IM q4–6h) or guanethidine (1–2 mg PO qd) can be considered when propranolol cannot be used. These drugs may promote hypotension, diarrhea, or mental status impairment [19].

    e. Specific therapy should be instituted in conjunction with the symptomatic management. These measures act together to inhibit peripheral enzymatic conversion of T_4 to T_3 and to limit thyroid hormone secretion.

      (1) Hydrocortisone sodium succinate, 100 mg IV or IM q6h, should be administered. Glucocorticoids are given to inhibit the conversion of T_4 to T_3.

      (2) Propylthiouracil (PTU), 1000 mg, or methimazole, 40 mg, should be given PO or by nasogastric tube. The thionamides act to inhibit T_4 to T_3 conversion and also inhibit the incorporation of iodide into hormonal precursors. Maintenance PTU (200–300 mg) or methimazole (20–40 mg) q6–8h should follow. PTU may be given IV if necessary.

      (3) Iodide. At 1 hour following thionamide therapy, a continuous infusion of sodium iodide, providing 1–2 gm/day IV, should be initiated. Iodide blocks the glandular release of thyroid hormone. Alternatively, patients who can take oral medication may be given a saturated solution of potassium iodide (SSKI), 5–10 drops PO tid.

    f. Precipitating factors should be sought. Since a stress leukocytosis occurs in the absence of infection, differential leukocyte counts and cultures of blood and urine are recommended.

H. Special considerations

    1. Surgical patients are treated as follows, anticipating thyroidectomy or extrathyroidal surgery.

    a. Elective surgery. In cases where surgery can be postponed, hyperthyroidism can be managed with administration of SSKI, 2 drops PO tid, for 1 week; outpatient treatment is acceptable. Timing of the administration of SSKI with planned surgery is important, as both latency and escape phenomena can complicate management. Treatment with thionamides or propranolol is acceptable concurrently. High initial dosages of propranolol, up to 40 mg PO qid, may be needed in preparation for surgery; hospitalization is usually preferable in these circumstances.

    b. Emergency surgery. Patients with severe trauma or acute nonthyroidal surgical emergency should be treated with propranolol, 0.5–1.0 mg IV q5–30minutes, titrating to a pulse of 100/minute. Hydrocortisone sodium succinate, 100 mg IV q6h, is recommended concurrently. A cooling blanket should be available to manage perioperative hyperthermia. Swan-Ganz catheterization is advised, and ECG monitoring for arrhythmias is needed. Atropine is not recommended. Since morphine may stimulate adrenergic activity, it should be used for severe pain only. A benzodiazepine or short-acting barbiturate is appropriate for preoperative sedation [18].

    2. Pregnant patients need specialized care [5]. Clinical diagnosis is essential, as serum T_4 levels may be increased due to elevated TBG. Propranolol may be used to achieve short-term symptomatic control, but long-term use should be avoided. If antithyroid drug therapy is required, PTU is preferred over methimazole. Radioiodine treatment is contraindicated. Surgery can be performed if necessary and is most acceptable in the second trimester. Transient thyrotoxicosis may occur in postpartum patients.

V. Thyroiditis. Although thyroid inflammation occurs with Graves' and Hashimoto's diseases, the clinical diagnosis of thyroiditis is often applied to disease processes that produce pain in the region of the thyroid gland or a transient fluctuation of thyroid function. Rarely, a thyroid abscess may produce pain and fever.

    A. Clinical manifestations. Neck pain and thyroid tenderness are common but are not always present. Subacute thyroiditis may follow a viral illness; malaise and low-grade fever may occur.

    1. Thyroid function. Mild hyperthyroidism often occurs early in the clinical course. Mild hypothyroidism may follow, leading to return of a euthyroid state within 4 weeks–8 months of initial derangement. Changing thyroid function, even without pain, should suggest thyroiditis.

2. **Thyroid enlargement** accompanying thyroiditis is generally diffuse. Discrete nodules are uncommon, but a painful nodule suggests an inflammatory etiology (see sec. **VI**).

B. **Laboratory evaluation.** The erythrocyte sedimentation rate (ESR) is mildly elevated in thyroiditis and may be helpful in distinguishing thyroiditis from chronic thyroid disease. A total T_4, TSH, and ESR are a useful diagnostic series. A very low radioiodine (RAI) uptake is common (see sec. **IV.B.2**).

C. **Treatment** of local manifestations is accomplished with an anti-inflammatory drug. Aspirin, 10 gr PO qid, is sufficient in most cases. With severe affliction, prednisone, 40 mg PO qd, is indicated, followed by prompt referral to an internist or endocrinologist. The symptomatic management of hyperthyroidism may be accomplished with propranolol, 10–20 mg PO qid. Hypothyroidism accompanying thyroiditis seldom needs treatment, but thyroxine, 50–100 μg PO qd, may be indicated.

D. **Suppurative thyroiditis and thyroid abscess** are caused by a bacterial infection, usually with a staphylococcal or streptococcal species. Severe pain, neck swelling, dysphagia, and fever are manifestations. Leukocytosis with a left shift is usually present. Definitive bacteriologic diagnosis is required. Aspiration or surgical drainage is important if an abscess is present. The disposition should be guided by clinical assessment of the severity and extent of infection. While awaiting culture results, a penicillinase-resistant penicillin or cephalosporin with a strong gram-positive spectrum should be given. Functional thyroid abnormality is uncommon.

VI. **Thyroid nodules.** The principal concern in evaluation of thyroid nodules is exclusion of malignancy. The incidence of malignancy in patients with solitary nodules is low; it is increased in patients with a history of neck irradiation in childhood [11]. Malignant disease is more common in young women. The prognosis is worse in older patients. Although multinodular glands are usually benign, malignancy should be suspected in an enlarging nodule

A. **Clinical manifestations.** Compressible midline nodules most likely represent thyroglossal duct cysts. Firm nodules are often adenomas and are more likely to contain malignancy. Fixed, hard nodules or cervical lymph nodes suggest cancer.

B. **Laboratory evaluation.** Findings from physical examination can be substantiated by **technetium pertechnitate or ^{123}I thyroid scanning.** Uptake of high amounts of isotope (a "hot nodule") in malignant disease is very uncommon with technetium pertechnitate and rare with ^{123}I. Low isotope uptake (a "cold nodule") is more common for both benign and malignant disease and suggests the need for further evaluation. A multifocal appearance suggests multinodularity or an inflammatory disease. The diagnosis of cystic nodules may be aided by **ultrasonography.** In some centers ultrasonography is preferred for initial evaluation. Measurement of thyroid hormones is of little help in evaluation of thyroid nodules unless symptoms indicate a functional thyroid abnormality.

C. **Disposition.** A high suspicion of malignancy is an indication for hospitalization to expedite a diagnostic evaluation and surgical treatment. Patients with constitutional symptoms or anatomic evidence of metastastic disease (most often in bone or lung) also warrant admission. The patient with a solitary nodule should be referred for diagnostic evaluation, including consideration of aspiration cytology [11].

VII. **Goiter.** Diffuse thyroid enlargement requires evaluation.

A. **Clinical manifestations.** Notice of a mass, dysphagia, or stridor may prompt presentation with a goiter. Examination of the mass may suggest a pathologic diagnosis. Multiple lobulations or nodules are typical of a multinodular goiter. The texture of the goiter in Graves' disease is soft and homogeneous. A firmer, rubbery texture is indicative of Hashimoto's disease. Tenderness to palpation suggests subacute thyroiditis. Lymphadenopathy or hard nodules may indicate a primary thyroid malignancy or a thyroid lymphoma.

B. **Laboratory evaluation.** Disturbances of thyroid function are common enough to warrant screening with a total T_4, T_3RU, and TSH, but patients are most often euthyroid. A technetium scan is indicated and may complement the physical findings.

C. **Disposition.** Patients who present with a simple goiter may be referred for outpatient evaluation. Dysphagia accompanying goiter is common but is usually not an indication for admission when patients can eat. Stridor from airway entrapment is rare but warrants admission for a subtotal thyroidectomy.

D. **Treatment** should be deferred to hospital or outpatient management. Thyroxine, 50–100 μg PO qd, is used to suppress TSH production and limit enlargement of a benign goiter.

Disorders of Adrenal Function

I. **Adrenal physiology and pathophysiology.** The adrenal glands produce hormones with diverse actions. Steroid hormones are produced by the adrenal cortex; catecholamines are products of the medulla. Cortisol is the most important glucocorticoid and is an important catabolic regulator. Aldosterone is the principal mineralocorticoid and is fundamental to sodium and potassium balance. Nonselective destruction of the adrenal cortex often affects both glucocorticoid and mineralocorticoid production. Cortisol, aldosterone, and the catecholamines are regulated by distinct physiologic mechanisms.

   A. **Cortisol production** is regulated directly by the pituitary, through secretion of adrenocorticotropic hormone (ACTH), and indirectly by hypothalamic control. Mean ACTH levels are influenced by glucocorticoid activity. ACTH is released in a pulsatile pattern, making a single ACTH measurement near the normal range difficult to interpret. Both ACTH and cortisol normally exhibit diurnal variation, with peak levels at roughly 8:00 A.M. and trough levels in the evening.

   B. **Aldosterone production** is regulated predominantly by angiotensin, which is responsive to fluctuations in volume status and is mediated by plasma renin activity. Aldosterone also responds to changes in plasma potassium.

   C. **Catecholamine production** normally results from sympathetic nervous system activity. Pathology may be recognized from autonomous or functionally accentuated hormonal secretion (e.g., pheochromocytoma) or from secretory impairment due to destruction of medullary tissue or loss of neural control.

II. **Adrenocortical insufficiency.** Insufficiency of cortisol and aldosterone may occur in patients with Addison's disease or after adrenalectomy. More commonly, cortisol deficiency occurs in patients treated with corticosteroids following interruption of treatment or a stress to which the chronically suppressed adrenal gland cannot respond. Recognition of adrenocortical insufficiency in the emergency department must be from clinical features.

   A. **Clinical manifestations.** Postural hypotension is an initial manifestation in many patients, particularly in those with a deficit in mineralocorticoid activity. Hypotension results from a loss of vascular tone and a volume deficit. Glucocorticoid insufficiency causes generalized abdominal pain, often with anorexia, nausea, and vomiting. Muscular aches may be present. A disturbance in temperature regulation may be seen; fever is common. Patients with long-standing Addison's disease may be recognized by the presence of skin and mucosal hyperpigmentation or by ear calcification.

   B. **Laboratory evaluation.** Hyponatremia and hyperkalemia are common in mineralocorticoid deficit but are less likely when only cortisol is deficient. Hypercalcemia and hypoglycemia occur with glucocorticoid deficiency. Serum cortisol and ACTH measurements are a useful diagnostic screen if performed at 8:00 A.M. after an overnight fast; the circumstances of collection should be recorded.

   ACTH stimulation testing is essential for the diagnosis of primary adrenocortical insufficiency and may be performed in the emergency department when patients can tolerate a delay in treatment. After collection of blood for a baseline serum cortisol, intravenous administration of cosyntropin (Cortrosyn), 25 units (0.25 mg), is followed by cortisol determinations at 30 and 60 minutes. Normal individuals should respond with at least a 6 μg/dl increment in serum cortisol to a maximum level of greater than 20 μg/dl [1].

   C. **Disposition.** When the history reveals interruption of chronic glucocorticoid therapy, patients may be discharged from the emergency department if the symptomatology is mild and no complicating illness is evident. When there is no recent history of glucocorticoid therapy, symptoms suggesting adrenocortical insufficiency warrant admission or prompt referral to an endocrinologist for further evaluation.

   D. **Outpatient therapy** for patients needing only physiologic replacement of adrenocorticoids may be accomplished with a number of different regimens (Table 9-4). Prednisone, 5 mg PO qd, is sufficient in unstressed individuals. Patients who have interrupted pharmacologic steroids should resume therapy as prescribed; hydrocortisone sodium succinate, 50–100 mg IM, may be given to ameliorate mild symptoms. Separate administration of glucocorticoids and mineralocorticoids may be preferable in patients with primary adrenal disease.

Table 9-4. Characteristics of some synthetic adrenocorticoids

Generic name	Glucocorticoid potency	Mineralocorticoid potency	Duration of action (hours)
Hydrocortisone	1.0	1.0	8–12
Cortisone	0.8	0.8	8–12
Prednisone	3.5	0.5	12–36
Prednisolone	4.0	0.5	12–36
Triamcinolone	5.0	0.0	24–48
Betamethasone	30.0	0.0	36–60
Dexamethasone	30.0	0.0	36–60
Fludrocortisone	10.0	125.0	24–48

1. **Instruction** for patients taking glucocorticoids should include provisions for increasing the dosage in situations of stress, including infection or trauma. A twofold increase in glucocorticoid dosage is usually sufficient.
2. **Identification** for patients at risk for adrenal crisis should describe the nature of their disorder.

E. **Adrenal crisis.** Adrenocortical insufficiency may cause shock, mental status aberration, or incapacitating gastrointestinal symptomatology. Stress from infection, trauma, pregnancy, or surgery may promote adrenal crisis in patients with inadequate adrenocortical secretory reserve.
   1. **Diagnosis** of adrenal crisis is often presumptive, particularly when shock or coma is present. Blood should be collected for cortisol and ACTH determinations before initiating therapy. Electrolytes and an ECG should be obtained to check for hyponatremia and hyperkalemia. Sepsis should be considered in the differential diagnosis.
   2. **Treatment** includes replacement of glucocorticoids and management of the clinical manifestations.
      a. **Hydrocortisone sodium succinate,** 100 mg IV q6h, should be given. Intramuscular administration should be avoided when hypotension is present.
      b. **Isotonic saline** should be used to replace the volume deficit. Potassium should be avoided in intravenous fluids until hyperkalemia is no longer evident.
      c. **Dopamine** may be needed for hypotension refractory to a saline infusion. Administration should be continued until the vascular tone responds to steroid treatment.
      d. **Correction of temperature disturbance** should be addressed. Hyperpyrexia may require treatment with a cooling blanket. Management of hypothermia should include warming measures (see Chap. 15).
      e. **Dextrose,** 50 ml of a 50% solution, should be given to comatose patients, and 5% dextrose should be added to maintenance IV fluids to prevent hypoglycemia (see **Hypoglycemia**).
   3. **Disposition.** Hospitalization is warranted. Patients who do not respond promptly to initial management with fluids and hydrocortisone are candidates for intensive care.
F. **Surgical patients.** Suspected adrenocortical insufficiency should be treated aggressively when emergency surgery is needed; hydrocortisone sodium succinate, 100 mg IV q6h, should be given. Hypotension, hypoglycemia, and abdominal symptoms warrant intensive management (see sec. **II.E**).
III. **Adrenocortical excess** (Cushing's syndrome) most often follows chronic, pharmacologic administration of glucocorticoids but also occurs spontaneously from adrenal or pituitary tumor.
   A. **Clinical manifestations** of glucocorticoid excess include obesity, with a predominance of facial and abdominal fat, hypertension, and glucose intolerance, leading to diabetes mellitus in some patients. The presence of pigmented striae is helpful toward a presumptive diagnosis, particularly among young patients. Dermal atrophy is common.
   B. **Laboratory evaluation** is necessary to establish the diagnosis of Cushing's syndrome only when an endogenous origin is suspected. Measurement of a random

serum cortisol alone is of little use in diagnosis. Assessment of a 24-hour urinary free cortisol is useful if urine collection is reliable.

Overnight dexamethasone suppression testing represents a useful screen for Cushing's syndrome. Dexamethasone, 1.0 mg, should be given at 12:00 midnight preceding a fasting 8:00 A.M. cortisol determination. Normal individuals should demonstrate a serum cortisol of less than 5.0 µg/dl, in contrast to patients with endogenous Cushing's syndrome, in whom suppression does not occur. Psychiatric depression and alcoholism also may produce abnormal responses [2].

C. Disposition. The initial screening evaluation for Cushing's syndrome does not require hospitalization, but admission for definitive diagnosis is prudent when the clinical presentation is overt and endogenous glucocorticoid excess is suspected.

D. Complications of glucocorticoid excess are numerous.

    1. Osteopenia is a frequent accompaniment to long-standing glucocorticoid excess. Treatment with calcium carbonate supplements (e.g., OsCal, 500 mg PO bid) and vitamin D (5000–10000 units/week) is appropriate for patients on long-term pharmacologic glucocorticoid therapy.

    2. Steroid psychosis may occur in patients treated with glucocorticoids and is an indication for hospitalization when manifestations are severe.

Pituitary Disorders

I. Pituitary physiology and pathophysiology. Pituitary hormones control varied metabolic processes. Anterior pituitary hormones are regulated by hypothalamic secretion, and most in turn regulate remote glandular activity, including thyroid, adrenal, gonadal, and breast function. Posterior pituitary hormones are themselves hypothalamic peptides; vasopressin (ADH) is the most important as a regulator of osmolarity. Sudden loss of pituitary function is rare but may result from hemorrhagic infarction. More often an expanding sellar mass may lead to deficient secretion of growth hormone, gonadotropins, ACTH, and TSH, often in that order, over months to years. Suprasellar expansion may lead to a visual field deficit. When the mass is a pituitary adenoma, hypersecretion of one hormone may occur. Prolactinoma is most common; in women, this tumor presents with amenorrhea and galactorrhea. Metabolic effects of a hormone-secreting pituitary tumor may occur without a mass effect or sellar enlargement.

II. Evaluation of an enlarged sella turcica. When the clinical diagnosis suggests hypopituitarism, sellar enlargement is indicative of a soft tissue mass. Sellar enlargement may also be an incidental finding on a skull radiograph obtained for other purposes; questioning and examination for an endocrinopathy should be prompted. The empty sella syndrome may account for an enlarged sella turcica without hormonal abnormality. Secondary sellar enlargement may occur in primary hypothyroidism. Unless illness suggests a need for admission, referral is appropriate.

III. Hypopituitarism

    A. Clinical manifestations. Pituitary hyposecretion should be suspected in patients with growth failure, delayed puberty, or changes in secondary sexual characteristics or sexual function not attributable to drugs, pregnancy, or menopause. Suspicion is also warranted in patients with nongoitrous hypothyroidism or symptoms of adrenal insufficiency. Symptoms of a sellar mass may include a global headache or bitemporal hemianopsia.

    B. Laboratory diagnosis may be expedited when hypopituitarism is suspected in the emergency department. Evaluation should address the function of glands under pituitary control.

        1. Adrenal function may be assessed by measurement of cortisol and ACTH at 8:00 A.M. after an overnight fast.

        2. Thyroid function assessment should include total T_4, T_3RU, and TSH (see **Thyroid Disorders,** sec. **II.B**). Secondary hypothyroidism is apparent when the total T_4 and T_3RU are low without compensatory TSH elevation.

        3. Gonadal function should be assessed by measurement of testosterone in men and estradiol in women. Low gonadotropin levels are of diagnostic utility only when gonadal hormones are deficient. When hypogonadism is suspected on clinical grounds, measurement of gonadal steroids may be accompanied by assays of luteinizing hormone (LH) and follicle-stimulating hormone (FSH).

        4. Growth hormone measurement is of little benefit, as the diagnosis of growth hormone deficiency is usually made after demonstration of a loss of stimulated secretion.

5. A lateral skull radiograph is sufficient for anatomic evaluation; computed tomography should be deferred to the follow-up physician.

C. Disposition in suspected hypopituitarism should include referral, unless complications warrant hospitalization.

IV. Pituitary apoplexy. Hemorrhage into the pituitary gland may complicate a pituitary adenoma or, more rarely, may be spontaneous.

A. Clinical manifestations include sudden onset of severe headache, visual disturbances, mental status aberration, vomiting, fever, and extraocular muscle paresis. Physical findings include pupillary asymmetry, nuchal rigidity, and optic atrophy, which may be important for diagnosis in the stuporous or comatose patient. Adrenocortical insufficiency is the first endocrine manifestation, appearing several hours after the onset of local symptoms.

B. Diagnostic evaluation. Clinical suspicion may be supported by findings of standard or high-resolution computed tomography. Skull radiography is nonspecific. Cerebrospinal fluid erythrocytosis or xanthochromia suggests hemorrhage and supports the diagnosis.

C. Emergency management should follow that outlined for subarachnoid hemorrhage (see Chap. 32) and for adrenal crisis (see **Disorders of Adrenal Function,** sec. **II.E.2**).

D. Disposition. Patients with suspected pituitary apoplexy should be hospitalized. Medical intensive care is advised for patients in shock or with mental status aberration. Neurologic impairment or an abnormal cerebrospinal fluid indicates the need for emergency surgical intervention [10].

V. Diabetes insipidus (DI) results from insufficient vasopressin (ADH) activity, due to either impaired pituitary secretion or renal resistance. In DI, the urine cannot be concentrated sufficiently to maintain a normal plasma osmolarity; excessive free water loss results. Partial deficits in ADH activity may be difficult to detect. ADH deficit may be idiopathic or follow destruction of the anatomic centers of hormone production due to surgery, a basilar skull fracture, suprasellar tumor, metastatic cancer, aneurysm, granulomatous disease, stroke, or pituitary infarction. ADH resistance may accompany renal tubular disease, hyponatremia, hypokalemia, hypercalcemia, or protein deficiency.

A. Clinical manifestations. Polyuria and volume depletion are usually present; hypovolemic shock may result. Polydipsia occurs when hypothalamic thirst centers are intact.

B. Laboratory diagnosis. Presentation with polyuria and polydipsia should first raise suspicion of diabetes mellitus. DI should be considered when plasma osmolarity is elevated without an appropriate compensatory urinary concentration, in the absence of an osmotic diuresis.

1. Plasma electrolytes are often abnormal. **Hypernatremia** is present when urinary free-water output exceeds oral intake. The diagnosis of DI should be presumed when hypernatremia accompanies polyuria. Life-threatening hypernatremia in DI may result from interference with thirst mechanisms or the inability to drink.

2. Plasma and urine osmolarities should be measured in all patients in whom the diagnosis of DI is suspected. Complete DI is suggested when an elevated plasma osmolarity is greater than the concurrent urine osmolarity. Low urinary specific gravity aids in developing a presumptive diagnosis.

3. Water deprivation testing may establish the diagnosis of complete or partial DI and also may distinguish between a central or nephrogenic origin. Volume-depleted patients should not be subjected to water deprivation. Oral intake should be withheld until polyuria produces a 3–5% loss of body weight. Plasma and urine osmolarities are then measured, and 5 units of aqueous vasopressin is given subcutaneously. After 1 hour, the urine osmolarity is remeasured. Water deprivation promotes normal urinary concentration to greater than 1000 mOsm/liter. Central DI is suggested when urine osmolarity rises to less than 500 mOsm/liter but rises further in response to exogenous ADH. Complete nephrogenic DI is diagnosed by an absent ADH response [15].

C. Compulsive water drinking may be difficult to distinguish from partial DI. Excessive water intake produces renal ADH resistance. A history of psychologic instability is often present. Water deprivation should concentrate the urine to 800 mOsm/liter, after which the ADH response is minimal [15].

D. Disposition. Patients who present with volume depletion or a plasma sodium of greater than 150 mEq/liter should be hospitalized, as this suggests inability to maintain free-water intake. Patients with less severe manifestations should be admitted when there is mental status impairment or when an illness may prevent oral intake in the face of continued polyuria. Since water deprivation testing is facilitated in the hospital, admission for diagnostic evaluation of partial DI may be warranted. Patients with polyuria and polydipsia who have no evidence of acute volume depletion, an unimpaired mental status, and plasma sodium of less than 150 mOsm/liter may be referred for outpatient evaluation.

E. **Treatment of diabetes insipidus**

1. **Treatment of decompensated patients** should be prompt, with initial attention toward replacement of volume deficit. After blood is taken for the measurement of electrolytes and osmolarity, isotonic saline should be administered. The first liter may be given within 2 hours, or faster if hypotension is present. Laboratory confirmation of hypernatremia may suggest the need for treatment with half-normal saline. Use of 5% D/W, however, should be avoided until intravascular volume is restored.

2. **Administration of vasopressin** to patients with a central ADH deficiency should accompany initial volume repletion; initially, 5 units of aqueous vasopressin should be given subcutaneously. Administration of vasopressin to hypotensive patients will result in poor absorption.

3. **Treatment of patients with chronic DI** has been facilitated by the ADH analog desmopressin (DDAVP, 1-[3-mercaptopropionic acid]-8-D-arginine vasopressin). Intranasal administration of 5–20 μg bid should be titrated to limit polyuria. Free-water retention associated with desmopressin treatment may produce serious hyponatremia; therefore, patients should be carefully instructed to normalize their water intake. A poor response to desmopressin may result from rhinitis or use of nasal decongestants; in these cases, desmopressin may be absorbed from a cotton swab placed against the mucosa of the oral vestibule. Desmopressin may also be administered by subcutaneous injection.

Disorders of Calcium, Magnesium, and Phosphate

I. **Disorders of calcium homeostasis**

A. **Maintenance of serum calcium.** Levels of ionized calcium in extracellular fluids are normally kept within narrow limits through the control of gastrointestinal absorption, urinary excretion, and bone deposition of calcium. Parathyroid hormone and vitamin D metabolites influence these processes. Disorders arise from a disturbance in hormonal regulation or from other events that overwhelm hormonal controls.

B. **Measurement of serum calcium and its interpretation.** Serum calcium is measured by a variety of methods in the clinical laboratory. Since circulating calcium is partly bound to albumin, serum albumin affects total calcium levels without substantially affecting the serum free (ionized) calcium. A rough correction of the total calcium level accounting for hypoalbuminemia may be made by adding 0.8 mg/dl to the reported value for each gm/dl of albumin deficit. Total calcium also may be influenced by serum lipids and immunoglobulins.

C. **Hypercalcemia** may be caused by hyperparathyroidism, malignancy, myeloma or lymphoma, sarcoidosis or other granulomatous diseases, vitamin D intoxication, hyperthyroidism, milk-alkalai syndrome, or acute adrenocortical insufficiency. Hypercalcemia may be worsened by the use of thiazide diuretics or prolonged immobilization. Knowledge of the cause affects management.

1. **Clinical manifestations** of hypercalcemia are both acute and chronic. Longstanding hyperparathyroidism may cause renal stones, chronic abdominal pain, and osteopenia. Acute hypercalcemia results in anorexia, nausea, vomiting, abdominal pain, volume depletion, and mental status aberration ranging from confusion to coma; psychosis or seizures may also occur.

2. **Laboratory evaluation** should establish a high serum calcium and assess associated abnormalities of phosphate and magnesium. The ECG often shows a short QT_c interval. Hyperparathyroidism may stimulate a renal bicarbonate loss and hyperchloremia. When the clinical diagnosis is not apparent, an appropriate laboratory screen includes measurement of ionized calcium and parathyroid hormone.

3. **Management**

a. **Acute, symptomatic hypercalcemia** should be managed as dictated by the severity of symptoms. Volume-depleted patients should be admitted; isotonic saline should be given to restore volume and initiate a calciuresis. A forced diuresis is established with isotonic saline at 150–350 ml/hour and promoted with furosemide, 10–40 mg IV, as needed. Monitoring of the saline infusion and urinary output is essential to minimize complications, particularly in patients with heart failure. Dialysis is indicated for patients with renal insufficiency. Intravenous phosphate should be avoided.

  b. Asymptomatic hypercalcemia should prompt referral for outpatient management. Thiazide diuretics should be discontinued; furosemide is a satisfactory substitute if a diuretic is indicated. Patients should maintain a liberal fluid intake and should restrict dietary calcium. Therapy with corticosteroids, oral phosphates, mithramycin, calcitonin, indomethacin, or diphosphonates should be deferred to follow-up [21].

D. Hypocalcemia may be caused by hypoparathyroidism, vitamin D deficiency, pseudohypoparathyroidism, hyperphosphatemia, renal tubular acidosis, or magnesium deficiency. Acute, life-threatening hypocalcemia may accompany pancreatitis.

  1. Clinical manifestations may include the development of circumoral paresthesias or muscle spasms in discerning patients, but often the first sign of acute hypocalcemia is tetany. Carpopedal spasm and positive Trousseau's and Chvostek's signs are important diagnostic aids.

  2. Laboratory evaluation should establish a low total and ionized calcium. The ECG often reveals QT_c prolongation. Serum magnesium and phosphate should be determined.

  3. Management

   a. Acute, symptomatic hypocalcemia warrants calcium replacement and hospitalization. Intravenous 10% calcium gluconate, 10–20 ml (100–200 mg Ca^{++}), should be given slowly over 15 minutes and repeated until symptoms respond. Subsequent replacement may include intravenous calcium with maintenance fluids or oral therapy with calcium carbonate to provide 50–100 mg of Ca^{++}/hour. Phosphate administration should be avoided and intravenous calcium limited in hyperphosphatemic patients to that needed for a symptomatic response. Vitamin D is not indicated in emergency treatment.

   b. Asymptomatic hypocalcemia may be managed according to chronicity. The acute hypocalcemia accompanying hemorrhagic pancreatitis should be treated with intravenous calcium gluconate. For chronic hypocalcemia, oral calcium supplements may be prescribed following measurement of ionized calcium and parathyroid hormone; follow-up should be arranged. Vitamin D should be given in the emergency department only when the etiology of hypocalcemia is established. Aggressive management of mild hypocalcemia may be indicated in patients with congestive heart failure because the inotropic effects of digitalis depend on a normal serum ionized calcium concentration.

II. Disorders of magnesium metabolism

 A. Hypermagnesemia is usually the result of intoxication in patients with renal failure. Massive tissue necrosis also may raise serum magnesium levels.

  1. Clinical manifestations include anorexia, nausea, vomiting, lethargy, muscular weakness, hyporeflexia, and hypotension. Extreme hypermagnesemia may produce coma, seizures, respiratory depression, or cardiac arrest.

  2. Laboratory evaluation establishes elevation of the serum magnesium, often to greater than 3 mEq/liter when symptoms are noted. The ECG may show PR and QT_c prolongation.

  3. Management

   a. Acute, symptomatic hypermagnesemia should be treated with 10–20 ml of 10% calcium gluconate IV over 15 minutes, which can reverse acute symptoms in anticipation of hemodialysis or peritoneal dialysis. Hypotension should be treated initially with isotonic saline; pressors may be necessary. Disposition can be influenced by the response to hemodialysis; admission is usually warranted.

   b. Management of asymptomatic hypermagnesemia may still require emergent dialysis if levels are in excess of 3 mEq/liter. In milder cases, the source of magnesium should be sought and eliminated and referral arranged.

 B. Hypomagnesemia may be related to intestinal malabsorption, chronic alcoholism, magnesium-losing nephropathy, or surgical hypoparathyroidism. Serum magnesium levels decline in polyuric states, including chronic diuretic therapy and the diuretic phase of acute renal failure.

1. **Clinical manifestations** include weakness, muscle spasm, mental status aberration, and seizure. Tetany occurs from accompanying hypocalcemia. Hypomagnesemia may cause cardiac arrhythmias and potentiate digitalis intoxication.

2. **Laboratory evaluation** should establish low serum magnesium and may also show low calcium. Ventricular arrhythmia may be evident on ECG monitoring.

3. **Management**

   a. **Symptomatic hypomagnesemia** should be treated promptly with magnesium and calcium supplementation. Magnesium sulfate, 1–2 gm IV over 15 minutes, should be given to patients with ventricular fibrillation, shock, or seizure; otherwise, 1–2 gm IM is preferred. Hypocalcemia should be treated as indicated (see sec. **I.D.3**). Hospitalization is prudent; intensive care may be needed.

   b. **Asymptomatic patients** may be treated with intramuscular magnesium sulfate (1–2 gm IM) if gastrointestinal absorption is questionable; however, oral therapy is generally acceptable. Magnesium oxide, 10–20 gr PO qd, is usually sufficient. Follow-up is important to ensure efficacy.

III. **Disorders of phosphate homeostasis**

   A. **Hyperphosphatemia** usually occurs in the setting of renal failure. Hypoparathyroidism, vitamin D excess, and tissue necrosis from trauma or cancer chemotherapy may raise serum phosphate levels. Intoxication may be caused by excessive phosphate absorption from laxatives or retention enemas.

   1. **Clinical manifestations** of acute hyperphosphatemia are related to accompanying hypocalcemia (see sec. **I.D.1**). Metastatic calcification may be seen with chronicity.

   2. **Laboratory evaluation** should establish elevation of serum phosphate, usually with a low serum calcium and magnesium.

   3. **Management**

      a. **Severe hyperphosphatemia** warrants dialysis and treatment of associated magnesium and calcium deficiencies. Intravenous administration of magnesium and calcium, however, should wait until acute dialysis is available, thus avoiding metastatic calcification and the precipitation of more severe renal failure.

      b. **Mild hyperphosphatemia** may be managed by phosphate restriction and the use of phosphate-binding antacids. Magnesium-containing antacids should be avoided in patients with renal failure. Aluminum hydroxide or calcium carbonate is preferred, given with meals [21].

   B. **Hypophosphatemia** may result from malabsorption, excessive use of phosphate-binding antacids, alcohol withdrawal, glucocorticoid excess, hyperparathyroidism, vitamin D deficiency, renal tubular acidosis, gram-negative sepsis, or respiratory alkalosis. Reduction of serum phosphate accompanies glucose-containing fluid administration, particularly in the treatment of diabetic ketoacidosis, alcoholism, and malnutrition.

   1. **Clinical manifestations** include weakness, hypotonia, seizure, and CNS aberration, including irritability, paresthesias, dysarthria, and coma. Hemolysis, rhabdomyolysis, or heart failure may occur.

   2. **Laboratory evaluation** reveals a low serum phosphate. Serum bicarbonate may also be low. There may be evidence of hemolysis or rhabdomyolysis. Hypercalcemia suggests hyperparathyroidism and should direct therapy toward correction of the elevated serum calcium.

   3. **Management**

      a. **Severe hypophosphatemia** associated with neurologic impairment is an indication for intravenous phosphate in anticipation of hospital admission. Sodium phosphate or potassium phosphate may be given; infusion should provide 30–40 mg/hour. Intravenous phosphate should be discontinued when symptoms respond to emergency treatment and oral therapy is tolerated [21].

      b. **Asymptomatic hypophosphatemia** should be treated with oral phosphate therapy only. Neutra-Phos, 2 capsules PO bid, or Phospho-Soda, 5 ml PO bid, is appropriate for initial supplementation. Oral phosphate therapy may be complicated by diarrhea. Outpatient follow-up should be prompt.

Bibliography

1. Byrny, R. L. Withdrawal from glucocorticoid therapy. *N. Engl. J. Med.* 295:30, 1981.
2. Crapo, L. Cushing's syndrome: A review of diagnostic tests. *Metabolism* 28:955, 1979.
3. Cryer, P. E. Glucose counterregulation in man. *Diabetes* 30:261, 1981.
4. Hershman, J. M. Clinical application of thyrotropin releasing hormone. *N. Engl. J. Med.* 290:886, 1974.
5. Hollingsworth, D. R. Graves' disease. *Clin. Obstet. Gynecol.* 26:615, 1983.
6. Genuth, S. Classification and diagnosis of diabetes mellitus. *Clin. Diabetes* 1:1, 1983.
7. Kahn, C. R., and Rosenthal, A. S. Immunologic reactions to insulin: Insulin allergy, insulin resistance, and the autoimmune insulin syndrome. *Diabetes Care* 2:283, 1979.
8. Kaplan, M. M. Interactions between drugs and thyroid hormones. *Thyroid Today* 4(5):1, 1981.
9. Lebovitz, H. E. Clinical utility of oral hypoglycemic agents in the management of patients with noninsulin-dependent diabetes mellitus. *Am. J. Med.* 75(5B):94, 1983.
10. Markowitz, S., et al. Acute pituitary vascular accident (pituitary apoplexy). *Med. Clin. North Am.* 65:105, 1981.
11. Molitch, M. E., et al. The cold thyroid nodule: An analysis of diagnostic and therapeutic options. *Endocr. Rev.* 5:185, 1984.
12. Nuttall, F. Q. Diet and the diabetic patient. *Diabetes Care* 6:197, 1983.
13. Scarlett, J. A. The Surgical Patient with Diabetes. In D. R. Goldman et al. (eds.), *Medical Care of the Surgical Patient*. Philadelphia: Lippincott, 1982.
14. Schade, D. S., et al. *Intensive Insulin Therapy*. New York: Medical Examination, 1983. Pp. 26–35.
15. Schreier, R. W., and Leaf, A. Effect of Hormones on Water, Sodium, Chloride, and Potassium Metabolism. In R. H. Williams (ed.), *Textbook of Endocrinology* (6th ed.). Philadelphia: Saunders, 1981.
16. Service, F. J. Clinical Presentation and Laboratory Evaluation of Hypoglycemic Disorders in Adults. In F. J. Service (ed.), *Hypoglycemic Disorders*. Boston: Hall, 1983. Pp. 73–95.
17. Seth, J., et al. A sensitive immunoradiometric assay for serum thyroid stimulating hormone: A replacement for the thyrotrophin releasing hormone test? *Br. Med. J.* 289:1334, 1984.
18. Slap, G. B. The Surgical Patient with Thyroid disease. In D. R. Goldman et al. (eds.), *Medical Care of the Surgical Patient*. Philadelphia: Lippincott, 1982.
19. Urbanic, R. C., and Mazzaferri, E. L. Thyrotoxic crisis and myxedema coma. *Heart Lung* 7:435, 1978.
20. Wartofsky, L., and Burman, K. D. Alterations in thyroid function in patients with systemic illness: The "euthyroid sick syndrome." *Endocr. Rev.* 3:164, 1982.
21. Whyte, M. Mineral, Parathyroid, and Metabolic Bone Disorders. In M. J. Orland and R. J. Saltman (eds.), *Manual of Medical Therapeutics* (25th ed.). Boston: Little, Brown, 1986.

Gastrointestinal Disorders

Fredric G. Regenstein

Hepatic Diseases

I. **Jaundice** can occur with either an impairment in the production of bile or an abnormality of biliary flow (i.e., cholestasis). Abnormalities of biliary flow may be due to either mechanical (e.g., extrahepatic obstruction) or nonmechanical etiologies (e.g., intrahepatic cholestasis due to hepatitis, biliary cirrhosis, or drugs). The initial evaluation needs to distinguish between intrahepatic cholestasis and mechanical obstruction.

   A. **Clinical features** suggesting extrahepatic obstruction include abdominal pain, a palpable abdominal mass or gallbladder, or evidence of cholangitis.

   B. **Laboratory features.** A disproportionate elevation of the alkaline phosphatase and bilirubin relative to the serum transaminase activity suggests mechanical obstruction. Marked elevations of the serum transaminases are indicative of hepatocellular disease (i.e., hepatitis).

   C. **Diagnosis.** In patients with suspected obstruction, ultrasonography (USN) is an excellent initial screening investigation. Patients with mechanical obstruction usually develop intrahepatic and extrahepatic bile duct dilation that is readily detectable on USN. Computed tomography (CT) is comparable in sensitivity to USN but is more expensive and involves some radiation exposure to the patient. In difficult cases, percutaneous transhepatic cholangiography or endoscopic retrograde pancreatocholangiography may be required to demonstrate mechanical obstruction.

   D. **Disposition.** Patients with suspected mechanical obstruction should be admitted to the hospital for further evaluation. If an obstruction is demonstrated, prompt surgical consultation is required.

II. **Viral hepatitis**

   A. **Etiologies.** Viral hepatitis can be caused by one of several different hepatotropic viruses: hepatitis A (HAV), hepatitis B (HBV), hepatitis non-A, non-B (NANB), and hepatitis D or delta hepatitis (HDV). Other viral agents can cause hepatitis, for example, cytomegalovirus (CMV) and Epstein-Barr virus (EBV), but they infect other organs in addition to the liver and thus are not hepatotropic. All of these viral agents can cause an icteric illness with similar clinical features; the specific viral diagnosis depends on the results of serologic testing [35]. Since serologic tests for NANB hepatitis are not available, infection with this agent is diagnosed by exclusion.

      1. **Hepatitis A (HAV).** Infection with this agent occurs by the fecal-oral route, usually through person-to-person contact. Episodic outbreaks due to ingestion of contaminated foodstuffs (especially shellfish) are occasionally seen. Since the heaviest fecal shedding of the virus occurs 2–3 weeks prior to the onset of jaundice, maximal viral exposure to contacts generally has occurred by the time the patient seeks medical attention. The onset of disease is usually abrupt, and most cases are mild. The case mortality is low (< 1%), and HAV does not cause chronic infection.

      2. **Hepatitis B (HBV).** Spread of infection occurs by both apparent parenteral transmission (i.e., direct percutaneous inoculation of contaminated blood or body fluid by a needle or a bite) and inapparent parenteral transmission (i.e., mucosal surface or skin abrasion exposed to contaminated blood or body fluid). Health care workers, male homosexuals, dialysis patients, drug addicts, Asian immigrants, and children born to hepatitis B surface antigen (HB_sAg)–positive mothers are at a high risk for acquiring infection. Symptoms are similar to those of HAV except for a more insidious onset and often a more severe course. HBV infections are associated with a higher case mortality (1–3%), and unlike HAV infection, a chronic HB_sAg carrier state develops in 5–10% of individuals following acute HBV infection. Some HB_sAg carriers develop chronic active

hepatitis, which can eventuate in cirrhosis, or hepatocellular carcinoma, while others remain asymptomatic and have no biochemical evidence of liver disease. The presence of the hepatitis B e antigen (HB_eAg) in the serum correlates with the presence of complete replicating virus particles (Dane particles), while antibody to HB_eAg (anti-HB_e) in the serum of an HB_sAg carrier indicates that there are few complete virus particles present. Thus, HB_eAg-positive individuals are more infectious than anti-HB_e-positive patients.

3. **Non-A, non-B hepatitis (NANB).** There are at least two and possibly more NANB agents. These viruses are responsible for 90–95% of all cases of posttransfusion hepatitis and approximately 20–40% of sporadic (i.e., nontransfusion related) hepatitis cases. The illness resulting from NANB infection is similar to HBV but generally is less severe. Transaminase fluctuations occur frequently with NANB infection, and evolution to chronic hepatitis may occur in up to 50% of cases.

4. **Hepatitis D (HDV)** is an incomplete virus particle that requires the presence of the HBV for infection to occur. Thus, HDV infection can only occur in HB_sAg carriers and in people simultaneously infected with both HBV and HDV. In the United States, most HDV infections occur in drug users and multiply transfused individuals.

B. **Historical features.** All patients presenting with apparent viral hepatitis should be queried about dietary habits, occupational exposure to blood or body fluids, possible laboratory accidents, recent needle sticks, blood transfusion, exposure to individuals with hepatitis, intravenous drug usage, tattoos, ear piercing, and homosexuality. In many cases, no apparent source of infection can be identified.

C. **Clinical features.** The clinical expression of acute viral hepatitis is varied, ranging from asymptomatic anicteric infection to fulminant hepatic necrosis and death. In general, the illness can be divided into three stages [35].

1. **Prodromal period.** Nonspecific symptoms such as fatigue, anorexia, nausea, arthralgias, and fever often occur in this period.

2. **Icteric period.** Dark urine (bilirubinuria), pruritus, and jaundice develop at this time. Abdominal pain with a tender liver and sometimes an enlarged spleen also may be present.

3. **Convalescence.** Symptoms resolve and the jaundice gradually abates during this period. Full clinical recovery with return of a normal energy level and regaining lost weight occurs over the next 3–6 months.

D. **Laboratory features**

1. **The hallmark** finding of acute hepatitis is an elevated aminotransferase level. Both serum glutamic-oxaloacetic transaminase (SGOT, or aspartate aminotransferase [AST]) and serum glutamic-pyruvic transaminase (SGPT, or alanine aminotransferase [ALT]) levels are elevated, but the SGPT levels usually exceed SGOT levels and remain elevated for longer than the SGOT. Both the SGPT and SGOT should be followed until the values are back to normal. The serum bilirubin is elevated in most patients, although in anicteric patients the bilirubin may be normal or only minimally elevated. Alkaline phosphatase levels usually are normal or mildly elevated.

2. **Serologic features** (Table 10-1). Specific serologic tests are now available that allow the accurate diagnosis of acute hepatitis A or hepatitis B infection [34, 35]. An acute viral hepatitis screening panel includes testing for (a) IgM antibody to hepatitis A virus **(IgM anti-HAV),** (b) hepatitis B surface antigen **(HB_sAg),** and (c) IgM antibody to hepatitis B core antigen **(IgM anti-HB_c). A positive test for IgM anti-HAV is diagnostic of acute hepatitis A, while a test panel positive for both IgM anti-HB_c and HB_sAg is virtually diagnostic of acute HBV infection.** Testing for IgM anti-HB_c is preferred over IgG anti-HB_c, since simultaneous detection of IgG anti-HB_c and HB_sAg does not distinguish recent from remote infection with HBV (Table 10-1). Testing for HB_sAg alone is inadequate, since a negative test does not exclude acute HBV infection. At the time of clinical presentation, some patients with HBV infection may be in the serologic "window" period; this period represents the time following disappearance of HB_sAg but prior to the appearance of antibody to HB_sAg (anti-HB_s). Patients in the window period for acute HBV infection can only be detected if testing for anti-HB_c is performed. Delta hepatitis should be suspected in patients with acute hepatitis who are HB_sAg-positive but IgM anti-HB_c-negative. Infection with HDV is confirmed when serologic tests reveal high titers of antibody against the delta agent. When serologic tests fail to indicate an acute

Table 10-1. Interpretation of serologic markers for viral hepatitis A and B

Marker	Interpretation
Hepatitis A	
Anti-HAV	Convalescent from HAV
IgM anti-HAV	Acute hepatitis A
Hepatitis B	
HB$_s$Ag	Acute hepatitis B or chronic hepatitis B
HB$_e$Ag	High titer of HBV in serum and high level of infectivity
Anti-HB$_s$	Convalescent from hepatitis B or following vaccination against hepatitis B
Anti-HB$_c$	Acute hepatitis B, chronic hepatitis B, or convalescent from hepatitis B
IgM, anti-HB$_c$	Acute hepatitis B or, rarely, chronic active hepatitis B
Anti-HB$_e$	Low titer of HBV in serum and low level of infectivity (in HB$_s$Ag-positive patients), or convalescent from hepatitis B (in HB$_s$Ag-negative patients)

infection, drug and alcohol exposure has been excluded, and there is no evidence of either CMV or EBV infection, the presumptive diagnosis of non-A, non-B hepatitis is made.

E. Management. Patients should be seen by a physician at least twice a week during the first 2 weeks of their illness. Thereafter, less frequent follow-up (e.g., 1–2 times/month) is required if the patient is improving. Liver function tests (i.e., SGOT, SGPT, bilirubin, alkaline phosphatase, and prothrombin time) should be performed at the initial visit and at least weekly until the tests are improving. Thereafter, liver function tests can be obtained every 2–4 weeks until resolution occurs. HB$_s$Ag-positive cases should be retested for HB$_s$Ag every 2–3 months until it is no longer detectable. Anti-HB$_s$ testing can be performed once HB$_s$Ag has disappeared. Patients with abnormal liver function tests or persistent HB$_s$Ag positivity at 6 months should be referred to a specialist for evaluation. During the acute illness, there is no evidence that enforced bed rest or a specialized (high-protein) diet will hasten recovery. Patients should avoid activities leading to overexertion and fatigue, and they may resume normal activities when they feel fit.

F. Disposition. Most patients can be managed on an outpatient basis. Hospital admission is indicated, however, for patients with severe vomiting, dehydration, or changes in mentation. Marked deterioration in liver function tests, especially when associated with a worsening of the patient's clinical status, is a further indication for admission. Hospitalized patients with suspected viral hepatitis should be maintained on stool and blood precautions until the serologic diagnosis is confirmed. Private rooms are indicated for patients who are incontinent of stool [9]. For patients with confirmed HAV infections, stool precautions only are necessary, while patients with HBV, HDV, or presumed NANB infections should be maintained on blood precautions. All laboratory specimens should be clearly marked "hepatitis" to minimize the risk of transmission to laboratory personnel.

G. Employment. Most patients with documented viral hepatitis should be allowed to return to work when they feel fit. Patients with HAV who are employed as food handlers should wait at least 2 weeks after the onset of jaundice to ensure clearance of virus from the stool before returning to work. Individuals with HBV or NANB infection who are employed in health-related fields should wait until jaundice subsides before returning to work. These individuals must be made aware of their potentially infectious status, and they should take appropriate measures (e.g., use of gloves) to avoid transmission of infection through blood or body fluids. Patients with HBV or NANB infection who are employed in non-health-related fields and in professions that do not involve close personal contact can return to work as soon as they feel back to normal. It is usually unnecessary to wait until clearance of HB$_s$Ag is documented before allowing people with acute HBV infection to return to work.

H. Preventive measures
   1. **Hepatitis A.** To minimize the spread of infection, patients should be instructed to use good handwashing techniques and refrain from sexual activity during the icteric phase of their illness.

2. **Hepatitis B.** Since transmission of infection requires intimate contact or exposure to the blood or body fluids of an infected individual, patients with hepatitis B infections should avoid sharing razors, toothbrushes, and eating utensils with other members of the household. Clothes, towels, and sheets should be machine laundered, and dishes and eating utensils should be thoroughly washed after meals. Sexual intercourse and sexual activities that involve the mixing of body fluids should be avoided during the acute stages of illness. Condoms are recommended for sexual intercourse during the convalescent period prior to the disappearance of HB_sAg from the blood.

3. **Non-A, non-B hepatitis.** Since NANB behaves epidemiologically in a fashion similar to hepatitis B, precautions to minimize the exposure of others are the same as for HBV (see sec. **II.H.2**).

4. **Hepatitis D.** See sec. **II.H.2**.

I. **Prophylaxis** is most effective when performed as soon as possible following exposure. When possible, decisions regarding prophylaxis should be based on the results of specific serologic tests (Table 10-2).

1. **Serologic status unknown**

   a. **Possible hepatitis A.** If serologic test results cannot be obtained within 72 hours and hepatitis A is suspected on clinical and epidemiologic grounds, immune globulin (IG), in a dosage of 0.02 ml/kg IM, may be administered to household and sexual contacts. Since IG is inexpensive, safe, and effective in preventing HAV infection when given early, it can be administered prior to making a specific serologic diagnosis.

   b. **Needlesticks.** When dealing with needlesticks and the lack of rapidly available serologic tests, decisions regarding prophylaxis need to consider the clinical characteristics of the donor. When needlesticks involve donors with a low probability for hepatitis (e.g., normal liver function tests, no history of hepatitis or liver disease), patients require no treatment other than appropriate wound care. Alternatively, when donors have a high probability for hepatitis (e.g., abnormal liver function tests, male homosexual, history of illicit drug usage), patients are best treated with a single dose of IG, 0.06 ml/kg IM. If, subsequently, the donor's serologic test returns positive for HB_sAg and the recipient is negative for anti-HB_s, hepatitis B immune globulin (HBIG) can be administered at that time. When needlesticks involve an unknown donor, a single dose of IG, 0.06 ml/kg IM, is optional [21].

2. **Donor with hepatitis A.** All household and sexual contacts of individuals with documented HAV infection should receive a dose of IG, 0.02 ml/kg IM [21]. Screening exposed individuals for antibody to HAV is not necessary. In daycare- or school-related epidemics, IG should be given only to individuals having close contact with the index case (particularly those individuals in contact with articles contaminated by feces); IG is not indicated for all members of the school.

3. **Donor with hepatitis B**

   a. **Mucosal and needlestick exposure.** Persons exposed to HB_sAg-positive material by percutaneous (e.g., needlestick or human bite), mucous membrane (e.g., ingestion of HB_sAg-positive material), or ocular exposure who either never received the hepatitis B vaccine or did not receive all three doses of the vaccine should be tested promptly for anti-HB_s. Those individuals seropositive for anti-HB_s with an adequate titer (i.e., S/N ratio > 10) are immune and need no further therapy. Susceptible, seronegative individuals should receive a dose of HBIG (0.06 ml/kg or 5 ml IM for most adults) as soon as possible. If the exposure occurred to a person likely to experience another exposure in the future (e.g. physician, dentist, nurse, laboratory worker), the individual should receive the hepatitis B vaccine (Heptavax-B) simultaneously with the HBIG. The first 20-µg dose of hepatitis B vaccine is administered in the arm opposite the HBIG, and the second and third doses of the vaccine are given 1 and 6 months later. Individuals not getting the hepatitis B vaccine should receive a repeat dose of HBIG, 0.06 ml/kg or 5 ml IM, 1 month later.

   b. **Intimate contacts.** Spouses or regular sexual partners of patients with acute or chronic HBV are at risk for infection. Optimal prophylaxis for these individuals has not been determined; however, the Advisory Committee on Immunization Practices for the Centers for Disease Control [21] has recommended administering a single dose of HBIG, 0.06 ml/kg or 5 ml IM, to spouses or regular sexual partners of heterosexuals with acute HBV, pro-

Table 10-2. Postexposure prophylaxis of hepatitis A and B

Circumstance/exposure	Globulin/vaccine preparation	Dosage	Frequency/timing of administration
Hepatitis A			
Close personal contact (e.g., members of household, sexual partners)	Immune globulin (IG)	0.02 ml/kg IM	Single dose as soon as possible
Hepatitis B			
Perinatal	HBIG[a]	0.5 ml IM	Within 12 hours of birth
	and Heptavax-B	0.5 ml (10 µg) IM	Within 7 days; repeat at 1 and 6 months
Percutaneous	HBIG	5 ml IM	Single dose within 24 hours
	and Heptavax-B[b]	1.0 ml (20 µg) IM	Within 7 days; repeat at 1 and 6 months
Sexual[c]	HBIG	5 ml IM	Single dose within 14 days of sexual contact

[a] Hepatitis B immune globulin.
[b] Those individuals who choose not to receive Heptavax-B should receive a repeat dose of HBIG at 1 month.
[c] Vaccine is recommended for active homosexuals, promiscuous heterosexuals, and sexual partners of chronic hepatitis B virus carriers.
Source: Adapted from F. G. Regenstein, Hepatic Diseases. In M. J. Orland and R. J. Saltman (eds.), *Manual of Medical Therapeutics* (25th ed.). Boston: Little, Brown, 1986. With permission.

vided that the HBIG can be administered within 14 days of the last sexual contact and the partner is susceptible (i.e., seronegative for anti-HB$_s$). Serologic screening of heterosexual partners for anti-HB$_c$ or anti-HB$_s$ prior to administering HBIG is desirable; however, screening should not delay administration of HBIG beyond 14 days from the last exposure. Exposed homosexual partners should be screened for anti-HB$_c$, and if negative, they should receive both HBIG and hepatitis B vaccine [21]. When the index hepatitis patient remains HB$_s$Ag-positive for longer than 3 months, a repeat dose of HBIG can be administered to the sexual partner. Due to the expense and limited availability of HBIG, a single dose of IG, 0.12 ml/kg, can be substituted if necessary.

  c. **Perinatal exposure.** Pregnant mothers with acute or chronic HBV infection can transmit infection to their children at either the time of delivery or shortly thereafter. Infants born to HB$_s$Ag-positive mothers should receive HBIG, 0.5 ml IM, within 12 hours of birth and hepatitis B vaccine, 10 μg IM, within the first 7 days. Subsequent doses of the hepatitis B vaccine should be given at 1 and 6 months [21].

  4. **Donor with hepatitis non-A, non-B.** Due to the lack of serologic tests for these agents, studies dealing with the prophylactic efficacy of IG are difficult to evaluate. Many investigators recommend administration of a single dose of IG, 0.06 ml/kg IM, to individuals exposed by needlestick and to sexual partners of patients with NANB hepatitis [41]. Infants born to mothers with NANB hepatitis should also receive IG, 0.5 ml IM.

III. **Alcoholic liver disease.** Chronic ingestion of large amounts of alcohol can lead to irreversible liver damage in susceptible individuals. The explanation for an individual's sensitivity to the effects of alcohol remains unclear; however, genetic and environmental factors probably are involved.

  A. **Historical features.** A daily consumption of alcohol in excess of 40–60 gm over many years is required for liver damage. Since patients often deny or underestimate the quantity of alcohol ingested, it is often necessary to query a person's family or friends to determine accurately the amount of alcohol consumed.

  B. **Clinical features.** There are three forms of alcoholic liver disease that can occur either separately or in combination.

  1. **Alcoholic fatty liver.** In most cases, uncomplicated fatty liver is asymptomatic, and patients frequently have neither clinical nor biochemical evidence of liver disease. Hepatomegaly with slight elevations of the serum bilirubin, alkaline phosphatase, and transaminases may be present. The presence of ascites, splenomegaly, varices, or encephalopathy suggests more serious disease. This lesion generally is considered to be reversible once alcohol ingestion has stopped.

  2. **Alcoholic hepatitis.** The diagnosis of alcoholic hepatitis should be suspected when an individual with a history of heavy alcohol usage presents with fever, leukocytosis, jaundice, hepatomegaly, and an elevated SGOT (with a SGOT/SGPT ratio > 1.0) [40]. Proof of the diagnosis of alcoholic hepatitis, however, requires a liver biopsy and pathologic confirmation. Alcoholic hepatitis may progress to cirrhosis or progressive hepatic fibrosis without cirrhosis. Mortality with this lesion is variable and depends both on the severity of the acute episode and the degree of underlying liver disease (cirrhosis or fibrosis). Features associated with an increased mortality include renal failure, encephalopathy, ascites, variceal hemorrhage, a prolonged prothrombin time, and a markedly elevated bilirubin.

  3. **Alcoholic cirrhosis.** Most patients with alcoholic cirrhosis have signs or symptoms of liver disease. Like alcoholic hepatitis, alcoholic cirrhosis may be suspected on clinical grounds; however, definitive diagnosis requires liver biopsy confirmation. Physical findings that are often present include hepatosplenomegaly (although a small liver may occur with advanced disease), ascites, edema, jaundice, hepatic encephalopathy, prominent venous collaterals (e.g., abdominal wall veins, hemorrhoids), spider angiomata, palmar erythema, and parotid gland enlargement. Laboratory features are similar to those in alcoholic hepatitis and include elevated transaminases, alkaline phosphatase, and bilirubin and a prolonged prothrombin time. Additional findings of note are elevated serum globulins and a depressed serum albumin level. The prognosis is worse in individuals who continue to drink.

C. **Management.** Patients with fever, dehydration, jaundice, hepatic encephalopathy, or the recent onset of ascites should be admitted to the hospital. Therapy is primarily supportive. These patients should receive multivitamin supplements (including thiamine, 100 mg/day PO or IM) and either enteral or parenteral alimentation if their oral caloric intake is inadequate. In patients with edema or ascites, sodium intake should be restricted to 1–2 gm/day of NaCl. Management of hepatic encephalopathy is discussed under sec. **V.B.** Therapy of acutely ill patients with androgens or corticosteroids remains controversial; they are not recommended for routine use. In-hospital therapy should include counseling about the importance of abstinence.

IV. **Fulminant hepatic failure** occurs following acute necrosis of large numbers of hepatocytes leading to severe impairment of liver function. Hepatic encephalopathy (see sec. **V.B**) must be present for the diagnosis to be made.

A. **Etiologies.** Viral hepatitis (i.e., HBV, HDV, NANB, and HAV) is the most common cause, but toxins, drugs, ischemia, and metabolic abnormalities can also cause fulminant liver damage.

B. **Management** is mainly supportive and requires good nursing care, with prompt recognition and management of treatable complications, which include encephalopathy, cerebral edema, coagulopathy with gastrointestinal bleeding, hypoglycemia, renal failure (hepatorenal syndrome), and infection. Heroic measures have not clearly been shown to benefit patients and in some cases may be harmful. Encephalopathy should be managed as outlined under sec. **V.B.** Cerebral edema may respond to intravenous mannitol. Transfusion of fresh frozen plasma should be reserved for patients with evidence of overt hemorrhage. Antacids or H_2 blockers should be administered prophylactically (to maintain the gastric pH > 5.0) to prevent upper gastrointestinal tract bleeding. Suspected or documented hypoglycemia should be treated with glucose infusions. Nosocomial infections occur frequently in these patients; prompt recognition and empiric antibiotic therapy are essential and may be lifesaving. Progressive azotemia associated with a urinary sodium below 10 mEq/ liter is usually indicative of the hepatorenal syndrome [48]; however, intravascular volume depletion should be excluded. Most cases of hepatorenal syndrome occurring in the presence of fulminant hepatic failure are progressive and indicate irreversible liver failure.

V. **Chronic liver disease**

A. **Cirrhosis** is the end result of a variety of chronic progressive liver diseases that cause hepatic scarring and lead to disorganization of both the lobular and vascular structure of the liver. In the United States, most cases of cirrhosis are related to either alcohol abuse or viral hepatitis.

1. **Clinical features.** Some patients are completely asymptomatic, while others present with a variety of nonspecific symptoms. The most frequent symptoms include fatigue, anorexia, weight loss, weakness, nausea, and vomiting. Physical examination may reveal evidence of palmar erythema, spider angiomata, gynecomastia, testicular atrophy, hepatic encephalopathy, and evidence of portal hypertension (e.g., splenomegaly, hemorrhoids, ascites, prominent abdominal veins, esophageal varices). The liver can be either large or small, and jaundice may be present. While the constellation of clinical features may suggest the presence of cirrhosis, the diagnosis can be made with certainty only by liver biopsy.

2. **Laboratory features.** No laboratory tests are diagnostic, but a variety of abnormalities may be seen. In patients with compensated, inactive cirrhosis, all liver function tests may be normal. In cirrhotics with active necroinflammatory disease, the alkaline phosphatase, bilirubin, and transaminases (SGOT and SGPT) may all be elevated. Individuals with cirrhosis and limited hepatic reserve frequently exhibit a depressed serum albumin and a prolonged prothrombin time.

3. **Treatment.** With the exception of Wilson's disease and hemochromatosis, there is no specific therapy available for individuals with cirrhosis. Most forms of treatment are directed at the complications of cirrhosis, which include ascites, variceal hemorrhage, hepatic encephalopathy, and infections.

4. **Disposition.** Individuals with the new onset of ascites or hepatic encephalopathy should be admitted for evaluation. Patients with chronic ascites or encephalopathy who develop a mild exacerbation can often be managed as outpatients. Severe decompensation is an indication for admission.

B. **Hepatic encephalopathy** is the hallmark finding in patients with severe liver dysfunction [19,20]. Precipitating or exacerbating factors include azotemia, gastro-intestinal hemorrhage, hypokalemia, alkalosis, infection, constipation, sedative or narcotic medication, surgery, deterioration of liver function, and an excessive dietary protein intake.

1. **Clinical features.** There are four stages of hepatic encephalopathy.

    a. **Stage 1.** Characteristic features include sleep disturbances, mood changes with emotional lability, slow mentation, and bizarre behavior.

    b. **Stage 2.** The above changes become more apparent. Gross mental confusion is usually apparent, and asterixis should be present.

    c. **Stage 3.** There is increasing obtundation with a loss of sphincter control and limited ability to cooperate.

    d. **Stage 4.** The patient is comatose but may be responsive to painful stimuli.

2. The **diagnosis** of hepatic encephalopathy is made clinically, based on the findings of abnormal mentation in a patient known to have severe liver disease. Laboratory tests are usually not helpful in making the diagnosis; however, electroencephalography (EEG) and arterial ammonia levels occasionally are useful.

3. **Treatment** should be directed toward elimination of the precipitating factors and reduction of the amount of nitrogenous substrates in the gut.

    a. **Lactulose** is a synthetic disaccharide effective in the treatment of hepatic encephalopathy. When given in adequate amounts, the compound causes diarrhea with an acidic pH. The drug can be administered either orally or as an enema of 300 ml of lactulose added to 700 ml of water. In most patients, the effective oral dosage is 30–45 ml bid–qid, but the dosage should be adjusted to produce two to three soft formed stools per day. When administered as an enema, lactulose can be given 2–4 times/day. To induce a rapid catharsis in patients with encephalopathy due to either constipation or blood in the gastrointestinal tract, lactulose can be given orally on an hourly basis for several doses. Lactulose administered in excess causes severe diarrhea that can lead to dehydration, hypokalemia, and hypernatremia. The drug should not be administered orally to individuals with an ileus or a possible bowel obstruction.

    b. **Neomycin** is a poorly absorbed aminoglycoside antibiotic. Oral administration reduces bacterial flora in the gastrointestinal tract and consequently decreases the production of putative bacterial toxins. The usual dosage is 1 gm PO qid, but it can be administered bid–tid as a retention enema consisting of 1–2 gm of neomycin added to 200 ml of saline. A small percentage of orally administered neomycin is absorbed with the attendant risk of both nephrotoxicity and ototoxicity. Since the potential for toxicity increases in patients with renal insufficiency, the drug should be used with caution in these individuals. In patients with encephalopathy refractory to either lactulose or neomycin alone, the two agents may be used together in combination.

    c. **Azotemia** associated with dehydration or excessive diuresis should be corrected. Diuretics should be discontinued or the dosages decreased. In some cases, a cautious IV fluid challenge will be needed.

    d. **Gastrointestinal hemorrhage** should be managed as outlined in the section **Gastrointestinal Bleeding.** Once bleeding has subsided, blood should be removed from the bowel by using either a cathartic or lactulose.

    e. **Narcotic and sedative drugs** should be used with caution or avoided entirely. If sedation is required, oxazepam or lorazepam are preferred because metabolism of these benzodiazepines is affected less by the presence of liver disease.

    f. **Electrolyte abnormalities** require prompt recognition and appropriate therapy. Hypokalemia occurs often and may require large amounts of potassium replacement.

    g. **Infections** often develop insidiously in these patients. Aspiration pneumonia, urinary tract infection, spontaneous bacterial peritonitis, and IV catheter–related sepsis commonly occur in this setting. A high index of suspicion is required to make the diagnosis, and appropriate antimicrobial therapy is indicated.

    h. **Dietary protein** should be restricted to 20–40 gm/day initially, while adequate calories (1800–2500 cal/day) are administered by either the enteral or parenteral route.

   i. **Constipation** should be treated initially with enemas and followed by either a laxative or lactulose orally.
C. **Ascites** and edema due to liver disease are the result of a complex series of interactions involving the liver and kidney. An elevated portal hydrostatic pressure, decreased plasma oncotic pressure, decreased effective intravascular volume, and avid sodium and water resorption by the kidney all contribute to the development of edema and ascites.
   1. **The diagnosis** of ascites can easily be made at the bedside in individuals with a distended abdomen and bulging flanks. When physical signs (e.g., shifting dullness, fluid wave) are equivocal, ultrasonography often facilitates localization of even small amounts of ascitic fluid, which can then be aspirated for laboratory analysis.
   2. **Evaluation.** All patients with liver disease presenting with either a new onset of ascites or a sudden increase in the amount of ascites need to be admitted to the hospital for evaluation. A paracentesis to determine the nature of the ascitic fluid should be performed on all patients. Enough fluid should be removed for a cell count with differential, total protein, albumin, amylase, and, depending on the situation, culture and cytology. In general, an ascitic fluid protein of less than 3.0 gm/dl is consistent with liver disease, while a protein greater than 3.0 gm/dl is often secondary to either neoplasm or an inflammatory process. These values are only arbitrary, and it is important to recognize that there may be overlap.
   3. **Treatment.** Since ascites itself is rarely life-threatening, treatment should proceed in a cautious manner. Salt restriction should be instituted in all patients. No more than 1–2 gm/day of NaCl should be allowed. Fluid restriction (i.e., 1000–1500 ml/day) should be reserved for those individuals with hyponatremia. Patients not responding to sodium restriction are started on a diuretic. Spironolactone is the preferred initial agent, administered in a dosage of 25–100 mg qid. The therapeutic goal should be a diuresis leading to the loss of 1–2 pounds/day in patients with edema and 0.5 pound/day in patients with ascites and no edema [28]. In patients with progressive azotemia and in those unresponsive to increasing doses of diuretics, a peritoneovenous (LeVeen) shunt should be considered.
   4. **Complications**
      a. **Tense ascites** may lead to respiratory compromise or rupture of the peritoneal membrane. In such situations, urgent paracentesis is indicated. Removal of 1–2 liters often provides substantial patient comfort; however, since fluid reaccumulates rapidly, therapy should be instituted as outlined in sec. **V.C.3.**
      b. **Spontaneous bacterial peritonitis** only develops in patients with preexisting ascites. This illness is characterized by the development of fever, abdominal pain or distention, and worsening encephalopathy. The diagnosis relies on finding ascitic fluid with greater than 500 polymorphonuclear leukocytes, an arterial-ascitic fluid pH gradient greater than 0.1, and isolation of organisms on culture [14]. Empiric therapy should be initiated promptly in suspected cases; an aminoglycoside in combination with either ampicillin or a second-generation cephalosporin is a reasonable initial antibiotic regimen.
VI. **Drug- and toxin-induced liver disease**
   A. **Classification.** Drug- and toxin-induced liver damage can be classified according to either the nature of the liver injury (i.e., acute, subacute, or chronic), the mechanism of injury (i.e., direct, indirect, or idiosyncratic), or the type of injury (i.e., cytotoxic, cholestatic, or mixed). Some drugs are unpredictable hepatotoxins (idiosyncratic), while others predictably cause liver damage (direct hepatotoxins) [49].
      1. **Direct hepatotoxins** can be divided into two groups: those toxins causing liver damage at any dosage and toxins that are damaging only when ingested in large amounts. Agents leading to direct hepatic damage at low dosages include carbon tetrachloride, trichloroethylene, phosphorous, arsenic, and the amatoxins and phallotoxins present in poisonous mushrooms *(Amanita phalloides)*. Hepatotoxic compounds that are damaging only when ingested in large amounts include acetaminophen, iron, and copper. Since other organ systems frequently are affected by exposure to many of these agents, close observation for evidence of damage to other systems is mandatory.
      2. **Indirect hepatotoxins** damage the liver by interfering with normal metabolic

and secretory function. Agents in this group include tetracycline, contraceptive and anabolic steroids, and many antineoplastic agents.

3. **Idiosyncratic hepatotoxins** cause hepatic damage in only a percentage of the recipients. Damage by these agents may be mediated either by a hypersensitivity type of reaction or by metabolic intermediates resulting from drug degradation through an unusual pathway. Hypersensitivity reactions typically are associated with a fever, rash, and eosinophilia. Drugs causing this type of reaction include phenytoin, sulfonamides, and halothane.

B. **Treatment.** Recent toxin ingestions, including acetaminophen and iron, should be managed as outlined in Chap. 16. In most cases, therapy is limited to supportive care and withdrawal of the offending agent; however, penicillamine may be of benefit in treating copper overdoses.

Gastrointestinal Bleeding

The symptoms and signs associated with gastrointestinal bleeding are dependent on the location of the bleeding site, the rate of blood loss, and the etiology of bleeding. Some patients present with few, if any, symptoms, while others may present in shock due to exsanguinating hemorrhage. Management of the patient with gastrointestinal bleeding depends on both the severity of the hemorrhage and the condition of the patient. The approach to each patient must be individualized. Despite marked improvements in the physician's diagnostic and therapeutic armamentarium, the mortality from gastrointestinal bleeding (approximately 10%) has changed little in the past 30 years [26].

I. **Assessment**

A. **Historical features.** Attention to historical details may help in assessing the location of gastrointestinal bleeding (i.e., upper versus lower tract). Hematemesis or coffee-ground emesis indicates bleeding from the upper gastrointestinal tract proximal to the ligament of Treitz, while hematochezia (bright red blood through the rectum) usually occurs with bleeding from the distal colon or rectum. Occasionally, when the bleeding is brisk and intestinal transit is rapid, an upper gastrointestinal bleed will present with hematochezia. Melena usually indicates that the source of bleeding is from a site proximal to the right colon; however, this is not always the case.

1. A **complete history** should be obtained in all patients, with special attention directed at obtaining a history of prior gastrointestinal bleeding or peptic ulcer disease. A history of abdominal vascular surgery should be sought in patients with abdominal surgical scars. Patients should also be questioned about the recent onset of symptoms, such as abdominal pain, nausea, vomiting, and weight loss.

2. **Drug usage.** All patients should be queried about the ingestion of alcohol, salicylates, nonsteroidal anti-inflammatory drugs, and anticoagulants, as these are drugs that can either cause or aggravate gastrointestinal bleeding.

B. **Physical examination**

1. **Vital signs.** The severity of bleeding can be estimated from the vital signs. In general, a pulse greater than 120/minute or a systolic blood pressure (BP) less than 90 mm Hg indicates significant (i.e., 20–25%) depletion of the intravascular volume. Patients with "normal" supine vital signs should be evaluated in the sitting or upright posture. An orthostatic drop in systolic BP of greater than 15 mm Hg or an increase in pulse of greater than 20/20/minute indicates at least a 10% depletion of circulating blood volume.

2. **General appearance** and condition of the patient should be assessed on the initial examination. Signs of portal hypertension (e.g., ascites, splenomegaly, prominent abdominal wall veins, hemorrhoids), previous abdominal surgery, and other organ system dysfunction should be noted.

C. **Laboratory studies**

1. A **hematocrit** should be obtained on all patients with gastrointestinal bleeding as soon as possible after their arrival. A spun hematocrit is preferable, as it can be obtained in 5 minutes. However, the magnitude of the blood loss may be underestimated if it is not appreciated that the hematocrit may not change for the first several hours following a hemorrhage. The hematocrit begins to fall when the extravascular fluid enters the intravascular space. The maximum fall in hematocrit may not occur for up to 72 hours following an acute hemorrhage.

2. **Type and cross-match.** Blood should be obtained for type and cross-match

immediately after the patient's arrival. To ensure availability of blood and blood products, the blood bank should be notified about all patients with massive gastrointestinal bleeding.

3. **Coagulation** and routine blood studies are indicated.

II. **Initial management**

A. **A large-bore** peripheral IV line is essential for infusion of crystalloid and blood. Additional IV lines should be established as needed, depending on the clinical situation.

B. **Normal saline** or Ringer's lactate solution should be infused initially to restore the vascular volume.

C. **Transfusions.** Generally, any patient who is symptomatic or hypotensive after infusion of 2 liters of crystalloid should be transfused. Packed red blood cells (RBCs) are preferred for individuals with an adequate intravascular volume and a low hematocrit (i.e., < 30%). Whole blood should be reserved for actively bleeding patients with a decreased blood volume. Fresh frozen plasma (FFP) should be infused after every 5–6 units of packed RBCs to correct for clotting factor depletion. Individuals on an oral anticoagulant should receive FFP as soon as possible; depending on the situation, vitamin K is usually given at the same time. Patients with liver disease and a prolonged prothrombin time should receive 2 units of FFP initially, followed by 1 unit of FFP for every 3 units of packed RBCs transfused. Platelet transfusions are indicated in patients with thrombocytopenia (i.e., < 80,000/mm^3) and in cases of massive hemorrhage after every 8–10 units of blood.

D. **Monitoring.** Careful monitoring of the vital signs, cardiac rhythm, and urinary output is necessary. In elderly patients and those with a history of cardiac disease, fluid replacement should be guided by either central venous pressure or preferably pulmonary capillary wedge pressure measurements.

E. **Disposition.** Every patient with significant gastrointestinal bleeding should be admitted to the hospital. Elderly patients and individuals with significant intravascular volume depletion should be admitted to an intensive care unit.

III. **Diagnostic studies.** Once the patient has been resuscitated and is hemodynamically stable, the distinction between upper and lower gastrointestinal tract bleeding needs to be made. The history is reliable in diagnosing upper gastrointestinal bleeding only if the patient is observed to have hematemesis or coffee-ground emesis. Hematochezia and melena, on the other hand, can be associated with either an upper or lower site of gastrointestinal bleeding.

A. The **nasogastric tube** test is often helpful in determining an upper gastrointestinal source of bleeding. In patients without hematemesis, a nasogastric tube should be passed (even in patients with known or suspected varices) and the stomach contents aspirated. If fresh or old blood is aspirated, the test is positive and the patient is probably bleeding from an upper gastrointestinal source. Small flecks of blood or brown particles mixed with mucus are nondiagnostic. Furthermore, a nondiagnostic or negative nasogastric tube test does not exclude an upper gastrointestinal bleed. Hemoccult testing should not be routinely performed on the nasogastric tube aspirate. Hemoccult testing of the gastric aspirate is indicated in the rare situations where the aspirated material is dark red or brown and it is unclear whether the aspirated material is blood; in that setting, if the aspirated substance is blood, the Hemoccult test will be strongly positive. In patients with a blood-filled stomach who are repeatedly vomiting, the stomach should be emptied using gentle gastric lavage with normal saline. The patient should be placed in the left lateral decubitus position with the head lowered and a large-bore Ewald (34 F) tube inserted. Once the tube is passed, the stomach is gently lavaged; vigorous aspiration should be avoided, as this damages the gastric mucosa. Smaller nasogastric tubes are not effective in evacuating blood and clot from the stomach. Iced-saline lavage is frequently employed; however, its effect on active bleeding remains questionable [16]. Continuous iced-saline lavage should be avoided because it can lead to hypothermia. The use of an indwelling nasogastric tube to monitor recurrent bleeding usually is unnecessary; resumption of bleeding is frequently evident by other means (e.g., change in vital signs, hematemesis, or hematochezia).

B. **Endoscopy.** Panendoscopy (esophagogastroduodenoscopy) has become the procedure of choice for evaluating patients with acute upper gastrointestinal bleeding [43]. In cases where the source of bleeding (i.e., upper or lower gastrointestinal tract) is unclear, endoscopy can quickly determine whether bleeding is coming from the upper gastrointestinal tract and usually can identify the bleeding lesion. However, endoscopy should not be attempted in individuals who are hemodynamically unstable or uncooperative, have life-threatening cardiac arrhythmias, or are suspected of having a perforated viscus. Furthermore, in patients with massive bleeding, endoscopy often is not helpful because the stomach and duodenum cannot be adequately visualized. Since early or emergent endoscopy does not alter mortality in patients who spontaneously stop bleeding [36], endoscopy can be safely performed in most patients as an elective procedure within 24 hours of admission. Endoscopy should be done as soon as possible on individuals who rebled, those who continue to bleed actively following admission, those with suspected variceal hemorrhage, and those with a history of abdominal aortic surgery with a possible aortoenteric fistula.

C. **Arteriography.** When bleeding is rapid (i.e., > 1.0 ml/minute) and the stomach cannot be cleared of blood or endoscopy was nondiagnostic, selective abdominal angiography may be helpful. However, **patients who are unstable or cannot be stabilized medically should never have surgery postponed until after an arteriogram is obtained; these individuals should proceed directly to surgery.** In patients with an angiogram revealing active bleeding, the catheter can be left in place and vasopressin infused; some patients will stop bleeding with an intraarterial vasopressin infusion [1].

D. **Barium radiography.** Upper GI radiographs are less sensitive than endoscopy in the diagnosis of bleeding lesions of the upper gastrointestinal tract [44]. However, in the evaluation of the patient who has stopped bleeding, an upper GI examination is an acceptable alternative to endoscopy. Of note, barium studies should not be performed if either early endoscopy or arteriography is anticipated, as the barium can interfere with these studies.

E. **Proctosigmoidoscopy.** All individuals with apparent lower gastrointestinal bleeding should undergo proctosigmoidoscopy [43]. Examination with a rigid instrument is preferred because the larger channel facilitates removal of blood. Flexible sigmoidoscopy is best performed after bleeding has stopped and the rectum has been prepped with enemas. In patients bleeding proximal to the rectosigmoid, either angiography or a nuclear medicine scan using technetium 99m–labeled red blood cells should be performed.

F. **Technetium 99m–labeled red blood cells** (^{99m}Tc-RBC). In patients with slow bleeding, ^{99m}Tc-RBC scanning often can help localize the site of bleeding in either the small bowel or colon [29]. Early scans are obtained routinely, while delayed scans should be obtained in patients with no evidence of bleeding on the early scans.

G. **Colonoscopy.** Endoscopic examination of the colon usually is not feasible during active bleeding. This procedure is best performed after bleeding has stopped or slowed and the colon can be cleaned with enemas or oral lavage solutions.

H. **Barium enema** should be reserved until after the episode of bleeding has stopped. There is no evidence that a barium enema will stop an active lower gastrointestinal hemorrhage.

IV. **Specific treatment**

A. **Upper gastrointestinal bleeding.** In the majority (85%) of cases, bleeding will stop without specific intervention. In patients who do not undergo early endoscopy or an upper GI series, it is reasonable to initiate therapy with any of the peptic ulcer regimens until the diagnosis is made and specific therapy instituted.

1. **Peptic ulcer disease**

   a. **Medical therapy.** Cimetidine, ranitidine, sucralfate, and large doses of antacids have all been demonstrated to increase the rate of healing of peptic ulcers; however, no agent alone or in combination has convincingly demonstrated efficacy in either stopping acute bleeding or in preventing rebleeding in patients with upper gastrointestinal bleeding [50]. Any of the ulcer regimens presented in Table 10-3 would be appropriate initial medical therapy for a patient with an acute upper gastrointestinal bleed presumed to be due to a peptic ulcer. Patients who are NPO can be given cimetidine or ranitidine IV. Vasopressin administered IV does not appear to stop hemorrhage in most patients with upper gastrointestinal bleeding [11].

   b. **Surgical therapy.** In patients with bleeding peptic ulcers, surgery is indicated for those who bleed massively and cannot be stabilized, those who continue bleeding, and those who have a second episode of bleeding after they are admitted to the hospital. Difficulty obtaining adequate amounts of compatible blood is also an indication for early operative intervention.

2. **Mild gastritis, duodenitis.** Bleeding from these lesions is usually self-limited, and treatment generally is the same as for peptic ulcer disease. Avoidance of irritating agents (e.g., alcohol, salicylates) is sometimes all that is needed.

Table 10-3. Medical regimens for peptic ulcer disease

Medication	Dosage
High-potency liquid antacid (Mylanta II, Maalox-TC)	30 ml (144 mEq) 1 hour and 3 hours after meals and hs
Cimetidine (Tagamet)	300 mg PO with meals and hs, 400 mg PO bid, 800 mg PO hs, or 300 mg IV q6h*
Ranitidine (Zantac)	150 mg PO bid, 300 mg PO hs, or 50 mg IV q6–8h*
Sucralfate (Carafate)	1.0 gm PO 1 hour before meals and hs

*Dosage should be reduced in the elderly and in the presence of renal insufficiency.

3. **Severe (hemorrhagic or erosive) gastritis and stress ulcers.** A combination of antacids and H_2 blocking agents may stop active bleeding and prevent re-bleeding. In refractory cases, selective infusion of vasopressin into the left gastric artery may help control the hemorrhage [1].

4. **Aortoenteric fistula.** Patients with a history of abdominal vascular surgery, especially with an aortic graft, are at risk for an aortoenteric fistula. Any patient suspected of having an aortoenteric fistula should undergo emergent endoscopy. If no source of bleeding is found, prompt surgical exploration should be performed to evaluate for the presence of an aortoenteric fistula. Arteriography is rarely helpful.

5. **Mallory-Weiss tear.** Most patients will stop bleeding without specific therapy [31]. In some patients, selective infusion of vasopressin into the left gastric artery will control the hemorrhage. Occasionally, surgery is required.

6. **Arteriovenous malformations** are becoming increasingly recognized as the etiology of recurrent upper gastrointestinal bleeding. No specific therapy is available.

7. **Esophagogastric varices.** Unlike most lesions of the upper gastrointestinal tract, bleeding from varices often persists or recurs after admission [10]. In-hospital mortality from variceal hemorrhage is approximately 30%, higher than for most other causes of gastrointestinal bleeding [13].

   a. **Vasopressin.** Continous infusion of low doses of vasopressin into a peripheral vein is often the initial therapy. A convenient formulation is 100 units of vasopressin in 100 ml of 5% D/W. Infusion is started at 0.3 units/minute (18 ml/hour), and the dosage is increased by 0.3 units/minute every 30–60 minutes until bleeding is controlled or a maximum dosage of 0.9 units/minute is reached. The dosage should be tapered from 0.9 units/minute within 2–4 hours. Once the dosage is at 0.6 units/minute, the infusion can be tapered by 0.2–0.3 units/minute every 12–24 hours. Bleeding that continues or recurs while the patient is on intravenous vasopressin may be managed with either intraarterial vasopressin, balloon tamponade, esophageal sclerotherapy, or portal-systemic shunt surgery. Due to vasopressin's potent vasoconstrictor properties, it should be used with caution in patients with congestive heart failure, coronary artery disease, peripheral vascular disease, or cerebrovascular disease.

   b. **Intraarterial vasopressin.** Infusion through the superior mesenteric artery is sometimes effective when the intravenous route fails [6]. The dosage is 0.1–0.5 units/minute.

   c. **Balloon tamponade** [13]. Either a Sengstaken-Blakemore (SB) tube (i.e., esophageal and gastric balloons with a tube for gastric suction) or a Linton-Nachlas (LN) tube (i.e., a large gastric balloon with gastric and esophageal ports for suction) may be used. The triple-lumen SB tube should be modified by attaching a nasogastric tube along its side with the nasogastric tip just above the esophageal balloon. The nasogastric tube should be attached to intermittent low suction; this prevents aspiration of secretions that accumulate in the esophagus when the gastric or esophageal balloon is inflated. This modification is not needed with the LN tube. Either tube can be passed through the mouth or nose (the mouth is preferred when there is any difficulty with nasal passage), and its passage can be facilitated by anesthetizing the oropharynx or nasal mucosa with a topical anesthetic. In all but the most critical situations, the position of the gastric balloon should be verified by x-ray or fluoroscopy both before and after inflation. The SB gastric balloon is inflated with 250 ml of air (the LN tube with 800 ml of air) and is doubly clamped. No more than 1 kg of tension is placed on the tube to pull the gastric balloon up against the cardia of the stomach. Continuous tension is maintained by using weights and orthopedic traction over the foot of the bed or by securing the tube to either a baseball catcher's mask or a football helmet. Blood is then removed from the stomach by lavage. If active bleeding persists or recurs after inflation of the gastric balloon, the SB esophageal balloon is inflated to a pressure of 30–45 mm Hg (using a sphygmomanometer), and the inlet is doubly clamped. Tamponade is continued for 24–36 hours; however, the esophageal balloon is intermittently deflated. If no bleeding occurs over the next 12–24 hours, the tube is removed. Patients who continue bleeding or rebleed after balloon deflation should be considered candidates for variceal sclerotherapy or shunt surgery. Patients treated with balloon tamponade should be kept under continuous observation in an intensive care unit. Scissors should be kept near the bedside, so that the SB tube can be cut and removed if the balloon slips into the pharynx.

B. Lower gastrointestinal bleeding

1. **Diverticulosis.** Most patients will stop bleeding without treatment. If the diagnosis is made at the time of angiography, selective arterial infusion of vasopressin frequently controls bleeding [1]. Surgery may be needed in patients in whom bleeding persists or the site of bleeding cannot be localized.

2. **Neoplasms.** Cancers and polyps uncommonly cause severe hemorrhage. These lesions can be removed either at endoscopy or surgery.

3. **Inflammatory bowel disease.** Severe hemorrhage is unusual, and most episodes are self-limited. If the hemorrhage is due to active disease, treatment is the same as that for active inflammatory bowel disease (see **Inflammatory Bowel Disease,** sec. I.D). Rarely, surgical resection is needed.

4. **Arteriovenous malformations** can occur throughout the gastrointestinal tract. They are often responsible for recurrent, self-limited episodes of lower gastrointestinal bleeding. The diagnosis usually is made by colonoscopy or arteriography. Surgical resection of the involved segment should be performed in patients in whom hemorrhage persists and the bleeding site can be identified. Thermocoagulation can be attempted in individuals who are poor surgical risks.

Disorders of the Esophagus

I. Gastroesophageal reflux disease

A. Clinical features. Heartburn is the symptom most often associated with gastroesophageal reflux disease; it is a symptom that occurs intermittently in greater than 30% of normal individuals [32]. Patients with significant gastroesophageal reflux disease usually complain of persistent or severe heartburn, which can be incapacitating. In addition to heartburn, patients with reflex esophagitis may complain of dysphagia, odynophagia, regurgitation, or chest pain [39]. Reflux symptoms often are worse after large meals (especially with fatty foods), when lying supine, and when bending over.

B. Pathophysiology. The following factors either alone or in combination are responsible for pathologic gastroesophageal reflux disease.

1. **Lower esophageal sphincter (LES) dysfunction** secondary to an abnormally low LES pressure or inappropriate LES relaxation.

2. **Reduced esophageal acid clearance** due to absent peristalsis (scleroderma), poor stripping waves (esophageal motility disorders), or decreased salivary flow (sicca syndrome).

3. **Excessive gastric acid secretion** secondary to peptic ulcer disease or the Zollinger-Ellison syndrome.

4. **Delayed gastric emptying** due to diabetic gastroparesis or gastric outlet obstruction.

C. The diagnosis of gastroesophageal reflux disease often is suspected after taking a history; however, upper endoscopy, a barium swallow, a Bernstein test, or esophageal pH monitoring may be necessary to confirm the diagnosis.

D. Therapy is directed at reducing the amount of gastric acid refluxing into the esophagus. Initial measures should include elevation of the head of the bed on blocks (6 inches), small meals, weight reduction, avoidance of reclining for at least 4 hours after meals, avoidance of alcohol and smoking, frequent administration of antacids, and administration of H_2 blockers (see Table 10-3).

II. **Esophageal motility disorders** represent a group of related disorders, many of which are poorly defined (i.e., nonspecific esophageal motility disorders). The best characterized of these disorders are achalasia and diffuse esophageal spasm [7].

   A. **Clinical features.** Most patients with esophageal motility disorders have symptoms of dysphagia or chest pain.

      1. **Dysphagia** due to a motility disorder needs to be distinguished from dysphagia due to a mechanical obstruction from a stricture or tumor. In general, dysphagia due to a motility disorder is present for both liquids and solids, while dysphagia secondary to a mechanical obstruction primarily involves solids.

      2. **Chest pain** of esophageal origin may be indistinguishable from pain due to angina pectoris or myocardial infarction. Esophageal pain, however, is not exertional, may be precipitated by cold beverages, and is often associated with dysphagia.

   B. **Evaluation** of the patient with dysphagia should consist of at least a barium swallow and an upper endoscopy to assess for mechanical obstruction. Patients presenting with only chest pain should have cardiac disease excluded before presuming the pain is of esophageal origin. An esophageal motility study may be needed to establish the diagnosis in individuals with noncardiac chest pain.

   C. **Management.** Patients with chest pain or dysphagia due to esophageal spasm or a nonspecific motility disorder usually are treated with nitroglycerin, a calcium channel blocking agent, or a tricyclic antidepressant. Many patients will benefit from one or a combination of these medications. Most individuals can be managed as outpatients, once it is clear that their chest pain is noncardiac. Patients with refractory symptoms and those with achalasia should be referred to specialists for evaluation and treatment.

Peptic Ulcer Disease

I. **Duodenal ulcer.** Approximately 10% of the population will experience a duodenal ulcer during their lifetime. Most individuals will suffer either a relapse of symptoms or an ulcer recurrence. Since the disease tends to be chronic, many patients will have symptoms for weeks to years prior to their seeking medical attention. Most will have found that antacid ingestion provides relief. Some patients are asymptomatic and never see a physician, while others only present when a complication (see sec. III) ensues.

   A. **Clinical features.** Patients typically complain of epigastric or upper abdominal pain that is burning or gnawing in nature. The pain usually occurs on an empty stomach 1–3 hours after meals and during sleep and is relieved by food or alkali. Symptoms generally are present for weeks or months before the patients seek medical attention. Patients often do not present with the "classic symptoms." In some people, the pain may be diffuse, worse with meals, or unrelieved with alkali, while other patients may have nausea and vomiting as their primary complaint. When diagnosing ulcer disease, it is important to recognize the variability in the clinical presentation.

   B. The **diagnosis** usually can be established in an outpatient setting using either upper endoscopy or an upper GI series.

   C. **Treatment.** Any of several different drug regimens (see Table 10-3) are equally effective for treating patients with duodenal ulcer disease [12,46]. Additional anti-ulcer agents will soon be on the market; however, they should be comparable in efficacy to the drugs already available [46]. Ulcer patients should be advised to stop smoking, reduce alcohol intake, and avoid salicylates and nonsteroidal anti-inflammatory agents. No special diets are necessary, but foods that precipitate symptoms should be avoided. Individuals with recurring episodes of pain while being treated should be given antacids ad lib. Treatment should continue for 6–8 weeks. Since duodenal ulcers are almost never malignant, they do not need to be biopsied or followed with healing with endoscopy or barium radiography. Only patients who continue to experience symptoms suggestive of a persistent ulcer need follow-up endoscopy or upper GI examination.

      Recurrence of symptoms months or years later is frequent, and virtually all of these people respond to a repeat course of treatment. Upper GI or endoscopic documentation of an ulcer recurrence is not always necessary in individuals with a documented previous history of peptic ulcer disease.

II. **Gastric ulcers** are less common than duodenal ulcers and usually occur in individuals over 40 years of age. Like duodenal ulcers, they tend to recur; but unlike duodenal ulcers, gastric ulcers may be malignant.
   A. **Clinical features.** Abdominal pain is the most frequent symptom; it tends to be a poorly localized dull or aching discomfort. The pain has a variable relationship to meals, with either worsening or improvement with eating. Often the pain is relieved with antacids. Anorexia, nausea, and weight loss can occur with both benign and malignant ulcers; however, early satiety is more often a feature of gastric malignancy.
   B. **Diagnosis.** Most patients are evaluated as outpatients using either upper endoscopy or an upper GI examination to establish the diagnosis.
   C. **Treatment** is essentially the same as for duodenal ulcer disease (see Table 10-3) [22]. Salicylates, nonsteroidal anti-inflammatory agents, alcohol, and smoking should be avoided, but no special diet is required. Gastric ulcers should be followed to healing with either endoscopy or an upper GI examination, and treatment should continue until complete healing has occurred.
III. **Complications of peptic ulcer disease.** All patients with known or suspected complications of peptic ulcer disease should be admitted to the hospital for further evaluation and treatment.
   A. **Perforation** can occur with both duodenal and gastric ulcers. Furthermore, the ulcer can perforate freely into the abdomen, or it can penetrate into an adjacent structure (e.g., pancreas, biliary tract, liver, omentum, or colon). Patients usually present with severe abdominal pain, and peritoneal signs may be present. The diagnosis is confirmed when either free intraperitoneal air is seen on an upright abdominal film or when contrast extravasation is noted on an upper GI series. Water-soluble contrast material (e.g., Hypaque) should be used if a perforation is suspected. In patients with a suspected or documented perforation, a nasogastric tube should be passed and attached to intermittent suction while surgical consultation is obtained. Endoscopy should never be attempted in the setting of a suspected perforation.
   B. **Obstruction** of the gastric outlet can occur in patients with either active or previous peptic ulcer disease. Vomiting and epigastric pain are the most frequent symptoms. Outlet obstruction should be suspected when patients present with volume depletion associated with a hypokalemic, hypochloremic alkalosis. The diagnosis usually can be made on an upper GI examination. Treatment consists of correction of fluid and electrolyte disturbances, gastric decompression with a nasogastric tube, and anti-ulcer therapy (see Table 10-3). Surgery may be necessary in patients not responding to medical treatment.
   C. **Hemorrhage.** See **Gastrointestinal Bleeding, sec. IV.A.1.**
   D. **Intractable pain.** Occasional patients will continue to have pain and active ulcer disease following a complete course of treatment. Factors associated with treatment failure include noncompliance, smoking, hypersecretion (e.g., Zollinger-Ellison syndrome), or ingestion of nonsteroidal anti-inflammatory agents. These patients should be referred to a specialist for further management and follow-up.

Gastritis

I. **Acute gastritis**
   A. **Clinical features.** Many patients with this disease are asymptomatic; however, gastrointestinal bleeding, abdominal discomfort (often ulcerlike), nausea, or vomiting may be present. Patients with acute gastritis frequently have a recent history of stress (e.g., surgery, infection) or drug ingestion (e.g., salicylates, alcohol).
   B. **The diagnosis** is made on the basis of endoscopic and histologic findings.
   C. **Treatment.** No good studies are available evaluating the effects of therapy on this lesion. Most patients are managed with either antacids or an anti-ulcer regimen (see Table 10-3). Patients with evidence of bleeding should be managed as outlined in the section on **Gastrointestinal Bleeding, sec. IV.A.3.**
II. **Chronic gastritis**
   A. **Clinical features.** More so than acute gastritis, chronic gastritis tends to be an asymptomatic illness that becomes clinically apparent only if a patient develops pernicious anemia (atrophic gastritis) or a gastric cancer. Occasionally, patients with dyspepsia or poorly defined upper abdominal pain are assumed to have symptoms due to gastritis.
   B. **Diagnosis.** See sec. **I.B.**
   C. **Treatment.** See sec. **I.C.**

Pancreatitis

Pancreatitis is typically subdivided into two forms of disease: acute and chronic. In acute pancreatitis, pancreatic function and histology return to normal following the acute attack. With chronic pancreatitis, irreversible damage to the gland has occurred, and both pancreatic histology and function are abnormal. The term *relapsing pancreatitis* is used to describe individuals with repeated attacks of pancreatic inflammation.

I. **Acute pancreatitis.** Alcohol and biliary tract disease account for the majority of cases of acute pancreatitis in the United States, while trauma, drugs, familial disease, viral infections, hyperlipidemia, vascular insufficiency, and vasculitis are implicated in most of the remaining cases (45).

A. **Clinical features.** Pain localized to the upper abdomen and epigastric area is the cardinal symptom, with pain radiating to the back being present less often. Fulminant cases may present in shock without an antecedent history of abdominal pain. Nausea, vomiting, fever, abdominal distention, and hypotension may also occur. In virtually all cases of acute pancreatitis, the amylase and lipase are elevated; in addition, the hemoglobin (due to hemoconcentration), white blood cell (WBC) count, glucose, SGOT, bilirubin, and lactic dehydrogenase (LDH) are often elevated as well. The serum calcium is frequently depressed.

B. The **diagnosis** is usually made when the amylase or lipase is elevated in a patient presenting with the characteristic clinical features. It is important to recognize, however, that not all amylase elevations are due to pancreatitis; amylase determinations, as routinely performed in most clinical laboratories, detect the total serum amylase, which actually represents a combination of both pancreatic and extrapancreatic (mostly salivary) amylase. Since patients with pancreatitis may have an elevated pancreatic amylase but a normal total amylase, simultaneous determination of both the serum amylase and lipase activities may improve the diagnostic yield in patients suspected of having acute pancreatitis [23].

C. **Initial studies** should include a complete blood count, serum electrolytes, creatinine, blood urea nitrogen (BUN), calcium, magnesium, SGOT, LDH, bilirubin, glucose, cholesterol, triglycerides, and arterial blood gases (except in very mild cases). Most patients admitted with acute pancreatitis should have a chest x-ray and upright and supine radiographs of the abdomen; these studies are necessary to assess for the presence of a perforated viscus, a pleural effusion, or a pulmonary infiltrate. Ultrasonography or CT scanning to evaluate for biliary tract disease or other pathology should be performed, especially in patients with (1) persistent fever or persistent symptoms (e.g., pain, nausea, or vomiting), (2) no history of alcohol usage, (3) a palpable abdominal mass, or (4) progressive clinical deterioration.

D. **The differential diagnosis** should consider peptic ulcer disease, perforated viscus, acute cholecystitis, myocardial infarction, mesenteric infarction, and intestinal obstruction.

E. **Complications** of acute pancreatitis vary in severity from a mild ileus to septic shock with the adult respiratory distress syndrome. Common complications include the following.

1. **Pseudocysts** are a fairly common complication and often resolve spontaneously. Patients with persistent symptoms of pain, nausea, or vomiting should be suspected of having a pseudocyst. The diagnosis can be confirmed by ultrasonography or CT scanning.

2. **A pancreatic abscess** occurs in about 5% of cases of acute pancreatitis. Patients usually have persistent pain, fever (> 101°C), a tender abdominal mass, leukocytosis, and an elevated left hemidiaphragm. The diagnosis can often be made on a CT scan or ultrasound study. Definitive treatment usually requires surgical drainage.

3. **Pancreatic ascites** develops as a result of either disruption of the pancreatic duct or pseudocyst rupture. The diagnosis is made when ascites fluid contains a markedly elevated amylase.

4. **Gastrointestinal bleeding** occurs frequently in patients with severe pancreatitis. Bleeding episodes are usually minor (with occult blood in the stools), but massive hemorrhage can occur when the inflamed pancreas erodes into either the stomach, duodenum, colon, or a major blood vessel. Bleeding into either the peritoneal cavity or the retroperitoneum can also occur. All patients with acute pancreatitis and occult blood present in the stools should receive either intravenous cimetidine or antacids by nasogastric tube to maintain the gastric pH greater than 4.0 (to prevent development of stress ulcers).

5. **Hyperglycemia** may require insulin therapy.
6. **Hypocalcemia** is common, and tetany may occur. Replacement with intravenous calcium is recommended. Magnesium deficiency, if present, should also be corrected.
7. **Respiratory insufficiency** is a major problem in severe pancreatitis. Pulmonary edema (with or without an elevated pulmonary capillary wedge pressure), atelectasis, pneumonia, and pleural effusions are the major causes of respiratory complications in these patients. Close patient observation, careful attention to fluid balance, and appropriate specific therapy may reduce the mortality from these complications.
F. **Prognosis.** Features present on admission that have been associated with an increased morbidity and mortality are age over 55 years, WBC count above 16,000/mm^3, SGOT greater than 250 units, and glucose greater than 200 mg/dl [38]. Any of the following features developing after 48 hours in the hospital may also be associated with an increased morbidity and mortality: a BUN rise greater than 5 mg/dl, serum calcium less than 8 mg/dl, PO$_2$ below 60 mm Hg, and third spacing more than 6000 ml [38].
G. **Management.** Virtually all patients with acute pancreatitis should be hospitalized.
   1. **Fluid replacement.** Most patients have some degree of intravascular volume depletion during the early stages of the disease. Isotonic salt solutions with or without dextrose should be infused to maintain the blood pressure and urinary output. Careful monitoring of input and output is essential. If questions arise about the patient's fluid status, a central venous or a Swan-Ganz catheter should be inserted.
   2. **Nutrition.** Patients should be maintained NPO until the abdominal pain abates. A nasogastric tube to decompress the stomach should be inserted in all patients with nausea, vomiting, severe abdominal pain, or a distended abdomen. Once abdominal pain has resolved, a clear liquid diet can be initiated. The diet can then be advanced as tolerated, but if abdominal pain recurs, the patient should be made NPO. In most cases, symptoms last no longer than 5–10 days. If patients are severely malnourished or do not respond to medical management within 7–10 days, total parenteral nutrition may be necessary.
   3. **Analgesia.** Pain severe enough to require opioids is usually present. Meperidine remains the preferred drug; it should be administered in appropriate dosages (e.g., 75–100 mg) q3–6h, to provide adequate pain relief.
   4. **Drug therapy.** A variety of agents (e.g., anticholinergics, aprotinin, glucagon, somatostatin, cimetidine) have been tried in acute pancreatitis in the hope that by either inactivating pancreatic enzymes or reducing gland secretion they would reduce the severity of an attack. Unfortunately, none of these agents clearly has been shown to be of any benefit.
   5. **Antibiotics** should not be administered routinely. However, patients who appear toxic or develop fever after being afebrile should be started on broad-spectrum antibiotics once appropriate cultures have been obtained.
II. **Chronic pancreatitis**
A. **Clinical features.** Abdominal pain is the dominant clinical feature with this disease, and the pain may be either constant or intermittent. The pain typically involves the upper abdomen, is precipitated by meals, and radiates to the back. Weight loss and diarrhea are frequent, and patients with destruction of greater than 90% of the pancreas may develop diabetes mellitus or steatorrhea. Pancreatic calcifications occur in approximately 30% of cases and are most often seen in association with alcohol-related chronic pancreatitis.
B. **Treatment.** Pain is the primary reason that patients seek medical attention, and many of these patients become addicted to narcotics. It is of the utmost importance that these patients be followed by a single physician, who controls the administration of all narcotic analgesics. Malnutrition is also a major problem; therefore, vitamins and dietary supplements are frequently required. Diarrhea and steatorrhea can usually be controlled with adequate dosages of pancreatic enzyme replacements. Absolute abstinence from alcohol is mandatory.

Diarrhea

I. **Definition and classification.** Diarrhea generally is defined as a stool weight in excess of 200 gm/day, associated with an increase in the liquidity of stool. Patients with acute diarrhea (i.e., <3 weeks' duration) should be distinguished from those with chronic

Table 10-4. Causes of acute and chronic diarrhea

Acute diarrhea	Chronic diarrhea
Viral, bacterial, or parasitic infections	Irritable bowel syndrome
Food poisoning	Inflammatory bowel disease
Drugs	Bacterial or parasitic infection
Food additives	Carbohydrate malabsorption
Fecal impaction	Pancreatic insufficiency
Inflammatory bowel disease	Bacterial overgrowth
	Drugs
	Food additives
	Gluten enteropathy
	Bile acid malabsorption
	Surreptitious laxative abuse
	Neuroendocrine tumors (carcinoid, medullary carcinoma of the thyroid, gastrinoma)

diarrhea (>3 weeks), since this can be helpful in determining the etiology (Table 10-4) [33]. Infectious etiologies are responsible for most cases of acute diarrhea.

II. **Pathophysiology.** It is useful to consider the underlying pathophysiology when evaluating patients with a diarrheal illness. Familiarity with the mechanisms involved will aid the physician in directing the patient workup in a logical, cost-effective manner. One of four possible mechanisms can be implicated in most cases of diarrheal illness.

   A. Ion secretion induced by humoral agents (vasoactive intestinal peptide), enterotoxins (*Escherichia coli, Vibrio cholerae*), bile acids, or neoplasm (villous adenoma).

   B. Reduced absorption due to mucosal disease (infectious agents, gluten enteropathy), pancreatic disease (chronic pancreatitis with pancreatic insufficiency), or previous surgery (gastroenterostomy, jejunoileal bypass).

   C. Increased luminal osmolality due to laxatives, maldigestion, or malabsorption.

   D. Altered motility (irritable bowel syndrome).

III. **Evaluation**

   A. **History.** All patients with diarrhea should be questioned about possible exposure to an infectious agent; specifically, a travel history, household or sexual exposure to an individual with diarrhea, or a history of homosexuality [2,17] should be sought. In addition, the character of the stools and the clinical features of the diarrheal illness often provide clues about the etiology. Large-volume, bulky stools imply malabsorption or maldigestion, usually seen with diseases involving the small bowel or pancreas. Rectal urgency with the passage of small-volume stools associated with red blood or mucus indicates an abnormality of the distal colon or rectum. Diarrhea that persists during a 24–36 hour fast and is large in volume (i.e., >2 liters/day) indicates a secretory type of diarrhea. Diarrhea that abates with fasting suggests an osmotic diarrhea, while diarrhea that diminishes with fasting (but does not stop completely) may be due to reduced absorption.

   B. **The physical examination** is often unremarkable or reveals findings that are nonspecific. Evaluation for abdominal tenderness and dehydration is necessary. Patients with a secretory-type diarrhea may present dehydrated, while individuals with malabsorption often appear chronically ill or cachectic.

   C. **Laboratory evaluation** should include routine electrolytes, a complete blood count, total protein, albumin, cholesterol, calcium, and prothrombin time (PT). Patients with chronic malabsorption frequently exhibit a depressed albumin and cholesterol along with a prolonged PT.

IV. **Acute diarrhea (<3 weeks' duration)**

   A. **Evaluation.** Since most cases are self-limited, the majority of patients do not require an extensive evaluation. A minimum workup should include proctosigmoidoscopy and examination of a stool specimen for fecal leukocytes. Stool specimens should be sent for culture whenever individuals present with bloody diarrhea, fever, and persistent diarrhea [24].

   B. **Management.** No specific therapy is necessary in the majority of cases because the illness usually is short-lived. Patients with an acute diarrheal illness who are other-

Table 10-5. Antidiarrheal and anticholinergic medications

Medication	Dosage*
Anticholinergics	
Tincture of belladonna	5–15 drops PO before meals or q4h
Dicyclomine (Bentyl)	10–20 mg PO tid–qid
Hyoscyamine (Levsin)	0.125–0.25 mg PO or SL tid–qid
Clindinium bromide and chlordiazepoxide (Librax)	1–2 capsules PO tid–qid
Belladonna alkaloids and phenobarbital (Donnatal)	1–2 tablets PO tid–qid
Antidiarrheals	
Codeine	15–30 mg PO tid–qid
Tincture of opium	5–15 drops PO tid–qid
Diphenoxylate (Lomotil)	1–2 tablets (2.5–5.0 mg) PO tid–qid
Loperamide (Imodium)	1–2 capsules (2–4 mg) PO bid–qid

*For patients with postprandial symptoms of diarrhea or abdominal pain, medication is best given 20–30 minutes before meals. For nocturnal symptoms, medication can be administered at bedtime.

wise healthy should be instructed to follow a predominantly clear-liquid diet (consisting mostly of fruit juice, broth, soft drinks, jello, and salted crackers) until symptoms resolve [15]. Oral rehydration solutions, such as Gatorade or Pedialyte, also can be used. Beverages containing caffeine should be avoided, as they may exacerbate diarrhea. Transition to solid food should proceed gradually, beginning with cookies and toast. Milk and foods with a high fat content should be avoided until the patient feels completely back to normal. Antidiarrheal and anticholinergic agents (Table 10-5) are best reserved for patients with severe symptoms; bismuth subsalicylate (Pepto-Bismol) may be helpful in individuals with mild to moderate symptoms. Antibiotics may be useful in selected situations (see sec. **IV.C.1**). Patients who are severely dehydrated, toxic appearing, or at the extremes of age may need hospital admission and intravenous hydration.

C. Specific entities

   1. Infectious diarrhea

      a. Viral gastroenteritis. A variety of different viral agents are associated with diarrhea. In adults, the Norwalk virus is the pathogen most often isolated in outbreaks of gastroenteritis [4]. The major features of viral gastroenteritis are vomiting and diarrhea, while myalgias, malaise, a low-grade fever, and anorexia also are common. The duration of symptoms tends to be short (i.e., 1–7 days). The diagnosis is made clinically, as no simple diagnostic tests are yet available. **Management** is supportive, with oral rehydration being the mainstay of therapy; antiemetics and antidiarrheals sometimes are helpful in severe cases. Rarely, patients who are severely dehydrated or unable to tolerate oral fluids require hospital admission and intravenous hydration.

      b. *Campylobacter fetus* is now one of the most commonly isolated enteric pathogens in hospital laboratories [5]. The organism most often causes an enteritis, but involvement of the colon also occurs. Symptoms usually begin acutely with periumbilical pain, fever, and a large-volume diarrhea. Patients with colonic involvement (i.e., colitis) may present with bloody diarrhea. The diagnosis rests on finding the organism on stool culture, and most microbiology laboratories now routinely culture for this agent. *Campylobacter* enteritis usually is self-limited, and antimicrobial therapy is not always needed. In severe or protracted cases, erythromycin, 250–500 mg PO qid for 7 days, appears effective.

      c. *Salmonella*. Most cases of *Salmonella* gastroenteritis are related to the ingestion of contaminated food, with symptoms beginning 8–48 hours after ingestion of the organisms [37]. Venereal transmission also has been reported. Nausea, vomiting, midabdominal cramping, and a large-volume diarrhea are the predominant symptoms; fever and bloody diarrhea are variably present. The organism typically invades the mucosa of the small intestine, resulting in an enteritis; however, a colitis can occur as well. The diagnosis requires isolation of the organism from stool or blood. **Treatment** is supportive, as most often the illness is self-limited. Antibiotics are indicated in patients with severe disease and those at risk for complications of bacteremia (i.e., neonates, the elderly, immunocompromised hosts, and patients with bone or vascular prostheses). Ampicillin, 4–8 gm/day in divided doses IV or PO for 10–14 days, or trimethoprim-sulfamethoxazole, 320–640 mg/day of trimethoprim in divided doses IV or PO for 14 days, is a reasonable antibiotic selection. Antidiarrheals should not be used routinely, as they may prolong the illness.

d. **Shigella** infections occur 36–72 hours following the ingestion of contaminated food or water. Venereal transmission also occurs. Initial symptoms include fever, periumbilical pain, and diarrhea. Later, patients may develop the full-blown syndrome of bacterial dysentery (shigellosis), which is characterized by bloody diarrhea mixed with mucus or pus, tenesmus, and rectal urgency. Early in the infection, symptoms may be due to the effects of an enterotoxin on the small bowel (enteritis); however, the dysentery syndrome is caused by bacterial invasion of the colonic mucosa. The diagnosis requires isolation of the organism from the stool. **Treatment** consists primarily of rehydration, with antibiotic therapy limited to those with severe infections. Depending on local patterns of resistance, either ampicillin, 2–4 gm/day IV or PO for 5 days; tetracycline, 2.5 gm PO as a single dose; or trimethoprim-sulfamethoxazole, 320 mg/day of trimethoprim PO for 5 days, is effective. Antidiarrheal agents may prolong the illness and should be avoided.

e. **Escherichia coli.** Infection with diarrheagenic types of *E. coli* occurs after the ingestion of contaminated food or water. This organism is responsible for most cases of traveler's diarrhea, a frequent cause of diarrhea in people visiting Africa and South and Central America [17]. At least two different types of infection can occur. The enterotoxigenic syndrome is characterized by the ingestion of an *E. coli*–associated enterotoxin that causes abdominal cramps and a secretory-type watery diarrhea; the symptoms usually last about 1 week. The syndrome caused by enteroinvasive *E. coli* is virtually identical to shigellosis (see sec. **IV.C.1.d**). The diagnosis of *E. coli* infection is made clinically on the basis of a compatible history and the absence of other detectable pathogens. The illness is almost always self-limited, and oral rehydration is the primary form of therapy. Bismuth subsalicylate, 30 ml every 30 minutes for 8 doses, may be effective in reducing the number of stools and relieving the symptoms of nausea and abdominal cramping [14]. Severe cases occurring in debilitated hosts may require antidiarrheal agents or antibiotics to reduce the severity and frequency of the diarrhea.

f. **Vibrio cholera.** Cholera is an acute diarrheal illness that begins several days after the ingestion of food or water contaminated with the organism. The illness begins acutely with the onset of severe watery diarrhea and sometimes vomiting. Fluid loss can be massive, leading to rapid dehydration and death if untreated. The diagnosis is usually made on clinical grounds, but finding the organism in the stool provides confirmation. **Treatment** consists of fluid replacement with either intravenous or oral fluids. Oral rehydration solutions are less expensive and utilize the fact that intestinal glucose-facilitated absorption of sodium and water is intact. Antimicrobial therapy shortens the duration of diarrhea and should be administered. Tetracycline, 3–4 gm/day PO in divided doses for 2 days, is usually given, while chloramphenicol remains an effective alternative. Household contacts should receive tetracycline, 1.0 gm/day PO in divided doses for 5 days.

g. **Yersinia enterocolitica.** Infection usually occurs in the pediatric population following ingestion of contaminated food or water. Most children present with abdominal pain (often localized to the right lower quadrant), diarrhea, and fever. Bloody diarrhea and vomiting can also occur. In many children, the disease mimics acute appendicitis. The diagnosis requires isolation of the organism from the stool. The disease is self-limited, and antibiotic therapy has not been shown to be of benefit.

h. **Clostridium difficile.** Antibiotic-associated (pseudomembranous) colitis occurs most often in patients recently treated with antibiotics [3]. Virtually all antibiotics have been implicated in the disease, but most cases follow treatment with ampicillin, clindamycin, and the cephalosporins. Primary symptoms include abdominal pain, fever, and watery stools (sometimes mixed with blood or mucus). A fulminant form of the disease resembling toxic megacolon can also occur. The diagnosis is made when either the characteristic pesudomembranes are seen on proctosigmoidoscopy, the *C. difficile* cytopathic toxin is isolated from the stool, or *C. difficile* is present in the stool cultures. In many patients, the illness is self-limited; however, severely ill patients or those with persistent symptoms should be treated with vancomycin, 125 mg PO qid. Relapse frequently occurs following successful therapy.

i. *Giardia lamblia* infection occurs following the ingestion of contaminated water or by venereal transmission (the major route of infection in homosexual males). Infections are common in hypogammaglobulinemic patients and male homosexuals [47]. The severity of symptoms varies; but in symptomatic patients, abdominal cramps, bloating, flatulence, and watery diarrhea occur less frequently. Identifying trophozoites or cysts in the stool establishes the diagnosis, but they are often difficult to find, and small-bowel aspiration or biopsy frequently is needed to make the diagnosis. Quinacrine, 100 mg PO tid, or metronidazole, 250 mg PO tid, for 5 days eradicates the organism in most cases [30].

j. *Entamoeba histolytica* infection occurs following ingestion of substances contaminated by cysts. In male homosexuals, infection usually occurs through oral-anal sexual contact [18]. The severity of illness ranges from a completely asymptomatic carrier to a patient presenting with fulminant colitis [25]. Symptoms vary depending on the location of the disease in the bowel; most symptomatic individuals experience crampy abdominal pain and diarrhea mixed with blood or mucus. Patients with rectal involvement may have tenesmus and urgency. Finding cysts or trophozoites in the stool establishes the diagnosis. Serologic tests usually are positive with invasive disease and are helpful in distinguishing amebic colitis from inflammatory bowel disease. Iodoquinol, 650 mg PO tid for 20 days, is effective in eradicating disease within the bowel lumen (asymptomatic carriers). Metronidazole, 750 mg PO tid for 5–10 days, plus iodoquinol, 650 mg PO tid for 20 days, is recommended for invasive disease [30].

2. **Food poisoning.** In most cases of food poisoning, illness occurs due to a combination of improper handling and storage of foodstuffs following the introduction of organisms. Attack rates are high, but the illness tends to be of short duration. The diagnosis usually is made clinically, and the treatment consists primarily of rehydration; an occasional patient will require antiemetics.

a. *Staphylococcus aureus.* Staphylococcal food poisoning is the second most common cause of food poisoning in the United States (next to *Salmonella*). It is caused by the ingestion of a preformed enterotoxin present in contaminated food. The illness occurs 3–6 hours following ingestion of contaminated food [37], and often several individuals in the same group or family are afflicted. Foods with custard or cream usually are implicated in outbreaks. Vomiting, diarrhea, nausea, and abdominal cramping are the primary symptoms. The diagnosis is made clinically, and the illness abates within 24–48 hours. **Therapy** is supportive.

b. *Clostridium perfringens.* Symptoms of diarrhea and severe crampy abdominal pain occur 8–24 hours after ingesting contaminated food. The disease is caused by an enterotoxin produced when the organisms sporulate in the small intestine. Outbreaks usually involve meat or poultry that is cooked and then reheated to a temperature that does not kill the spore form of the organism. Symptoms usually abate after 24 hours, and therapy is limited to rehydration.

c. *Bacillus cereus* is responsible for two syndromes of food poisoning, a vomiting syndrome and a diarrhea syndrome. The diagnosis of each illness is established on clinical grounds. **Treatment** is supportive.

(1) **The vomiting syndrome** has a short incubation period (2–4 hours) and a brief duration (8–10 hours). Most cases are associated with the ingestion of reheated or fried rice.

(2) **The diarrhea syndrome** is characterized by watery diarrhea, abdominal cramps, and occasionally vomiting. This illness usually occurs 8–12 hours after eating contaminated food and persists for up to 36 hours. A variety of foodstuffs have been associated with disease transmission.

d. *Salmonella.* See sec. **IV.C.1.c.**

e. *Shigella.* See sec. **IV.C.1.d.**

V. Chronic diarrhea

A. Clinical features. Patients with chronic diarrhea associated with malabsorption usually have some degree of weight loss and, depending on the specific etiology, associated metabolic abnormalities or malnutrition. These people often have large-volume, greasy, malodorous stools that should decrease in frequency and volume during fasting. In patients with pancreatic insufficiency, there often is a history of alcohol abuse or diabetes mellitus, while individuals with inflammatory bowel disease often have a history of abdominal pain, fever, nightsweats, and diarrhea associated with blood and/or mucus in the stool. Diarrhea due to a gastrinoma (i.e., the Zollinger-Ellison syndrome) typically is associated with concurrent symptoms of peptic ulcer disease. In patients with irritable bowel syndrome, diarrhea may alternate with constipation and usually is not associated with weight loss.

B. Evaluation. The minimum evaluation should include a complete history and physical examination, proctosigmoidoscopy, and stool specimens for culture and cyst and trophozoite examination. Barium studies should never be performed prior to or in place of proctoscopy, and stool specimens must always be obtained before barium studies. **All patients with chronic diarrhea should have an infectious etiology excluded prior to undergoing a more extensive evaluation.** Patients with suspected malabsorption should have a 72-hour stool fat collection on a 100 gm/day fat intake. Other studies available for evaluating patients with chronic diarrhea include the D-xylose absorption test, a small-bowel biopsy, pancreatic function tests, and radiographic studies of the small bowel and colon.

C. Treatment is adjusted according to the underlying disease.

Inflammatory Bowel Disease

I. Ulcerative colitis

A. Clinical features. Patients with ulcerative colitis most often present with the insidious onset of crampy abdominal pain, rectal urgency, and bloody stools mixed with mucus. Fever, chills, malaise, anorexia, nightsweats, and tenesmus are variably present [8]. Extracolonic disease (e.g., arthritis, uveitis, pyoderma gangrenosum) occurs in 10–20% of cases. In the typical cases, symptoms are present for several weeks before the patient seeks medical attention. Once diagnosed, the disease tends to run a chronic course characterized by remissions and exacerbations; most patients are successfully managed as outpatients. Approximately 10–15% of patients present with a fulminant disease accompanied by fever, abdominal pain (with peritoneal signs), and toxemia. In patients with fulminant disease, sepsis, bowel perforation, and even death can occur if appropriate therapy is delayed.

B. Diagnosis. Ulcerative colitis should be suspected when a patient presents with persistent bloody diarrhea, and the characteristic changes of mucosal edema, erythema, friability, and ulceration are seen on proctosigmoidoscopy. Confirmation of the diagnosis requires exclusion of infectious etiologies. Pathologic features on rectal biopsy are not specific for ulcerative colitis, but they do provide supportive information. Colonoscopy and a barium enema are useful in determining the extent of colonic involvement; however, these tests should not be performed when the disease is very active.

C. Differential diagnosis. Major diseases to exclude are the infectious causes of colitis (e.g., *Shigella, Campylobacter, Salmonella,* gonococcal proctitis, amebiasis). Sometimes differentiating ulcerative colitis from Crohn's disease can be extremely difficult.

D. Management is designed to control symptoms [27].

1. Patients with primarily **mild crampy abdominal pain or diarrhea** can be adequately managed with anticholinergics or antidiarrheal agents (Table 10-5).

2. Patients with **mild to moderate disease** associated with bloody stools should be treated with sulfasalazine [42]. Treatment is started with 500 mg bid, and the dosage should be increased slowly in 500-mg increments every 3–5 days to a total dosage of 2–6 gm/day, administered qid. If nausea, anorexia, or dyspepsia occurs, the dosage can be reduced or an enteric-coated preparation (Azulfidine EN) can be substituted.

3. **Moderately severe disease** or ulcerative colitis not responding to sulfasalazine is managed with oral corticosteroids. Therapy with 40–60 mg/day of prednisone in divided doses usually will induce a remission.

4. **Localized disease** involving only the rectum or the left colon can be effectively

managed with either a hydrocortisone-containing foam preparation (e.g., Proctofoam-HC) bid–qid or a steroid retention enema (e.g., Cortenema) hs–bid.

   5. Patients with **severe disease** (see sec. **I.E**) and those unresponsive to outpatient medical therapy should be admitted to the hospital and placed NPO. Corticosteroids should be administered parenterally (hydrocortisone, 100 mg q6h or equivalent) along with intravenous fluids; total parenteral nutrition may also be of some benefit. Patients who appear toxic should be treated with broad-spectrum antibiotics after appropriate cultures have been obtained.

   6. Once a **remission** has been induced with any of the above regimens, maintenance therapy with sulfasalazine, 2 gm/day, appears effective in preventing relapse [27].

E. Complications. Most complications occur in the small group of patients with severe disease. Severe disease can occur with either the initial presentation or a disease relapse. These individuals present with severe bloody diarrhea, abdominal pain, fever, leukocytosis, dehydration, and/or sepsis. Some of these patients will develop **colonic dilatation, toxic megacolon,** and **colonic perforation.** All patients with evidence of severe disease should be admitted to the hospital and closely observed.

   1. **Initial evaluation** includes routine blood work, a type and cross-match, blood cultures (for febrile patients), and supine and upright abdominal radiographs to exclude perforation and evaluate the degree of colonic dilatation.

   2. **Initial management** consists of the following:

      a. Making the patient **NPO,** and passing a nasogastric tube.

      b. **Intravenous hydration** and correction of any identifiable electrolyte disturbances.

      c. Administration of broad-spectrum **antibiotics** and parenteral **steroids.**

      d. Absolute **avoidance of antimotility drugs** (i.e., narcotics or anticholinergics), as these may precipitate toxic megacolon.

      e. Early **surgical consultation** in the event that a colectomy is needed.

II. Crohn's disease is a chronic illness that can involve any area of the gastrointestinal tract, with the colon and terminal ileum being involved most often. The disease is characterized by transmural inflammation of the bowel wall leading to ulceration, abscess formation, fistulae, and strictures. Crohn's disease involving only the colon may be impossible to distinguish from ulcerative colitis; however, focal areas of involvement with normal intervening segments (skip areas) and disease involving the perianal region are more typical of Crohn's disease.

A. Clinical features. Most patients present with an insidious history of weight loss, anorexia, malaise, abdominal pain, and diarrhea (with or without blood and mucus). Some individuals present with fever, perianal lesions, an abdominal mass, or extraintestinal disease (e.g., arthritis, uveitis) [8].

B. The **diagnosis** is based on the constellation of radiographic and endoscopic findings, once an infectious etiology has been excluded. Histologic sections from bowel biopsies revealing granulomas confirm the diagnosis, but they are frequently absent.

C. Treatment

   1. Patients whose primary symptoms are **diarrhea or crampy abdominal pain** can be managed with anticholinergic or antidiarrheal agents (see Table 10-5), as long as they are not acutely ill.

   2. Patients with disease of **mild to moderate severity** are managed with oral corticosteroids (e.g., 20–60 mg/day of prednisone). Sulfasalazine is less effective for Crohn's disease than it is for ulcerative colitis [28,42].

   3. **Severely ill or toxic-appearing patients** experiencing either a disease flare-up or an apparent complication (see sec. **II.D**) should be admitted to the hospital for further evaluation and observation. Emergency management of the toxic patient with Crohn's disease is similar to that outlined for patients with severe ulcerative colitis (see sec. **I.E**).

D. Complications

   1. **Obstruction.** Patients with involvement of the small bowel (usually the distal ileum) can develop luminal narrowing with signs and symptoms of a small-bowel obstruction. Mild episodes (e.g., partial obstruction, food bolus obstruction) can be managed on an outpatient basis with the institution of either a liquid or a low-residue diet. Persistent symptoms or radiographic findings suggestive of a high-grade obstruction necessitate hospital admission. **Initial treatment** includes the following:

      a. Making the patient **NPO,** and instituting nasogastric suction.

b. **Intravenous hydration** and correction of electrolyte abnormalities.

c. Administration of parenteral steroids (usually the equivalent of 40–100 mg/day of prednisone in divided doses.

d. Administration of **broad-spectrum antibiotics** in patients who appear toxic (after obtaining appropriate cultures).

e. Total parenteral nutrition in patients who are severely malnourished or debilitated.

f. Early **surgical consultation.** Patients with a solitary stenotic segment and recurrent episodes of obstruction usually are good candidates for surgical resection. Patients with several stenotic segments or a history of multiple previous surgical procedures are best managed with medical therapy.

2. **Fistulae.** Fistulous tracts may develop between involved loops of bowel and areas of uninvolved bowel, the mesentery, skin, ureters, bladder, or vagina. Most patients require surgical resection, but occasional cases respond to medical therapy in conjunction with total parenteral nutrition.

3. **Abscess.** Patients presenting with pain, fever, and an abdominal mass should be suspected of having an abscess; however, distinguishing an abscess from a disease recurrence can be difficult. Individuals suspected of having an abscess should be admitted to the hospital and managed as outlined for patients with obstruction (see sec. **II.D.1**); in particular, treatment with broad-spectrum antibiotics is essential.

4. **Perforation.** Free intraabdominal perforation occurs infrequently with Crohn's disease. Any patient with Crohn's disease who develops the acute onset of abdominal pain or abdominal distention should be suspected of having a perforation. An upright or left lateral decubitus radiograph of the abdomen to evaluate for free intraperitoneal air is mandatory. Patients suspected of having a perforation should be admitted to the hospital, even if the x-rays are negative. These patients are managed as outlined for obstruction (see sec. **II.D.1**). Broad-spectrum antibiotics and early surgical consultation are essential.

5. **Bleeding.** Most episodes of bleeding due to Crohn's disease are self-limited and not severe. Moderate bleeding frequently abates with an increase in steroid dosage to 40–60 mg/day of prednisone. Since gastrointestinal bleeding in these patients is not always due to Crohn's disease, evaluation should proceed as outlined in the section **Gastrointestinal Bleeding.**

Constipation and Fecal Impaction

I. **Constipation** implies a reduction in stool frequency, and in general, passage of fewer than three stools per week is considered abnormal. Patients with constipation may also complain of hard stools or difficulty in expelling stools (straining). Most patients with chronic constipation have a history of chronic laxative usage. While the majority of cases are idiopathic, it is important to recognize that a variety of disorders may present with constipation as an early manifestation (Table 10-6).

A. **Evaluation.** The minimum evaluation includes a thorough history, a rectal examination (including stool for occult blood), and proctosigmoidoscopy. Patients with the recent onset of constipation, blood in the stool, or signs and symptoms suggestive of an associated disorder require further evaluation (e.g., a barium enema or colonoscopy).

B. **Treatment.** Increasing the amount of dietary fiber will help some patients, but since most patients fail to increase consumption of foods with a high fiber content (e.g., fruits, vegetables, bran), a fiber supplement like psyllium (Metamucil) is recommended. Patients should be instructed to take this supplement daily in a dosage of 1 heaping teaspoon–tablespoon bid–tid whether or not they feel constipated. Laxatives and enemas should be stopped or tapered, and patients should be informed that it is perfectly normal not to have a bowel movement every day. Some individuals continue to require laxatives, but they should be encouraged to use them infrequently (i.e., once a week or less, if possible).

II. **Fecal impaction**

A. **Clinical features.** Fecal impaction usually occurs in elderly or bedridden individuals. These patients frequently have multiple medical problems and are often receiving a variety of medications, some of which may be constipating (see Table 10-6). When patients develop an impaction, they may complain of either constipation or diarrhea (i.e., liquid stool passing around the impaction). They can develop abdominal distention, pain, and findings that can mimic a bowel obstruction.

Table 10-6. Conditions associated with constipation

Drugs	Spinal cord injury
Anticholinergics	Hirschsprung's disease
Antacids (calcium and aluminum	Multiple sclerosis
compounds)	Parkinson's disease
Antidepressants	Cerebrovascular accident
Barium sulfate	Colorectal disorders
Iron	Tumor
Opioids	Stricture
Metabolic disorders	Rectal prolapse
Diabetes mellitus	Rectocele
Hypothyroidism	Hernia
Panhypopituitarism	Thrombosed hemorrhoid
Hypokalemia	Anal fissure
Hypercalcemia	Miscellaneous
Neuromuscular disorders	Irritable bowel syndrome
Dermatomyositis	Pregnancy
Scleroderma	Psychogenic constipation

B. Evaluation. Patients who have not had a bowel movement in several days and who do not appear to be responding to gentle laxatives should undergo a rectal examination to check for an impaction. If no stool is present in the rectum, but an impaction is suspected, a plain film of the abdomen should be obtained to exclude a bowel obstruction.

C. Treatment. Several hypertonic or oil retention enemas usually are effective in dislodging the impaction and evacuating the distal colon. Manual disimpaction can be extremely uncomfortable for the patient and is not recommended. An oral laxative should be administered once the impaction has been dislodged to empty the remainder of the colon.

Gastrointestinal Foreign Bodies

The esophagus is the most frequent site of acute foreign body obstruction. Once objects have traversed the esophagus, most will pass through the entire gastrointestinal tract; occasionally, objects get stuck at either the pylorus or the ileocecal valve. The major complication associated with foreign body ingestion is perforation, and the risk of perforation is increased when sharp objects (e.g., needles, razors, scissors) are ingested.

I. **Esophagus.** Acute foreign body obstruction in the esophagus can occur in either the normal esophagus or above a partially obstructing lesion (e.g., a stricture or ring).

  A. Clinical features. Patients usually complain of the acute onset of odynophagia, chest pain, choking, or regurgitation. Symptoms typically occur during or shortly after a meal.

  B. Diagnosis. Soft-tissue films of the neck or a barium swallow (barium-soaked cotton pledgets are useful for demonstrating a partial esophageal obstruction) can be used to establish the diagnosis.

  C. Management. Sharp objects (e.g., needles, bones, toothpicks) are associated with a significant risk of perforation and should be extracted endoscopically, if possible. Patients with a large food bolus obstruction may respond to medical therapy with glucagon, 1.0 mg IV, or diazepam, 2.0–10.0 mg IV. Some authors recommend papain (meat tenderizer) for meat impactions; however, this is rarely helpful and can lead to severe complications if the papain is aspirated or if a perforation occurs.

II. **Stomach and small intestine**

  A. The diagnosis is usually made on the basis of the patient's history; however, children and patients with a psychiatric illness may be unable to supply reliable historical information. Plain radiographs of the chest and abdomen will reveal ingested radiopaque objects. Barium studies are indicated to demonstrate objects not visualized on plain films.

  B. Management depends on both the nature of the foreign body and its location in the alimentary tract.

    1. Since **sharp objects** run the risk of perforating the bowel, an attempt should be made to remove these objects endoscopically while they are still in the upper

gastrointestinal tract. If extraction is unsuccessful or not possible due to passage of the foreign body distally, the patient should be hospitalized and observed closely for signs of perforation. The course of the foreign body should be monitored, as necessary, with periodic radiographs. If pain or fever develops, radiographic studies using water-soluble contrast may be obtained to document the site of perforation prior to surgery.

2. **Since blunt objects** generally pass without difficulty, patients ingesting a blunt object can be managed conservatively as outpatients while the object passes through the gastrointestinal tract. Periodic radiographs should be obtained to monitor the progress of the foreign body. For objects remaining in the stomach or duodenum for more than 2–3 days, endoscopic extraction should be attempted.

Bibliography

1. Athanasoulis, C. A., et al. Angiography: Its contribution to the emergency management of gastrointestinal hemorrhage. *Radiol. Clin. North Am.* 14:265, 1976.
2. Baker, R. W., and Peppercorn, M. A. Gastrointestinal ailments of homosexual men. *Medicine* 61:390, 1982.
3. Bartlett, J. G. Antibiotic-associated pseudomembranous colitis. *Hosp. Pract.* 16:85, 1981.
4. Blacklow, N. R., and Cukor, G. Viral gastroenteritis. *N. Engl. J. Med.* 304:397, 1981.
5. Blaser, M. J., et al. Campylobacter enteritis in the United States: A multicenter study. *Ann. Intern. Med.* 98:360, 1983.
6. Chojkier, M., et al. A controlled comparison of continuous intraarterial and intravenous infusions of vasopressin in hemorrhage from esophageal varices. *Gastroenterology* 77:540, 1979.
7. Cohen, S. Motor disorders of the esophagus. *N. Engl. J. Med.* 301:184, 1979.
8. Farmer, R. G. Clinical features and natural history of inflammatory bowel disease. *Med. Clin. North Am.* 64:1103, 1980.
9. Favero, M. S., et al. Guidelines for the care of patients hospitalized with viral hepatitis. *Ann. Intern. Med.* 91:872, 1979.
10. Fleischer, D. Etiology and prevalence of severe persistent upper gastrointestinal bleeding. *Gastroenterology* 84:538, 1983.
11. Fogel, M. R., et al. Continuous intravenous vasopressin in active upper gastrointestinal bleeding. *Ann. Intern. Med.* 96:565, 1982.
12. Freston, J. W. Cimetidine: I. Developments, pharmacology, and efficacy. *Ann. Intern. Med.* 97:573, 1982.
13. Galambos, J. T. Esophageal variceal hemorrhage: Diagnosis and an overview of treatment. *Semin. Liver Dis.* 2:211, 1982.
14. Garcia-Tsao, G., et al. The diagnosis of bacterial peritonitis: Comparison of pH, lactate concentration and leukocyte count. *Hepatology* 5:91, 1985.
15. Gertler, S., et al. Management of acute diarrhea. *J. Clin. Gastroenterol.* 5:523, 1983.
16. Gilbert, D. A., and Saunders, D. R. Iced saline lavage does not slow bleeding from experimental canine gastric ulcers. *Dig. Dis. Sci.* 26:1065, 1981.
17. Gorbach, S. L., et al. Traveler's diarrhea and toxigenic *Escherichia coli. N. Engl. J. Med.* 292:933, 1975.
18. Heller, M. The gay bowel syndrome: Common problem of homosexual patients in the emergency department. *Ann. Emerg. Med.* 9:487, 1980.
19. Hoyumpa, A. M., et al. Hepatic encephalopathy. *Gastroenterology* 76:184, 1979.
20. Hoyumpa, A. M., and Schenker, S. Perspectives in hepatic encephalopathy. *J. Lab. Clin. Med.* 100:477, 1982.
21. Immunization Practices Advisory Committee of the Centers for Disease Control. Recommendations for protection against viral hepatitis. *Morbid. Mortal. Weekly Rep.* 34:313, 1985.
22. Isenberg, J. I., et al. Healing of benign gastric ulcer with low-dose antacid or cimetidine: A double-blind, randomized, placebo-controlled trial. *N. Engl. J. Med.* 308:1319, 1983.
23. Kolars, J. C., Ellis, C. J., and Levitt, M. D. Comparison of serum amylase pancreatic isoamylase and lipase in patients with hyperamylasemia. *Dig. Dis. Sci.* 29:289, 1984.
24. Koplan, J. P., et al. Value of stool cultures. *Lancet* 2:413, 1980.
25. Krogstad, D. J., et al. Current concepts in parasitology: Amebiasis. *N. Engl. J. Med.* 298:262, 1978.
26. Larson, D. E., and Farnell, M. B. Upper gastrointestinal hemorrhage. *Mayo Clin. Proc.* 58:371, 1983.

27. Lennard-Jones, J. E., and Powell-Tuck, J. Drug treatment of inflammatory bowel disease. *Clin. Gastroenterol.* 8:187, 1979.
28. Linas, S. L., et al. The Rational Use of Diuretics in Cirrhosis. In M. Epstein (ed.), *The Kidney and Liver Disease* (2nd ed.). New York: Elsevier, 1983. Pp. 555–567.
29. Markisz, J. A., et al. An evaluation of ^{99m}Tc-labeled red blood cell scintigraphy for the detection and localization of gastrointestinal bleeding sites. *Gastroenterology* 83:394, 1982.
30. Medical Letter. Drugs for parasitic infections. *Med. Lett. Drugs Ther.* 26:27, 1984.
31. Michel, L., et al. Mallory-Weiss syndrome: Evolution of diagnostic and therapeutic patterns over two decades. *Ann. Surg.* 192:716, 1980.
32. Nebel, O. T., et al. Symptomatic gastroesophageal reflux: Incidence and precipitating factors. *Dig. Dis. Sci.* 21:953, 1976.
33. Netchvolodoff, C. V., and Hargrove, M. D. Recent advances in the treatment of diarrhea. *Arch. Intern. Med.* 139:813, 1979.
34. Perrillo, R. P. Differentiation between recent and remote hepatitis infections. *Intern. Med.* 5:123, 1984.
35. Perrillo, R. P., and Aach, R. A. Acute viral hepatitis: Current concepts and practical guidelines for the primary physician. *Pract. Gastroenterol.* 5:9, 1981.
36. Peterson, W. L., et al. Routine early endoscopy in upper gastrointestinal tract bleeding: A randomized, controlled trial. *N. Engl. J. Med.* 304:925, 1981.
37. Plotkin, G. R., et al. Gastroenteritis: Etiology, pathophysiology, and clinical manifestations. *Medicine* 58:95, 1979.
38. Ransom, J. H. C., et al. Prognostic signs and nonoperative peritoneal lavage in acute pancreatitis. *Surg. Gynecol. Obstet.* 143:209, 1976.
39. Richter, J. E., and Castell, D. O. Gastroesophageal reflux: Pathogenesis, diagnosis, and therapy. *Ann. Intern. Med.* 97:93, 1982.
40. Sabesin, S., et al. Alcoholic hepatitis. *Gastroenterology* 74:276, 1978.
41. Seeff, L. B., and Koff, R. S. Passive and active immunoprophylaxis of hepatitis B. *Gastroenterology* 86:958, 1984.
42. Singleton, J. W. Medical therapy of inflammatory bowel disease. *Med. Clin. North Am.* 64:1117, 1980.
43. Steer, M. L., and Silen, W. Diagnostic procedures in gastrointestinal hemorrhage. *N. Engl. J. Med.* 309:646, 1983.
44. Theoni, R. F., and Cello, J. P. A critical look at the accuracy of endoscopy and double-contrast radiography of the upper gastrointestinal (UGI) tract in patients with substantial UGI hemorrhage. *Radiology* 135:305, 1980.
45. Toskes, P. P., and Greenberger, N. J. Acute and chronic pancreatitis. *D.M.* 5:5, 1983.
46. Tytgat, G. N. J., et al. Sucralfate, bismuth compounds, substituted benzimidazoles, trimipramine and pirenzepine in the short- and long-term treatment of duodenal ulcer. *Clin. Gastroenterol.* 13:543, 1984.
47. Wolfe, W. S. Current concepts in parasitology: Giardiasis. *N. Engl. J. Med.* 298:319, 1978.
48. Wong, P. Y., et al. The hepatorenal syndrome. *Gastroenterology* 77:1326, 1979.
49. Zimmerman, H. J. Drug-induced liver disease: An overview. *Semin. Liver Dis.* 1:93, 1981.
50. Zuckerman, G., et al. Controlled trial of medical therapy for active upper gastrointestinal bleeding and prevention of rebleeding. *Am. J. Med.* 76:361, 1984.

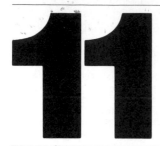

Hematologic and Oncologic Emergencies

Alan P. Lyss

Hematologic Emergencies

I. Red blood cell (RBC) disorders

A. Anemia is a condition of deficient RBC mass.

1. **General principles**

   a. **Classification**

   (1) **Physiologic classification.** Anemia may result from blood loss or under-production (e.g., secondary to toxic suppression, nutritional deficiency, or stem cell hypoproliferation) or increased destruction (hemolysis) of RBCs. A reticulocyte count and serum bilirubin level should be obtained to classify the basis for the anemia. Since approximately 1% of the RBC mass dies each day, the normal reticulocyte count of 1% represents the bone marrow's compensation for this loss. The reticulocyte percentage decreases or remains at 1% when there is underproduction of RBCs in spite of anemia; in contrast, the reticulocyte percentage increases when RBC loss increases through destruction or hemorrhage. Since 85% of the serum bilirubin is attributable to hemoglobin catabolism, an increased indirect bilirubin level in the absence of severe liver dysfunction implies augmented erythrocyte destruction.

   (2) **Morphologic classification.** A review of the peripheral blood smear is a mandatory part of the initial data base. Microcytic and hypochromic RBCs suggest chronic iron deficiency on hemoglobinopathy (thalassemia). The latter may also be suspected when target cells or bizarre erythrocyte forms (e.g., sickle cells) are observed. Macrocytic and hyperchromic RBCs are seen when nutritional deficiencies (e.g., folate or B_{12} deficiency) are responsible for the anemia. Normochromic and normocytic erythrocytes are seen in the anemia of chronic disease and acute blood loss. Dimorphic (mixed) populations of cells occur in sideroblastic anemias and disorders of marrow invasion by malignancy or infection; marrow invasion may also be suspected when a leukoerythroblastic smear is observed. Fragmented RBCs are seen in severe vascular disease (e.g., thrombotic thrombocytopenic purpura [TTP], disseminated intravascular coagulation [DIC], malignant hypertension) or in the presence of valvular prostheses. The differential diagnosis of all of these morphologic pictures is quite broad beyond the most common etiologies noted here.

   b. **Clinical effects.** In anemia, several changes occur to maintain normal tissue oxygenation.

   (1) **Mild anemia** (hemoglobin of 10–14 gm/dl). Symptoms are usually detected only on exercise and reflect the augmented cardiopulmonary burden to meet tissue oxygen requirements. Subjective complaints of dyspnea, diaphoresis, and palpitations may be accompanied by tachycardia and/or tachypnea. The clinical manifestations of mild anemia are more pronounced when the RBC deficiency develops acutely (i.e., over minutes to days).

   (2) **Moderate anemia** (hemoglobin of 7–10 gm/dl). Symptoms and signs are present with minimal exertion and may include generalized fatigue and pallor.

   (3) **Severe anemia** (hemoglobin of 3–7 gm/dl). Subjective complaints include insomnia, orthostatic dizziness, syncope, pounding headache, and anorexia. Signs of specific organ dysfunction (e.g., myocardial or peripheral ischemia) may be evident, especially in elderly patients.

c. **Management.** The therapy of anemia depends on the physiologic mechanism responsible for the erythrocyte deficiency.

   (1) **Underproduction of red blood cells.** The etiology is established by obtaining a blood level of the factor that is suspected to be deficient; however, if the blood test is unrevealing, bone marrow aspiration may be necessary. Treatment involves supplying the deficient factor in the case of iron-, folate- or vitamin B_{12}-deficiency.

   (2) Anemic patients with an **elevated reticulocyte count** require a detailed investigation of the etiology. In addition to a careful history, physical examination, and inspection of the peripheral blood smear, a Coombs' test (direct and indirect) is always part of the initial workup. More specific tests (e.g., cold agglutinin titer, glucose 6-phosphate dehydrogenase [G-6-PD] level, DIC screen) depend on the physician's index of suspicion. While many patients with brisk acute hemolysis or chronic hemolysis will require folic acid supplementation and discontinuation of potentially offending drugs, other interventions require a specific diagnosis. Transfusion may be dangerous in the patient with a positive Coombs' test and should not be performed without prompt consultation with an internist or hematologist.

   (3) **Transfusions.** Patients with evidence of organ ischemia (e.g., shock, angina pectoris, neurologic symptoms, dyspnea at rest, peripheral ischemia) must be transfused in lieu of establishing the diagnosis; however, blood should be drawn for specific tests prior to the transfusion. Patients with recurrent refractory anemia may also benefit from transfusions. Packed RBCs usually are administered over 3–4 hours unless the clinical situation demands more rapid correction of the anemia. **The use of whole blood should be restricted to urgent situations requiring concomitant repletion of clotting factors, RBCs, and volume** (e.g., traumatic blood loss, massive gastrointestinal hemorrhage). (For a more detailed discussion of blood component therapy of anemia, see sec. **IV.A.**)

d. **Disposition.** Patients with active, uncontrolled hemorrhage require admission for stabilization and transfusion. Any patient with moderate or severe anemia (see sec. **I.A.1.b**) may also benefit from hospitalization for diagnosis and initial treatment. Lesser degrees of anemia may be investigated in the outpatient setting after referral to a family physician, pediatrician, internist, or hematologist.

2. **Sickle cell anemia.** Sickle hemoglobin results from substitution of valine for glutamic acid in the sixth position of the beta chain of the globin molecule, resulting in cyclization of the beta chain and interdigitation with alpha chains. The net effect is a rigid structure that forms irreversibly sickled cells when the heme moiety is deoxygenated. This leads to small-vessel occlusion, stasis, and further deoxygenation. When the patient is heterozygous for hemoglobin S (10% of black Americans), symptoms occur under conditions of severe oxygen lack. Sickle cell anemia patients, on the other hand, are homozygous for hemoglobin S and are incapable of hemoglobin A production; they are severely affected.

   a. **Clinical effects**

      (1) Moderate to severe **hemolytic anemia** occurs and is manifest by a hemoglobin of 6–9 gm/dl, reticulocytosis of 15–30%, and hyperbilirubinemia. Autosplenectomy from splenic infarction leads to peripheral blood signs of hyposplenism (i.e., poikilocytosis, Howell-Jolly bodies, target cells, siderocytes, and basophilic stippling). These findings are superimposed on a smear showing polychromasia and variable percentages of irreversibly sickled cells.

      (2) **Organ damage** from infarction leads to skin ulceration, especially over the malleoli; renal damage resulting in a concentration defect, papillary necrosis, and chronic pyelonephritis; splenic infarction causing functional asplenia and splenic pain; bone infarction leading to painful crises and aseptic necrosis of the femoral head; central nervous system thromboses; pulmonary infarction; hepatitis and hepatic infarction; cardiac disease, including myocardial ischemia secondary to thrombosis and chronic high-output cardiac failure secondary to the anemia; and/or abortion due to infarction of the decidua.

      (3) **Crises. Painful crises** due to small-vessel occlusion are the most common. The pain is dramatic, diffuse, and migrating; it can mimic appen-

dicitis, cholecystitis, and pulmonary infarction. Other types of crises are **aplastic** (i.e., transient marrow aplasia usually induced by viral infection), **hyperhemolytic** (i.e., sudden RBC sequestration in a rapidly enlarging spleen in a child), and **dactylitic** (i.e., painful and swollen hands and feet in children).

(4) Infection. Patients with sickle cell disease are predisposed to infection because of vascular stasis and organ infarction, as well as impaired granulocyte function. Furthermore, adult sickle cell patients are functionally asplenic and are at risk for serious pneumococcal and meningococcal sepsis. In addition, periodic red cell transfusions expose patients to an increased risk of infectious hepatitis.

b. Treatment. There is no generally accepted way to prevent crises or organ damage safely and effectively. Partial exchange transfusions at 4- to 6-week intervals may prevent painful crises, fetal wastage during pregnancy, recurrent cerebrovascular events, and complications of surgery. However, exchange transfusions deliver a large iron load, leading to iron deposition and hemochromatosis; thus they carry substantial risks if not combined with a careful program of iron chelation. During painful crises, appropriate therapy consists of the following:

(1) Hydration with oral fluids or intravenous crystalloid solutions (e.g., 0.9% saline at a rate of 150–200 ml/hour) to decrease blood viscosity.

(2) Administration of supplemental oxygen.

(3) Administration of narcotic analgesics (e.g., meperidine, 1.0–1.5 mg/kg of body weight IM q2–4h).

(4) Correction of acid-base and electrolyte imbalances, especially acidosis.

(5) Administration of appropriate antibiotics for documented infections.

c. Disposition. Patients with painful crises require hospitalization if the above measures are unsuccessful within a specified time period (e.g., 6–12 hours) or if complications (e.g., infection, cerebrovascular accident) are suspected. In addition, patients with aplastic crises require hospitalization.

B. Polycythemia (erythrocytosis)

1. Definition and classification

a. Relative polycythemia occurs when the plasma volume is decreased and the erythrocyte mass is normal; an elevated hematocrit (exceeding 48% in females and 54% in males) results from dehydration or from unclear mechanisms in certain nervous, tense individuals.

b. Absolute polycythemia refers to a condition in which the erythrocyte mass is increased, as determined by chromium 51 (^{51}Cr) RBC labeling; it arises from increased RBC production and can be classified as secondary or primary.

(1) Secondary polycythemia. Many stimuli cause erythrocytosis without leukocytosis or thrombocytosis, including

(a) Arterial hypoxemia when the oxygen saturation is less than 92%.

(b) Certain abnormal hemoglobins that have a high affinity for oxygen.

(c) Certain drugs, such as cobalt and androgens.

(d) Particular neoplasms (e.g., renal carcinoma, cerebellar hemangioblastoma, and uterine fibromas) that produce an erythropoietin-like substance.

(e) Certain benign renal conditions (e.g., cysts, tuberculosis, hydronephrosis).

(2) Primary polycythemia (polycythemia rubra vera). Panmyelosis (increased production of all marrow elements) results in excess numbers of circulating leukocytes, platelets, and especially erythrocytes. The erythrocytosis causes hyperviscosity, leading to tissue hypoxia, thrombosis, and hemorrhage due to stasis. Prominent features are an elevated hematocrit and pruritus after bathing. Other complaints include headache, dizziness, dyspnea, fatigue, and generalized muscle aches. Physical examination discloses a ruddy complexion, splenomegaly in 75% of patients, and, less frequently, hepatomegaly. In uncontrolled disease, serious complications may arise, such as thrombosis (e.g., cerebrovascular accident, hepatic or portal venous thrombosis) or hemorrhage (e.g., gastrointestinal bleed).

2. Therapy

a. Relative polycythemia is treated with intravascular volume expansion.

    b. Treatment of **secondary polycythemia** is directed at the underlying cause, but phlebotomy may relieve symptoms of hyperviscosity in selected patients.

    c. Treatment of **primary polycythemia** is as follows.

        (1) Phlebotomy is the only therapeutic maneuver that has a role in the emergency treatment of absolute polycythemia. Phlebotomy of 1 unit of blood at monthly or bimonthly intervals relieves symptoms and reduces complications but will induce or aggravate iron deficiency and thrombocytosis.

        (2) Phosphorus 32 (^{32}P) and alkylating agent **chemotherapy** are helpful for patients who cannot be managed with phlebotomy alone because of worsening thrombocytosis or excessive phlebotomy requirements (i.e., greater than 1 unit/month).

  3. Disposition. All patients with polycythemia should be referred to a hematologist for definitive diagnosis and consideration of long-term management. Hospitalization is indicated for patients with signs or symptoms of thrombosis, hemorrhage, or tissue hypoxia (e.g., angina pectoris, alteration of consciousness).

II. Coagulation disorders. Bleeding may result from a local lesion (e.g., trauma) in a hemostatically normal patient or from dysfunction of the hemostatic system. Judicious use of the coagulation laboratory will enable the correct diagnosis to be made and the proper therapy to be instituted.

  A. Evaluation

    1. History and physical examination. In evaluating hemostatic function, the emergency department physician should determine the amount and duration of blood loss, whether there is a history of similar bleeding problems in the patient and family members, and whether there has been excessive blood loss after minor surgical procedures (e.g., tooth extraction, tonsillectomy). Objective measures of bleeding events should be emphasized (e.g., the need for further surgery, blood transfusion, or hospitalization as a result of bleeding). Furthermore, a careful history of drug ingestion should be obtained, with particular attention to the use of alcohol, aspirin-containing compounds, and oral anticoagulants. Certain physical findings tend to characterize particular hemostatic deficiencies: Petechiae are often associated with thrombocytopenia or thrombocytopathy; spontaneous hemarthroses and intramuscular hematomas occur in inherited clotting factor deficiencies; and excessive bleeding from venipuncture sites characterizes DIC.

    2. Laboratory studies. Screening tests of hemostatic function that should be obtained in the emergency department include the following.

      a. Platelet count (normal 140,000–350,000 mm^3) is a measure of platelet number.

      b. Prothrombin time (PT) (normal range established for each laboratory) is a measure of the "extrinsic" coagulation system.

      c. Partial thromboplastin time (PTT) (normal range established for each laboratory) is a measure of the "intrinsic" coagulation system.

      d. Bleeding time (normal approximately 3–8 minutes) is a measure of platelet function.

      e. Fibrinogen level (normal 100–300 mg/dl). Causes of an abnormally low fibrinogen level include DIC, hereditary dysfibrinogenemia, and hepatic failure.

      f. Fibrin degradation products (normal level established for each laboratory). Abnormal elevation occurs in DIC, primary fibrinolytic states, and hepatic failure.

  B. Platelet disorders

    1. Thrombocytopenia. When platelet count is low (i.e., less than 140,000 mm^3), it should be verified by inspecting the peripheral blood smear and repeating the platelet count. If the blood specimen has been inadequately anticoagulated, platelet clumps will form, resulting in artifactual thrombocytopenia. These patients lack the ecchymoses, petechiae, and history of bleeding that characterize true thrombocytopenia. True thrombocytopenia is classified by the physiologic disturbance responsible for the low platelet count.

      a. Disorder of platelet production. The number of platelets leaving the marrow and entering the circulation can be fewer than expected because of hypoproliferation of megakaryocytes (due to aplastic anemia, infection, toxin exposure, congenital abnormalities, or myelophthisis) or because of ineffective thrombopoiesis (due to megaloblastic anemia, preleukemic conditions, or familial thrombocytopenia). Both types of "production disorders" require a bone marrow examination for diagnosis. Inadequate platelet production should be managed by treating the primary disease or by withdrawing potentially offending drugs; bleeding or marked thrombocytopenia (i.e., a platelet count < 10,000/mm³) may require platelet transfusion (see sec. **IV.B**). Bleeding, thrombocytopenic patients require hospitalization.

   b. Disorders of platelet distribution. In conditions associated with splenomegaly (e.g., congestive heart failure, portal hypertension, myelofibrosis), thrombocytopenia can develop because of pooling of platelets in the enlarged spleen. While platelet transfusions (see sec. **IV.B**) are necessary for bleeding patients, their effectiveness is limited because of splenic pooling.

   c. Accelerated platelet destruction. Platelet destruction is augmented in several disorders (e.g., DIC, immune thrombocytopenic purpura, drug-induced thrombocytopenia, eclampsia). Despite augmented platelet production by the bone marrow, thrombocytopenia results. Bone marrow examination is required to establish the diagnosis. Treatment of these conditions involves prompt therapy of the primary disease and withdrawal of potentially offending drugs. Platelet transfusions are of limited or no benefit in the management of thrombocytopenia due to accelerated platelet destruction.

   2. Thrombocytosis. Increased platelet counts may result from either benign or malignant processes.

   a. Reactive thrombocytosis. An increase in platelet count (up to 1,000,000 mm³) may be a physiologic response to stress, such as infection, trauma, surgery, inflammatory conditions, or iron deficiency. In addition, following splenectomy, the usual postoperative thrombocytosis is exaggerated because of the elimination of splenic pooling. In reactive thrombocytosis, the rise in platelet numbers is usually not harmful and requires no specific therapy. This condition is benign.

   b. Essential thrombocytosis. In these disorders, platelet production is independent of normal control mechanisms, resulting in very high (sometimes > 1,000,000/mm³) numbers of circulating platelets. Autonomous thrombocytosis is most commonly seen in hematologic malignancies such as polycythemia vera, chronic myelogenous leukemia, myelofibrosis, and essential thrombocythemia. A bone marrow examination is required for diagnosis. Although thrombosis is a potential complication, a bleeding diathesis is more common. Prolonged bleeding times can be corrected by reducing the platelet count to the normal range through plateletpheresis, administration of ³²P, or alkylating agent chemotherapy. Prompt referral to a primary care physician or hematologist is essential to diagnose and manage these disorders correctly. Immediate hospitalization is not needed, in the absence of thrombosis or hemorrhage.

C. Coagulation factor deficiencies

   1. Inherited clotting disorders

   a. Hemophilia. Congenital factor VIII deficiency or factor IX deficiency (hemophilia A or B, respectively) are sex-linked recessive diseases and, therefore, occur in males only; the former is much more common. The clinical manifestations (i.e., excessive bleeding with or without antecedent trauma) are similar in hemophilia A and B and are directly proportional to the degree of factor VIII or factor IX deficiency, respectively, as determined by quantitative factor levels. It is important to differentiate between hemophilia A and B because of differences in blood component therapy. For both disorders, avoidance of injury and early treatment following trauma are important. The ongoing care of hemophiliacs should be delegated to specialized centers so that the medical, surgical, dental, and psychologic needs of patients can be well coordinated.

   (1) Treatment of factor VIII deficiency. Fresh frozen plasma (see sec. **IV.C.2.a**) can be used, but it contains little of the necessary factor in a large volume of fluid (1 unit/ml); thus, fluid overload is a hazard. Cryoprecipitate and commercial factor VIII concentrates (see sec. **IV.C.2b and c**) are more appropriate and can be given according to the equation:

   Units of factor VIII activity to be given
   = (desired VIII concentration − observed VIII concentration)
   × 41 ml/kg × body weight in kg

The factor VIII activity units to be given depend on the nature and location of the hemorrhage and the severity of the patient's factor deficiency. For example, minor lacerations may necessitate no therapy. Hemarthroses or symptomatic hematomas may require that a factor VIII level of 50% be achieved and maintained by factor transfusion q12h for 2–4 days. Major surgery and life-threatening hemorrhage demand initial achievement of a factor VIII level of 100% and administration of half of the initial dose q8h for 48 hours, as well as maintenance of 50% levels for a few days thereafter. Factor VIII levels should be monitored daily and treatment adjusted to maintain the desired factor VIII concentration. Furthermore, prior to initiating concentrate transfusion, the physician needs to ensure that the patient lacks antibodies against factor VIII (determined by a "inhibitor screen"), since these patients are refractory to conventional treatment; management of these patients is most appropriately directed by a specialist in hematology.

(2) **Treatment of factor IX deficiency.** Minor hemorrhage can be controlled with fresh frozen plasma (15–20 ml/kg of body weight), but more severe bleeding events necessitate use of commercial factor IX concentrates (see sec. **IV.C.2c**). Guidelines for emergency therapy are similar to those for hemophilia A, although transfused factor IX has a more prolonged half-life than factor VIII, and therefore maintenance transfusions need not be given as often (e.g., q12h instead of q8h).

(3) **Treatment of hemarthroses.** See **Chap. 14**.

b. **Von Willebrand's disease.** An autosomal dominant pattern of inheritance results in von Willebrand's disease is both males and females. This congenital disorder is characterized by platelet dysfunction (i.e., poor adsorption to endothelial surfaces) and deficient factor VIII production. The clinical severity and onset of manifestations are variable. In contrast to patients with classic hemophilia A, patients with von Willebrand's disease respond to fresh frozen plasma, cryoprecipitate, or factor VIII concentrate transfusion with a prolonged, progressive rise in factor VIII activity. In general, bleeding episodes are easily controlled, the major surgery can be treated prophylactically with 10–15 ml/kg/day of fresh frozen plasma or an equivalent amount of cryoprecipitate (see sec. **IV.C.2**). The bleeding time, PTT, and factor VIII activity require monitoring.

c. **Other inherited disorders.** Only rare patients have coagulation factor deficiencies other than hemophilia and von Willebrand's disease. Consultation with a hematology specialist is important in their management.

2. **Acquired clotting disorders**

a. **Vitamin K deficiency.** Severe liver disease, malabsorption, coumarin therapy, malnutrition. and prolonged antibiotic therapy can lead to decreased levels of factors II, VII, IX, and X, with hemorrhagic manifestations. Under most circumstances, the prothrombin time is an adequate test for vitamin K–dependent factor deficiency. Therapy consists of administration of parenteral vitamin K (phytonadione, 10–20 mg IM or slowly IV q12–24h) and/or fresh frozen plasma in an initial dosage of 15–20 ml/kg of body weight if rapid correction is desired. The treatment chosen depends on the severity of the hemostatic defect and on the extent, if any, of hepatocellular disease, since vitamin K will not correct deficiencies in the presence of profound liver disease.

b. **Coagulopathy secondary to hepatic disease.** Uncontrolled hemorrhage in a setting of liver disease presents a very difficult diagnostic and therapeutic dilemma. Severe hepatocellular dysfunction results in many potential factor deficiencies (I, II, V, VII, IX, X, XII) and may be complicated by concomitant DIC or fibrinolysis (see sec. **II.C.2.c** and **d**). A microangiopathic blood smear, thrombopenia, and factor VIII deficiency suggest that DIC is contributing to the hemostatic defect. All bleeding patients with liver disease should be given a therapeutic trial of vitamin K, although the majority will not benefit. Transfusion with fresh frozen plasma should be part of the initial management of fulminant bleeding episodes, and if there is evidence of fibrinolysis (see sec. **II.C.2.d**) but not DIC, antifibrinolytic agents (e.g., ε-aminocaproic acid [EACA]) may be helfpul.

c. **Disseminated intravascular coagulation** can be an acute or chronic asymptomatic or fulminant phenomenon resulting in intravascular activation of the coagulation sequence and thrombosis and/or hemorrhage. Overwhelming infections (especially gram-negative or anaerobic sepsis), cardiovascular collapse, obstetric or surgical complications, snakebites, and transfusion or anaphylactic reactions account for the majority of cases. Laboratory findings include a microangiopathic blood smear, thrombopenia, hypofibrinogenemia, and an elevated titer of fibrin degradation products. **Treatment of the underlying condition is the major therapeutic approach to DIC.** Bleeding patients who require urgent correction of the hemostatic defect may benefit from fresh frozen plasma and platelet transfusions (see sec. **IV.B–C**) while the etiologic disorder is being treated. Patients with thrombosis and occasional patients with exsanguinating hemorrhage may respond to heparinization. In bleeding patients, heparin should not be used until transfusion of clotting factors and platelets has failed to control the bleeding.

   d. **Primary fibrinolysis** is a rare disorder that can present laboratory and clinical manifestations identical to those of DIC; it is seen most commonly in patients with liver disease or prostate cancer. Since antifibrinolytic therapy with EACA can aggravate DIC if heparin therapy has not been used initially, most patients should be treated initially for DIC. If evidence of fibrinolysis continues (i.e., persistently low fibrinogen levels), antifibrinolytic therapy with 5 gm of EACA (PO or IV over 1 hour) should be initiated. If successful, EACA, 1 gm/hour for 8 hours, will maintain hemostasis.

   e. **Heparin overdose or covert abuse.** Heparin is a sulfated mucopolysaccharide that acts in part by potentiating the action of antithrombin III against thrombin and factors IXa, Xa, and XIa. Heparin administration therefore prolongs the PT, PTT, thrombin time, and whole-blood clotting time. Abnormalities of all of these tests suggest that heparin is present. Further confirmation can be obtained by ordering a reptilase time or repeating the above tests in the presence of a heparin-binding resin. Four hours after cessation of therapy, no heparin is detectable in normal patient plasma. If anticoagulation must be reversed more rapidly, protamine sulfate, at an initial dosage of 50 mg in a solution of normal saline given slowly IV over 10 minutes may be used; no more than 200 mg of protamine sulfate should be given within a 2-hour interval. The dosage varies with the amount of heparin present and the time interval after heparin administration. The correction of heparin effect can be ascertained by monitoring the PTT.

   f. **Coumarin overdose or covert abuse.** The coumarin derivatives interfere with the synthesis of the vitamin K–dependent factors II, VII, IX, and X and prolong the PT to a greater extent than they affect the PTT. Anticoagulation by these drugs depends on the integrity of liver function, access to vitamin K, and interaction between the coumarins and many other drugs. Except for the risk of hemorrhage, toxicity is unusual. The diagnosis of coumarin overdose is suggested by a markedly prolonged (i.e., greater than twice the control) PT in a patient with a normal PTT and platelet count and low levels of vitamin K–dependent factors. The PT gradually returns to normal over several days following drug withdrawal, but more rapid correction can be accomplished by transfusing with fresh frozen plasma (10–15 ml/kg). Vitamin K, 5–15 mg PO or IV at a rate not greater than 5 mg/minute, will correct the hemostatic defect as well but will take at least 6–12 hours to begin to correct the deficiency. Furthermore, renewed oral anticoagulation will be very difficult for several days, Caution is advised in the intravenous administration of vitamin K to avoid a hypotensive episode. Generally, hospitalization is indicated if there is evidence of hemorrhage or recent trauma.

III. **Leukocyte disorders.** Leukopenia is defined as a total white blood cell (WBC) count less than 4000/mm^3 and leukocytosis as a total WBC count greater than 11,000/mm^3. It is critical to determine which of the WBC lineages is responsible for the decrease or increase in the total count. Concomitant anemia and thrombocytopenia usually indicate more serious disorders and provide important data toward the differential diagnosis.

   A. **Granulocytopenia (neutropenia)**
      1. **Definition and clinical significance.** Although neutropenia exists when there are fewer than 2500 polymorphonuclear leukocytes (PMNs)/mm^3, a significantly increased risk of infection does not exist until a level of 500–1000 PMNs/mm^3 is reached. Among Yemenite Jews and American blacks, mild

neutropenia is not uncommon; otherwise, neutropenia implies that disease is present. There are patients with moderately severe neutropenia who do not have infections, implying that other factors may modify susceptibility to infection, such as the monocyte count, granulocyte function, presence of underlying disease, and additional immunologic defects. However, **fever in a patient with neutropenia must be regarded as a medical emergency.**

2. **Etiology.** Increased peripheral utilization in association with hypersplenism, sepsis, immunologic conditions, and the use of certain drugs may produce granulocytopenia. In addition, reduction of neutrophils may be secondary to decreased production due to maturation defects (e.g., vitamin B_{12} or folic acid deficiency), marrow infiltration (with carcinoma, leukemia, fibrosis, or granulomatous processes), or marrow hypoplasia (from drugs, alcohol, radiation, or undetermined causes).

Drugs are an especially important cause of agranulocytosis. Phenothiazines, antithyroid drugs, sulfonamides, nonsteroidal anti-inflammatory drugs (e.g., phenylbutazone), and antibiotics (e.g., chloramphenicol, trimethoprim-sulfamethoxazole) are the most common drugs causing idiosyncratic neutropenia. Dose-related agranulocytosis occurs with use of chemotherapeutic agents, certain antibiotics (e.g., chloramphenicol), pyrazolones, hydantoins, sulfonylureas, and gold compounds.

3. **Management.** The febrile neutropenic patient must be closely observed or hospitalized. The use of "reverse isolation" is controversial. A source of infection and organism must be sought; therefore, blood (for bacterial and fungal organisms), urine, throat, sputum, and wound cultures should be obtained after a thorough history and physical examination (including careful rectal and pelvic examinations) are performed. An aggressive radiographic investigation of any suspicious site should also be undertaken. A lumbar puncture must be strongly considered in all patients and is mandatory if there is encephalopathy or suspicion of meningitis. Empiric use of a broad-spectrum antibiotic combination, such as an aminoglycoside and a semisynthetic penicillin or cephalosporin derivative, is justified in toxic neutropenic patients, but a more judicious approach involving appropriate therapy for any positive culture results is encouraged. Empiric use of oral antibiotics on an outpatient basis is seldom appropriate. Prompt consultation with a hematologist/oncologist is encouraged to determine the cause of the neutropenia and to assess for an underlying bone marrow disease.

B. **Granulocytosis**

1. **Definition and clinical significance.** When there are more than 8000 neutrophils/mm^3, neutrophilic leukocytosis exists. Bacterial infections produce the most striking elevations of granulocyte counts, especially in children; in some older adults, only a "shift to the left" (due to release of immature neutrophil precursors) may provide a clue that infection is present. The presence of toxic granulations and Doehle bodies offers further evidence of infection. Under severe stress (e.g., burns, trauma), the marrow may release early WBC forms, including, rarely, myeloblasts, resulting in a leukemoid peripheral blood picture.

2. **Etiology.** In addition to bacterial infections, viral illnesses, metabolic disorders (e.g., acidosis, uremia), acute inflammation (e.g., rheumatoid arthritis), toxins, pregnancy, glucocorticoid or epinephrine administration, and myeloproliferative diseases (e.g., leukemia, myelofibrosis) can cause granulocytosis.

3. **Therapeutic approach**

   a. Patients with mild to moderate leukocytosis (i.e., WBC count of 11,000–50,000/mm^3) should be treated for the underlying condition in the appropriate fashion. Toxic, febrile patients require hospitalization.

   b. Patients with a more marked leukocytosis (i.e., WBC count > 50,000/mm^3), especially when persistent or when associated with anemia, thrombocytopenia, erythrocytosis, thrombocytosis, lymphadenopathy, or hepatosplenomegaly, should be referred promptly to a hematologist or internal medicine specialist for diagnosis. When more than 100,000 WBCs/mm^3 are seen, especially if the majority are blast forms, the patient requires hospitalization and urgent treatment. Treatment alternatives include leukopheresis, definitive chemotherapy, and radiotherapy. A hematologist/oncologist must be consulted promptly to aid in the treatment plan.

   c. **Eosinophilia** (i.e., an absolute eosinophil count > than 600/mm^3) may be attributable to allergic conditions (e.g., allergic rhinitis, asthma, drug allergy), parasitic infestation, dermatologic disorders (such as pemphigus), vasculitis, or myeloproliferative diseases. Extensive testing may not reveal a cause. Such patients do not require emergency hospitalization unless they are clinically ill.

    d. Basophilia is usually caused by a myeloproliferative syndrome. If the basophilia is reproducible, the patient requires hematologic consultation.

IV. Blood component therapy
A. Red blood cell transfusions

    1. Indications for an RBC transfusion include anemia associated with angina pectoris or ischemic electrocardiographic (ECG) changes, high-output congestive heart failure, or changes in mental status and acute blood loss sufficient to cause shock (in this setting, the hematocrit will not accurately reflect the amount of blood loss for 24–72 hours). However, patients with chronic anemia tend to tolerate the anemia well and generally are best served not with transfusion but rather with therapy tailored to the specific cause of their RBC deficiency. In hemolytic anemias, transfusion should be avoided, if possible.

    2. Red blood cell components

        a. Whole blood. Since whole-blood transfusions provide the patient with more unnecessary components (plasma, platelets, leukocytes) than desired components (erythrocytes), indications for their use are few. However, the actively bleeding patient with hypovolemia, especially after major trauma, will benefit from whole-blood transfusions.

        b. Packed red blood cells. This product has a hematocrit of approximately 70% in volume of 200–250 ml. It is prepared from individual patients, and much of the platelet-rich plasma has been removed. **Packed RBCs are the standard component to be used in transfusing the anemic patient.**

        c. Leukocyte-poor red blood cells. WBCs can be removed from packed erythrocytes by various techniques (i.e., freezing and washing, buffy coat separation). This component is indicated when it is important to avoid leukoagglutinin-type febrile reactions in multiply transfused patients. The expense and laboriousness of preparing this product make it impractical for the transfusion requirements of most patients.

        d. Fresh blood is blood that has been stored less than 6 hours. It is given to avoid storage injury to platelets, loss of coagulation factors V and VIII, excess extracellular potassium, and significant loss of RBCs per volume. It may be useful in transfusions in newborns and in patients with thrombotic thrombocytopenic purpura.

        e. Type-specific, uncross-matched blood. Although it takes less than 5 minutes to determine a patient's ABO and Rh type, a complete cross-match takes at least 45–60 minutes. When urgent transfusion is needed, type-specific packed cells may be administered. In rare circumstances, when even the 5-minute blood typing cannot be tolerated, type O, Rh-negative packed cells can be given to the exsanguinating patient.

    3. Complications

        a. Febrile reactions. With an incidence of approximately 3%, fever and chills are the most common adverse reaction to transfusions. Since febrile reactions usually result from sensitivity to donor WBCs, platelets, and plasma proteins in patients who have received multiple transfusions, they can be prevented by giving leukocyte-poor erythrocytes to patients with a history of such reactions. If a febrile reaction occurs, the transfusion should be discontinued transiently, the patient's and the blood unit's identification rechecked, and a urine and plasma sample examined for color (i.e., red or brown, indicative of hemoglobin or methemoglobin, respectively). If no evidence of hemolysis exists, the transfusion may be continued after an antipyretic agent has been administered. In addition, administration of an antipyretic (e.g., acetaminophen, 325 mg PO) and an antihistamine (e.g., diphenhydramine, 50 mg IV) prior to the transfusion may prevent these reactions.

        b. Hemolytic reactions. Fortunately, hemolytic reactions due to RBC incompatibility are rare. Because the consequences are serious (i.e., cardiovascular collapse and renal failure), prompt diagnosis and treatment are required.

            (1) Clinical manifestations. The first symptoms, which usually appear after 50 ml or less of blood has been given, include a throbbing headache, severe back and/or precordial pain, dyspnea, and anxiety. On examination, cyanosis or facial flushing, diaphoresis, and a rapid, thready pulse may be the initial signs of a severe reaction. In the anesthetized or obtunded patient, shock or DIC may be the first manifestation of hemolysis. For an interval of days after the transfusion has been discontinued, the patient may appear well; nonetheless, hemoglobinuria, hemoglobinemia, and an elevated serum bilirubin may progress to jaundice and oliguric renal failure. With proper initial management, however, these complications can be avoided.

(2) **Laboratory investigation.** The transfusion should be discontinued if a hemolytic-type reaction is suspected. As noted in sec. **IV.A.3.a,** a plasma and urine sample should be checked immediately for free hemoglobin (the semiquantitative urine "dipsticks" are adequate for this test). In addition, the patient's type and cross-match should be rechecked on a fresh sample of blood, and the cross-match on the original patient specimen and the donor unit should be reconfirmed as well. If more than 6 hours has elapsed, increased serum bilirubin and decreased (or absent) serum haptoglobin levels may be noted as confirmatory evidence of a hemolytic reaction.

(3) **Management.** If a major transfusion reaction is even a remote consideration, immediate management is indicated. Crystalloid solution (e.g., normal saline) should be administered at a rate sufficient to produce a urine flow of at least 100 ml/hour. Mannitol, 25 gm, should be infused over 5 minutes and repeated if the urine output falls, but no more than 100 gm of mannitol should be administered within 24 hours. If hypotension supervenes, plasma expanders or vasopressors may be necessary. If bleeding develops, DIC should be suspected and appropriate documentation and therapy begun (see sec. **II.C.2.c**). In the event that renal failure supervenes, appropriate management (including short-term dialysis, if necessary) should be instituted.

c. **Allergic reactions.** Urticaria is common, but vascular collapse and asthma are rare in multiply transfused recipients. Administration of an antihistamine (e.g., diphenhydramine, 50 mg PO or IV) prior to the transfusion will usually abrogate such allergic reactions. Transient discontinuation of the transfusion while allergic manifestations are treated with an antihistamine is advised.

d. **Cardiac failure.** Despite slow, cautious administration of packed RBCs, patients with borderline cardiac compensation may develop congestive heart failure. In such patients, administration of a diuretic (e.g., furosemide) prior to, during, or after the transfusion is recommended.

e. **Citrate intoxication.** In adults who are massively transfused at a rate exceeding 100 ml of blood/minute or have severe hepatic dysfunction, clinical signs of hypocalcemia (e.g., arrhythmia, hypotension, or tetany) may be observed. This problem is more common in infants receiving exchange transfusions and is rarely observed in adults. In adults, calcium gluconate, 10 ml of a 10% solution, should be injected slowly IV at a site remote from the transfusion to correct such reactions.

f. **Excessive bleeding.** Since stored blood contains diminished numbers of competent platelets and variable amounts of coagulation factors, thrombocytopenia and excessive bleeding may occur after massive (i.e., > 10 units) transfusion. To combat this complication, 1 unit of fresh frozen plasma may be administered for every 5 units of packed cells and 10 units of random donor platelets given for every 10 units of packed RBCs. An alternative regimen involves transfusion of a freshly drawn (i.e., < 4 hours old) RBC unit for every 4–5 stored units given.

B. **Platelet transfusion**

1. **Indications.** Definitive treatment of thrombocytopenia depends on the mechanism responsible for producing the platelet deficiency. Platelet transfusions are given to patients experiencing serious hemorrhage when the platelet count is less than 10,000 mm^3 and as an adjunct to major surgery when the platelet count is less than 100,000 mm^3 (which is the count at which most patients have a prolongation of the bleeding time).

2. **Platelet components**

a. **Random donor platelets** are harvested by centrifugation from a single unit of fresh blood; the platelets are suspended in 30–50 ml of donor plasma and, therefore, are essentially devoid of RBC-associated ABO and Rh antigens. A pool of random single-donor units can then be prepared and administered as a rapid infusion. Ordinarily, this product is given in a dosage of 1 unit/10 kg of body weight and can be expected to produce an increment of 5000–10,000 platelets/mm^3/M^2 body surface area/unit transfused. However, increments are lower in the setting of fever, infection, splenomegaly, or sensitization from prior transfusions. **In emergencies, random donor platelets are the appropriate platelet product for the thrombocytopenic patient.** If the patient has a history of febrile transfusion reactions, premedication with an antipyretic and antihistamine should be given.

   b. HLA-compatible platelets. In the multiply transfused thrombopenic patient who no longer achieves a significant increment in the platelet count from random donor units, the blood bank should arrange for HLA-compatible platelet products. These are obtained by plateletpheresis of compatible donors.

   3. **Complications.** Febrile and allergic reactions may accompany platelet transfusion and should be treated in the same fashion as similar reactions from RBC transfusion. With repeated use of random donor platelets, most patients will become "refractory," that is, will not achieve adequate increments of platelet numbers. Therefore, conservative use of repeated platelet transfusions is advised.

C. **Plasma and plasma-component transfusion**
   1. **Indications.** The proper treatment of a coagulopathy depends on the etiology of the clotting disorder. Plasma and plasma-fraction transfusions are appropriate for hemorrhaging or preoperative patients with coagulation abnormalities due to intrinsic disease or anticoagulant therapy.
   2. **Available plasma products**
      a. **Fresh frozen plasma** is useful to prevent dilution of clotting factors in the massively transfused patient, to correct rapidly coagulation abnormalities due to anticoagulant therapy, and to treat various congenital factor deficiencies, including von Willebrand's disease. It contains active coagulation factors in a volume of 200–250 ml/unit from a single donor. When indicated, 2 units of fresh frozen plasma are given at a rapid rate and the effect on the coagulation parameters is assessed. **Fresh frozen plasma is the most commonly used product for the hemorrhaging, nonthrombocytopenic patient in the emergency setting.**
      b. **Cryoprecipitate** transfusion is appropriate for bleeding patients with hypofibrinogenemia, von Willebrand's disease, or factor VIII deficiency (when commercially prepared factor VIII concentrate is unavailable). It contains high concentrations of fibrinogen and factor VIII in a volume of less than 50 ml. For hypofibrinogenemia or von Willebrand's disease, an initial priming dose of 2 units/10 kg of body weight should be followed by maintenance therapy of one-half the priming dosage q12h. Further therapy should be adjusted depending on the coagulation parameters and the effect on hemorrhage.
      c. **Commercial concentrates of factor VIII or factor IX.** When hemorrhaging or in preparation for surgery, patients with hemophilia A or B are appropriately treated with commercial products. Dosages should be guided by the manufacturer's recommendations. The prolonged PTT will normalize if the depressed factor level has been raised to 40–60% of the normal value. Risk of joint damage from hemarthrosis is reduced if the affected joint is aseptically aspirated only after corrective therapy has been administered.

Oncologic Emergencies

I. **Patients with suspected neoplasms.** Occasionally, a patient presents to the emergency department with symptoms or signs suggestive of a malignancy (e.g., weight loss, an abdominal mass, unexplained lymphadenopathy, vaginal bleeding in a postmenopausal female, an unexplained density on a chest radiography, a leukoblastic peripheral smear). Whenever carcinoma is part of the differential diagnosis in the emergency department, the **abnormalities identified must be followed to resolution,** either by admitting the patient to the hospital or by arranging close follow-up on an outpatient basis. Hospitalization is indicated if the patient is systemically ill, there is evidence or the possibility of a potentially serious complication (e.g., spinal cord compression), or there are concerns about patient compliance with outpatient follow-up.

II. Tumor-related emergencies

A. Obstruction. Both malignant and benign tumors can cause obstruction of normal organs. In some cases, this may be the first manifestation of neoplasia.

1. **Bowel obstruction.** Both intrinsic and extrinsic masses can result in partial or complete intestinal obstruction.

   a. **Clinical manifestations.** Initially, in bowel obstruction, severe cramping pain occurs synchronously with hyperperistalsis. As the obstruction progresses, colicky discomfort may be replaced by generalized dull pain as the bowel distention becomes extreme. Vomiting may occur early, late, or not at all depending on the site of obstruction. Failure to pass gas or feces is a valuable diagnostic clue, as is abdominal distention. The clinical manifestations of obstruction due to tumor do not distinguish this etiology from other causes of mechanical obstruction.

   b. **Roentgenographic and laboratory findings.** Supine and upright abdominal plain films should be obtained as soon as the diagnosis is suspected. Gas-fluid levels in the small intestine and, perhaps, proximal colon in a "stair-step" pattern, with less than normal gas in the distal colon, are important diagnostic signs. Additional radiographic studies, such as a sodium diatrizoate (Hypaque) enema (sodium diatrizoate is preferable to barium because the latter is not water-soluble), are sometimes indicated immediately to localize and outline the area of obstruction. Serum electrolytes may show evidence of intravascular dehydration as fluid is sequestered within the bowel. A complete blood count may show evidence of hemoconcentration and a mild leukocytosis; extreme leukocytosis implies bowel strangulation. Serum amylase levels may be elevated because of back pressure in the duodenum or peritoneal absorption after leakage from necrotic bowel.

   c. **Management.** Essentially all patients with intestinal obstruction due to tumor require hospitalization. Urgent consultation with a general surgeon is mandatory. The principles of emergency management include correcting any fluid and electrolyte abnormalities, bowel decompression with a nasogastric or, preferably, nasointestinal tube, and timed surgical intervention.

2. **Urinary obstruction.** Obstruction of urine flow can involve any level of the urinary tract. Obstructive uropathy due to tumor must always be included in the differential diagnosis of hematuria, bladder distention, and acute renal failure.

   a. **Clinical manifestations.** Obstructive uropathy may present with total anuria and bladder distention, fluctuating urine output and colicky flank pain, polyuria, hematuria, infection, or unexplained renal failure. The clinical manifestations depend on the level and cause of the obstruction.

   b. **Roentgenographic and laboratory findings.** Ultrasonography and intravenous pyelography should be the initial radiographic studies obtained. A sonogram of both kidneys will show dilatation of the collecting system proximal to the site of obstruction, bilaterally if the bladder outlet is the location of the obstruction. An intravenous pyelogram with delayed films will usually visualize the collecting system well, if the creatinine clearance exceeds 20 ml/minute, and confirm the presence and location of the blockage. Although needless instrumentation of the urinary tract should be avoided, in some cases retrograde pyelography may be necessary to demonstrate the patency of at least one ureter. Laboratory abnormalities (e.g., pyuria, hematuria, proteinuria, bacteriuria) are variable and depend on the etiology, duration, and completeness of obstruction.

   c. **Management.** If obstructive uropathy is documented, recovery of renal function in the affected kidney(s) depends on relief of the obstruction. Furthermore, if infection or pain is part of the presenting manifestations, management will be facilitated by drainage. Prompt consultation with a urologist is important in determining the urgency and nature of surgical intervention. Generally, such patients require hospitalization.

3. **Superior vena cava (SVC) syndrome.** In the antibiotic era, the most common cause of the SVC syndrome is malignant disease, with extrinsic compression of the SVC by nodal metastases from bronchogenic carcinoma or lymphoma predominating. The syndrome represents an acute or subacute emergency that requires prompt diagnosis and treatment.

a. **Clinical manifestations.** The SVC syndrome develops insidiously and then progresses rapidly as obstruction becomes more complete. Symptoms include dyspnea and swelling of the face, upper extremities, and/or trunk. Chest pain, cough, dysphagia, and headache or other neurologic symptoms are less frequent complaints. Venous distention of the thorax, neck, and upper extremities; facial edema and plethora or cyanosis; and tachypnea are among a variety of physical findings. Confinement of these signs to the upper part of the body differentiates the SVC syndrome from constrictive pericarditis and cor pulmonale. The development of these signs is attributable to obstruction of venous drainage of the upper body, resulting in elevated venous pressure leading to venous dilatation of collaterals and increased intracranial pressure. Prolonged obstruction leads to irreversible thrombosis, with vascular and central nervous system complications.

b. **Roentgenographic and laboratory findings.** The diagnosis is usually made clinically without extensive diagnostic testing. A chest x-ray reveals a superior mediastinal mass, usually on the right side, in almost all patients. Pulmonary parenchymal lesions, a pleural effusion, and hilar adenopathy may also be noted. Further radiographic tests to delineate the mass lesion, however, should not be pursued at the expense of prompt therapy.

c. **Management.** All patients with suspected SVC syndrome require hospitalization and early consultation with those experienced in managing the problem (e.g., a thoracic surgeon, radiation oncologist, and medical oncologist). Invasive diagnostic procedures such as bronchoscopy, mediastinoscopy, and/or a scalene node biopsy are often necessary to establish a tissue diagnosis. However, since the SVC syndrome may require urgent therapy (e.g., when there is severe dyspnea or neurologic signs), attempts to obtain tissue for diagnosis may have to be deferred until after appropriate therapeutic management is underway. The primary treatment is radiation therapy, although chemotherapy has also been successfully employed. Medical measures including anticoagulation, diuresis, and steroid administration have not been studied in a controlled fashion and cannot be recommended for routine use, but they may be helpful in selected patients.

4. **Increased intracranial pressure.** Neurologic deterioration in patients with primary or metastatic brain tumors is secondary to elevated intracranial pressure (ICP), resulting in uncal or cerebellar tonsil herniation or vascular compression. Prompt diagnosis and therapy are essential to prevent irreversible neurologic damage.

a. **Clinical manifestations.** Increased ICP should be suspected when there is headache, vomiting (with or without nausea), and a change in the level of consciousness in a patient known (or suspected) to have cancer. The major early feature is an alteration in mental status. Bradycardia, hypertension, pupillary dilatation (unilateral or bilateral), and focal neurologic signs suggest more advanced ICP elevation. Papilledema is an important clue to the diagnosis but is subtle or absent early in the disorder; it suggests that the pressure is dangerously elevated.

b. **Roentgenographic and laboratory findings.** A computerized tomographic (CT) scan showing one or more mass lesions and/or shift of midline structures establishes the diagnosis. The CT scan conveys additional important information about tumor location and the presence or absence of hydrocephalus and thus has valuable therapeutic implications. **If there is any suggestion of intracranial metastasis and/or elevated ICP by CT scan, a lumbar puncture is contraindicated.** However, if the CT scan is unrevealing, a lumbar puncture may be necessary to establish the diagnosis (e.g., meningeal carcinomatosis). Laboratory tests are not particularly germane to the diagnosis of increased ICP, but hyponatremia and hypoosmolality in the presence of a less than maximally dilute urine suggest the presence of syndrome of inappropriate antidiuretic hormone (SIADH), which requires management. Furthermore, metabolic causes of an altered consciousness (e.g., hypercalcemia) require exclusion.

c. **Management.** All patients with elevated ICP require hospitalization and prompt consultation with a radiation oncologist. An IV line should be established, but fluids and sodium chloride should be restricted. Administration of corticosteroids in large doses (e.g., dexamethasone, 10 mg q6h) should be begun promptly. A nonsedative anticonvulsant, such as phenytoin, should be considered for administration. In mild cases, these medical measures (i.e., fluid and salt restriction, corticosteroid therapy), combined with radiation therapy, will be sufficient treatment. The use of intravascular dehydration (e.g., with glycerol, mannitol, or furosemide) may be necessary in advanced cases but should not be undertaken without neurosurgical consultation, since these agents produce a tendency for "rebound" increases in ICP within 4–7 hours; therefore, their use should be coordinated with neurosurgical intervention. Emergency neurosurgical techniques include ventricular drainage and shunting, bony decompression, and/or tumor resection. All patients require careful monitoring with frequent attention to the vital signs, level of consciousness, and the neurologic and funduscopic examinations. Select patients may require continuous invasive monitoring of the ICP using a pressure transducer.

5. Spinal cord and cauda equina compression. Extradural spinal cord compression is among the most common neurologic complications of malignant tumors. Both extradural and intramedullary tumor, which is rare, will produce permanent neurologic damage if not recognized and treated urgently.

    a. Clinical manifestations. The clinical presentation of spinal cord compression is typified by pain at the level of the lesion, autonomic dysfunction of the bowel and/or bladder, extremity weakness, and sensory loss distal to the level of lesion. The pain may be localized or radicular and may differ from the pain of a herniated intervertebral disk by exacerbation upon assuming the supine position. Bowel and bladder dysfunction may take the form of either retention or incontinence (secondary to loss of sphincter control). Careful neurologic testing will document motor weakness of the extremities below the site of the lesion in the vast majority of cases. Sensory loss is not usually a presenting complaint but is often documented on examination, nonetheless. Loss of rectal sphincter tone and perineal hypesthesia are important diagnostic signs.

    b. Roentgenographic and laboratory findings. Most of the solid tumors that produce epidural cord compression arise in a vertebral body, although lymphomas may cause this syndrome by direct extension through the intervertebral foramina from paraspinous nodal masses. Therefore, plain films of the spine at the level of the neurologic dysfunction are indicated and are frequently positive for bone destruction. However, myelography is necessary in all cases; a myelogram will delineate the upper and lower margins of the lesion and determine whether there is an additional asymptomatic lesion elsewhere along the spinal cord. If a complete block is found, cisternal myelography will be necessary to determine the cephalad margin of the lesion. At the time of myelography, spinal fluid examination should be performed to identify malignant cells and/or infectious organisms. A CT scan of the area of compression may yield valuable information but has not replaced myelography as the diagnostic test of choice.

    c. Management. Hospitalization and urgent consultation with a radiation oncologist and neurosurgeon are required. This neurologic emergency is usually aggressively treated with intravenous corticosteriods (e.g., dexamethasone, 4–10 mg q6h), in addition to radiation therapy and/or decompressive neurosurgery. Treatment of the individual case is based on considerations of tumor type, the level of the block, and the rapidity of onset and duration of symptoms. Pain relief, bladder catheterization, and relief of constipation are important ancillary management considerations. The role of chemotherapy in the treatment of spinal cord compression is that of adjuvant, rather than primary, treatment.

B. Secretion. Many tumors secrete fluid, protein, or other soluble factors that produce symptoms and suggest the diagnosis of a malignancy. Serosal fluid accumulation results in ascites or pericardial or pleural effusion. Protein secretion can produce the hyperviscosity syndrome. Several different mechanisms are responsible for the "hypercalcemia of malignancy" and other metabolic disorders.

    1. The hyperviscosity syndrome develops when the size, shape, and concentration of an abnormal protein cause an increase in plasma viscosity. The syndrome is associated most often with macroglobulins from lymphoma or Waldenström's disease but has been reported with IgG and IgA aggregates in multiple myeloma.

        a. Clinical manifestations. Symptoms usually do not develop until the plasma viscosity rises above three times the viscosity of water. Under these circumstances, visual disturbances, central nervous system symptoms (e.g., weakness, confusion, headache, somnolence), cardiac failure, and a bleeding diathesis may occur. As the syndrome progresses, cardiovascular catastrophes, such as stroke and myocardial or peripheral infarction, develop. Physical findings include retinal vein distention, tortuosity and "beading," and retinal hemorrhage. Epistaxis, mucosal hemorrhage, and peripheral ischemia may also be seen.

   b. **Roentgenographic and laboratory findings.** The erythrocyte sedimentation rate is prolonged and the serum viscosity elevated in patients with the hyperviscosity syndrome. Serum protein electrophoresis, serum and urine immunoelectrophoresis, and quantitative immunoglobulin levels should be ordered in all patients to ascertain the type and concentration of the offending protein, since definitive treatment is influenced by this information. A lateral skull film and x-rays of painful bones may show osteolytic lesions characteristic of multiple myeloma.

   c. **Management.** All patients with the hyperviscosity syndrome require hospitalization and hematologic consultation. Fluids should be administered cautiously, since most patients present with an expanded intravascular volume. Therefore, blood transfusion should be avoided until the serum viscosity has been lowered toward normal. Plasmapheresis should be undertaken and continued daily until the serum viscosity is less than or equal to three times that of water. Chemotherapy directed at the underlying disease will prevent a recurrence of the hyperviscosity syndrome but has no role in the emergency management of the syndrome.

2. **Hypercalcemia of malignancy.** Neoplastic disease is the most common etiology of hypercalcemia.

   a. The **clinical and laboratory manifestations** are indistinguishable from hypercalcemia secondary to endocrine or other diseases (see Chap. 9).

   b. **Management.** Hospitalization is always indicated. Prompt consultation with an internist or medical oncologist is encouraged.

      (1) **General measures.** Since all forms of hypercalcemia are characterized by extracellular volume contraction, rehydration with a crystalloid solution (e.g., 0.9% saline) is the cornerstone of treatment. Since most symptomatic patients are lethargic or somnolent, sedatives, hypnotics, and analgesics should be discontinued. Similarly, any medications that might exacerbate hypercalcemia (e.g., thiazide diuretics) should be eliminated. Immobilization should be avoided, since it will contribute to leaching of calcium from bone.

      (2) **Saline diuresis.** Since sodium competitively inhibits calcium resorption by the renal tubules, therapeutic measures that augment renal sodium clearance will increase calcium clearance as well. If cardiac function is normal, 0.9% saline should be given aggressively (e.g., at a rate of 200–500 ml/hour). If there is concern about myocardial dysfunction, the central venous pressure should be monitored. Furosemide, 20–40 mg IV q2–6h, will increase the tubular sodium load and prevent intravascular volume overload. The serum electrolytes must be assessed frequently, and potassium should be replaced as needed. With appropriately aggressive saline diuresis, serum calcium may decrease by 2–4 mg/dl/day.

      (3) **Corticosteroids.** Glucocorticoids (e.g., hydrocortisone 250–500 mg IV q8–12h, followed by maintenance with prednisone, 10–30 mg/day) promote calciuresis, decrease intestinal absorption of calcium, and decrease bone turnover. However, the hypocalcemic effect is delayed by several days. Furthermore, while corticosteroids may be helpful for hypercalcemia associated with lymphoma or multiple myeloma, the hypocalcemic effect is unpredictable with solid tumors.

      (4) **Mithramycin** is a cytotoxic antibiotic that directly inhibits bone resorption. It is administered in a dosage of 15–25 μg/kg of body weight IV and produces a fall in serum calcium within 12–24 hours that may be durable for 3–7 days. Toxic effects, such as thrombocytopenia and renal and/or hepatic damage, limit its use and are dose- and frequency-related. Nausea, vomiting, postural hypotension, a bleeding diathesis, and hypocalcemic tetany may also complicate its use. Despite these dis-

advantages, mithramycin is an important agent in the treatment of hypercalcemia of malignancy.

(5) **Calcitonin** is a biologic product of the C cells of the thyroid gland, produced in human, salmon, or porcine sources. Its hypocalcemic effect is secondary to inhibition of bone resorption. Salmon calcitonin is the most potent and long-acting of the available preparations. Intramuscular administration of 25–50 MRC units q6–8h (or 2–8 MRC units/kg of body weight SQ q4–6h) will lower the serum calcium by 1–4 mg/dl within a few hours. Allergic reactions, development of tolerance to its hypocalcemic effect, and unpredictability limit its usefulness. Nevertheless, it remains an important agent in the initial treatment of malignant hypercalcemia.

(6) **The diphosphonates** are analogs of inorganic pyrophosphate and selectively inhibit osteoclastic resorption of bone. Ethane-1-hydroxy-1-diphosphonate and dichloromethylene diphosphonate have been evaluated most extensively; the former is approved for the therapy of Paget's disease of bone. In preliminary studies, both agents appear effective in the treatment of hypercalcemia of malignancy and have minimal toxicity. The diphosphonates act within 48 hours and control calcium levels for 5–10 days. Controlled clinical trials are ongoing and will establish the appropriate role of these agents in the therapeutic armamentarium.

(7) **Phosphate supplementation.** The hypocalcemic effect of inorganic phosphate results from acute precipitation of calcium phosphate salt in bone and soft tissues. Because phosphate administration can initiate and potentiate calcium deposition in the heart, kidneys, lens, and other tissues, it should be avoided in hyperphosphatemic and dehydrated patients. Oral Phospha-Soda, 600 mg tid–qid, or Neutra-phos, 500–750 mg tid–qid, are useful adjuncts to therapy but may cause intolerable diarrhea. Oral phosphates, therefore, are of limited value; intravenous phosphate is not recommended.

(8) **Prostaglandin synthesis inhibitors.** In general, the use of prostaglandin synthesis inhibitors in hypercalcemia of malignancy has been disappointing. They may be of benefit when prostaglandin production is etiologic in producing hypercalcemia. Since the toxicity of aspirin (in sufficient dosage to result in a salicylate level of 20 mg/dl) or indomethacin (100–150 mg/day in divided doses) is limited, a therapeutic trial may be worthwhile.

III. **Treatment-related emergencies**
  A. **Leukopenia and fever.** (See **Hematologic Emergencies,** sec. III.A.3.)
  B. **Tumor lysis syndrome.** In lymphoproliferative and myeloproliferative diseases, augmented cell turnover results in increased synthesis and catabolism of nucleic acids. Uric acid is a product of purine degradation and is released from cells in a great quantity when they are lysed by cytotoxic chemotherapy. Hyperuricemia can result in severe renal disease (secondary to acute hyperuricemic nephropathy or uric acid nephrolithiasis) and gouty arthritis, if not managed promptly. When massive tumor lysis occurs, other metabolic abnormalities may accompany hyperuricemia, including hyperphosphatemia, hypocalcemia, hyperkalemia, hypoglycemia, and azotemia; as a group, this metabolic emergency is called the tumor lysis syndrome.
    1. **Clinical manifestations.** When a patient with leukemia or lymphoma who has recently been treated with chemotherapy presents to the emergency department with oliguria, the tumor lysis syndrome should be strongly suspected. Renal stones, gouty arthritis, tetany, and cardiac arrhythmias may be other presenting features. If hyperuricemia, azotemia, hyperphosphatemia, and hypocalcemia are present, treatment should be initiated immediately. If uric acid and phosphate measurements are not available routinely, uric acid crystalluria in an azotemic patient with lymphoma or leukemia may be regarded as presumptive evidence of the tumor lysis syndrome.
    2. **Management.** All patients require hospitalization and immediate consultation with a nephrologist, medical oncologist, or internist. The treatment of the tumor lysis syndrome is directed toward prevention of renal failure. Prophylactic measures include establishing an alkaline diuresis by administering a bicarbonate-rich crystalloid solution (e.g., 5% D/W plus 50–100 mEq/liter of sodium bicarbonate). Every effort should be made to achieve a dilute urine (to lower the uric

acid concentration in the renal tubules) with a pH of 7.0 or greater (to promote conversion of uric acid to the more soluble urate salt). Allopurinol, a xanthine oxidase inhibitor, is a valuable adjunct to therapy; it should be given in initial dosages of 500 mg/m²/day. Both the alkaline diuresis and allopurinol doses can be deescalated as the clinical condition improves. Hyperkalemia, hypocalcemia, hyperphosphatemia, and hypoglycemia should be treated according to conventional guidelines. If the urine output and azotemia do not improve with an alkaline diuresis, the administration of mannitol should be tried. If these measures fail, hemodialysis can remove uric acid, improve metabolic factors, and prevent permanent renal damage.

Bibliography

1. Cassileth, P. A., et al. *Practical Approaches to Hematology-Oncology: A Guideline to Diagnosis and Therapy with Supplemental Case Problems.* Garden City, N.Y.: Medical Examination, 1982.
2. Cohen, L. F., et al. Acute tumor lysis syndrome. *Am. J. Med.* 68:486, 1980.
3. DeVita, V. T., Hellman, S., and Rosenberg, S. A. *Cancer: Principles and Practice of Oncology.* Philadelphia: Lippincott, 1982.
4. Mazzaferri, E. L., O'Dorisio, T. M., and LoBuglio, A. F. Treatment of hypercalcemia associated with malignancy. *Semin. Oncol.* 5:141, 1978.
5. Perez, C. A., Presant, C. A., and Van Amburg, A. L. Management of superior vena cava syndrome. *Semin. Oncol.* 5:123, 1978.
6. Posner, J. B. Management of central nervous system metastases. *Semin. Oncol.* 4:81, 1977.
7. Rodriguez, M., and Dinapoli, R. P. Spinal cord compression. *Mayo Clin. Proc.* 55:442, 1980.
8. Schwartz, G. R., Safar, P., Stone, J. H., et al. *Principles and Practice of Emergency Medicine* (2nd ed.). Philadelphia: Saunders, 1986.
9. Waterbury, L. *Hematology for the House Officer.* Baltimore: Williams & Wilkins, 1982.
10. Williams, W. J., et al. *Hematology.* New York: McGraw-Hill, 1977.

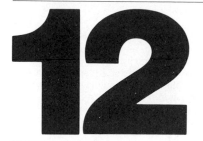

Infectious Diseases

William G. Powderly and
J. William Campbell

General Principles

Infection results from a disturbance of the equilibrium between humans and their microbiologic environment. Either an individual's ability to resist microorganisms (i.e., host factors) or a change in the microbial milieu, or both, may result in clinical infection.

I. Host Defenses

A. General factors

1. **Age.** The very young and the elderly are more susceptible to infection than the normal adult. This increased susceptibility reflects both qualitative and quantitative alterations in the immune system.

2. **Nutrition.** Malnutrition predisposes to infection not only in situations of poverty but also in patients with chronic debilitating diseases (e.g., liver failure, alcoholism).

B. Nonspecific local mechanisms

1. **Skin.** Intact skin provides a physical obstacle to infection. Breaches of this barrier (e.g., by trauma, surgery, intravenous catheterization) are associated with infection, often with organisms normally resident in the skin.

2. **Mucous membranes.** Although less effective than skin as a physical barrier, mucous membranes do offer some resistance to direct invasion. In addition, the secretions of the glands located beneath the mucosa have antimicrobial properties.

3. **Respiratory tract.** The inspired air is filtered, with the larger particles being coated with mucus and transported away from the lungs by ciliary action. Within the alveoli, respiratory macrophages act to clear foreign material. Respiratory diseases, especially those caused by cigarette smoking, impair these respiratory defenses.

4. **Genitourinary system.** Micturition through an unobstructed lower urinary tract provides a constant cleansing mechanism. In males, the length of the urethra is an additional defense mechanism. Obstruction, as in prostatic hypertrophy, predisposes to infection.

5. **Gastrointestinal tract.** Gastric acidity and the alkaline bile and pancreatic juices are antimicrobial. Achlorhydric patients are prone to tuberculosis and salmonella infections. Normal bowel flora provides competition to foreign organisms and acts as a host defense mechanism. Antibiotic administration interferes with this ecologic protection.

6. **Eye.** Tears protect the eye by constant bathing and by their lysozyme content.

C. Specific defense mechanisms

1. **Granulocytes.** Leukocytes act by the phagocytosis of organisms and are particularly important in defense against bacteria and fungi. Granulocytopenia, most commonly seen in patients receiving myelosuppressive chemotherapy for malignancy, predisposes to disseminated bacterial and fungal infections. Congenital defects of white blood cell function are associated with increased staphylococcal and fungal infections.

2. **Humoral immunity.** Antibodies are particularly important in protection against bacterial pathogens. Congenital or acquired (e.g., multiple myeloma) reduction in circulating immunoglobulin is associated with an increase in pyogenic infections. IgA is important in local mucosal defenses; its deficiency is associated with increased sinopulmonary infections.

3. **Complement.** The complement system is a group of serum proteins closely

linked to humoral immunity and phagocytosis. The rare deficiencies in complement are associated with increased susceptibility to *Neisseria*.

4. **Spleen.** The spleen acts as a filter in conjunction with humoral immune mechanisms. An increased incidence of bacteremia with encapsulated bacteria, especially *Streptococcus pneumoniae*, is characteristic of asplenic patients.

5. **Cellular immunity.** The intact T lymphocyte–macrophage system provides the normal protection against tissue invasion. Patients with impaired cellular immunity (e.g., glucocorticoid therapy, reticuloendothelial malignancy, acquired immunodeficiency syndrome) are more susceptible to opportunistic infections with viruses, fungi, mycobacteria, and protozoa.

II. **Microbial factors.** Microorganisms produce disease in two major fashions.
 A. **Toxin production**
   1. An organism that may transiently colonize a host may liberate a toxin responsible for the clinical syndrome. Such syndromes include tetanus, diphtheria, pertussis, and the toxic shock syndrome
   2. Preformed toxins may be ingested without any direct contact between the human and the microbe (e.g., botulism).
 B. **Direct invasion.** Organisms generally produce symptoms by gaining access to and damaging host cells. Some organisms are always pathogenic to humans and always produce disease (e.g., rabies virus, *Salmonella typhi*). Many organisms, innocuous in their normal habitat, may be pathogenic if they gain access to tissues that are normally sterile (e.g., *Escherichia coli* in the urine) or if the host's ability to respond to invasion is impaired. The isolation of organisms from clinical specimens, however, does not always indicate infection. Colonization may follow the introduction of new flora, for example, bacteriuria or candiduria in a patient with a long-standing indwelling urinary catheter or the presence of gram-negative bacilli in the respiratory secretions of a patient on a ventilator. Diagnosis of infection in these and similar situations requires a careful clinical evaluation of the patient for signs of inflammation.

III. **Evaluation of the patient with suspected infection**
 A. **Presenting features.** Patients with infection usually present with signs of inflammation, such as fever, local pain, erythema, and/or swelling.
 Unexplained fever should always suggest the possibility of infection. The normal body temperature ranges from 36.0–37.8° C (97–100° F) orally, with rectal temperatures about 0.6°C greater. Temperatures above this range are abnormal. Very high temperatures may be associated with rigors, which often reflect bacteremia. In contrast, some patients may be unable to mount a febrile response to infection (e.g., the elderly, neonates, patients with uremia, and patients receiving corticosteroids or antipyretics). In these cases, infection should be suspected if there is any deterioration, however subtle, in the patient's well-being. In addition, a subnormal body temperature may be a sign of sepsis.
 B. **History.** The tempo of the illness gives important information on the possible etiology and also on the urgency of therapeutic intervention. In addition, epidemiologic features, such as age, sex, sexual practices, occupation, and travel, are useful in the evaluation of a patient with possible infection. In particular, the presence of an illness in the community or in family members may be useful diagnostically.
 C. **Physical examination.** Anatomic localization of infection is important diagnostically and therapeutically. Thus, a thorough physical examination, including a careful rectal and vaginal examination, is essential. In particular, patients should be examined for signs of inflammation. Findings such as jaundice or nuchal rigidity warrant close attention. The skin, mucous membranes, and retinae may reflect systemic infection.
 D. **Diagnostic tests**
   1. The presence of a **leukocytosis** confirms inflammation, although a normal white blood cell count does not exclude infection.
   2. **Blood cultures** should be performed in the presence of undiagnosed fever or suspected septicemia.
   3. Appropriate **specimens** should be obtained and inspected both grossly and microscopically. Gram stains should be performed and the material submitted for appropriate cultures. Additional stains may be useful in specific circumstances.
   4. **Serology** may often be diagnostic, but in general, paired sera (acute and convalescent) are needed. If the etiology is in doubt, a serum specimen should be obtained and stored for future diagnostic tests.

Table 12-1. Common microbial pathogens associated
with community-acquired infection

Infection	Pathogens
Cellulitis	*Streptococcus pyogenes* *Staphylococcus aureus* Clostridia
Phlebitis	*S. aureus*
Pharyngitis	Adenovirus Group A streptococcus Herpes simplex virus Ebstein-Barr virus *Neisseria gonorrhoeae*
Pneumonia	*Streptococcus pneumoniae* *Haemophilus influenzae* *Mycoplasma pneumoniae* *Legionella* sp. Influenza virus
Biliary tract infection, intraabdominal sepsis	*Escherichia coli* Enterococcus *Klebsiella pneumoniae* *Bacteroides fragilis*
Pelvic abscess	Anaerobic streptococci *B. fragilis* *E. coli* *N. gonorrhoeae* *Actinomyces* (associated with IUD)
Urinary tract infection	*E. coli* *Proteus mirabilis* *Staphylococcus saprophyticus*
Meningitis	*S. pneumoniae* *H. influenzae* *Neisseria meningitidis*
Septic arthritis	*S. aureus* *N. gonorrhoeae*

Antimicrobial Agents

I. **Principles of use.** Antimicrobials are indicated for the treatment of proven or probable infection with susceptible organisms. Empiric antimicrobial usage is warranted in patients with clear signs of focal infection (responsive to such agents) or sepsis, patients with serious underlying disease, and the elderly. In other patients, therapy may be delayed pending the results of diagnostic studies. This approach avoids the inappropriate use of antimicrobials in situations where there is no infection or where infection is caused by organisms unresponsive to antibiotics (e.g., viruses). In addition, drug costs and toxicity are reduced. Finally inappropriate antimicrobial usage may obscure or delay the diagnosis of a serious illness (e.g., infective endocarditis). When empiric antibiotics are necessary, it is essential to obtain all appropriate clinical specimens for smears and culture prior to the initiation of therapy. In many cases, the examination of a Gram stain of these specimens will aid in the choice of an appropriate antimicrobial agent.

II. **Choosing an antimicrobial.** The choice of therapy is guided by the likely pathogen(s) and by host factors.

A. **Microbe.** If the clinical findings do not suggest a likely pathogen, therapy should be directed against those pathogens commonly associated with the clinical situation (Table 12-1). Organisms causing infection acquired in a hospital or in a nursing home are more likely to be resistant to antimicrobials than those pathogens acquired in the community. When a pathogen is identified, therapy should be specific (Table 12-2), preferably guided by susceptibility results.

Table 12-2. Antimicrobials of choice for particular bacteria*

Organism	Drug of first choice	Alternate(s)
1. Gram-positive cocci		
Streptococci		
Group A, group B, *Streptococcus viridans*	Penicillin G	Cephalosporin Vancomycin Erythromycin
Group D (enterococcus)	Penicillin G or ampicillin, plus gentamicin	Vancomycin plus gentamicin
Streptococcus pneumoniae	Penicillin G	Cephalosporin Erythromycin Chloramphenicol
Staphylococci		
Staphylococcus aureus		
Non–penicillinase producer	Penicillin G	Cephalosporin Vancomycin
Penicillinase producer	Oxacillin Nafcillin	Vancomycin Clindamycin
Staphylococcus epidermidis	Vancomycin	
2. Gram-positive bacilli		
Listeria monocytogenes	Ampicillin	TMP-SMZ
Clostridia	Penicillin G	Chloramphenicol Clindamycin
Clostridium difficile	Vancomycin	Metronidazole
3. Gram-negative cocci		
Neisseria gonorrhoeae	Penicillin G	Tetracycline
Neisseria meningitidis	Penicillin G	Chloramphenicol
4. Gram-negative bacilli		
Bacteroides fragilis	Clindamycin Metronidazole	Chloramphenicol Cefoxitin
Campylobacter jejuni	Erythromycin	Tetracycline
Enterobacter	Aminoglycoside	
Escherichia coli		
UTI	Ampicillin TMP-SMZ	
Systemic	Aminoglycoside	Cefamandole Cefotaxime
Francisella tularensis (tularemia)	Streptomycin	Tetracycline Gentamicin
Haemophilus influenzae	Ampicillin (mild) Chloramphenicol (severe) TMP-SMZ	Cefuroxime Cefotaxime
Klebsiella pneumoniae	Aminoglycoside and/or cephalosporin	
Legionella	Erythromycin	Rifampin
Proteus mirabilis	Ampicillin	TMP-SMZ
Proteus (other sp.)	Aminoglycoside	
Pseudomonas aeruginosa	Aminoglycoside plus antipseudomonal beta-lactam (e.g., ticarcillin)	
Salmonella typhi	Chloramphenicol	TMP-SMZ Ampicillin
Salmonellae	Ampicillin	TMP-SMZ Chloramphenicol
Shigellae	TMP-SMZ	Ampicillin
5. Other organisms		
Chlamydia trachomatis	Doxycycline Tetracycline	Erythromycin
Mycoplasma pneumoniae	Erythromycin	Tetracycline
Rickettsiae	Tetracycline	Chloramphenicol

*The choice of antimicrobial therapy should always be reviewed in light of results of susceptibility testing.
Source: Adapted from *Medical Letter,* The choice of antimicrobial drugs. *Med. Lett. Drugs Ther.* 26:19, 1984.

B. Host factors
1. Patients with **underlying diseases** that impair their ability to respond to infection (e.g., leukopenia, corticosteroid therapy) generally require therapy with broad-spectrum bactericidal agents.
2. A history of **allergy** to antimicrobials should be sought before starting therapy.
3. Underlying **renal insufficiency** necessitates alterations in dosages of many antimicrobials (see Chap. 13) [5].
4. **Liver disease,** unless severe, rarely necessitates adjustments of dosages. Drugs excreted by the liver, however, should be avoided in the presence of hepatic insufficiency.
5. **Pregnancy.** No antimicrobial is known to be completely safe. Tetracyclines and metronidazole are contraindicated, and sulfonamides should be avoided in the third trimester. Most antimicrobials are detectable in human colostrum.
6. **Genetic factors.** Sulfonamides and primaquine should be avoided in patients with glucose 6-phosphate dehydrogenase (G-6-PD) deficiency.
C. Route of administration. Patients with serious infections should be treated with intravenous agents. In less acute situations, oral therapy can be used if gastrointestinal absorption of the antimicrobial is adequate.
D. Combinations. Combination therapy should be reserved for situations where antimicrobial synergy is advantageous or where multiple pathogens are likely; the latter, however, is uncommon. Antimicrobial combinations may also be necessary if the cause of infection is unclear, but single-drug therapy usually is initiated once the etiology is certain.
E. Cost. The least expensive of equally efficacious agents should be chosen.
F. Toxicity. If equally effective alternatives exist, the least toxic antimicrobial should be used in the lowest appropriate dosage and for the minimum time required to treat the infection.
G. Reassessment. The initial choice of an antimicrobial should always be reviewed in the light of subsequent clinical response and laboratory data.
III. Individual antimicrobial agents
A. Beta-lactam antibiotics include the penicillins and the cephalosporins.
1. **Mode of action.** The beta-lactam antibiotics act by binding with specific proteins in the bacterial cell membrane and interfering with cell-wall synthesis. Resistance to these agents is either intrinsic (possibly due to lack or unavailability of binding proteins) or mediated by beta-lactamases, enzymes that split the beta-lactam molecule, rendering it inactive.
2. **Individual agents** [55]
   a. **Penicillin G** is the drug of choice for many infections, including infections due to streptococci, *Neisseria meningitidis, Pasteurella multocida*, actinomycosis, and syphilis. In addition, most anaerobes are susceptible, with the exception of *Bacteroides fragilis*. Penicillin G is administered parenterally as a potassium salt in dosages ranging from 600,000–2,000,000 units IV q2–4h. Rapidly excreted by the kidney, the drug must be given at least q4h to be effective. Dosages should be reduced in renal failure. **Benzathine penicillin,** 1.2 million units, is a depot preparation that provides detectable drug levels for 3–4 weeks. **Phenoxymethyl penicillin** (penicillin V) is active orally; a 125-mg dose is equivalent to 200,000 units of penicillin G.
   b. **Beta-lactamase–stable penicillins** are indicated for the treatment of infections due to beta-lactamase–producing staphylococci. Parenteral preparations (with dosages) include **nafcillin** (2–3 gm IV q6h), **oxacillin** (1–2 gm IV q4h), and **methicillin** (1–2 gm IV q4h). **Dicloxacillin** (250–500 mg PO q6h) is an orally active agent.
   c. **Ampicillin** has a spectrum of activity against gram-positive organisms similar to that of penicillin G but is also active against many gram-negative bacilli. It is susceptible to beta-lactamases. **Amoxicillin** is an analog of ampicillin with similar activity; it may be preferable as an oral form because of less gastrointestinal upset. The usual dosage of ampicillin for mild infections is 500 mg PO q6h and for serious infections, 1–2 gm IV q4–6h. The dosage of amoxicillin is 250–500 mg PO q8h. Single-dose preparations are effective for gonorrhea and uncomplicated urinary tract infections in women. Ampicillin is also useful in the treatment of respiratory tract infections, chronic bronchitis, and infections due to salmonella.
   d. **Antipseudomonal penicillins.** There are now available several penicillins whose major indication is the treatment of infection due to *Pseudomonas*

aeruginosa. These agents include **carbenicillin** (100–600 mg/kg/day IV in 6 divided doses), **ticarcillin** (200–300 mg/kg/day IV in 6 doses), **piperacillin** (3–4 gm IV q4h), **mezlocillin** (3–4 gm IV q4–6h), and **azlocillin** (3–4 gm IV q4–6h). The spectrum of activity of these agents is otherwise similar to ampicillin. They remain susceptible to staphylococcal beta-lactamases.

e. Cephalosporins

(1) First-generation cephalosporins are active against most gram-positive organisms, including beta-lactamase–producing staphylococci, and against many gram-negative bacilli including *Klebsiella pneumoniae* [29]. *Pseudomonas,* anaerobes, *Haemophilus influenzae,* and enterococci, however, usually are resistant. These drugs are widely distributed in the body but do not enter the cerebrospinal fluid (CSF); they should not be used in the treatment of meningitis. Commonly used examples include **cefazolin** (0.5–2.0 gm IV q8h), **cephalothin** (1–2 gm IV q4–6h), and **cephalexin** (250–500 mg PO q6h).

(2) Second-generation cephalosporins offer selected expanded gram-negative coverage [29].

(a) Cefamandole, 1–2 gm IV q4–6h, is active against *H. influenzae* and most *Enterobacteriaceae.* It is widely used in surgical prophylaxis. It does not enter the CSF.

(b) Cefuroxime, 1–2 gm IV q8h, is similar to cefamandole but is also active against *Neisseria gonorrhoeae* and *Bacteroides.* It crosses the blood-brain barrier and can be used in meningitis.

(c) Cefoxitin, 1–2 gm IV q4–6h, it particularly useful in the treatment of anaerobic infections.

(3) Third-generation cephalosporins [34] have an expanded activity against gram-negative organisms but tend to be less active against gram-positive cocci, especially staphylococci. Problems have included superinfection with resistant organisms (e.g., enterococci) and bleeding diatheses.

There is not sufficient clinical experience with these agents to define their precise role in the treatment of infection. **Cefotaxime,** 1–2 gm IV q4–6h, or **moxalactam,** 1–2 gm IV q6h, is indicated in the treatment of gram-negative bacillary meningitis due to susceptible organisms. **Cefoperazone,** 1–2 gm IV q8–12h, and **ceftazidime,** 1–2 gm IV q8h, are more active against *P. aeruginosa.*

f. Imipenem, 500 mg IV q6–12h, is a newly introduced beta-lactam antibiotic with a broad range of activity against most gram-positive, gram-negative, and anaerobic bacteria. Its place in therapy has yet to be established, but its use should be limited to treatment of infections with susceptible organisms for which alternative therapy is not available.

g. Inhibitors of beta-lactamase. Clavulanic acid is a beta-lactam which has minimal intrinsic antibacterial activity but is a potent inhibitor of many beta-lactamases, including some of those produced by *S. aureus, H. influenzae, E. coli,* and *K. pneumoniae.* The enzymes produced by *P. aeruginosa, Serratia,* and *Enterobacter,* however, are resistant to these drugs. Further evaluation is needed, but this agent may prove useful in combination with amoxicillin (Augmentin) in the treatment of urinary tract infections, respiratory infections (including sinusitis), otitis media, and soft-tissue infections. The combination of clavulanic acid and ticarcillin (Timentin) is also available. Since CSF penetration is unreliable, these agents should not be used to treat meningitis. Methicillin-resistant staphylococci are resistant to these combinations.

3. Toxicity [15]

a. The principal side effect is **hypersensitivity** [45]. Hypersensitivity to penicillin occurs in about 0.1–1.0% of patients. Reactions are primarily caused by the immunogenicity of the metabolic by-products of penicillin. These form strong covalent bonds with tissue and serum proteins. The principal metabolite is benzyl penicilloyl, which is known as the major antigenic determinant. Other breakdown products (minor antigenic determinants) are important because they generally are responsible for anaphylactic reactions to penicillin. All penicillins share common immunogenicity. Although experience with the newer agents is limited, there is no evidence that they can be used safely in allergic patients. A patient with a history of a major reaction to penicillin should also be presumed allergic to cephalosporins.

Table 12-3. Aminoglycoside dosages in patients with normal renal function

Agent	Loading Dose	Maintenance dosage
Gentamicin	1.5–2.0 mg/kg	3–5 mg/kg/day
Tobramycin	1.5–2.0 mg/kg	3–5 mg/kg/day
Amikacin	7.5 mg/kg	15 mg/kg/day
Streptomycin		0.5–2.0 gm/day
Netilmicin	2 mg/kg	4–6 mg/kg/day
Kanamycin	7.5 mg/kg	15 mg/kg/day

   (1) Types of reactions
   　(a) Anaphylaxis occurs within 2–30 minutes of oral or parenteral administration of penicillin. It is characterized by erythema, urticaria, angioedema, bronchospasm, hypotension, and/or shock. Therapy includes administration of antihistamines, epinephrine, and/or corticosteroids (see Chaps. 3 and 31).
   　(b) Accelerated (cytotoxic) reaction. Mediated by IgG and complement, this reaction occurs 1–72 hours after administration of the drug. Clinically it is similar to anaphylaxis but usually less severe and responds to the administration of antihistamines.
   　(c) Late reactions are the most common form of reaction to penicillin. They occur days to weeks after initiation of the drug. Overt immunologic mechanisms (e.g., serum sickness or urticaria) are less common than nonspecific skin rashes (see Chap. 31).
   (2) Approach to the patient with a history of penicillin allergy
   　(a) An effective non–beta-lactam alternative drug should be used, if available.
   　(b) If the patient has a history of a minor reaction (e.g., skin rash after 1 week of ampicillin therapy), a cephalosporin may be considered. However, there is still a potential risk of anaphylaxis, and if a cephalosporin is used, the patient should be observed after the initial dose.
   　(c) If the patient cannot characterize the allergy, beta-lactams should be avoided.
   　(d) In specialized circumstances, skin testing with the antigenic determinants may be performed. A negative reaction makes anaphylaxis unlikely if the beta-lactam is given immediately but does not preclude other allergic reactions or the occurrence of an anaphylactic reaction in the future.
   b. Coombs'-positive hemolytic anemia, neutropenia, and thrombocytopenia are rare and probably immunologic in origin.
   c. Neurotoxicity (e.g., seizures) occurs with very high blood concentrations.
   d. Interstitial nephritis may occur, especially with methicillin.
   e. Bleeding problems have been observed with the newer beta-lactams; these include interference with the action of platelets by carbenicillin, ticarcillin, and piperacillin and prolongation of the bleeding time with moxalactam, cefamandole, and cefoperazone.
B. Aminoglycosides are bactericidal antibiotics that act through irreversible inhibition of bacterial protein synthesis by interference with ribosomal activity [35].
   1. Spectrum. The aminoglycosides are active against aerobic gram-negative cocci and bacilli and staphylococci. Other gram-positive organisms and anaerobes are resistant.
   2. Pharmacology. All aminoglycosides are poorly absorbed from the gastrointestinal tract and must be given parenterally. After administration, the aminoglycosides are rapidly distributed throughout the extracellular fluid compartment but do not cross the blood-brain barrier.
   3. Indications [35]
   　a. Infections caused by gram-negative bacilli. Gentamicin is the aminoglycoside of choice for proven or suspected serious systemic gram-negative infections. It should be combined with a beta-lactam in septicemia of unknown origin. Tobramycin and netilmicin are equivalent to gentamicin. Amikacin should be used if there is a high prevalence of gentamicin resistance.
   　b. Endocarditis. The aminoglycosides can be combined with a penicillin in the

management of streptococcal (especially enterococcal) and staphylococcal endocarditis.

    c. Streptomycin can be used in tuberculosis, tularemia, plague, and (in conjunction with a tetracycline) brucellosis.

   4. Dosages. The aminoglycosides have a low therapeutic index, and the dosage (Table 12-3) must be adjusted in each individual patient to account for age, sex, creatinine clearance, and body weight. In patients with renal failure, a normal loading dose is given, with an appropriate reduction made in maintenance doses [5]. Serum concentrations should be monitored in patients receiving prolonged therapy.

   5. Toxicity. The major disadvantages of the aminoglycosides are ototoxicity and nephrotoxicity.

    a. Ototoxicity, manifested by high-frequency hearing loss, vertigo, and ataxia, is more common in patients with renal impairment, those receiving the drug for a prolonged period, and those receiving other ototoxic agents. Damage to the eighth nerve may be irreversible.

    b. Nephrotoxicity [32] is due to tubular necrosis and is more likely to occur in patients exposed to other renal insults (e.g., dehydration, hypotension, other nephrotoxic agents) and in patients with preexisting renal disease.

C. Erythromycin [25]. This bacteriostatic agent acts by inhibiting ribosomal protein synthesis.

   1. The **spectrum** of activity includes gram-positive bacteria, *Legionella,* mycoplasmas, chlamydiae, and rickettsiae.

   2. Indications. Erythromycin is the drug of choice for infections due to *Mycoplasma pneumoniae, Legionella, Bordetella pertussis* (whooping cough), and *Campylobacter fetus.* It is a therapeutic alternative to penicillin in patients with streptococcal infections.

   3. Dosages. Erythromycin is generally administered orally in a dosage of 250–500 mg q6h; however, intravenous preparations are available. Because the drug is metabolized by the liver, its use should be avoided in the presence of liver disease. Dosage reduction is not necessary in patients with renal failure.

   4. Toxicity. The most common side effects are gastrointestinal upset with the oral form and thrombophlebitis with the intravenous preparation. Hepatotoxicity has been most commonly associated with the estolate preparation.

D. Chloramphenicol [25]

   1. Spectrum. Although bacterial resistance is an increasing problem, chloramphenicol is bacteriostatic against most bacteria, both aerobic and anaerobic, with the exception of *P. aeruginosa.* In addition, the spirochetes, mycoplasmas, rickettsiae, and chlamydiae are usually susceptible.

   2. Pharmacology. Administered orally or intravenously, chloramphenicol is widely distributed throughout the body, including the CSF. The drug is metabolized by the liver and does not accumulate in the presence of renal failure.

   3. Indications include typhoid fever, bacterial meningitis of unknown origin or due to *H. influenzae,* and brain abcess (in combination with penicillin G). Because of its toxicity, widespread empiric use of chloramphenicol is contraindicated. Effective alternative antimicrobials are usually available.

   4. The usual adult **dosage** is 0.5–1.0 gm PO or IV q6h.

   5. The most important **toxicity** is bone marrow suppression, of which there are two forms. Reversible hemopoietic toxicity is dose-related and can be detected by monitoring the complete blood count (CBC) and drug levels during therapy; in contrast, irreversible aplastic anemia is an idiosyncratic late reaction to the drug and is usually fatal.

E. Tetracyclines [25] are bacteriostatic agents that act by inhibiting ribosomal protein synthesis.

   1. Spectrum. Although possessing a wide spectrum of activity, including chlamydiae and rickettsiae, resistance is widespread, especially among the staphylococci and gram-negative bacteria.

   2. Pharmacology. The tetracyclines generally are administered orally. Absorption is improved if the drug is taken when fasting. Widely distributed throughout the body, the drug is excreted in the urine and the bile. Accumulation occurs in renal failure, and with the exception of doxycycline, tetracyclines should not be used in renal failure.

   3. The principal **clinical uses** of tetracyclines are treating nongonococcal urethritis, Rocky Mountain spotted fever, Lyme disease, and chronic bronchitis.

They are alternatives in the penicillin-allergic patient with syphilis or *P. multocida* infection and may be used for infections with mycoplasma.

4. **Dosages.** Tetracycline HCl, 250–500 mg PO q6h, is the preparation of choice. Doxycycline, 100 mg PO q12–24h, is excreted by the liver and is preferred in renal failure.

5. **Toxicity.** Gastrointestinal upset is common. Photosensitivity may be induced in susceptible individuals. The tetracyclines should not be administered to pregnant women or to children under 12 years of age because of their effect on bone growth and tooth pigmentation.

F. **Vancomycin** [25]

1. **Spectrum.** Vancomycin is a bactericidal agent active against most gram-positive bacteria.

2. **Indications.** Systemic vancomycin is the agent of choice in infections caused by methicillin-resistant staphylococci. It is also indicated for the treatment of staphylococcal and enterococcal infections in patients allergic to penicillin. Oral vancomycin, 125 mg PO q6h, is indicated in the treatment of colitis caused by *Clostridium difficile* (pseudomembranous colitis).

3. **Dosages.** The drug is generally administered IV in a dosage of 500 mg q6h. Infusion should be slow over a period of 30–60 minutes, as rapid infusion is associated with a histaminelike reaction (the "redneck syndrome"). Vancomycin is excreted by the kidneys, and the dosage must be reduced in renal insufficiency.

4. **Toxicity.** The major side effect of vancomycin is ototoxicity. Serum levels should be monitored during prolonged usage. Skin rashes and phlebitis also occur.

G. **Sulfonamides** [38] are bacteriostatic drugs that interfere with folic acid synthesis in bacteria.

1. **Indications.** Although bacterial resistance has limited the clinical usefulness of the sulfonamides, they are used in the treatment of uncomplicated urinary tract infection (UTI), nocardiosis, chancroid, and when combined with pyrimethamine, toxoplasmosis.

2. **Dosages.** Sulfisoxazole, 1 gm PO q6h, is used in the treatment of UTI; alternatively, a single dose of 2 gm may be given. Sulfadiazine, 1 gm PO or IV q4–6h, is used in the treatment of nocardiasis.

3. **Toxicity**

   a. Hypersensitivity reactions are common and include skin rashes, vasculitis, erythema multiforme, and the Stevens-Johnson syndrome. These are more frequent with the long-acting sulfonamides.

   b. The sulfonamides are contraindicated in the latter part of pregnancy and in neonates because of the increased risk of neonatal kernicterus.

   c. The sulfonamides should be avoided in patients with G-6-PD deficiency, because of the increased risk of hemolysis.

H. **Trimethoprim** [38] has a slow bactericidal effect against many gram-negative bacilli. It acts by inhibiting bacterial dihydrofolate reductase. Although currently approved only for the treatment of UTI in a dosage of 100 mg PO qd, it has been available combined with sulfamethoxazole for many years (see sec. I). Side effects of trimethoprim include megaloblastic anemia, bone marrow suppression, and skin rashes.

I. **Trimethoprim-sulfamethoxazole (TMP-SMZ, co-trimoxazole)** is a fixed-dose combination of trimethoprim and sulfamethoxazole in a ratio of 1:5 [38, 39]. In theory, the combination is synergistic and bactericidal and has the advantage of less bacterial resistance.

1. **Spectrum.** TMP-SMZ is active against many gram-positive cocci and most gram-negative bacilli, except *P. aeruginosa.*

2. **Indications.** TMP-SMZ is useful in the treatment of UTI, prostatitis, chronic bronchitis, acute otitis media, sinusitis, and shigella and salmonella infections. TMP-SMZ in a dosage of 20 mg of trimethoprim/kg/day is the treatment of choice for pneumonia due to *P. carinii.*

3. **Dosages.** TMP-SMZ is administered orally or intravenously. The oral preparation contains 80 mg of trimethoprim and 400 mg of sulfamethoxazole in the single-strength formulation, and the usual dosage is 2 single-strength tablets bid. Reduction in dosage or avoidance of the drug is recommended in patients with renal insufficiency.

4. **Toxicity**

   a. As the combination contains a sulfonamide, it shares the hypersensitivity reactions of that class of agents and **should not be administered to patients with a history of sensitivity to sulfonamides.**

    b. Megaloblastic anemia can occur due to folate deficiency. This can be circumvented (without interfering with the antibacterial action) by the administration of folinic acid.

    c. Bone marrow suppression can occur, especially at high dosages. Patients with the acquired immunodeficiency syndrome seem particularly susceptible to this complication [22].

J. Clindamycin [26]

  1. Spectrum. Clindamycin is active against many gram-positive organisms and most anaerobic bacteria.

  2. Indications. Clindamycin is used in anaerobic infections, especially where *B. fragilis* is suspected. It is an alternative to penicillin in the treatment of lung abcesses.

  3. Dosages. Both oral and parenteral preparations are available. The usual adult dosage is 300–600 mg PO or IV q6h. Dosages do not have to be reduced in the presence of renal failure; however, dosage reduction may be necessary in the presence of severe liver disease.

  4. Toxicity. The most important side effect of clindamycin is diarrhea. A minority of patients may develop pseudomembranous colitis, which is caused by a toxin produced by *C. difficile*. Other side effects are rare and include allergic reactions and hepatotoxicity.

K. Metronidazole [19]

  1. Spectrum. Metronidazole is active against most anaerobic bacteria, *Trichomonas vaginalis, Giardia lamblia,* and *Entamoeba histolytica*.

  2. Indications

    a. The major indication is anaerobic infection where *B. fragilis* is the significant pathogen. It is particularly useful in cases of bacteremia and intravascular infection (e.g., endocarditis, infected shunt) with this organism. Metronidazole is also useful in the management of brain abscesses.

    b. Metronidazole can also be used to treat trichomoniasis, nonspecific vaginitis, amebiasis, and giardiasis.

  3. Dosages. Metronidazole is administered orally or intravenously, in a dosage of 250–750 mg q6–8h. The drug is distributed throughout the body, including the CSF. Metabolism is by the liver, with excretion of metabolites by the kidneys.

  4. Toxicity

    a. Mild gastrointestinal upset and a metallic taste are common with the oral preparation.

    b. Alcohol should be avoided because of a disulfiram-like reaction.

    c. A peripheral neuropathy may occur with prolonged use.

    d. The mutagenicity of the drug contraindicates its use in pregnancy. Metronidazole is carcinogenic in rodents, but there is no evidence of carcinogenicity in humans.

L. Antifungal agents [9, 30]

  1. Amphotericin B is a polyene antibiotic that acts by binding ergosterol, the principal sterol of fungal cell walls.

    a. Indications. Because of its toxicity, its use is reserved for the treatment of documented or probable systemic fungal infections.

    b. Administration. Amphotericin B can only be administered intravenously. A test dose of 1 mg in 100 ml of 5% dextrose is given initially, and if tolerated, the drug is gradually increased to its maintenance dosage, 0.3–1.0 mg/kg/day.

    c. Toxicity includes immediate hypersensitivity reactions, fever, hypotension, nausea and vomiting during administration, hypokalemia, and nephropathy that may be irreversible.

  2. Nystatin is a polyene antibiotic that is given topically or orally for the treatment of localized cutaneous or mucosal candidiasis.

  3. Ketoconazole is an orally active imidazole agent that is fungistatic for a wide variety of fungi. It is useful in chronic mucocutaneous candidiasis, localized pulmonary histoplasmosis, localized cryptococcosis, and paracoccidiomycosis. The usual dosage is 200–600 mg daily. Absorption is dependent on gastric acidity and may be impaired in achlorhydric patients or patients taking concurrent antacids or H_2-blockers. Drug levels should be monitored. Side effects include nausea, gynecomastia, and hepatitis.

  4. Miconazole is a parenteral imidazole used in the treatment of systemic candidal infections. It is primarily used when amphotericin B cannot be given. The dosage is 400–1200 mg IV q8h.

5. **Clotrimazole** is an imidazole available in topical form for the treatment of candidiasis and some dermatophytoses.
6. **5-fluorocytosine** (5-FC) is a semisynthetic pyrimidine derivative that acts by interfering with fungal nucleic acid synthesis. Its usefulness, when used alone, is limited by the rapid development of resistance. However, when combined with amphotericin B, 5-FC is useful in the treatment of cryptococcal meningitis and possibly systemic candidiasis. The oral dosage (150 mg/kg/day) must be reduced in patients with renal failure. Toxicity includes significant gastrointestinal upset and bone marrow suppression.
7. **Griseofulvin** is an antibiotic active against most dermatophytes. The dosage is 0.5–1.0 gm/day PO given for a prolonged period (e.g., 1–3 months for skin and hair infections and up to 1 year for toenail infections).
M. **Antiviral agents**
   1. **Amantadine** is useful in the treatment and prophylaxis of infection with the influenza A virus [12]. It acts by blocking early viral replication. Treatment is reserved for patients with underlying cardiopulmonary disease and for the seriously ill. To be effective, amantidine must be given early in the infection. The dosage is 200 mg PO qd. Side effects of neurologic dysfunction (e.g., confusion, slurring of speech, and blurred vision) are seen more frequently in the elderly.
   2. **Acyclovir** acts against DNA viruses by inhibiting DNA synthesis.
      a. **Spectrum.** It is highly active against herpes simplex virus and to a lesser extent against varicella-zoster virus [21]. It is ineffective against cytomegalovirus.
      b. **Indications and dosages.** Acyclovir, 5 mg/kg IV q8h, is useful in the treatment of herpes simplex infections in immunosuppressed hosts and may also be used in severe symptomatic primary infections with herpes simplex virus. Higher dosages, 10 mg/kg IV q8h, are used in the management of herpes zoster [21] and in herpes simplex encephalitis [40]. Oral acyclovir, 200 mg PO 5 times/day, is effective in genital herpes. Topical acyclovir (5% ointment) reduces viral shedding and symptoms in primary herpes simplex infections; gloves should be worn when applying the ointment to prevent autoinoculation.
   3. **Vidarabine** (adenine arabinoside) acts by inhibiting DNA synthesis. It is most active against herpes simplex and varicella-zoster viruses [21]. Its usefulness is limited by significant toxicity, particularly gastrointestinal and neurologic, and by the need to give the drug in a large volume of fluid. Vidarabine is currently reserved for the treatment of herpes simplex encephalitis and disseminated herpes simplex infection in neonates.
   4. Ophthalmic preparations of **trifluorothymidine** and **idoxuridine** are available for the treatment of herpes simplex keratitis.

Specific Infections

I. **Septicemia** occurs when the presence of microorganisms in the bloodstream is associated with signs of toxemia. Gram-negative bacilli are the most frequent pathogens causing septicemia, but a similar clinical picture may be seen in infections with gram-positive bacteria (e.g., *Staphylococcus aureus*), rickettsiae, and fungi (e.g., *Candida*). Early initiation of appropriate antimicrobial therapy is vital in reducing the high mortality associated with septicemia [24].
A. **Clinical features.** Patients usually present with fever and tachycardia, although some patients may have a subnormal temperature. Respiratory alkalosis is often an early sign. Hypotension may be present, and septic shock may ensue. Since elderly or immunosuppressed patients may exhibit few signs of infection, sepsis should be considered in such patients presenting with hypotension or unexplained clinical deterioration. Since most blood-borne infections originate from an extravascular focus, careful consideration of the epidemiology, history, and physical findings may be extremely valuable in localizing the source.
   1. **Normal hosts.** Usually localization is possible. In the absence of such findings, a travel history should be sought. Typhoid fever (septicemia with *S. typhi*) is endemic in many underdeveloped countries. Rocky Mountain spotted fever and tularemia should be considered in patients recently in rural areas, especially if there is a history of tick bite. Contact with wild mammals in the southwest should suggest the possibility of plague. Ectopic pregnancy and septic abortion should be considered in young women with septicemia without an obvious cause.

Table 12-4. Antimicrobial therapy of septicemia

Underlying patient problem	Antimicrobials
Leukopenia	Ticarcillin, 3 gm q4h, plus gentamicin*
Splenectomy	Ampicillin, 2 gm q4h
Drug addict	Nafcillin, 2 gm q6h, plus gentamicin*
Probable pelvic or abdominal focus	Ampicillin, 2 gm q4h, plus clindamycin, 600 mg q6h, plus gentamicin*
Urinary tract source	Ampicillin, 2 gm q4h, plus gentamicin*
Pulmonary source	Ampicillin, 2 gm q4h, plus gentamicin*
No obvious source	Cefazolin, 2 gm q8h, plus gentamicin*

*The appropriate dosage of gentamicin is a 2 mg/kg IV loading dose, followed by a 5 mg/kg/day IV maintenance dose (in 3 divided doses), provided renal function is normal.

   2. Abnormal hosts
   a. Recent abdominal surgery may result in abscess formation with gram-negative and anaerobic organisms.
   b. Urinary catheterization predisposes to UTI with resultant gram-negative septicemia.
   c. Granulocytopenic patients commonly develop gram-negative sepsis. *P. aeruginosa* is a notable pathogen in these patients.
   d. Patients who have had a splenectomy are at risk of infection with encapsulated bacteria, especially *S. pneumoniae* and *H. influenzae.*
   e. Intravenous drug abusers develop bacteremia with staphylococci and gram-negative bacilli.
B. Diagnosis. Septicemia is a clinical diagnosis, which is confirmed by the presence of microorganisms in the bloodstream. Blood cultures should always be performed prior to the initiation of antimicrobial therapy.
C. Treatment
   1. Supportive measures to maintain blood pressure and tissue oxygenation and to reverse acidosis and coagulopathies are extremely important.
   2. Appropriate **antimicrobial therapy** should be directed against the probable source, as outlined in Table 12-4.
   3. When indicated, appropriate **surgical therapy** (e.g., incision and drainage) of infection is essential.
D. Disposition. Hospitalization, often in an intensive care unit, is mandatory.
II. Infections of the respiratory system
A. Acute rhinitis (the common cold) is usually viral in origin; the common pathogens include rhinoviruses, coronaviruses, and adenoviruses. Infection is most common in winter and is characterized by a mild, self-limited, and usually afebrile course lasting 4–7 days. Purulent sinusitis is a rare complication. Symptoms include nasal discharge or obstruction, sneezing, pharyngeal discomfort, cough, and malaise. The physical examination is unremarkable, apart from rhinorrhea. Treatment is symptomatic.
B. Acute pharyngitis
   1. Etiology. Acute infection of the throat can be caused by many bacteria and viruses. Important viral pathogens include the Epstein-Barr virus, herpes simplex virus, adenoviruses, and enteroviruses. Among the bacterial pathogens are group A beta-hemolytic streptococci (which account for 5–10% of adult pharyngitis), *Corynebacterium diphtheriae, M. pneumoniae, N. gonorrhoeae,* and *Chlamydia trachomatis.*
   2. Clinical features. Symptoms include a sore throat, fever, chills, myalgias, and headache. The physical examination may be normal; however, most commonly the throat is erythematous, and in severe cases, a white exudate may be present on the tonsils or posterior pharyngeal wall. Generally, this exudate is easily removable; however, a thick gray membrane that is difficult to remove suggests diphtheria. Vesicles in the pharynx indicate herpes simplex or herpangina. Cervical adenopathy may be present; generalized adenopathy or splenomegaly suggests infectious mononucleosis. Skin rashes occur in many pharyngeal infections; a scarlatiniform rash is associated with infection with beta-hemolytic streptococci. Viral infections usually cause diffuse erythema or urticaria.

3. **Complications** of pharyngitis include otitis media, sinusitis, peritonsillar abscess, and retropharyngeal space infections.
4. **Diagnosis.** The history and examination may allow the physician to identify those patients in whom further investigation is necessary.
   a. **Throat cultures** are indicated in certain situations.
      (1) The primary purpose of throat cultures has been the identification of group A beta-hemolytic streptococci to prevent acute rheumatic fever. However, with the rarity of rheumatic fever, throat cultures for this purpose can be reserved for the small subset of patients at major risk of streptococcal infection. These include patients with a previous history of rheumatic fever, symptomatic patients exposed to a patient with streptococcal pharyngitis, and patients with significant infection (e.g., fever, pharyngeal exudate, and cervical adenopathy).
      (2) Patients who fail to clear a pharyngeal infection despite symptomatic therapy should be cultured.
      (3) Specific cultures for *N. gonorrhoeae* are performed if indicated by history.
      (4) If diphtheria is suspected, specific cultures are required.
   b. **Serology** (i.e., a Monospot test for heterophil agglutinin) is useful when infectious mononucleosis is suspected. A differential white blood cell count (looking for atypical lymphocytes) should also be performed.
5. **Management.** Most cases of pharyngitis do not require antibiotic therapy, as the condition is self-limited and benign. Treatment for group A beta-hemolytic streptococci should be given if the culture is positive, the patient is at high risk of developing rheumatic fever, or the diagnosis is strongly suspected pending the results of culture. Treatment schedules include penicillin VK, 250 mg PO qid for 10 days; benzathine penicillin, 1.2 million units IM; or erythromycin, 250 mg PO qid, for 10 days. Hospitalization and parenteral therapy are indicated when the patient is unable to take oral fluids or there is impending airway obstruction. Surgical drainage of abscesses may be necessary.
C. **Influenza**
   1. **Pathogens.** The syndrome of influenza is caused by the enveloped RNA viruses, influenza viruses types A, B, and C [14]. Influenza A causes the major and usually annual epidemics; influenza B contributes to significant endemic infection, while influenza C is unimportant in human disease.
   2. **Clinical features.** Infection is acquired by inhalation of respiratory droplets from affected individuals. After an incubation period of 1–3 days, the patient suddenly experiences a **systemic illness** with high fevers, myalgias, headache, dry cough, and nasal discharge. Ocular symptoms of photophobia and conjunctival irritation also occur. The duration of the illness is usually 3–5 days with a gradual but complete recovery within 7–10 days.
   3. **Diagnosis** can be confirmed by viral cultures or serology. If epidemiologic evidence indicates the presence of influenza A in the community, diagnostic procedures are unnecessary.
   4. **Treatment**
      a. **Symptomatic treatment** with antipyretics usually is sufficient. The use of salicylates in children with influenza is not recommended because of the association with Reye's syndrome.
      b. Amantadine, 200 mg PO qd, may be used for seriously affected patients or those with underlying cardiopulmonary disease. Effective therapy requires early initiation of the drug within 24 hours of the onset of symptoms [13]. Treatment should be continued for 48 hours after defervescence.
      c. A vaccine is available for prophylaxis of those at high risk. Amantadine, 200 mg PO qd, is useful in preventing influenza in unvaccinated susceptible patients, particularly in the presence of an epidemic.
   5. **Complications.** The major complication is pneumonia, which may be primary viral or secondary to bacteria, especially *S. aureus, H. influenzae,* or *S. pneumoniae.* Since distinction between primary and secondary forms of infection of the lung is difficult, antibacterial therapy is usually indicated. The initial choice, pending bacteriologic identification, is ampicillin, 1–2 gm IV q6h, plus oxacillin, 2 gm IV q6h. Cefuroxime, 1.5 gm IV q8h, or cefamandole, 2 gm IV q6h, is an alternative.
   6. **Disposition.** Hospitalization is indicated in the presence of complications.
D. **Pneumonia**
   1. **Etiology.** Infection of the lung parenchyma may be caused by many pathogens.

Important bacterial causes include *S. pneumoniae* (pneumococcus), *H. influen-zae*, *M. pneumoniae*, *Legionella pneumophila*, *K. pneumoniae*, *S. aureus*, and *Mycobacterium tuberculosis*. Among the nonbacterial etiologies of pneumonia are viruses (e.g., influenza virus, adenoviruses), fungi (e.g., *Histoplasma cap-sulatum, Coccidiodes immitis,* and aspergilli), and protozoa (e.g., *P. carinii*).

2. **Clinical approach.** The diagnosis of pneumonia is suspected in patients com-plaining of fever, chest pain, and the production of purulent sputum and is supported by the presence of pulmonary consolidation or an abnormal chest radiograph. Because of the diverse potential pathogens, an etiologic diagnosis should be made to direct appropriate therapy.

   a. **Epidemiologic considerations** may aid in making an etiologic diagnosis; the following points should be considered.

      (1) **Normal hosts**

         (a) Community-acquired pneumonia is most commonly due to the pneumococcus. In young adults, infection due to *M. pneumoniae* should be considered. *Legionella* infections are more likely in older patients, as are gram-negative bacillary infections [48].

         (b) A travel history should be obtained. Histoplasmosis and coccidi-oidomycosis are endemic to the Mississippi Valley and the south-west, respectively.

         (c) A recent contact with wild mammals raises the possibility of plague or tularemia. Tularemia should also be suspected if there is a history of a tick bite. Psittacosis is a chlamydial infection acquired from birds.

      (2) **Abnormal hosts**

         (a) Institutionalized or recently hospitalized patients are prone to infec-tion with gram-negative bacilli.

         (b) Alcoholics are prone to aspiration pneumonia. They are also apt to be infected with *K. pneumoniae* or *M. tuberculosis*.

         (c) Patients with a seizure disorder, disorders of swallowing, poor denti-tion, or esophageal problems are likely to develop aspiration pneu-monia.

         (d) Diabetics are susceptible to staphylococcal infections.

         (e) Immunosuppressed patients (e.g., patients with neutropenia or on steroid therapy) are susceptible to infection with many opportunistic organisms [28].

         (f) Male homosexuals may be infected with unusual pathogens (e.g., *P. carinii*).

   b. **Investigations**

      (1) **Sputum analysis.** A sputum sample should be obtained for Gram stain and culture. An adequate sputum sample (i.e., few epithelial cells and many leukocytes) determines the initial choice of antimicrobial therapy. The usefulness of sputum examination correlates directly with the ade-quacy of the specimen. If tuberculosis is a consideration, an acid-fast stain of the sputum should be performed.

      (2) **Blood cultures** should be performed in febrile or septic patients.

      (3) **Chest radiograph.** Although certain pathogens have characteristic radiologic patterns (e.g., cavitary disease with *Klebsiella*), often the ra-diographic features are not diagnostic.

      (4) Acute and convalescent **serology** may aid in the diagnosis of many infections (e.g., mycoplasma and *Legionella* infections, histoplasmosis, coccidioidomycosis, psittacosis, and tularemia).

      (5) Invasive studies (e.g., bronchoscopy, lung biopsy) may be required in the diagnosis of pneumonia in immunocompromised hosts.

      (6) If a pleural effusion is present, thoracentesis (see Chap. 38) should be performed and a specimen submitted for analysis, Gram stain, and cul-ture (see Chap. 7).

3. **Differential diagnosis** of pneumonia includes pulmonary embolism, allergic alveolitis, interstitial fibrosis, and malignancy.

4. **Treatment**

   a. **Antimicrobial therapy.** Selection of antimicrobial therapy should be based on the clinical presentation and the findings on Gram stain of the sputum and subsequently adjusted according to culture results.

      (1) **Gram-positive cocci** in pairs (diplococci) suggest pneumococcal infec-tion. Treatment of choice is penicillin G, 1 gm PO qid, or 2.4–12.0

million units IV qd. Erythromycin, 500 mg PO or IV qid, is used in patients allergic to penicillin.

(2) **Gram-positive cocci** in clusters suggest staphylococcal infection for which the therapy is a beta-lactamase stable penicillin (e.g., oxacillin, 2 gm IV q4–6h).

(3) If **gram-negative bacilli** are identified, the patient should be treated with a combination of an aminoglycoside plus a cephalosporin, pending identification of the organism.

(4) **Gram-negative coccobacilli** suggest *H. influenzae.* The treatment of choice is ampicillin, 1–2 gm IV q4h, or cefamandole, 1–2 gm IV q6h.

(5) **Mixed flora** in an adequate sample suggests aspiration pneumonia. The treatment of choice is penicillin, 2 million units IV q4h, or clindamycin, 600 mg IV qid.

(6) If **no organism** is seen or no sample is obtained but bacterial infection is suspected, therapy should be directed against the most likely pathogen. Erythromycin, which is effective against gram-positive organisms, *M. pneumoniae,* and Legionnaires' disease, is the drug of choice in treating community-acquired pneumonia; the dosage is 500 mg IV or PO qid. Ampicillin, 0.5–1.0 gm PO q6h, or TMP-SMZ, 2 single-strength tablets bid, is useful in the outpatient with underlying chronic obstructive pulmonary disease. TMP-SMZ, 5 mg TMP/kg IV q6h, should be started empirically for the treatment of *P. carinii* in patients at risk for the acquired immunodeficiency syndrome (AIDS) who present with pneumonia and associated hypoxia. Pneumonia in patients immunocompromised by age, alcoholism, diabetes mellitus, or steroid therapy should be treated initially with a combination of gentamicin, 1.5 mg/kg IV q8h, and cefazolin, 2 gm IV q8h. Gentamicin, 1.5 mg/kg IV q8h, and ticarcillin, 3 gm IV q4h, should be commenced empirically to treat pneumonia in the granulocytopenic patient. Amphotericin B may also be necessary if fungal infection is a consideration.

b. Supportive care. Oxygen should be given when indicated. Chest physiotherapy aids in drainage of secretions. Potentially infected pleural spaces should be drained.

5. Disposition. Many patients, particularly young adults, may be managed in the community provided adequate follow-up is available. Hospitalization is indicated for the elderly, immunocompromised patients, patients with signs of sepsis or respiratory distress, and those patients who are unable to tolerate oral medications or who fail outpatient therapy.

E. Lung abscess

1. The **diagnosis** of a lung abscess is made by observing a cavitary lesion on a chest radiograph.

2. Etiology

a. Mixed **anaerobic aspiration** is the most common cause [3] and occurs in those patients prone to aspiration of pharyngeal and gastric contents.

b. Necrotizing pneumonia due to *K. pneumoniae* or *S. aureus* may produce a similar picture to that of a primary abscess.

c. Septic emboli may cause abscesses. *S. aureus* is the common pathogen in intravenous drug addicts. Anaerobic organisms (e.g., *B. fragilis*) are associated with emboli from pelvic thrombophlebitis.

3. Microbial diagnosis is determined on the clinical presentation. The sputum Gram stain and culture may be unrewarding in abscesses secondary to aspiration. Blood cultures should be performed.

4. Management

a. Hospitalization is warranted.

b. Drainage either by physiotherapy or bronchoscopy should be performed.

c. Penicillin, 2 million units IV q4h, or clindamycin, 600 mg IV q6h, is appropriate for the usual abscesses acquired by aspiration [27]. If specific organisms are isolated, treatment should be modified appropriately.

F. Tuberculosis

1. Pathogenesis. Tuberculosis (TB) is caused by an aerobic bacterium, *M. tuberculosis,* and is spread by infected patients by small-particle aerosolization. These aerosols are inhaled, with primary infection occurring in the respiratory tract. Local lymph nodes are subsequently infected, and dissemination may ensue. Control of the infection is achieved by cellular immunity, with hypersensitivity being a feature of the immune response. A major feature of tuberculous infection is its ability to remain dormant, with possible reactivation many years later. The organism is a slow-growing, obligate aerobe that possesses the ability to survive in an intracellular environment, remain metabolically inert, and tolerate unfavorable conditions (such as are found in caseous material).

2. **Presentation.** TB has many clinical manifestations, both pulmonary and extrapulmonary.

   a. **Pulmonary TB** can present in several ways.

      (1) **Tuberculous pneumonia** is newly acquired TB, which characteristically affects the middle and lower lobes and is highly infectious.

      (2) **Tuberculous pleural disease** occurs in the early post-primary phase, causes an isolated pleural effusion, and is associated with low infectivity.

      (3) **Cavitary TB** is reactivated tuberculosis. The features are those classically associated with TB, that is, fever, night sweats, and weight loss. Cavitary lesions usually occur in the apices and are highly infectious.

   b. **Extrapulmonary TB,** which is always reactivated disease, can involve many sites: lymph nodes, liver, urinary tract, bones, gastrointestinal tract, skin, and meninges. None is associated with high infectivity.

   c. **Miliary TB** reflects bacteremic dissemination and is characterized by the occurrence of multiple, widespread, small nodules of infection. It can occur in either primary or reactivation TB.

3. The **diagnosis** of TB is suggested by the radiographic appearance (e.g., apical cavitary lesions), particularly in individuals at high risk for the disease (e.g., the elderly, alcoholics, patients with underlying malignancy, American Indians, immigrants from underdeveloped countries). The diagnosis is established by culturing the organism. The demonstration of typical acid-fast bacilli in appropriate clinical specimens is sufficient to justify therapy pending final identification. A tuberculin skin test may be performed. Its interpretation, however, depends on intact cellular immunity, does not reflect current disease activity, and requires 48 hours to be read. Consequently, its usefulness in the emergency setting is limited.

4. **Management**

   a. **Antituberculous therapy.** Patients in whom active pulmonary tuberculosis is suspected are usually hospitalized for verification of the diagnosis, initiation of therapy, patient education, and isolation. Patients who are believed to be infectious should wear masks while therapy is initiated. Standard treatment is with isoniazid, 5–10 mg/kg PO qd up to 300 mg qd, and rifampin, 10 mg/kg PO qd up to 600 mg qd [1].

   b. **Prophylaxis.** Preventive therapy is recommended for household members and other close contacts of infected patients, patients with a tuberculin skin test conversion within the past 2 years, persons with positive reactions to tuberculin and abnormal chest radiographs, and previously untreated tuberculin skin test reactors under the age of 35 years [1]. Chemoprophylaxis with isoniazid, 300 mg PO qd, is administered for 1 year.

III. **Urinary tract infections**

   A. **Pathogenesis.** The most common mode of acquisition of UTI is ascending infection from the urethra through the bladder and ureter to the kidney. Hematogenous infection affecting the kidney and subsequently the lower tract is less common but should be considered with infections due to *S. aureus.* Females are affected more commonly than males, although the sex difference is less marked in neonates and the elderly. Other predisposing factors include obstruction (at any level of the urinary tract), the presence of foreign bodies (i.e., catheters, stones), vesicoureteral reflux, and sexual intercourse in women.

   B. **Microbiology.** Most UTIs are caused by the enterobacteriaceae, especially *E. coli. Staphylococcus saprophyticus* is an important pathogen in young, sexually active women. Enterococci, *S. aureus,* and *Candida albicans* are important nosocomial pathogens.

   C. **Clinical features.** UTIs can be divided into two categories: (1) infection in the parenchyma and pelvis of the kidney (pyelonephritis or upper-tract disease) and (2) infection confined to the bladder and urethra (lower-tract disease). Upper-tract disease and lower-tract infection, however, are difficult to distinguish on clinical grounds alone. Urinary frequency, dysuria, and suprapubic discomfort are symptoms of lower-tract infection but do not exclude upper-tract involvement. Dysuria may also be caused by urethritis and in women by vaginitis. Classic features of upper-tract disease include high fever, shaking chills, and lumbar pain; nausea and vomiting may also occur. However, all these features may also be seen in severe cystitis.

D. Diagnosis. The diagnosis of UTI is based on the demonstration of a significant number of microorganisms in a clean specimen of urine obtained from a symptomatic patient.

1. **Urine culture.** The classic criterion for the diagnosis of significant bacteriuria (i.e., > 100,000 organisms/ml) was determined in studies on women with acute pyelonephritis. Recent investigations [43], however, have shown that this criterion is not sufficiently sensitive to diagnose many patients with lower-tract infections. Consequently, the value and interpretation of a urine culture reflect the clinical situation from which it was obtained. A culture may not be necessary in young, sexually active women whose urinalysis suggests infection; however, a urine culture is necessary in other patients.

2. **Urinalysis.** Microscopic examination of an unspun specimen of urine may show pyuria (i.e., 8 leukocytes/high-power field) or bacteria (under oil immersion). Both of these findings indicate infection in a symptomatic patient.

E. Management

1. **Treatment of UTI in women. Single-dose antibiotic therapy** is appropriate for women with lower-tract symptoms and signs and a urinalysis suggestive of infection, provided there are no complications or contraindications [23]. Therapy includes amoxicillin, 3 gm; sulfisoxazole, 2 gm; or TMP-SMZ, 2 double-strength tablets.

   a. Contraindications to single-dose therapy

   (1) Women in whom acute pyelonephritis is suspected require 7–14 days of antibiotic therapy.

   (2) Patients with suspected bacteremia, the elderly, and patients with serious underlying disease need a 14- to 21-day course of therapy.

   (3) Patients with a prior history of genitourinary tract abnormalities or known calculous disease should be treated for 7–14 days and referred for evaluation.

   (4) Pregnant women should be treated for 7–14 days and referred to an obstetrician. Sulfonamides and tetracylines are contraindicated during pregnancy.

   b. Failure of single-dose therapy. A urine culture should be obtained from all patients who remain symptomatic despite therapy, and a more prolonged course of antibiotics administered based on the results of the culture. Some of these patients may have subclinical pyelonephritis and require prolonged therapy. Urethral infection with *C. trachomatis* or *N. gonorrhoeae* should be considered in patients with pyuria and negative routine cultures [42].

2. **Treatment of UTI in men.** There is no evidence to support the use of single-dose therapy for UTI in men. A culture should be obtained and patients treated for at least 7–14 days. Referral to a urologist is necessary.

3. **"Recurrent urinary infections"** may be (a) relapses with the same organism (usually due to uneradicated tissue infection), which justifies prolonged antibiotic treatment, or (b) true recurrences with different organisms, which may necessitate further investigation and/or prophylaxis. Patients who present with recurrent UTIs should be treated in the usual manner and referred for assessment.

4. **Patients with indwelling urinary catheters.** Bacteriuria is inevitable in patients with chronic catheterization. Consequently, catheterization should be undertaken only when absolutely required and with strict aseptic technique. Prophylactic antibiotics are of no value and merely select for bacterial resistance. Antimicrobial therapy should be given only for known or suspected systemic infection, presumed secondary to urinary infection. Since bacterial resistance is common, urine cultures and susceptibilities should be sought as an aid in the choice of antibiotics.

F. Disposition. With single-dose therapy, patients need only return if failure or relapse occurs. Other patients should be seen 2–3 days after start of therapy. Hospitalization is indicated for patients with complicated infections (e.g., immunocompromised patients, pregnant patients with upper-tract disease, patients with nephrolithiasis and upper-tract infection, patients unable to take oral medications) or suspected bacteremia.

IV. Sexually transmitted diseases

A. Gonorrhea is caused by a gram-negative diplococcus, *N. gonorrhoeae,* which is a fastidious organism with specific growth requirements.

1. **Clinical features**

   a. Asymptomatic carriage on the pharynx, urethra, rectum, and cervix is common.

b. Urethritis is the most common presentation in men, who complain of dysuria and a mucoid discharge 2–5 days after exposure. A concomitant nongonococcal urethritis is common.

c. Endocervicitis is the usual form of infection in women. Symptoms are often mild and nonspecific, such as dysuria, urinary frequency, and an abnormal discharge. Infection may extend to cause salpingitis and chronic pelvic inflammatory disease, and sterility may ensue.

d. Anorectal infection, which is seen in male homosexuals and in females with contiguous genital infection, may be asymptomatic, cause nonspecific symptoms (e.g., pruritus ani), or present with severe proctitis.

e. Pharyngitis occurs in those who engage in orogenital sexual contact.

f. Disseminated infection occurs in less than 1% of patients and presents with a petechial or vesicopustular rash, fever, tenosynovitis, and arthralgias. A septic arthritis (usually monoarticular) may ensue. However, some patients may present with arthritis without a prodrome. Endocarditis and meningitis are rare complications of dissemination.

2. Diagnosis

a. Gram stains should be performed on urethral exudates in men. Gram-negative intracellular diplococci, in contrast to extracellular organisms, are diagnostic. Gram stains of cervical, rectal, and pharyngeal secretions are unreliable.

b. Culture proof should always be sought, and cultures should be plated directly in the emergency department on prewarmed specific media (e.g., Thayer-Martin). If such media are not available, transport media are an alternative, but cultures should be dispatched promptly to the laboratory. All exudates should be cultured. In addition, rectal and pharyngeal cultures should be routinely performed in women and homosexual men.

c. Blood cultures should be performed and the laboratory notified if disseminated infection is suspected.

d. Serology for syphilis should be performed.

3. Therapy [7]

a. Urethritis and cervicitis should be treated with ampicillin, 3.5 gm PO; amoxicillin, 3 gm PO; or procaine penicillin G, 4.8 million units IM at two injection sites; each plus probenecid, 1 gm PO; or ceftriaxone, 250 mg IM. Each of these regimens is followed by tetracycline, 500 mg PO qid for 7 days, or doxycycline, 100 mg PO bid for 7 days, or (in patients unable to take tetracyclines) erythromycin, 500 mg PO qid for 7 days, to provide therapy for possible coincident chlamydial infection. Tetracycline, 500 mg PO qid, or doxycycline, 100 mg PO bid, for 7 days alone is an alternative for patients allergic to penicillins or cephalosporins. For pregnant women, erythromycin should be used instead of tetracycline in conjunction with one of the above regimens. Spectinomycin, 2.0 gm IM, plus erythromycin, is used in patients allergic to penicillins or cephalosporins and unable to take tetracyclines (e.g., pregnant women).

b. The therapy of **salpingitis** is discussed in Chap. 33.

c. Pharyngeal gonorrhea. Ceftriaxone, 250 mg IM, is preferred. Procaine penicillin G, 4.8 million units IM, plus probenecid, 1.0 gm PO, is alternative therapy.

d. Anorectal gonorrhea. See Chap. 30.

e. Disseminated infection. The initial phase of rash, fever, and arthralgias is extremely sensitive to antimicrobials and may be managed with ampicillin, 3.5 gm PO; amoxicillin, 3 gm PO; or procaine penicillin, 4.8 million units IM; each plus probenecid, 1.0 gm PO, followed by ampicillin, 500 mg PO qid for 7 days. Patients who are toxic, have purulent arthritis, or may be noncompliant require hospital admission. Treatment of these patients is penicillin G, 2 million units IV q4h, followed by ampicillin, 500 mg PO qid for a 7-day course. Alternative regimens, which may also be used in the treatment of disseminated disease caused by penicillinase-producing organisms, include ceftriaxone, 1.0 gm IV daily for 7 days; cefoxitin, 1.0 gm IV q6h for 7 days; or cefotaxime, 500 mg IV q6h for 7 days. Except for homosexual men, patients with disseminated gonococcal infection should also be treated for concomitant chlamydial infection with tetracycline, doxycycline, or erythromycin (see sec. **IV.A.3.a**). Patients allergic to penicillins or cephalosporins may be treated with tetracycline, 500 mg PO qid for 7 days, or doxycycline, 100 mg PO bid for 7 days. Repeated joint aspiration or drainage may be necessary.

     f. Treatment failures. There are a number of causes of apparent treatment failure of gonorrhea.

       (1) Nongonococcal coinfection, particularly with chlamydia (see sec. **IV.B**), is a common cause of apparent treatment failure.

       (2) Reinfection, particularly if contacts are not treated, can lead to early relapse.

       (3) Resistance to antibiotics is the least likely cause in the United States. Penicillinase-producing gonococci are prevalent in Southeast Asia and occasionally cause infection in the West, especially in seaports. These patients should be treated with spectinomycin, 2 gm IM, or ceftriaxone, 250 mg IM, each followed by a 7-day course of tetracycline, doxycycline, or erythromycin. Pharyngitis due to resistant organisms should be treated with ceftriaxone, 250 mg IM, or TMP-SMZ, 9 single-strength tablets daily for 5 days.

B. Chlamydial disease. *C. trachomatis* is an obligate intracellular parasite that is a common cause of sexually acquired infection [42].

     1. Diagnosis can be made by direct examination of the discharge by cytology or using immunofluorescent techniques. Cultivation of the organism requires specialized media and is not commonly performed.

     2. Clinical features. Patients present with urethritis or cervicitis. It is impossible to distinguish on clinical grounds chlamydial infection from other causes of urethritis, such as gonorrhea, and both may coexist. Pelvic inflammatory disease in women and epididymitis in men may be caused by *C. trachomatis*. These infections may be an important contribution to future infertility.

     3. Treatment is with tetracycline, 500 mg PO qid, or doxycycline, 100 mg PO bid for 7 days [7, 41]. Erythromycin, 500 mg PO qid, is an alternative.

C. Syphilis is caused by a spirochete, *T. pallidum.*

     1. Pathogenesis. Syphilis is transmitted sexually by contact with moist skin lesions. After 3–6 weeks of incubation, a **primary** stage (chancre) occurs at the site of inoculation. A **secondary** stage of disseminated disease occurs 6–8 weeks later as the result of bacteremia. Both the primary and secondary stages are infectious. A **latent** period of variable length follows untreated syphilis. This may be followed by a **tertiary** phase, characterized by endarteritis and granuloma formation. Although rarely seen, this stage accounts for aortitis and the chronic neurologic forms of syphilis.

     2. Clinical features. (Gloves should always be worn during examination of potentially infectious lesions.)

       a. A **primary lesion** occurs at the site of inoculation. It starts as a papule and develops into an indurated ulcer with associated lymphadenopathy. Genital and oral ulcers are typically painless; however, pain is a feature of rectal syphilis in homosexuals.

       b. Secondary syphilis

         (1) The highly infectious **mucocutaneous manifestations** include a diffuse erythematous or maculopapular rash, often involving the palms and soles; condylomata lata, which are red-brown erosions in the perineum, perirectal, and perivulvar areas; mucous patches (i.e., shallow erosions in the oral cavity); and patchy alopecia.

         (2) Systemic manifestations such as fever, malaise, and headache are usual. Meningismus is common, although frank meningitis is rare. Unusual features include hepatitis, arthritis, and uveitis.

     3. Diagnosis. Because the organism cannot be isolated on artificial media, direct visualization or serology is necessary to diagnose the infection.

       a. Dark-field microscopy of fresh serum exudates or skin lesions should be performed. Failure to demonstrate treponemes does not exclude the diagnosis.

       b. Serology

         (1) Tests for a nonspecific antigen, serum syphilitic reagin, are used as a screening test. The commonly available methods (VDRL and RPR) become positive after 2–4 weeks. Consequently, false-negative results are possible in primary infection. However, all patients with secondary syphilis have positive serology. Because false-positive results may occur, a positive test should be verified using more specific methods.

         (2) FTA-ABS and TPHA are specific antitreponemal antibody tests. Once positive they remain so for life.

     4. Treatment. Penicillin is the drug of choice for all stages of syphilis [7]. Benzathine penicillin G, 2.4 million units IM, is given for primary or secondary syphilis or latent syphilis of less than 1 year's duration. Tetracycline, 500 mg PO qid for 15 days, or erythromycin, 500 mg PO qid for 15 days, is used in the penicillin-allergic patient. Syphilis of more than 1 year's duration may be treated with benzathine penicillin G, 2.4 million units IM weekly, for 3 weeks. A lumbar puncture is unnecessary in patients with latent syphilis who have no neuropsychiatric symptoms or signs.

D. Herpes simplex. Genital infection can be caused by either type 1 or type 2 herpes simplex virus. The major problem with infection with this DNA virus is its ability to become latent and cause recurrent infection. This occurs in about 60% of patients.

1. **Clinical features.** Infection presents as tender vesicles or ulcers [11]. Most commonly, these affect the genitalia, but they may also be seen in the anorectal area and in the oropharynx. Systemic symptoms (e.g., fever, malaise) secondary to viremia, local symptoms of dysuria, urinary frequency or dysfunction, and tender adenopathy are common, particularly in primary infections. The symptoms of recurrent herpes usually are less severe.

2. The **diagnosis** is usually suspected clinically in the presence of multiple painful vesicles and ulcers. A positive Tzanck preparation strongly suggests herpes simplex. A viral culture confirms the diagnosis.

3. **Treatment.** Acyclovir, 200 mg PO 5 times daily for 7–10 days, accelerates healing and reduces local and systemic symptoms in primary disease. Chronic treatment with oral acyclovir also reduces the frequency of recurrences [44]. Intravenous therapy in a dosage of 5 mg/kg q8h should be reserved for patients with primary disease and severe constitutional symptoms or complicated infection [10]. Topical acyclovir, 5% ointment, reduces the duration of viral shedding in initial attacks and may reduce local symptoms [10].

E. Acquired immunodeficiency syndrome (AIDS) [17] is characterized by multiple opportunistic infections and unusual malignancies occurring in patients less than 60 years of age and without obvious predisposing causes for such infections and tumors. Although 70% of cases have occurred in male homosexuals, intravenous drug users, hemophiliacs, and Haitian immigrants (usually homosexual) are also at increased risk. Occasional cases have been seen in sexual contacts of index cases, children born to mothers with AIDS, and patients exposed to multiple blood transfusions. A retrovirus, human T-cell lymphotropic virus III (HTLV-III), is the cause [6]. The main immunologic defect is in cell-mediated immunity. A number of markers of the depressed immunologic state have been described. These include lymphopenia, a selective defect in the helper subset of T lymphocytes, defective killer-cell function, and cutaneous anergy.

1. **Clinical features**
   a. **Opportunistic infections.** The pathogens involved are those usually contained by intact cell-mediated immunity.
      (1) **Pneumonia** due to *P. carinii* is common. Infection is characterized by fever, dyspnea, hypoxemia, and diffuse pulmonary infiltrates. Diagnosis is made by lung biopsy. Treatment is with TMP-SMZ or pentamidine.
      (2) Other pathogens include viruses (e.g., cytomegalovirus [CMV] and herpes simplex), fungi (e.g., *Candida* and *Cryptococcus neoformans*, the latter causing meningitis), protozoa (e.g., toxoplasmosis causing central nervous system lesions and cryptosporidiosis causing diarrhea), and mycobacteria (causing disseminated infection with bacteremia).
   b. An unusual tumor, **Kaposi's sarcoma**, is commonly seen in patients with AIDS. It usually presents as a pigmented nodule on the skin or mucous membranes, rapidly disseminates both cutaneously and systemically, and is resistant to chemotherapy.
   c. HTLV-III infection has also been associated with a syndrome of recurrent fevers and lymphadenopathy. In some cases, this may progress to true AIDS.

2. **Therapy**. There is no specific treatment. Opportunistic infections require prompt and aggressive intervention, both diagnostic and therapeutic, similar to those in other immunocompromised patients.

3. **Precautions.** The current recommendations are similar to those for hepatitis B carriers, that is, care with blood and body fluids. In addition, because of the high incidence of CMV carriage, pregnant women should avoid close contact with patients with AIDS.

V. Central nervous system infections
 A. Meningitis
  1. **Pathogenesis.** Inflammation of the meninges is usually infectious in origin [46]. Most microorganisms have been associated with meningitis. Acute bacte-

rial infection is particularly important, because untreated cases have a high and rapid mortality.

In normal hosts, infection is usually acquired through the bloodstream. Important bacterial pathogens include *S. pneumoniae, N. meningitidis, H. influenzae,* and *M. tuberculosis.* Enteroviruses, mumps virus, and herpes zoster virus are the most common viral causes. Fungal meningitis due to *Cryptococcus neoformans, Coccidiodes immitis,* and *Histoplasma capsulatum* is rare, as is protozoan meningitis (e.g., due to *Naegleria fowleri*).

Certain patients are predisposed to menigeal infection. The elderly are prone to infection with gram-negative bacilli as well as with pneumococci. Patients with cancer, especially those receiving chemotherapy, tend to develop infections with *Listeria monocytogenes* and fungi. Staphylococcal infections are common following neurosurgery or trauma to the head. Patients with CSF leaks are prone to develop recurrent pneumococcal meningitis.

2. **Clinical features.** Meningitis should be considered in any patient with fever and even minimal neurologic symptoms or signs. Most patients with acute bacterial infections present with fever, headache, confusion, lethargy, and nuchal rigidity within 24 hours of the onset of infection [46]. A purpuric skin rash may be seen with meningococcal infection. Viral infections also present acutely, although the patient usually is less ill. Fungal and mycobacterial infections may be acute but more commonly present with a subacute or chronic history of progressive neurologic dysfunction.

3. **Diagnosis**
   a. The diagnosis of meningitis is based on the demonstration of signs of inflammation in the CSF (Table 12-5). A **lumbar puncture** should be performed whenever the diagnosis is considered. CSF samples should be submitted routinely for the following analyses: cell count and differential, protein, glucose, Gram stain, India ink preparation, VDRL serology, and bacterial culture. If indicated, the following tests may also be performed: countercurrent immune electrophoresis (CIE) or latex agglutination for antigens of *S. pneumoniae, N. meningitidis,* and *H. influenzae*; latex agglutination for cryptococcal antigen; cytology to detect meningeal carcinomatosis; fungal and mycobacterial cultures; and viral cultures.
   b. **Blood cultures** should be obtained when the diagnosis of bacterial meningitis is considered.
   c. Blood should be drawn to measure a leukocyte count and glucose.
   d. Throat washings and stool may be cultured for enterovirus if indicated. Acute and convalescent serologies are useful in making a specific viral diagnosis.

4. **Differential diagnosis.** Noninfectious causes of meningitis include vasculitis, sarcoidosis, and carcinoma. Parameningeal infections (e.g., subdural empyema, paraspinal abscess, complicated sinusitis) may result in a clinical picture similar to meningitis.

5. **Treatment**
   a. **Bacterial infection.** Early initiation of therapy is mandatory, and treatment should be initiated immediately if the CSF findings suggest acute bacterial infection. If a lumbar puncture is delayed, empiric institution of therapy prior to CSF analysis may be necessary.
      (1) **If the Gram stain of the CSF is positive,** specific therapy is directed accordingly.
      (2) **If the pathogen is unknown,** patients should be treated with penicillin G, 2 million units IV q2h plus an agent effective against *H. influenzae,* that is, chloramphenicol, 1 gm IV or PO q4–6h; cefuroxime, 2 gm IV q8h; or cefotaxime, 2 gm IV q4h. Chloramphenicol, 1 gm IV or PO q4–6h, is used in the patient allergic to penicillin.
      (3) **If staphylococcal infection is suspected** (e.g., prior head trauma), nafcillin, 2 gm IV q4h, should be added to penicillin. Cefotaxime, 2 gm IV q4h, is used with penicillin if gram-negative infection is likely (e.g., elderly patient with concomitant UTI, alcoholic). Treatment should be modified according to the results of culture and susceptibility testing and continued for a total of 10–14 days.
      (4) Patients with meningitis of unknown origin or due to *N. meningitidis* or *H. influenzae* should be isolated for the first 24 hours of treatment.
   b. **Viral meningitis** is treated symptomatically. Patients with minimal symptoms and adequate home circumstances do not require hospitalization.

Table 12-5. Diagnostic features in the cerebrospinal fluid

Disease	White blood cell count	Cell type	Glucose (mg/dl)	Protein (mg/dl)	Gram stain
Normal	1–6	Mononuclear cells	40–75	15–55	–
Bacterial meningitis	↑ ↑	>75% polymorphonuclear leukocytes	↓ (<45)[a]	↑ (>80)	+/–
Viral meningitis	↑	Lymphocytes[b]	Normal	Normal, slightly ↑	–
TB meningitis	↑	Lymphocytes	↓	↑	–
Fungal meningitis	↑	Lymphocytes	Normal, slightly ↓	↑	–
Meningeal carcinomatosis	↑	Lymphocytes Abnormal cells	Normal, ↓	↑	–

Key: ↑ = increase; ↓ = decrease; + = positive; – = negative
[a] CSF glucose must be compared to a concomitant blood glucose. In bacterial meningitis, the CSF glucose is generally less than 40% of the blood glucose.
[b] A polymorphonuclear reaction can be seen in early viral meningitis [18]. This usually converts in 6–12 hours to a mononuclear predominance.

    c. Patients with **equivocal CSF findings** may present with clinical and CSF features of a viral meningitis except for a predominance of polymorphonuclear leukocytes. In these cases, the differential is between an early bacterial and an early viral infection. Therapy may be delayed if the following conditions are met: (1) the patient is stable without any underlying disease, (2) the patient has not received previous antimicrobial therapy, (3) there is no associated skin rash, (4) the CSF white cell elevation is moderate (i.e., < 1000 cells/ml), (5) there are adequate facilities in which to observe the patient, and (6) the CSF glucose and protein are normal. A repeat lumbar puncture should be performed in 8–12 hours. Ninety percent of viral meningitides will have converted to a lymphocytic predominance by this time [18]. Empiric antibiotic therapy should be started after cultures are obtained if any of the above criteria cannot be met, if the physician or patient is unwilling to wait, or if a neutrophil leukocytosis persists on repeat lumbar puncture.

    d. Patients who have previously received antibiotics. Although antimicrobials may interfere with subsequent cultures, they rarely affect the CSF parameters of a bacterial meningitis. If there is any doubt, the patient should be treated empirically for a bacterial infection. CSF antigen detection techniques are useful in these patients.

B. Encephalitis. Inflammation of the brain parenchyma is usually of viral origin. Other causes of encephalitis include nonviral pathogens (e.g., malaria and rickettsiae) and vasculitis. Reye's syndrome may be a postviral encephalitis.

    1. Etiology

        a. Herpes simplex virus is the most common cause of nonepidemic infective encephalitis. Infection occurs most frequently in patients over 50 and under 20 years of age. Early initiation of treatment significantly alters the course of illness [20].

        b. Arboviruses causing encephalitis are transmitted to humans by the bite of arthropods (mosquitoes). Consequently, infection occurs during the seasons of vector activity.

        c. Rabies causes a severe encephalitis.

        d. Epstein-Barr virus and mumps are rare causes of encephalitis.

    2. Clinical features. Patients usually present with an abrupt illness characterized by headache and neurologic dysfunction (e.g., seizures, drowsiness, coma, hallucinations, and behavioral disturbance). Although difficult to diagnose clinically, herpes encephalitis is suggested by subtle behavioral changes noted in the days prior to presentation and the presence of focal temporal lobe signs. A prodrome of malaise, myalgias, and gastrointestinal symptoms is suggestive of arbovirus infection.

    3. Diagnosis. Although most investigations are nonspecific in patients with encephalitis, they should be performed because of other diagnostic possibilities (e.g., meningitis, brain abscess).

        a. A **lumbar puncture** usually shows a mild pleocytosis with an elevated protein and a normal glucose. The opening pressure is usually raised.

        b. A **brain scan** may show the earliest evidence of temporal lobe damage in herpes encephalitis. An electroencephalogram and computed tomography (CT) scan may also localize abnormalities to the temporal lobe.

        c. A **brain biopsy** is necessary to make a definitive diagnosis of herpes simplex encephalitis [52].

    4. Treatment. Supportive care in the hospital with particular attention to fluid and electrolyte management is essential. Acyclovir, 10 mg/kg IV q8h, is indicated for the treatment of herpes encephalitis [40].

    5. Prognosis. Untreated cases of herpes simplex encephalitis have a 60–80% mortality. The mortality in other cases of encephalitis is variable and dependent on the etiologic agent.

C. Brain abscess

    1. Pathogenesis. Brain abscesses develop secondary to infection elsewhere, that is, local chronic infection with direct extension (e.g., otitis media, sinusitis, mastoiditis), head trauma with wound infection, or distant infection with bacteremia (e.g., bacterial endocarditis, congenital heart disease, chronic suppurative lung disease).

    2. Etiology. The bacteriology is dependent on the source of infection [12]. In local disease, a mixed infection with streptococci and anaerobic bacteria is most likely. Abscesses associated with head trauma and metastatic abscesses commonly are caused by *S. aureus*.

Table 12-6. Guidelines for tetanus prophylaxis

History of tetanus immunization (doses)	Clean minor wounds		All other wounds	
	Td	TIG	Td	TIG
Uncertain	Yes	No	Yes	Yes
0–1	Yes	No	Yes	Yes
2	Yes	No	Yes	No[a]
3 or more	No[b]	No	No[c]	No

Key: Td = tetanus and diphtheria toxoid; TIG = human tetanus immune globulin, 250 units IM.
[a] Unless wound is more than 24 hours old.
[b] Unless it is more than 10 years since last toxoid dose.
[c] Unless it is more than 5 years since last toxoid dose.
Note:
1. Prior history. Any patient who cannot give a clear, reliable history should be considered unimmunized.
2. Nature of wound. A clean, minor wound is one that is less than 6 hours old, nonpenetrating, and not associated with tissue damage.
3. Mode of acquisition of wound. Relatively trivial wounds caused by contaminated material should not be regarded as clean. In narcotic addicts, the practice of skin-popping has been associated with tetanus.
Source: Adapted from Centers for Disease Control, Diphtheria and tetanus toxoids and pertussis vaccine. *M.M.W.R.* 26:401, 1977.

   3. Clinical features. A brain abscess presents most commonly as an intracranial mass lesion. The presentation may be indolent; however, an abscess should be suspected in the presence of headache and lethargy, particularly if there is fever or a predisposing cause. Death is by herniation.
   4. Diagnosis
      a. A **CT scan** should be performed, preferably with contrast, in all patients in whom a brain abscess is suspected.
      b. Blood cultures and **sinus radiographs** are useful.
      c. A lumbar puncture is contraindicated in the presence of a brain abscess; it is nondiagnostic and may precipitate herniation.
   5. Management. Hospital admission and immediate antimicrobial therapy are mandatory. The choice of antibiotics depends on the likely source of infection. Neurosurgical consultation is necessary.
D. Tetanus is a disease of the nervous system caused by an exotoxin produced by an anaerobic gram-positive rod, *Clostridium tetani* [51]. The disorder is characterized by tonic muscle spasms.
   1. Clinical features. After an incubation period of 7–21 days, patients develop painful tonic muscle spasms (e.g., trismus, opisthotonus). Progressive spasms lead to seizures, and respiration may be impaired.
   2. The **diagnosis** is clinical.
   3. Treatment is mainly supportive, with rest in a quiet hospital environment and elective tracheostomy for airway support [14]. Antitoxin (500–3000 units IM) is given. Wound debridement should be performed and penicillin, 2 million units IV q4h, administered to prevent further toxin production.
   4. Prophylaxis. Prevention of tetanus is closely associated with the management of wounds. Two factors should be considered when managing a patient with a wound: the nature of the wound and the degree of personal immunity. Current guidelines are given in Table 12-6.
E. Botulism is a life-threatening neurologic disorder caused by a toxin produced by *Clostridium botulinum*. The disease results from the ingestion of food contaminated with preformed toxin. Canned food, in particular, is associated with infection if the temperature of the canning process is not high enough to kill the bacterial spores [31].
   1. Clinical features. The signs of botulism appear 12–36 hours after ingestion of the toxin. A **descending paralysis** with progressive respiratory failure is the primary manifestation. Bilateral ptosis and cranial nerve pareses are common initial signs. Involvement of the autonomic nervous system may be manifested by dilated, nonreactive pupils, postural hypotension, and drying of the mouth and mucous membranes.
   2. The **differential diagnosis** includes Guillain-Barré syndrome, poliomyelitis, and other polyneuropathies.
   3. Diagnosis. Electromyography may be diagnostic. The toxin may be isolated from blood, stool, or gastric contents.

    4. Treatment is supportive. Equine antitoxin (1 vial IV and 1 vial IM) should be administered, with anticipation of hypersensitivity reactions. Health authorities should be notified of all cases of botulism.

F. Rabies is a viral infection of the nervous system acquired by direct inoculation or inhalation of the rabies virus [2]. Exposure to the virus is usually by an animal bite but may be by direct contact with mucous membranes or an open wound. The disease is manifested by a progressive and fatal encephalitis, characterized by hyperactivity, hydrophobia, delirium, and paralysis. Treatment is supportive. However, mortality approaches 100%.

  1. Prevention. Although vaccination is available for those at high risk, prophylaxis of rabies is generally postexposure. The decision to give prophylaxis for an animal bite is dependent on several factors.

    a. Species of the biting animal. Wild carnivores and bats are most likely to be rabid. Domestic cats and dogs are less likely to be infected, particularly if vaccinated. Rodents do not transmit rabies.

    b. The presence of rabies in the region. A significant prevalence rate increases the risk that the animal is rabid.

    c. Circumstances of the biting incident. An unprovoked attack increases the likelihood that the animal is rabid.

  2. Management of a possible rabies exposure

    a. The wound should be thoroughly cleansed with soap and water, followed by ethanol (of at least 43% concentration).

    b. Tetanus prophylaxis (see Table 12-6) and measures to control potential bacterial infections (see Chap. 22) should be instituted.

    c. The suspected animal should be caught. If wild or ill, it should be sacrificed and the brain examined for rabies virus. Domestic pets are observed for 10 days.

    d. Rabies prophylaxis is administered as in Table 12-7.

VI. Infective endocarditis

A. Pathogenesis. Although natural heart valves may become infected, endocarditis most commonly involves abnormal valves (e.g., congenitally diseased valves, valves damaged by rheumatic heart disease, prolapsed mitral valves, prosthetic valves). After initial microbial invasion, a vegetation of organisms, platelets, and fibrin is formed on the valve surface. Within this vegetation, the organism is relatively protected from host defenses and from administered antimicrobials. Progressive valvular damage leads to destruction with resultant valvular incompetence. Direct invasion of the myocardium may occur, resulting in abscess formation and conduction defects. Embolization from the vegetation causes cutaneous, retinal, and neurologic manifestations of endocarditis. Systemic effects, including glomerulonephritis, are secondary to immune complex deposition.

B. Microbiology [4]. Almost all bacteria have been associated with endocarditis. *Streptococcus viridans*, which is part of the normal mouth flora, accounts for the majority of cases of endocarditis. *S. aureus* is increasingly common, particularly in intravenous drug abusers and the elderly. Infection with enterococcus, the primary gut streptococcus, is also seen with increasing frequency in the elderly. *Staphylococcus epidermidis* frequently infects prosthetic valves, especially during the first 6 weeks after surgery. Additional pathogens commonly infecting prosthetic valves include gram-negative bacilli and *C. albicans* [54]. The valves of intravenous drug abusers are more likely to be infected with *S. aureus* and gram-negative bacilli. With the decline in prevalence of rheumatic heart disease, endocarditis has increasingly become a disease of the elderly. In this population, one streptococcal organism, *Streptococcus bovis*, should be highlighted because of the frequent association between endocarditis due to this organism and neoplastic bowel disease.

C. Clinical features. Endocarditis may present acutely or subacutely.

  1. Acute endocarditis is seen in certain patient groups, particularly intravenous drug abusers with left- or right-sided endocarditis and patients with early prosthetic valve endocarditis. In these groups, the onset is rapid, and the patient presents with fever and a changing cardiac status. Acute heart failure is common.

  2. The features of **subacute endocarditis** are more subtle. Fever is generally low-grade and constant. Associated night sweats, malaise, and loss of energy are frequent. Cardiac examination demonstrates new murmurs or documented changes in old murmurs. There may be peripheral manifestations of embolization, such as Osler's nodes, splinter hemorrhages, or Roth's spots. Splenomegaly and finger clubbing are late findings. An acute change in neurologic function

Table 12-7. Guidelines for rabies prophylaxis

Species of animal	Condition of animal at time of attack	Treatment of exposed person
Domestic: cat, dog	Healthy and available for 10 days of observation	None, unless animal develops rabies
	Rabid or suspected rabid	RIG[a] and HDCV[b]
	Unknown	Contact public health officials
Wild: skunk, bat, fox, coyote, raccoon, other carnivores	Regard as rabid unless proved negative by laboratory tests	RIG[a] and HDCV[b]
Other: livestock, rodents (e.g., chipmunks, gerbils, guinea pigs, hamsters, mice, rats, squirrels), lagomorphs (e.g., rabbits, hares)	Bites of rodents and lagomorphs virtually never require antirabies prophylaxis	Consider individually; contact public health officials

[a] RIG (rabies immune globulin) is given once only, 10 units/kg at the wound site and 10 units/kg IM at a distant site.
[b] HDCV (human diploid cell vaccine) is given in five 1-ml doses IM on days 0, 3, 7, 14, and 28.
Source: Adapted from Centers for Disease Control. Rabies prevention. *M.M.W.R.* 33:393, 1984.

Table 12-8. Endocarditis prophylaxis

Procedure	Treatment
Dental	Penicillin V, 2 gm PO 1 hour prior to the procedure and 1 gm PO 6 hours after initial dose Alternate: Erythromycin, 1 gm PO prior to the procedure and 500 mg PO 6 hours after initial dose
Lower gastrointestinal or genitourinary	Ampicillin, 2 gm IV or IM, plus gentamicin, 1.5 mg/kg IV or IM. Both are administered 30 minutes before the procedure and 8 hours after initial dose. Alternate: Vancomycin, 1 gm infused over 1 hour, plus gentamicin, 1.5 mg/kg IV or IM

Source: Adapted from *Medical Letter*, Prevention of bacterial endocarditis. *Med. Lett. Drugs Ther.* 26:3, 1984.

(e.g., confusion, cerebrovascular accident, seizures) may be a manifestation of endocarditis [36].

  D. Diagnosis

    1. Since endocarditis produces a constant bacteremia, the cardinal diagnostic feature is the demonstration of **positive blood cultures** in the appropriate clinical setting. Antimicrobials should not be administered until blood cultures (three sets) have been obtained.

    2. Urinalysis may reveal microscopic hematuria or red cell casts.

    3. Echocardiography is a useful adjunct in the management of patients known to have endocarditis. However, its role in diagnosis is more limited, and a normal echocardiograph does not exclude endocarditis.

    4. An **electrocardiogram** should be obtained because of the possibility of conduction defects.

  E. Treatment [53]. Infective endocarditis is treated with bactericidal antimicrobials, given parenterally in large dosages for a prolonged period. Surgical removal of the infected valve is indicated in the presence of fulminant heart failure, persistent embolization, significant conduction abnormalities, and fungal endocarditis.

    1. Patients who present with **acute endocarditis** should be treated with empiric antimicrobials as soon as blood cultures are obtained. The appropriate regimen should contain an antistaphylococcal beta-lactam (nafcillin, 2 gm IV q4–6h) and an aminoglycoside (gentamicin, 1.5 mg/kg IV q8h). Early surgical intervention may be necessary.

    2. Immediate initiation of empiric antibiotics is unnecessary in the management of **subacute endocarditis.** However, if the diagnosis is clinically evident and all necessary blood cultures have been obtained, therapy can be initiated with penicillin, 2 million units IV q4h, and gentamicin, 1.5 mg/kg IV q8h, and adjusted according to culture results.

  F. Prophylaxis. Antimicrobial prophylaxis (Table 12-8) may prevent endocarditis in patients who have cardiac valvular abnormalities, including mitral valve prolapse and prosthetic valves, and are about to undergo procedures that are associated with a transient bacteremia.

VII. Osteomyelitis is best classified on the basis of the origin of the infection, that is, hematogenous, acquired from contiguous foci, or associated with peripheral vascular disease [49, 50].

  A. Hematogenous osteomyelitis

    1. Pathogenesis. Hematogenous osteomyelitis usually presents as an acute infection of young people, affecting rapidly growing long bones. Because of the anatomy of these bones and their blood supply, infection in children occurs at the metaphysis; the epiphyseal plate protects the neighboring joint from infection. However, this does not apply to adults or neonates, and an associated septic arthritis may occur. If acute infection is untreated, persistent inflammation leads to bony destruction. Dead bone remains as a sequestrum and provides a nidus for continued infection. Tracking of the infection to the skin may occur and lead to sinus formation.

    2. Microbiology. *S. aureus* is the most common pathogen in all age groups. *H. influenzae* is an important pathogen in children. Gram-negative bacilli are frequent causes of infection in intravenous drug abusers. *Salmonella* osteomyelitis is associated with sickle cell disease.

3. Clinical features

a. **Local.** Bone pain is prominent. Local signs of inflammation (i.e., tenderness, immobility, and erythema), although common, may be absent.

b. **Systemic.** Bacteremia is common, usually with fever and rigors.

c. **Laboratory data.** Leukocytosis is usually present. The erythrocyte sedimentation rate is usually elevated and can be a useful marker of disease activity.

d. Although **radiographs** generally show periosteal elevation or bone loss, they may be normal early in the course. Scintigraphy, using technetium or gallium, may be abnormal preceding radiographic abnormalities, but normal scans do not exclude the diagnosis.

4. Diagnosis.
Osteomyelitis is diagnosed by culturing pathogens from bone. Microbiologic information must be obtained before antimicrobials are begun. Blood cultures should be taken and may be diagnostic. However, bone aspirate or biopsy usually is necessary.

5. Management.
Hospitalization is required for the administration of parenteral antimicrobials for a prolonged period. Empiric antibiotics generally are not required before obtaining cultures. Once the necessary measures to acquire a microbial diagnosis have been performed, therapy may be initiated. In normal hosts, an antistaphylococcal penicillin (e.g., oxacillin, 2 gm IV q4–6h) is usually necessary. In patients allergic to penicillin, vancomycin, 500 mg IV q6h, or clindamycin, 600 mg IV q6h, is an alternative. If gram-negative infection is suspected, an aminoglycoside should be added. Once the culture results and susceptibilities are known, antimicrobial therapy should be adjusted accordingly.

B. **Vertebral osteomyelitis** is usually seen in patients over 50 years of age. The origin may be hematogenous or from a urinary source through the contiguous venous plexuses. Consequently, either *S. aureus* or a gram-negative enteric bacillus may be the pathogen. The presentation is often subacute. The diagnosis should be considered in patients with the recent onset of back pain or pain referred along the nerve roots, particularly if fever is present. Establishing the diagnosis is important because of the risk of spinal abscess formation. Treatment is with the appropriate parenteral antimicrobial administered for 4–6 weeks.

C. **Osteomyelitis associated with contiguous foci**

1. **Predisposing conditions** include previous orthopedic procedures (e.g., following repair of a fracture or insertion of a prosthesis), soft-tissue infections adjacent to bone, infected decubitus ulcers, and infected teeth or sinuses.

2. **Microbiology.** Mixed infection is usual. *S. aureus* is common. Gram-negative bacilli and anaerobes are also frequently found. *S. epidermidis* is a particular problem in infection of prosthetic joints.

3. **Clinically** the disease is indolent and may present as chronic pain or persistent fever, or it may be recognized on routine radiographs.

4. The **diagnosis** is difficult. Blood cultures are usually negative. Radiographs are often normal and scans difficult to interpret. Cultures of the contiguous wound or sinus are of little value unless *S. aureus* is isolated. A bone biopsy and culture remain essential.

5. **Treatment** is primarily surgical debridement. Appropriate antimicrobials are administered parenterally for a prolonged period.

D. **Osteomyelitis and peripheral vascular disease.** Infection of poorly vascularized bone is a common problem in patients with peripheral vascular disease, especially diabetics. The pathogens usually are polymicrobial, and surgery is frequently required. An empiric trial of antimicrobial therapy is worthwhile but often fails.

VIII. Rocky Mountain spotted fever

A. **Pathogenesis.** Rocky Mountain spotted fever is a tick-borne illness caused by *Rickettsia rickettsii* [33]. The tick serves as a reservoir and as a vector. The disease is endemic to much of the United States. Infection usually occurs between April and September, the period of maximum tick activity. The organism invades endothelial cells and causes an intense vasculitis, which may result in shock and death.

B. **Clinical features.** Most patients will have a history of a tick bite, but the exposure may be inapparent, especially in children. Fever is a constant finding and headache is a major symptom. There is often associated malaise, myalgias, and nausea. An erythematous maculopapular or petechial rash occurs at any time during the first 10 days; this rash characteristically starts on the wrists, ankles, palms, and soles but may in fact be seen anywhere on the body. Neurologic complications (e.g., meningismus, seizures, hemiplegia, ascending paralysis) may occur.

C. The **diagnosis** is clinical and based on a high index of suspicion, particularly in endemic areas during the appropriate season.
  1. **Skin biopsies** should be performed. Vasculitis may be demonstrated, and occasionally the rickettsiae seen. Direct immunofluorescence, when available, is diagnostic.
  2. **Specific serology** confirms the diagnosis but usually is retrospective. The Weil-Felix test for OX2 and OX19 agglutinins (a nonspecific reaction) is rarely positive before 7 days.
D. **Differential diagnosis.** The major differential diagnosis is that of an acute vasculitis. In a patient with neurologic or meningeal signs, meningococcal meningitis should be excluded by a lumbar puncture. Tularemia should be considered if there is a history of a tick bite.
E. **Therapy** with tetracycline, 25 mg/kg PO qd, or chloramphenicol, 50 mg/kg PO qd, should be begun when the diagnosis is suspected. Hospitalization is indicated.

IX. **Infectious mononucleosis** is a disease of the reticuloendothelial system caused by the Epstein-Barr (EB) virus, a DNA virus of the herpes group. The majority of cases occur in persons 15–25 years old.
A. **Clinical features.** The incubation period is 30–40 days; this is followed by a prodrome lasting 3–7 days, consisting of fatigue, malaise, myalgias, and a mild pharyngitis. Characteristic features suggestive of mononucleosis include severe pharyngitis and tonsillitis with palatal petechiae, lymphadenopathy (especially posterior cervical), splenomegaly, hepatomegaly without jaundice, periorbital and eyelid edema, and fever often persisting for 7–10 days.
B. **Complications** include neurologic syndromes (e.g., aseptic meningitis, mild encephalitis), hemolytic anemia, thrombocytopenia, a compromised airway due to enlarged tonsils, and splenic rupture (excessive palpation of the spleen should be avoided).
C. **Diagnosis** [37]
  1. **White blood cell count.** The total white blood cell count is variable, but an absolute ($>4500/mm^3$) and relative ($>50\%$) lymphocytosis occurs. Atypical phocytes (i.e., large cells with abundant cytoplasm) constitute 10–20% of the circulating white blood cells.
  2. **Heterophil antibodies** are antibodies that react with antigens of other mammals. Their production is a response to EB virus infection, and their detection is a clue to the diagnosis. Elevation, although not invariable, usually occurs 2–3 weeks after initial infection.
  3. The detection of a fourfold rise in **specific antibodies** to EB virus is diagnostic.
D. **Differential diagnosis**
  1. **Mononucleosis syndromes.** Other pathogens (e.g., cytomegalovirus and *Toxoplasma gondii*) may produce a syndrome of pharyngitis, lymphadenopathy, and hepatosplenomegaly associated with atypical lymphocytosis. In these cases, the heterophil antibody will be negative.
  2. Specific features of mononucleosis may be mimicked by other pathogens (e.g., viral hepatitides, leptospirosis, and rubella).
  3. Hematologic malignancies (e.g., acute leukemia) should be excluded.
E. **Treatment.** Symptomatic therapy only is indicated for the majority of cases. Corticosteroids (e.g., prednisone, 60 mg PO qd) may be used for the treatment of severe pharyngitis and airway compromise. Antimicrobials play no role in the treatment of infectious mononucleosis; the use of ampicillin may lead to the complication (often diagnostic) of a maculopapular rash.

X. **Toxic shock syndrome** is a disorder seen primarily in menstruating women who use tampons. Its incidence is currently declining.
A. **Etiology.** The cause is an exotoxin produced by *S. aureus*. Most cases have occurred in women using tampons after vaginal colonization by the staphylococcus. However, since the syndrome is secondary to staphylococcal colonization, it may be seen in men and children.
B. **Clinical features** [45]. The disorder has a dramatic onset with fever (often exceeding 39°C); a diffuse erythematous rash, often involving the palms and soles, that desquamates 7–14 days after the onset of the illness; hypotension; conjunctivitis; pharyngitis; vomiting; and diarrhea. The most severe complication is shock. Disorders of consciousness and focal neurologic signs may also occur.
C. The **diagnosis** is clinical.
D. **Treatment** [8]
  1. **Supportive care,** particularly to maintain blood pressure, is essential.

Table 12-9. Diseases in travelers

Presentation after travel	Disease
Early (1–7 days)	Traveler's diarrhea; dysentery (bacillary); yellow fever; dengue; malaria
Intermediate (7 days–4 weeks)	Malaria; typhoid; Lassa fever
Late (weeks to years)	Amebiasis; trypanosomiasis

2. **Antistaphylococcal therapy** (e.g., nafcillin, 2 gm IV q6h), although not of immediate benefit as the disease is secondary to a toxin, is indicated to prevent progression and relapse. Antimicrobials should also be considered if other infectious conditions associated with profound shock and a skin rash (e.g., Rocky Mountain spotted fever, meningococcemia) cannot be excluded.
3. Relapse may also be prevented by avoiding further use of tampons.

   E. Disposition. Hospitalization is mandatory.

XI. Fever in travelers. Some of the diseases that may present as fever in a person returning from the tropics and their relationship to the time of travel are listed in Table 12-9.

   A. Arboviral infections are transmitted to humans by mosquitoes.

1. **Yellow fever** presents acutely after an incubation period of 4–5 days with high fever, headache, jaundice, oliguria, and abdominal symptoms. Treatment is supportive. Vaccination is available for travelers to endemic areas (tropical Africa and Central America).
2. **Dengue** occurs between the latitudes 30°N and 30°S. After an incubation period of 5–7 days, sudden fever with severe headache and myalgias occur. Treatment is supportive.

   B. Malaria is a protozoan infection transmitted to humans by mosquitoes. It is caused by parasites of the genus *Plasmodium* and is endemic in Southeast Asia, tropical Africa, and South America. The incubation period is 12–28 days depending on the species. **Malaria should be considered in any patient with unexplained fever and a history of recent travel to an endemic area.** The diagnosis is made by demonstrating malarial parasites on a Giemsa's stain of a peripheral blood smear. Treatment depends on the likelihood of chloroquine resistance, and this information should be sought from local health authorities or the Centers for Disease Control (CDC). If the parasite is susceptible, chloroquine phosphate, 1000 mg PO, is the initial dose, followed in 6 hours by 500 mg PO and then by 500 mg PO qd for 2 days. Resistant *Plasmodium falciparum* organisms require initial therapy with quinine sulfate, 650 mg PO q8h. Severe *P. falciparum* infection may require intravenous quinine, 10 mg/kg IV infused over 4 hours q8h.

Bibliography

1. American Thoracic Society. Treatment of tuberculosis and other mycobacterial diseases. *Am. Rev. Respir. Dis.* 127:790, 1983.
2. Anderson, L. J., et al. Human rabies in the United States, 1960–1979: Epidemiology, diagnosis and prevention. *Ann. Intern. Med.* 100:728, 1984.
3. Bartlett, J. G., et al. Bacteriology and treatment of primary lung abscess. *Am. Rev. Respir. Dis.* 109:510, 1974.
4. Bayliss, R., et al. The microbiology and pathogenesis of infective endocarditis. *Br. Heart J.* 50:513, 1983.
5. Bennett, W. M., et al. Drug therapy in renal failure: Dosing guidelines for adults. Part 1: Antimicrobial agents, analgesics. *Ann. Intern. Med.* 86:754, 1977.
6. Broder, S., and Gallo, R. C. A pathogenic virus (HTLV-III) linked to AIDS. *N. Engl. J. Med.* 311:1292, 1984.
7. Centers for Disease Control. 1985 STD treatment guidelines. *Morbidity Mortality Weekly Report.* 34(Suppl. 4):75S, 1985.
8. Chesney, P. J., et al. Toxic shock syndrome: Management and long-term sequelae. *Ann. Intern. Med.* 96:847, 1982.
9. Cohen, J. Antifungal chemotherapy. *Lancet* 2:532, 1982.
10. Corey, L., and Holmes, K. K. Genital herpes simplex virus infections: Current concepts in diagnosis, therapy and prevention. *Ann. Intern. Med.* 98:973, 1983.

11. Corey, L., et al. Genital herpes simplex infections: Clinical manifestations, course and complications. *Ann. Intern. Med.* 98:958, 1983.
12. de Louvois, J. The bacteriology and chemotherapy of brain abscess. *J. Antimicrob. Chemother.* 4:395, 1978.
13. Douglas, R. G. Amantadine as an antiviral agent in influenza. *N. Engl. J. Med.* 307:617, 1982.
14. Douglas, R. G., and Betts, R. F. Influenza Virus. In G. L. Mandell, R. G. Douglas, and J. E. Bennett (eds.), *Principles and Practice of Infectious Diseases.* New York. Wiley: 1984. Pp. 846–866.
15. Edmondson, R. S., and Flowers, M. W. Intensive care in tetanus: Management, complications and mortality. *Br. Med. J.* 1:1401, 1979.
16. Erffmeyer, J. E. Adverse reactions to penicillin. *Ann. Allergy* 47:288, 1981.
17. Fauci, A. S., et al. Acquired immunodeficiency syndrome: Epidemiologic, clinical, immunologic and therapeutic considerations. *Ann. Intern. Med.* 100:92, 1984.
18. Feigin, R. D., and Shackleford, P. G. Value of repeat lumbar puncture in the differential diagnosis of meningitis. *N. Engl. J. Med.* 289:571, 1973.
19. Goldman, P. Metronidazole. *N. Engl. J. Med.* 303:1212, 1980.
20. Griffith, J. F., and Ch'ien, L. T. Herpes simplex virus encephalitis: Diagnostic and treatment considerations. *Med. Clin. North Am.* 67:991, 1983.
21. Hirsch, M. S., and Schooley, R. T. Treatment of herpesvirus infections. *N. Engl. J. Med.* 309:963, 1034, 1983.
22. Jaffe, H., et al. Complications of cotrimoxazole in the treatment of AIDS-associated *Pneumocystis carinii* pneumonia in homosexual men. *Lancet* 2:1109, 1983.
23. Komaroff, A. L. Acute dysuria in women. *N. Engl. J. Med.* 310:368, 1984.
24. Kreger, B. E., Craven, D. E., and McCabe, W. R. Gram-negative bacteremia: IV. Reevaluation of clinical features and treatment in 612 patients. *Am. J. Med.* 68:344, 1980.
25. Kucers, A. Chloramphenicol, erythromycin, vancomycin, tetracyclines. *Lancet* 2:425, 1982.
26. LeFrock, J. L., Moldavi, A., and Prince, R. Clindamycin. *Med. Clin. North Am.* 66:103, 1982.
27. Levison, M. E., et al. Clindamycin compared with penicillin for the treatment of anaerobic lung abscess. *Ann. Intern. Med.* 98:466, 1983.
28. Matthay, R. A., and Greene, W. H. Pulmonary infections in the immunocompromised patient. *Med. Clin. North Am.* 64:529, 1980.
29. Medical Letter. Choice of cephalosporins. *Med. Lett. Drugs Ther.* 25:57, 1983.
30. Medoff, G., and Kobayashi, G. S. Strategies in the treatment of systemic fungal infections. *N. Engl. J. Med.* 302:145, 1980.
31. Merson, M. H., et al. Current trends in botulism in the United States. *J.A.M.A.* 229:1305, 1974.
32. Moore, R. D., et al. Risk factors for nephrotoxicity in patients treated with aminoglycosides. *Ann. Intern. Med.* 100:352, 1984.
33. Murray, E. S. Rickettsial Diseases. In R. D. Feigin and J. D. Cherry (eds.). *Textbook of Pediatric Infectious Diseases.* Philadelphia: Saunders, 1981. Pp. 1437–1449.
34. Neu, H. C. The new betalactamase-stable cephalosporins. *Ann. Intern. Med.* 97:408, 1982.
35. Phillips, I. Aminoglycosides. *Lancet* 2:311, 1982.
36. Pruitt, A., et al. Neurologic complications of bacterial endocarditis. *Medicine* (Baltimore) 57:329, 1978.
37. Radetsky, M. A diagnostic approach to Epstein-Barr virus infections. *Pediatr. Infect. Dis.* 1:425, 1982.
38. Reeves, D. Sulphonamides and trimethoprim. *Lancet* 2:370, 1982.
39. Rubin, R. H., and Swartz, M. N. Trimethoprim-sulfamethoxazole. *N. Engl. J. Med.* 303:426, 1980.
40. Skoldenberg, B., et al. Acyclovir versus vidarabine in herpes simplex encephalitis. *Lancet* 2:707, 1984.
41. Stamm, W. E., et al. Treatment of the acute urethral syndrome. *N. Engl. J. Med.* 301:956, 1979.
42. Stamm, W. E., et al. Causes of the acute urethral syndrome in women. *N. Engl. J. Med.* 303:409, 1980.
43. Stamm, W. E., et al. Diagnosis of coliform infection in acutely dysuric women. *N. Engl. J. Med.* 307:463, 1982.
44. Straus, S. E., et al. Suppression of frequently recurring genital herpes. *N. Engl. J. Med.* 310:1545, 1984.

45. Sullivan, T. J. Pathogenesis and management of allergic reactions to penicillin and beta-lactam antibiotics. *Pediatr. Infect. Dis.* 1:344, 1982.
46. Swartz, M. N., and Dodge, P. R. Bacterial meningitis: A review of selected aspects. *N. Engl. J. Med.* 272:725, 779, 842, 898, 954, 1003, 1965.
47. Tofte, R. W., and Williams, D. N. Clinical and laboratory manifestations of the toxic shock syndrome. *Ann. Intern. Med.* 96:843, 1982.
48. Verghese, A., and Berk, S. Bacterial pneumonia in the elderly. *Medicine* (Baltimore) 62:271, 1983.
49. Waldvogel, F. A., Medoff, G., and Swartz, M. N. Osteomyelitis: A review of clinical features, therapeutic considerations and unusual aspects. *N. Engl. J. Med.* 282:198, 260, 316, 1970.
50. Waldvogel, F. A., and Vasey, H. Osteomyelitis: The past decade. *N. Engl. J. Med.* 303:360, 1980.
51. Weinstein, L. Tetanus. *N. Engl. J. Med.* 289:1293, 1973.
52. Whitley, R., et al. Herpes simplex encephalitis: Vidarabine therapy and diagnostic problems. *N. Engl. J. Med.* 304:313, 1981.
53. Wilson, W., et al. General considerations in the diagnosis and treatment of infective endocarditis. *Mayo Clin. Proc.* 57:81, 1982.
54. Wilson, W., et al. Prosthetic valve endocarditis. *Mayo Clin. Proc.* 57:155, 1982.
55. Wright, A. J., and Wilkowske, C. J. The penicillins. *Mayo Clin. Proc.* 58:21, 1983.

13 Renal Disorders

L. Lee Hamm III

Renal Physiology

The kidneys are involved in at least three major functions: (1) control of extracellular ionic composition, (2) excretion of various metabolic end products and toxins, and (3) metabolism of certain hormones.

I. **Control of extracellular ionic composition** involves the filtration of plasma across the glomeruli and subsequent resorption and secretion of the involved ions in a precise and regulated manner. Disorders of water metabolism, acid-base balance, and plasma ionic composition (Na^+, K^+, Ca^{2+}, Mg^{2+}, and $PO_4^=$) occur with renal failure; these problems are discussed in detail in Chaps. 8 and 9, since they frequently occur with other illnesses.

II. The **excretory function of the kidney** first involves glomerular filtration. Other processes, such as direct cellular uptake of some substances from the peritubular capillaries, cellular catabolism, and tubular secretion, also contribute to the renal elimination of toxins and metabolic end products.

   A. Normal **glomerular filtration** occurs at a rate exceeding 100 ml/minute for a young adult but decreases with advancing age. Glomerular filtration can be estimated by the **creatinine clearance** (C_{cr}) as follows:

   $$C_{cr} = \frac{\text{urine Cr concentration (mg/dl)} \times \text{urine volume (ml)}}{\text{plasma Cr concentration (mg/dl)} \times \text{time of urine collection (minutes)}}$$

   Usually collections are made for 24 hours; however, shorter periods can be used if the urine volume is collected reliably. A complete collection is essential and should contain at least 700 mg or 900 mg of creatinine/24 hours for females or males, respectively, with a stable plasma creatinine concentration.

   B. **Blood urea nitrogen (BUN) and plasma creatinine** can also be used as indices of renal function. However, both are affected by certain factors. The BUN is affected by dietary nitrogen (protein) intake, the catabolic rate, steroid administration, blood in the gastrointestinal tract, and severe liver disease. Plasma creatinine is a better index; however, it is affected by the muscle mass, muscle catabolism, and use of certain drugs (e.g., cimetidine) that interfere with creatinine handling by the kidney without altering glomerular filtration. Thus, both the BUN and creatinine, as indices of renal function, can be falsely low in small persons or malnourished patients with a decreased muscle mass.

III. **Hormonal functions.** The kidneys are a predominant target organ of certain hormones, such as aldosterone, antidiuretic hormone (ADH), and parathyroid hormone. In addition, the kidneys are also involved in the production, metabolism, and/or catabolism of certain hormones. The kidneys are the major site of production of erythropoietin and the active form of vitamin D; in contrast, the kidneys are involved in the degradation of certain hormones, such as insulin. Hormonal functions of the kidneys are altered by both acute and chronic renal failure.

Acute Renal Failure

The patient with acute renal failure may or may not be oliguric. Conversely, the patient with oliguria may or may not have acute renal failure. Certain aspects of the evaluation of these patients are common to both. The evaluation of both types of patients will be described together and the differences noted.

I. **Clinical features.** Patients with renal failure may present with oliguria or anuria; a change in pattern of urination (e.g., nocturia, frequency, hesitancy, decrease in urinary stream); dark urine; signs and symptoms of volume overload, including peripheral and/

or pulmonary edema; or a variety of nonspecific symptoms, including weakness, easy fatigability, and dyspnea. Occasionally, patients may be asymptomatic with severe renal insufficiency. On the other hand, patients may present severely ill from hyperkalemia, a metabolic acidosis, and/or volume overload. Few if any physiologic derangements are present in adults with glomerular filtration rates greater than 50 ml/minute, and patients with glomerular filtration rates above 20 ml/minute are usually asymptomatic.

II. The **diagnosis** of acute renal failure is established by a rising BUN or plasma creatinine or by a falling urine output. However, the elevation of plasma creatinine and BUN lag behind the fall in glomerular filtration; for example, with complete cessation of glomerular filtration, plasma creatinine usually rises only 1.2–2.5 mg/dl/day. Also, urine output does not necessarily fall with some forms of acute renal failure.

III. **Assessment.** The initial evaluation of patients with acute renal failure, oliguria, worsening of chronic renal insufficiency, or conditions with a strong possibility of causing acute renal failure (e.g., hypotension, sepsis, major trauma, chemical intoxication) includes a thorough history and physical examination, determination of serum electrolytes and plasma BUN and creatinine, and a urinalysis. In addition, an initial assessment of the urine volume is essential. Complete anuria should raise the suspicion of obstruction or loss of renal blood flow.

   A. The **history** should include a family history of renal disease, exposure to potential toxic medications, any changes in the pattern of urination, and any cardiovascular symptoms such as chest pain and dyspnea. In addition, a history of prior renal disease, hypertension, urinary tract obstruction, or diabetes mellitus is of importance.

   B. The **physical examination** should emphasize the following:
   1. Measurement of the **pulse and blood pressure,** both supine and standing.
   2. **Funduscopic examination** for signs of diabetes mellitus or hypertension.
   3. A thorough **abdominal examination,** including checks for tender or palpable kidneys and a palpable bladder.
   4. Scrutiny for signs of **intravascular volume overload** (including peripheral and pulmonary edema) or volume depletion.
   5. Careful evaluation for **pericarditis.**
   6. A careful **neurologic examination** for such signs as asterixis and peripheral neuropathy.
   7. **Examination of the extremities,** which should include not only an evaluation of muscle strength but also an assessment of muscle tenderness, looking for rhabdomyolysis.

   C. **Radiologic evaluation** should be obtained in nearly all cases of oliguria or acute renal failure. However, radiocontrast studies can be detrimental and should only be used in selected circumstances. Radiologic studies are useful to demonstrate obstruction, identify vascular problems, demonstrate kidney size, and check for the presence of two kidneys. The last is important, since pathologic processes involving a single kidney usually do not cause major decrements in renal function unless only one functioning kidney was initially present.
   1. **Plain abdominal films** can demonstrate radiopaque stones (most kidney stones) and kidney size and number in many patients. In some patients, the kidneys are not visualized well with plain films.
   2. **Renal sonography** is very useful in detecting obstruction as a cause of renal failure; its sensitivity and specificity are high.
   3. **Radionuclide scans** are best suited to establish the integrity of blood flow to the kidneys.
   4. **Radiocontrast studies** (e.g., renal arteriogram, intravenous pyelogram [IVP]) should only be obtained with clear indications. **In most cases of oliguria or acute renal failure, the administration of a radiocontrast agent is a high risk for additional renal damage.** However, certain circumstances require a radiocontrast study. An IVP is generally indicated in the trauma patient when damage to the kidneys or ureters is suspected. A strong possibility of obstruction amenable to surgery should lead to an IVP or retrograde pyelogram.

   D. **Consideration of obstructive uropathy.** Sonography is usually the best method to screen for ureteral obstruction. In addition, obstruction at the level of the bladder or urethra should be addressed; a post-void residual urine volume of less than 200 ml usually eliminates this possibility. In patients with an indwelling bladder catheter, the catheter should be irrigated to ensure patency.

Table 13-1. Urinary indices in oliguria

Urinary index	Prerenal azotemia	"Paranchymal" acute renal failure
Urine Na$^+$ (mEq/liter)	<20	>40
FE$_{Na^+}$*	<1	>2
Urine/plasma creatinine	>40	<20

*Fractional excretion of Na$^+$: $FE_{Na^+} = \dfrac{\text{urine Na}^+ \times \text{plasma creatinine}}{\text{plasma Na}^+ \times \text{urine creatinine}} \times 100.$

E. The **urine composition** (Table 13-1) can be very helpful in differentiating causes of oliguria or renal failure. In the oliguric patient, a low urinary sodium, a low fractional excretion of sodium, and a high urine-plasma creatinine ratio usually indicate a prerenal cause of azotemia. Conversely, a high urinary sodium, a high fractional excretion of sodium, and low urine-plasma creatinine ratio generally indicate parenchymal renal damage in the oliguric patient. Urinary indices, however, are more variable in nonoliguric patients, patients with obstruction, and patients with preexisting kidney disease. The recent use of diuretics or a metabolic alkalosis may also alter the pattern of the urinary indices; the urinary sodium may be high despite volume depletion and prerenal azotemia. In patients with a metabolic alkalosis, the excretion of large amounts of bicarbonate in the urine obligates the excretion of sodium; however, the urinary chloride will still be low in patients with a prerenal cause of azotemia. In addition, the urine in patients with parenchymal acute renal failure may contain numerous epithelial cells, cellular debris, and casts.

F. **Fluid challenge.** In some patients with oliguria where differentiation of parenchymal renal damage and prerenal azotemia is difficult, a fluid challenge may be indicated (in the absence of intravascular volume overload). Usually, 500–1000 ml of normal saline is administered over 1–2 hours. Caution must be exercised in administering fluid, however, since patients with parenchymal renal damage may be unable to excrete the administered volume.

IV. **Specific types of acute renal failure**

A. **Prerenal azotemia**

1. **Etiology.** Prerenal azotemia is most often caused by volume depletion or hypotension. Some states of whole-body sodium excess, such as the nephrotic syndrome, cirrhosis, and severe congestive heart failure, can also cause prerenal azotemia; these conditions represent examples of low plasma volume or low "effective arterial volume." In these conditions, the kidneys avidly retain sodium and water (presumably because of hemodynamic or humoral factors). Some states of severe vasoconstriction can also cause prerenal azotemia without either hypotension or volume depletion.

2. **Differential diagnosis.** Malignant hypertension and some cases of acute glomerulonephritis can mimic many aspects of prerenal azotemia, particularly the urinary indices. The hepatorenal syndrome seen in severe liver disease also mimics prerenal azotemia in urinary indices and other functional abnormalities.

3. **Diagnosis.** Prerenal azotemia is suggested by a history and physical examination consistent with volume depletion, hypotension, or one of the conditions mentioned in sec. **IV.A.1.** Samples of urine and plasma should be obtained before any therapy, especially administration of diuretics or fluid. A plasma BUN/creatinine ratio greater than 10–15:1 often indicates prerenal azotemia. The urinary indices are usually as described in Table 13-1. The urine volume is usually (but not invariably) low.

4. **Treatment** should be directed at the cause of the prerenal azotemia. With volume depletion, fluid should be administered in the form of normal saline, Ringer's lactate, or blood (if needed). Prerenal azotemia caused by hypotension, shock, and those conditions associated with overall volume excess (e.g., nephrotic syndrome, cirrhosis, congestive heart failure) requires treatment of the underlying illness to improve renal function; in difficult cases, a Swan-Ganz catheter may be needed to assess adequately the intravascular volume, left

Table 13-2. Causes of acute renal failure

Prerenal azotemia

Obstruction

Parenchymal renal damage
   Ischemia
   Exogenous nephrotoxins (e.g., aminoglycosides, nonsteroidal anti-inflam-
     matory drugs, amphotericin, radiographic contrast agents, ethylene glycol)
   Endogenous nephrotoxins (myoglobin, hemoglobin, uric acid)
   Acute interstitial nephritis
   Acute glomerulonephritis
   Hepatorenal syndrome
   Postpartum renal failure, hemolytic uremic syndrome, thrombotic throm-
     bocytopenic purpura
   Sepsis
   Collagen-vascular diseases, vasculitis
   Malignant hypertension

ventricular filling pressure, and cardiac output. Contrast agents, prostaglandin inhibitors (i.e., nonsteroidal anti-inflammatory drugs), and other potential nephrotoxins should be avoided in these patients, if possible. Dialysis may be required if parenchymal renal damage and renal failure ensue; but even without "parenchymal" renal failure, the azotemia may occasionally require dialysis when the condition is not quickly reversible.

B. Parenchymal renal failure

  1. Etiology. Important causes of acute renal failure are listed in Table 13-2.

  2. Diagnosis. In patients presenting with renal failure, parenchymal renal failure is presumed when obstruction and prerenal azotemia have been excluded. Parenchymal renal failure may or may not produce oliguria or anuria. Parenchymal renal disease is sometimes indicated by an abnormal urine sediment (e.g., numerous casts, cellular debris, red or white cells) in contrast to either pre- or postrenal causes of azotemia in which these abnormalities are not usually found.

  3. Classification. Parenchymal renal failure should be classified as either acute renal failure or chronic renal failure. This separation is important in defining the etiology, therapy, and prognosis for recovery. Although this differentiation can often be difficult, clues to the presence of chronicity of the renal failure include evidence of small kidneys, anemia, and metabolic bone disease on x-rays. A history of chronic renal disease or a lack of history of an acute renal insult is also important.

  4. Prevention or amelioration of acute renal failure. Certain measures may help prevent or ameliorate parenchymal renal failure. Careful following of aminoglycoside levels may lessen the occurrence of aminoglycoside nephrotoxicity. Nonsteroidal anti-inflammatory drugs generally should be avoided in patients with impaired renal function. The use of mannitol and hydration prior to the use of radiographic contrast agents may decrease the incidence of contrast-induced acute renal failure. Acute uric acid nephropathy from tumor lysis may be preventable with hydration and administration of allopurinol prior to chemotherapy. Prompt treatment of any underlying illness (e.g., hypotension, sepsis, major trauma, chemical intoxication) may ameliorate developing renal failure. In addition, acute renal failure secondary to ischemia, rhabdomyolysis, or hemolysis may be ameliorated with the use of mannitol and maintenance of a good urine flow rate. The usual dosage of mannitol in the prophylaxis of acute renal failure is 25 gm IV over 15–30 minutes; furosemide, 80–320 mg IV, may also be used in an attempt to establish a high urine flow rate.

  5. Treatment

    a. General measures. In patients presenting with renal failure, careful attention to fluid and electrolyte administration should be observed. Potassium, magnesium, or phosphate should not be given unless there is a documented deficiency. Salt and water administration should be limited. In the oliguric patient without volume depletion, 1000–1500 ml of fluid/day usually replaces insensible and urinary losses; in the nonoliguric patient, fluid and salt intake can be greater than in the oliguric patient. In either case, good nutritional support is necessary. Drug administration in patients with renal failure frequently has to be altered because of the renal failure (see **Chronic Renal Failure**, sec. **V**). In the patient with acute renal failure, careful and strict precautions against nosocomial or iatrogenic infections and gastrointestinal bleeds must be observed, since much of the high morbidity and mortality from acute renal failure results from these two complications.

b. Dialysis. In addition to careful management of fluid and electrolytes, dialysis may be necessary for complications of azotemia. Patients in a catabolic state (e.g., from severe sepsis, heat injury, surgery, or trauma), in particular, should undergo dialysis before the onset of complications and at frequent intervals.

(1) Indications for emergency dialysis include neurologic signs (e.g., lethargy, asterixis), severe symptoms (e.g., nausea, vomiting), symptomatic volume overload (i.e., pulmonary edema), refractory acidosis, pericarditis, and severe electrolyte disturbances (e.g., hyperkalemia, hypermagnesemia). Ideally, dialysis should be initiated before the onset of these severe problems.

(2) Choice of dialysis. Either peritoneal dialysis or hemodialysis may be used.

(a) Peritoneal dialysis (see **Chronic Renal Failure**, sec. **II.B.2**) has the advantages of slower fluid and electrolyte shifts (which may avert the disequilibrium syndrome) and avoidance of systemic heparinization. The disadvantages of peritoneal dialysis include the risk of peritoneal infection, slower removal of toxins, and technical difficulty in patients with prior abdominal surgery. Moreoever, peritoneal dialysis generally is not effective in the catabolic patient with acute renal failure.

(b) Hemodialysis (see **Chronic Renal Failure**, sec. **II.B.1**) is very efficient in removing small-molecular-weight uremic toxins (e.g., urea) and electrolytes (e.g., potassium). It requires blood access and usually systemic heparinization during dialysis. Temporary access can be obtained by catheterization of femoral or subclavian veins or placement of an external shunt in the forearm or leg. Heparinization is problematic in the presence of gastrointestinal bleeding and uremic pericarditis.

(c) Ultrafiltration is the use of a hemodialysis setup (i.e. vascular access, machine) to remove liters of extracellular fluid rapidly with less hypotension than with regular hemodialysis. Although ultrafiltration is very inefficient in removing uremic toxins, it can be used sequentially with hemodialysis to remove both toxins and fluid.

C. Postrenal obstruction. Identifying obstruction as the cause of azotemia is particularly important, since obstruction can often be relieved surgically or by other maneuvers, thus preventing permanent renal damage.

1. Etiology. Causes of obstruction are listed in Table 13-3. Since obstruction of

Table 13-3. Causes of postrenal obstruction

Ureteral obstruction
  Extraureteral
    Tumors
    Postsurgical
  Intraureteral
    Stones
    Blood clots
    Papillary necrosis (e.g., especially in diabetes mellitus, analgesic nephropathy, sickle cell disease)
Bladder neck obstruction
  Prostatic disease
  Bladder tumor
  Functional (e.g., diabetic autonomic neuropathy)
Urethral obstruction (e.g., blocked urinary catheter)

---

only one of two functioning kidneys does not cause azotemia, azotemia results only when both kidneys are obstructed, a solitary kidney is obstructed, one kidney is obstructed in combination with other renal functional impairment, or obstruction occurs at the level of the bladder or below.

2. **Clinical features.** Patients with urinary tract obstruction may present with symptoms referable to the urinary output, such as hesitancy or inability to empty the bladder completely. Alternating oliguria and polyuria or polyuria alone can be seen in patients with obstruction. Complete anuria should raise a strong suspicion of obstruction. The physical examination may reveal a distended bladder in cases of urethral or bladder neck obstruction.

3. **Diagnosis.** Methods to assess for obstruction usually include sonography (looking for a dilated renal calyceal system) and an estimation of residual urine with bladder catheterization after voiding. A radiocontrast study is often needed to identify the exact site and nature of the obstruction.

4. **Treatment** usually involves either surgical placement of a temporary drainage device (e.g., stint) or corrective surgery.

V. **Disposition.** Hospital admission is always indicated in patients with acute renal failure.

Chronic Renal Failure

Chronic renal failure implies irreversible renal injury and includes two groups of patients. The first group of patients consists of those with severe chronic renal insufficiency that is not yet to the point of requiring chronic dialysis. The second group includes patients who have very little or no renal function and therefore require chronic dialysis to replace the excretory functions of the kidney.

I. Frequent **etiologies** of chronic renal failure are listed in Table 13-4.

II. **Management principles**

A. **Conservative management of chronic renal insufficiency**

1. **Preservation of remaining renal function.** The goal of management of patients with chronic renal insufficiency is to slow or halt the progression to end-stage renal disease. These efforts include good control of hypertension, prevention or early treatment of urinary tract infection, and avoidance of other renal insults, such as obstruction, volume depletion, and nephrotoxic drugs (including nonsteroidal anti-inflammatory agents). A low-protein diet is well known to lessen azotemia and hence is prescribed for many patients with chronic renal insufficiency. In addition, recent suggestions have been made that a very low protein diet may slow the progression of renal insufficiency. With certain forms of kidney disease, medications may be used to treat the renal disease directly, such as steroids in membranous nephropathy and steroids or cytotoxic agents in lupus erythematosus.

2. **Maintenance care.** When creatinine clearance is less than 20–30 ml/minute (usually a plasma creatinine > 3 mg/dl), dietary restriction of potassium, phosphate, magnesium, protein, salt, and fluid may be required. Phosphate binders, such as aluminum hydroxide or calcium carbonate, and alkalinizing agents (i.e., sodium bicarbonate or Shohl's solution) may be necessary in some patients with chronic renal insufficiency. Patients with chronic renal insufficiency are also followed for symptoms or signs of severe azotemia that indicate the need for institution of dialysis; these include lassitude, lethargy, extreme fatigue, anorexia, nausea, pericarditis, weight loss, refractory fluid retention, and encephalopathy.

Table 13-4. Important causes of chronic renal failure

Chronic glomerulonephritis

Secondary glomerular injury (e.g., diabetes mellitus, lupus erythematosus)

Hypertensive nephrosclerosis

Hereditary renal disease (e.g., polycystic kidney disease, Alport's syndrome)

Chronic obstruction or reflux

Renal artery stenosis (bilateral)

Interstitial renal disease (e.g., analgesic nephropathy, chronic pyelonephritis)

B. Dialysis
1. **Hemodialysis** basically involves the pumping of heparinized blood through a dialyzer and returning the blood to the patient. Small molecules, such as potassium and uremic toxins, are removed in the dialyzer by diffusion across a semipermeable membrane. Most patients with chronic renal failure undergo hemodialysis 3 times/week for 3–5 hours/treatment. Blood access may be obtained through an external Scribner shunt, a surgically created arteriovenous fistula, or a subcutaneous bovine or Gortex graft. The use of dialysis, however, does not eliminate the need for dietary restrictions. In general, the well-dialyzed patient who is adhering to a prescribed diet should not develop severe complications of azotemia or uremia. Therefore, the new onset of a problem, such as encephalopathy, should prompt the physician to look for causes other than azotemia or uremia, such as infection.
2. **Peritoneal dialysis** involves instillation of an aqueous solution into the peritoneal cavity, diffusion of uremic toxins and other small molecules into this solution, and removal and discarding of the fluid. The principle by which uremic toxins, potassium, and other small molecules are removed by peritoneal dialysis is the same as for hemodialysis, that is, passive diffusion of molecules down a concentration gradient across a semipermeable membrane, which in the case of peritoneal dialysis is the peritoneal lining. Chronic peritoneal access is obtained through a surgically placed Silastic tube, a Tenchoff catheter. The dialysis fluid contains electrolytes, such as sodium and chloride, and is hypertonic with dextrose to remove fluid. Chronic peritoneal dialysis can be done intermittently (commonly only at night) or continuously as continuous ambulatory peritoneal dialysis (CAPD). With CAPD, 1.5–2.0 liters of dialysis fluid is instilled into the peritoneal cavity, kept there for several hours, and then drained; usually this procedure is repeated 4 times/day by the patient.

III. Complications of renal failure. Only severe or frequent complications are mentioned.
A. Anemia is almost invariably found in patients with chronic renal failure. Patients on hemodialysis usually have a hematocrit of 20–30%. Patients are usually transfused only for specific symptoms or problems, such as progressive weakness or chest pain.
B. Pericarditis (see Chap. 5) can occur in patients with severe uremia and in those seemingly well dialyzed. The etiology in the latter group is not clear. Chest pain and a pericardial friction rub may not be present. Pericardial effusions are usually small and sometimes loculated. However, pericardial tamponade (see sec. **IV.B**) can occur. The usual therapeutic approach is to institute more frequent dialysis with minimal heparinization. Administration of steroids or surgical pericardial stripping is generally reserved for refractory or recurrent cases.
C. Hyperkalemia is a common and serious complication of chronic renal failure. Dietary indiscretion, iatrogenic potassium loads, and endogenous cellular potassium release following surgery are common causes. Clinical features and therapy are discussed in Chap. 8.
D. Vascular access complications. Access problems probably represent the most frequent cause for hospitalization in hemodialysis patients.
1. **Infections** in and around the vascular access are common. The most frequent organism is *Staphylococcus aureus*. Bacteremia from these infections is common and may not be attended by the usual manifestations of bacteremia (e.g., fever, hypotension). Although some access infections can be managed on an outpatient basis, physicians experienced in the care of hemodialysis patients should be involved in this decision. Vancomycin, which needs to be given IV only once per week in patients with no renal function, or a cephalosporin is often good initial therapy for access infections.
2. **Clotted vascular accesses** also account for a significant number of hospitalizations in hemodialysis patients. Clots frequently can be removed surgically and a functioning access preserved if therapy is initiated early.
3. **Bleeding** may occur at the vascular access site. Application of direct pressure generally will control the bleeding.
E. Peritonitis is a very frequent problem in patients on peritoneal dialysis. Common organisms include *Staphylococcus epidermidis*, other gram-positive cocci, *Escherichia coli, Pseudomonas,* and other gram-negative rods. Abdominal pain and a cloudy dialysis fluid are almost invariably present. However, fever is often absent. Hospitalization is not necessary unless the infection is prolonged or accompanied by

severe pain or systemic manifestations. A sample of the dialysis drainage should be sent for a cell count and culture. The patient should then be started on an antibiotic. Pending culture results, a good antibiotic regimen is the instillation of a cephalosporin into the dialysis fluid (e.g., 250 mg of cephalothin/liter of dialysis fluid). Frequent (hourly) dialysis exchanges are performed until the pain is relieved and the dialysis drainage is clear. Indications for removal of the peritoneal catheter include frequent infections with the same organisms, infection of the catheter tract, fungal peritonitis, and peritonitis resistant to appropriate antibiotics.

F. **Other complications.**

1. **Ischemic heart disease** is a frequent occurrence in patients on chronic hemodialysis.
2. **Hypertension** is common and frequently results from volume overload.
3. **Excessive bleeding** may occur because of coagulation disturbances that accompany chronic renal failure.
4. **Infections.** Patients with chronic renal failure are predisposed to a number of infections (e.g., cryptococcal meningitis, tuberculosis) and may have more subtle manifestations than usual (e.g., lack of fever) from almost any infection. A chronic carrier state of **hepatitis B** antigen is not infrequent, although symptomatic hepatitis is more unusual.

IV. **Dialysis emergencies**

A. **Hypotension** is a common occurrence during hemodialysis and results from fluid removal and a variety of other phenomena, such as osmotic shifts. Hypotension usually responds to the administration of fluid, hypertonic saline, mannitol, or albumin. Hypotension unresponsive to these agents may require discontinuation of dialysis and a search for other causes, such as intrinsic cardiac problems or pericardial tamponade.

B. **Pericardial tamponade** (see Chap. 5) is not common during dialysis but is frequently fatal when it occurs. Patients may or may not have been recognized as having had pericarditis prior to the tamponade. This complication is undoubtedly promoted by the systemic administration of heparin during dialysis. Emergency treatment consists of fluid administration, isoproterenol infusion, and pericardiocentesis. Definitive therapy, however, is necessary on an emergent basis and involves surgical placement of a pericardial window.

C. **Bleeding** is a predictable complication of dialysis and renal failure, particularly acute renal failure. Not only do patients with renal failure have recognized coagulation defects, but also hemodialysis requires the systemic administration of heparin to prevent clotting of the dialyzer. Bleeding complications can be lessened by administering lower doses of heparin during dialysis; this can be accomplished by carefully monitoring clotting times during dialysis. When bleeding occurs, fresh frozen plasma may be of some benefit. Occasionally, administration of protamine may be necessary to reverse the heparin effect.

D. **Technical problems** that arise during hemodialysis should be managed by someone experienced in the technique of hemodialysis. Such complications include air embolism (the patient should be placed on the left side with the head down and feet up), blood leaks, dialysate solution errors (hypotonic or hypertonic dialysate can produce hemolysis and central nervous system manifestations), and the use of over- or underheated dialysate.

E. **Complications of peritoneal dialysis** that should be considered include infection (see sec. **III.E**), hyperglycemia, hypo- and hypernatremia, and fluid imbalances (i.e., excess fluid retention or depletion).

V. **Medication modifications.** The dosages or dosing intervals of many medications need to be adjusted in patients with chronic renal disease. Loading doses, however, usually do not need to be adjusted. Drugs that are metabolized or excreted primarily by the kidneys obviously require dosage adjustments as renal function decreases. Also, drugs removed by hemodialysis or peritoneal dialysis need to be adjusted accordingly. Table 13-5 lists common medicines that need to be adjusted in patients with renal disease. For a more complete and detailed summary of drug modification in patients with renal failure, the reader is referred to reviews on the subject [2, 4].

Nephrotic Syndrome

The nephrotic syndrome is characterized by heavy proteinuria (i.e., >3–5 gm of protein/24 hours), hypoalbuminemia, edema, and hypercholesterolemia.

I. **Etiology.** Frequent causes of the nephrotic syndrome include diabetic nephropathy,

Table 13-5. Common drugs requiring major adjustments with renal failure[a]

Antimicrobials	Cardiovascular agents/antihypertensives
Aminoglycosides	Atenolol
Acyclovir	Nadolol
Cephalosporins[b]	Bretylium
Tetracyclines (should be avoided)	Disopyramide
Penicillins[b]	Procainamide
Sulfonamides	Digoxin
Vancomycin	Miscellaneous
Sedatives, psychotropics, anticonvulsants	Allopurinol
Lithium	Cisplatin
Some sedatives	Methotrexate
Primidone	Acetohexamide
	Chlorpropamide
	Clofibrate
	Pancuronium
	Cimetidine

[a]See a more complete list for specific information, including dosage guidelines, and drugs not listed [2, 4].
[b]Only a small modification needed with some of these drugs.

membranous glomerulonephritis, minimal change disease (the most common lesion in the pediatric population), and other glomerular diseases, including those caused by certain systemic illnesses (e.g., lupus erythematosus, amyloidosis).

II. **Pathophysiology.** The nephrotic syndrome originates from an excess leakage of plasma proteins (chiefly albumin) across the glomerulus into the tubular fluid. As more plasma albumin is lost in the urine, the capacity of the liver to produce albumin eventually is exceeded and hypoalbuminemia ensues. Hypoalbuminemia results in edema from the reduced plasma oncotic pressure in systemic capillaries and from salt retention by the kidneys secondary to the reduced effective arteriolar volume.

III. **Clinical features.** The primary manifestation is edema. Ascites and pleural effusions may also occur. The intravascular volume is usually low or normal. Infections are not infrequent, particularly cellulitis and peritonitis. Renal vein thrombosis may occur secondary to the nephrotic syndrome, particularly when caused by membranous glomerulonephritis; occasionally, renal vein thrombosis may be associated with pulmonary embolism. Renal insufficiency and urinary sediment abnormalities frequently are absent in patients with the nephrotic syndrome.

IV. The **differential diagnosis** of the nephrotic syndrome includes the other major diseases that cause edema: congestive heart failure and other heart conditions (e.g., constrictive pericarditis), cirrhosis, and renal insufficiency with volume overload. The heavy proteinuria and hypoalbuminemia serve to distinguish the nephrotic syndrome from the other conditions. The nephrotic syndrome also needs to be distinguished from other causes of proteinuria, such as myeloma and certain renal interstitial diseases that cause "tubular proteinuria"; in these conditions, profound hypoalbuminemia is usually absent.

V. Symptomatic **treatment** of the edema is usually the goal (in the absence of specific treatment of the primary disease process). Salt restriction and the judicious use of diuretics are usually indicated. Bed rest (with precautions against venous thrombosis) can also be used. However, diuresis may be difficult because of the low intravascular volume. Dietary protein should be sufficient to replace urinary losses and provide nutritional requirements. Corticosteroids (and occasionally cytotoxic agents) are used in several types of glomerulonephritis that lead to the nephrotic syndrome; steroids not only frequently lessen proteinuria but in some cases may decrease the progression to renal insufficiency.

VI. **Disposition.** The new presentation of the nephrotic syndrome deserves a thorough evaluation for an etiologic diagnosis; this frequently requires hospitalization. Patients with the nephrotic syndrome (with an established etiology and treatment plan) who present with progressive edema generally require hospitalization because of the risk of intravascular volume depletion and electrolyte abnormalities with diuresis. On the other hand, a new discovery of mild, isolated proteinuria can be worked up initially on an outpatient basis.

Renal Transplantation

I. **Cadaveric donor kidney procurement.** Many aspects of the management of the potential organ donor should be guided by an experienced procurement team, which should be notified as soon as a potential donor (see sec. I.A) is identified. However, initial screening and management are often instituted in the emergency department.

   A. **Criteria for potential cadaveric donors.** In general, kidneys are best procured from donors who have irreversible brain damage but are otherwise free of potential insults to the kidneys. Such conditions include head trauma and cerebrovascular accidents. Brain death (see Chap. 32) is required, and the cause of death needs to be known with certainty. The potential donor can be from 6 (occasionally younger) to 55 years old. The potential donor should have normal kidney function as assessed by a plasma BUN or creatinine, occasionally some elevation of the BUN or creatinine is allowed when the cause is thought to be volume depletion or mild prerenal azotemia. However, there can be no evidence of diseases likely to involve the kidneys (e.g., diabetes mellitus, hypertension, severe atherosclerotic disease) and no evidence of potentially transmissible diseases (i.e., bacterial, viral, or fungal infections and most malignancies except for solitary nonmetastasizing brain tumors). Appropriate consent for organ donation needs to be obtained.

   B. **Medical treatment of the cadaveric donor.** Pending organ procurement, the potential cadaveric donor should be maintained to ensure well-functioning kidneys. Generous hydration needs to be provided by intravenous fluids; this should also provide an adequate diuresis. The blood pressure should be maintained near normal; if a vasopressor is necessary, one that does not adversely affect renal blood flow (e.g., dopamine) should be used. Some centers may also give cyclophosphamide and/or prednisone prior to harvesting the kidneys.

II. **Complications in renal transplant patients.** A variety of medical illnesses are frequent complications in the renal transplant recipient after the initial posttransplant period. Many of these complications are chronic and will not be discussed further. Rejection of the transplanted organ and acute infections, however, need to be recognized early.

   A. **Acute renal transplant rejection** is usually indicated by a fever, reduced renal function, and frequently graft tenderness. Acute rejection (to be differentiated from gradually occurring chronic rejection) usually occurs within the first 6 months of transplantation and is frequently treatable with additional immunosuppression. A sudden decline in renal function, a rise in serum BUN or creatinine, or other problems raising suspicion of acute rejection should prompt immediate hospitalization and further evaluation (e.g., renal sonogram, renal scan). Obstruction of the transplanted kidney, arterial stenosis, cyclosporine toxicity, and other conditions are included in the differential diagnosis of acute rejection in the transplant patient.

   B. **Infections.** Immunosuppressed transplant recipients are predisposed to life-threatening infections but may not show typical signs of serious infection. Urinary tract infection, pneumonia, sepsis, and wound infection represent common infections in renal transplant recipients. In addition to ordinary infections, immunosuppressed transplant recipients are particularly susceptible to a variety of opportunistic infections, such as cryptococcal meningitis, *Listeria* meningitis, cytomegalovirus, and pneumocystis pneumonia. Furthermore, such common diagnoses as appendicitis may be difficult because of the immunosuppression. Transplant patients presenting with fever should be hospitalized and extensively evaluated.

Bibliography

1. Anderson, R. J., et al. Nonoliguric acute renal failure. *N. Engl. J. Med.* 296:1134, 1977.
2. Bennett, W. M., et al. Drug prescribing in renal failure: Dosing guidelines for adults. *Am. J. Kidney Dis.* 3:155, 1983.
3. Bennett, W. M., Plamp, C., and Porter, G. A. Drug-related syndromes in clinical nephrology. *Ann. Intern. Med.* 87:582, 1977.
4. Bennett, W. M., et al. Drug therapy in renal failure: Dosing guidelines for adults. *Ann. Intern. Med.* 93:62, 286, 1980.
5. Fer, M. F., et al. Cancer and the kidney: Renal complications of neoplasms. *Am. J. Med.* 71:704, 1981.
6. Harrington, J. T., and Cohen, J. J. Acute oliguria. *N. Engl. J. Med.* 292:89, 1975.
7. Harter, H. R., and Martin, K. J. Acute renal failure. *Postgrad. Med.* 72:175, 1982.
8. Madais, M. P., and Harrington, J. T. The diagnosis of acute glomerulonephritis. *N. Engl. J. Med.* 309:1299, 1984.
9. Schrier, R. W. Acute renal failure. *Hosp. Pract.* 16:93, 1981.

Rheumatologic Disorders

Jeffrey L. Kaine

General Principles

I. Evaluation

A. History and physical examination. The protean nature of the rheumatic diseases makes a careful medical history and physical examination essential in the initial patient management.

   1. Extraarticular symptoms are often the key to the diagnosis. Fever, constitutional symptoms, alopecia, symptoms of the sicca syndrome, oral and nasal ulcers, a photosensitive skin rash, and pleurisy suggest systemic lupus erythematosus (SLE). Subcutaneous nodules occur in 20% of rheumatoid arthritis (RA) patients. Genital lesions associated with arthritis may provide evidence for Behçet's disease or Reiter's syndrome, while a vaginal discharge associated with skin lesions and arthritis is nearly pathognomonic of disseminated gonococcal infection. Jaw claudication, headache, and associated visual complaints strongly suggest giant-cell arteritis.

   2. Detailed **characterization of arthritis** is critical in the initial patient evaluation. Acute onset of arthritis suggests an infectious or crystal-induced arthritis. Morning stiffness is characteristic of the synovial based arthritides (e.g., rheumatoid arthritis), while pain with exercise suggests degenerative joint disease (DJD).

     a. Acute monarthritis. Traumatic, infectious, and crystalline-induced arthritides are the most commonly encountered forms of acute monarthritis. Chronic monarticular arthritis is most commonly degenerative in nature, although tumors and indolent infections may cause diagnostic dilemmas.

     b. Oligoarthritis (i.e., involvement of 2–4 joints) and **polyarthritis** (i.e., involvement of 5 or more joints) are seen in a wide variety of rheumatic diseases, including the classic "connective tissue diseases," viral arthritis, crystalline arthritis, the vasculitides, and serum sickness. Among infectious arthritis, gonococcal arthritis is frequently oligoarticular, while nongonococcal arthritis is usually monarticular.

B. Laboratory tests. A variety of sophisticated immunologic tests are available to characterize various aspects of rheumatic disease; however, these complex tests generally have no role in emergency patient management.

   1. A complete blood count, urinalysis, erythrocyte sedimentation rate (ESR), and serum creatinine are the only routinely required tests. Uric acid determination is often helpful, although not essential in emergency department management.

   2. Synovianalysis. The evaluation of acute arthritis demands a detailed analysis of the synovial fluid, whenever possible. In acute monarthritis, synovianalysis can establish the diagnosis in a majority of patients. In oligo- and polyarthritis, synovianalysis is required to exclude infection, as well as to assess the degree of synovial inflammation. Analysis of the synovial fluid involves determination of a cell count with differential, a Gram stain and culture, a glucose determination, and crystal examination with polarizing microscopy. If only a small quantity of synovial fluid is obtained, 1 drop can be examined microscopically for the presence of crystals and degree of inflammation (inflammatory versus noninflammatory); a second drop is used for a Gram stain, and the remainder is sent for bacterial culture. Synovial fluid is classified as shown in Table 14-1.

C. Radiographic studies generally are indicated in evaluating patients with rheumatic symptoms. They may establish or confirm a suspected diagnosis (e.g., RA, DJD, osteomyelitis), although radiographs frequently are normal (e.g., SLE, many cases of gout, early RA).

Table 14-1. Classification of synovial effusions

Gross examination	Normal	Noninflammatory (Group I)	Inflammatory (Group II)	Septic (Group III)
Volume (ml), knee	<3.5	Often >3.5	Often >3.5	Often >3.5
Viscosity	High	High	Low	Variable
Color	Colorless to straw	Straw to yellow	Yellow	Variable
Glucose	Similar to serum	Similar to serum	Variable	Low
WBCs (/mm^3)	<200	200–1999	2000–75,000	Often >100,000*
PMN leukocytes (%)	<25	<25	Often >50	>75*
Culture	Negative	Negative	Negative	Often positive
Differential diagnosis		Osteoarthritis	RA	Bacterial infections
		Traumatic arthritis	Gout	
		Avascular necrosis	Pseudogout	
		SLE	SLE	
		ARF	ARF	
		PSS	PSS	
			Vasculitides	
			Spondyloarthropathies	
			Infectious arthritis	

Key: WBCs = white blood cells; PMN = polymorphonuclear; RA = rheumatoid arthritis; SLE = systemic lupus erythematosus; ARF = acute rheumatic fever; PSS = progressive systemic sclerosis.
*WBC count and percent PMN leukocytes will be less if infection is partially treated.

D. For patients with established rheumatic disease, the primary physician should be contacted. Useful information regarding prior drug therapy or complications of disease will often influence the emergency department physician's choice of therapy.

II. Drug therapy in rheumatic diseases. The nonsteroidal anti-inflammatory agents (NSAIDs) and glucocorticoids are rapidly acting anti-inflammatory drugs. Initiation of therapy with these drugs is appropriate in the emergency setting. In contrast, the slow-acting antirheumatic agents (e.g., gold, D-penicillamine, alkylating agents) must be administered for weeks to months before clinical efficacy becomes apparent. Initial administration of these agents should be limited to physicians providing primary care.

A. NSAIDs include salicylate derivatives and other inhibitors of prostaglandin biosynthesis.

   1. Salicylates represent the initial drug of choice for most rheumatic complaints. Various preparations are listed in Table 14-2. In addition to being less expensive than the other NSAIDs, serum levels (the therapeutic level is 15–25 mg/dl) may be obtained to monitor compliance. The major disadvantages of salicylate therapy are the larger dosage of medication required and an increased incidence of gastrointestinal discomfort. Nausea and occult blood loss frequently occur. Enteric coated aspirin or sustained-release salicylate preparations are well absorbed, provide steady state levels, and are associated with less gastrointestinal disturbances than acetylsalicylic acid (ASA). Under most circumstances, salicylates should not be administered to patients taking anticoagulants because of an increased risk of bleeding. Magnesium or choline salicylate or salsalate may be used in patients "allergic" to ASA; although these nonacetylated derivatives are probably less potent than ASA, they have the advantage of decreased gastrointestinal toxicity. Salicylates may be used during pregnancy, although increased bleeding at parturition may occasionally present problems.

   2. Nonsalicylate anti-inflammatory agents clinically are considered equally potent as anti-inflammatory agents. However, patients often note varying clinical responses, and a trial with different drugs is frequently warranted. Dosages of the various nonsalicylate NSAIDs are given in Table 14-2. Overall their similarities are more striking than their differences. The nonsalicylate NSAIDs should be avoided during pregnancy. All these drugs may interact with warfarin-type anticoagulants, demanding careful monitoring of coagulation indices in patients taking such drugs. Patients allergic to ASA are generally allergic to all the nonsalicylate NSAIDs; however, the nonacetylated salicylates (see sec. **II.A.1**) may be used with caution. If a nonsalicylate NSAID is required, desensitization is necessary.

   Common **side effects** include gastrointestinal intolerance, central nervous system symptoms (especially with indomethacin), fluid retention, constipation, and skin rash. Hepatic and renal dysfunction may occur in individuals with preexisting disease; thus, these patients require careful follow-up. Bronchospasm, angioedema, and urticaria are rare side effects. Unique adverse reactions include: (a) aplastic anemia and agranulocytosis associated with phenylbutazone (which, if administered at all, should be for less than 1 week), (b) confusion and hallucinations in the elderly associated with indomethacin, and (c) diarrhea associated with mefenamic acid.

B. Corticosteroids are potent anti-inflammatory and immunosuppressive agents useful in treating both the articular and systemic manifestations of rheumatic diseases. They may be used safely during pregnancy.

   1. Drug selection. Prednisone is the drug of choice for oral administration; alternative compounds, such as prednisolone and dexamethasone, are substantially more expensive without substantial advantages. For intravenous administration, methylprednisolone is the preferred agent.

   2. The myriad **side effects** of glucocorticoids are in Table 14-3. Adverse reactions may be related to both the cumulative drug dose and the daily dosage.

   3. Dosage and route of administration. In all rheumatic diseases, the lowest dose of drug required to obtain disease control is the required dosage. Alternate-day corticosteroids are less suppressive of the hypothalamic-pituitary-adrenal axis but often do not provide adequate disease control. Twice daily administration is required for severe systemic disease and is the most suppressive of adrenal function. High-dose pulse steroids are occasionally used in life-threatening disease (see **Systemic Lupus Erythematosus**). Drug regimens are discussed in the individual disease sections. In general, initially a large dosage is used to control disease manifestations, and once this is accomplished, the dosage is tapered.

Table 14-2. Nonsteroidal anti-inflammatory agents

Generic name	Trade name	Tablet size (mg)	Starting adult dosage (mg)	Maximal daily dose (mg)
Salicylates				
Acetylsalicylate[a]	Aspirin	325	650–1300 q4–6h	b
	Encaprin	500	1000 q6–8h	b
	Zorprin	800	1600 q12h	b
Magnesium salicylate	Mobidin	600	600–1200 tid–qid	b
	Magan	545	545–1090 tid–qid	b
Choline salicylate[a]	Arthropan liquid	1 tsp = 650 mg acetylsalicylate	1 tsp q3–4h	b
Choline magnesium trisalicylate[a]	Trilisate	500, 750	1000–1250 bid	b
	Trilisate liquid	1 tsp = 500 mg salicylate	1000–1250 bid	b
Salsalate	Disalcid	500	1000 bid–1500 tid	b
Nonsalicylates				
Diflunisal	Dolobid	250, 500	250 bid	1500
Fenoprofen calcium	Nalfon	200, 300, 600	300–600 qid	3200
Ibuprofen	Motrin, Rufen	400, 600, 800	400 qid	3200
Indomethacin	Indocin	25, 50, 75	25 tid–qid	150
	Indocin suppositories	50	50 bid	150
Meclofenamate sodium	Meclomen	50, 100	50 tid–qid	400
Naproxen[a]	Naprosyn	250, 375, 500	250–375 bid	1000
Naproxen sodium	Anaprox	275	275 q6–8h	1375
Phenylbutazone	Butazolidin	100	100 tid	600
Piroxicam	Feldene	10, 20	20 qd	20
Sulindac	Clinoril	150, 200	150–200 bid	400
Tolmetin sodium[a]	Tolectin	200, 400	400 tid	1600

[a] Approved for use in children:
Acetylsalicylate: Children < 25 kg body weight: 80–100 mg/kg/day in 4 divided doses. Children > 25 kg body weight: 2400–3600 mg/day in 4 divided doses.
Naproxen (children 2 years and older): 10–15 mg/kg/day in 2–3 divided doses.
Tolmetin (children 2 years and older): Starting dosage, 20 mg/kg/day in 3–4 divided doses. Maintenance, 15–30 mg/kg/day in 3–4 divided doses.
Choline salicylate: See acetylsalicylate for childhood dosage.
Choline magnesium trisalicylate: Children < 37 kg body weight: 50 mg/kg/day in 2 divided doses. Children > 37 kg body weight: 2250 mg/day in 2 divided doses.
[b] Determined by measurement of serum salicylate level.
Source: Adapted from J. L. Kaine, Arthritis and Rheumatologic Diseases. In M. J. Orland and R. J. Saltman (eds.), *Manual of Medical Therapeutics* (25th ed.). Boston: Little, Brown, 1986.

Table 14-3. Glucocorticoid side effects

Cosmetic: moon face, buffalo hump, abdominal paunch, striae, weight gain, acne, hirsutism, fragile skin, poor wound healing

Cardiopulmonary: salt retention, hypertension, type IV hyperlipidemia with accelerated atherosclerosis, increased thromboembolic disease

Skeletal: osteopenia, vertebral and rib fractures, aseptic necrosis of hips and shoulders, other fractures

Metabolic: diabetes mellitus, hypokalemia, amenorrhea, adrenal insufficiency, altered drug metabolism

Ocular: cataracts, glaucoma

Central nervous system: depression, mania, psychosis, seizures, sleep disturbance

Gastrointestinal: gastritis, pancreatitis, peptic ulcer disease, gastrointestinal bleeding

Infections: decreased host resistance, opportunistic infections

---

The use of intraarticular corticosteroids is discussed under **Arthrocentesis** in Chap. 38.

   C. **Disease-modifying antirheumatic drugs** are used primarily in rheumatoid arthritis. They include parenteral gold compounds (aurothioglucose, aurothiomalate), D-penicillamine, and hydroxychloroquine; oral gold (auranofin) should be available in the near future. Prolonged therapy is required for clinical efficacy. All of these agents have substantial toxicity and do not represent initial therapy in rheumatoid arthritis; initiation of therapy should be made only by the primary care physician. None of these agents are approved for use during pregnancy. Approximately 30% of patients treated with parenteral gold experience toxicity; in D-penicillamine–treated patients, side effects are even more common (50%). Adverse reactions are similar and include (1) skin rash and oral mucosal lesions, both treated with transient cessation of the drug, followed by resumption at a lower dosage; (2) renal dysfunction with the nephrotic syndrome (i.e., >2 gm of protein/24-hour urine collection), which requires discontinuation of therapy; and (3) hematologic abnormalities (i.e., agranulocytosis, thrombocytopenia, and, rarely, aplastic anemia), which require immediate and permanent cessation of therapy. Hydroxychloroquine therapy requires routine ophthalmologic follow-up. An unusual retinopathy primarily affecting the macula is the major toxicity and is related to the cumulative dose; other adverse reactions include gastrointestinal side effects and skin rashes.

   D. **Immunosuppressive agents** (e.g., methotrexate, cyclophosphamide, chlorambucil, azathioprine) are used in severely ill patients with RA, SLE, polymyositis, and the vasculitic syndromes. All are myelosuppressive, and careful hematologic monitoring is essential. These drugs are all contraindicated during pregnancy. Immunosuppressive therapy is initiated by the primary physician, not by the emergency physician. Informed consent and detailed explanation of the risks and benefits are mandatory. The dosage is generally adjusted to maintain a leukocyte count greater than 3500 cells/mm^3, with an absolute lymphocyte count of less than 500 cells/mm^3. Unpredictable rapid declines in the leukocyte count occasionally occur, and patients may present acutely with infectious complications secondary to neutropenia. Temporary cessation of therapy will usually allow the white blood cell (WBC) count to return to normal. Additional side effects include hepatotoxicity, alopecia, sterility, amenorrhea, and possible delayed development of neoplasia. Hemorrhagic cystitis secondary to cyclophosphamide therapy may be severe and usually requires hospitalization with close observation.

   E. **Colchicine, allopurinol,** and the **uricosuric agents** are discussed under **The Arthritides,** sec. II.A.4.

  III. **Disposition.** Patient disposition depends on the diagnosis and clinical status of the patient. Systemically ill patients with suspected or documented rheumatic disease require hospitalization. Patients with septic arthritis (with the possible exception of gonococcal arthritis) also require hospitalization. Other patients generally can be discharged with referral to an internist or rheumatologist. Since rheumatic diseases are difficult to diagnose early in their disease course and responses to therapy are highly variable, careful follow-up is essential.

The Arthritides

I. **Infectious arthritis** is a critically important condition to recognize because rapid diagnosis and specific therapy can prevent permanent joint damage. Most nongonococcal bacterial infections are monarticular; most viral arthritides are polyarticular and difficult to diagnose.

   A. **Epidemiology.** With the exception of gonococcal arthritis, infectious arthritis tends to occur predominantly in two patient subgroups.

      1. **Prior joint damage** (e.g., RA, prior joint surgery or infection, DJD). The injured joint may be "seeded" during an episode of bacteremia.

      2. **Compromised host defenses** from any cause. Patients with malignancies, diabetes mellitus, chronic renal or hepatic disease, or parenteral drug abuse or receiving chronic glucocorticoid or immunosuppressive therapy constitute this subgroup of patients.

   B. **Etiologies.** *Neisseria gonorrhoeae* is responsible for half of all cases of septic arthritis in adults but is uncommon in children. Among nongonococcal arthritis, staphylococcal infection accounts for 50–65% of bacterial arthritis. Other less common gram-positive organisms include *Streptococcus pneumoniae* and other streptococcal species. Gram-negative bacillary arthritis makes up 12% of all nongonococcal infections and is most commonly seen in adults with compromised immune defenses. *Haemophilus influenzae* may cause septic arthritis in young children. Joint infections predominantly arise from hematogenous bacterial dissemination, and any site of extraarticular infection may lead to septic arthritis.

   C. **Clinical features** suggesting infectious arthritis include the rapid development of a painful inflamed joint associated with systemic symptoms (e.g., fever, chills, malaise). Any joint may be affected, although the knees and hips predominate. Pustulovesicular skin lesions in conjunction with tenosynovitis suggest disseminated gonococcal arthritis; this most typically occurs in women within 1 week of the onset of menses or during pregnancy. Monarticular and polyarticular gonococcal arthritides occur with equal frequency. Skin overlying an infected joint may be warm and erythematous, suggesting cellulitis.

   D. **Unusual infectious arthritides** include arthritis associated with infectious endocarditis, hepatitis B, rubella, and occasionally mumps. These diseases typically produce an oligoarthritis. Tuberculosis and fungal arthritides are rare and usually present as a chronic monarthritis; these are diagnosed by culture of the synovial fluid or synovium. Extraarticular manifestations of granulomatous infection (e.g., pulmonary infiltrates, skin rash, systemic symptoms) are not consistently present.

   E. Emergency department **evaluation** should include a diligent search for evidence of any primary infection.

      1. **Cultures** of blood, urine, sputum, skin lesions, oral lesions, urethra, cervix, and rectum are obtained, depending on the clinical situation. Synovial fluid cultures are usually diagnostic in nongonococcal septic arthritis but positive in only 50% of cases of gonococcal arthritis.

      2. **Gram stains** of any skin lesions and any primary sites of infection (except for the female gynecologic tract) are indicated.

      3. **Radiographs** are usually normal but are required for baseline evaluation and to assess for adjacent osteomyelitis.

      4. **Arthrocentesis** with drainage, culture, and a Gram stain is essential. Both routine agar and chocolate or Thayer-Martin agar are used. A large-bore needle (16–18 gauge) should be used if fluid is difficult to aspirate. Fluoroscopic guidance generally is required for aspiration of the hip. **Synovianalysis** reveals findings presented in Table 14-1. The higher the WBC count in synovial fluid, the greater is the likelihood of infection. Gram stains are often positive in nongonococcal septic arthritis but are rarely helpful in patients with gonococcal arthritis.

   F. **Treatment**

      1. **Antibiotic therapy.** Initial choice of drug therapy is based on the clinical situation and the results of the Gram stain of the joint fluid (Table 14-4).

         a. **Gonococcal arthritis** may be treated (see Chap. 12) with one of the following regimens: (1) amoxicillin, 3.0 gm PO, or ampicillin, 3.5 gm PO, each with probenecid, 1.0 gm PO, followed by amoxicillin or ampicillin, 500 mg PO qid for 7 days; (2) aqueous penicillin G, 2 million units IV q4h, followed by amoxicillin or ampicillin, 500 mg qid to complete a 7-day course; (3) cefoxitin, 1.0 gm IV qid for 7 days; (4) cefotaxime, 500 mg IV qid for 7 days; or (5) ceftriaxone, 1.0 gm IV daily for 7 days. The last three regimens are also

Table 14-4. Choice of initial antibiotic therapy in adults with septic arthritis

Gram stain	Presumed organism(s)	Antimicrobial agents
Gram-positive cocci	*Staphylococcus aureus*—common *Streptococcus*—uncommon	Oxacillin or nafcillin
Gram-negative cocci	*Neisseria gonorrhoeae*	Penicillin G
Gram-negative bacilli	*Escherichia coli* *Pseudomonas aeruginosa*	Tobramycin and ticarcillin
Gram stain negative Normal host	*N. gonorrhoeae* or *S. aureus*	Treat for both until cultures available: penicillin G and oxacillin
Compromised host	*S. aureus* or gram-negative bacilli	Treat for both until cultures available: oxacillin, tobramycin, and ticarcillin

effective against penicillinase-producing strains of *N. gonorrhoeae*. Patients who are toxic or have purulent synovial fluid require parenteral therapy. For patients allergic to penicillins or cephalosporins, tetracycline, 500 mg PO qid for 7 days, or doxycycline, 100 mg PO bid for 7 days, may be used.

   b. **Nongonococcal septic arthritis.** High-dose intravenous antibiotics provide adequate antimicrobial coverage against most pathogenic bacteria. The initial Gram stain and clinical likelihood determine the choice of antibiotics (Table 14-4). If the etiologic agent is in question, antistaphylococcal therapy is initially included because of the organism's incidence and virulence; oxacillin or nafcillin in dosages of 8–12 gm/day, given IV, provides acceptable coverage. In neutropenic patients or intravenous drug abusers, anti-*Pseudomonas* therapy (e.g., ticarcillin) is required initially in addition to an aminoglycoside antibiotic.

   c. Special guidelines apply to **children.** Since neonates develop infection from group B streptococci, staphylococci, or gram-negative organisms, initial therapy with parenteral penicillin, methicillin, and an aminoglycoside is appropriate. Infants (< 2 years old) develop infection from staphylococci or *H. influenzae*; thus, ampicillin (150–200 mg/kg/day) and chloramphenicol (50–75 mg/kg/day) IV provide adequate coverage. Older children require oxacillin or nafcillin, 50 mg/kg IV q8h.

   2. **Additional therapy. Repeated arthrocentesis** is performed frequently to prevent synovial fluid from reaccumulating. Splinting and analgesia are important ancillary measures. Septic arthritis of the hip requires prompt surgical drainage. Infected prosthetic joints usually require surgical removal of the infected prosthesis.

G. **Disposition.** All patients suspected of having nongonococcal septic arthritis require hospital admission. Normal immune hosts with gonococcal arthritis who are reliable and "nontoxic" may be treated as outpatients as long as their joint fluid is nonpurulent.

II. Crystalline arthropathies

A. **Acute gout.** Gout is a common metabolic disease characterized by chronic hyperuricemia. Primary gout (90% of cases) results from as yet unexplained abnormalities in purine metabolism; only rarely (1%) can genetic defects responsible for uric acid overproduction be identified. Secondary gout (10%) is a consequence of overproduction or underexcretion of uric acid resulting from underlying disease. Causes of hyperurecemia are summarized in Table 14-5.

   1. **Clinical features**
      a. **Classic podagra** is the acute onset of pain and swelling in the first metatarsophalangeal joint. Knees, ankles, wrists, and elbows are also frequent sites of acute gouty attacks. Polyarticular disease is rare at the time of diagnosis but becomes increasingly more common with long-standing disease. Ninety percent of patients with gout are male and older than 40 years. Fever, severe pain, and erythema are common; by mimicking cellulitis or infectious ar-

Table 14-5. Common causes of hyperuricemia

Overproduction of uric acid
  Primary gout (1% of cases)
  Lymphoma and myeloproliferative disorders
  Sickle cell disease and other hemolytic anemias
  Severe psoriasis
  Cancer chemotherapy
Underexcretion of uric acid
  Chronic renal failure
  Chronic lead intoxication (saturine gout)
  Drugs (diuretics except spironolactone, ethambutol, low-dose aspirin)
  Lactic and other types of organic acidosis
  Ketosis (diabetes, starvation)
  Hyperparathyroidism
  Hypertension
Mechanism unknown
  Sarcoidosis
  Obesity
  Paget's disease

---

thritis, they may produce diagnostic confusion. Untreated, a typical attack resolves in 3–5 days.

  b. Inciting events include diuretic or salicylate use, alcohol abuse, or dietary indiscretion.

2. The **diagnosis** is established by identifying crystals of monosodium urate monohydrate in the synovial fluid. Characteristic needlelike crystals with strongly negative elongation (birefringence) are seen in 85% of cases. Under polarized light, urate crystals appear yellow when parallel to the axis of the red compensator and blue when perpendicular to the axis.

3. **Laboratory findings.** An inflammatory synovial fluid is present (see Table 14-1). With serial determinations, uric acid is elevated in 90% of patients, but only 70% have hyperuricemia at the time of the initial attack.

4. **Therapy.** Management of gout has two independent aspects: treatment of the acute gouty attack and prophylaxis against long-term side effects of chronic hyperuricemia (e.g., tophi, destructive polyarthritis, nephrolithiasis). Acute gouty arthritis may be treated with an NSAID (except salicylates) or colchicine.

  a. Maximal doses of any of the nonsalicylate **NSAIDs** provide rapid relief of an acute attack within several hours. The dosage may then be gradually tapered over the ensuing week. Absolute contraindications against NSAID therapy include drug allergy and active gastrointestinal bleeding. Relative contraindications include congestive heart failure (fluid retention), chronic renal disease, and peptic ulcer disease.

  b. Colchicine is used to treat acute and chronic gouty arthritis. Although the precise mechanism of action is not well understood, colchicine interferes with polymorphonuclear leukocyte function, including inhibition of chemotaxis. For an acute attack, intravenous administration of colchicine is advised; 2 mg in 15 ml of saline is infused IV over 15 minutes with care to avoid extravasation of the drug into the subcutaneous tissue, which is painful and dangerous. If no response occurs within 1–2 hours, an additional 1-mg dose is administered. The earlier treatment is initiated, the greater is the likelihood of clinical improvement. This approach has the advantages of a rapid response, relative specificity for the crystalline arthritides, and lack of gastrointestinal distress or salt retention. Oral colchicine should then be administered prophylactically in a dosage of 0.6 mg bid until a decision about chronic therapy is reached.

  c. Chronic treatment of gout revolves around treatment of the hyperuricemia with allopurinol or an uricosuric agent (probenecid, sulfinpyrazone). **Allopurinol and the uricosuric agents, however, have no role in the management of an acute gouty attack.** Initiation of therapy during an acute episode may paradoxically exacerbate the attack. (For further discussion of the use of these agents, see ref. 8.)

    5. Disposition. Refractory pain, a question of concomitant infection, or inability to tolerate medication occasionally will necessitate admission and observation of patients with acute gouty arthritis. The majority of patients, however, can be successfully managed as outpatients. Patients need to be referred to their primary physician for chronic treatment of hyperuricemia.

B. Pseudogout is an inflammatory arthropathy caused by polymorphonuclear leukocyte ingestion of intraarticular calcium pyrophosphate dihydrate (CPPD) crystals. Chondrocalcinosis (calcified cartilage) is the radiographic hallmark of pseudogout and is seen in most patients.

    1. Pathogenesis. Multiple disease states are associated with pseudogout, including hyperparathyroidism, hemochromatosis, hypophosphatasia, gout, hypothyroidism, neuropathic arthritis, and hypomagnesemia. An association between pseudogout and osteoarthritis is postulated.

    2. Clinical features. Pseudogout is primarily a disease of the elderly. Both sexes are equally affected. The disease occurs as an acute monarthritis or oligoarthritis or as a chronic polyarthritis.

        a. Acute pseudogout is the most common clinical presentation and is indistinguishable from acute gout. The knee is usually affected, although any synovial based joint may be involved. Dehydration, an acute illness, and surgery (especially parathyroidectomy) are notorious for precipitating acute attacks of pseudogout.

        b. Chronic pseudogout is present in less than 10% of patients. The small joints of the hands and wrists are commonly affected. This syndrome creates diagnostic confusion, as it mimics both osteoarthritis (OA) and RA.

    3. Diagnosis

        a. Synovianalysis is the only method for establishing a precise diagnosis. Polarizing microscopy reveals predominantly intracellular rhomboid-shaped crystals with weak positive elongation (birefringence), that is, the crystals appear blue when parallel to the axis of the red compensator. Since the crystals are difficult to visualize, high-power oil magnification ($1000 \times$) may be needed. Synovianalysis simultaneously reveals a typical sterile inflammatory fluid (see Table 14-1).

        b. Radiographic studies demonstrate chondrocalcinosis in 75% of pseudogout patients. Typical findings include linear calcification involving the knee menisci, symphysis pubis, and the triangular cartilage of the wrist.

        c. Biochemical evaluation demonstrates no characteristic abnormalities except those related to pseudogout-associated diseases (see sec. **II.B.1**). Routine biochemical evaluation eventually should include a serum calcium, phosphate, magnesium, iron studies, and evaluation of thyroid function.

    4. Therapy

        a. Acute pseudogout is treated similarly to acute gouty arthritis. Both the NSAIDs (other than salicylates) and colchicine are useful, although intravenous colchicine is most effective if administered early in the course of an attack. Joint aspiration alone will often produce prompt relief of symptoms. A Gram's stain and bacterial culture routinely should be performed, as pseudogout may accompany infectious arthritis.

        b. Chronic pseudogout is treated with anti-inflammatory dosages of salicylate or another NSAID. Colchicine, 0.6 mg PO bid, can also be used for prophylaxis.

    5. Disposition. Indications for hospital admission are identical to those of acute gouty arthritis (see sec. **II.A.5**).

III. Osteoarthritis (OA, DJD, or osteoarthrosis) represents the most common rheumatic disease. Prevalence increases with longevity, such that 90% of the population has radiographic evidence of the disease by age 40. However, only a small percentage of these individuals are clinically affected. With the exception of OA involving the hips and knees, radiographic changes correlate poorly with symptomatology.

A. Pathogenesis. OA is divided into primary and secondary disease, depending on whether an inciting agent is identified. In both forms, progressive destruction and loss of cartilage initially are noted. These are followed by reactive changes in the joint margin and subchondral bone. Known risk factors for development of secondary OA include altered joint biomechanics, trauma, intraarticular hemorrhage, neuropathic joint disease, joint infection, synovial-based arthritis, and metabolic diseases (e.g., Wilson's disease, alkaptonuria, acromegaly, and hemochromatosis).

B. **Clinical presentation**

1. **Symptoms.** The insidious onset of aching pain associated with joint movement and relieved by rest is typical. As the disease progresses, exercise tolerance dramatically decreases. Crepitance, a feeling of crackling inside the joint, is common. Morning stiffness of short duration is frequently noted. The distal interphalangeal joints and the first carpometacarpal joint of the hand commonly are affected. Other common sites include the hips, knees, and the lumbosacral and cervical spines.

2. **Signs.** Joint tenderness is more striking than synovial thickening. Heberden's and Bouchard's nodes are common chronic findings. Patients occasionally may present acutely with inflammation mimicking a synovial-based arthritis; however, signs of inflammation are relatively uncommon. In contrast to rheumatoid arthritis, grip strength and dexterity tend to be preserved. Hip involvement leads to reduced internal rotation and an antalgic gait. Knee disease may present with bland effusions or ligamentous laxity.

C. **Laboratory findings**

1. **Biochemical studies** are characteristically normal. The ESR is normal to slightly elevated.

2. **Synovianalysis** usually reveals a noninflammatory fluid (see Table 14-1).

D. **Radiographic studies** reveal a spectrum of findings. Radiographs may be normal in early disease. More advanced findings include joint space narrowing secondary to cartilage loss, subchondral bony sclerosis, marginal osteophyte formation, and periarticular bony cysts. Ankylosis and osteopenia, however, are not radiographic features of OA.

E. **Differential diagnosis.** Since OA is ubiquitous, it frequently occurs in conjunction with other forms of arthritis. In addition, infection, synovial-based arthritis, seronegative spondyloarthropathies, and crystalline arthropathies may all masquerade as OA. Thus, in the emergency department setting, OA must be approached as a diagnosis of exclusion; otherwise, cases of infectious and crystalline arthritis may be missed. Careful history taking, examination, and synovianalysis are required to arrive at the correct diagnosis.

F. **Acute therapy**

1. **Drugs.** Salicylates and the other NSAIDs are equally effective in treating the pain and inflammation associated with OA. Salicylates are generally preferred initially because of their lower cost. Concomitant administration of acetaminophen or propoxyphene may provide additional analgesia. Although intraarticular steroids benefit some patients with synovitis of the knees, there is no indication for systemic corticosteroid therapy.

2. **Nonmedical therapy** includes physical therapy, local application of heat, and avoidance of weight bearing. Strengthening and prevention of muscle atrophy are particularly useful in OA involving the knee. When pain is unrelieved by conservative measures, orthopedic consultation should be considered.

IV. **Rheumatoid arthritis (RA),** a systemic disease of unknown etiology, produces a symmetric polyarthritis as its major clinical manifestation. Occurring in 1–2% of the population in the United States, it has a widely variable clinical course, ranging from mild arthritis in 70% of patients to a severe crippling form in 15%.

A. **Diagnosis** of new-onset RA in the emergency department setting is difficult. Although 80% of RA patients have detectable rheumatoid factor, this test is not routinely available on an emergency basis. Radiographs early in the course of the disease are normal or demonstrate nonspecific findings of soft-tissue swelling and periarticular osteopenia. Physical findings early in the disease usually reveal fusiform swelling of the proximal interphalangeal (PIP) and metacarpophalangeal (MCP) joints of both hands. Subcutaneous nodules and typical hand deformities (i.e., swan-neck and boutonnière deformities, ulnar deviation) usually are evidence of long-standing disease. Laboratory analysis reveals evidence of a chronic inflammatory state with an elevated ESR and a mild anemia. Other rheumatic syndromes such as SLE, scleroderma, rheumatic fever, and the vasculitic syndromes may present in an identical fashion, and a precise diagnosis can only be made with additional laboratory data and serial observation.

B. **Treatment**

1. **Initial treatment** of acute inflammation utilizes the salicylates and other NSAIDs. Maximal anti-inflammatory effects with the salicylates are obtained

only when the salicylate level is in the therapeutic range. Although the NSAIDs are considered equipotent, individual responses vary, and failure with one particular drug does not preclude use of another drug.

2. Slow-acting remittive agents have no role in the emergency department setting. Detailed patient education, as well as the need for frequent chronic care, dictates that the decision to use these agents be made by the patient's primary physician. No benefit of therapy is evident for at least 1–2 months after initiation of therapy.

3. **Corticosteroids** are indicated for patients with disabling arthritis, despite adequate therapy with the salicylates or NSAIDs.

   a. **Systemic administration** of corticosteroids is required for patients with severe polyarthritis, disabling constitutional symptoms (e.g., fever, weight loss), or associated systemic vasculitis. Arthritis and constitutional symptoms will usually respond dramatically to 20 mg/day of prednisone; this can then be rapidly tapered to a chronic dose of 5–10 mg/day. Cutaneous vasculitis such as nail fold infarcts or ulcers may portend more serious visceral involvement and requires close observation. Systemic vasculitis, manifested by mononeuritis multiplex, gastrointestinal bleeding, or cardiac involvement, requires high dosages of prednisone (1 mg/kg/day or higher) for a prolonged period of time.

   b. **Intraarticular corticosteroids** are useful adjunctive therapy for suppression of synovitis when only a few peripheral joints are inflamed. These may be used concomitantly with other modes of therapy. Systemic absorption of intraarticular corticosteroids is minimal. Techniques and dosages are discussed in Chap. 38. All patients should be warned that a self-limited crystalline-induced synovitis may occur within 12–48 hours of injection. A successful injection may produce relief for weeks to several months. Injections probably should not be repeated more frequently than every 3–4 months.
   Caution. Patients with RA are prone to develop septic arthritis. Thus, any joint substantially more inflamed than other joints should be aspirated for synovianalysis and culture, and intraarticular corticosteroids should be withheld until infection is ruled out.

C. **Disposition.** Hospitalization generally is warranted for patients with severe polyarthritis, disabling constitutional symptoms, associated vasculitis, or a question of septic arthritis. In such situations, hospitalization is useful for close observation, systemic and articular rest, physical and occupational therapy, and patient and family education.

V. **Rheumatoid variants**

A. **Syndromes.** Several other rheumatic diseases have many similarities to RA. Included among these are **juvenile rheumatoid arthritis, Felty's syndrome,** and **Sjögren's syndrome.** Juvenile RA varies from a chronic oligoarthritis in young children to Still's disease, a multisystem disorder presenting with fever, arthritis, and skin rash in children and young adults. Felty's syndrome is the constellation of RA, neutropenia, splenomegaly, and lower extremity cutaneous ulcers. It occurs in rheumatoid factor–positive individuals with long-standing disease. Sjögren's syndrome (accompanying RA in 20–30% of cases) is manifest by decreased salivary and lacrimal gland secretions, leading to complaints of dry eyes and mouth (sicca syndrome).

B. **Treatment.** Acute arthritic manifestations of these syndromes are treated identically to RA (see **IV.B**). NSAIDs approved for use in preadolescents include salicylates, tolmetin, and naproxen. Extraarticular manifestations of these syndromes often require specialized care. Corticosteroid eyedrops and mydriatics/cycloplegics are administered for the anterior uveitis in juvenile RA. Artificial tears are helpful in Sjögren's syndrome for corneal protection and symptomatic relief.

VI. **Traumatic arthritis** is easily diagnosed by its history. After bony fracture has been excluded radiographically, treatment consists of immobilization, avoidance of weight bearing, and analgesia with acetaminophen (in conjunction with a narcotic, if required). A joint effusion that is large should be aspirated for symptomatic relief. Synovianalysis reveals hemorrhagic or noninflammatory fluid.

VII. **Osteonecrosis** (avascular necrosis, aseptic necrosis) is focal ischemic death of bone secondary to decreased blood flow. It is a noninflammatory process that most commonly involves the femoral heads but may also affect the knees, shoulders, or any other joint. The pathogenesis is complex; multiple disease states, including alcoholism, steroid therapy, hemoglobinopathies, trauma, SLE, and diabetes mellitus, are all associated with the development of osteonecrosis. Patients present with the insidious onset of pain but well-preserved joint motion. Osteonecrosis is diagnosed by the characteristic late radiographic features of increased density, focal collapse, patchy bone loss, and microfractures. Acute treatment is symptomatic, while chronic therapy frequently involves joint replacement.

VIII. **Other crystalline arthropathies** include apatite deposition arthropathy and calcium oxalate disease. These syndromes clinically produce an acute arthritis or periarthritis similar to gout and pseudogout. Patients generally have underlying OA, connective tissue disease, or chronic renal failure. Since the crystals can only be identified using electron microscopy, establishing the diagnosis is both difficult and impractical. Empiric treatment with joint aspiration and administration of an NSAID and colchicine occasionally may be useful.

Systemic Lupus Erythematosus (SLE)

I. **Clinical features.** SLE, a common rheumatic disease of young women, is a chronic inflammatory syndrome with protean manifestations, including fever, skin rash with photosensitivity, arthritis, glomerulonephritis, central nervous system (CNS) manifestations, and pleuropulmonary and hematologic abnormalities. At the time of diagnosis, the most common presenting symptoms are arthritis and a skin rash. This disease typically has an unpredictable course with periods of remission and exacerbation.

II. **Diagnosis.** Recognition of a multisystem disease state without other recognizable disease processes should alert the physician to consider the diagnosis of SLE. Antinuclear antibody (ANA) determination is the single most useful screening test. While not specific, it is positive in greater than 95% of patients with active disease. Other tests that should be obtained in a suspected SLE patient include a complete blood count, platelet count, urinalysis, liver function tests, and serum creatinine. In the emergency department, SLE can be clinically suspected but rarely diagnosed, as the requisite immunologic tests are not ordinarily available on an emergency basis. Emergency decision making, however, requires only the routinely available hematologic and biochemical tests.

III. **The differential diagnosis** is extensive and includes much of internal medicine. Scleroderma, RA, chronic active hepatitis, and idiopathic pulmonary fibrosis are among the most common diseases with positive ANAs masquerading as SLE.

IV. **Treatment** of SLE is largely symptomatic, since no curative therapy is known.

A. **Conservative therapy** is used for patients with mild disease.

1. Generalized **bed rest** is advisable for patients with symptomatic fatigue.

2. **Topical therapy** for patients with photosensitive skin includes avoiding sun exposure and the liberal use of a sunscreen lotion; para-aminobenzoic acid with a sun protection factor of 15 (SPF-15) is effective. Topical fluorinated corticosteroid skin creams may be effective for cutaneous lesions but generally should be avoided on the face.

3. The **NSAIDs** (including salicylates) are commonly used to treat myalgias, arthralgias, arthritis, tendinitis, and fevers. Mild pleuritis and pericarditis may also respond to conservative therapy. Since all the NSAIDs (including salicylates) inhibit synthesis of renal prostaglandins and may consequently reduce renal blood flow, patients with lupus nephritis should be carefully monitored for an increase in serum creatinine within 1 week of starting therapy. Since sulindac may have less effect on renal blood flow than the other NSAIDs, it is the initially preferred agent. Symptomatic patients taking greater than 20 mg of prednisone daily are unlikely to be helped by the addition of NSAIDs to their medical regimens. Special toxicities of the NSAIDs in SLE patients include occasional reports of hepatoxicity and, rarely, aseptic meningitis.

4. **Hydroxychloroquine,** an antimalarial drug, is useful in the treatment of skin and joint manifestations. However, because of its delayed onset of action, it has no role in the emergency medical armamentarium. Long-term side effects other than a retinopathy with visual field defects are extremely rare.

B. **Corticosteroid therapy** is indicated for patients with potentially life-threatening disease (see sec. **V**). Dosage is individualized, depending on the clinical setting, and the primary care physician should routinely be involved in these decisions. **Fulminating disease,** such as rapidly progressive renal failure, pulmonary hemorrhage, or lupus cerebritis with cranial neuropathies and seizures (see sec. **V**) may be treated initially with intravenous **pulse therapy** of methylprednisolone; 500 mg is infused over 30 minutes q12h for 6–10 doses. Identical therapy is used occasionally in patients refractory to therapy with lower steroid dosages. Although no controlled data demonstrate that this therapy is more effective than conventional high-dose steroid therapy (i.e., prednisone, 1–2 mg/kg/day PO), many physicians feel that more rapid control of the disease may be obtained with intravenous pulse therapy.

V. Complications

   A. Pleuropericarditis responds to low to moderate dosages of prednisone. Initially, 20 mg bid usually provides rapid disease control. Cardiac tamponade in treated pericarditis has been reported, although it is quite unusual.

   B. Hematologic abnormalities include lymphopenia, hemolytic anemia, and thrombocytopenia. Lymphopenia requires no specific therapy. Coombs-positive hemolytic anemia and thrombocytopenia vary from mild to life-threatening; prednisone in a dosage of 30–50 mg bid is often required for disease control.

   C. Pneumonitis presents most commonly as fleeting pulmonary infiltrates. Difficulty in ruling out associated infection is frequent. No specific therapy is required. Rarely, a fulminant form of alveolitis occurs. Pulmonary hemorrhage is treated with high dosages of corticosteroids; the mortality is substantial.

   D. Neurologic abnormalities are common and exceedingly varied.

   1. Seizures are treated initially with anticonvulsants. If uncontrollable, high-dose corticosteroids are added.

   2. Peripheral and central nervous system disease require high dosages of corticosteroids (i.e., pulse therapy or prednisone, 60–100 mg/day PO in divided doses). Since an altered mental status in steroid-treated patients may be secondary to infection, underlying disease, or drug therapy, each patient must be evaluated individually. The diagnosis of **CNS lupus** is one of exclusion. Emergency department evaluation includes a lumbar puncture and head computed tomography (CT) scan. Lumbar punctures are abnormal only in one-third of patients with active cerebritis; typically, the cerebrospinal fluid protein is minimally elevated, and a mild pleocytosis is noted. A CT or brain scan detects nonspecific abnormalities in a minority of patients

   E. Lupus nephritis. Patients present with proteinuria, an active urine sediment, and/or decreased creatinine clearance. Treatment is highly controversial. Active disease is generally treated with prednisone, 60–100 mg/day in divided doses. In some institutions, pulse steroids and cytotoxic agents are routinely used, but this decision is best made by a rheumatologist or nephrologist. A patient with active nephritis should avoid the NSAIDs.

   F. Less common manifestations of SLE include an inflammatory myositis and vasculitis involving the skin, adipose tissue, mesentery, or bowel. High dosages of corticosteroids are used for all of these disease manifestations.

   G. Drug-induced lupus may result from chronic administration of hydralazine (usually in dosages exceeding 200 mg/day) or procainamide. Arthritis and pleuropericarditis predominate. Treatment consists of withdrawal of the offending drug. The NSAIDs often provide symptomatic relief. In severe cases, low dosages of prednisone, 10–25 mg/day, may be required transiently for several months. This disease does not evolve into classic SLE.

VI. Disposition. For patients with mild disease, conservative therapy can be prescribed on an outpatient basis. However, initiation of aggressive therapy (e.g., pulse therapy, high-dose glucocorticoids, or other immunosuppressive therapy) in newly diagnosed patients or patients with potentially life-threatening complications of the disease requires hospital admission. In addition, new pleuropericarditis or hematologic abnormalities in a known SLE patient are best treated in the hospital to be sure of a rapid response to glucocorticoid therapy. Likewise, patients with active nephritis or CNS disease are usually acutely ill and demand close inpatient observation. Patients with mild drug-induced lupus can be treated safely as outpatients if the diagnosis is certain.

Progressive Systemic Sclerosis (PSS)

PSS, or scleroderma, is a rare systemic disease characterized by Raynaud's phenomenon (RP) and fibrosis of the skin. The pathogenesis is unknown, although a diffuse vasculopathy associated with increased collagen synthesis is consistently observed. Multiple abnormalities of the humoral and cellular immune systems are present.

   I. Diagnosis. The characteristic taut, hidebound skin is diagnostic of PSS. Initially, the fingers and hands become puffy (edematous phase), followed by tightening and thickening producing typical sclerodactyly. RP is seen in greater than 90% of patients. Demonstration of visceral involvement is not required for diagnosis.

II. Management. Because no specific curative therapy is known, treatment is largely symptomatic.

   A. Raynaud's phenomenon. Exposure of the entire body or an isolated extremity to cold is contraindicated in patients suffering from RP. Nicotine from cigarette smoking produces peripheral vasoconstriction and must be avoided. Vasodilator therapy has met with limited success but is often poorly tolerated because of hypotensive side effects; the most commonly used drugs include prazosin, captopril, reserpine, and the calcium channel antagonists. Patients are instructed to begin with a small dose and advance the dosage as tolerated. The long-term benefits of this therapy, however, are unknown. Occasionally, a patient will develop acute, painful, severe vasospasm involving one or more digits. This can progress to gangrene. These patients should be hospitalized, kept warm, and started on rapidly increasing dosages of vasodilators.

   B. The **skin disease** of PSS is treated with moisturizing creams and proper hygiene. D-Penicillamine may be useful in long-term therapy for softening the skin. Low-dose prednisone and colchicine, 0.6 mg bid, are also occasionally used, although no long-term benefit has been demonstrated. None of these measures is appropriate for the emergency department.

   C. Renal disease represents a true medical emergency. Scleroderma renal crisis most commonly is an acute hypertensive state with markedly elevated plasma renin levels. It may be accompanied by a microangiopathic hemolytic anemia. Scleroderma patients with new-onset hypertension or an increasing serum creatinine require hospitalization and aggressive blood pressure control (with lowering of the diastolic blood pressure to < 85 mm Hg). Intensive care monitoring and nitroprusside infusion generally are required initially. Captopril therapy (up to 400 mg/day) may abort acute renal failure. Diuretics should be avoided whenever possible. Some patients develop progressive azotemia despite therapy, and these patients may ultimately require nephrectomy and hemodialysis.

   D. Gastrointestinal involvement. PSS may affect all aspects of the gastrointestinal tract. Esophageal involvement varies from reflux esophagitis (treated with antacids or H_2 antagonists) to esophageal stricture (treated with dilatation, antacids, and elevation of the head of the bed) to aperistalsis (generally unresponsive to medical drug therapy). Abnormal motility in the small- and large-bowel segments may lead to malabsorption, bacterial overgrowth, and weight loss; oral antibiotics occasionally are useful.

   E. Other manifestations include myositis, myocarditis, and pericarditis. All may respond to 20–40 mg of prednisone daily. Cardiac arrhythmias are common and may require specific therapy. Pulmonary hypertension and interstitial lung disease are generally refractory to therapy. Myopathy and arthritis are generally treated with the NSAIDs. D-Penicillamine therapy has recently been reported to prolong life and decrease visceral involvement in PSS patients; because long-term therapy is required, initiation of therapy should be performed by the primary care physician.

Polymyositis

Polymyositis (PM) is an inflammatory disease of the proximal skeletal muscles. The etiology is unknown. It may be associated with a specific skin rash (i.e., dermatomyositis [DM]) or with malignancy, and it may occur in childhood.

I. Clinical and laboratory features

   A. Proximal muscle weakness is insidious in onset but usually striking at the time of diagnosis. Muscle pain and elevation of the serum aldolase and creatine phosphokinase are routinely seen. Dysphagia, shortness of breath, and aspiration pneumonia are evidence of advanced disease. Electromyelogram testing and muscle biopsy confirm the diagnosis.

   B. The skin rash of DM may consist of a heliotrope (reddish-purple discoloration of the eyelids associated with periorbital edema), Gottron's papules (scaly erythematous lesions over the dorsum of the MCP and PIP joints), or an erythematous scaly rash involving the upper torso or face. Biopsies are nonspecific.

   C. Less common features include arthritis, interstitial lung disease, myocarditis, Raynaud's phenomenon, and esophageal dysmotility.

II. Differential diagnosis. Diseases mimicking PM include hyperthyroid myopathy, the muscular dystrophies, trichinosis, McArdle's disease, and acid maltase deficiency.

III. **Treatment**
   A. **Prednisone,** 1–2 mg/kg/day in divided doses, constitutes initial therapy. Typically, muscle strength improves over several weeks. Serum enzymes decline more slowly and may take 2–3 months to normalize.
   B. **Methotrexate and cytotoxic drugs** are reserved for patients with refractory disease or with fulminant, rapidly progressive disease.
   C. **Intensive rehabilitation** with physical and occupational therapy is usually helpful.
IV. **Disposition.** Hospitalization is usually required for initial evaluation and therapy of fulminant disease states.

Polymyalgia Rheumatica and Temporal Arteritis

I. **Clinical features. Polymyalgia rheumatica** (PMR) and **temporal arteritis** (TA) are both diseases of the elderly. PMR is a syndrome of proximal shoulder and pelvic girdle myalgias associated with normal muscle enzymes. TA is an inflammatory arteritis affecting the cranial arteries; it is characterized by a bitemporal headache, claudication of the jaw muscles, visual disturbances, and rarely cerebrovascular accidents. Both diseases commonly occur together and have greatly elevated ESRs.
II. **Diagnosis.** PMR is a clinical diagnosis (of exclusion), while TA is diagnosed by a temporal artery biopsy. Diseases mimicking PMR in the elderly include hyperthyroidism, hypercalcemia, RA, depression, malignancy, other rheumatic diseases, and fibromyalgia.
III. **Management.** Patients suspected of having TA should be started on 60 mg/day of prednisone prior to biopsy in an attempt to prevent irreversible blindness. Biopsies should be performed within 3–4 days. Patients with suspected PMR will have dramatic improvement on 15–20 mg/day of prednisone. This lower dosage, however, will not protect against visual loss if both diseases are present. Hospitalization is required only for patients who appear systemically ill.

Necrotizing Vasculitis

Systemic necrotizing vasculitis comprises a heterogeneous group of disease states. All are characterized by inflammation and necrosis of bood vessels. Involvement varies from a large-vessel arteritis in Takayasu's disease to a small venulitis seen in hypersensitivity vasculitis. The size of the involved blood vessel partially determines the disease manifestations. A clinical diagnosis of vasculitis is suspected in any patient with multisystem disease, especially those with arthritis, skin lesions (e.g., purpura, nodules, ulcers, urticaria), myalgias, renal disease, abdominal pain, and unexplained neurologic symptoms. Ultimately, vasculitis remains a pathologic diagnosis. Exact classification of the vasculitic syndromes (Table 14-6) is imprecise and impossible in the emergency department setting. These patients are usually quite ill and require hospital admission. If skin lesions are present, biopsies should be performed. Corticosteroids and cytotoxic agents are beneficial in most patients but are not initiated until a complete diagnostic workup is completed. Mild cutaneous disease may not require any therapy other than topical care.

Seronegative Spondyloarthropathies

Seronegative spondyloarthropathies (SNSAs) comprise a group of interrelated enthesopathies (i.e., syndromes associated with inflammation at the sites of ligamentous insertion into bone). The most common SNSAs are ankylosing spondylitis, Reiter's syndrome, and psoriatic arthritis. All are rheumatoid factor- and ANA-negative but tend to occur within certain families and are associated with HLA-B27 positivity. The SNSAs involve both the axial skeleton and peripheral joints. Males are predominantly affected and have more disabling disease.
I. **Ankylosing spondylitis** (AS) is the most common SNSA with a prevalence of 1% of the general population. The average age of onset is between 15 and 40 years.
   A. **Symptoms and signs.** The insidious onset of low back pain, worse in the morning and relieved with exercise, is typical. This is markedly different from pain associated with muscle strain. Spinal examination confirms the loss of mobility with associated sacroiliac tenderness. Peripheral asymmetric oligoarthritis involving the hips, shoulders, and knees occurs commonly. Radiographs may confirm sacroilitis and syndesmophyte formation (bony bridging of adjacent vertebra). Extraskeletal

Table 14-6. Major forms of systemic vasculitides

Type of vasculitis	Common clinical manifestations	Therapy
Hypersensitivity vasculitis (includes serum sickness, Henoch-Schönlein purpura, cutaneous vasculitis)	Purpura, arthritis, GN	None or prednisone
Systemic lupus erythematosus	Rash, GN, arthritis, cytopenias, CNS dysfunction, pleuropericarditis	Prednisone/immunosuppressive
Rheumatoid vasculitis	Arthritis, neuropathy, bowel infarction, skin ulcers	Prednisone/immunosuppressive
Polyarteritis nodosa	Vascular infarcts (CNS, cardiac, GI, renal)	Prednisone/immunosuppressive
Cryoglobulinemia	Purpura, arthritis, GN	Prednisone/immunosuppressive
Wegener's granulomatosis	Sinusitis, pneumonitis, GN	Cyclophosphamide
Allergic granulomatosis	Asthma, eosinophilia, pulmonary infiltrates	Prednisone
Temporal arteritis	Visual loss, arthralgias, proximal myalgias	Prednisone

Key: GN = glomerulonephritis.

manifestations include acute iritis (25%), restrictive pulmonary disease with apical infiltrates, and aortic insufficiency (rare). Other late complications include cauda equina syndrome, amyloidosis, and myopericarditis.

B. **Diagnosis** is suspected clinically and confirmed by the characteristic radiographic findings. HLA-B27 testing usually is unnecessary.

C. **Therapy** has several goals.

1. **Pain relief.** Indomethacin in maximal dosages is the drug of choice. For patients intolerant of or not responding to indomethacin, phenylbutazone may offer relief. However, this drug is not advised for chronic therapy due to its hematologic toxicity. The other NSAIDs (including salicylates) are generally less effective.

2. **Maintenance of skeletal mobility** and **prevention of deformity** are both long-term therapeutic goals. Treatment primarily involves physical therapy and avoidance of smoking.

II. **Reiter's syndrome** (RS) is a common disease of young men. It consists of the clinical association of arthritis with urethritis and conjunctivitis.

A. **Clinical features.** The syndrome in the United States most commonly follows extramarital sexual intercourse. In Europe, RS occasionally follows infectious dysentery. Nongonococcal mucopurulent urethritis is often followed by arthritis, tendinitis, and back pain. Conjunctivitis is usually mild and bilateral, but chronic iritis occasionally occurs. Other disease manifestations include circinate balanitis, keratoderma blenorrhagica, fever, pericarditis, iritis, and painless oral ulcers. Patients with severe arthritis typically follow a relapsing course with each episode lasting several months.

B. **Diagnosis** is based on a typical clinical presentation. Initially, RS can be confused with gonococcal arthritis, rheumatoid arthritis, psoriatic arthritis, or Behçet's disease. HLA testing may be helpful in difficult cases, as approximately 80% of patients are B27-positive.

C. **Therapy** is supportive with the NSAIDs. Ophthalmologic manifestations usually remit spontaneously, although corticosteroid and immunosuppressive therapy is indicated for severe cases.

III. **Psoriatic arthritis** (PA) occurs in 6% of patients with psoriasis and varies from an indolent oligoarthritis to a severe destructive polyarthritis. Spinal involvement mimicking AS occurs in a small percentage of patients. It may easily be confused with RS, RA, or even gout. Treatment initially involves administration of NSAIDs. More severe cases are treated with hydroxychloroquine or methotrexate. Corticosteroids are used very rarely.

Acute Rheumatic Fever (ARF)

ARF is an inflammatory syndrome of acute polyarthritis, fever, and carditis that in recent years has become distinctly uncommon, particularly in adults. Other early manifestations include subcutaneous nodules and chorea. Later manifestations of this disease are aortic and mitral valvular heart disease. The acute syndrome is self-limited and invariably preceded by group A streptococcal pharyngitis. The diagnosis is based on the characteristic clinical features and documentation of a prior streptococcal infection (i.e., positive throat culture, rising antistreptolysin O[ASO] or antihyaluronidase titers). **Therapy** consists of (1) eradication of the streptococcal infection, (2) prevention of recurrent attacks with long-term penicillin prophylaxis, and (3) salicylate therapy for symptomatic arthritis and/or fever. Severe carditis requires corticosteroid therapy.

Nonarticular Rheumatism

I. **Fibromyalgia (fibrositis)** is a clinical syndrome of reproducible localized muscle pain in an anxious or depressed individual. Patients typically complain of exhaustion and difficulty sleeping. The only positive physical findings are localized points of pain known as trigger points (Fig. 14-1). Laboratory and radiographic studies are consistently normal. Therapy is primarily supportive. Explanation of fibromyalgia's benign course coupled with drug therapy utilizing salicylates, anxiolytic agents, and the tricyclic antidepressants generally provides adequate relief.

II. **Bursitis and tendinitis**

A. **Traumatic bursitis and tendinitis.** Chronic local irritation or direct trauma to a bursal sac or tendon sheath may produce a marked local inflammatory response with pain and erythema. Although over 150 anatomic bursae are described, clinical involvement occurs most commonly at only a few sites: the subacromial and subdel-

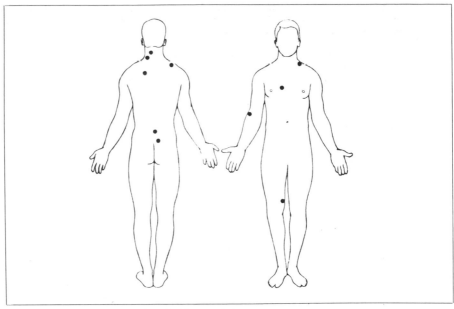

Fig. 14-1. Common trigger points in fibromyalgia.

toid bursae of the shoulder, the olecranon bursa of the elbow, the trochanteric bursa of the hip, the anserine bursa of the knee, and several bursae surrounding the Achilles tendon. Common sites of tendinitis include the bicepital groove of the humerus and the medial and lateral epicondyles of the elbow. Bursitis is distinguished from synovitis by the finding of localized pain (point tenderness), as opposed to generalized tenderness with reduced range of motion. Traumatic bursitis or tendonitis is treated with localized rest, salicylates, or other NSAIDs. For more severe cases, aspiration and injection of the offending bursa with a lidocaine-glucocorticoid suspension mixture are often useful.

B. **Infectious bursitis.** Bursae may become secondarily infected, usually following cellulitis or puncture wounds. *Staphylococcus aureus* is the most frequent causative agent. Bursal fluid should always be examined for evidence of infection (i.e., Gram stain) and sent for culture. Septic bursitis is treated by aspiration and administration of dicloxacillin, 500 mg PO qid for 10 days. In the immunocompromised host or the systemically ill patient, hospitalization and parenteral antibiotic therapy are advisable. Purulent tenosynovitis is discussed in Chap. 23.

C. **Gout and pseudogout** may occasionally cause chronic bursitis. Bursal fluid, whenever obtained, should be examined for crystals. If the patient does not improve with NSAIDs, a local bursal corticosteroid injection is effective.

III. The **carpal tunnel syndrome** (see Chap. 32) results from entrapment of the median nerve at the wrist. Although usually idiopathic, it may be associated with obesity, pregnancy, hypothyroidism, acromegaly, rheumatoid arthritis, amyloidosis, or SLE. Patients complain of wrist pain and also of clumsiness and paresthesias of the thumb, index, and long fingers. Acute compression of the median nerve at the palmar aspect of the wrist produces complaints of shooting pain in the index or long finger (Tinel's sign). The diagnosis is confirmed by demonstrating delayed nerve conduction. The syndrome is treated with wrist splints, local corticosteroid injections, and frequently surgical release.

Bibliography

1. Arthritis Foundation. *Primer on the Rheumatic Diseases* (8th ed.). Atlanta: Arthritis Foundation, 1983.
2. Cupps, T. R., and Fauci, A. S. *The Vasculitides.* Philadelphia: Saunders, 1981.
3. Goldenberg, D. L., and Cohen, A. S. Acute infectious arthritis: A review of patients with non-gonococcal joint infections (with emphasis on therapy and prognosis). *Am. J. Med.* 60:369, 1976.

4. Hunder, G. G., and Bunch, T. W. Treatment of rheumatoid arthritis. *Bull. Rheum. Dis.* 32(1):1, 1982.
5. Keat, A. Reiter's syndrome and reactive arthritis in perspective. *N. Engl. J. Med.* 309:1606, 1983.
6. Kelley, W. N., et al. (eds.). *Textbook of Rheumatology* (2nd ed.). Philadelphia: Saunders, 1985.
7. Schur, P. H. *The Clinical Management of Systemic Lupus Erythematosus.* New York: Grune & Stratton, 1983.
8. Simkin, P. Management of gout. *Ann. Intern. Med.* 90:812, 1979.
9. Simon, L. S., and Mills, J. A. Nonsteroidal anti-inflammatory drugs. *N. Engl. J. Med.* 302:1179, 1237, 1980.
10. Spencer-Green, G. Raynaud's phenomenon. *Bull. Rheum. Dis.* 33(5):1, 1983.

Environmental Emergencies

Robert J. Stine

Accidental Hypothermia

Accidental hypothermia is a disorder in which the core or internal body temperature is less than 35°C as a result of exposure to cold. The disorder results from loss of body heat to the environment. Extreme environmental conditions, however, are not required; accidental hypothermia has been reported under relatively mild conditions. High-risk groups for development of the disorder include the elderly, infants, outdoor workers and enthusiasts, and alcoholics. Factors predisposing to hypothermia include those that enhance loss of body heat (e.g., excessive exposure to cold due to environmental exposure, inadequate clothing and heating, drug intoxication, and acute and chronic incapacitating illnesses and injuries; dermal disorders), decrease heat production (e.g., hypothyroidism, hypopituitarism, hypoadrenalism, malnutrition), and impair thermoregulation (e.g., certain drugs such as phenothiazines, barbiturates, and alcohol; hypoglycemia; central nervous system [CNS] disorders; sepsis). To establish the diagnosis requires a high index of suspicion and a low-reading rectal (or tympanic membrane) thermometer or thermistor probe.

I. **Pathophysiology.** Exposure to cold invokes compensatory responses in an attempt to preserve the body temperature. These include intense peripheral vasoconstriction to hinder heat loss from the body and shivering to increase metabolic heat production by up to five-fold. Prolonged exposure to cold, however, may override these compensatory mechanisms and lead to a progressive decline in core temperature. At approximately 32°C, shivering ceases and is replaced by muscular rigidity. Continued cold exposure will then result in a rapid fall in body temperature and metabolic rate (the latter declining by about 13%/1°C).

A. **Cardiovascular effects.** Initially, with a decline in core temperature, the heart rate and cardiac output increase as a result of increased sympathetic activity and metabolic rate. A progressive decline in core temperature below 32°C, however, is associated with progressive decreases in heart rate and cardiac output. The reduction in cardiac output is due to bradycardia, depressed left ventricular function, and hypovolemia resulting from shift of plasma from the intravascular to the extravascular space [18]. Although peripheral resistance is elevated, hypotension may occur due to reduced cardiac output; generally, hypotension is severe at temperatures below 25°C [50].

A decline in core temperature below 30°C is associated with a variety of arrhythmias (usually a sinus bradycardia or atrial fibrillation with a slow ventricular response but also a junctional rhythm, ventricular arrhythmias, or asystole) as a result of increased myocardial irritability and depression of intracardiac conductivity and impulse formation. In addition to arrhythmias, the electrocardiogram (ECG) may reveal prolongation of all intervals, conduction defects, T-wave inversion (not necessarily due to ischemia), muscle tremor artifact, and the characteristic J or Osborn wave (Fig. 15-1), an abnormal terminal deflection of the QRS complex.

B. The **pulmonary responses** to a decline in core temperature include an initial increase in minute ventilation in response to an elevated metabolic rate, followed by a progressive decrease in minute volume (secondary to a decline in metabolic rate and depression of the medullary respiratory center) as the core temperature falls below 32°C. In addition, cold-induced bronchorrhea is common. Hypoxemia and a respiratory acidosis may occur, and respiration may cease at temperatures below 24°C [50].

C. **CNS effects.** A progressive decline in core temperature below 32°C is associated with progressive depression of coordination, mental status, and reflexes. Below 27°C, most patients are verbally unresponsive [12], and below 19°C, the electroen-

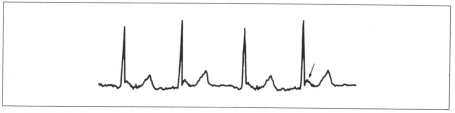

Fig. 15-1. ECG of a hypothermic patient demonstrating atrial fibrillation, muscle tremor artifact, and J or Osborn waves (*identified by the arrow*).

cephalogram (EEG) generally is without activity [3]. The reduced cerebral metabolism, however, protects the brain against hypoxic-induced injury.

D. Blood effects. The effects of hypothermia on the blood include hemoconcentration secondary to loss of plasma from the intravascular space and increased blood viscosity leading to intravascular sludging and impaired tissue perfusion. Leukopenia and thrombocytopenia may occur from sequestration of those components in the spleen, liver, and splanchnic bed.

E. Other **common physiologic responses** to a decline in core temperature include a metabolic acidosis secondary to tissue hypoxia and decreased hepatic metabolism of lactate, a diuresis (contributing to hypovolemia) due to renal tubular dysfunction, shift of the oxyhemoglobin dissociation curve to the left with resultant impaired oxygen release to the tissues, hyperglycemia secondary to decreased insulin release and impaired glucose utilization, elevated plasma cortisol levels due to impaired utilization, and elevated serum enzymes reflecting cellular injury. Oliguria and hypoglycemia, however, may be encountered.

II. The **clinical features** of hypothermia depend on the level of decline in the core temperature, the duration of hypothermia, and the presence of underlying disease. Generally, the following features are common: **CNS depression, hypovolemia** (with orthostatic or sustained hypotension), **acidosis** (usually metabolic), and **arrhythmias.** The state of profound hypothermia, manifested by a cold, rigid, apneic, pulseless, areflexic, unresponsive patient with fixed dilated pupils, may be indistinguishable from death. In such a situation, death should be defined as failure to revive with rewarming and appropriate resuscitative measures.

III. **Complications** of hypothermia include respiratory or cardiac arrest, arrhythmias, aspiration or bronchopneumonia, pulmonary edema, acute renal failure (acute tubular necrosis), pancreatitis, intravascular thrombosis (e.g., cerebrovascular accident, myocardial infarction, disseminated intravascular coagulation), gastrointestinal bleeding, and local cold injury (frostbite). The mortality in accidental hypothermia is high, averaging nearly 50% in the cases appearing in the medical literature [7, 14], and is primarily related to the presence of underlying disease [7, 34]. Increased severity and duration of hypothermia also appear to contribute to increased mortality [7, 34, 55].

IV. **Evaluation.** Once the diagnosis is established by a low-reading thermometer, it is important to determine the circumstances leading to the hypothermic state. In particular, because of therapeutic implications, it is important to identify underlying and associated conditions, such as acute and chronic illnesses and injuries, alcohol and drug intoxication, and metabolic disorders. Clinical assessment should include the following: a thorough history (including social aspects); a thorough but gentle (to avoid precipitating ventricular fibrillation) physical examination; arterial blood gases (ABGs), which must be corrected to the patient's body temperature (Table 15-1); a complete blood count (CBC); serum glucose, blood urea nitrogen or creatinine, electrolytes, and enzymes; coagulation indices; a urinalysis; an ECG; and a chest x-ray. Depending on the circumstances, the following tests also might be indicated: additional x-rays (e.g., abdominal films, cervical spine films), toxicologic analyses, blood cultures, thyroid function studies, and a serum cortisol.

V. **Treatment** of hypothermia consists of intensive supportive care, rewarming, and treatment of underlying and complicating disorders.

A. Intensive supportive care

1. **Careful monitoring** of the vital signs; cardiac rhythm; and fluid, acid-base, and electrolyte status of the hypothermic patient is essential because of the cardiovascular and respiratory instability inherent in the disorder. In particular,

Table 15-1. Temperature correction factors for arterial blood gases

Temperature		Correction*		
°F	°C	PCO_2	PO_2	pH
108	42.2	1.25	1.35	−.08
106	41.1	1.19	1.26	−.06
104	40.0	1.14	1.19	−.04
102	38.9	1.08	1.11	−.03
98.6	37.0	1.00	1.00	0
95	35.0	.92	.89	+.03
90	32.2	.82	.76	+.07
88	31.1	.78	.72	+.09
86	30.0	.74	.67	+.10
84	28.9	.71	.63	+.12
82	27.8	.68	.59	+.14
80	26.7	.64	.56	+.15
78	25.6	.61	.52	+.17
76	24.4	.59	.49	+.18
74	23.3	.56	.46	+.20
72	22.2	.53	.43	+.22

*Corrected PO_2 and PCO_2 are obtained by multiplying the measured values by the appropriate factors, and corrected pH is obtained by adding the appropriate correction factor to the measured value.
Source: R. L. Wears, Blood gases in hypothermia. *J.A.C.E.P.* 8:247, 1979. With permission.

continuous cardiac monitoring and recording of the core temperature (with a rectal or tympanic membrane thermistor probe) are important. Central venous pressure (CVP) monitoring with the catheter tip located in the superior vena cava is a safe and useful means of assessing the fluid status of the hypothermic patient. Swan-Ganz catheterization, however, should be avoided, because it may precipitate ventricular fibrillation in a cold, irritable heart. In the unstable patient, an arterial line will enable continuous and accurate recording of the blood pressure and facilitate blood sampling. Foley catheter insertion is indicated to monitor the urine output.

2. **Respiratory care.** Heated humidified oxygen at 40°C should be administered by mask or endotracheal tube. **Tracheal intubation** is indicated in comatose patients and patients with respiratory insufficiency. To avoid precipitating ventricular fibrillation, tracheal intubation must be performed skillfully and be preceded by oxygenation by mask. If assisted ventilation is required, it should be initiated at a rate of 8–10/minute and adjusted to avoid producing a respiratory acidosis or alkalosis, both of which appear to be arrhythmogenic [47]. Gentle suctioning should be performed as indicated.

3. **Management of cardiovascular disturbances**
   a. **External cardiac massage** at a rate of 80 compressions/minute is indicated if there is cardiac arrest (i.e., ventricular fibrillation or asystole) or if there is no palpable pulse in a central artery and the core temperature exceeds 30°C. However, in the pulseless hypothermic patient with a core temperature less than 30°C, external cardiac massage should be avoided if there is organized electrical activity on the ECG because of the risk of inducing ventricular fibrillation.
   b. **Intravenous fluids,** initially normal saline, should be heated to 40°C (with a blood warming device) and administered (preferably with CVP monitoring) at a rate to correct hypovolemia and achieve adequate hydration. Vasopressors should be avoided until a core temperature of 32°C is exceeded and the intravascular volume has been repleted.
   c. **Since a cold heart is relatively unresponsive to cardiac drugs, countershock, and electrical pacing, these measures generally should be avoided in the hypothermic patient** except when confronted with car-

diac arrest (i.e., ventricular fibrillation or asystole). Most arrhythmias, such as bradycardia and atrial fibrillation, require no specific therapy; they usually revert to normal sinus rhythm with rewarming. In particular, it is important to resist the temptation to treat bradycardia by pacemaker insertion because of the high risk of inducing ventricular fibrillation. Lidocaine in a dosage of 1 mg/kg, however, probably is indicated for suppression of ventricular premature contractions unresponsive to correction of hypoxia and acid-base disturbances. If ventricular fibrillation occurs, defibrillation should be attempted and repeated, if necessary, with incremental increases in the core temperature but is unlikely to be successful until the core temperature exceeds 28°C. Bretylium in a dosage of 5–10 mg/kg may aid defibrillation. Maintenance dosages of antiarrhythmic drugs must be markedly reduced because of the hypometabolic state of hypothermia.

4. **Sodium bicarbonate** should be administered IV as needed to correct a metabolic acidosis. Such therapy should be guided by temperature-corrected ABGs (Table 15-1) to avoid creating a metabolic alkalosis.

5. **General measures**
   a. **Gentle handling** of hypothermic patients is imperative, since at core temperatures less than 30°C any sudden or rough manipulation of the patient may precipitate ventricular fibrillation.
   b. **Immediate determination of the blood glucose** (with Dextrostix) or administration of 50% dextrose is indicated. If there is any suspicion of alcohol or drug abuse, thiamine, 100 mg IM or IV, or naloxone hydrochloride, 0.4–2.0 mg IV, respectively, should be administered.
   c. Since hyperglycemia usually reverts to normal with rewarming and insulin is ineffective below 31°C [6], insulin should be avoided until the patient is rewarmed to avert the risk of inducing hypoglycemia during rewarming.
   d. Prophylactic antibiotics are not indicated; however, if there is a reasonable suspicion of an infectious process, antibiotic therapy should be initiated after appropriate cultures have been obtained.
   e. Thyroid hormone (levothyroxine, 500 μg IV) should not be administered unless there is strong suspicion of an underlying hypothyroid or myxedematous state (see Chap. 9).
   f. Steroids have no role in the routine management of hypothermia and should only be used if there is evidence of underlying adrenal insufficiency.

B. **Rewarming** is an essential aspect of the therapy of hypothermia.
   1. **Rewarming methods** include passive, active external, and active core rewarming.
      a. **Passive rewarming** involves insulating the patient with blankets (preferably in a warm environment) and using the patient's endogenous metabolic heat production to effect rewarming. This method is most effective when the patient is shivering; however, it may not be effective at core temperatures below 30°C because of the low metabolic rates associated with such temperatures.
      b. **Active external rewarming** involves application of heat to the surface of the body by immersing the patient (preferably just the trunk) in a hot bath at 40–45°C or applying heated objects or a hyperthermic blanket to the patient. However, by causing peripheral vasodilatation and increasing the metabolic needs of the periphery, this method has the disadvantage of producing a decline in blood pressure (rewarming shock), serum pH, and core temperature (after drop, presumably due in part to shunting of cold blood from the periphery to the core). Since rewarming shock generally requires underlying volume depletion for its occurrence, it is most pronounced when the duration of hypothermia is prolonged (i.e., >8 hours).
      c. **Active core rewarming** or application of exogenous heat to the body's core, on the other hand, has distinct advantages over the other rewarming methods; it preferentially warms the heart with resultant increase in cardiac output and decrease in cardiac irritability and averts the problems associated with surface rewarming. Active core rewarming methods include central venous infusion of heated fluids; inhalation rewarming; heated peritoneal lavage; extracorporeal blood rewarming (using hemodialysis or cardiopulmonary bypass); heated gastric lavage, colonic irrigation, or bladder irrigation; and heated mediastinal irrigation via a thoracotomy or tube thoracostomy. Administration of heated humidified oxygen and heated in-

travenous fluids should be the routine adjunctive measures in all cases of hypothermia. Of the invasive procedures, heated peritoneal lavage has the advantage of being readily available and very effective at rewarming. The technique involves inserting a dialysis catheter (or preferably two catheters, one for inflow and one for outflow) into the peritoneal space and rapidly administering standard 1.5% dextrose dialysate solution heated to 40–45°C (by passing it through a blood-warming coil immersed in water at about 54°C) [42]. Peritoneal dialysis also has the advantage of correcting fluid, electrolyte, and acid-base disturbances and removing toxic drugs. In the cardiac arrest situation, cardiopulmonary bypass for rewarming is the method of choice, if available. Heated mediastinal lavage through a thoracotomy should be used as a last resort, and heated gastric lavage should be avoided because of the risk of precipitating ventricular fibrillation.

   d. For the various rewarming methods, the following **warming rates** generally can be expected: passive rewarming, 0–1°C/hour; inhalation rewarming, 0.5–1°C/hour; active external rewarming, 1–3°C/hour; heated peritoneal dialysis, 3–5°C/hour; and extracorporeal blood rewarming, 5–15°C/hour [34, 42].

2. **Rewarming selection.** Since there have been no controlled studies in humans with moderate and severe hypothermia, the optimal method and rate of rewarming remain controversial. However, from a review of hypothermia cases in the medical literature, it appears that active external rewarming has a higher mortality than passive rewarming [7, 14] and generally should be avoided, except possibly for acute hypothermia of short duration (e.g., acute immersion hypothermia) where the circulatory volume is maintained. Whatever rewarming method is chosen, it must be effective, yielding at least a 0.5°C/hour rise in core temperature; if not, an alternate method should be selected. It is recommended that the choice of a particular rewarming method be based on the clinical status of the patient. The following guidelines are suggested.

   a. **Hypothermia with stable cardiovascular status.** Passive rewarming using blankets for insulation (plus the routine use of heated oxygen and intravenous fluids) generally suffices.

   b. **Hypothermia with cardiovascular insufficiency or instability** (i.e., persistent hypotension or serious arrhythmias). Active core rewarming using heated peritoneal lavage or extracorporeal blood rewarming is indicated.

   c. **Hypothermia with cardiovascular collapse** (i.e., ventricular fibrillation or asystole). Rapid core rewarming is indicated. Cardiopulmonary bypass, if readily available, is the method of choice. Alternatively, heated peritoneal dialysis with concomitant cardiopulmonary resuscitation (CPR) in progress may be used. Because hypothermic patients may tolerate prolonged cardiac arrest due to the CNS protective effect of hypothermia, this technique may be successful even when cardiac arrest persists for hours [47].

   d. **Hypothermia with an associated toxic ingestion.** If a dialyzable drug is involved, hemodialysis or peritoneal dialysis may be preferred, depending on the severity of intoxication and the clinical status of the patient.

C. Underlying disorders must be actively sought and, when identified, aggressively treated, since they contribute significantly to the high mortality associated with hypothermia. Appropriate treatment of the complications of hypothermia is also important.

VI. Disposition. Hypothermic patients with core temperatures exceeding 32°C may be discharged from the emergency department following rewarming, provided they are free of underlying disease and social problems. All others require hospitalization. Patients with core temperatures less than 30°C, cardiovascular instability, or significant underlying or complicating disease require admission to an intensive care unit. No patient should be pronounced dead if the core temperature is less than 32°C. Such a determination can be made only after the patient fails to revive with rewarming to 32°C and appropriate resuscitative measures.

Heat Illness

Heat illness is a spectrum of disease arising from heat stress (i.e., endogenous and exogenous heat load). The illness includes heat cramps, a benign disorder; heat exhaustion, the most common syndrome; and heat stroke, a true life-threatening emergency.

I. **Pathophysiology.** Under normal conditions, the human body's metabolic processes continuously produce heat that is dissipated to the usually cooler environment, resulting in a steady state with a core body temperature of about 37°C. When the body gains heat (with a resultant increase in core temperature) due to increased metabolic production (from 70 kcal/hour at basal levels to 900 kcal/hour with maximal work [25]), absorption from a hot environment, impaired dissipation to the environment, or a combination of these, compensatory cooling processes are initiated. These include (1) an increased cutaneous circulation secondary to cutaneous vasodilatation and an increased cardiac output (if the heart is able to respond appropriately) resulting in increased heat loss from the surface of the body through radiation and convection, and (2) sweating with resultant heat loss (of 580 kcal/liter of sweat [51]) through evaporation. Sweating, however, may lead to considerable losses of sodium, potassium, and body water. If the heat stress is severe or prolonged, the capacity of these cooling mechanisms may be exceeded, resulting in an increase in core body temperature. Since cellular metabolism increases 13%/1°C rise in body temperature, a vicious cycle is produced, contributing to a rise in body temperature. Cellular hypoxia may result if the increased oxygen demand exceeds the supply. In addition, at core temperatures exceeding 42°C, direct cellular thermal injury may occur [46]. The net result is widespread cellular necrosis.

II. **Acclimatization,** achieved by daily exposure to heat stress for at least 10 days, is the process of adaption that enables humans to tolerate heat stress. Several physiologic responses occur with acclimatization. These include increased metabolic efficiency, increased sweating efficiency (i.e., sweating is initiated at a lower elevation in the core temperature and the sweat rate is doubled from 1.5 liters/hour to 3 liters/hour), increased myocardial efficiency characterized by an increase in stroke volume and cardiac output, and increased plasma volume resulting in part from sodium conservation by the kidneys and sweat glands (the sodium concentration in sweat decreases from 30–50 mEq/liter to 2–5 mEq/liter) [25, 51]. The net effect of these adaptive processes is decreased metabolic heat production and enhanced heat dissipation, thus protecting the human body against a rise in core temperature.

III. **The heat syndromes**

A. **Heat cramps** are painful skeletal muscle cramps affecting heavily exercised muscles, usually the lower extremity and abdominal muscles. They occur during or after strenuous exertion in the heat in individuals who sweat profusely and replace losses with hypotonic fluids. Although never proved, it is believed that heat cramps are due to sodium depletion and declining serum sodium levels secondary to sweat losses. Clinically, skeletal muscle spasms are evident, the body temperature is normal, and the serum sodium level (which does not need to be measured) is low or normal.

Treatment consists of rest in a cool environment and salt replacement with salt tablets, electrolyte solutions, or intravenous saline. Since this is a benign disorder, patients may be discharged and return to their usual activities, with instructions to increase their salt intake, unless contraindicated.

B. **Heat exhaustion** or heat prostration occurs as a result of salt and water depletion secondary to sweating in response to heat stress. Depending on the patient's oral intake, the heat exhaustion may be classified as primarily water depletion, salt depletion, or, most commonly, both.

1. The **manifestations** are nonspecific and include gastrointestinal upset (e.g., anorexia, nausea, vomiting), mild CNS dysfunction (e.g., headache, dizziness, faintness, irritability, lassitude, weakness), volume depletion (e.g., thirst, orthostatic or sustained hypotension, tachycardia, syncope), hyperventilation, and diaphoresis. Muscle cramps may occur if there is significant sodium loss. Usually, the body temperature is normal or mildly elevated, but it may be as high as 41°C.

2. **Laboratory examination,** although generally not necessary, may reveal a variable serum sodium, hemoconcentration, and respiratory alkalosis.

3. The **differential diagnosis** primarily includes an infectious (usually viral) illness and heat stroke. Rapid improvement and defervescence with therapy and an intact sensorium help differentiate heat exhaustion from those disease processes, respectively.

4. **Treatment** consists of rest in a cool environment, rehydration, and salt replacement. In the emergency department, rehydration and salt repletion are best achieved by administration of intravenous saline. If it is not possible to differentiate heat exhaustion from heat stroke, active cooling measures should be

instituted as in the management of heat stroke. Patients with heat exhaustion generally can be discharged to home with instructions to increase their salt and water intake, unless contraindicated, during periods of heat stress. Hospitalization, however, is indicated for those patients not responding to emergency department therapy, elderly patients with significant underlying disease or a poor home situation (e.g., no air conditioning), and patients for whom the diagnosis is in doubt.

C. **Heat stroke,** the least common but most serious of the heat syndromes, is characterized by the triad of **hyperpyrexia** (with a core temperature usually exceeding 40.6°C), **severe CNS dysfunction** (manifested by delirium, psychosis, stupor, or coma), and often **anhidrosis** (however, sweating may be present in exertional heat stroke of rapid onset). It is due to excessive body heat as a result of overloading or impairment of the body's heat dissipating mechanisms. Predisposing factors for heat stroke include those that (1) lead to exogenous heat gain (i.e., an ambient temperature greater than the body temperature), (2) increase endogenous heat production (e.g., physical exertion, infection, hypermotor activity, hyperthyroidism, certain drugs—amphetamines, phencyclidine, LSD), and (3) impair heat dissipation (e.g., lack of acclimatization, high ambient temperature, high humidity, obesity, heavy clothing, cardiovascular disease, dehydration, extremes of age, CNS lesions involving the hypothalamus, sweat gland dysfunction, prior heat stroke, potassium depletion, certain drugs—anticholinergics, phenothiazines, diuretics, propranolol).

1. **Pathophysiology.** Heat stroke is characterized by widespread cellular dysfunction and damage, primarily due to direct thermal injury, and the extent of damage appears to be related to both the degree and duration of the temperature elevation [46]. In addition, cellular hypoxia secondary to inability to meet the elevated metabolic demand for oxygen is likely a contributing factor to cellular injury. Thus, dysfunction or failure of any organ system may occur. Typical pathologic findings include widespread cellular degeneration and necrosis (with associated edema) and petechial and gross hemorrhages [45, 46].

2. The **diagnosis** of heat stroke generally is established when the clinical features of hyperpyrexia (usually >40.6°C), marked CNS dysfunction, and possibly anhidrosis occur under conditions of heat stress (i.e., an elevated ambient temperature and/or strenuous exercise). The diagnosis is supported by the finding of elevated serum enzymes reflecting cellular damage. Since sufficient cooling by endogenous or exogenous means may have ameliorated a marked hyperpyrexia and since the sweating mechanism may not have ceased functioning (secondary to fatigue or thermal injury), the absence of marked hyperpyrexia or anhidrosis does not exclude the diagnosis. Thus, a high index of suspicion is required to establish the diagnosis of heat stroke.

3. The **differential diagnosis** includes the other causes of a febrile state and CNS dysfunction, principally severe heat exhaustion and infection (particularly CNS infection and sepsis). Other entities in the differential diagnosis are epilepsy, severe head trauma, cerebrovascular accident, drug intoxication (particularly with amphetamines and phencyclidine), delirium tremens, malignant hyperthermia, and thyroid storm. If the diagnosis is in doubt, the patient should be treated for heat stroke by immediate active cooling (see sec. **III.C.5.a**), and then other possible diseases should be actively pursued.

4. **Clinical features.** There are two types of heat stroke (Table 15-2). Classical heat stroke primarily involves sedentary elderly people and is due to their inability to handle an exogenous heat load; in contrast, exertional heat stroke usually afflicts young people participating in strenuous physical activity and results from their inability to dissipate an endogenous heat load. Despite the different etiologies of these two forms of heat stroke, the clinical features are generally similar.

   a. **Signs and symptoms.** Marked hyperpyrexia, severe CNS dysfunction (e.g., marked altered mental status, seizures, focal neurologic deficits), and usually anhidrosis are the cardinal manifestations. The cardiovascular response in heat stroke may be either hyperdynamic with an increased cardiac output (if the cardiovascular system is able to respond appropriately to heat stress) or hypodynamic with a decreased cardiac output secondary to hypovolemia, peripheral pooling of blood, and/or myocardial dysfunction [40, 48]; a sinus tachycardia is common, and hypotension may be present. Also common to heat stroke are hyperventilation, vomiting, and diarrhea.

Table 15-2. Clinical characteristics of the two forms of heat stroke

Characteristic	Classical	Exertional
Age group affected	Older	Young
Activity	Sedentary	Physical exertion
Occur in epidemics	Yes	No
Predisposing illnesses	Often	No
Prevailing weather	Prolonged heat wave	Variable
Prodromal symptoms	Yes	Transient
Sweating	Often absent	May be present
Acid-base disturbance	Respiratory alkalosis common	Lactic acidosis common
Rhabdomyolysis	Rare	Common
Disseminated intravascular coagulation	Rare	Common
Acute renal failure	Rare	Common

Source: Adapted from G. R. Hart et al., Epidemic classical heat stroke: Clinical characteristics and course of 28 patients. *Medicine* (Baltimore) 61:189, 1982. Copyright 1982 by Williams & Wilkins.

    b. Common **laboratory features** include a leukocytosis, acid-base disturbances (particularly a respiratory alkalosis or metabolic acidosis), elevated serum enzymes, electrolyte disturbances (particularly hypokalemia, hypocalcemia, and hypophosphatemia), azotemia, hyperuricemia, myoglobinuria, and coagulation abnormalities.

    c. **Complications** are frequent and may involve any organ system. They include aspiration and bronchopneumonia, arrhythmias, cardiac failure and pulmonary edema, myocardial infarction, bleeding diatheses (including disseminated, intravascular coagulation), rhabdomyolysis, renal failure, hepatic failure, gastrointestinal ulcers, neurologic deficits, sepsis, and intravascular coagulation (e.g., pulmonary embolism, cerebrovascular accident). The mortality of heat stroke is considerable and is primarily related to the magnitude and duration of the hyperthermia [51].

  5. **Treatment** of heat stroke is directed at immediate elimination of hyperpyrexia and support of vital organ systems.

    a. **Immediate and rapid reduction of the hyperpyrexia** by immediate institution of active cooling measures is essential. It is imperative that the body temperature be reduced to near normal within 1 hour of the onset of heat stroke to effect a successful outcome. The best method of cooling is to immerse the patient in an ice-water bath. If this is not possible, continuous application of ice water to the patient may be used; this may be accomplished by covering the patient with a sheet and continuously pouring ice water on the patient. It is important, however, to avoid having ice come into direct contact with the patient's skin to prevent local cold injury to the skin. The extremities should be massaged during cooling to reduce cold-induced cutaneous vasoconstriction. Chlorpromazine, 10–25 mg IM or IV at a rate of 1 mg/minute, may be administered as needed to stop shivering. To avoid hypothermia, active cooling should be discontinued when the core (rectal) temperature reaches 39°C.

    b. **Supportive measures**

      (1) **Careful monitoring,** particularly of the vital signs, cardiac rhythm, ABGs corrected to the body temperature (see Table 15-1), and fluid status, is essential. In particular, the temperature should be monitored with a rectal or tympanic membrane thermistor probe and the cardiac rhythm with a cardiac monitor. CVP monitoring or Swan-Ganz catheterization (when there is persistent hemodynamic compromise) is useful in assessing the patient's fluid status. The urinary output also should be monitored. In addition, the CBC, coagulation indices, and serum chemistries should be followed.

(2) Because of the **altered mental status,** immediate determination of the blood glucose with Dextrostix or administration of 50% dextrose is indicated, even though hypoglycemia is uncommon in heat stroke.

(3) **Oxygen** should be administered by mask or endotracheal tube to supply the hypermetabolic tissue needs. **Tracheal intubation** is indicated if the patient is comatose (to protect the airway), repetitively seizing, or ventilating inadequately.

(4) **Intravenous fluids** (initially, normal saline or Ringer's lactate solution) are administered, with CVP or pulmonary wedge pressure monitoring as needed, to replace fluid losses, correct hypotension, and maintain an adequate urinary output. Fluid requirements, however, generally are modest, averaging 1200–1400 ml during the first 4 hours [40].

(5) A persistent **hypodynamic state,** characterized by hypotension and a low cardiac output despite adequate volume repletion, requires administration of an inotropic agent. Although isoproterenol has been used successfully in managing this state [40], dobutamine, 2–40 μg/kg/minute may be preferable. Alpha-adrenergic agents, however, should be avoided during the hyperthermic period because they impair heat dissipation.

(6) **Sodium bicarbonate** should be given IV as needed to correct a metabolic acidosis. This should be guided by temperature-corrected ABGs (see Table 15-1).

(7) **Mannitol,** 12.5–25.0 gm IV as needed to promote renal blood flow and urinary output, is beneficial in treating oliguria not responding to hydration and myoglobinuria secondary to rhabdomyolysis.

(8) **Seizures** require aggressive treatment with diazepam and phenytoin to avoid the heat production associated with seizure activity.

(9) The management of the **bleeding diatheses** of heat stroke is controversial. If treatment is required, most authorities recommend administration of clotting factors (e.g., fresh blood, fresh frozen plasma, platelets) rather than heparin.

(10) Prophylactic antibiotics are not indicated. However, if there is significant concern regarding the possibility of infection, antibiotic therapy should be initiated after appropriate cultures have been obtained.

(11) Corticosteroids are of no benefit in managing heat stroke and of questionable benefit in treating cerebral edema.

6. Disposition. Hospitalization, preferably in an intensive care unit, is indicated for all patients with heat stroke.

Near-Drowning

Drowning is death due to asphyxiation as a result of submersion in a liquid medium. Near-drowning, on the other hand, refers to initial survival following submersion. However, death may later ensue (secondary drowning), usually as a result of respiratory failure or anoxic encephalopathy. Both drowning and near-drowning can be classified as wet (80–90% of cases), in which aspiration of fluid occurs, or dry (10–20% of cases), in which aspiration is prevented by laryngospasm [37]. Drowning is the fourth leading cause of accidental mortality in the United States [26]. Each year there are approximately 8000 drownings in the United States, with several times as many near-drownings [20]. Predisposing factors include inability to swim, poor judgment regarding water activities, inadequate supervision of children, alcohol and drug intoxication, acute illnesses (e.g., seizures) and injuries (e.g., head and cervical spine injuries), water sports and automobile accidents, hypothermia, hyperventilation preceding underwater swimming, and suicide and homicide attempts.

I. Pathophysiology. The underlying pathophysiologic insult in drowning and near-drowning is **hypoxia** secondary to asphyxia (following submersion) or pulmonary insufficiency (following aspiration of the fluid medium). Both freshwater and saltwater aspiration commonly lead to pulmonary insufficiency and the adult respiratory distress syndrome (ARDS, or noncardiogenic pulmonary edema—see Chap. 7), although by different mechanisms. When freshwater is aspirated, the hypotonic fluid is rapidly absorbed from the alveoli into the circulation; but washout of pulmonary surfactant occurs, leading to alveolar collapse [37]. Aspirated saltwater by its hypertonic properties, on the other hand, draws fluid from the circulation into the alveoli, yielding fluid-filled but perfused alveoli. In addition, injury to the alveolar capillary membrane by hypertonic fluid or contaminants present in the aspirate can lead to exudation of protein-rich fluid into the alveoli. The net result of these processes is ventilation-perfusion mismatching and intrapulmonary shunting leading to hypoxemia that may be profound. Also, pulmonary compliance decreases and airway resistance increases. The resultant tissue hypoxia is mainly responsible for the features of near-drowning.

Much has been written about the differences between freshwater and seawater drowning and near-drowning in terms of fluid and electrolyte disturbances. Aspiration and subsequent absorption of large volumes (i.e., >22 ml/kg) of freshwater through the alveoli into the circulation may lead to hypervolemia, hemodilution (with decreased serum electrolyte concentrations), and hemolysis (with hemoglobinuria and hyperkalemia). On the other hand, aspiration of large volumes of hypertonic seawater may result in hypovolemia and increased concentrations of salts due to shift of fluid out of the circulation into the alveoli and absorption of salts from the seawater. In reality, serious fluid and electrolyte disturbances are distinctly uncommon, since aspiration of more than 22 ml/kg usually does not occur (only about 15% of drowning victims in one series) [36, 37].

II. **Clinical features. Hypoxemia** due to asphyxia or pulmonary insufficiency is the hallmark of near-drowning. Noncardiogenic pulmonary edema (ARDS) is common, but its appearance may be delayed up to 3 days. **Acidosis** is also common and is primarily metabolic secondary to tissue hypoxia, but there may be an associated respiratory component. Arrhythmias and hypotension may occur and are usually related to hypoxia and acidosis. Hypothermia due to immersion in cold water may be present; although hypothermia can lead to adverse physiologic effects, particularly life-threatening arrhythmias, it protects the CNS against hypoxic injury. Anoxic encephalopathy, however, is an all too common complication of near-drowning. Other complications include bacterial pneumonia; acute renal failure secondary to hypoxia and hypotension (acute tubular necrosis) and, uncommonly, hemoglobinuria resulting from freshwater-induced hemolysis; and disseminated intravascular coagulation. The morbidity and mortality of near-drowning are primarily related to the resultant degree of pulmonary insufficiency and hypoxic CNS insult.

III. **Evaluation** of the near-drowning victim entails a thorough history and physical examination, ABGs, chest x-ray(s), cervical spine films (if indicated), a CBC, serum chemistries, coagulation indices, toxicologic analyses (if indicated), and other appropriate studies as dictated by the clinical circumstances.

IV. **Treatment**
   A. **Careful monitoring** of clinical and pertinent laboratory parameters (e.g., vital signs, ABGs, ECG) is essential. Hemodynamic and intracranial pressure monitoring may also be indicated depending on the clinical situation.
   B. If there is any suspicion of **cervical spine injury** (e.g., a diving accident), the cervical spine must be immobilized and evaluated by neurologic examination and appropriate x-rays.
   C. **Basic and advanced cardiac life support** (see Chap. 2) should be instituted as indicated.
   D. **Aggressive treatment of hypoxia** is the mainstay of management. Initially, 100% **oxygen** should be administered by mask or endotracheal tube (the latter is indicated in patients with a depressed mental status or inadequate ventilation). Inability to maintain a PaO_2 in excess of 60 mm Hg with an FiO_2 of 40% is an indication for the application of continuous positive airway pressure (CPAP) or positive end-expiratory pressure (PEEP) to the airway (see Chap. 7). In an awake, spontaneously breathing patient, CPAP with a tight-fitting face mask may be tried; otherwise or if unsuccessful, endotracheal intubation is required. Use of CPAP or PEEP generally increases the functional residual capacity (FRC) and reduces the ventilation-perfusion mismatching and intrapulmonary shunting with consequent improved PaO_2, but a decrease in cardiac output and oxygen delivery to tissues may occur. The goal of therapy is to achieve a PaO_2 greater than 60 mm Hg with an FiO_2 of 40% or less, while maintaining an acceptable cardiac output. This requires titrating the level of CPAP or PEEP, FiO_2, and fluid status of the patient (see sec. **IV.E**) to achieve the desired effect.
   E. Initially, regardless of whether near-drowning occurs in freshwater or seawater, **normal saline or Ringer's lactate solution** is administered IV at a rate commensurate with the clinical situation. **Swan-Ganz catheterization** may be needed to measure and monitor the left ventricular filling pressure, cardiac output, and intrapulmonary shunting.

    F. Nasogastric intubation, with prior protection of the airway if needed, is indicated to empty the stomach.

    G. Sodium bicarbonate should be administered IV as needed to reverse a metabolic acidosis.

    H. Bronchodilators (i.e., aminophylline and beta-adrenergic agents) may be used to treat bronchospasm. If aspiration of particulate matter occurred, **bronchoscopy** may be used for removal.

    I. Prophylactic administration of antibiotics is not indicated. If possible, daily sputum samples for Gram's stain and culture should be obtained and antibiotic therapy initiated at the first sign of infection.

    J. Corticosteroids have not been shown to be effective in treating the pulmonary injury in near-drowning [5], and their use is not recommended. In addition, they are likely of little benefit in reducing cerebral edema secondary to hypoxia [13].

    K. Hypothermia may accompany near-drowning. Since hypothermia protects against hypoxic cerebral injury, vigorous resuscitation is indicated for all hypothermic immersion victims. Appropriate therapy of hypothermia (see **Accidental Hypothermia,** sec. **V**) is indicated.

    L. To lessen neurologic sequelae, **intensive cerebral resuscitative measures** are indicated. Accepted therapeutic measures include intracranial pressure monitoring and use of hyperventilation (to lower the $PaCO_2$ to 25–30 mm Hg), fluid restriction, loop diuretics, and/or osmotic agents (e.g., mannitol, glycerol) to lower intracranial pressure. Controversial measures include use of controlled hypothermia, corticosteroids, and barbiturates [39].

V. Disposition. Asymptomatic patients with a normal ABG and chest x-ray may be discharged from the emergency department after a 6-hour period of observation if all parameters remain normal. Because of the possibility of delayed appearance of respiratory failure, all near-drowning victims with any suggestion of aspiration require hospitalization and careful observation for at least 24 hours.

Dysbaric Diving Illnesses

Dysbaric diving illnesses include the effects of barotrauma and decompression sickness.

I. Barotrauma is the most common medical problem of divers. It refers to bodily injury resulting from changes in ambient pressure. Barotrauma commonly involves the air spaces of the middle ear (see Chap. 28), sinuses, and lungs, although any closed air space may be involved.

    A. Barotrauma of descent. Unless equilibration occurs, air within the middle ear and sinuses is compressed during descent. The result is pain, edema formation, hemorrhage into the air space, and/or rupture of the tympanic membrane. **Treatment** includes administration of systemic and nasal decongestants, antibiotic therapy if there is perforation of the tympanic membrane, and otolaryngologic referral. An uncommon injury related to Valsalva attempts to equalize the middle ear pressure during descent is rupture of the round window. This is manifested by tinnitus, vertigo, and a neurosensory hearing loss (see Chap. 28). Management includes hospitalization, bed rest with the head elevated, and otolaryngologic consultation regarding the need for surgical repair of a perilymph fistula.

    B. Barotrauma of ascent. Pulmonary barotrauma can occur during ascent from depths exceeding 1 meter if exhalation does not take place during ascent or if there is pulmonary air-trapping secondary to lung disease. Under these conditions, as a result of decreasing ambient pressures encountered during ascent, overdistention of the lungs occurs. At transpulmonic pressure gradients in excess of 80 mm Hg, rupture of the lung parenchyma and pulmonary vasculature may occur [52]. This can result in four syndromes, singly or in combination, that usually are present upon surfacing. Each generally requires hospitalization.

        1. Pulmonary tissue damage is manifested by cough, dyspnea, and hemoptysis. Treatment includes supportive measures, particularly administration of oxygen by mask. Positive-pressure ventilation generally should be avoided because of the risk of causing further damage to the lungs.

        2. Soft-tissue emphysema may involve the subcutaneous tissues, the mediastinum, and the pericardium. Physical examination and radiologic evaluation will establish the diagnosis. Treatment is supportive care, including administration of oxygen by mask.

        3. Pneumothorax is manifested by cough, dyspnea, and pain. The diagnosis is confirmed by a chest x-ray. Treatment generally involves tube thoracostomy, although small pneumothoraces may be managed by careful observation.

4. **Air embolism** occurs when pulmonary air enters injured pulmonary vessels and gains access to the systemic circulation through the left heart. Air emboli block distal circulation, producing ischemia and infarction of the involved tissue. Any organ may be involved, but the most serious syndromes are as follows.

   a. **Coronary air embolism** produces typical signs and symptoms of myocardial ischemia and infarction. Management involves treating the myocardial infarction (see Chap. 5) and air embolism (see sec. **I.B.4.b**).

   b. **Cerebral air embolism**

      (1) **Manifestations** appear abruptly upon surfacing and include headache, dizziness, visual disturbances, sensory disturbances, monoplegia, hemiplegia, an altered mental status (e.g., personality change, confusion, coma), seizures, and death.

      (2) **Treatment**

         (a) The patient is placed in the **Trendelenburg and left lateral decubitus positions** to lessen the risk of additional cerebral emboli and improve the cerebral circulation.

         (b) Administration of 100% **oxygen** by mask or endotracheal tube will enhance oxygenation of tissues and increase the gradient for nitrogen elimination from the emboli.

         (c) **Intravenous fluids** are administered as needed to achieve adequate hydration.

         (d) **Recompression in a hyperbaric chamber** is definitive therapy. If a hyperbaric chamber is unavailable, the patient must be transferred to a facility having a chamber. If air transport is required, it must be in an aircraft pressurized to 1 atm, or the aircraft must maintain the lowest possible flying altitude.

II. **Decompression sickness** (the bends, caisson disease) is caused by formation of nitrogen bubbles in the blood and tissue following ascent from a dive. At increased ambient pressures, the inert nitrogen gas from the compressed air that the diver breathes is dissolved in various body tissues with a predilection for tissues high in lipid content. The amount of nitrogen dissolved during a dive is a function of both the ambient pressure and the time at that pressure, that is, the depth and duration of the dive. The U.S. Navy Standard Decompression Tables specify safety limits regarding times at various depths and the rate of ascent (i.e., the number and duration of decompression stops) from such depths [53]. Generally, decompression sickness does not occur with dives to depths less than 10 m (33 feet) but may occur with deeper dives when the Decompression Tables are not followed and, uncommonly, even when they are followed because of individual variability [44]. In such situations, various body tissues are saturated with nitrogen; and with too rapid a decline in ambient pressure upon ascent, nitrogen bubbles form in those tissues and in the blood, giving rise to the manifestations of decompression sickness (due to the mechanical effects of the bubbles themselves or resultant tissue ischemia).

   A. **Clinical features.** The manifestations of decompression sickness generally appear during the first hour after surfacing but may occur during ascent or be delayed up to 36 hours [23, 44]. Decompression sickness is usually divided into two types based on the clinical features.

      1. **Type I** decompression sickness refers to skin and/or musculoskeletal involvement only, manifested as pruritus with or without a rash (usually mottling) and pain, respectively.

      2. **Type II** decompression sickness refers to involvement of critical organs, particularly the CNS and lungs.

         a. **CNS manifestations** arise from involvement of the brain and spinal cord. Involvement of the brain may give rise to nausea and vomiting; visual disturbances; tinnitus, vertigo, and nystagmus (the "staggers"); dysarthria, an altered mental status; seizures; and hemiparesis. Spinal cord involvement may yield extremity weakness or numbness, paresthesias, paraparesis, ataxia, and bladder dysfunction.

         b. **Pulmonary involvement** (the "chokes") is manifested as chest pain, cough, and dyspnea.

         c. In very severe cases, **shock** (presumably due to obstruction of the pulmonary circulation by nitrogen bubbles or hypovolemia secondary to increased vascular permeability) and even death may ensue.

B. Treatment

1. In type II decompression sickness, **the patient should be placed on the left side with the head 30 degrees lower than the feet** to decrease the risk of cerebral air embolism and improve the cerebral circulation.

2. To improve tissue oxygenation and enhance nitrogen elimination from the body, 100% **oxygen** by face mask or endotracheal tube is administered.

3. **Recompression** in a hyperbaric chamber is essential and should be performed as soon as possible in all suspected cases of decompression sickness with the exception of isolated, mild skin manifestations [44, 52]. If air transport to a facility having a hyperbaric chamber is necessary, the aircraft should be pressurized to 1 atm or fly at the lowest possible altitude.

4. **Ringer's lactate** solution or normal saline is administered IV to achieve and maintain an adequate circulatory volume.

5. **Diazepam** is the drug of choice for termination of seizures.

6. The role of corticosteroids is controversial, although one retrospective review suggests a beneficial effect [23].

7. Narcotic analgesics and sedatives should be avoided, if possible, because of their respiratory depressant effects.

C. Disposition. In general, hospitalization for at least 24 hours is indicated for persons with decompression sickness.

III. **Consultation** regarding the management of dysbaric diving illnesses can be obtained from the National Diving Accident Network at Duke University (telephone: 919-684-8111).

High-Altitude Illness

Acute exposure to altitudes in excess of 2000 meters (6560 feet) may result in high-altitude illness. This illness encompasses a spectrum of clinical entities that likely represent different manifestations of the same disease process [15]. The clinical syndromes of high-altitude illness may overlap and range from mild to severe. Acute mountain sickness, peripheral edema, and retinal hemorrhages generally are mild forms of this illness, whereas pulmonary edema and cerebral edema are severe forms and may be fatal. Both the incidence and severity of high-altitude illness appear to be directly related to the altitude attained, the speed of ascent, and the amount of physical exertion expended at the high altitude, but inversely correlated to age and the time taken to acclimatize en route to the high altitude [17]. Thus, high-altitude illness commonly afflicts young people who rapidly ascend or reascend (following loss of acclimatization) to a high altitude, particularly if they undergo physical exertion at the high altitude. Manifestations of acute altitude illness generally appear from 6–96 hours after arrival at the high altitude [15].

I. **Pathophysiologic mechanisms.** The pathophysiology of high-altitude illness is not well understood. It is clear, however, that **hypoxia** is the key factor behind the illness and its various clinical syndromes. Although altitude-related hypoxia leads to compensatory hyperventilation in an attempt to improve arterial oxygen saturation, the hypocarbia and respiratory alkalosis produced tend to counteract this ventilatory response to hypoxia. In addition, the alkalosis-induced leftward shift of the oxygen-hemoglobin dissociation curve further impairs oxygen delivery to tissues. Tissue hypoxia may lead to malfunction of the cellular adenosine triphosphate (ATP)–dependent sodium pump, particularly in the CNS, resulting in intracellular sodium accumulation and cellular edema [21]. In addition, hypoxia-induced cerebral vasodilatation is thought to play a role in the development of cerebral edema and retinal hemorrhages [27]. In the lung, hypoxia has been demonstrated to increase pulmonary vascular resistance; nonuniform arteriolar vasoconstriction likely occurs and results in shunting of excessive blood through other areas of the lung with resultant capillary injury culminating in patchy, noncardiac pulmonary edema [24]. Thus, it appears that tissue hypoxia is principally responsible for high-altitude illness and its various clinical entities. Recent evidence, however, suggests that antidiuresis and fluid retention occur and play a role in the production of the various edema states [16].

II. In **acclimatization,** which may be achieved by spending 2–4 days at intermediate altitudes en route to a high altitude, physiologic adaptive processes occur that protect against high-altitude illness [17]. These physiologic processes principally involve renal excretion of bicarbonate, which reverses the systemic alkalosis, and an increase in red blood cell 2,3-diphosphoglycerate (DPG) [27]. The resultant effects are an increase in ventilatory drive and enhanced oxygen delivery to tissues, the latter due in part to a rightward shift of the oxyhemoglobin dissociation curve.

III. **Clinical features.** High-altitude illness likely represents a single disease with a variety of manifestations, which can be organized into five syndromes as follows

A. **Acute mountain sickness** is a symptom complex that occurs with increased frequency at increasing altitudes above 2000 m (6560 feet) following rapid ascent. Physical exertion at high altitude appears to be a contributing factor. Signs and symptoms, which usually begin within hours of arrival at the high altitude, include headache, malaise, anorexia, nausea, vomiting, dizziness, fatigue, lassitude, poor concentration, insomnia, mild dyspnea, hypernea, tachycardia, irritability, and Cheyne-Stokes respirations. For individuals remaining at the high altitude, symptoms generally resolve within 3–5 days as acclimatization occurs.

B. **High-altitude pulmonary edema,** which is a form of noncardiogenic pulmonary edema, generally occurs 1–3 days after rapid ascent to altitudes in excess of 2500 m (8200 feet). There appears to be a predilection for young people and previously acclimatized people reascending to a high altitude following a stay at low altitude, and physical exertion at high altitude frequently precedes its onset. Pulmonary signs and symptoms (e.g., cough, dyspnea progressing to severe respiratory distress, tachypnea, frothy pink sputum, rales, cyanosis) predominate, but manifestations of acute mountain sickness may also be present. A low-grade fever, tachycardia, respiratory alkalosis, and leukocytosis are other common features of the syndrome. The chest x-ray reveals patchy infiltrates with a predilection for the right midlung field but no cardiomegaly. With progression of the disease, an altered mental status, hypotension, and death may ensue.

C. **Cerebral edema** generally requires altitudes in excess of 3500 m (11,480 feet) for it to occur. Its onset generally is 2–3 days after arrival at such altitudes. Again, rapid ascent is a predisposing factor. Neurologic signs and symptoms are prominent and include a severe headache, vertigo, ataxia, an altered mental status, papilledema, and focal neurologic deficits. Nausea and vomiting are common. With progression of the disease, seizures, depression of consciousness, and death may ensue. Permanent neurologic deficits may be present in survivors.

D. **Peripheral edema** may occur 2–4 days after rapid ascent to altitudes above 2500 m (8200 feet). It is more common in women. The edema generally involves the face initially, progresses to involve the hands and lower extremities, and is associated with a weight gain. Manifestations of acute mountain sickness may also be present.

E. **Retinal hemorrhages** may occur at high altitudes (e.g., 4000 m or 13,120 feet), increasing in frequency the higher the altitude. Physical exertion at high altitude appears to be a predisposing factor. Symptoms referable to the eyes generally are minimal, but visual blurring and scotoma may be noted. Associated features of acute mountain sickness may be present.

IV. **Treatment** of high-altitude illness depends on the severity of the disease.

A. Mild manifestations of **acute mountain sickness** may be treated by rest at the altitude (until acclimatization occurs), fluid replacement as needed, and administration of a mild analgesic. More severe or persistent manifestations require administration of oxygen and descent to a low altitude.

B. Treatment of **high-altitude pulmonary edema** includes bed rest, administration of oxygen, and generally descent to a lower altitude [32]. Severe pulmonary edema may necessitate mechanical ventilation with PEEP.

C. **Cerebral edema** requires administration of oxygen and immediate and rapid descent to a low altitude. Corticosteroids generally are administered but are of questionable benefit. In severe cases, use of a hyperosmolar agent (e.g., mannitol, glycerol) may be of benefit.

D. **Peripheral edema** generally may be treated by rest at the high altitude. Severe edema, however, should prompt descent to a low altitude. A diuretic in a low dosage may also be administered.

E. Asymptomatic **retinal hemorrhages** require no treatment other than rest for a few days at the high altitude. Symptomatic retinal hemorrhages should prompt administration of oxygen, descent to a lower altitude, and ophthalmologic referral.

V. **Prophylaxis.** Staging of ascent to allow for acclimatization will help prevent high-altitude illness. Acetazolamide, which is a carbonic anhydrase inhibitor with diuretic properties, has been demonstrated to prevent and ameliorate the manifestations of acute mountain sickness when taken in a dosage of 250 mg q8h or 500 mg qd [2, 28]. By enhancing renal bicarbonate excretion and inducing a metabolic acidosis, acetazolamide increases the ventilatory response to hypoxia and improves arterial oxygenation [2, 28]. This drug is recommended for the prophylaxis of high-altitude illness, but it may also be of benefit in treating high-altitude illness, particularly acute mountain sickness and peripheral edema. In one study, dexamethasone, 4 mg PO q6h, prevented the symptoms of acute mountain sickness in subjects exposed to a simulated high altitude [22a]; thus, it may also prove to be an effective prophylactic agent.

VI. **Disposition.** Hospitalization is mandatory when cerebral edema is present and generally warranted in the presence of pulmonary edema. The other syndromes, however, usually can be managed on an outpatient basis.

Radiation Injuries

Short of a nuclear war, radiation injuries may result from exposure to or contamination by radioactive sources. Accidents involving radioactive sources can occur at hospitals, research laboratories, industries, and nuclear power plants and during transport of radioactive materials.

I. **Radiation physics and pathophysiology of radiation injuries.** A radioactive substance is one that emits ionizing radiation. Radiation is energy in the form of particles or electromagnetic waves (Table 15-3). Alpha particles, beta particles, and gamma rays are the three common types of radiation emitted from the nuclei of radioactive atoms during radioactive decay. Neutrons, protons, and x-rays are forms of radiation usually derived from nuclear reactors, accelerators, and x-ray machines, respectively. For radiation to affect the human body, it must gain access to the body. Thus, radiation that readily penetrates tissues (e.g., gamma rays, x-rays, neutrons) constitutes a significant external biologic threat to the human body. On the other hand, poorly penetrating radiation (e.g., alpha particles) generally requires incorporation into the body to be harmful. The biologic effects of radiation are a result of ionization produced by the radiation. Free radicals are formed from water; these then react with DNA and RNA molecules with resultant disruption of those molecules. Depending on the dose and time relationships, the effects of radiation may be acute or delayed (not appearing for up to several generations) and minor or major.

A. **Radiation dose units**

1. A **roentgen** (R) is the unit of exposure defined as the quantity of x or gamma radiation that will produce 1 electrostatic unit of electricity when passing through 1 cc of air under standard conditions of temperature and pressure.

2. A **rad** (radiation absorbed dose) is the unit of absorbed radiation defined as the absorption of 100 ergs of radiation energy per gram (or 10^{-2} joules/kg) of absorbing material.

3. A **rem** (roentgen equivalent man) refers to the biologic effect of radiation; it is the unit of radiation dose equivalent and is equal to the absorbed dose in rads multiplied by the relative biologic effectiveness (quality factor) of the radiation in question. For most beta, gamma, and x radiation, the quality factor is 1, and the rem and rad are equivalent.

B. **Radiation surveys.** The Geiger-Müller (GM) counter is the standard device used for detecting and measuring beta and gamma radiation. Personnel dosimeters, such as pocket chambers, film badges, and thermoluminescent dosimeters (TLD), are useful in detecting external radiation, principally gamma and x radiation. Because of the limited range and poor penetrating ability of alpha particles, careful technique and special devices must be used to measure this type of radiation. Once external contamination is removed from the body, radiation counters available in hospital nuclear medicine departments may be used to detect and measure internal radioactivity that emits penetrating radiation capable of escaping from the body, principally gamma radiation. The detection and measurement of internal radioactive contaminants emitting low-penetrating radiation (i.e., alpha and beta particles), however, requires the analysis of body excrements.

II. **Clinical situations.** Three clinical situations may occur singly or in combination. These include irradiation, external contamination, and incorporation (internal contamination).

A. **Irradiation** refers to exposure to ionizing radiation, principally gamma or x-rays. Unless simultaneously contaminated with a radioactive substance or exposed to neutrons that can induce radioactivity, the victim is not radioactive and presents no hazard to medical or other personnel. Irradiation may be whole-body or local, and the biologic effects may be acute or delayed.

Table 15-3. Types of ionizing radiation

Type	Usual source	Properties	Biologic hazard
Alpha particles	Heavy radioactive elements (e.g., plutonium, radium, uranium)	A particle composed of 2 protons and 2 neutrons with a mass of 4 and charge of +2. Range of a few centimeters in air. Very poor tissue penetration (limited to about the thickness of the epidermis).	Little or no external hazard. Serious internal hazard
Beta particles	Most radioisotopes Electron accelerators	A singly positively or negatively charged particle with the mass of an electron (positron or electron). Range of a few meters in air. Poor tissue penetration (usually <8 mm).	An external hazard An internal hazard
Neutrons	Nuclear reactors and accelerators	An uncharged particle with a mass of 1. Range of many meters in air. Deep tissue penetration. Resultant induced radioactivity.	Serious external hazard
Protons	Nuclear accelerators	A singly positively charged particle with a mass of 1. Variable tissue penetration.	Serious external hazard
Gamma rays	Most radioisotopes	High-energy electromagnetic radiation. Range of many meters in air. Deep tissue penetration (many centimeters)	Serious external hazard An internal hazard
X-rays	X-ray machines and nuclear accelerators	Electromagnetic radiation. Range of many meters in air. Deep tissue penetration.	Serious external hazard

Source: Adapted from G. A. Andrews and R. J. Cloutier, Accidental acute radiation injury. *Arch. Environ. Health* 10:498, 1965; and L. L. Richter et al., A systems approach to the management of radiation accidents. *Ann. Emerg. Med.* 9:303, 1980.

1. The **acute radiation syndrome** results from acute whole-body irradiation, usually by gamma or x-rays. The clinical features (Table 15-4) are a function of the delivered radiation dose, dose rate, dose distribution, and organ sensitivity. The greater and more acute the exposure to radiation, the earlier manifestations appear and the more severe the syndrome. Gastrointestinal effects, initially manifested by anorexia, nausea, and vomiting, occur following acute exposure to 100 rem or more; vomiting appearing within 1 hour of exposure signifies a potentially lethal exposure and from 1–5 hours after exposure, serious radiation illness [29]. Diarrhea, which may be severe (with associated fluid and electrolyte disturbances) and bloody, generally indicates a dose greater than 400 rem. Bone marrow depression generally occurs with acute exposure exceeding 100 rem; a lymphocyte count of less than 1200/mm³ 48 hours after exposure indicates serious radiation illness, and a count of less than 300/mm³ at 48 hours, likely a fatal outcome [1]. Radiation exposure exceeding 300 rem generally produces skin erythema within a few hours and epilation in about 2 weeks [1]. Radiation doses exceeding 1000 rem produce CNS signs and symptoms (e.g., headache, vomiting, an altered mental status, vertigo, ataxia, seizures) within

Table 15-4. Physiologic responses to acute whole-body irradiation

Whole-body dose (rem)	Response
5–100	Asymptomatic. Minor depression of leukocytes and platelets* in a few persons. Chromosome aberrations.
100–200	Mild anorexia, nausea, vomiting, and fatigue of <24 hours' duration in most persons. Depression of leukocytes and platelets* in most persons, with lymphocytes declining by about 50% within 48 hours.
200–400	Symptomatic course with nausea and vomiting lasting 2–4 days in most persons. Skin erythema and subsequent epilation. Marked reduction in leukocytes and platelets.* Some deaths within 60 days due to infection.
400–600	Serious illness with nausea and vomiting occurring within a few hours and diarrhea. Severe hematopoietic changes.* Approximately 50% mortality, usually within 30 days (LD_{50} = 450 rem).
600–1000	Accelerated version of acute radiation syndrome with severe nausea, vomiting, and diarrhea starting within a few hours and culminating in gastrointestinal hemorrhage and severe fluid and electrolyte loss. Lymphocyte depression to <500/mm^3 by 48 hours. High mortality, usually within 14 days.
>1000	Fulminant course with rapid onset of gastrointestinal and CNS manifestations and complications. Lymphocytes decline to 0 within 48 hours. Mortality of 100%, usually within 72 hours.

*Maximum depression of lymphocytes usually occurs within 48 hours, whereas maximum depression of neutrophils and thrombocytes usually takes 3–4 weeks.
Source: Adapted from G. R. Meckstroth, Preparedness for radiation injuries: A guide to initial treatment. *E.R. Reports* 3:79, 1982; F. A. Mettler, Jr., Emergency management of radiation accidents. *J.A.C.E.P.* 7:302, 1978; and L. L. Richter, et al., A systems approach to the management of radiation accidents. *Ann. Emerg. Med.* 9:303, 1980.

minutes. The median lethal radiation dose (LD_{50}) is approximately 450 rem [33]. With whole-body exposure exceeding 1000 rem, mortality approaches 100%.

   2. **Localized radiation effects** may appear following local exposure to ionizing radiation in excess of 300 rem. Depending on the dose, dose rate, quality of radiation, and anatomic location, the radiation effects may be acute or delayed (often taking weeks to reach full extent) in onset and include pain, burns (ranging from erythema to full thickness), epilation, and tissue necrosis.
   B. **External contamination** refers to the presence of radioactive material on the surface of the body (and the victim's clothes). In this situation, there is the risk of radiation exposure to the victim and attending personnel and the risk of spread of radioactive contamination both internally and externally.
   C. **Incorporation or internal contamination** denotes the presence of radioactive material within the body as a result of inhalation, ingestion, or contamination of an open wound. The radionuclide may be distributed throughout the body or concentrated in a particular organ (the critical organ) or tissue. In addition, the radionuclide may become permanently biochemically incorporated within the body. Although representing less of a radiation risk to attending personnel than when there is external contamination, internal contamination is a serious situation for the victim. The radioactive material will continue to irradiate internal tissues, with the potential for causing extensive cellular damage, until it is excreted or removed (by treatment) or becomes inactive through radioactive decay.
   III. **Management of radiation accidents. A radiation accident plan** is essential for the efficient and proper management of radiation accidents and their victims. The plan should specify the following: individuals to be notified; the roles of medical and ancillary personnel involved; the area to be used for decontamination; and the procedures, particularly regarding decontamination, to be followed. Key individuals involved include the physician-in-charge (team leader) responsible for directing patient care and decontamination and the radiation safety officer (health physicist) responsible for monitoring radiation levels and decontamination procedures, analyzing specimens for radioactivity

and isotope identification, disposing of radioactive wastes and contaminated materials, and advising the physician-in-charge regarding patient decontamination and decorporation. The goals of management are to provide for the victim's immediate and subsequent medical needs and to effect decontamination and decorporation of the victim, while at the same time preventing spread of contamination and protecting medical and other personnel from contamination and the hazards of radiation exposure.

A. **Stabilization.** Management of associated, potentially life-threatening conditions takes immediate precedence. In such situations, life-supportive measures should be initiated immediately. It is very unlikely that the level of radiation from radioactive contamination would constitute an immediate health hazard to medical personnel. General medical care, however, generally should be delivered following decontamination.

B. **Assessment.** Determination of the nature and extent of radioactive contamination and radiation exposure is of therapeutic and prognostic significance. In particular, the following information regarding the accident should be sought: the means of radioactive contamination (if any), an estimate of its severity and the suspected radionuclide(s) involved, the type of radiation involved and an estimate of the absorbed dose, whether there are associated injuries or medical illnesses involved, and the treatment and decontamination measures rendered at the scene and en route to the hospital. If a health physicist was at the scene of the accident, he or she should be able to provide such information. At the hospital, the patient's medical condition is assessed (while emergency treatment is rendered as necessary), and the patient is surveyed by the radiation safety officer with a Geiger-Müller counter (and an alpha-monitoring device if indicated) for external radioactivity. Cotton swab samples of the nares, ear canals, mouth, contaminated areas, and wounds are obtained, surveyed for radioactivity, placed in separate containers, appropriately labeled, and saved for later analysis. Nasal mucus (obtained by having the patient blow his nose into paper tissue) is also collected, surveyed, and saved for analysis. Likewise, any debrided tissue or foreign bodies removed are surveyed and saved for analysis. If there is any suspicion of internal contamination, all feces, urine, and vomitus must be collected and refrigerated for later analysis. The patient's clothing and metal accessories (in case of neutron-induced radioactivity) also should be saved for analysis. Blood should be sent for a CBC, differential count, platelet count, reticulocyte count, serum chemistries, chromosome analysis, radioisotope analysis, and human lymphocyte antigen (HLA) typing; in addition, a urinalysis should be performed. Once external decontamination is complete, radiation counters in the nuclear medicine department may be used to detect and measure internal contamination.

C. **Containment of radioactive contamination** is a vital aspect of managing radiation accidents. This can be accomplished by carefully monitoring radioactivity, decontamination procedures, the handling of contaminated materials, and personnel activities. A designated decontamination (radiation emergency treatment) area is essential. Ideally, this is a separate area within the emergency department with its own entrance and ventilation system. If it does not have a separate ventilation system, the ventilation should be turned off to prevent spread of airborne contamination. The route from the ambulance drop-off to the decontamination area and the floor of the decontamination area should be covered with plastic sheets or paper. Entrance to and exit from the decontamination area must be strictly monitored (by the radiation safety officer). Entrance to the decontamination area is to be limited to essential personnel wearing protective clothing, and exit only to personnel shown to be free of contamination. Decontamination should follow accepted procedures (see sec. **III.E**); and radioactive materials, contaminated clothing, and waste materials are to be collected in receptacles (e.g., plastic bags) for appropriate disposal. The victim should not be removed from the decontamination area until determined to be essentially free of external contamination.

D. **Protection of attending personnel** from radioactive contamination and radiation exposure is an important aspect of managing radiation accidents. Attending personnel are required to wear protective clothing (i.e., surgical gowns, caps, boots, masks, and gloves) and a dosimeter when entering the decontamination area. This clothing will protect personnel from radioactive contamination but not from radiation exposure. Protection from the latter may be provided by reducing the time spent in the area, increasing the distance from the source, and using of appropriate shielding. The radiation safety officer should monitor the radiation levels in the decontamination area and, if necessary, rotate personnel to lessen each person's exposure. Generally, personnel should be rotated after a dose of 5 rem (or less if possible) is received

[38]. The maximum allowable radiation dose is 100 rem [43]. If radioiodine may be involved, attending personnel should take 8–10 drops of a saturated solution of potassium iodide (SSKI) to block uptake of radioiodine by the thyroid gland.

E. **Decontamination** is the process of removing external radioactive contamination from the victim. Decontamination should be performed as soon as possible following initial stabilization. Careful technique should be used, so as not to spread contamination, particularly internally. Generally, removing the victim's clothes will remove most of the surface contamination. Obvious debris and devitalized tissue must be removed. Generally, decontamination is performed in the following order to prevent incorporation of radioisotopes: contaminated body orifices, open wounds, and intact skin. Gentle and careful swabbing and irrigation of body orifices and open wounds with copious amounts of normal saline (with suction and protection of adjacent areas to prevent spread of contamination) and gentle washing of intact skin with soap and tepid water generally will effect decontamination. If not, repeat of the procedure, irrigation with 3% hydrogen peroxide or an appropriate chelating agent, wound debridement, and more vigorous (but not abrasive) washing of the skin may be tried. Hair usually can be decontaminated by shampooing with soap and water, repeated as necessary; however, if contamination persists, the hair should be removed with clippers. Contaminated clothing should be deposited in receptacles or plastic bags for appropriate disposal. Debris and debrided tissues should be saved for analysis. Ideally, irrigating and wash solutions should be collected in receptacles for appropriate disposal. The usual principles of wound management should be followed.

F. **Decorporation** is the process of removing internal radioactive contamination due to ingestion, inhalation, or wound contamination. Internal contamination represents a true emergency, and therapy directed at removing the contaminant must be initiated immediately to lessen the radiation exposure and prevent permanent incorporation of the radioisotope in the body. Therapeutic measures directed at reducing absorption and enhancing elimination of the radionuclide include the following: gastric emptying by lavage or induced emesis with ipecac for ingested and inhaled substances (in the latter situation because inhaled particles tend to reach the gastrointestinal tract eventually); use of cathartics to hasten gastrointestinal elimination; administration of binding (e.g., aluminum-containing antacids), diluting, blocking (e.g., SSKI), chelating (e.g., DTPA), and mobilizing agents as appropriate; use of forced diuresis when indicated; bronchopulmonary lavage for inhaled radionuclides; and thorough decontamination of open wounds [33, 38]. Specific therapy, however, depends on the specific radionuclide involved [30, 38]. It is important to collect all body excrements and waste materials for analysis. Nuclear medicine radiation counters may be useful in assessing and following internal radioactivity.

G. **Management of the acute radiation syndrome** consists of mainly supportive care, that is, administration of antiemetics, maintenance of fluid and electrolyte balance, blood and platelet transfusions as needed, reverse (protective) isolation if the granulocyte count is less than $500/mm^3$, and administration of antibiotics upon signs of infection. Bone marrow transplantation may be needed if there is persistent, severe pancytopenia. Radiation burns should be treated in the same manner as thermal burns (see Chap. 21).

H. **Hospital admission** or transfer to a radiation treatment center is indicated in the presence of a whole-body radiation dose exceeding 100 rem (manifested by nausea and vomiting), significant residual external contamination (following attempted decontamination), significant internal contamination, or serious associated injuries. Isolation is required for contaminated patients and patients with severe acute radiation syndrome.

I. **Consultation** regarding the handling of radiation accidents is available from the Radiation Emergency Assistance Center/Training Site (REAC/TS) in Oak Ridge, Tennessee (telephone: 615-576-1004).

Bibliography

1. Andrews, G. A., and Cloutier, R. J. Accidental acute radiation injury. *Arch. Environ. Health* 10:498, 1965.
2. Birmingham Medical Research Expeditionary Society Mountain Sickness Study Group. Acetazolamide in control of acute mountain sickness. *Lancet* 1:180, 1981.
3. Black, P. R., Van Devanter, S., and Cohn, L. H. Effects of hypothermia on systemic and organ system metabolism and function. *J. Surg. Res.* 20:49, 1976.

4. Boysen, P. G. Dispelling the myths and controversies of near-drowning. *Emerg. Med. Reports* 5:23, 1984.
5. Calderwood, H. W., Modell, J. H., and Ruiz, B. C. The ineffectiveness of steroid treatment of fresh-water near drowning. *Anesthesiology* 43:642, 1975.
6. Carden, D., et al. Hypothermia. *Ann. Emerg. Med.* 11:497, 1982.
7. Chinard, F. P. Accidental hypothermia: A brief review. *J. Med. Soc. N.J.* 75:610, 1978.
8. Coniam, S. W. Accidental hypothermia. *Anesthesia* 34:250, 1979.
9. Conn, A. W., Edmonds, J. F., and Barker, G. A. Cerebral resuscitation in near-drowning. *Pediatr. Clin. North Am.* 26:691, 1979.
10. Eiseman, B., and Bond, V. Surgical care of nuclear casualities. *Surg. Gynecol. Obstet.* 146:877, 1978.
11. Evans, W. O., et al. Amelioration of the symptoms of acute mountain sickness by staging and acetazolamide. *Aviat. Space Environ. Med.* 47:512, 1976.
12. Fischbeck, K. H., and Simon, R. P. Neurological manifestations of accidental hypothermia. *Ann. Neurol.* 10:384, 1981.
13. Fishman, R. A. Brain edema. *N. Engl. J. Med.* 293:706, 1975.
14. Gregory, R. T., and Doolittle, W. H. Accidental hypothermia: Part II. Clinical implications of experimental studies. *Alaska Med.* 15:48, 1973.
15. Hackett, P. H., and Rennie, D. Rales, peripheral edema, retinal hemorrhage and acute mountain sickness. *Am. J. Med.* 67:214, 1979.
16. Hackett, P. H., et al. Acute mountain sickness and the edemas of high altitude: A common pathogenesis? *Respir. Physiol.* 46:383, 1981.
17. Hackett, P. H., Rennie, D., and Levine, H. D. The incidence, importance, and prophylaxis of acute mountain sickness. *Lancet* 2:149, 1976.
18. Harari, A., et al. Haemodynamic study of prolonged deep accidental hypothermia. *Eur. J. Intens. Care Med.* 1:65, 1975.
19. Hart, G. R., et al. Epidemic classical heat stroke: Clinical characteristics and course of 28 patients. *Medicine* (Baltimore) 61:189, 1982.
20. Hoff, B. H. Multisystem failure: A review with special reference to drowning. *Crit. Care Med.* 7:310, 1979.
21. Houston, C. S. High altitude illness: Disease with protean manifestations. *J.A.M.A.* 236:2193, 1976.
22. Houston, C. S., and Dickinson, J. Cerebral form of high-altitude illness. *Lancet* 2:758, 1975.
22a. Johnson, T. S., et al. Prevention of acute mountain sickness by dexamethasone. *N. Engl. J. Med.* 310:683, 1984.
23. Kizer, K. W. Delayed treatment of dysbarism: A retrospective review of 50 cases. *J.A.M.A.* 247:2555, 1982.
24. Kleiner, J. P., and Nelson, W. P. High altitude pulmonary edema: A rare disease? *J.A.M.A.* 234:491, 1975.
25. Knochel, J. P. Environmental heat illness. *Arch. Intern. Med.* 133:841, 1974.
26. Knopp, R. Near drowning. *J.A.C.E.P.* 7:249, 1978.
27. Larson, E. B. Recognizing, treating, and preventing high-altitude illness. *Emerg. Med. Reports* 4:121, 1983.
28. Larson, E. B., et al. Acute mountain sickness and acetazolamide: Clinical efficacy and effect on ventilation. *J.A.M.A.* 248:328, 1982.
29. Leonard, R. B., and Ricks, R. C. Emergency department radiation accident protocol. *Ann. Emerg. Med.* 9:462, 1980.
30. Lincoln, T. A. Importance of initial management of persons internally contaminated with radionuclides. *Am. Ind. Hyg. Assoc. J.* 37:16, 1976.
31. Marcus, P. The treatment of acute accidental hypothermia: Proceedings of a symposium held at the RAF institute of aviation medicine. *Aviat. Space Environ. Med.* 50:834, 1979.
32. Marticorena, E., and Hultgren, H. N. Evaluation of therapeutic methods in high altitude pulmonary edema. *Am. J. Cardiol.* 43:307, 1979.
33. Meckstroth, G. R. Preparedness for radiation injuries: A guide to initial treatment. *E. R. Reports* 3:79, 1982.
34. Miller, J. W., Danzl, D. F., and Thomas, D. M. Urban accidental hypothermia: 135 cases. *Ann. Emerg. Med.* 9:456, 1980.
35. Modell, J. H. Biology of drowning. *Annu. Rev. Med.* 29:1, 1978.
36. Modell, J. H., and Davis, J. H. Electrolyte changes in human drowning victims. *Anesthesiology* 30:414, 1969.
37. Modell, J. H., Graves, S. A., and Ketover, A. Clinical course of 91 consecutive near-drowning victims. *Chest* 70:231, 1976.

38. National Council on Radiation Protection and Measurements. *Management of Persons Accidentally Contaminated with Radionuclides.* Washington D.C.: N.C.R.P. Report No. 65, 1979.
39. Oakes, D. D., et al. Prognosis and management of victims of near-drowning. *J. Trauma* 22:544, 1982.
40. O'Donnell, T. F., Jr., and Clowes, G. H., Jr. The circulatory abnormalities of heat stroke. *N. Engl. J. Med.* 287:734, 1972.
41. Reuler, J. B. Hypothermia: Pathophysiology, clinical settings, and management. *Ann. Intern. Med.* 89:519, 1978.
42. Reuler, J. B., and Parker, R. A. Peritoneal dialysis in the management of hypothermia. *J.A.M.A.* 240:2289, 1978.
43. Rivera, J. C. Decompression sickness among divers: An analysis of 935 cases. *Milit. Med.* 129:314, 1964.
44. Richter, L. L., et al. A systems approach to the management of radiation accidents. *Ann. Emerg. Med.* 9:303, 1980.
45. Shibolet, S., et al. Heatstroke: Its clinical picture and mechanism in 36 cases. *Q. J. Med.* 36:525, 1967.
46. Shibolet, S., Lancaster, M. C., and Danon, Y. Heat stroke: A review. *Aviat. Space Environ. Med.* 47:280, 1976.
47. Southwick, F. S., and Dalglish, P. H., Jr. Recovery after prolonged asystolic cardiac arrest in profound hypothermia: A case report and literature review. *J.A.M.A.* 243, 1250, 1980.
48. Sprung, C. L. Hemodynamic alterations of heat stroke in the elderly. *Chest* 75:362, 1979.
49. Sprung, C. L., et al. The metabolic and respiratory alterations of heat stroke. *Arch. Intern. Med.* 140:665, 1980.
50. Stine, R. J. Accidental hypothermia. *J.A.C.E.P.* 6:413, 1977.
51. Stine, R. J. Heat illness. *J.A.C.E.P.* 8:154, 1979.
52. Strauss, R. H. Diving medicine. *Am. Rev. Respir. Dis.* 119:1001, 1979.
53. *U.S. Navy Diving Manual* (NAVSHIPS 0994-001-9010). Washington, D.C.: Government Printing Office, 1973.
54. Whitcraft, D. D., and Karas, S. Air embolism and decompression sickness in scuba divers. *J.A.C.E.P.* 5:355, 1976.
55. White, J. D. Hypothermia: The Bellevue experience. *Ann. Emerg. Med.* 11:417, 1982.

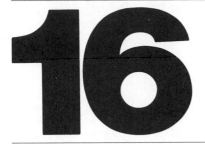

Toxicologic Emergencies

Robert J. Stine and
Robert H. Marcus

Drug Overdosage/Poisoning

Poisoning is a morbid condition produced by exposure to a toxic agent that by its chemical action causes damage to structure or disturbance of function. Drug overdosage refers to the state produced by an excess or abuse of a drug or substance. Poisoning connotes clinical symptomatology and generally implies that the toxic exposure was accidental or unknown to the recipient [49]. In contrast, drug overdosage generally infers an intentional toxic exposure. For simplicity, these terms shall be used interchangeably throughout this chapter. Accidental exposure to toxic agents commonly afflicts children; intentional overdoses, on the other hand, predominate in adults and have an associated higher mortality rate.

During the past three decades, major advances in the management of poisonings have occurred. These include adoption of the Scandinavian method stressing intensive supportive care in place of analeptic therapy [21], the advent of poison control centers and their active role in guiding therapy, and the use of dialytic measures. Primarily as a result of the first of these advances, the mortality for poisonings requiring hospitalization has declined from 20% to the current less than 1% [21, 115]. Severe overdoses, however, likely are associated with a higher mortality rate [115].

I. **Management principles.** The management of drug overdosage can be divided into seven phases. The actual order of these steps in patient management will vary depending on the clinical circumstances and the toxic agent(s) involved. Obviously, use of intensive supportive measures to stabilize the patient always takes precedence.

  A. **Clinical assessment** involves a thorough history and physical examination and pertinent laboratory tests.

   1. **Establishing the diagnosis.** Generally, the diagnosis of drug overdosage is evident from the history or the clinical presentation. The emergency physician, however, must maintain a high index of suspicion because the history may be unavailable or unreliable and the clinical features nonspecific. In particular, poisoning should be suspected in patients with psychiatric disturbances; patients with an altered mental status (including coma); trauma, near-drowning, and burn victims; young patients with arrhythmias; hypothermic patients; and patients with an unexplained metabolic acidosis. Conversely, the differential diagnosis of drug overdosage includes psychiatric disorders, meningitis and encephalitis, sepsis, metabolic disorders, head trauma, cerebrovascular accidents, hypertensive encephalopathy, hypo- and hyperthermia, and postictal states. In instances where the diagnosis of drug overdosage is uncertain, specimens of urine, gastric contents, and blood should be sent for toxicologic analysis, additional diagnostic maneuvers undertaken as indicated, and appropriate supportive therapy administered while awaiting confirmation of the diagnosis.

   2. **Identification of the toxic agent(s)** and determination of the extent of intoxication are essential, since such knowledge may influence therapy. Frequently, this information can be obtained from the history and clinical features. However, the history is notoriously unreliable [116], and the clinical findings may be obscured by multiple ingestions. Toxicologic analysis is useful in establishing the identity of the offending toxic agent(s) and in quantifying the severity of intoxication. However, since this information influences management only in certain situations, the use of toxicologic studies should be selective, that is, generally limited to serious and potentially life-threatening poisonings (particularly those presenting with a rapid onset of signs and symptoms) and those poisonings in which early specific treatment is required to prevent serious complications (e.g., acetaminophen, methanol, ethylene glycol, paraquat) [104]. For

Table 16-1. Radiopaque tablets

Acetazolamide	Methotrexate	Pyrvinium pamoate
Acetylsalicyclic acid	Metyrapone	Quadrinal
Amitriptyline HCl	Nystatin	Sodium chloride
Ammonium chloride	Pancreatin	Sodium salicylate
Busulfan	Penicillin G	Spironolactone
Chloral hydrate	Penicillin K	Trifluoperazine
Chlorpromazine HCl	Potassium chloride	Trihexyphenidyl
Chlorprothixene	Potassium iodide	Triiodothyronine
Ferrous sulphate	Potassium permanganate	Vitamins—multiple
Iopanoic acid	Prochlorperazine	Vitamins—prenatal
Methantheline bromide	Pseudoephedrine HCl	

Source: J. Greensher, H. C. Mofenson, and W. J. Gavin, The usefulness of abdominal x-rays in the diagnosis of poisoning. *Vet. Hum. Toxicol.* 21(Suppl.):45, 1979. With permission.

ingestions of solid agents, quantitative serum levels should be obtained 4 or more hours after the ingestion; otherwise, spurious low values may be obtained due to incomplete absorption of the agent. Supportive therapy, however, should not be delayed while awaiting drug identification.

3. **Ancillary measures.** It is important to determine whether there are concomitant (i.e., preexisting or drug-induced) conditions that will either affect the management of the poisoning or need specific treatment. In particular, the history, physical examination, and appropriate laboratory and radiologic tests should be directed at determining whether there is associated trauma (particularly head trauma) and assessing the status of the various body systems. Depending on the clinical situation, the following tests may be needed: a complete blood count (CBC); arterial blood gas (ABG); serum electrolytes, glucose, and creatinine; hepatic function tests; coagulation indices; urinalysis; electrocardiogram (ECG); chest x-ray; and other x-rays as indicated. An abdominal x-ray is useful in identifying radiopaque agents (Table 16-1), drug masses, and concretions and in following the course of intoxications with such agents [44].

B. **A knowledge of the toxic agent's pharmacology and pharmacokinetics** is essential in guiding management. Once the agent is identified, appropriate reference sources [49, 97] should be consulted for such information (and specific therapeutic measures). The regional **poison control center** is an invaluable source of vital information and should be readily contacted about any significant poisoning.

In addition to specific information pertinent to the involved toxic agent, a basic knowledge of pharmacology and pharmacokinetics is necessary for the rational management of drug overdosage. Excellent reviews [38, 49, 96] are available. However, a brief discussion of general principles is in order.

1. **Absorption of toxic agents** may occur through the gastrointestinal tract, skin, or respiratory tract. The gastrointestinal tract is the major site of absorption for most substances. The skin usually presents an effective barrier; however, certain highly lipid-soluble substances, such as organophosphate insecticides, are readily absorbed. Only gases and particles less than 1 μ in diameter are capable of being absorbed from the respiratory tract [49].

Since absorption from the gastrointestinal tract involves diffusion across lipid membranes of the epithelium, absorption occurs most readily with nonionized lipid-soluble substances. Because of the large surface area of the small intestine, that area is the primary site of absorption for most substances. Several factors affect the absorption of substances from the gastrointestinal tract [38, 49]. These include the following:

   a. **State of the substance.** Generally, liquids are better absorbed than solids, which require a certain degree of aqueous solubility for absorption.

   b. **Rate of gastric emptying.** Drugs that delay gastric emptying, such as the anticholinergics, tend to delay drug absorption.

   c. **Concentration of the agent** at the absorption site. A high concentration favors absorption, whereas the presence of food or binding substances tends to retard absorption.

      d. Intestinal motility. Drugs that impair intestinal motility, such as the anticholinergics, tend to enhance absorption from the small intestine; conversely, agents that increase intestinal motility (e.g., cathartics) may decrease absorption.

      e. Gastrointestinal blood flow. Shock states likely are associated with a decrease in drug absorption.

  2. Distribution of drugs within the body varies from drug to drug. Each drug has a definite distribution pattern that is established when drug concentrations in the various tissues are in equilibrium. The distribution pattern is affected by the following [38, 49].

      a. Blood flow to various organs. The early phase of drug distribution is determined primarily by the rate of blood flow to the various organs. Later, redistribution may occur from highly perfused organs, such as the brain, to more slowly perfused organs, such as adipose tissue and muscle.

      b. The relative partitioning between blood and tissues. Partitioning is determined largely by the agent's ability to cross capillary and cell membranes. Lipid-soluble drugs readily diffuse across these membranes. Thus, these drugs may readily distribute into the central nervous system (CNS) and other tissues, principally adipose tissue. Binding to plasma proteins, however, limits movement of drugs across capillary and cell membranes. Thus, protein-bound drugs are confined mainly to the plasma compartment. In drug overdosage, protein-binding sites may become saturated, resulting in an increased concentration of unbound drug that may distribute into the tissues. Since only nonionized agents can cross cell membranes, weak acids and bases distribute according to the relative pHs of blood and tissue fluids, becoming concentrated and trapped in the body fluids where they are more ionized. Later, redistribution from tissue or cellular reservoirs may occur in response to concentration gradients created by removal of the drug from the plasma.

      The **volume of distribution** is the apparent volume in which the drug is distributed. It is the volume the drug would occupy if distributed at the same concentration as measured in the plasma. Drugs that are sequestered in the plasma, such as highly protein-bound drugs, have a low volume of distribution, whereas drugs that are tissue-bound have large (i.e., >1 liter/kg) volume of distribution.

  3. Pharmacologic or toxicologic activity occurs when the drug becomes attached to specific tissue receptors. Since the drug generally must cross cell membranes to reach such receptors, only unbound (free) drug is the active moiety [49].

  4. Drug elimination involves the processes of metabolism and excretion. The liver with its enzyme systems is the principal organ of metabolism. Metabolites may be active or inactive. The kidneys serve as the major route for excretion of the parent drug and its metabolites. Some drugs and their metabolites are excreted into the bile and subsequently into the gastrointestinal tract, from which they may be resorbed (enterohepatic recirculation) or eliminated in the feces.

      a. Drug elimination may occur by **first-order or zero-order processes** [38, 49, 96]. Most drugs are eliminated by first-order kinetics, which are exponential processes in which a constant fraction or percentage of the drug is removed per unit time. In zero-order or linear processes, a constant amount of the drug is removed per unit time; this type of process is often associated with saturation of the metabolic mechanism(s) for drug elimination. Thus, a change from first-order kinetics to zero-order kinetics may occur when a drug that is normally eliminated by the former process has its metabolizing enzyme systems saturated, as may occur in overdosage.

      b. Measures of elimination

         (1) Clearance is the volume of plasma that can be cleared of the drug per unit time. Clearance involves both metabolic and excretory processes, and the total clearance is the sum of the various modalities of drug elimination.

         (2) The **half-life** is the time required to eliminate one-half of the drug from the body. The half-life is directly proportional to the volume of distribution and inversely proportional to the clearance [49]. For first-order processes, drug elimination is virtually complete in 5 half-lives [49].

C. Intensive supportive care is the mainstay of poison management. Such measures have been responsible for reducing the mortality associated with poisonings to the current less than 1% [115].

1. **Maintenance of ventilation**
   a. **Assessment of respiratory status.** The physical examination and, when indicated, chest x-ray and ABGs are important in assessing and monitoring the status of the respiratory system.
   b. **Establishing and maintaining a patent airway.** Initially, the standard airway maneuvers (see Chap. 2) should be performed as needed to open the airway. Intoxicated patients, if not tracheally intubated, should be placed in the left lateral decubitus and Trendelenburg positions to lessen the risk of aspiration. **Endotracheal intubation** by either the oral or nasal route is indicated in any patient with inadequate ventilation, loss of consciousness, impaired or absent gag reflex, or status epilepticus. For the lethargic or stuporous patient, clinical judgment will determine whether tracheal intubation is necessary. Loss of the lash reflex (i.e, involuntary blinking when the eyelash is gently stroked) is a useful sign indicating that endotracheal intubation should be attempted [92]. If there is doubt regarding the necessity for tracheal intubation, the emergency physician generally should attempt to insert an endotracheal tube. If the patient permits tracheal intubation, it was needed; if not, the patient likely does not require establishment of an artificial airway at that time. In the responsive, spontaneously breathing patient, the nasal route for tracheal intubation generally is preferred.
   c. **Respiratory insufficiency** is common in drug overdosage. Many drugs, particularly the opioids and sedative/hypnotics, cause respiratory depression with resultant hypercapnea and hypoxemia. In addition, certain drugs (e.g., opioids, salicylates, several sedative/hypnotics, certain hydrocarbons) can cause the adult respiratory distress syndrome (ARDS) secondary to damage to the alveolocapillary membrane. Respiratory insufficiency may also result from pulmonary aspiration. **Treatment** consists of administration of oxygen; a trial of naloxone hydrochloride, 0.4–2.0 mg IV, repeated as needed, in an attempt to reverse respiratory depression; institution of mechanical ventilation, including use of positive end-expiratory pressure (PEEP) as needed; vigorous pulmonary toilet; and careful fluid management.

2. **Maintenance of circulation**
   a. **Assessment of cardiovascular status.** The physical examination (particularly the vital signs) and ECG are important parameters to follow. In hemodynamically unstable patients, central venous or preferably Swan-Ganz catheterization should be performed.
   b. **Hypotension**
      (1) **Etiology.** Hypotension in overdoses may occur for various reasons [9].
         (a) Relative hypovolemia secondary to venous pooling.
         (b) Absolute hypovolemia resulting from vascular injury and fluid loss from the vascular compartment.
         (c) Peripheral vasodilatation secondary to drug-induced vascular relaxation, adrenergic receptor blockade, or depression of central vasomotor tone.
         (d) Myocardial depression due to direct drug effect, hypoxia, or acidosis.
         (e) Arrhythmias with inadequate cardiac output.
      (2) **Treatment** initially consists of correction of hypoxia, acidosis, and arrhythmias and **volume expansion** with normal saline, usually in increments of 200 ml up to 2 liters. In the absence of pulmonary edema, the Military Anti-Shock Trousers (MAST) suit may also be used. If these measures fail, hemodynamic monitoring (with central venous or preferably Swan-Ganz catheterization) should be instituted and a vasopressor administered. In most cases of drug overdose, **dopamine**, 2–50 μg/kg/minute, is the vasopressor of choice. However, in drug overdoses characterized by alpha-adrenergic receptor blockade (e.g., phenothiazine or tricyclic antidepressant overdoses), vasoactive drugs with predominantly alpha-adrenergic agonistic activity (i.e., norepinephrine or phenylephrine) are preferred.
   c. **Hypertension** due to drug overdosage is usually transient and usually does not require treatment. Sudden, marked, and sustained elevation of the blood pressure, however, may occur with overdoses of sympathomimetic drugs (e.g., amphetamines, cocaine, phencyclidine) and constitutes a hypertensive

urgency (see Chap. 6), especially in otherwise normotensive individuals. Useful therapeutic agents in such circumstances include **sodium nitroprusside**, sodium diazoxide, propranolol, and phentolamine.

    d. Arrhythmias in drug overdosage may occur as a result of autonomic and direct myocardial effects. Hypoxia, acid-base and electrolyte disturbances, and hypotension may be contributing factors and require correction. Specific **antiarrhythmic therapy**, if needed according to the clinical situation, should be guided by the toxic arrhythmogenic mechanism (Table 16-2).

    e. Cardiogenic pulmonary edema is uncommon in drug overdosage. When it occurs, it is usually the result of fluid overload in a patient with limited cardiac reserve. Drug-induced myocardial depression, increased peripheral vascular resistance (afterload), and arrhythmias may be contributing factors. Treatment is the same as that presented in Chap. 5.

3. Central nervous system depression is a common feature of many overdoses, particularly of the sedative/hypnotics and opioids. Staging (Table 16-3) is of some prognostic significance; stage IV coma appears to be associated with higher morbidity and mortality [115]. Initial **therapeutic endeavors** should be directed at establishing a protected airway (see sec. **I.C.1.b**) and achieving adequate oxygenation. In addition, any patient with a depressed level of consciousness requires either immediate determination of the blood glucose (with Dextrostix) or administration of 25 gm of 50% **dextrose**. A trial of **naloxone hydrochloride**, 0.4–2.0 mg IV, repeated as needed, should be attempted in an effort to reverse the CNS depressant effects of possible opioid overdosage. Although supportive care is the mainstay of management, hemoperfusion or hemodialysis generally is indicated in treating stage IV overdosage. Analeptic agents are contraindicated, since they have been associated with an increase in mortality.

4. Seizures (Table 16-4) may complicate poisonings. An isolated seizure or two requires no treatment other than correction of hypoxia, electrolyte disturbances, and metabolic disorders, if present. Sustained or repetitive seizures, however, require anticonvulsant therapy (see Chap. 32). **Diazepam** in repetitive doses of 2.5–5.0 mg IV as needed to a maximum of 30 mg (with appropriate airway management) is the anticonvulsant of choice for terminating drug-induced seizures. Persistent or recurrent seizure activity, however, requires the administration of phenytoin, 18 mg/kg IV, or phenobarbital, 15 mg/kg IV. The former is preferred because of its lesser CNS depressant effects, but the latter may be more effective in certain overdoses. The choice should be based on the toxic agent involved. If this therapy is unsuccessful, paraldehyde or general anesthesia is required, and hemoperfusion or hemodialysis generally is indicated, when applicable.

5. Acidosis, not uncommon in poisonings, may be either respiratory, metabolic (Table 16-5), or a combination of both. **Treatment** of respiratory acidosis includes establishing an airway, reversing respiratory depression with naloxone hydrochloride (if opioid overdosage), and assisting ventilation as needed. For metabolic acidosis, correcting hypotension and hypoxia, terminating seizures and muscle hyperactivity, and administering sodium bicarbonate IV (if pH < 7.2) as needed are appropriate therapeutic measures. For severe metabolic acidosis unresponsive to bicarbonate therapy, hemodialysis generally is indicated.

6. Thermal derangements may complicate drug overdosage. **Treatment** of hyperpyrexia, usually associated with sympathomimetic or anticholinergic overdoses, includes terminating seizures and hypermotor activity (the latter may require paralysis with pancuronium bromide) and cooling with ice-water sponge baths or submersion in an ice-water bath depending on the severity of hyperpyrexia (see Chap. 15). Hypothermia, common to sedative/hypnotic overdoses, usually can be managed with passive rewarming (see Chap. 15).

D. Prevention of drug absorption. Active measures to prevent absorption of toxic agents are of paramount importance to lessen the severity of intoxication.

    1. Skin and eye decontamination. Lipid-soluble substances, particularly the organophosphate and carbamate insecticides, may be absorbed through the skin; they require immediate removal. Contaminated clothing should be removed carefully, so as not to contaminate medical personnel, and sealed in plastic bags. The skin should then be thoroughly washed with soap and water to remove the toxic agent. Eye contaminants (particularly caustic agents) and caustic skin

Table 16-2. Management of drug-related arrhythmias[a]

Mechanism	Drugs	Arrhythmias[b]	Treatment[c]
Sympathetic stimulation	Amphetamines, caffeine, cannabis agents, chloral hydrate, cocaine, ethanol, fluorocarbons, hydrocarbon solvents, LSD (and related hallucinogens), monoamine oxidase inhibitors, phencyclidine, phenylpropranolamine (and other sympathomimetics), sedative drug abstinence, theophylline	Sinus tachycardia Atrial tachycardia Atrial fibrillation/flutter Ventricular arrhythmias	None, propranolol Verapamil, propranolol, DC cardioversion Propranolol, verapamil, digitalis, pace termination (atrial flutter), DC cardioversion Lidocaine, propranolol, bretylium, DC cardioversion/defibrillation
Sympathetic inhibition	Clonidine, guanethidine, methyldopa, propranolol (beta-blockers), reserpine	Bradyarrhythmias (including atrioventricular block)[d]	None, atropine, isoproterenol, glucagon (particularly with beta-blocker overdosage), cardiac pacing
Cholinergic stimulation	Bethanechol, carbamates, neostigmine, nicotine, organophosphates, physostigmine, pilocarpine, pyridostigmine	Bradyarrhythmias (including atrioventricular block)[d,e]	None, atropine, cardiac pacing
Anticholinergic effect	Antihistamines, antipsychotics, antispasmodics, belladonna alkaloids, plants (Jimson weed, mushrooms), tricyclic antidepressants	Sinus tachycardia Atrial tachycardia Ventricular arrhythmias	None, physostigmine, propranolol Physostigmine, verapamil, propranolol, DC cardioversion Lidocaine, phenytoin, bretylium, DC cardioversion/defibrillation
Membrane depression	Disopyramide, phenothiazines (and related antipsychotics), procainamide, propranolol (membrane-depressant beta-blockers), quinidine, tricyclic antidepressants	Bradyarrhythmias (including atrioventricular block)[d,f] Ventricular arrhythmias	None, isoproterenol, cardiac pacing Lidocaine, phenytoin, isoproterenol (with prolonged QT only), bretylium, overdrive pacing, DC cardioversion/defibrillation

[a]This table is only a guide. The need for and choice of a particular antiarrhythmic agent should be based on the clinical situation and the toxic mechanism involved, respectively.

[b]Ventricular arrhythmias secondary to myocardial ischemia may occur in patients with underlying coronary artery disease; treatment is the same as that employed in the setting of acute myocardial ischemia, except that antiarrhythmic agents with effects similar to those of the toxic agent are to be avoided.

[c]Correction of hypoxia, hypotension, and acid-base and electrolyte disturbances is required.

[d]Ventricular escape rhythms may occur; treatment is to increase the basic rate, as described.

[e]Sinus tachycardia may be an early manifestation secondary to ganglionic stimulation; usually no treatment is required.

[f]Sinus tachycardia may result from a vagolytic effect, reflex sympathetic stimulation, or associated anticholinergic activity; propranolol is the drug of choice if treatment is required.

Source: Adapted from N. L. Benowitz and N. Goldschlager, Cardiac Disturbances in the Toxicologic Patient. In L. M. Haddad and J. F. Winchester (eds.), *Clinical Management of Poisoning and Drug Overdose.* Philadelphia: Saunders, 1983.

Table 16-3. Staging of CNS depression

Stage 0	Asleep Arousable
Stage I	Comatose Withdrawal from painful stimuli
Stage II	Comatose No withdrawal from painful stimuli Most reflexes intact
Stage III	Comatose Most reflexes absent No respiratory or circulatory depression
Stage IV	Comatose Most reflexes absent Respiratory and/or circulatory failure

Source: Adapted from C. E. Reed, M. F. Driggs, and C. C. Foote, Acute barbiturate intoxication: A study of 300 cases based on a physiologic system of classification of the severity of the intoxication. *Ann Intern. Med.* 37:290, 1952.

Table 16-4. Poisonings associated with seizures*

Amphetamines	Hypoglycemic agents	Phencyclidine
Antihistamines	Isoniazid	Phenol
Beta-blockers	Jimson weed	Phenothiazines
Caffeine	Lead	Propoxyphene
Camphor	Lithium	Salicylates
Carbon monoxide	Methanol	Strychnine
Cocaine	Methaqualone	Theophylline
Cyanide	Monoamine oxidase inhibitors	Toxic mushrooms
Ethylene glycol	Opioids	Tricyclic antidepressants
Hydrocarbons	Organophosphates	Venomous snakes

*Seizures may also result from drug-induced metabolic and electrolyte disturbances (e.g., hypoxia, hypoglycemia) and sedative/hypnotic withdrawal.

Table 16-5. Poisonings commonly associated with a metabolic acidosis

Amonium chloride	Ethylene glycol	Isoniazid	Phenol
Carbon monoxide	Formaldehyde	Isopropyl alcohol	Salicylates
Carbon tetrachloride	Hydrogen sulfide	Methanol	Strychnine
Cyanide	Iron	Paraldehyde	Toluene
Ethanol			

contaminants should be removed immediately by irrigating with saline or water for 20–30 minutes.

2. **Prevention of drug absorption from the gastrointestinal tract**
    a. **Gastric emptying** can be achieved by induced emesis (with syrup of ipecac) or gastric lavage. Although controversial, it appears that induced emesis is slightly more effective than gastric lavage [29, 74]. The effectiveness of each procedure, however, decreases with increasing time lapse, with generally less than one-third of the ingestant being recovered 1 hour after ingestion [29, 74]. Since the history is often unreliable and many drugs delay gastric emptying, induced emesis or gastric lavage should be performed in all significant overdoses regardless of the time interval since ingestion, unless the procedure is contraindicated (see sec. **I.D.2.a.(1)–(2)**). Gastric emptying should also be undertaken even if the patient has spontaneously vomited,

since studies have shown that spontaneous emesis is associated with ineffective removal of the ingestant [29].

(1) Induced emesis is the preferred means of emptying the stomach in awake and fully responsive patients. The method of choice involves the administration of **syrup of ipecac**, 30 ml PO, followed by at least 16 oz of water, which facilitates vomiting and drug removal. Syrup of ipecac is a highly effective emetic agent whose emetic action is primarily mediated by stimulation of the medullary chemoreceptor trigger zone, but direct gastric irritation may also play a role. It is more than 90% effective in producing emesis within 30 minutes and is even effective in inducing emesis in antiemetic overdoses [29, 74]. However, if emesis does not occur within 20–30 minutes of administration of ipecac, the dose may be repeated. If there still is no response, gastric lavage is indicated to remove the ingested agent(s). Syrup of ipecac is essentially nontoxic in therapeutic doses and does not have to be removed if emesis does not ensue [29, 74, 91].

Apomorphine, on the other hand, although a very effective emetic agent, has significant toxic side effects, notably CNS depression, respiratory depression, and hypotension, that surprisingly may not be reversed by naloxone hydrochloride [101]. Its use is not recommended. Mechanical stimulation of the posterior pharynx, by itself, is not an effective means of producing emesis with sufficient volumes of vomitus; it should not be relied on [74].

Contraindications to inducing emesis include CNS depression, an impaired gag reflex, status epilepticus, caustic ingestions, and ingestions of certain hydrocarbons.

(2) Gastric lavage is a useful means of gastric emptying. In particular, it is indicated for drug removal in patients with a depressed level of consciousness or impaired gag reflex after the airway has been protected as needed by either proper positioning of the patient or insertion of a cuffed endotracheal tube (see sec. **I.C.1.b**). Patients with mild CNS depression but an intact gag reflex may be lavaged in the left lateral decubitus position with the head down. Patients with more severe CNS depression or loss of the gag reflex, however, require airway protection with a cuffed naso- or orotracheal tube. The gastric tube must be large-bore, at least 28 F and preferably 36 F, to remove ingested pills. The tube may be inserted by the nasal or oral route, but preferably by the oral route, especially if a 36-F tube is used. The preferred lavage solution is isotonic saline, but tap water is satisfactory. For certain overdoses, lavage with neutralizing solutions (e.g., sodium bicarbonate or potassium permanganate in iron or strychnine poisoning, respectively) is indicated. Use of warm lavage fluids and external massage of the epigastrium may augment the removal of pills [72]. From 100–400 ml (300 ml is ideal) of lavage fluid should be instilled at any one time before withdrawing fluid. Smaller or larger volumes may lead to ineffective removal or loss of the ingested agent(s) into the duodenum, respectively. Lavage is continued until the return is clear.

Contraindications to gastric lavage include CNS depression, an impaired gag reflex, status epilepticus, and hydrocarbon ingestions, unless the airway is properly protected (see above) to prevent aspiration. In addition, gastric lavage is contraindicated in caustic ingestions, with the possible exception of acid ingestions of less than 90 minutes' duration.

b. Activated charcoal is a fine powder composed of small particles that present a large surface area capable of adsorbing and nearly irreversibly binding a wide variety of substances. Since activated charcoal is not absorbed from the gastrointestinal tract, substances bound to the activated charcoal are retained within the gastrointestinal tract and prevented from being absorbed. Activated charcoal clearly has been demonstrated to decrease effectively the gastrointestinal absorption of many toxic agents [29, 45]. Exceptions include alkalis, cyanide, ferrous sulfate, and mineral acids [45]. Except for these substances, activated charcoal is indicated for all significant toxic ingestions. The dosage is 50–100 gm (or 10 times the amount of the ingested drug), administered orally or through a gastric tube as a slurry in approximately 8 oz of water. The effectiveness of this procedure is enhanced by early administration of the activated charcoal. Additives to increase the palatability of the charcoal appear to decrease its effectiveness and should be avoided, if possible [29]. Although unproved, concomitant administration of a cathartic may also decrease the effectiveness of the charcoal [69]. Since activated charcoal is an inert and nontoxic substance, there are no contraindications to its use. However, since activated charcoal effectively adsorbs and binds ipecac and orally administered antidotes, it should not be administered until after emesis has been induced and should be avoided if an oral antidote is required. Current practice in potentially toxic ingestions is to administer activated charcoal (often with a cathartic) following gastric emptying, unless it is not indicated or should be avoided (see above). However, because of the efficacy of activated charcoal in preventing gastrointestinal absorption of most drugs, its use may obviate in the future (when more data is available) the need for gastric emptying in many overdose situations [64a].

    c. A **cathartic** generally is administered either with or following administration of activated charcoal, with the rationale that by decreasing the intestinal transit time, absorption of an ingested toxic agent will be diminished. The efficacy of catharsis, however, has never been demonstrated [29, 94]. Suitable agents, administered orally or by gastric tube, include magnesium citrate, 5–10 oz; 70% sorbitol, 50–150 ml; and magnesium or sodium sulfate, 15–30 gm. Oil-based cathartics (e.g., mineral oil, castor oil) are contraindicated because of the risk of lipoid pneumonia if aspiration occurs. Although gastrointestinal absorption of cathartics is low, magnesium- and sodium-containing cathartics should be avoided in patients with renal failure (or at risk of developing renal failure) and congestive heart failure, respectively. Cathartics also should not be used in patients who have undergone recent bowel surgery, require the administration of an oral antidote, have a severe ileus or gastrointestinal bleeding, or ingested a corrosive agent or an agent with severe gastrointestinal toxicity.

E. Administration of an antidote. An antidote is an agent that prevents or counteracts the toxic effects of a poison. Each antidote has a specific mechanism of action (e.g., chelation, competitive inhibition at receptor sites) that varies from antidote to antidote. Antidotes are invaluable in treating specific poisonings. Unfortunately, there are very few available antidotes (Table 16-6). Since administration of an antidote is not necessarily benign, the decision to use a specific antidote should carefully weigh the benefits versus the risks. Generally, an antidote is indicated in specific poisonings as a diagnostic maneuver (e.g., naloxone hydrochloride in suspected opioid overdosage) or to prevent or reverse significant toxic effects.

F. Removal of absorbed substances. The method chosen, if any, to enhance elimination of an absorbed toxic agent from the body will depend on the pharmacology of the toxic agent involved, its toxicity, and the severity of intoxication.

    1. **Forced diuresis** may be useful in treating poisonings when the active agent (either parent drug or metabolites) is distributed largely to the extracellular fluid compartment, is minimally protein-bound, and has as a major mode of elimination renal excretion [49]. However, with rare exceptions (e.g., bromides), forced diuresis by itself is of limited usefulness; but, for weak acids and bases satisfying the above-mentioned criteria, when combined with altering the urinary pH to increase the ionized fraction of the drug in the urine thereby decreasing its renal tubular resorption (by ion trapping), forced diuresis may play a significant role in enhancing drug elimination. Because of the risk of causing acid-base and electrolyte disturbances and pulmonary and cerebral edema, forced diuresis should not be used unless specifically indicated. The urinary output and pH, serum electrolytes and pH, and the patient's fluid status must be carefully monitored. **Contraindications** to the procedure include cardiac disease, renal insufficiency, hypokalemia, ARDS, and cerebral edema.

    a. **Forced alkaline diuresis** is effective in enhancing elimination of certain weak acids (e.g., barbital, phenobarbital, salicylates). Urinary alkalinization usually can be achieved by administering sodium bicarbonate, 1 mEq/kg IV, as needed. Diuresis is accomplished by administering saline IV in combination with a diuretic (furosemide, 10–20 mg IV, or mannitol, 12.5–25 gm IV) as needed. A useful technique is to add 1–2 ampules of sodium bicarbonate to a liter of 0.45% saline and administer the solution at a rate of 250–500 ml/hour. Potassium should be given as needed. The goal of this therapy is to achieve a urinary flow of 3–6 ml/kg/hour and a pH of 7.5–9.0.

Table 16-6. Antidotes

Poison/toxic sign	Antidote	Adult dosage
Acetaminophen	N-Acetylcysteine	140 mg/kg PO, followed by 70 mg/kg q4h × 17 doses
Anticholinergics	Physostigmine salicylate	0.5–2 mg IV (IM) over 2 min q30–60min prn
Anticholinesterases	Atropine sulfate	1–5 mg IV (IM, SQ) q15min prn
	Pralidoxime (2-PAM) chloride[a]	1 gm IV (PO) over 15–30 min q8–12h × 3 doses prn
Carbon monoxide	Oxygen	100%, hyperbaric
Cyanide	Amyl nitrite[b]	Inhalation pearls for 15–30 sec qmin
	Sodium nitrite[b]	300 mg (10 ml of 3% solution) IV over 3 min, repeated in half dosage in 2 hr if persistent or recurrent signs of toxicity
	Sodium thiosulfate	12.5 gm (50 ml of a 25% solution) IV over 10 min, repeated in half dosage in 2 hr if persistent or recurrent signs of toxicity
Ethylene glycol	Ethanol	0.6 gm/kg of ethanol in 5% D/W IV (PO) over 30–45 min, followed initially by 110 mg/kg/hr to maintain a blood level of 100–150 mg/dl
Extrapyramidal signs	Diphenhydramine hydrochloride	25–50 mg IV (IM, PO) prn
	Benztropine mesylate	1–2 mg IV (IM, PO) prn
Heavy metals (e.g., arsenic, copper, gold, lead, mercury)	Chelator[c] Calcium disodium edetate (EDTA)	1 gm IV (IM) over 1 hr q12h
	Dimercaprol (BAL)	2.5–5 mg/kg IM q4–6h
	Penicillamine	250–500 mg PO q6h
Iron	Deferoxamine mesylate	1 gm IM (IV at a rate ≤15 mg/kg/hr if hypotension) q8h prn
Methanol	Ethanol	See Ethylene glycol
Methemoglobinemia	Methylene blue	1–2 mg/kg (0.1–0.2 ml/kg of 1% solution) IV over 5 min, repeated in 1 hr prn
Opioids	Naloxone hydrochloride	0.4–2 mg IV (IM, SQ, endotracheally) prn

[a]Pralidoxime is indicated in severe organophosphate poisoning with muscle weakness or fasciculations or respiratory depression.
[b]Nitrites probably have an antidotal effect in hydrogen sulfide poisoning.
[c]The use of a specific chelating agent or combination of agents will depend on the heavy metal involved and on the clinical situation.
Note: This table is only a guide. Antidote usage and dosage will depend on the specific clinical situation. The regional poison control center should be contacted for specific therapeutic recommendations.
Source: R. J. Stine and R. H. Marcus, Medical Emergencies. In M. J. Orland and R. J. Saltman (eds.), *Manual of Medical Therapeutics* (25th ed.). Boston: Little, Brown, 1986. With permission.

   b. Forced acid diuresis is of benefit in increasing the renal excretion of certain
      weak bases (e.g., amphetamines, phencyclidine, quinine). The technique in-
      volves administering saline IV; a diuretic (furosemide or mannitol); and
      ascorbic acid, 1–2 gm IV or PO q4h, and/or ammonium chloride, 1–2 gm IV
      or PO q6h, as needed. Ammonium chloride is more effective but also more
      toxic. The desired end point is a urinary output of 3–6 ml/kg/hour and a pH
      of 4.5–6.0.
 2. Extracorporeal removal of certain drugs and toxins may be achieved by dialy-
      sis or hemoperfusion (Table 16-7). For these procedures to be effective, the drug
      or toxin must be distributed in the plasma or be able to equilibrate readily with
      plasma, not be tissue-bound to any significant extent (i.e., have a relatively
      small volume of distribution), and have a low intrinsic body clearance so that
      the procedure can significantly enhance its elimination [115]. For dialysis to be
      effective, the substance must also be capable of diffusing from the blood across a
      semipermeable membrane (synthetic material or peritoneum) into a dialysate
      solution at a sufficient rate to yield a significant rate of removal from the
      plasma; this requires that the substance be relatively water-soluble, have a
      relatively low molecular weight, and be minimally bound to plasma proteins.
      On the other hand, the technique of hemoperfusion, which effects drug removal
      through adsorption to the large surface area of a sorbent material (either ac-
      tivated charcoal or a polystyrene Amberlite resin) as anticoagulated blood is
      passed through a column of such material, is not limited by a high molecular
      weight, water insolubility, or plasma protein binding of the substance [89].
   a. Indications for use. The decision to use dialysis or hemoperfusion in treat-
      ing poisonings must be individualized. The decision should be based on the
      agent involved, its toxicity, the plasma concentration of the substance, the
      clinical status of the patient, and the procedure's ability to enhance removal
      of the substance (Table 16-8). Although controversial [65], dialysis or
      hemoperfusion generally is considered to be indicated in the management of
      life-threatening poisonings due to dialyzable or hemoperfusable agents, re-
      spectively.
   b. Selection of method. Hemodialysis is more effective than peritoneal dialy-
      sis and is preferred when dialysis is indicated. However, hemoperfusion
      is generally more effective than hemodialysis in terms of drug clearances
      and plasma extraction ratios [49]. Hemodialysis, however, has the advan-
      tage of correcting acid-base, electrolyte, and osmolar disturbances. The
      choice between hemodialysis and hemoperfusion should be based on the
      relative effectiveness of the procedures in removing the involved agent and
      whether there are associated acid-base and electrolyte disturbances that
      require correction. Generally, when indicated, hemodialysis is preferred for
      intoxications with bromides, ethanol, ethylene glycol, lithium, methanol,
      and salicylates; and hemoperfusion, for overdoses with the barbiturates,
      other sedative/hypnotics, and lipid-soluble drugs [49]. Hemoperfusion may
      be performed using either an activated charcoal or polystyrene Amberlite
      resin column. The former is capable of removing both polar and nonpolar
      substances; the latter, however, is limited to binding nonpolar (lipid-soluble)
      drugs but is superior to activated charcoal in removing these drugs [89].
 3. Activated charcoal in repetitive doses of 20 gm PO q6h or 30 gm PO q2h has
      been demonstrated to increase the clearance from the body of phenobarbital [10]
      and theophylline [67], respectively. Presumably, the activated charcoal, by
      binding the drug in the gastrointestinal tract, creates a concentration gradient
      across the bowel wall, resulting in a net efflux of the drug from the blood into
      the bowel, where it is bound by the activated charcoal and then excreted [10].
      This procedure may be useful in enhancing the clearance from the body of other
      drugs, particularly those that undergo enterohepatic recirculation (e.g., tricyclic
      antidepressants, glutethimide).
 4. Exchange blood transfusion and plasmapheresis (plasma exchange) can remove
      drugs or toxins that are distributed mainly to the circulatory compartment.
      Since these procedures have been used infrequently in managing poisonings
      (e.g., exchange blood transfusion to treat severe methemoglobinemia), their role
      remains to be defined [49]. They appear, however, to be of limited use in treat-
      ing poisonings.
G. Disposition of poisoned patients depends on the following: the circumstances surrounding the poisoning, the toxicity of the involved agent(s), the clinical status of

Table 16-7. Substances removed by hemodialysis or hemoperfusion[a]

Hemodialyzable

Acetaminophen	Cyclophosphamide	Methaqualone[b]
Aluminum	Cycloserine	Methotrexate[b]
Amanita toxins[b]	Demeton	Methyldopa
Amikacin	Diazoxide[b]	Methylprednisolone[b]
Ammonia	Dimethoate	Methyprylon
Amobarbital	Diquat[b]	Metronidazole
Amoxicillin	Disopyramide	Monoamine oxidase
Amphetamines	Ethambutol	inhibitors[b]
Ampicillin	Ethanol	Neomycin
Aniline	Ethchlorvynol	Nitrofurantoin
Arsenic (arsine)	Ethinamate	Ouabain[b]
Azathioprine	Ethylene glycol	Paraquat[b]
Barbital	Flucytosine	Penicillin
Borate	Fluoride	Phenobarbital
Bromide (carbromal)	5-Fluorouracil	Phosphate
Butabarbital[b]	Fosfomycin	Potassium
Calcium	Gallamine	Primidone
Camphor	Gentamicin	Procainamide
Carbenicillin	Glutethimide[b]	Quinidine[b]
Carbon tetrachloride[b]	Hydrogen ions	Quinine[b]
Cephalosporins (most)	Iodide[b]	Salicylates
Chloral hydrate	Iron deferoxamine[b]	Sodium
(trichloroethanol)	Isoniazid	Streptomycin
Chloramphenicol	Isopropyl alcohol	Strontium[b]
Chlorate[b]	Kanamycin	Sulfonamides
Chloride	Lactate	Theophylline
Chromate[b]	Lead edetate[b]	Thiocyanate
Cimetidine	Lithium	Ticarcillin
Cisplatin[b]	Magnesium	Tobramycin
Citrate	Mannitol	Trichloroethylene[b]
Colistin[b]	Meprobamate	Urea
Creatinine	Methanol	Uric acid
Cyclobarbital[b]		Water

Hemoperfusable

Acetaminophen	Digoxin[b]	Parathion
Amanita toxins[b]	Dimethoate	Pentobarbital
Ammonia[b]	Diquat	Phenobarbital
Amobarbital	Disopyramide	Phenytoin
Barbital	Ethanol	Procainamide[b]
Bromide (carbromal)	Ethchlorvynol	Quinalbital
Butabarbital	Glutethimide	Quinidine[b]
Camphor	Heptabarbital	Salicylates
Carbon tetrachloride[b]	Meprobamate	Secobarbital
Chloral hydrate	Methaqualone	Theophylline
(trichloroethanol)	Methotrexate	Thyroxine
Chloroquine[b]	Methyprylon	Tricyclic antidepressants[b]
Creatinine	Nitrostigmine	Triiodothyronine
Cyclobarbital	Paraquat	Uric acid
Demeton		

[a]This table is only a guide. The need for hemodialysis or hemoperfusion should be based on the toxicity of the substance, the effectiveness of the procedure, and the clinical state.
[b]Possibly removed (but insufficient data).
Source: Adapted from J. R. Winchester et al., Dialysis and hemoperfusion of poisons and drugs—update. *Trans. Am. Soc. Artif. Intern. Organs* 23:762, 1977; W. M. Bennett et al., Drug therapy in renal failure: Dosing guidelines for adults. *Ann. Intern. Med.* 93:62, 286, 1980; and L. M. Haddad and J. F. Winchester (eds.), *Clinical Management of Poisoning and Drug Overdose.* Philadelphia: Saunders, 1983.

Table 16-8. Clinical considerations for extracorporeal drug removal

1. Intoxication with an extractable drug or poison that can be removed at a rate exceeding endogenous elimination.
2. Progressive deterioration despite intensive supportive therapy.
3. Severe intoxication with depression of midbrain function, characterized by respiratory and/or circulatory failure (stage IV coma).
4. Significant intoxication with agents with severe metabolic and/or delayed toxic effects (e.g., *Amanita phalloides*, ethylene glycol, methanol, paraquat).
5. Development of serious complications of coma (e.g., pneumonia) and/or the presence of significant underlying conditions (e.g., chronic obstructive pulmonary disease) predisposing to such complications.
6. Potentially lethal plasma drug concentration (e.g., ethylene glycol: >50 mg/dl; lithium: >4 mEq/liter; methanol: >50 mg/dl; salicylate: >100 mg/dl).
7. Significant intoxication complicated by impairment of endogenous drug elimination secondary to hepatic and/or renal insufficiency.

Source: Adapted from J. F. Winchester, Active Methods for Detoxification: Oral Sorbents, Forced Diuresis, Hemoperfusion, and Hemodialysis. In L. M. Haddad and J. F. Winchester (eds.), *Clinical Management of Poisoning and Drug Overdose.* Philadelphia: Saunders, 1983.

the patient, and the ability to observe the patient in the emergency department. For a few overdoses (e.g., acetaminophen, salicylates), quantitative blood levels may assist in determining the appropriate disposition. General guidelines regarding disposition are as follows:

1. For apparently **minor overdoses,** characterized by exposure to low doses of relatively nontoxic agents and by little or no signs of toxicity, observation in the emergency department for at least 4–6 hours, if possible, generally is warranted to determine whether more serious signs of toxicity will develop. When patients are determined to be essentially free from toxic effects, not at significant risk of developing delayed toxic manifestations, and not dangerous to themselves or others, they may be discharged home from the emergency department with appropriate arrangements for follow-up. Patients with intentional overdoses (but not possessing suicide ideation) should be referred for psychiatric evaluation, and patients with substance abuse generally should be referred for psychiatric or drug abuse counseling.

2. For **significant poisonings** characterized by exposure to particularly toxic agents or dosages or by the presence of more than minor toxic manifestations, hospitalization on a medical service is indicated. Patients requiring monitoring, intensive nursing care, or respiratory or cardiovascular support should be admitted to an intensive care unit.

3. For **patients judged to be a danger to themselves or others,** psychiatric hospitalization is necessary; but if ongoing medical attention is needed, medical admission and subsequent transfer to a psychiatric facility following resolution of drug toxicity are indicated.

II. **Specific overdoses/poisonings**
A. **Acetaminophen** is a common ingredient in many analgesic and antipyretic preparations. Chronic use of acetaminophen generally is not associated with toxicity, but an acute overdosage of more than 140 mg/kg (or 10 gm in a 70-kg adult) may lead to serious hepatotoxicity [87]. Rarely, cardiac or renal toxicity also occurs.
1. **Mechanism of toxicity.** Under normal conditions, most acetaminophen is metabolized in the liver to nontoxic sulfate and glucuronide compounds that are excreted in the urine; and a small fraction of acetaminophen is metabolized by the hepatic cytochrome P-450 mixed-function oxidase pathway to a toxic reactive intermediate, which is detoxified by conjugation with hepatic glutathione to form a mercapturate metabolite that is excreted in the urine [87]. In overdosage, hepatic glutathione stores become depleted; consequently, the reactive intermediate accumulates and becomes covalently bound to hepatic cellular protein macromolecules, resulting in hepatocellular necrosis [87].
2. The **clinical course** of acetaminophen overdosage involves four stages [99]. During the first 24 hours postingestion, patients may experience gastrointestinal symptoms (e.g., anorexia, nausea, vomiting), malaise, and diaphoresis. Dur-

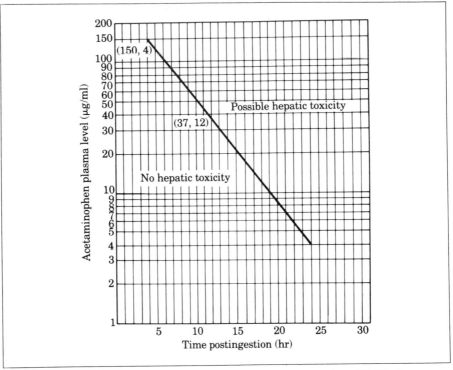

Fig. 16-1. Nomogram for acetaminophen toxicity. (From B. H. Rumack and H. Matthew, Acetaminophen poisoning and toxicity. *Pediatrics* 55:871, 1975. Reproduced by permission of *Pediatrics*, copyright 1975.

ing the next 24 hours, patients are clinically improved, but abnormal hepatic function tests appear. Peak hepatotoxicity generally occurs from 72–96 hours postingestion and is followed by recovery in 7–8 days or death from hepatic failure.

3. Management

a. **Gastric emptying** by gastric lavage or induced emesis with ipecac should be undertaken. Activated charcoal and a cathartic should be avoided, since they impair absorption of the antidote. However, if there is coingestion of another toxic agent, activated charcoal should be administered (following gastric emptying) and later removed by gastric lavage prior to administration of the antidote.

b. The **risk of hepatic toxicity** should be determined by plotting a plasma acetaminophen level obtained 4 or more hours postingestion versus time on the nomogram (Fig. 16-1). A level drawn less than 4 hours postingestion may yield a spurious low value due to incomplete absorption. A plasma acetaminophen level in the potentially toxic range is an indication for antidotal therapy.

c. **N-acetylcysteine (Mucomyst),** presumably by acting as a glutathione substitute or precursor, has been demonstrated to be an effective antidote in acetaminophen overdosage [99]. It is indicated for potentially toxic acetaminophen ingestion (as determined from the nomogram). Therapy with *N*-acetylcysteine is more effective the earlier it is started. For best results, therapy should be initiated within 16 hours of a potentially toxic ingestion but is indicated up to 24 hours postingestion [99]. If the result of the plasma acetaminophen level can be readily obtained, antidotal therapy can be withheld pending receipt of the level; otherwise, it is best to initiate therapy while awaiting the result of the acetaminophen level. If the plasma level returns in the potentially toxic range, antidotal therapy must be continued; if the level is nontoxic, antidotal therapy is discontinued.

The dosage of *N*-acetylcysteine is 140 mg/kg as an initial dose, followed by 70 mg/kg q4h for 17 doses, given PO or by gastric tube as a 5% solution in water or, preferably, a cola beverage. If emesis occurs within 1 hour of administration of a dose, the dose should be repeated.

   d. Although effective in removing acetaminophen from the body, hemoperfusion or hemodialysis is not indicated. Effective treatment of acetaminophen overdosage is early administration of the antidote.

   4. Disposition. Hospitalization, a complete course of antidotal therapy, and monitoring of hepatic function tests are indicated if the plasma acetaminophen level is in the potentially toxic range. If the level is nontoxic, the patient may be discharged from the emergency department (unless psychiatric admission is warranted).

B. Amphetamines include amphetamine sulfate (Benzedrine), dextroamphetamine (Dexedrine), and methamphetamine (Methedrine). Ingestion of 20–25 mg/kg in adults is potentially lethal, although death has been reported with smaller doses [49, 115]. Blood levels vary widely in fatal intoxication and correlate poorly with the clinical status. Chronic users may take potentially lethal doses without serious side effects due to development of tolerance to amphetamines; as a result, most cases of fatal intoxication occur in relatively recent users.

   1. Pathophysiologic mechanism. Amphetamines are sympathetic stimulants that function via norepinephrine- and dopamine-mediated systems by release of catecholamines stored in neurons, direct stimulation of postsynaptic adrenergic receptors, and possible inhibition of monoamine oxidase (the enzyme responsible for the degradation of catecholamines). Amphetamines are weak bases with a pK_a of about 9.9. They are metabolized in the liver, and active metabolites as well as free amphetamines are excreted by the kidneys.

   2. Clinical features are related to the adrenergic effect of amphetamines.

   a. Minor toxic manifestations include tachypnea, tachycardia, mild hypertension, mild hyperpyrexia, dry mouth, dizziness, chest pain, palpitations, abdominal cramps, nausea, vomiting, diarrhea, mydriasis, diaphoresis, flushing, hyperreflexia, hyperactivity, irritability, confusion, and a panic state.

   b. Major toxic manifestations include severe hypertension (which has been associated with intracranial hemorrhage), significant tachyarrhythmias (which may degenerate to ventricular tachycardia or fibrillation), severe hyperthermia (which has been associated with coagulopathies, rhabdomyolysis, and renal failure), convulsions, systemic acidosis, delirium, psychosis, coma, hypotension, and cardiovascular collapse.

   c. Amphetamine **psychosis** is usually seen in chronic abusers and is apparently caused by excess dopamine in the CNS. It is characterized by paranoia, delusions, and hallucinations, with preservation of orientation and memory. This syndrome may be differentiated from psychiatric conditions (e.g., paranoid schizophrenia) by a history of drug abuse, a premorbid personality not suggestive of a primary psychiatric disorder, a more appropriate and outgoing affect, and the identification of amphetamines on drug screening.

   3. Treatment

   a. Once stabilized, the patient should be moved to a cool, **quiet environment** minimizing external stimulation.

   b. Gastric emptying, followed by charcoal and cathartic administration, is indicated for oral ingestions. Since amphetamines delay gastric emptying, these maneuvers may be effective for prolonged periods postingestion.

   c. Forced acid diuresis (see sec. **I.F.1.b**) increases renal excretion and is recommended for overdoses with evidence of major toxicity.

   d. Psychosis and agitation are best treated with haloperidol (a dopamine antagonist). Chlorpromazine, 1 mg/kg IM, is also effective but may increase the half-life of amphetamines [4] and has greater respiratory depressive and hypotensive effects than haloperidol. Diazepam may also be useful, especially for nonpsychotic agitated patients.

   e. For terminating **seizures,** diazepam is the drug of choice; for prolonged or recurrent seizures, phenytoin should be administered.

   f. Amphetamine-induced **arrhythmias** are often responsive to beta-blockers, such as propranolol.

   g. Hypertension may be treated with haloperidol or chlorpromazine. Severe, sustained hypertension, however, may require phentolamine or nitroprusside.

    h. Hyperthermia is an ominous sign and temperatures above 102°F (especially if there has been a rapid rise) should be treated with haloperidol or chlorpromazine and active cooling measures.

    i. Since **hypotension** may be secondary to catecholamine depletion, a direct-acting agent (e.g., norepinephrine) should be used, if necessary, once an adequate intravascular volume has been achieved with intravenous fluids.

    j. Hemodialysis may be of benefit in life-threatening intoxications not responsive to supportive care and in patients with renal compromise.

    k. Vital signs must be monitored closely, since life-threatening complications, which usually are heralded by hyperthermia or a change in cardiovascular indices, may occur.

  4. Disposition. All patients with major toxic manifestations require hospitalization. Patients with minor toxic manifestations should be admitted to the hospital or observed in the emergency department (for at least 4 hours) until toxic signs resolve.

C. Barbiturates can be classified as **ultra short-acting** with a duration of action of about 20 minutes (e.g., thiopental), **short-acting** with a duration of action of about 3 hours (e.g., pentobarbital, secobarbital), **intermediate-acting** with a duration of action of about 3–6 hours (e.g., amobarbital, butabarbital), and **long-acting** with a duration of action of about 6–12 hours (e.g., barbital, phenobarbital). The activity of these drugs is related to their lipid solubility, with the more lipid-soluble drugs having a faster onset of action (related to their cerebral uptake) and a shorter duration of action (due to redistribution) [38]. The duration of action, however, does not correlate with the elimination half-life, making the above classification somewhat artificial [38]. Ingestion of more than 5 gm of a long-acting barbiturate or 3 gm of a short-acting drug may be fatal; potentially lethal levels are 8 mg/dl and 3.5 mg/dl, respectively [115]. The amount ingested and the blood level, however, may not correlate with the clinical presentation, since chronic abusers may develop tolerance allowing for minimal toxic effects with potentially lethal levels and some patients with low levels may be critically ill due to augmenting factors such as mixed-drug ingestions. The morbidity and mortality are more closely related to the patient's clinical status, with mortality principally confined to deeply comatose patients. Early deaths are usually due to cardiopulmonary depression.

  1. Pharmacology and toxicology. The barbiturates are weak organic acids with pK_a values of 7.2–8.0. They are CNS depressants and in toxic doses may depress the activity of other excitable tissue (e.g., skeletal, cardiac, and smooth muscle). The short-acting barbiturates are more potent hypnotic agents, more toxic, and more commonly abused. They are more lipid-soluble, more highly protein-bound, poorly filtered by the renal glomerulus, and readily resorbed from the renal tubular lumen; elimination is primarily by hepatic metabolism, with the inactive metabolites excreted through the kidneys. The long-acting barbiturates and, to a lesser extent, the intermediate-acting barbiturates are primarily eliminated unchanged in the urine.

  2. Clinical manifestations

    a. Central nervous system. Mild to moderate intoxication may exhibit CNS depression, slurred speech, ataxia, nystagmus, and miosis. Severe intoxication may exhibit extraocular motor palsies, absent corneal reflexes, sluggishly reactive pupils (usually the pupillary reflex is preserved), absent deep tendon reflexes, a positive Babinski sign, and coma.

    b. Respiratory depression is the major life-threatening manifestation of barbiturate overdose. Other pulmonary complications include aspiration pneumonia, atelectasis, pulmonary edema, and bronchopneumonia.

    c. Cardiovascular depression is characterized by hypotension, a low cardiac output, and an absolute or relative hypovolemia secondary to a decrease in plasma volume or expansion of the vascular capacity [115].

    d. Other manifestations include hypothermia (due to depressed temperature regulation in the brainstem), cutaneous bullae (predominantly over pressure areas), and renal failure (secondary to shock or rhabdomyolysis).

  3. Treatment. Supportive care is the mainstay of therapy.

    a. Gastric emptying, followed by charcoal and cathartic administration, is indicated.

    b. Repeated doses of **charcoal** PO or by gastric tube at 4-hour intervals may significantly enhance nonrenal elimination of phenobarbital [10].

    c. Hypotension is usually responsive to administration of oxygen and intravenous fluids. If an adequate blood pressure cannot be achieved with this therapy, dopamine should be given.

    d. Alkaline diuresis (see sec. **I.F.1.a**) is indicated for long-acting barbiturate overdoses in stage III or IV coma. However, injudicious use of forced diuresis must be avoided because of the risk of deterioration of the cardiovascular status.

    e. Extracorporeal removal. Charcoal hemoperfusion is the preferred procedure for both long- and short-acting life-threatening barbiturate overdoses not responding to intensive supportive measures. Hemodialysis is ineffective in removing short-acting barbiturates but may be useful in long-acting barbiturate overdoses.

  4. Disposition. Patients with mild barbiturate overdosage may be observed in the emergency department (for at least 4 hours) until toxic signs resolve and then referred to a detoxification unit (when appropriate). Severe barbiturate overdoses require admission to an intensive care unit.

D. Benzodiazepines (e.g., chlordiazepoxide, diazepam, flurazepam, and oxazepam) are CNS depressants with a half-life that varies (generally increasing with age) from 5–10 hours for oxazepam to 14–100 hours for diazepam. The benzodiazepines are metabolized in the liver, with active and inactive metabolites excreted in the urine; some benzodiazepines (e.g., diazepam) are also excreted in the bile and may undergo enterohepatic circulation [38]. These drugs are relatively safe, with overdoses generally manifested by drowsiness, dysarthria, ataxia, dizziness, weakness, and confusion. Since severe overdoses characterized by coma and respiratory and/or circulatory depression seldom are seen with orally ingested benzodiazepines alone, mixed overdoses should be suspected in such situations. Drug levels may not correlate with the patient's clinical status but can help confirm the diagnosis. **Treatment** consists of gastric emptying, followed by charcoal and cathartic administration, and supportive care. For nonsevere overdoses, observation in the emergency department (for at least 4 hours) until toxic manifestations subside is recommended. Hospitalization is indicated for severe overdoses.

E. Carbon monoxide is a colorless, odorless gas produced by incomplete combustion of carbon-containing fossil fuels. Carbon monoxide poisoning commonly occurs in confined, poorly ventilated spaces in which carbon monoxide is released by fires, combustion engines, faulty stoves or heating systems, or gas or kerosene space heaters. Generally, carboxyhemoglobin saturation is 0.85% in normal nonsmokers, may be raised up to 5% during prolonged exposure to freeway air [5], is under 10% during normal occupational exposure, and is under 15% for smokers [40].

  1. Pathophysiology. Carbon monoxide toxicity causes hypoxia by three mechanisms:

    a. Reduction of the oxygen-carrying capacity in the blood by displacing oxygen from hemoglobin because of its 250 times greater affinity than oxygen for hemoglobin.

    b. Shift of the oxyhemoglobin dissociation curve to the left with resultant impaired release of oxygen to the tissues.

    c. Depression of cellular respiration through inhibition of the cytochrome oxidase system.

  2. Clinical manifestations

    a. Acute poisoning. The CNS and heart are the organs most affected by carbon monoxide poisoning. **CNS manifestations** include headache, dizziness, visual disturbances, diminished hearing, an altered mental status, and seizures. **Cardiac manifestations** include arrhythmias, ischemia, and infarction, with patients with underlying coronary artery disease being particularly sensitive to the effects of carbon monoxide. Other manifestations include a cherry-red appearance to the skin or mucosae, weakness, nausea, vomiting, retinal hemorrhages or venous engorgement, rhabdomyolysis, and a metabolic acidosis. A low measured oxygen saturation may be present, but the PaO_2 (a measure of dissolved and not hemoglobin-bound oxygen) is often normal.

    Although carboxyhemoglobin levels may not correlate with clinical manifestations, the following generalizations can be made. Patients with carboxyhemoglobin levels below 10% usually are asymptomatic. Minor symptoms (e.g., headache, giddiness) generally occur with levels from 10–30%, and more serious manifestations (e.g., visual disturbances, tachycardia, tachypnea, syncope) with levels from 30–50%. Carboxyhemoglobin levels above 50% are often associated with severe toxicity, characterized by stupor, coma,

seizures, respiratory failure, or cardiovascular collapse. Death is likely at levels above 70%.
b. **Subacute carbon monoxide poisoning** may present with a flulike syndrome (with nausea, vomiting, headache, dizziness, and malaise) [42], usually in members of the same household during the winter months.
c. A **post–carbon monoxide syndrome**, characterized by headache, nausea, weakness, and dizziness, may be present up to 3 weeks postexposure [97]. Serious neuropsychiatric sequelae may occur between 2 and 40 days postexposure and include mental deterioration, fecal or urinary incontinence, gait disturbance, and mutism [20].

3. **Treatment** consists of intensive supportive care and providing **high tissue oxygen levels** to reduce cellular hypoxia and promote the elimination of carbon monoxide. When a person is breathing air, the half-life of carbon monoxide is about 5–6 hours; the half-life, however, can be reduced to about 90 minutes by breathing 100% oxygen and to less than 30 minutes by utilizing hyperbaric oxygen at 3 atm [42].
a. **Endotracheal intubation** is recommended for obtunded or comatose patients. Assisted ventilation should be provided as needed.
b. **Oxygen** in a concentration of 100% should be administered until the carboxyhemoglobin level declines below 10% [49, 76].
c. **Hyperbaric oxygen** is recommended for patients in coma and patients with a significant metabolic acidosis, myocardial ischemia, or significant neurologic deficits [97].

4. **Disposition.** Patients with mild manifestations may be discharged from the emergency department when the carboxyhemoglobin level is less than 10% and they are asymptomatic. Hospitalization, however, generally is advised for patients with a carboxyhemoglobin level above 30% and patients with cardiac manifestations, significant neurologic manifestations (e.g., an altered mental status, seizures), or a metabolic acidosis.

F. **Caustic ingestions. Alkalis** are common ingredients in cleaning agents, washing powders, and paint removers. Significant tissue injury is generally related to solutions with a pH equal to or greater than 12.5 [110]. These substances characteristically produce a liquification necrosis principally affecting the esophagus. **Acids** may be found in toilet bowl cleaners, disinfectants, and automobile batteries. Serious acid ingestions are uncommon due to the severe pain produced when strong acids come into contact with the oral mucosa. The severity of injury generally is related to the concentration of the acid and the duration of exposure. These substances characteristically produce a coagulation necrosis principally involving the stomach.

1. **Clinical manifestations** include pain in the oropharynx, chest, or abdomen; oropharyngeal burns; dysphagia; drooling; nausea; retching; and vomiting. In addition, respiratory distress secondary to upper airway edema or tracheal aspiration may occur. Gastrointestinal hemorrhage, perforation with mediastinitis or peritonitis, sepsis, and shock are other serious complications. Death is usually due to circulatory collapse or airway obstruction. Esophageal strictures in alkali ingestions and pyloric stenosis in acid ingestions are the most common long-term sequelae.

2. **Treatment**
a. **Dilution.** The caustic agent should be diluted in the oral cavity by copiously rinsing the mouth with cold water. In acid ingestions, swallowed diluents are not recommended due to the potential for an exothermic reaction [84]. In alkali ingestions , 6–8 oz of water or preferably milk should be swallowed, if tolerated [97, 98]. This should be followed by having the patient take nothing by mouth.
b. **Induced emesis and administration of charcoal and a cathartic are contraindicated in caustic ingestions.** Gastric lavage is also contraindicated in alkali ingestions. Although controversial, gastric lavage is probably beneficial in acid ingestions if performed within 90 minutes of ingestion [49, 84]; as much acid as possible should be removed from the stomach and followed by ice-water lavage.
c. Although controversial, early endoscopy is a means to document injury.
d. Airway management, adequate fluid replacement, and careful monitoring for perforation, hemorrhage, and infection are essential. Steroids and prophylactic antibiotics are controversial and of questionable benefit.

3. **Disposition.** Hospitalization is recommended for patients with a definite history of observed ingestion of a caustic material or signs or symptoms of a caustic ingestion. Otherwise, patients may be released from the emergency department after a 4-hour observation period with arrangements for follow-up in 24 hours.

G. **Cocaine** is an expensive and popular recreational drug. The purity of street samples may vary from 15–60% [33], and it is usually adulterated with a sugar (e.g., mannitol, lactose, glucose), local anesthetic (e.g., lidocaine, procaine), or another recreational drug (e.g., amphetamine, phencyclidine, heroin). Cocaine is absorbed by all mucous membranes and is most commonly administered by nasal insufflation but may be smoked, injected intravenously, or taken orally (although oral absorption is significantly diminished due to gastric hydrolysis). Death can occur by all routes of administration; however, the parenteral route and "freebasing" (i.e., the use of purified cocaine, usually by smoking) [2] are particularly dangerous. For a 70-kg individual, the fatal dose is about 1400 mg when taken orally and 750 mg when taken parenterally or inhaled; however, death may occur with much smaller doses [33]. Lethal blood levels vary widely. Blood and urine determinations are useful in confirming the diagnosis.

1. **Pharmacology and toxicology.** Cocaine is a powerful CNS and sympathetic stimulant and an effective local anesthetic. Cocaine may also sensitize the myocardium to epinephrine and norepinephrine [39], as well as have a direct cardiotoxic effect [33]. Cocaine is rapidly metabolized in the liver and by plasma cholinesterase, and metabolites as well as up to 20% of unchanged cocaine are excreted in the urine [49]. The time to peak action depends on the route of administration, varying from 3–5 minutes (for IV administration) to 60–90 minutes (for PO administration). Cocaine has a brief duration of action with a plasma half-life of about 1 hour.

2. **Clinical manifestations** generally are secondary to adrenergic stimulation, with effects similar to those seen with amphetamine toxicity. Recently, a purified, smokable form of cocaine (alkaloidal cocaine) known as "crack" has become increasingly popular [73a]. Because of its purity and rapid absorption through the pulmonary vasculature, its effects are intensified, and it can readily cause lethal overdosage. In addition, use of the drug can rapidly lead to addiction. Chronic abusers of cocaine may exhibit an ulcerated or perforated nasal septum or a toxic psychosis.

    a. **Mild to moderate toxicity** is manifested by increased respiration, tachycardia (or, occasionally, transient bradycardia), increased blood pressure, nausea, vomiting, skin pallor, mydriasis, diaphoresis, headache, hyperreflexia, excitability, apprehension, dysphoria, confusion, and hallucinations.

    b. **Severe intoxication** is characterized by a psychotic reaction, seizures, ventricular arrhythmias, myocardial ischemia or infarction, hyperthermia, severe hypertension (which may cause an intracranial hemorrhage), pulmonary edema, respiratory depression, hypotension, coma, and/or circulatory collapse. Death, which usually occurs rapidly [46, 114], is usually secondary to respiratory depression (often preceded by a grand mal seizure) and, less commonly, circulatory collapse [46].

3. **Treatment. Supportive care** is the mainstay of therapy, with careful attention to maintaining ventilation and cardiovascular monitoring.

    a. **Seizures.** Diazepam should be used to terminate seizures. Recurrent or prolonged seizures may require administration of phenytoin.

    b. Since cardiac **arrhythmias** usually are secondary to adrenergic stimulation, propranolol is the drug of choice when treatment is necessary.

    c. **Hyperthermia** is treated with external cooling.

    d. **Hypertension** is usually transient; however, severe, sustained hypertension may occur and require administration of propranolol or, in more resistant cases, nitroprusside.

    e. **Hypotension** is treated with intravenous fluids. Dopamine or norepinephrine may be needed for fluid-resistant hypotension.

    f. Significant **behavioral disturbances** may be treated with diazepam.

    g. **Cocaine-filled condom ingestions** for the purpose of transporting cocaine is a potentially lethal situation due to the risk of condom leakage or rupture. Early surgical removal generally is recommended. However, the use of a mild cathartic and careful monitoring may be warranted if the ingestion is recent, the cocaine container appears to be resistant to leakage or rupture, there is no evidence of cocaine toxicity, and the cocaine-filled condom is in the lower gastrointestinal tract [71].

   4. **Disposition.** All severely intoxicated patients should be admitted to the hospital. If emergency department policy permits, mildly to moderately toxic patients may be observed in the emergency department (for at least 4 hours) and discharged when free of toxic manifestations).

H. **Cyanide** is a rapidly acting, very potent poison. Common sources of cyanide include fumigants, silver polishes, rodenticides, burning plastics, and amygdalin (Laetrile), a substance contained in several fruit pits. Poisoning may occur from inhalation of hydrogen cyanide gas or ingestion of hydrocyanic acid, its sodium or potassium salt, or amygdalin. Cyanide toxicity may also result from prolonged or excessive use of sodium nitroprusside. Lethal doses are approximately 50 mg of the gas or acid and 200–300 mg of the salt [49]. Lethal blood levels generally exceed 3 μg/ml [43].

   1. **Mechanism of toxicity.** Cyanide paralyzes cellular respiration by reversibly binding and inhibiting cytochrome oxidase (and possibly other ferric-containing enzymes) of the mitochondrial electron transport chain [19]. The result is cellular and tissue anoxia.

   2. **Clinical features** of cyanide poisoning appear rapidly following ingestion, skin application, or, particularly, inhalation. CNS manifestations are prominent and include headache, dizziness, confusion, ataxia, seizures, and coma. Dyspnea (hyperpnea), nausea, and vomiting are other common features. Arrhythmias, lactic acidosis, pulmonary edema, and respiratory or cardiac arrest may also complicate the poisoning. The victim's breath may reveal an odor of bitter almonds or silver polish, and the venous blood may resemble arterial blood in color and oxygen saturation (because of impaired cellular utilization of oxygen).

   3. **Treatment**

      a. **Intensive supportive measures,** particularly administration of 100% oxygen and assisted ventilation as needed, are essential to support the patient until the cyanide can be eliminated from the body. Appropriate treatment of arrhythmias, pulmonary edema, and lactic acidosis is indicated. In severe poisoning unresponsive to therapy, a trial of hyperbaric oxygen may be attempted [97].

      b. **Amyl nitrite, sodium nitrite, and sodium thiosulfate** are specific antidotes for cyanide poisoning and are of paramount importance in its management [19]. The nitrites convert hemoglobin (Fe^{2+}) to methemoglobin (Fe^{3+}), which competes with cytochrome oxidase for the cyanide ion; the result is the binding of cyanide as cyanmethemoglobin, thus sparing cytochrome oxidase for its vital cellular respiratory function. The thiosulfate serves as a substrate for the conversion of cyanide to the relatively nontoxic thiocyanate, which is renally excreted.

      It is essential that these antidotes be administered as early as possible to improve the chance for survival. Antidotal therapy is initiated by administering amyl nitrite by inhalation for 15–30 seconds of each minute until 10 ml of a 3% solution (300 mg) of sodium nitrite can be given IV at a rate of 2.5–5.0 ml/minute. Following the sodium nitrite injection, 50 ml of a 25% solution (12.5 gm) of sodium thiosulfate is administered IV over 10 minutes. (These are adult dosages; appropriate adjustments in dosages must be made in children.) For recurrent or persistent signs of cyanide toxicity, the sodium nitrite and sodium thiosulfate may be repeated in half dosages in 2 hours. The goal of nitrite therapy is reversal of cyanide toxicity with a methemoglobin level (which requires monitoring) of less than 30%.

      c. **Measures to lessen the intoxication** should be performed as indicated. These include decontaminating the skin (by removing contaminated clothing and thoroughly washing the skin with soap and water) and lavaging the stomach to remove unabsorbed, ingested poison. Activated charcoal and a cathartic, however, are of questionable benefit.

   4. **Disposition.** Any symptomatic patient with suspected or known cyanide exposure should be hospitalized. Asymptomatic patients may be discharged from the emergency department after a 4-hour period of observation if still asymptomatic.

I. **Ethanol** is the most widely abused drug worldwide, and problems associated with ethanol abuse are commonly seen in most emergency departments. In a 70-kg patient, one oz of 80-proof ethanol (40% ethanol by volume), one glass of wine, or a 12-oz bottle of beer will increase the blood ethanol level by about 25 mg/dl [26].

Blood levels greater than 100 mg/dl generally define legal intoxication, levels above 150 mg/dl usually produce clinical intoxication, and levels exceeding 350 mg/dl may be fatal [26]. However, there is marked individual variation in clinical intoxication at various blood levels, with chronic alcoholics generally tolerating higher levels better and metabolizing alcohol at an increased rate.

1. **Pharmacology.** About 25% of ethanol is absorbed from the stomach, with the rest absorbed from the upper small intestine. Absorption is rapid, and ethanol may be detected in the blood within 5 minutes after ingestion, with a maximum concentration reached in 30–90 minutes. Ethanol is metabolized in the liver to carbon dioxide and water, with about 10% excreted unchanged through the kidneys, sweat glands, and respiratory tract. Blood levels decline at variable rates, averaging about 15 mg/dl/hour for a 70-kg person [26].

2. **Clinical features**
   a. **Acute ethanol intoxication.** The odor of an ethanolic beverage on the patient's breath along with CNS manifestations is characteristic. CNS signs include an altered sensorium, nystagmus, ataxia, slurred speech, confusion, transient amnesic events, toxic psychosis, and, with severe intoxication, stupor or coma. Other features include nausea, vomiting, diarrhea, esophagitis, Mallory-Weiss tears, gastritis (which may cause gastrointestinal hemorrhage), acute pancreatitis, peripheral vasodilatation (which may cause flushing or orthostatic hypotension), lactic or ketoacidosis, hypo- or hyperglycemia, dehydration or fluid overload, hypokalemia, hyperuricemia, hyperosmolality, antidiuretic hormone (ADH) suppression (responsible for a urinary diuresis), ventricular dysfunction, cardiac arrhythmias or conduction blocks, hypothermia (also a predisposition for hyperthermia), and rhabdomyolysis. Ethanol abuse is also associated with an increased incidence of suicide, violent behavior, accidental injuries, mixed-drug overdoses, infectious complications (e.g., pneumonia, meningitis), aspiration pneumonitis, and fetal malformations (with maternal ethanol abuse during pregnancy). In acute ethanol poisoning, death is usually due to respiratory depression and, less commonly, cardiovascular collapse.
   b. **Chronic ethanol abuse** may affect practically any organ, with the primary effect on the liver, leading to a fatty liver, alcoholic hepatitis, and cirrhosis. Liver damage may progress to portal hypertension (with esophageal varices) and hepatic failure. Other manifestations of chronic ethanolism include chronic relapsing pancreatitis, cardiomyopathy, noncardiac myopathy, peripheral neuropathy, bone marrow suppression, nutritional deficiencies (e.g., Wernicke's disease from thiamine deficiency, folate deficiency, hypomagnesemia, hypocalcemia, hypophosphatemia), and CNS injury (e.g., alcoholic dementia, cerebellar degeneration).

3. **Treatment.** The mainstay of therapy is **supportive care.** A thorough history and physical examination are essential to assess for treatable complications (e.g., hypoglycemia, traumatic injuries, pneumonia). For patients with a significant alteration in mental status, a blood ethanol level and glucose determination should be obtained, with other studies performed as indicated.
   a. **Thiamine**, 100 mg IM or IV, generally should be given; if the patient has evidence of Wernicke's disease, intravenous administration is recommended. If hypoglycemia is a possibility, 25–50 gm of dextrose should be given IV.
   b. For **comatose patients**, airway protection by endotracheal intubation should be performed and followed by gastric lavage and charcoal and cathartic administration. Although alcohol is rapidly absorbed from the gastrointestinal tract, gastric lavage may be effective if performed within 2 hours of ingestion (as well as treating mixed-drug ingestions).
   c. Hemodialysis is rarely necessary but may be beneficial in life-threatening ethanol intoxications not responding to conservative measures (especially intoxications with blood levels exceeding 600 mg/dl or 400 mg/dl with associated severe acidosis).

4. **Disposition.** Patients with evidence of mild to moderate intoxication generally can be discharged from the emergency department once the intoxication is resolved or if accompanied by a responsible individual. Since intoxicated patients may be unable to make rational decisions and thus are a potential danger to themselves or others, they should not be allowed to leave the emergency department unaccompanied by a responsible individual. Thus, the emergency physician should attempt to convince the patient to remain in the emergency

Table 16-9. Intoxications associated with an osmolal gap*

Ethanol	Glycerol	Mannitol
Ethylene glycol	Isopropyl alcohol	Methanol

*Osmolal gap is the difference between the measured and calculated serum osmolalities; it is abnormal when

$$\text{Measured osmolality} - (2\,[\text{Na}^+] + \frac{[\text{Blood glucose}]}{18} + \frac{[\text{BUN}]}{2.8}) > 10\ \frac{\text{mOsm}}{\text{kg H}_2\text{O}}.$$

department until no longer intoxicated. If this fails, reasonable physical restraint may be necessary to prevent the patient from eloping [37]. On discharge, referral to a detoxification unit or rehabilitation program should be arranged, when appropriate. Hospitalization is recommended for patients with severe intoxication or significant complications, including coma, respiratory depression, significant acid-base or electrolyte abnormalities, pancreatitis, gastrointestinal hemorrhage, or pneumonia.

J. Ethylene glycol may be present in detergents, paints, lacquers, polishes, coolants, and, most commonly, antifreeze. It is one of the most serious poisonings encountered in clinical toxicology, with the lethal dose being about 100 ml in adults [49].

1. **Pharmacology and toxicology.** Ethylene glycol is rapidly absorbed from the gastrointestinal tract and has a plasma half-life of about 3 hours. Ethylene glycol in itself appears to be nontoxic; however, its metabolites (i.e., aldehydes, glycolate, oxalate, and lactate) are highly toxic and responsible for the life-threatening manifestations of the poisoning. Metabolism takes place primarily in the liver, and the metabolites as well as free ethylene glycol are excreted in the urine.

2. **Clinical manifestations.** The **diagnosis** of ethylene glycol poisoning should be suspected from four major signs: (a) apparent ethanol intoxication with no odor of an ethanolic beverage on the patient's breath and a zero blood ethanol level (unless ethanol was also ingested), (b) a metabolic acidosis with a large anion gap, (c) an osmolal gap (Table 16-9), and (d) calcium oxalate crystals in the urine. The clinical presentation can be divided into three stages [49].

   a. **Stage 1,** which occurs within 30 minutes–12 hours postingestion, is characterized predominantly by **CNS manifestations,** including features similar to ethanol intoxication (see sec. **II.I.2**), optic signs (e.g., ophthalmoplegia, papilledema, optic atrophy), depressed deep tendon reflexes, and myoclonic jerks. Severe poisoning may exhibit focal or generalized seizures, stupor, or coma and culminate in death. Other manifestations include mild hypertension, tachycardia, low-grade fever, nausea, vomiting, and abdominal pain. Laboratory studies may reveal a metabolic acidosis (predominantly from glycolic and lactic acids), hypocalcemia (due to calcium precipitation with oxalate), hyperkalemia, a mild leukocytosis, an abnormal urinalysis (e.g., proteinuria, hematuria, pyuria, oxalate crystals), and, occasionally, an abnormal cerebrospinal fluid analysis (e.g., increased protein, a polymorphonuclear pleocytosis).

   b. **Stage 2** begins 12–24 hours postingestion. **Cardiopulmonary manifestations** predominate and include a tachycardia, mild hypertension, and tachypnea. Severe poisoning may exhibit cyanosis, congestive heart failure, pulmonary edema, and bronchopneumonia.

   c. **Stage 3** appears 24–72 hours postingestion. **Renal manifestations** predominate, including flank pain and tenderness, an elevated BUN and creatinine, and oliguria or anuria (acute tubular necrosis).

3. **Treatment** consists of gastric emptying and intensive supportive care, with attention to correction of acidosis and hypocalcemia as indicated. Specific therapy includes the following.

   a. Administration of **thiamine,** 100 mg IM or IV, and **pyridoxine,** 100 mg IM or IV, daily is recommended [97]. Although not of proved benefit, thiamine and pyridoxine act as cofactors in ethylene glycol degradation and thus may shunt metabolism to less toxic metabolites.

   b. It is important to maintain a **diuresis** until crystalluria disappears to enhance the renal clearance of ethylene glycol and its metabolites [14]. This may be accomplished by the administration of saline IV along with the use of furosemide or mannitol as needed. Close monitoring is essential to avoid electrolyte disturbances, fluid overload, and pulmonary edema.

   c. Ethanol should be administered early, since it competes for alcohol dehydrogenase used to convert ethylene glycol to its toxic metabolites. Initially, 0.6 gm/kg (about 0.75 ml/kg of 100% ethanol) should be given IV (or PO) over about 30–45 minutes and followed by an infusion of 109 mg/kg/hour [86]. If dialysis is being performed, the maintenance dosage must be increased to 237 mg/kg/hour [86]. Ethanol should be mixed with 5% D/W to form a 5–10% solution when given IV; for PO administration, a 50% solution for loading and a 20% solution for maintenance may be used. Ethanol levels need to be carefully monitored to assure levels of 100–150 mg/dl.

   d. Hemodialysis effectively removes ethylene glycol and several of its metabolites and should be considered early in all ethylene glycol poisonings. Indications for its use include an ethylene glycol level exceeding 50 mg/dl; the presence of acid-base, fluid, or electrolyte imbalance; and renal failure [97].

   4. Disposition. Patients with evidence of ethylene glycol poisoning require hospitalization.

K. Hallucinogens (or more properly psychedelic drugs) and cannabinoids (marijuana). The psychedelic drugs include lysergic acid diethylamide (LSD), morning glory seeds, mescaline, the psychotomimetic amphetamines (e.g., DOM, MDA), psilocybin, dimethyltryptamine (DMT), nutmeg, and Jimson weed. Psychic (rather than physiologic) manifestations are most prominent, and clinical differentiation of the various psychedelic drugs is often unreliable. Generally, the differences among the psychedelic drugs are related to the potency and duration of action. The durations of action are 8–12 hours for LSD (the most potent psychedelic agent), 30–60 minutes for DMT, 5–6 hours for psilocybin, 5–8 hours for the cannabinoids, up to 14 hours for mescaline, and up to 60 hours for nutmeg. Adverse reactions, however, may be prolonged for days; also, acute recurrences of psychedelic-like states (flashbacks) may occur for several months. These drugs may be smoked, taken orally, or administered parenterally or by nasal insufflation, depending on the particular psychedelic agent used.

   1. Clinical manifestations characteristically include visual illusions, sensory perceptual disturbances, synesthesias, depersonalization, and derealization. Other manifestations may include dysphoria, confusion, disorientation, hallucinations, hyperactivity, an acute anxiety state (panic reaction), an acute psychotic reaction, and delusional behavior (which increases the potential for accidental injury and, less commonly, suicide or homicide). Physiologic manifestations include a slightly increased blood pressure, tachycardia, tachypnea, mydriasis (often resulting in photophobia), cutaneous flushing, conjunctival injection, nausea, vomiting, salivation, lacrimation, tremors, incoordination, hyperreflexia, and diaphoresis. Hyperthermia, convulsions, coma, coagulopathy, and respiratory arrest have been reported with massive LSD overdoses [49]. Unique manifestations include anticholinergic effects with Jimson weed; orthostatic hypotension (with large doses), normal size pupils, and a dry mucosa with the cannabinoids; and decreased salivation, miosis, hypothermia, and hepatic damage with nutmeg ingestions.

   2. Treatment
   a. The patient should be placed in a **quiet, dim room.** The patient should not be left unattended, and verbal attempts to reassure and calm the patient should be undertaken.
   b. Gastric emptying and administration of a cathartic generally should be avoided unless there is concomitant ingestion of a toxic substance or the patient exhibits manifestations of severe physiologic toxicity.
   c. Diazepam may be useful in severely anxious patients, but phenothiazines should be avoided, since they may worsen toxicity if anticholinergic substance was taken. Physical restraints should be avoided unless the patient cannot be controlled by other means.

   3. Disposition. Patients should be observed in the emergency department, if possible, until the acute toxic reaction has subsided. Hospitalization is recommended for patients with significant toxic manifestations (e.g., toxic psychosis, seizures, coma, respiratory depression, hyperthermia) or prolonged toxic symptoms or signs.

L. Hydrocarbons are a diverse group of compounds that may cause direct pulmonary or cutaneous injury, as well as being absorbed through the lungs, skin, or gastrointestinal tract or, rarely, by intravenous injection in drug abusers. Accidental ingestion by children is the most common mode of poisoning. Generally, ingestions of more than 1 ml/kg are considered potentially toxic.

1. **Pharmacology and toxicology.** Hydrocarbons are organic substances that contain only carbon and hydrogen. They are divided into aliphatic compounds (containing straight chains) and containing aromatic compounds (containing a benzene ring). Petroleum distillates are hydrocarbons produced by fragmentation of crude petroleum oil. In hydrocarbon ingestions, the principal effects are pulmonary aspiration, gastrointestinal upset, and CNS alteration. Less frequently, myocardial, renal, hepatic, and hematologic complications occur. Morbidity and mortality are usually due to pulmonary aspiration, with low-viscosity hydrocarbons (e.g., mineral seal oil, petroleum ether, petroleum naphtha, mineral spirits, gasoline, kerosene) commonly involved. Systemic toxicity is related to the amount ingested, the ability of the hydrocarbon to be absorbed, the presence of toxic additives, and the volatility of the hydrocarbon, with the more volatile hydrocarbons (e.g., benzene, petroleum ether) generally being more toxic [117].

2. **Clinical manifestations** usually occur within 6 hours after ingestion [3] and include the odor of hydrocarbons on the patient's breath or vomitus, a tachycardia, tachypnea, low-grade fever, mucous membrane irritation, cyanosis, cough, dyspnea, rales, rhonchi, wheezing, stridor, hemoptysis, nausea, vomiting, diarrhea (which occasionally is bloody), chest or abdominal discomfort, an altered sensorium, vertigo, ataxia, seizures, arrhythmias, leukocytosis, and/or cutaneous injury (with skin contact). Acute radiographic changes usually occur from 30 minutes to 12 hours following ingestion [28, 117] and include infiltrates, atelectasis, pulmonary edema, and rarely a pneumothorax or pneumomediastinum. Radiographic changes, however, may not correlate with the clinical manifestations. A double gastric fluid shadow on an upright abdominal x-ray after giving the patient 4–8 oz of water may detect as little as 5 ml of a petroleum distillate in the stomach [49]. Late effects include bacterial pneumonia, hematologic abnormalities, hepatic or renal injury, radiographic evidence of pneumatoceles or a pleural effusion, and chronic abnormalities on pulmonary function tests.

3. **Treatment.** Since the hydrocarbons are a diverse group of compounds with controversy regarding treatment (especially concerning gastric emptying), it is important to contact the regional **poison control center** for information regarding toxicity and specific therapeutic guidelines.

   a. **Skin decontamination.** To prevent dermatitis and percutaneous absorption, all contaminated clothing should be removed and the skin washed.

   b. Supplemental **oxygen** is recommended in all significant aspiration injuries.

   c. Although controversial, **gastric emptying** is recommended for ingestions of **toxic hydrocarbons**, including halogenated hydrocarbons (e.g., carbon tetrachloride, trichloroethane), aromatic hydrocarbons (e.g., benzene, xylene, toluene), and hydrocarbons with toxic additives (e.g., heavy metals, insecticides, camphor). In awake patients, gastric emptying should be performed by induced emesis with ipecac; gastric lavage should not be used because of an associated increased incidence of aspiration [79]. However, in patients with CNS depression, a depressed gag reflex, or seizures, gastric lavage with a cuffed endotracheal tube in place is indicated. Gastric emptying is not recommended for ingestions of low-toxicity hydrocarbons (e.g., high-viscosity products such as grease, petroleum jelly, paraffin wax, lubricating oils, fuel oil, diesel oil, mineral oil, baby oil, rubber cement, glues, tars, or asphalt) or hydrocarbons in which the risk of aspiration outweighs the risk of systemic toxicity (e.g., mineral seal oil) [34].

   d. Although not of proved benefit, **cathartics** may decrease gastrointestinal absorption of hydrocarbons. **Charcoal** administration is recommended for ingestions of hydrocarbons with toxic additives that are absorbed by the charcoal (e.g., heavy metals, insecticides, camphor).

   e. Epinephrine generally should be avoided because of the risk of inducing arrhythmias. Corticosteroids and prophylactic antibiotics should not be used.

4. **Disposition.** Observation for at least 6 hours is required for all patients who have ingested hydrocarbons. Hospital admission is indicated for patients who are symptomatic or have pulmonary abnormalities detected on physical examination, ABGs, or a chest radiograph.

M. Iron. Iron-containing preparations are often used to treat iron-deficiency anemia and pregnant women and as supplements in vitamins. Fatalities usually occur as a result of accidental ingestions in children or suicide attempts in adults. Toxicity is related to the amount of elemental iron ingested. The content of elemental iron varies with different iron preparations, being 20% in ferrous sulfate, 12% in ferrous gluconate, and 33% in ferrous fumarate [49].

1. **Physiology.** Iron is absorbed from the duodenum and jejenum in the ferrous form and then oxidized to the ferric state. It is transported in the plasma bound to transferrin (a beta-globulin). The iron is then stored as ferritin and hemosiderin in the liver, spleen, and bone marrow or is transported to the reticuloendothelial cells of the bone marrow for hemoglobin synthesis. There are limited physiologic losses of iron, with excretion occurring through sweat, bile, and desquamation of skin and mucosal surfaces (with menses in females being the greatest normal source of iron loss). The normal body iron content is about 4–5 gm, with about two-thirds present in hemoglobin, about one-third in iron stores, and a small fraction in myoglobin, catalase, and the cytochrome system and bound to transferrin. Normal serum iron levels are 50–150 µg/dl, and the total iron-binding capacity is 300–400 µg/dl, with plasma transferrin normally about one-third saturated.

2. **Clinical manifestations**
   a. **Early changes** occur from 30 minutes–6 hours postingestion and include corrosive injury to the gastrointestinal tract resulting in abdominal pain, vomiting, and diarrhea; the vomitus and stools may be bloody or iron-stained. Corrosive gastrointestinal injury may progress to necrosis of the bowel wall. A metabolic acidosis may occur due to the release of hydrogen ions resulting from the conversion of ferrous iron to ferric iron. Interruption of the Krebs cycle and lactate and citrate accumulation due to poor tissue perfusion may add to the metabolic acidosis. Hypotension or shock may occur from dehydration, gastrointestinal blood loss, or possibly the direct effect of iron or ferritin on the vasculature. Other manifestations include fever, leukocytosis, hyperglycemia, hepatic damage, pancreatic damage, and pulmonary injury.
   b. **Intermediate changes.** From 6–48 hours postingestion, a period of improvement may occur and be followed by massive hepatic failure (with jaundice), coagulopathies, hypo- or hyperglycemia, a metabolic acidosis, seizures, coma, shock, and vascular collapse. Other manifestations include renal impairment, diffuse vascular congestion, pulmonary edema, and pulmonary hemorrhage.
   c. **Late changes** occur from 3 days–3 weeks following ingestion and include pyloric stenosis or gastric strictures as a result of the corrosive gastrointestinal injury.

3. **Treatment** consists of **intensive supportive care** with careful attention to the correction of acidosis, electrolyte abnormalities, hypovolemia, and coagulation abnormalities.
   a. **Gastric emptying,** followed by administration of a cathartic, is indicated. If ipecac is used, 50–100 ml of a 2% bicarbonate solution should be given along with the ipecac and followed by a repeat dose of bicarbonate after cessation of emesis. If gastric lavage is performed, the initial 250–500 ml of lavage should be with a 2% bicarbonate solution; and following lavage, 50–100 ml of the 2% bicarbonate solution should be instilled into the stomach [97]. Bicarbonate and iron form a ferrous carbonate salt that is poorly absorbed and less irritating to the gastrointestinal tract. Following gastric emptying, an abdominal x-ray should be obtained to look for retained iron in the stomach, which will necessitate a repeat attempt at removal (with gastric lavage). The usual measures of gastric emptying may not be effective due to the formation of iron aggregates that may adhere to the stomach mucosa. If these measures fail in cases of severe iron poisonings, emergency gastrostomy should be considered [85].
   b. **Deferoxamine** chelates free serum iron and is specific therapy for serious iron poisonings. Deferoxamine therapy is indicated in the presence of free serum iron (i.e., elevation of the serum iron above the iron-binding capacity) or a serum iron level exceeding 350 µg/dl [97]. If the serum iron or iron-binding capacity is not readily available, deferoxamine therapy should be initiated in the presence of a potentially lethal ingestion (i.e., > 300 mg/kg

of elemental iron) or in patients exhibiting shock, coma, or seizures. The deferoxamine challenge test is a quick method of determining the need for deferoxamine therapy. This test is performed by administering 25–50 mg/kg (up to 1 gm) of deferoxamine IM; the presence of a vin rose color to the urine (signifying the excretion of the iron-ferrioxamine complex) indicates the presence of free serum iron and the need for deferoxamine therapy [49]. Deferoxamine is administered in a dosage of 90 mg/kg (up to 1 gm) IM or, in hypotensive patients, IV (infused at a rate of less than 15 mg/kg/hour) q8h until the vin rose color of the urine clears [97].

   c. Dialysis is indicated in the presence of renal failure. Deferoxamine therapy is necessary during dialysis, since the iron-ferrioxamine complex is dialyzable, whereas iron is not.

  4. Disposition. Hospitalization is indicated if the patient is symptomatic, iron pills are identified on an abdominal radiograph, or the serum iron level exceeds 300 μg/dl. If a serum iron level is not readily available, hospitalization is also indicated if there is a history of ingesting more than 75 mg/kg of elemental iron, the white blood cell count exceeds 15,000/mm^3, or the blood sugar is greater than 150 mg/dl, since these factors tend to correlate with serum iron levels exceeding 300 μg/dl [49]. Other patients who are asymptomatic after a 6-hour period of observation may be released from the emergency department with instruction to return if they become symptomatic.

N. Lithium, used primarily in the treatment of manic-depressive illness, is rapidly and completely absorbed from the gastrointestinal tract. The drug is distributed in whole-body water, with a slow uptake and release by CNS tissue [49]. Excretion is almost entirely renal, with a half-life of elimination of about 29 hours [49]. The drug has a narrow therapeutic index. Toxicity may result from chronic administration of the drug or acute overdosage. In the former situation, which is more common, deficits in body sodium and/or water secondary to inadequate intake or increased loss (e.g., due to gastroenteritis, diuretic therapy) are frequent factors predisposing to toxicity by impairing renal excretion of lithium. Blood levels exceeding 1.5 mEq/liter correlate with toxicity, and levels greater than 3.5 mEq/liter are life-threatening [52].

  1. Toxic manifestations. Neurologic signs and symptoms are prominent and include dysarthria, ataxia, an altered mental status (e.g., confusion, delirium, lethargy, stupor, coma), coarse tremors, muscle rigidity, muscle fasciculations, myoclonus, hyperreflexia, and seizures. Severe gastroenteritis, characterized by nausea, vomiting, and profuse diarrhea, is common. Cardiovascular disturbances may occur and include arrhythmias, conduction disturbances, hypotension, and circulatory failure. Impaired renal function, particularly nephrogenic diabetes insipidus, may also be associated with lithium toxicity [52].

  2. Treatment

    a. In acute overdosage, **gastric emptying** by induced emesis (with ipecac) or gastric lavage is indicated. Activated charcoal (but no cathartic) should then be administered.

    b. Correcting sodium and water deficits (if present) and maintaining a good urinary output are important. However, forced diuresis is of questionable efficacy in enhancing renal excretion of lithium and is not recommended [49]. In addition, diuretics should be avoided (or discontinued).

    c. Hemodialysis is very effective in removing lithium from the body. It is indicated if there are potentially life-threatening complications of the intoxication (e.g., severe neurologic impairment, cardiotoxicity), the serum level exceeds 4 mEq/liter [59], or renal clearance of lithium is impaired.

  3. Disposition. Hospital admission is indicated whenever lithium toxicity is suspected or confirmed. Cardiac monitoring during the period of intoxication is recommended because of the risk of arrhythmias.

O. Methanol may be an ingredient in cleaning agents, paints, shellacs, solvents, windshield-washing fluids, solid canned fuels, liquid fuels, and illegal whiskeys. The minimal lethal dose in an adult is about 30 ml [41], but as little as 4 ml has caused blindness [97].

  1. Pharmacology and toxicology. Methanol may be absorbed through the skin, lungs (by inhalation), or the gastrointestinal tract, with oral ingestion being the most frequent route. The plasma half-life of methanol varies from 28–62 hours [41]. Approximately 30% of methanol is excreted unchanged through the respiratory tract and less than 5% through the kidneys [49]. The remaining methanol is biotransformed, principally in the liver, with complete metabolism and excretion taking several days. The significant morbidity and mortality associated with methanol poisoning are due to its metabolites (i.e., formaldehyde, formate, and lactate).

2. **Clinical manifestations.** Initially, there is a mild inebriation similar to that seen with ethanol intoxication but with no odor of an ethanolic beverage on the patient's breath and a zero blood ethanol level (unless ethanol was also ingested). Due to a delay in production of toxic metabolites, there is a latency period of about 6–30 hours before the following significant toxic manifestations occur.

   a. **Retinal toxicity,** a characteristic manifestation, may be manifested by photophobia, blurred vision, poorly reactive dilated pupils, hyperemic disks, and papilledema. Optic atrophy and blindess may be late sequelae.

   b. **Gastrointestinal toxicity,** characterized by nausea, vomiting, and severe abdominal pain, may occur, possibly due to acute pancreatitis induced by methanol poisoning.

   c. **CNS toxicity** may be manifested by headache, vertigo, restlessness, delirium, seizures, obtundation, and coma. Cerebral edema is frequently found at autopsy.

   d. A large **anion-gap metabolic acidosis,** predominantly from formic and lactic acids, and an **osmolal gap** (see Table 16-9) are characteristic features.

3. **Treatment** consists of gastric emptying and intensive supportive care, with attention to correction of acidosis, which may be severe and require large amounts of sodium bicarbonate. Specific therapy includes the following:

   a. **Ethanol** administration (see sec. **II.J.3.c**) is indicated if the methanol level exceeds 20 mg/dl (or while awaiting the results of the level); this treatment should continue until the level falls below 20 mg/dl.

   b. **Hemodialysis** is effective in removing methanol and its toxic metabolites. It is recommended if the blood methanol level exceeds 50 mg/dl; acidosis is present; mental status, visual, or funduscopic abnormalities develop [41]; or renal failure occurs [97].

   c. Folic acid acts as a cofactor in the detoxification of methanol and may be useful. Leucovorin (folinic acid) is the active form of folic acid and may also be useful in symptomatic methanol intoxication [97].

4. **Disposition.** Hospitalization is indicated for patients with evidence of methanol poisoning.

P. **Methemoglobinemia** may be caused by many oxidizing agents, including nitrites, nitrates, chlorates, sulfonamides, aniline dyes, nitrobenzene, phenazopyridine, phenacetin, acetanilid, and local anesthetics. These substances oxidize hemoglobin to its ferric state, thereby limiting its oxygen-carrying capacity and producing symptoms of anemia. The diagnosis is suggested in patients with generalized cyanosis (unrelieved with oxygen) and a normal PaO_2.

1. **Clinical features.** Methemoglobin levels above 15% usually produce cyanosis. Symptoms (e.g., fatigue, weakness, dizziness, dyspnea, headache, tachycardia) usually are present at levels above 30%. Serious toxicity (characterized by an altered mental status, metabolic acidosis, cardiac arrhythmias, or seizures) is associated with levels above 55%, and death (from cellular hypoxia) often occurs with levels above 70%.

2. **Treatment** includes administration of supplemental oxygen. Methylene blue, 1–2 mg/kg IV over 5 minutes, is indicated if there are signs of hypoxia or the methemoglobin level exceeds 30%; a repeat dose should be given in 1 hour for persistent cyanosis or signs of hypoxia [25].

3. **Disposition.** Hospitalization generally is indicated for patients exhibiting symptoms or signs of methemoglobinemia.

Q. **Nonbarbiturate sedative/hypnotics** (other than the benzodiazepines) include a variety of drugs used to produce drowsiness and promote sleep. Intoxication with these drugs produces similar clinical manifestations characterized by CNS depression. This section will deal specifically with methaqualone, ethchlorvynol, glutethimide, and chloral hydrate.

1. **Clinical manifestations** of overdosage with these sedative/hypnotics commonly include CNS depression, slurred speech, nystagmus, and ataxia. In severe overdosage, respiratory depression, coma, hypotension, and pulmonary edema may occur.

2. **Unique features**
   a. **Methaqualone (Quaalude)** has a duration of action of 6–8 hours, which may be prolonged in overdosage. Overdosage is marked by pyramidal signs (e.g., hypertonicity, hyperreflexia, myoclonus). Overdoses may also exhibit excitation, delirium, or seizures. In general, doses exceeding 8 gm [97] or blood levels greater than 3 mg/dl [49] are potentially fatal. Deaths, however, are frequently due to traumatic events rather than the direct result of overdosage [113].
   b. **Ethchlorvynol (Placidyl).** In general, ingestions of more than 10 gm are potentially lethal, and blood levels greater than 10 mg/dl during the first 12 hours postingestion indicate severe intoxication [49]; however, there is a variable response to ethchlorvynol dosages. Overdoses are characterized by prolonged coma (up to 288 hours) [49]. Other manifestations include the presence of a pungent, aromatic odor on the patient's breath, bradycardia, and hypothermia. The primary characteristic of oral overdosage is CNS depression, whereas intravenous usage usually produces noncardiogenic pulmonary edema [102].
   c. **Glutethimide (Doriden).** In general, ingestions exceeding 10 gm and serum levels greater than 3 mg/dl are potentially lethal [49]; however, smaller ingestions may be lethal, and blood levels may not correlate with clinical manifestations. Overdoses are characterized by prolonged coma (because the serum half-life in overdosage is about 40 hours) and a fluctuating level of consciousness. Other manifestations include hypothermia; seizures; the development of sudden, unexpected apnea; and anticholinergic effects, such as dilated pupils (which may be fixed unilaterally or bilaterally) and hyperthermia.
   d. **Chloral hydrate** is rapidly metabolized to trichloroethanol, which is probably responsible for its CNS and cardiac toxicities [49, 115]. The half-life of trichloroethanol is about 8 hours but may be prolonged during overdosage. In general, ingestions of more than 2 gm produce toxic symptoms, and blood levels (measured as trichloroethanol) exceeding 5 mg/dl are potentially lethal. Chloral hydrate is a gastric irritant, with nausea and vomiting often occurring after ingestions; in addition, gastric necrosis has been reported [49]. Cardiac toxicity (i.e., depression of myocardial contractility, sensitization of the myocardium to catecholamines, and ventricular and supraventricular arrhythmias) commonly occurs following overdoses. Other manifestations include hypothermia, miosis, and hepatic or renal injury.
3. **Treatment**
   a. **Gastric emptying,** followed by charcoal and cathartic administration, is indicated.
   b. **Supportive care** is the mainstay of therapy.
      (1) **Seizures.** Diazepam is the drug of choice for terminating seizures.
      (2) For **hypotension** unresponsive to fluid administration, dopamine or norepinephrine may be used.
      (3) **Arrhythmias.** Lidocaine, phenytoin, and beta-adrenergic antagonists have been used to terminate arrhythmias due to chloral hydrate [9].
      (4) **Hemoperfusion** is more effective than hemodialysis and is preferred for life-threatening overdoses not responding to supportive therapy.
4. **Disposition.** In general, hospitalization is recommended for overdoses with these sedative hypnotic drugs because of their prolonged durations of action. Cardiac monitoring is indicated for significant chloral hydrate intoxications and overdoses exhibiting cardiovascular toxicity.
R. **Opioids** are drugs with morphinelike properties. They can be divided into drugs derived from opium (e.g., codeine, morphine), semisynthesized from opium (e.g., heroin, oxycodone, oxymorphine), and completely synthesized (e.g., diphenoxylate, meperidine, methadone, pentazocine, propoxyphene). Although the manifestations and treatment of opioid overdoses are similar, individual drugs may have unique features. **Propoxyphene** has a direct cardiodepressant effect that may not be reversed with narcotic antagonists administered in the usually recommended doses [53, 58]. **Diphenoxylate** (Lomotil) has a delayed onset of toxic manifestations with the onset of respiratory depression occurring up to 14 hours postingestion, and **methadone** has a prolonged duration of action that may last up to 72 hours. **Pentazocine** (Talwin) has been abused in combination with tripelennamine (Pyribenzamine) to form a substance known as "Ts and Blues"; however, pentazocine tablets

have been reformulated and now contain naloxone (which is not active orally) to discourage illicit parenteral use of the tablets [18]. Blood and urine determinations are helpful in confirming the diagnosis of opioid intoxication.

1. **Clinical manifestations.** Opioid overdosage is characterized by the triad of a depressed mental status, respiratory depression, and miosis (mydiasis, however, may be present with meperidine overdose, hypoxia, or mixed-drug usage). Other features include the presence of needle marks and sclerosed vessels, hypo- or hyperthermia, hypo- or hyperglycemia, lymphadenopathy, lymphedema, amenorrhea, flushing, pruritus, and urticaria (due to opioid-induced histamine release). Death is usually due to respiratory depression.

2. **Complications of opioid overdosage**
   a. **Pulmonary complications. Pulmonary edema** is seen in virtually all fatal opioid overdoses [49]. It usually occurs soon after opioid use but may be delayed for up to 48 hours. Pulmonary embolism may occur secondary to right-sided endocarditis, thrombophlebitis, or injection of insoluble materials. Recurrent pulmonary emboli may lead to the syndrome of angiothrombotic pulmonary hypertension [105]. Aspiration pneumonitis is also a common complication of opioid overdose.
   b. **Infectious complications** include hepatitis, tetanus, cutaneous abscesses, cellulitis, lymphangitis, septic thrombophlebitis, endocarditis, pneumonia, osteomyelitis, septic arthritis, malaria, mycotic aneurysms, septic embolism, and necrotizing fasciitis.
   c. **Neurologic complications** include CNS depression, traumatic or atraumatic mononeuropathy, polyneuritis, transverse myelitis, Horner's syndrome (from neck injections), anoxic encephalopathy, and seizures (usually with meperidine or propoxyphene overdosage).
   d. **Cardiovascular complications** include hypotension (due to peripheral vasodilatation) and vagally-mediated bradycardia. Less commonly, arrhythmias (usually atrial fibrillation) and conduction disturbances may occur [9]. Vascular insufficiency may occur due to peripheral embolization, arterial injections, or vasculitis.
   e. **Muscular complications** include crush injuries (from prolonged rest on an extremity), compartment syndromes, and rhabdomyolysis.
   f. **Renal complications** include urinary retention and heroin nephropathy (e.g., focal-segmental glomerulosclerosis, epimembranous nephropathy, type I membranoproliferative glomerulonephritis, acute glomerulonephritis).
   g. Other complications associated with opioid abuse include an increased incidence of traumatic injuries and mixed-drug usage. Addicts may also present to emergency departments feigning pain syndromes (e.g., nephrolithiasis, migraine headache) to obtain opioids.

3. **Treatment.** The mainstay of therapy is **supportive care** with attention to providing a patent airway and adequate ventilation. Gastric emptying, followed by charcoal and cathartic administration, is indicated in oral ingestions.
   a. **Naloxone hydrochloride** is a useful diagnostic and therapeutic agent for opioid overdosage. Naloxone is a specific opioid antagonist effective in reversing the CNS and respiratory depression of opioids; it also reverses opioid-induced peripheral vasodilatation [22]. The initial dose is 0.4–2.0 mg IV; the higher dose is recommended in the presence of respiratory depression. If an IV line cannot be readily established, naloxone may be given IM or SQ; endotracheal administration is also effective [106]. If there is no response to the initial dose of naloxone, 2 mg should be given at 2- 3-minute intervals as needed; if there is no response to 10 mg of naloxone, the diagnosis of opioid overdose should be questioned. Large doses of naloxone may be needed to reverse the effects of propoxyphene, pentazocine, and large overdoses of other opioids. Since the half-life of naloxone is short (approximately 60 minutes), repeated doses or a naloxone drip may be required. A drip infusion is prepared by adding 4 mg of naloxone to 1 liter of 5% D/W and titrating to the desired effect, which usually requires 0.4 mg of naloxone/hour (100 ml/hour).
   b. **Pulmonary edema** is treated with oxygen, mechanical ventilation, and PEEP as needed; in addition, naloxone may be administered to reverse respiratory depression.
   c. **Hyperthermia** may be secondary to infection or injection of pyrogens. It is essential to obtain appropriate cultures, since infection with unusual organ-

isms may be involved. Appropriate antibiotic therapy is indicated when infection is present.

4. **Disposition.** All significant opioid overdoses should be admitted to the hospital, since these patients are at risk of developing delayed pulmonary edema. Also, if naloxone is used, symptoms may recur once the effects of the naloxone wear off. Patients who awaken after naloxone administration often are combative and agitated and want to leave the hospital. Attempts should be made to persuade these patients to be hospitalized; furthermore, if these patients are suicidal or deemed incapable of making rational decisions, they should not be allowed to leave the hospital, and reasonable physical restraint should be employed as needed.

S. **Phencyclidine** (PCP) is an illicit drug of abuse. It is sold on the street under a variety of names, the most common of which are PCP and angel dust. It is commonly smoked but may be snorted, ingested, or injected intravenously. Smoking or snorting the drug generally leads to absorption of less than 5 mg and results in low-dose intoxication (with serum levels < 30 ng/ml) in which behavioral disturbances predominate [6]. On the other hand, ingestion or intravenous injection of phencyclidine generally gives rise to severe intoxication characterized by prominent physiologic disturbances that may be life-threatening. Morbidity and mortality, however, generally are secondary to the drug's behavioral effects [49].

1. **Pharmacology and pharmacokinetics.** Phencyclidine is a highly lipid-soluble weak base (with a pK_a of 8.5) that is rapidly absorbed from the gastrointestinal tract [83]. Following absorption, phencyclidine readily distributes into various tissues, particularly the CNS and adipose tissue, with tissue levels greatly exceeding plasma levels [49]. It produces CNS stimulation or depression depending on the dose, has potent sympathomimetic and psychotomimetic properties, and is a dissociative anesthetic [90]. It also appears to have cholinergic properties [7]. Phencyclidine is eliminated from the body primarily by hepatic metabolism and by renal excretion of inactive metabolites and, to a lesser extent, by renal excretion of free phencyclidine. In addition, the drug is secreted into the stomach and later absorbed from the alkaline small intestine [6]. The half-life of phencyclidine is from 7–46 hours, depending on the dosage [7].

2. The **cardinal features** of phencyclidine intoxication encompass the triad of an altered mental status (e.g., agitation, confusion, violent or bizarre behavior, psychosis, catatonia, stupor, coma), hypertension (which may be severe), and horizontal or vertical nystagmus. Tachycardia, hyperpyrexia, diaphoresis, ataxia, sensory anesthesia, hyperreflexia, hypertonicity, hypersecretions, bronchospasm, and seizures are other features of phencyclidine intoxication. With massive overdosage, hypotension, apnea, areflexia, and status epilepticus may occur. Rhabdomyolysis (with myoglobinuria) from involuntary hypermotor activity and resultant renal failure are common complications of severe overdosage.

3. **Treatment**
   a. **Gastric emptying is not recommended in conscious patients,** unless there is evidence of a substantial ingestion. For severe overdosage with coma, gastric lavage (after the airway has been protected by tracheal intubation, which must be performed with care to avoid inducing laryngospasm) should be undertaken and followed by administration of activated charcoal and a cathartic.
   b. Because of the gastric secretion of phencyclidine, repetitive administration of **activated charcoal** in a dosage of 50 gm q2–4h is indicated in severe overdosage to enhance gastrointestinal clearance of the drug.
   c. Since phencyclidine is a renally excreted weak base, **forced acid diuresis** (see sec. **I.F.1.b**) markedly increases urinary clearance of the drug [6]. However, because of the marked tissue distribution (i.e., large volume of distribution) of the drug and the fact that most of the drug undergoes hepatic metabolism, the efficacy of forced acid diuresis in removing the drug from the body is in doubt. Until this issue is clarified (through clinical studies), forced acid diuresis probably should be attempted unless the risks of the procedure outweigh the potential benefits. In low-dose intoxications, urinary acidification may be attempted with oral ascorbic acid and cranberry juice. In severe overdoses, the standard procedure (see sec. **I.F.1.b**) may be followed. Urinary acidification, however, must be avoided in the presence of rhabdomyolysis because of the tendency to increase renal deposition of

myoglobin. Hemodialysis is not indicated unless there is renal insufficiency.

  d. Appropriate **supportive measures** should be instituted as indicated.
    (1) The **behavioral toxicity** of phencyclidine is best managed by providing a **quiet, nonthreatening, protective environment** and minimizing sensory input. For low-dose intoxications, this may be all that is required. If necessary, diazepam may be used to manage agitation, and haloperidol, the psychotomimetic drug effects.
    (2) Propranolol may be used to reverse serious **adrenergic effects.**
    (3) Diazoxide, nitroprusside, or phentolamine may be used to treat severe **hypertension.**
    (4) Diphenhydramine may be used to treat **dystonic reactions.**
    (5) Diazepam is the drug of choice for terminating **seizures.**
    (6) Pancuronium bromide may be required to manage uncontrollable **motor activity.**
    (7) Aminophylline is the drug of choice for treating **bronchospasm.**
    (8) **Hyperpyrexia** should be treated with appropriate cooling measures.
  4. **Disposition.** Patients with low-dose intoxication, characterized primarily by behavioral disturbances, generally can be discharged from the emergency department after symptoms resolve (unless psychiatric admission is warranted). These patients should be instructed to take ascorbic acid tablets and drink cranberry juice. In addition, a short course of diazepam or haloperidol (with diphenhydramine) and propranolol may be beneficial. Patients with more severe intoxication, characterized by significant physiologic disturbances, however, generally should be admitted to a medical service.
T. **Phenothiazines** generally are used as antipsychotic and antiemetic agents. They can be divided into three categories: (1) **aliphatic derivatives** (e.g., chlorpromazine, promazine, trifluopromazine), which produce the highest incidence of autonomic effects (e.g., hypotension, miosis, dry mucous membranes); (2) **piperidyl derivatives** (e.g., thioridazine, mesoridazine), which have the lowest incidence of extrapyramidal and anticholinergic side effects but the highest frequency of adverse electrophysiologic cardiotoxic effects (with thioridazine being the phenothiazine most commonly responsible for cardiac complications); and (3) **piperazine derivatives** (e.g., prochlorperazine, trifluoperazine, fluphenazine), which produce the greatest incidence of extrapyramidal reactions and may produce agitation before CNS depression occurs but are the least likely of the phenothiazines to produce hypotension and sedation. Overdoses with as little as 2 gm can cause death, with thioridazine, mesoridazine, and chlorpromazine being the agents most commonly implicated in lethal overdoses. The phenothiazines, however, generally are safe agents with a high therapeutic index, and death from overdosage is rare [49]. The biologic effects of a single dose of phenothiazines usually persist for at least 24 hours [38]. Phenothiazine levels may help confirm the diagnosis but often do not correlate with the clinical presentation due to variations in individual responses and the presence of active metabolites.
  1. **Clinical manifestations** of overdosage include a spectrum from confusion, agitation, and delirium to CNS depression. Other manifestations include respiratory depression, hypotension (commonly orthostatic hypotension due to alpha-adrenergic blockade), anticholinergic signs, extrapyramidal reactions (e.g., dystonic reactions, akathisia, parkinsonian syndrome), obstructive jaundice, photosensitivity, loss of thermoregulation (which may be responsible for hypo- or hyperthermia), and seizures. Cardiovascular toxicity is related to anticholinergic properties, alpha-adrenergic blockade, and a quinidinelike effect of the phenothiazines [9, 78]. Arrhythmias and conduction disturbances may occur; the ECG may show prolongation of the PR, QT, and QRS intervals, as well as slurring or notching of the T wave and ST-segment depression. Chronic phenothiazine usage has been associated with cardiac arrhythmias and conduction disturbances, as well as a tardive dyskinesia (especially in older patients).
  2. **Treatment**
    a. Although the phenothiazines have antiemetic properties, **ipecac** generally is effective in inducing vomiting [39]. In patients who are unresponsive to ipecac or have contraindications to induced emesis, gastric lavage should be performed. Gastric emptying should be followed by administration of charcoal and a cathartic.
    b. **Extrapyramidal reactions** may be treated with diphenhydramine hydro-

chloride, 25–50 mg IV (IM or PO), or benztropine mesylate, 1–2 mg IV (IM or PO), as needed. Patients who are discharged from the emergency department should receive continued outpatient therapy for 48–72 hours [24] with diphenhydramine hydrochloride, 25–50 mg PO q6h, or benztropine mesylate, 1–2 mg PO q12h.

   c. Hypotension is treated with intravenous saline. If a vasopressor is needed, norepinephrine is recommended. Drugs with beta-adrenergic activity generally should be avoided, since they may worsen the hypotension [9].

   d. Because of the potential for **cardiac arrhythmias,** patients with significant phenothiazine overdosage, especially those with acute ECG changes, should be monitored for at least 24 hours. Lidocaine and phenytoin are the agents of choice for treating ventricular arrhythmias. Quinidine and procainamide, however, are contraindicated. Cardiac pacing may be useful in managing high-degree atrioventricular block or refractory ventricular tachycardia [49, 66].

U. The **salicylates** include acetylsalicylic acid (aspirin), sodium salicylate, salicylic acid, and methyl salicylate (oil of wintergreen). Overdosage, which is most often due to ingestion of acetylsalicylic acid, may be accidental, intentional, or the result of unintentional excessive administration of a salicylate-containing preparation. Acute ingestion of greater than 150 mg/kg (or 10 gm in an adult) generally leads to toxic manifestations, and a dose of more than 500 mg/kg is potentially lethal [107]. Toxicity is generally associated with plasma levels exceeding 30 mg/dl. In acute overdosage, the severity of intoxication correlates well with plasma salicylate levels, but in chronic intoxication (salicylism) the correlation is poor [107].

  1. Pharmacokinetics

    a. Absorption and distribution. In usual dosages, salicylates are rapidly absorbed from the gastrointestinal tract, but in overdosage, absorption may be markedly delayed due to impaired gastric emptying [96]. During absorption through the intestinal mucosa and first-pass through the liver, salicylates are rapidly hydrolyzed to salicylic acid, which is a weak acid with a pK_a of 3.0 [57]. Salicylic acid readily distributes into various tissues, including the CNS; and partition into these tissues is enhanced by acidemia [57].

    b. Elimination from the body is by hepatic metabolism of salicylic acid and renal excretion of the metabolites and free salicylate. At higher doses and particularly in overdosage, the two major hepatic metabolic pathways become saturated, and the elimination kinetics change from first-order to zero-order [49, 97]. As a result, the half-life of salicylate is increased from 2–6 hours to 20–30 hours at toxic levels, and the percentage of free salicylate excreted in the urine is increased.

  2. Major pathophysiologic effects of toxic doses of salicylates include the following [107, 108]:

    a. Initial stimulation and terminal depression of the CNS (including the respiratory center).

    b. Uncoupling of oxidative phosphorylation, leading to increased carbohydrate metabolism with resultant increased utilization of oxygen and glucose (glycolysis) and increased production of carbon dioxide and heat.

    c. Stimulation of lipid metabolism with formation of ketone bodies.

    d. Inhibition of Krebs cycle enzymes, leading to increased production of pyruvic and lactic acids.

    e. Inhibition of amino acid metabolism, resulting in increased blood levels of amino acids and aminoaciduria.

    f. Increased fluid and electrolyte losses, leading to dehydration, sodium, and potassium depletion, and loss of buffer capacity.

    g. Interference with hemostatic mechanisms due to increased capillary fragility, impaired platelet adhesiveness, and although usually insignificant, decreased synthesis of coagulation factors.

    h. Noncardiogenic pulmonary edema.

  3. Clinical features. Nausea, vomiting, and diaphoresis are common. **CNS manifestations** are prominent and include tinnitus, decreased auditory acuity, an altered mental status (e.g., agitation, disorientation, lethargy, coma), and seizures. **Acid-base disturbances** are common. Whereas infants and young children commonly develop a metabolic acidosis, adults usually develop a respiratory alkalosis or a combined respiratory alkalosis and metabolic acidosis. Hyperpyrexia and hypovolemia are other features of salicylate intoxication.

Electrolyte disturbances, particularly hypokalemia and hyper- or hypoglycemia, may also be encountered. Significant coagulation abnormalities, however, are unusual. Gastrointestinal bleeding (although usually not serious), pulmonary edema, and, rarely, renal failure may complicate the poisoning. Death, when it occurs, is usually due to respiratory failure or cardiovascular collapse and in animals has been shown to correlate with CNS salicylate levels [57]; acid-base and metabolic disturbances (particularly hypoglycemia) likely are contributing factors.

4. **Treatment**
   a. **Gastric emptying** by either induced emesis or lavage, followed by administration of activated charcoal and a cathartic, is indicated.
   b. **Salicylate levels** should be monitored. It should be remembered, however, that levels obtained less than 6 hours postingestion may be spuriously low due to incomplete absorption, and in chronic intoxication, levels correlate poorly with the severity of intoxication.
   c. **Correction of systemic acidosis,** if present, with sodium bicarbonate IV is particularly important to increase the ionized fraction of salicylic acid and thus decrease CNS levels and the CNS toxicity of the drug [57]. In addition, hypovolemia, hypoglycemia, hypokalemia, hyperpyrexia, and, uncommonly, hypoprothrombinemia require correction if present.
   d. **Forced alkaline diuresis** (see sec. I.F.1.a) is indicated, since it markedly accelerates elimination of salicylic acid [107]. Urinary alkalinization should be attempted with sodium bicarbonate (initially, 1–2 ampules in a liter of 0.45% saline). Acetazolamide should not be used, since it produces systemic acidosis and thus increases salicylate toxicity [108]. Potassium repletion is required to alkalinize the urine.
   e. **Hemodialysis and hemoperfusion** are both effective in eliminating salicylate from the body, but the former is preferred because of its ability to correct acid-base and electrolyte disturbances. Extracorporeal removal of salicylate is indicated in the following situations: life-threatening intoxication (e.g., coma, status epilepticus, respiratory or cardiovascular insufficiency, unresponsive acidosis, plasma salicylate level exceeding 100 mg/dl [49]), renal insufficiency, or inability to achieve or perform an alkaline diuresis when needed.
5. **Disposition.** The decision to hospitalize a patient with salicylate overdosage depends on the clinical status of the patient, the plasma salicylate level, and the ability to treat the intoxication in the emergency department. Generally, patients with a plasma salicylate level greater than 50 mg/dl, serious acid-base or electrolyte disturbances (particularly a metabolic acidosis), and prominent toxic signs and symptoms warrant hospitalization. The last is particularly important in determining the need for hospitalization in chronic salicylism because of the poor correlation between plasma levels and the severity of intoxication. For acute intoxications treated in the emergency department, patients may be discharged when the plasma level declines to approximately 30 mg/dl.

V. **Theophylline** is used primarily as a bronchodilator in the therapy of asthma and chronic obstructive pulmonary disease. Since the drug has a narrow therapeutic window, toxicity commonly results from inadvertent excessive therapeutic doses, particularly in the presence of factors that impair its plasma clearance (e.g., hepatic disease, congestive heart failure). In addition, intentional overdoses may lead to severe toxicity.
   1. **Pharmacology and pharmacokinetics**
      a. **Absorption and elimination.** Short-acting preparations (e.g., aminophylline) are rapidly and nearly completely absorbed from the gastrointestinal tract, with peak blood levels occurring within 2 hours of ingestion [49]. On the other hand, sustained-release preparations (e.g., Theo-Dur) generally attain peak blood levels from 5–10 hours postingestion [49]. Theophylline is metabolized in the liver to relatively inactive metabolites that are excreted in the urine; less than 15% of theophylline is excreted unchanged in the urine [56]. Elimination is generally by first-order kinetics; but in higher doses and particularly in overdosage, saturation of metabolic pathways may occur with resultant decrease in the drug's clearance and prolongation of its half-life, which in adults normally averages about 8 hours [56, 112]. Numerous other factors including age, diet, certain drugs (e.g., cimetidine, erythromycin, marijuana, phenobarbital, phenytoin, propranolol), cigarette smok-

ing, hepatic disease, and congestive heart failure affect the clearance of theophylline and consequently its half-life [49, 56].

    b. Bronchodilatation is directly proportional to the logarithm of the plasma concentration of theophylline over a range of 5–20 µg/ml [75]. Although further bronchodilatation likely occurs at concentrations exceeding 20 µg/ml, the progressive increase in toxicity at these concentrations outweighs any added bronchodilator effect and precludes use of these concentrations. Since maximal bronchodilatation with minimal toxicity occurs at concentrations of 10–20 µg/ml, this narrow range is considered the therapeutic range of theophylline.

  2. Toxic manifestations. Although toxic manifestations may occur at theophylline plasma concentrations less than 20 µg/ml, they are common at concentrations exceeding this level, increasing in frequency and severity the higher the plasma level. Toxicity may be classified as minor or major. **Minor toxicity** includes mild CNS disturbances (e.g., headache, anxiety, nervousness, tremulousness, insomnia), gastrointestinal upset (e.g., anorexia, nausea, vomiting, diarrhea, abdominal pain), and a sinus tachycardia. **Major toxicity,** which frequently is not heralded by signs of minor toxicity [55, 118], includes seizures, serious cardiac arrhythmias (e.g., supraventricular tachycardia, ventricular arrhythmias, asystole), hypotension, and cardiac arrest. Although seizures have been reported at a theophylline level of 25 µg/ml [118], they usually are associated with levels exceeding 30 µg/ml [81]; they frequently are refractory to therapy and thus have a high mortality [81, 118]. A sinus tachycardia usually is present in theophylline toxicity, whereas serious cardiac arrhythmias generally occur at theophylline levels exceeding 35 µg/ml [55]. A distinction should be made between **chronic and acute theophylline intoxication,** since in the former situation seizures and serious arrhythmias are more likely to occur at lower serum levels than in the latter [79a]. In one study, patients with theophylline overdose caused by chronic repeated overmedication frequently developed seizures and serious arrhythmias with serum levels of 40-70 µg/ml, whereas those with acute single ingestion were unlikely to suffer these serious complications until serum levels exceeded 100 µg/ml; in addition, hypotension occurred only in association with acute intoxication and then much more commonly at serum levels exceeding 100 µg/ml [79a].

  3. Management

    a. Cardiac monitoring is indicated in the presence of a theophylline plasma level exceeding 35 µg/ml or signs of major toxicity.

    b. For oral overdoses of theophylline, **gastric emptying** by induced emesis with ipecac or gastric lavage, followed by administration of activated charcoal and a cathartic, is indicated.

    c. Repetitive doses of **activated charcoal,** 30 gm PO or by gastric tube q2h, has been demonstrated to increase the plasma clearance of theophylline [67] and is recommended.

    d. Diazepam is the drug of choice for treating **seizures**. Phenytoin and phenobarbital may be added as needed.

    e. Lidocaine is the drug of choice for treating ventricular **arrhythmias;** procainamide may also be used. Serious supraventricular arrhythmias may be treated with propranolol (unless contraindicated) or verapamil.

    f. Hemoperfusion is more effective than hemodialysis and is indicated in potentially life-threatening intoxications (i.e., presence of intractable seizures, resistant serious arrhythmias, or hypotension not responding to fluids; or serum level > 60 µg/ml in chronic overdose or > 100 µg/ml in acute overdose) and serious intoxications in which there is impaired clearance of the drug (i.e., serum level > 40 µg/ml in the presence of liver disease, congestive heart failure, or respiratory failure) [79a].

  4. Disposition. Patients with a plasma theophylline level exceeding 25 µg/ml should be observed in the emergency department (if possible) or hospitalized until the level declines below that value. If the level exceeds 35 µg/ml or there are signs of major toxicity, admission to an intensive care unit is warranted.

W. Toxic inhalants include a wide variety of noxious gases and particulate matter. The toxic mechanisms of these inhalants include local irritation, systemic toxicity, asphyxiation, and hypersensitivity reactions. The toxic inhalants may exhibit any combination of these mechanisms. In managing victims of toxic inhalant exposure,

it is important to **identify the offending inhalant** and **contact the regional poison control center** for specific therapeutic guidelines.
1. **Irritant gases**
   a. **Clinical manifestations** of irritant gas exposure include cutaneous burns, mucosal irritation, laryngotracheitis, bronchitis, pneumonitis, bronchospasm, and pulmonary edema (which may be delayed up to 24 hours after exposure). In general, the more water-soluble gases (e.g., chlorine, ammonia, formaldehyde, sulfur dioxide, ozone) are very irritating to mucous membranes, causing inflammation of the eyes, throat, and upper respiratory tract. In contrast, the less soluble gases (e.g., phosgene, nitrogen dioxide) are less irritating to the mucosae but tend to cause more damage to the peripheral airways and alveoli.
   b. **Evaluation.** In addition to the physical examination, an ABG and chest x-ray should be obtained initially and repeated in 12–24 hours. Other tests (e.g., ECG, spirometry, xenon ventilation-perfusion lung scan, carbon monoxide level) should be obtained as indicated.
   c. **Treatment.** General management principles are as follows:
      (1) **Airway.** Patients who develop significant oropharyngeal or laryngeal edema need a patent airway established, preferably by endotracheal intubation. If endotracheal intubation is not possible, transtracheal catheter ventilation (see Chap. 38), cricothyrotomy (see Chap. 38), or tracheostomy should be performed.
      (2) Symptomatic patients should receive humidified **oxygen.**
      (3) The treatment of noncardiogenic **pulmonary edema** consists of respiratory support with oxygen, mechanical ventilation, and the use of PEEP as needed (see Chap. 7).
      (4) **Bronchospasm** is treated with bronchodilators (see Chap 7).
      (5) In chemical **contamination of the skin,** the clothing should be removed and the residual chemical washed off the patient's body. Cutaneous skin burns may be treated by local cleansing, application of a topical burn cream (e.g., silver sulfadiazine), and administration of tetanus prophylaxis (if needed).
      (6) **Chemical contact with the eye** should be treated with immediate eye irrigation. For treatment of corneal abrasions or caustic eye burns (as may occur from ammonia exposure), see Chap. 35.
      (7) In general, routine use of steroids is not recommended; however, in certain toxic inhalations (e.g., nitrogen dioxide), the use of steroids may be warranted. Routine use of prophylactic antibiotics is not indicated.
   d. **Disposition.** Patients who are asymptomatic or have minor symptoms (e.g., conjunctivitis, minor skin burns) may be discharged from the emergency department after an observation period of at least 6 hours if still essentially asymptomatic. These patients should be referred for follow-up in 24 hours and be given instructions to return to the emergency department if symptoms develop. In general, patients with pulmonary symptoms or signs, a new infiltrate on a chest radiograph, or hypoxemia should be admitted to the hospital (particularly in nonsoluble gas inhalations) due to the risk of serious, delayed pulmonary complications.
2. **Systemic toxicity** may occur from a variety of inhaled agents. Specific systemic toxins include the following:
   a. **Hydrogen sulfide** gas has the odor of rotten eggs. Exposure may occur in people who work with decaying organic material (e.g., decomposing fish, sewage) or in workers in the petrochemical or tanning industries. Hydrogen sulfide toxicity is thought to be due to inhibition of cytochrome oxidase (as in cyanide toxicity).
      (1) **Clinical manifestations** include keratoconjunctivitis, rhinitis, pharyngitis, bronchitis, pneumonia, pulmonary edema, metabolic acidosis, cardiac arrhythmias, mental status changes (including coma), and respiratory arrest.
      (2) **Treatment** consists of vigorous **supportive care.** Severe cases are treated similarly to cyanide poisoning (see sec. **II.H.3**) with the use of nitrite-induced methemoglobinemia. However, there is no need to give sodium thiosulfate [63].

b. Methyl bromide is used as a fumigant for grain, fruit, and other produce.

    (1) Clinical manifestations of toxicity may occur after a latency period of up to 12 hours and include dizziness, ataxia, tremor, headache, nausea, vomiting, abdominal pain, malaise, blurred vision, and dyspnea. Severe poisoning may exhibit a polyneuropathy, hallucinations, a toxic psychosis, seizures, and coma.

    (2) Treatment consists of removing the patient's clothes and cleansing contaminated skin. Further treatment consists of symptomatic and supportive care.

c. Metal fume inhalation may occur during the smelting, galvanizing, or welding of metals. A syndrome known as metal fume fever commonly occurs after inhalation of fumes from a variety of metals.

    (1) Clinical manifestations of metal fume fever usually occur within 4–8 hours after exposure and include a sense of thirst, a metallic taste in the mouth, rigors, fever, diaphoresis, weakness, and myalgias. Less commonly, cough, dyspnea, rales, wheezing, leukocytosis, and pulmonary infiltrates may occur. The course is usually benign, with resolution of symptoms occurring within 24–48 hours.

    (2) Treatment includes **symptomatic care** (e.g., administration of supplemental oxygen and bronchodilators) as needed. Steroids may be of benefit if respiratory tract injury occurs [27].

    (3) Disposition. Hospitalization is recommended for toxic patients and patients with evidence of significant pulmonary involvement (e.g., dyspnea, pulmonary infiltrates, hypoxemia). Asymptomatic or mildly symptomatic patients should be observed for at least 6 hours prior to discharge and should return for a follow-up visit 24 hours after release.

d. Organophosphates (e.g., chlorthion, parathion, malathion) are used as pesticides. Their toxicity is due to inhibition of acetylcholinesterase.

    (1) Clinical manifestations result from increased cholinergic activity and include the following [38, 49]:

        (a) Muscarinic effects (from stimulation of postganglionic autonomic effector cells): salivation, lacrimation, urinary and fecal incontinence, vomiting, diarrhea, diaphoresis, miosis, bronchospasm, bradycardia.

        (b) Nicotinic effects (from stimulation of autonomic ganglion cells and skeletal muscle end plates): muscle fasciculations, weakness, paralysis, hypertension, tachycardia.

        (c) CNS signs: anxiety, ataxia, tremor, slurred speech, restlessness, confusion, seizures, coma, cardiopulmonary depression.

    (2) Treatment. In significant organophosphate poisonings, **atropine,** 1–5 mg IV, should be administered and repeated q15 minutes until muscarinic signs are relieved (e.g., decreased secretions, reversal of miosis and bradycardia); large doses of atropine may be necessary. In severe poisonings with muscle weakness or fasciculations, **pralidoxime** (2-PAM) chloride in a dosage of 1 gm (diluted in 100 ml of normal saline) should be given IV over 15–30 minutes and repeated q8–12h for up to 3 doses, as needed.

    (3) Disposition. Hospitalization is warranted for all patients with evidence of organophosphate poisoning.

e. Other systemic toxic inhalants include cyanide (see sec. **II.H**), carbon monoxide (see sec. **II.E**), and hydrocarbons (see sec. **II.L**).

3. Simple asphyxiants (e.g., acetylene, helium, hydrogen, nitrogen, methane, butane, neon, nitrous oxide, carbon dioxide, natural gas) are physiologically inert gases that deprive the tissues of oxygen by displacement of oxygen from the inspired air. Generally, symptoms occur when these gases comprise 20–30 ml/dl of the inspired air. Morbidity and mortality are related to the degree and duration of the hypoxia. Symptomatic patients should be evaluated for hypoxic injury (e.g., with an ECG, chest x-ray, ABG) as indicated. **Treatment** consists of administering supplemental oxygen to symptomatic patients and providing supportive care as needed. Hospitalization is indicated for patients with evidence of significant hypoxic complications (e.g., cardiac ischemia, mental status changes, metabolic acidosis).

4. Hypersensitivity reactions may occur from inhalation of an antigen causing a humoral immune response. This immunologic reaction may cause release of vasoactive substances (asthma), formation of an antigen-antibody complex (hypersensitivity pneumonitis), or a combination of these responses.

a. **Occupational asthma** (immediate hypersensitivity reaction) may occur secondary to inhalation of a variety of antigens, including dust from cotton, hemp, grain, and wood. Inhalation of toluene diisocyanate used in the manufacture of polyurethane foams, adhesives, insulation fibers, and other plastic materials may also cause an immediate hypersensitivity reaction, as well as causing mucosal irritation and gastrointestinal and CNS toxicity. **Management** consists of avoiding reexposure and treating the bronchospasm as an acute asthma attack (see Chap. 7).

b. **Hypersensitivity pneumonitis** (extrinsic allergic alveolitis) occurs from exposure to organic dusts such as that found in moldy hay (farmer's lung), thermophilic molds found in air conditioning or humidification equipment (humidifier lung), mushroom compost, and droppings of parakeets, pigeons, and budgerigars (bird-breeder's lung).

   (1) **Clinical manifestations** of hypersensitivity pneumonitis usually occur within 4–8 hours after exposure and include fever, chills, malaise, anorexia, nausea, headache, chest tightness, nonproductive cough, dyspnea, and, occasionally, an infiltrate on chest radiograph. Improvement usually occurs within 12–24 hours after the patient is removed from the antigenic source. Repeated exposures may cause a productive cough, dyspnea, easy fatigability, and weight loss. In chronic exposures, pulmonary fibrosis may occur.

   (2) **Treatment is** aimed at avoidance of exposure. Acute symptoms are treated symptomatically (e.g., with bronchodilators, oxygen), as needed. The use of steroids may decrease systemic toxicity and hasten resolution of the pulmonary disease [47].

5. **Pneumoconiosis** is a fibrorestrictive disease of the lungs caused by chronic exposure to inorganic dusts. It is characterized by the gradual onset of a cough and progressive dyspnea. Disease entities caused by specific exposures include silicosis (which is commonly complicated by a mycobacterium superinfection of the lungs), asbestosis (which is associated with an increased incidence of bronchogenic carcinoma, mesothelioma, and gastrointestinal tract neoplasms), and coal worker's pneumoconiosis (miner's lung). Treatment is primarily symptomatic.

6. **Smoke inhalation** (see Chap. 21) can cause injury by a combination of thermal damage (usually confined to the upper respiratory tract), simple asphyxiation, and inhalation of noxious fumes. Smoke is composed of carbon particles that are coated with products of combustion (e.g., organic acids and aldehydes) and suspended in a heated gas. The gaseous fraction consists of carbon monoxide, carbon dioxide, and a variety of toxic gases that may be released from thermal degradation of man-made and natural materials (e.g., hydrogen chloride, phosgene, chlorine, benzene, isocyanate, hydrogen cyanide, aldehydes, oxides of sulfur and nitrogen, ammonia, and numerous organic acids). These toxins produce epithelial injury with resultant airway edema, increased capillary permeability, and mechanical obstruction from desquamated tissue and secretions. Bronchoscopy and xenon lung scanning are useful in confirming the diagnosis.

a. **Clinical features.** Expectoration of carbonaceous sputum and respiratory distress from asphyxiation, upper airway edema, bronchospasm, and/or noncardiogenic pulmonary edema are characteristic features. In addition, upper airway burns may be noted.

b. **Treatment** of victims of smoke inhalation involves **supportive care,** including ensuring a patent airway and adequate ventilation, administering humidified oxygen (to symptomatic patients), and treating specific toxic inhalants (e.g., carbon monoxide, cyanide), as needed.

c. **Disposition.** Hospitalization is indicated for all patients with evidence of significant smoke inhalation (e.g., symptoms, signs, or laboratory evidence of cardiac, CNS or pulmonary dysfunction; a carbon monoxide level greater than 20%). Patients with a history of smoke inhalation who are asymptomatic or have minimal symptoms may be observed in the emergency department for at least 6 hours and discharged if still essentially asymptomatic, with a follow-up visit in 24 hours.

X. The **tricyclic antidepressants** (TCAs) include tertiary amines (imipramine, amitriptyline, and doxepin) and secondary amines (desipramine, nortriptyline, and protriptyline). Desipramine and nortriptyline are pharmacologically active metabolites of imipramine and amitriptyline, respectively. The TCAs, which possess antidepressant, sedative, and anticholinergic properties, have a narrow therapeutic index. Although total tricyclic antidepressant serum levels have been reported to correlate with severity of intoxication in overdosage, with levels exceeding 1000 ng/ml signifying severe intoxication [11, 88], the electrocardiogram appears to be a better predictor of clinical severity in acute antidepressant overdose [11a]. In a recent study, the maximum limb-lead QRS duration predicted the risk of seizures (QRS $\geq$ 0.10 second) and ventricular arrhythmias (QRS $\geq$ 0.16 second), with all seizures and ventricular arrhythmias occurring within 6 hours of overdose, whereas serum drug levels failed to accurately predict the risk of these serious complications [11a]. The lethal dose is generally greater than 35 mg/kg [97]. In one study, virtually all fatalities from direct tricyclic antidepressant toxicity occurred within 24 hours of drug ingestion and were heralded by the appearance of major signs of toxicity (i.e., depressed level of consciousness, depressed respirations, hypotension, arrhythmias, conduction disturbances, or seizures) within 2 hours of presentation [17].

  1. Pharmacology, pharmacokinetics, and toxicology. The tricyclic antidepressants are lipid-soluble weak bases with a pK_a of 9.5 [16].

    a. Absorption and distribution. In therapeutic dosages, the tricyclic antidepressants are rapidly absorbed from the gastrointestinal tract, but in overdosage, absorption may be markedly delayed due to the anticholinergic effect of the drugs. Following absorption, the tricyclic antidepressants are 85–95% bound to plasma proteins (with the unbound drug being pharmacologically active) and extensively distributed and bound to various tissues, with tissue levels about 10 times plasma levels [16]. Both plasma protein binding and tissue distribution are affected by the pH, with both increasing with an increase in pH [49].

    b. Elimination is by hepatic metabolism and renal excretion of metabolites. The tertiary amines are metabolized to pharmacologically active secondary amines that are then inactivated in the liver. In addition, the tricyclic antidepressants are excreted into the biliary tract and stomach and later resorbed from the small bowel (enterohepatic recirculation) [49]. The half-lives of these drugs vary from 10–80 hours in therapeutic dosages [38] but generally are much longer in overdosage.

    c. The **pharmacologic and toxic actions** of the tricyclic antidepressants are due to four mechanisms [16, 68]:

      (1) Blockade of norepinephrine reuptake by adrenergic nerve endings (the amine pump), leading to sympathomimetic and presumably antidepressant effects.

      (2) Inhibition of acetylcholine at neuroreceptor sites, resulting in central and peripheral anticholinergic effects.

      (3) A direct quinidine-like action on the myocardium that may lead to impaired intracardiac conduction, depression of myocardial contractility, and arrhythmias.

      (4) Peripheral alpha-adrenergic receptor blockade contributing to hypotension.

  2. Clinical manifestations of tricyclic antidepressant overdoses result from the drugs' CNS effects, peripheral anticholinergic properties, and the direct and indirect (autonomic) cardiovascular effects.

    a. CNS signs include an altered mental status (e.g., agitation, disorientation, hallucinations, stupor, coma), myoclonus, seizures, respiratory depression, and pyramidal signs (e.g., clonus, hyperreflexia).

    b. Peripheral anticholinergic signs are tachycardia, hypertension, mydriasis, dry mucous membranes and skin, hyperpyrexia, ileus, and urinary retention.

    c. Cardiovascular effects include supraventricular and ventricular arrhythmias, conduction disturbances, hypotension, and pulmonary edema.

  3. Treatment

    a. Gastric emptying by induced emesis or gastric lavage is required and should be followed by administration of activated charcoal and a cathartic.

    b. Repetitive doses of **activated charcoal**, 50 gm PO or by gastric tube q2–4h, may be of benefit in enhancing elimination of the tricyclic antidepressants because of their biliary and gastric excretion.

  c. **Management of cardiovascular complications. Alkalinization of the blood** to a pH of 7.5 by administration of **sodium bicarbonate** IV or induced hyperventilation is the therapy of choice for reversing arrhythmias [15], conduction disturbances, and hypotension of tricyclic antidepressant overdoses. The mechanism is unclear but may be related to increasing the plasma protein binding of the drug, thereby decreasing the proportion of the pharmacologically active component in the circulation [16]. Additional therapy of cardiovascular disturbances, however, may be required as follows.

  (1) For **hypotension** unresponsive to alkalinization and a fluid challenge, norepinephrine is the vasopressor of choice.

  (2) For **serious supraventricular tachyarrhythmias** requiring specific antiarrhythmic therapy, physostigmine, 1–2 mg IV slowly q30–60 minutes, propranolol, or verapamil may be used. These drugs, however, generally should be avoided in the presence of conduction disturbances.

  (3) For **ventricular arrhythmias,** lidocaine or phenytoin is indicated. Overdrive pacing may be of benefit in terminating ventricular tachycardia, and bretylium tosylate should be considered for refractory ventricular tachycardia or fibrillation. Although electrical cardioversion may be ineffective, it should be attempted when indicated. Quinidine, procainamide, and disopyramide are contraindicated because of their membrane-depressant effects.

  (4) **Conduction disturbances and bradycardia.** Phenytoin in a dosage of 5–7 mg/kg IV at a rate of 50 mg/minute has been shown to be effective in reversing the conduction disturbances of tricyclic antidepressant overdoses [50]. Isoproterenol and/or cardiac pacing, however, may be needed to manage bradycardia and high-grade atrioventricular block. Atropine should be avoided because of the anticholinergic effects of the tricyclic drugs.

  d. Diazepam is the drug of choice for terminating **seizures**; physostigmine may also be used. Phenytoin or phenobarbital should be used to treat sustained or repetitive seizures.

  e. Physostigmine salicylate generally will reverse the **coma** and **delirium** of tricyclic antidepressant overdose but should be used only if these manifestations become life-threatening to the patient.

  f. Dialysis and hemoperfusion generally are considered not to be of benefit in the management of tricyclic overdose because of the marked tissue binding and large volume of distribution of these drugs [49].

  4. **Disposition.** Patients with a history of tricyclic antidepressant overdose require observation for at least 6 hours. If at any time a major sign of toxicity (i.e., decreased level of consciousness, respiratory depression, hypotension, arrhythmias including a sinus tachycardia with a rate of 120/minute or more, conduction disturbances, or seizures) develops, admission to an intensive care unit for monitoring and intensive supportive care is required [17]. However, if after 6 hours of observation, no major signs of toxicity have developed and the patient is on an improving or stable course, the patient may be discharged with psychiatric follow-up, unless there are complicating factors warranting hospitalization (e.g., an ileus, suicide ideation).

Drug Withdrawal

Drug withdrawal is a syndrome characterized by a constellation of clinical manifestations of a psychic and physical nature following the abrupt discontinuation of a drug that causes physical dependence and is taken in large doses over a prolonged period of time. Drug withdrawal manifestations are thought to result from CNS counteradaptation to the agonist actions of a drug; when the drug is discontinued or antagonized, rebound phenomena occur that generally affect the same physiologic systems that were modified initially by the drug (e.g., withdrawal of a sedative/hypnotic, which elevates the seizure threshold, may cause spontaneous seizures) [38]. Drug withdrawal syndromes are associated with ethanol, opioids, barbiturates, benzodiazepines, nonbarbiturate sedative/hypnotics, and amphetamines.

I. **Ethanol withdrawal syndromes** characteristically occur in patients who have consumed large quantities of alcohol over a prolonged period of time.

A. Clinical syndromes
  1. **The minor ethanol withdrawal syndrome** usually occurs about 6 hours after cessation or reduction of alcohol consumption and subsides within 7 days. The minor alcohol withdrawal syndrome is characterized by a coarse tremor, anorexia, nausea, vomiting, malaise, generalized weakness, anxiety, depression, irritability, tendency to startle easily, insomnia, hyperreflexia, headache, flushed facies, conjunctival injection, and autonomic hyperactivity (e.g., tachycardia, elevated blood pressure, diaphoresis). Illusions and brief, poorly formed hallucinations may also occur during this stage but usually are not as prominent as in the alcohol hallucinosis stage.
  2. **Alcohol hallucinosis** usually occurs within 48 hours after alcohol withdrawal (but may occur while the patient is still drinking) and characteristically persists for up to 1 week. However, in about 10% of cases, the syndrome may last up to several months, and, occasionally, chronic hallucinosis develops; this stage is usually heralded by illusions or perceptual disorders. Alcohol hallucinosis is characterized by hallucinations that usually are auditory (but may be visual, tactile, olfactory, or mixed) in the presence of a clear consciousness.
  3. **Alcohol withdrawal seizures** usually occur in patients between 25 and 60 years old. The seizures occur from 7–48 hours after cessation of drinking in more than 90% of cases [111]. Characteristically, the seizures are generalized and brief with a low incidence of morbidity and mortality [60]. A majority of patients have one to four seizures; however, about 10% of patients have more than four seizures, and in about 3% of cases, status epilepticus occurs. If more than one seizure occurs, the time interval between the first and last seizure is usually less than 6 hours [111]. Almost one-third of patients with alcohol withdrawal seizures progress to delirium tremens, in which case the seizures invariably precede the delirium tremens. When this occurs, there is usually a lucid interval of 12 hours to 5 days between the seizures and the onset of delirium tremens, although in some cases the seizures may progress directly to delirium tremens without a lucid interval [13].
  4. **Delirium tremens** usually occurs from 3–5 days after ethanol withdrawal, and once delirium occurs, more than 80% of cases resolve within 3 days [13]. Delirium tremens is characterized by delirium (i.e., clouding of consciousness, global confusion, perceptual disturbances, memory impairment, insomnia, and increased psychomotor activity) and marked autonomic hyperactivity (e.g., fever, hypertension, tachycardia, diaphoresis, tremor, mydriasis). Delirium tremens is a medical emergency with a mortality of about 5–15% [1]. The high morbidity and mortality of this condition are related to associated infections, trauma, and hepatic disease, as well as to dehydration, electrolyte abnormalities, hyperthermia, cardiac arrhythmias, aspiration of gastric contents, nutritional deficiencies, self-inflicted injuries, and oversedation or undersedation (with uncontrolled agitation).
B. Management. A careful examination is essential to assess for associated treatable medical or surgical conditions (e.g., hypoglycemia, infections, subdural hematoma). Since malnutrition is often associated with chronic ethanol abuse, thiamine, 100 mg IM or IV, is recommended to prevent development of Wernicke's disease; if the patient has evidence of Wernicke's disease, intravenous administration is preferred.
  1. **Minor alcohol withdrawal syndrome.** Emergency department management includes administration of chlordiazepoxide, 50–100 mg PO, or diazepam, 5–10 mg PO, and observation for at least 4 hours. If the signs and symptoms remain minor, the patient may be discharged with a 4-day supply of chlordiazepoxide, 25 mg PO q6h, or diazepam, 5 mg PO q6h [103]. The patient should be accompanied by a responsible individual willing to stay with the patient during the withdrawal period. Close follow-up with referral to a detoxification unit or rehabilitation program, when appropriate, should be arranged. Hospitalization is recommended for patients who cannot care for themselves, have persistent hallucinations or delusions, are significantly agitated, or are confused.
  2. **Alcohol hallucinosis.** Hospitalization is recommended for patients with alcohol hallucinosis to prevent self-injury or injury to others (as a result of the acting out of hallucinations), to substantiate the diagnosis, and to observe the patient for development of more serious alcohol withdrawal problems (i.e., seizures, delirium tremens). Haloperidol, initiated at 1–5 mg/day and titrated to up to 20 mg/day as needed, may be beneficial in keeping these patients calm and comfortable.

3. **Alcohol withdrawal seizures**
   a. **Emergency department management** consists of observing these patients for a seizure-free period of at least 6 hours (if emergency department policy permits) with appropriate seizure precautions. Anticonvulsant therapy (see Chap. 32) is not indicated unless there is an underlying seizure disorder, repetitive (i.e., more than three) seizures, or status epilepticus.
   b. **Disposition.** Generally, patients may be discharged when free of seizures for 6 or more hours, if accompanied by a responsible individual willing to stay with the patient during the withdrawal period. In addition, seizure precautions (e.g., no driving, swimming, or walking in high places) should be given, a sedative prescribed (as for the minor alcohol withdrawal syndrome), and close follow-up arranged. Hospitalization is indicated if inpatient evaluation for an underlying seizure disorder is deemed necessary or if there are complicating factors (e.g., persistent seizures, impending delirium tremens, electrolyte abnormalities, infectious complications, possible head injury).

4. **Delirium tremens** requires a careful examination to assess for associated treatable medical or surgical conditions. A chest x-ray and lumbar puncture (unless contraindicated) are recommended. Attention to fluid requirements and electrolyte balance is essential. Patients should be treated in a well-lighted room in a calm, reassuring manner. If physical restraints are necessary, these patients should be restrained in the prone or lateral decubitus position to lessen the risk of aspiration. **Sedation** may be achieved by administering diazepam, 5–10 mg IV, followed by 5 mg IV q5minutes until the patient is calm but awake [109]. This is followed by diazepam, 5 mg IV q1–4h, as needed. Admission to an intensive care unit is recommended.

II. The **opioid withdrawal syndrome** occurs in patients who are physically dependent on opioids and abruptly discontinue usage or receive an opioid antagonist. While uncomfortable, opioid withdrawal generally is not life-threatening.
   A. **Clinical manifestations** of opioid withdrawal evolve over a period of days, with variations in the timing and severity according to the opioid involved and the degree of physical dependence developed. Generally, symptoms subside within 7–10 days.
      1. **Early manifestations** include yawning, lacrimation, rhinorrhea, restless sleep, and diaphoresis.
      2. **Intermediate manifestations** include mydriasis, piloerection, flushing, tachycardia, muscle twitching, tremors, restlessness, irritability, anorexia, insomnia, and abdominal cramps.
      3. **Late manifestations** include muscle spasms, fever, nausea, vomiting, diarrhea, hypertension, and hyperglycemia. In severe cases, dehydration may develop.
   B. **Management.** Generally, these patients may be treated on an outpatient basis unless thay have a concomitant illness necessitating hospital admission. **An attempt should be made to treat narcotic withdrawal problems in conjunction with an established narcotic treatment program; furthermore, if the patient is enrolled in a treatment program, an attempt should be made to contact the patient's drug counsellor.** If narcotic treatment program personnel are unavailable, the following general guidelines are suggested.
      1. Patients exhibiting no objective signs of withdrawal should be referred to a narcotic treatment center.
      2. Patients exhibiting objective signs of withdrawal may receive symptomatic treatment with librium, 10–25 mg PO q8h, and, if necessary, compazine suppositories, 25 mg q12h, for nausea and vomiting.
      3. No attempt should be made to detoxify patients admitted to the hospital for other significant illnesses. Such patients with objective signs of narcotic withdrawal may be given methadone, 10 mg PO, with additional doses q8–12h as needed; if the oral form cannot be tolerated, methadone may be given SQ or IM in a dose of 5–10 mg [32]. For pain or refractory withdrawal syndrome, morphine, 15 mg IM, may be added as needed.

III. The **barbiturate withdrawal syndrome** is a potentially life-threatening condition that is similar clinically to the alcohol withdrawal syndrome.
   A. **Clinical manifestations**
      1. **Minor manifestations** usually occur within 48 hours after barbiturate withdrawal and include a coarse tremor, weakness, insomnia, diaphoresis, restlessness, depression, anorexia, nausea, vomiting, headache, malaise, restless

sleep, dehydration, postural hypotension, apprehension, an acute anxiety state, irritability, dyspnea, tachycardia, and hyperreflexia. The minor manifestations usually subside within 1 week.

2. **Major manifestations** occur from 24 hours to 8 days after barbiturate withdrawal and include myoclonus, grand mal seizures (which may progress to status epilepticus), hyperpyrexia, hallucinations, and delirium. The major manifestations usually subside within 2 weeks [61].

B. **Management.** Hospitalization is recommended for patients undergoing barbiturate withdrawal. Treatment is initiated by administering a test dose of 200 mg of pentobarbital IM or PO to addicts not exhibiting evidence of barbiturate toxicity. If there is no evidence of barbiturate toxicity after 1 hour, it can be concluded that the patient has developed physical dependence to the barbiturates [61]. Once physical dependence is verified, the patient's daily habitual dose is estimated by history and is converted to an equivalent dose of phenobarbital (with 100 mg of a short-acting barbiturate being equivalent to 30 mg of phenobarbital). The estimated phenobarbital dosage is then administered PO q8h, with a maximum daily dosage of 500 mg of phenobarbital. If barbiturate toxicity develops, the daily dose is halved. If symptoms of withdrawal develop, 200 mg of phenobarbital is given IM, and the daily dose is increased by 25%. Once a stable dose is achieved, withdrawal of 30 mg/day of phenobarbital is undertaken [12, 61].

IV. The **nonbarbiturate sedative/hypnotic withdrawal syndrome** is similar to the barbiturate withdrawal syndrome. The degree of physical dependence can be gauged by the response to a test dose of about twice the recommended hypnotic dose of the drug being abused. Detoxification may be achieved by gradual reduction of the dependent drug or by gradual reduction of a withdrawal equivalent of phenobarbital (see sec. **III.B**), estimated as 30 mg of phenobarbital per hypnotic dose of the sedative/hypnotic agent; specific withdrawal equivalents are 30 mg of phenobarbital/500 mg of chloral hydrate, 350 mg of ethchlorvynol, 250 mg of glutethimide, or 250–300 mg of methaqualone [61].

V. **Benzodiazepine withdrawal syndrome**

A. **Clinical features** are similar to those of barbiturate withdrawal except that they usually are less severe. The syndrome usually occurs from 3–10 days following benzodiazepine withdrawal and lasts about 5–20 days. It is more likely to occur in patients who have been taking a short-acting benzodiazepine (e.g., oxazepam, lorazepam) in a high dose for more than 4 months and then suddenly discontinue the drug [80].

B. **Treatment** consists of reinstituting the benzodiazepine and slowly tapering the dose over a 1- to 2-week period. Alternatively, gradual reduction of a withdrawal equivalent of phenobarbital (see sec. **III.B**) may be undertaken [80]. Specific withdrawal equivalents are 30 mg of phenobarbital/100 mg of chlorodiazepoxide or 50 mg of diazepam [61]. Minor benzodiazepine withdrawal may be managed on an outpatient basis, but patients with more severe withdrawal manifestations should be admitted to the hospital.

VI. The **amphetamine withdrawal syndrome** consists of lethargy, lassitude, sleep disturbance, and severe depression (often with suicidal ideation) that may last for months. **Management** consists of administration of a tricyclic antidepressant to patients with significant depression and close psychiatric follow-up. Hospitalization is indicated for patients with severe or prolonged depression and patients considered a danger to themselves [61].

Bibliography

1. Adams, R. D., and Victor, M. *Principles of Neurology* (2nd ed). New York: McGraw-Hill, 1981.
2. Allred, R. J., and Ewer, S. Fatal pulmonary edema following intravenous "freebase" cocaine use. *Ann. Emerg. Med.* 10:441, 1981.
3. Anas, N., et al. Criteria for hospitalizing children who have ingested products containing hydrocarbons. *J.A.M.A.* 246:840, 1981.
4. Angrist, B. M. Toxic manifestations of amphetamines. *Psychiatr. Ann.* 8:443, 1978.
5. Arnow, W. S., et. al. Effects of freeway traffic on angina pectoris. *Ann. Intern. Med.* 77:669, 1972.
6. Aronow, R., and Done, A. K. Phencyclidine overdose: An emerging concept of management. *J.A.C.E.P.* 7:56, 1978.
7. Bayer, M. J., and Norton, R. L. Solving the clinical problems of phencyclidine intoxication. *E.R. Reports* 4:7, 1983.

8. Bennett, W. M., et al. Drug therapy in renal failure: Dosing guidelines for adults. *Ann. Intern. Med.* 93:62, 286, 1980.
9. Benowitz, N. L., Rosenberg, J., and Becker, C. E. Cardiopulmonary catastrophes in drug-overdosed patients. *Med. Clin. North Am.* 63:267, 1979.
10. Berg, M. J., et al. Acceleration of the body clearance of phenobarbital by oral activated charcoal. *N. Engl. J. Med.* 307:642, 1982.
11. Biggs, J. T., et al. Tricyclic antidepressant overdose: Incidence of symptoms. *J.A.M.A.* 238:135, 1977.
11a. Boehnert, M. T., and Lovejoy, F. H., Jr. Value of the QRS duration versus the serum drug level in predicting seizures and ventricular arrhythmias after an acute overdose of tricyclic antidepressants. *N. Engl. J. Med.* 313:474, 1985.
12. Bourne, P. E. (ed.). *A Treatment Manual for Acute Drug Abuse Emergencies.* Rockville, Md.: National Institute on Drug Abuse, 1974.
13. Brown, C. G. The alcohol withdrawal syndrome. *Ann. Emerg. Med.* 11:276, 1982.
14. Brown, C. G., et al. Ethylene glycol poisoning. *Ann. Emerg. Med.* 12:501, 1983.
15. Brown, T. C. Tricyclic antidepressant overdosage: Experimental studies on the management of circulatory complications. *Clin. Toxicol.* 9:255, 1976.
16. Callaham, M. Tricyclic antidepressant overdose. *J.A.C.E.P.* 8:413, 1979.
17. Callaham, M., and Kassel, D. Epidemiology of fatal tricyclic antidepressant ingestion: Implications for management. *Ann. Emerg. Med.* 14:1, 1985.
18. Carlson, C. Talwin 50 reformulated to avert "T's and blues" abuse. *J.A.M.A.* 249:1689, 1983.
19. Chen, K. K., and Rose, C. L. Nitrite and thiosulfate therapy in cyanide poisoning. *J.A.M.A.* 149:113, 1952.
20. Choi, S. Delayed neurologic sequelae in carbon monoxide intoxication. *Arch. Neurol.* 40:433, 1983.
21. Clemmesen, C., and Nilsson, E. Therapeutic trends in the treatment of barbiturate poisoning: The Scandinavian method. *Clin. Pharmacol. Ther.* 2:220, 1961.
22. Cohen, R. A., and Coffman, J. D. Naloxone reversal of morphine-induced peripheral vasodilation. *Clin. Pharmacol. Ther.* 28:541, 1980.
23. Coleman, D. L. Smoke inhalation. *West. J. Med.* 135:300, 1981.
24. Corre, K. A., et al. Extended therapy for acute dystonic reaction. *Ann. Emerg. Med.* 13:294, 1984.
25. Cury, S. Methemoglobinemia. *Ann. Emerg. Med.* 11:214, 1982.
26. Done, A. K. The toxic emergencies: Not "just a drunk." *Emerg. Med.* 12:77, 1980.
27. Dula, D. J. Metal fume fever. *J.A.C.E.P.* 7:448, 1978.
28. Eade, N. R., et al. Hydrocarbon pneumonitis. *Pediatrics* 54:351, 1974.
29. Eason, J. M., and Lovejoy, F. H. Efficacy and safety of gastrointestinal decontamination in the treatment of oral poisoning. *Pediatr. Clin. North Am.* 26:827, 1979.
30. Ettlinger, P. O., et al. Arrhythmias and the "holiday heart": Alcohol-associated cardiac rhythm disorders. *Am. Heart J.* 95:555, 1978.
31. Farrow, J. Major tranquilizers: The phenothiazines. *Tex. Med.* 68:51, 1972.
32. Fultz, J. M., and Senay, E. C. Guidelines for the management of hospitalized narcotic addicts. *Ann. Intern. Med.* 82:815, 1975.
33. Gay, G. R. Clinical management of acute and chronic cocaine poisoning. *Ann. Emerg. Med.* 11:562, 1982.
34. Geehr, E. Management of hydrocarbon ingestion. *Top. Emerg. Med.* 1:97, 1979.
35. Gelfand, M. C., and Winchester, J. F. Hemoperfusion in drug overdosage: A technique when conservative management is not sufficient. *Clin. Toxicol.* 17:583, 1980.
36. Gelfand, M. C., et al. Treatment of severe drug overdosage with charcoal hemoperfusion. *Trans. Am. Soc. Artif. Intern. Organs* 23:599, 1977.
37. George, J. E. The alcoholic patient in the E.D. *Emerg. Phys. Legal Bull.* 6(4):1, 1980.
38. Gilman, A. G., Goodman, L. S., and Gilman, A. (eds.). *The Pharmacological Basis of Therapeutics* (6th ed.). New York: Macmillan, 1980.
39. Goldfrank, L. R. (ed.). *Toxicologic Emergencies I: A Comprehensive Handbook in Problem Solving.* New York: Appleton-Century-Crofts, 1982.
40. Goldsmith, J. R. Contributions of motor vehicle exhaust, industry, and cigarette smoking to community carbon monoxide exposures. *Ann. N.Y. Acad. Sci.* 174:122, 1970.
41. Gonda, A., et al. Hemodialysis for methanol intoxication. *Am. J. Med.* 64:749, 1978.
42. Grace, T. W., and Platt, F. W. Subacute carbon monoxide poisoning: Another great imitator. *J.A.M.A.* 246:1698, 1981.
43. Graham, D. L., et al. Acute cyanide poisoning complicated by lactic acidosis and pulmonary edema. *Arch. Intern. Med.* 137:1051, 1977.

44. Greensher, J., Mofenson, H. C., and Gavin, W. J. The usefulness of abdominal x-rays in the diagnosis of poisoning. *Vet. Hum. Toxicol.* 21(suppl.):45, 1979.
45. Greensher, J., et al. Activated charcoal updated. *J.A.C.E.P.* 8:261, 1979.
46. Grinspoon, L., and Bakalar, J. B. Adverse effects of cocaine: Selected issues. *Ann. N.Y. Acad. Sci.* 362:125, 1981.
47. Guenter, C. A., and Welch, M. H. *Pulmonary Medicine* (2nd ed.). Philadelphia: Lippincott, 1982.
48. Haddad, L. M. Iron poisoning. *J.A.C.E.P.* 5:691, 1976.
49. Haddad, L. M., and Winchester, J. F. (eds.). *Clinical Management of Poisoning and Drug Overdose.* Philadelphia: Saunders, 1983.
50. Hagerman, G. A., and Hanashino, P. K. Reversal of tricyclic-antidepressant-induced cardiac conduction abnormalities by phenytoin. *Ann. Emerg. Med.* 10:82, 1981.
51. Handal, K. A., Schauben, J. L., and Salamone, F. R. Naloxone. *Ann. Emerg. Med.* 12:438, 1983.
52. Hansen, H. E., and Amdisen, A. Lithium intoxication (report of 23 cases and review of 100 cases from the literature). *Q. J. Med.* 47:123, 1978.
53. Heaney, R. M. Left bundle branch block associated with propoxyphene hydrochloride poisoning. *Ann. Emerg. Med.* 12:780, 1983.
54. Hedges, J. R., et al. Acute chlorine gas exposure. *J.A.C.E.P.* 8:59, 1979.
55. Hendeles, L., et al. Frequent toxicity from IV aminophylline infusions in critically ill patients. *Drug Intell. Clin. Pharmacy* 11:12, 1977.
56. Hendeles, L., and Weinberger, M. Theophylline: A "state of the art" review. *Pharmacotherapy* 3:2, 1983.
57. Hill, J. B. Salicylate intoxication. *N. Engl. J. Med.* 288:1110, 1973.
58. Holland, D. R., and Steinberg, M. I. Electrophysiologic properties of propoxyphene in canine cardiac conducting tissue in vitro and in vivo. *Toxicol. Appl. Pharmacol.* 47:123, 1979.
59. Jefferson, J. W., and Greist, J. H. Lithium intoxication. *Psychiatr. Ann.* 8:458, 1978.
60. Josepheson, G. W., and Sabatier, H. J. Rational management of alcohol withdrawal seizures. *South. Med. J.* 71:1095, 1978.
61. Khantzian, E. J., and McKenna, G. J. Acute toxic and withdrawal reactions associated with drug use and abuse. *Ann. Intern. Med.* 90:361, 1979.
62. Kilham, H. A. Hospital management of severe poisoning. *Pediatr. Clin. North Am.* 27:603, 1980.
63. Kizer, K. W., and Naccari, P. F. Recognizing and managing common toxic inhalants. *E.R. Reports* 4(9):51, 1983.
64. Knopp, R. Caustic ingestions. *J.A.C.E.P.* 8:329, 1979.
64a. Kulig, K., et al. Management of acutely poisoned patients without gastric emptying. *Ann. Emerg. Med.* 14:562, 1985.
65. Lorch, J. A., and Garella, S. Hemoperfusion to treat intoxications. *Ann. Intern. Med.* 91:301, 1979.
66. Lumpkin, J., et al. Phenothiazine-induced ventricular tachycardia following acute overdose. *J.A.C.E.P.* 8:476, 1979.
67. Mahutte, C. K., et al. Increased serum theophylline clearance with orally administered activated charcoal. *Am. Rev. Respir. Dis.* 128:820, 1983.
68. Marshall, J. B., and Forker, A. D. Cardiovascular effects of tricyclic antidepressant drugs: Therapeutic usage, overdose, and management of complications. *Am. Heart J.* 103:401, 1982.
69. Mayersohn, M., Perrier, D., and Picchioni, A. Evaluation of a charcoal-sorbitol mixture as an antidote for oral aspirin overdose. *Clin. Toxicol.* 11:561, 1977.
70. McCarron, M. M., et al. Acute phencyclidine intoxication: Clinical patterns, complications, and treatment. *Ann. Emerg. Med.* 10:290, 1981.
71. McCarron, M. M., and Wood, J. D. The cocaine body packer syndrome: Diagnosis and treatment. *J.A.M.A.* 250:1417, 1983.
72. McDougal, C. B., and Maclean, M. A. Modifications in the technique of gastric lavage. *Ann. Emerg. Med.* 10:514, 1981.
73. Medical Letter. Diagnosis and management of reactions to drug abuse. *Med. Lett. Drugs Ther.* 22:73, 1980.
73a. Medical Letter. "Crack." *Med. Lett. Drugs. Ther.* 28:69, 1986.
74. Meester, W. D. Emesis and lavage. *Vet. Hum. Toxicol.* 22:225, 1980.
75. Mitenko, P. A., and Ogilvie, R. I. Rational intravenous doses of theophylline. *N. Engl. J. Med.* 288:600, 1973.
76. Myers, R. A., et al. Carbon monoxide poisoning: The injury and its treatment. *J.A.C.E.P.* 8:479, 1979.

77. Nelson, R., et al. Caustic ingestions. *Ann. Emerg. Med.* 12:559, 1983.
78. Neimann, J. T. Cardiac conduction and rhythm disturbances following suicidal ingestions of mesoridazine. *Ann. Emerg. Med.* 10:585, 1981.
79. Ng, R. C., et al. Emergency treatment of petroleum distillate and turpentine ingestion. *Can. Med. Assoc. J.* 111:537, 1974.
79a. Olson, K. R., et al. Theophylline overdose: Acute single ingestion versus chronic repeated overmedication. *Am. J. Emerg. Med.* 3:386, 1985.
80. Owen, R. T., and Tyrer, P. Benzodiazepine dependence: A review of the evidence. *Drugs* 18:385, 1983.
81. Park, G. D., et al. Use of hemoperfusion for treatment of theophylline intoxication. *Am. J. Med.* 74:961, 1983.
82. Parry, M. F., and Wallack, R. Ethylene glycol poisoning. *Am. J. Med.* 57:143, 1974.
83. Pearlson, G. D. Psychiatric and medical syndromes associated with phencyclidine (PCP) abuse. *Johns Hopkins Med. J.* 148:25, 1981.
84. Penner, G. E. Acid ingestion toxicology and treatment. *Ann. Emerg. Med.* 9:374, 1980.
85. Peterson, C. D., and Fifield, G. C. Emergency gastrostomy for acute iron poisoning. *Ann. Emerg. Med.* 9:262, 1980.
86. Peterson, C. D., et al. Ethylene glycol poisoning: Pharmacokinetics during therapy with ethanol and hemodialysis. *N. Engl. J. Med.* 304:21, 1981.
87. Peterson, R. G., and Rumack, B. H. Toxicity of acetaminophen overdose. *J.A.C.E.P.* 7:202, 1978.
88. Petit, J. M., et al. Tricyclic antidepressant plasma levels and adverse effects after overdose. *Clin. Pharmacol. Ther.* 21:47, 1977.
89. Pond, S., et al. Pharmacokinetics of haemoperfusion for drug overdose. *Clin. Pharmacokinet.* 4:329, 1979.
90. Rappolt, R. T., Sr., Gay, G. R., and Farris, R. D. Emergency management of acute phencyclidine intoxication. *J.A.C.E.P.* 8:68, 1979.
91. Rauber, A. The cardiac safety of ipecac used as a therapeutic emetic. *Vet. Hum. Toxicol.* 20:166, 1978.
92. Redding, J. S., Tabeling, B. B., and Parham, A. M. Airway management in patients with central nervous system depression. *J.A.C.E.P.* 7:401, 1978.
93. Reed, C. E., Driggs, M. F., and Foote, C. C. Acute barbiturate intoxication: A study of 300 cases based on a physiologic system of classification of the severity of the intoxication. *Ann. Intern. Med.* 37:290, 1952.
94. Riegel, J. M., and Becker, C. E. Use of cathartics in toxic ingestions. *Ann. Emerg. Med.* 10:254, 1981.
95. Rosenbaum, J. L., et al. Current status of hemoperfusion in toxicology. *Clin. Toxicol.* 17:493, 1980.
96. Rosenberg, J., Benowitz, N. L., and Pond, S. Pharmacokinetics of drug overdose. *Clin. Pharmacokinet.* 6:161, 1981.
97. Rumack, B. (ed.). *Poisindix.* Englewood, Colo.: Micromedix, 1984.
98. Rumack, B. H., and Burrington, J. D. Caustic ingestions: A rational look at diluents. *Clin. Toxicol.* 11:27, 1977.
99. Rumack, B. H., et al. Acetaminophen overdose: 662 cases with evaluation of oral acetylcysteine treatment. *Arch. Intern. Med.* 141:380, 1981.
100. Schlueter, D. P. Response of the lung to inhaled antigens. *Am. J. Med.* 57:476, 1974.
101. Schofferman, J. A. A clinical comparison of syrup of ipecac and apomorphine use in adults. *J.A.C.E.P.* 5:22, 1976.
102. Schottstaedt, M. W., et al. Placidyl abuse: A dimorphic picture. *Crit. Care Med.* 9:677, 1981.
103. Sellers, E. M., and Kalant, H. Alcohol intoxication and withdrawal. *N. Engl. J. Med.* 294:757, 1976.
104. Sohn, D., and Byers, J., III. Cost effective drug screening in the laboratory. *Clin. Toxicol.* 18:459, 1981.
105. Sternbach, G., et al. Heroin addiction: Acute presentation of medical complications. *Ann. Emerg. Med.* 9:161, 1980.
106. Tandberg, D., and Abercrombie, D. Treatment of heroin overdose with endotracheal naloxone. *Ann. Emerg. Med.* 11:443, 1982.
107. Temple, A. R. Acute and chronic effects of aspirin toxicity and their treatment. *Arch. Intern. Med.* 141:364, 1981.
108. Temple, A. R. Pathophysiology of aspirin overdosage toxicity, with implications for management. *Pediatrics* 62(suppl):873, 1978.
109. Thompson, L. W., et al. Diazepam and paraldehyde for treatment of severe delirium tremens: A controlled trial. *Ann. Intern. Med.* 82:175, 1975.

110. Vancura, E. M., et al. Toxicity of alkaline solutions. *Ann. Emerg. Med.* 9:118, 1980.
111. Victor, M. A Study of Epilepsy in the Alcoholic Patient. In L. Simmeon (ed.), *Modern Neurology.* Boston: Little, Brown, 1969.
112. Weinberger, M., and Ginchansky, E. Dose-dependent kinetics of theophylline disposition in asthmatic children. *J. Pediatr.* 91:820, 1977.
113. Wetli, C. V. Changing patterns of methaqualone abuse: A survey of 246 fatalities. *J.A.M.A.* 249:621, 1983.
114. Wetli, C. V., and Wright, R. K. Death caused by recreational cocaine use. *J.A.M.A.* 241:2519, 1979.
115. Winchester, J. F., et al. Dialysis and hemoperfusion of poisons and drugs—update. *Trans. Am. Soc. Artif. Intern. Organs* 23:762, 1977.
116. Wright, N. An assessment of the unreliability of the history given by self-poisoned patients. *Clin. Toxicol.* 16:381, 1980.
117. Zieserl, E. Hydrocarbon ingestion and poisoning. *Compr. Ther.* 5:35, 1979.
118. Zwillich, C. W., et al. Theophylline-induced seizures in adults: Correlation with serum concentrations. *Ann. Intern. Med.* 82:784, 1975.

Surgical Emergencies

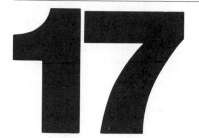

Trauma

Robert J. Stine

In the United States, trauma is the leading cause of death of people between the ages of 1 and 44 years and for all ages, the third leading cause of death, surpassed only by cardiovascular disease and cancer [11]. Each year trauma is responsible for the deaths of more than 150,000 individuals in the United States [11]. An additional 10–17 million people are disabled, 380,000 of them permanently [11]. Annually, the cost to society exceeds $83 billion in medical and insurance costs, lost wages and productivity, and property damage [42]. Trauma is so devastating because it commonly afflicts young people, with resultant loss of years of productivity and earnings, not infrequently replaced by years of dependency.

I. **Pathogenesis of injury**
  A. **Bodily injury** results when physical forces impart sufficient energy to the body to cause structural damage. Energy can be chemical, electrical, kinetic, radiation, or thermal. This chapter discusses injuries resulting from the body's absorption of kinetic energy, which is proportional to the mass of the moving object (e.g., automobile, missile, human body) and the square of its velocity (i.e., kinetic energy = $0.5 \times \text{mass} \times \text{velocity}^2$). The absorption of kinetic energy by the human body is associated with forces acting on the body's tissues and organs. The primary forces tending to produce tissue and organ damage are those of tension (pulling apart), compression (pushing together), and shearing (causing adjacent parts of a tissue to slide with respect to each other) [26]. These forces act singly or in combination to produce tissue and organ strain, contusion, laceration, fracture, and/or rupture. In **blunt trauma**, injury can occur in any area of the body where the forces are applied. In **penetrating trauma**, structural damage occurs along the paths of the penetrating missiles; in addition, high-velocity missiles, by virtue of the shock wave or cavity they create, may produce injury remote from their paths. This blast effect of penetrating missiles is common in war but is uncommon in civilian acts of violence where lower-velocity missiles generally are involved. The primary determinant of the severity of injury produced by the forces applied to the human body is the amount of kinetic energy absorbed by the body. Other factors involved are the location of the applied forces (e.g., critical organ involvement), the duration of action of the forces, and the ability of the body to dissipate the applied energy (e.g., use of protective devices, tissue strength) [26].
  B. When **death** results from trauma, it tends to follow a trimodal distribution [42]. The first death peak occurs within minutes of injury and is due to severe injury to critical organs (e.g., laceration of the brainstem, heart, or great vessels). The second death peak occurs within 2 hours of injury and is due to potentially treatable severe injuries (e.g., intracranial hematoma, hemopneumothorax, ruptured spleen, liver laceration, fractured pelvis with associated hemorrhage). The third peak occurs days or weeks after injury and is usually due to sepsis or multiple organ failure.

II. **The pathophysiology of trauma** is complex. It depends on the nature and extent of the patient's injuries and, to a large extent, is that of hemorrhagic shock (see Chap. 3) and the attendant state of impaired tissue perfusion. In response to tissue injury, pain, emotion, or hemorrhagic shock, several responses occur in an attempt by the human body to maintain homeostasis. These responses include the following: (1) activation of the clotting sequence in order to retard blood loss; (2) release of hormones (e.g., adrenocorticotropic hormone, catecholamines, cortisol, antidiuretic hormone, renin, angiotensin, aldosterone, growth hormone, glucagon, insulin) to effect cardiac stimulation, constriction of peripheral arterioles and venules, shunting of blood to the heart and brain, renal conservation of salt and water, plasma refilling by movement of interstitial fluid and protein into the vascular space, glycogenolysis, lipolysis, protein catabolism, and gluconeogenesis; and (3) increased extraction of oxygen by tissues [26, 44]. The net effect of these responses is an attempt to preserve life by maintaining adequate perfusion of vital structures and providing them with the required metabolic substrates [26]. If these compensatory responses, aided by treatment, prove inadequate, an irreversible state of shock may result, leading to multiple organ failure and death.

III. **Management of trauma.** The successful management of trauma requires a rapid, aggressive, organized, systematic, and thorough approach to the traumatized patient with proper setting of priorities. The primary priority is to preserve life; thus, throughout the management of the traumatized patient, immediate attention must be directed at detecting and correcting the most life-threatening physiologic derangements facing the patient [26]. The secondary priority is to preserve function; thus, only when the potential threats to life have been stabilized is this priority given attention [26]. Management of the traumatized patient can be divided into five phases: organization (determined prior to patient arrival), primary survey, resuscitation, secondary survey, and definitive care [9]. Although these phases will be discussed in the above-mentioned sequence, it is essential that resuscitative efforts be initiated during the primary survey. Prompt recognition of potentially life-threatening disorders (including occult injuries) and equally prompt, aggressive, and appropriate therapy of such disorders is the mainstay of successful trauma management.

A. **Organization.** It has been demonstrated that trauma victims are best managed with **an organized team approach** [11]. The team approach is necessary because of the frequent need to rapidly perform several procedures simultaneously in trauma victims.

1. The key to a smooth and successful resuscitation is the **team leader.** This person should be the physician with the most experience in trauma management. The team leader is responsible for directing the resuscitation. His or her duties include preparing for the patient's arrival (by assembling the team, assigning roles and tasks to various team members, and directing the setup of the resuscitation area), assessing the patient, directing diagnostic procedures and therapeutic interventions, determining management priorities, requesting specialty consultations as needed and coordinating the activities of these consultants, monitoring the patient's progress, obtaining consent for procedures, and informing the family of the patient's status. Since the team leader is responsible for coordinating the resuscitative efforts, he or she generally should be free from having to perform procedures.

2. The **other members** of the team usually include physicians, nurses, and aids. The physicians generally are responsible for performing diagnostic and therapeutic procedures at the direction of the team leader. The nurses generally are responsible for monitoring the patient's vital signs and status, delivering medications, documenting the progress of the resuscitation, setting up equipment, and assisting with or performing procedures at the direction of the team leader. The aides and other personnel perform assigned tasks as directed.

B. The **primary survey** involves a rapid assessment of the patient's status and identification of immediately and potentially life-threatening problems. (Appropriate resuscitation also should be initiated at this time.) When the patient arrives in the receiving area, the paramedics or accompanying personnel should be questioned regarding the circumstances and magnitude of the event(s) leading to the injury, prehospital care administered, and the patient's status at the scene and en route to the hospital. On arrival, the patient is immediately transferred to a stretcher (taking care to immobilize the cervical spine as indicated), and all clothing is removed (by cutting away if necessary). Vital signs are obtained, and cardiac monitoring is initiated. A rapid (< 2-minute), prioritized total-body assessment, including the patient's back (by logrolling the patient), is conducted while resuscitative therapy [see C] is instituted as needed. Using the skills of observation, palpation, and auscultation as appropriate, particular attention is directed at assessing the status of the respiratory, cardiovascular, and central nervous systems. Additional history, particularly regarding the patient's underlying medical problems, medications, allergies, and time of last meal, should be obtained (if possible).

1. **Assessment of ventilation. Inadequate ventilation** in trauma victims may be indicated by poor air movement, respiratory distress (e.g., anxiety, tachypnea or bradypnea, intercostal retractions, use of accessory muscles), stridor, or cyanosis. Impaired ventilation may be due to the following: (1) **upper airway obstruction** secondary to the tongue (in an unconscious patient), foreign bodies (including teeth and dentures), body secretions (including blood and vomitus), or direct maxillofacial or neck injuries; (2) **altered chest wall mechanics**

caused by a tension pneumothorax, open pneumothorax (sucking chest wound), massive hemothorax, or flail chest; (3) **respiratory depression** resulting from central nervous system (CNS) depression (secondary to head injury or drug intoxication); and (4) direct **pulmonary injury** (e.g., pulmonary contusion). Generally, the mechanism of injury and physical findings (e.g., stridor, unilateral absence of breath sounds, percussion tympany or dullness, paradoxical chest wall motion) will identify the cause of ventilatory impairment.

2. **Assessment of the circulatory status** involves interpreting the vital signs and evaluating the status of the peripheral pulses and circulation. In the absence of peripheral vascular disease, the **quality of the peripheral pulses and circulation** is a more reliable indicator of the circulatory status than is the blood pressure. Strong peripheral (e.g., pedal) pulses and good capillary refilling are reliable indicators of an adequate circulatory status. On the other hand, thready or absent peripheral pulses, delayed capillary refilling (i.e., >2 seconds), a narrow pulse pressure, relative hypotension (with respect to the baseline blood pressure), coolness of the extremities, collapse of peripheral veins, an altered mental status, and oliguria are signs of shock (i.e., perfusion failure).

The most common cause of shock in trauma is blood loss (external or internal), which should be actively sought. Generally, acute blood loss of less than 15% of the blood volume (750 ml in a 70-kg person) is well tolerated with minimal physiologic manifestations; a blood loss of between 15 and 25% of the blood volume is characterized by tachycardia, tachypnea, and orthostatic hypotension; and blood loss exceeding 25% of the blood volume (1250 ml) is manifested by frank shock. Shock in trauma, however, may have causes other than blood loss. These causes include tension pneumothorax, cardiac tamponade, myocardial contusion or infarction, spinal cord injury, and air embolism. Generally, the mechanism of injury and the physical findings will identify the etiology. A useful clue is that hemorrhagic shock generally is associated with flat neck veins (or a low central venous pressure) [CVP]), whereas cardiac and pulmonary etiologies usually are associated with distended neck veins (or a high CVP).

3. **CNS assessment** involves evaluating and closely observing the neurologic status of the patient. Initially, a brief neurologic examination assessing the patient's level of consciousness, pupillary size and reactivity, and motor activity is performed. The development of lateralizing signs and a deteriorating level of consciousness are ominous signs. Any trauma victim complaining of neck pain; having an altered mental status or other neurologic findings; having sustained head, maxillofacial, or neck trauma; or having been subjected to acceleration or deceleration forces should be assumed to have sustained a cervical spine injury until proved otherwise (and appropriate immobilization should be instituted [see **C.3.a**]).

C. Resuscitation

1. **Maintenance of ventilation**

   a. **Establishing an airway.** The first priority in managing a trauma victim is to establish an airway. **Extreme caution must be exercised, however, if there is any possibility of a cervical spine injury.** In such a situation, hyperextension of the neck is contraindicated; the neck must be maintained in axial orientation by manual in-line traction or a semirigid collar until radiologic clearance is obtained.

   (1) **Opening the airway.** The first maneuver in establishing an airway is to **clear the oropharynx** of foreign bodies and secretions manually or with suction (preferably with a tonsil sucker). Next a **standard airway maneuver,** such as the chin lift or jaw thrust with or without head tilt, may be performed to move the tongue anteriorly and open the airway. If there is any suspicion of a cervical spine injury, the chin lift or jaw thrust without head tilt should be used. Then an oropharyngeal or nasopharyngeal airway may be inserted to maintain an open airway; the former, however, must be avoided in conscious patients. With severe facial fractures, it may be necessary to grasp the tongue with a towel clip or a suture and pull it forward in order to establish an airway.

   (2) **Tracheal intubation** is indicated in comatose patients, patients in severe shock, patients with inadequate ventilation, and patients with airway compromise or the potential for airway compromise (secondary to maxillofacial or neck trauma). Endotracheal intubation (see Chap. 38) may be attempted via the oral or nasal route. The latter, however, generally

should be avoided in nonbreathing patients and patients with suspected fracture of the cribriform plate (to avoid intracranial intubation). In patients with suspected or confirmed cervical spine injury, nasotracheal (or possibly orotracheal) intubation may be attempted; however, care must be taken to maintain the neck in a neutral position.

(3) **Surgical airway.** If an airway cannot be established by one of the preceding techniques because of facial or neck injuries precluding their use or because of technical failure, the establishment of a transtracheal airway below the level of the vocal cords is indicated. In emergent situations, percutaneous transtracheal ventilation (see Chap. 38) may be used as a temporizing measure until a cricothyrotomy (see Chap. 38) can be performed. In general, tracheostomy should be avoided (except under well-controlled, relatively elective conditions).

(4) **Alternative means of establishing an airway** include use of the esophageal obturator airway (EOA), unless precluded by maxillofacial or neck trauma, and insertion of an endotracheal tube by passing it over a fiberoptic bronchoscope or laryngoscope.

b. **Ventilation**

(1) Initially, administration of **oxygen** by nasal prongs, face mask, or tracheal tube is indicated for all seriously injured patients. If ventilation is inadequate, assisted ventilation must be provided, initially with a bag-valve device and later with a ventilator. Positive end-expiratory pressure (PEEP) should be added as indicated for management of respiratory insufficiency.

(2) In order to achieve adequate ventilation, **altered chest wall mechanics must be corrected,** often immediately.

(a) **Tube thoracostomy** (see Chap. 38) via the fifth or sixth intercostal space in the midaxillary line is indicated for the treatment of pneumothoraces or hemothoraces (see Chap. 18). If the patient is in cardiopulmonary distress, tube thoracostomy must be performed immediately on the basis of the physical findings, without delaying to obtain a chest x-ray. For a suspected tension pneumothorax, needle thoracostomy via the second intercostal space in the midclavicular line is recommended, pending insertion of a chest tube. Prophylactic chest tubes generally are placed in trauma victims who are about to undergo positive-pressure ventilation and are at high risk of developing a pneumothorax (e.g., patients with rib fractures or a possible penetrating thoracic wound).

(b) An **open pneumothorax** (sucking chest wound) (see Chap. 18) is managed by prompt closure of the defect with a sterile occlusive dressing, followed immediately by tube thoracostomy. Later, definitive surgical repair usually is required.

(c) A **flail chest** (see Chap. 18) can be temporarily stabilized by placing the patient on the affected side or by placing sandbags against the flail segment. Flail chests of significant proportions, however, generally require internal stabilization with endotracheal intubation and volume-cycled ventilation.

2. **Maintenance of circulation**

a. **Control of hemorrhage.** External hemorrhage is arrested by application of direct pressure (e.g., hand-applied pressure, pressure dressing, packing). Pneumatic splints and the military antishock trousers (MAST suit) can also be used to control external hemorrhage. Because of the high incidence of complications associated with the use of tourniquets (e.g., increased venous bleeding, limb ischemia), they should not be used, except possibly for traumatic amputations. Blind clamping in a wound is to be condemned because of the risk of injuring vital structures. Direct clamping of identified bleeding vessels, however, is acceptable if time permits, but noncrushing vascular clamps must be used unless the vessels can be sacrificed. For control of internal bleeding involving the lower half of the body, particularly when associated with pelvic or femoral fractures, the MAST suit (see Chap. 38) has been shown to be beneficial [16].

b. **Venous access** is critical in the management of the trauma victim. The size, number, and location of venous lines are dictated by the nature and severity of the patient's injuries. If it is anticipated that rapid volume expansion will be required, short, large-bore catheters should be used, since resistance to flow is directly proportional to the length of the catheter and inversely proportional to the fourth power of its radius [26].

(1) For potentially serious trauma, one or more **peripheral IV lines** must be established using 14- or 16-gauge catheters. Several lines may be required, depending on the magnitude of the patient's hemodynamic instability. For patients with severe trauma to the torso, it is recommended that venous access involve at least one vein above and one vein below the diaphragm so as to ensure fluid access to the heart. If possible, injured extremities should be avoided, particularly if there is any possibility of venous disruption proximally. Venous access may be achieved by percutaneous venipuncture or by venesection (cutdown) (see Chap. 38). Generally, the former is attempted first, but the latter may be required if vascular collapse is severe. Veins readily accessible for cutdown include the basilic and cephalic veins in the antecubital fossa, the cephalic vein at the shoulder, the external jugular vein in the neck, and the saphenous vein at the groin or ankle. An advantage of performing a venous cutdown is that a sterile pediatric feeding tube (size 8–12F) or even the IV tube itself may be placed in the vein for rapid infusion of fluids.

(2) Although not essential, a **central line** inserted via the jugular, subclavian, basilic, or femoral vein is useful for monitoring the CVP. Although not as reliable as left heart pressure measurements obtained via Swan-Ganz catheterization, CVP monitoring is useful in assessing the volume status of trauma victims and in detecting cardiac tamponade. A central line may also be used for volume infusion, although peripheral lines usually are superior for this purpose. Generally, insertion of a central line should follow establishment of peripheral lines and initial volume expansion. If the jugular or subclavian route is used and the patient has sustained thoracic trauma, the line should be placed on the same side as the injury unless there is concern regarding proximal injury to the vasculature.

c. **Administration of IV fluids**

(1) Initially, a **crystalloid solution** (Ringer's lactate solution or normal saline, preferably the former) is infused at a rate commensurate with the clinical situation and the hemodynamic status of the patient. Although there has been much debate regarding the use of crystalloid versus colloid in the resuscitation of trauma victims, the latter has never been demonstrated to be superior to the former and is much more expensive [44]. For patients with head injuries, fluid restriction is indicated unless the patient is in shock (which is rarely due to head injury and then only as a manifestation of a terminal insult); a balanced salt solution should be administered at a rate of 50–75 ml/hour. For patients in shock, rapid administration of crystalloid is indicated.

(2) **Blood.** Persistence of a shock state after the infusion of 2 liters of crystalloid is an indication for administration of blood (i.e., if the shock is due to blood loss and if reversible causes of shock, such as a tension pneumothorax and cardiac tamponade, have been ruled out or corrected). Cross-matched whole blood is preferred. If unavailable, the following may be given in decreasing order of preference: cross-matched packed cells, type-specific whole blood or packed cells, O–Rh-negative packed cells, and O–Rh-positive packed cells. The last has the disadvantage of sensitizing women of childbearing age who are Rh-negative; in such situations Rh immune globulin may be administered within 48 hours of the transfusion. Generally, administered blood, in addition to passing through a macropore filter, should pass through a blood-warming device to prevent the occurrence of hypothermia, but use of this device may slow the rate of administration. Ideally, the patient's hematocrit should be kept above 30%.

With **massive blood transfusion** (generally, involving the infusion of more than 10 units within a 24-hour period), coagulopathies, usually on a dilutional basis, may result because bank blood is deficient in clotting factors (particularly factors V and VIII) and functioning platelets. With massive transfusion, it is important to monitor the coagulation indices.

Transfusion of platelets or fresh-frozen plasma is indicated when severe thrombocytopenia ($< 50,000/mm^3$) or significant prolongation of the prothrombin or partial thromboplastin time, respectively, is associated with bleeding [11, 44]. In the absence of the ability to rapidly determine the coagulation indices, 1 unit of group-specific fresh-frozen plasma and 10 platelet packs may be administered to the bleeding patient following infusion of 5 and 10 units of blood, respectively.

   d. The MAST suit is a useful device in the treatment of shock. By effecting an autotransfusion of 100–300 ml of blood from the venous capacitance system to the central circulation [3] and by increasing the afterload [18, 31], the MAST suit raises the systemic blood pressure [18, 31, 46] and augments blood flow to the heart and brain [27]. In addition, the MAST suit tamponades lower-extremity and intraabdominal hemorrhage and splints lower-extremity and pelvic fractures [16, 27]. Use of this device is indicated in trauma victims with a systolic blood pressure less than 90 mm Hg. It may also be used to control hemorrhage and immobilize fractures in the lower half of the body and generally will facilitate gaining venous access in the upper half of the body. Use of the MAST suit is discussed in Chap. 38.

   e. Autotransfusion is a useful means of repleting the patient's blood volume with autologous blood with minimal delay. It has the advantage of ready availability of fresh blood and avoidance of the complications associated with transfusion of homologous blood (e.g., transfusion reactions, hypothermia, disease transmission). Autotransfusion is particularly useful for patients with a traumatic hemothorax, since pooled blood within the chest cavity is readily available by tube thoracostomy and is usually not contaminated. The procedure is presented in Chap. 38.

   f. In trauma victims with cardiac tamponade (Chaps. 5 and 18) and shock (despite volume infusion), emergent **pericardiocentesis** (see Chap. 38) may be performed in the receiving area as a temporizing measure, pending **definitive surgical therapy** [6]. Generally, the subxiphoid approach is used, and a catheter may be left in the pericardial space for continued aspiration of blood. Removal of as little as 5–10 ml of blood may lead to hemodynamic improvement. If at any point in time the patient's clinical status markedly deteriorates, with impending cardiovascular collapse, immediate thoracotomy (see Chap. 38) is required.

   g. External cardiac massage should be initiated immediately if cardiac arrest ensues in the trauma victim, unless there is a justifiable reason to withhold resuscitation (see Chap. 2). Other critical measures include rapid volume infusion (including administration of blood as indicated), correction of reversible entities such as a tension pneumothorax or cardiac tamponade, and appropriate use of cardiac drugs and defibrillation (see Chap. 2). However, since external cardiac massage generally is ineffective in the presence of hypovolemia or cardiac tamponade, consideration should be given to performing an immediate thoracotomy in these situations.

   h. The decision of whether to perform an **emergent thoracotomy** (see Chap. 38) in the receiving area depends on both the clinical status of the trauma victim and the available resources (i.e., physician experience and backup availability of the operating suite). Generally, an emergent thoracotomy is indicated in trauma victims in cardiac arrest with recent signs of life (unless there is evidence of a terminal head injury) or in extremis and unable to be stabilized. Objectives of an emergent thoracotomy include immediate relief of cardiac tamponade, control of intrathoracic hemorrhage and air embolism, cross-clamping of the descending aorta to control hemorrhage below the diaphragm and enhance perfusion of the heart and brain, and performing internal cardiac massage (if needed) in an attempt to improve the cardiac output. The results are best for patients sustaining penetrating thoracic injuries (a 24.4% survival rate associated with penetrating cardiac injuries from a review of the medical literature) but poor for patients sustaining penetrating abdominal wounds (a 5.7% survival rate) or blunt thoracoabdominal trauma (a 5.2% survival rate) [4]. If an emergent thoracotomy (see Chap. 38 for the procedure) in the receiving area is successful, the patient is taken immediately to the operating suite for definitive surgical repair.

   i. Emergent laparotomy in the receiving area is to be condemned. Such a procedure, which is accompanied by relief of tamponade of intraabdominal hemorrhage and poor visibility, is associated with essentially a 100% mortality [25].

   j. **Vasoactive drugs** (inotropic drugs, vasopressors, vasodilators) may be useful in augmenting cardiac output and perfusion of vital organs. They generally should be used, however, only after an adequate circulating volume is established. A particular indication of the use of a vasopressor in the trauma victim is spinal (neurogenic) shock in which loss of vasomotor tone occurs; in such a situation dopamine is a useful drug. Hypotension and arrhythmias following massive blood transfusion may be due to hypocalcemia secondary to binding by citrate; in such a situation, slow IV administration of 10 ml of 10% calcium chloride may be useful.

   k. **Cardiac monitoring** is indicated for all significantly injured patients.

3. **CNS resuscitation** (see Chap. 25) is directed at both ensuring that the brain and spinal cord's metabolic needs are met and avoiding further insults to already compromised, traumatized tissue. To accomplish these goals requires appropriate spinal immobilization (as needed), proper fluid administration, appropriate blood pressure control, maintenance of adequate ventilation, and avoidance of hyperthermia. In particular, it is essential to maintain adequate oxygenation (i.e., $PaO_2 > 80$ mm Hg) and cerebral perfusion (i.e., systolic blood pressure between 100 and 170 mm Hg and intracranial pressure < 15 mm Hg) [11].

   a. **Immobilization of the spine.** Because of the potential for mortality and devastating, permanent morbidity, it is absolutely imperative that the cervical spine be immobilized (preferably in a neutral position) in any trauma victim with any possibility of a cervical spine injury (see **B.3**) until radiologic clearance is obtained. Cervical spine immobilization may be achieved by application of a semirigid cervical collar and by placing sandbags against the victim's head and securing the head to a spine board with tape. In patients with potential injury to the thoracic or lumbar spine, the spine must be immobilized by placing the victim on a firm surface (preferably a backboard) and preventing flexion, extension, and lateral movement (but logrolling may be performed, if needed) until radiologic clearance is obtained.

   b. **Hyperventilation** with reduction of the carbon dioxide tension (PCO_2) to 25–30 mm Hg to reduce the intracranial pressure is indicated in trauma victims with severe head injury. This procedure usually requires tracheal intubation and assisted ventilation.

   c. **Mannitol,** 1 gm/kg IV, is indicated to decrease the intracranial pressure when there is deterioration of the neurologic status suggestive of CNS herniation or impending herniation. Ideally, mannitol should be administered in consultation with a neurosurgeon while preparations are made for surgical decompression. A loop diuretic, such as furosemide, may also be given. In addition, fluid restriction is indicated (unless the patient is in hypovolemic shock).

   d. **Corticosteroids** (e.g., dexamethasone, 10–100 mg IV) are commonly administered to patients with severe CNS injury, but their efficacy in improving outcome has not been clearly demonstrated [5, 10].

   e. **Emergent burr holes.** The need to perform emergent burr holes in the receiving area (prior to computed tomographic [CT] scanning or transport to the operating suite) is rare. However, if a patient with a head injury rapidly deteriorates with signs of CNS herniation and is unresponsive to hyperventilation and administration of mannitol, an emergent temporal burr hole may be placed on the same side of the head as the abnormal pupil. If a clot is found, the patient is transferred immediately to the operating suite for a decompressive craniotomy; if no clot is found, the patient undergoes CT scanning [11].

D. **Secondary survey.** This stage of trauma management involves a more detailed evaluation of the trauma victim and the performance of certain nonresuscitative procedures. It is during this phase of care that the nature and extent of the patient's injuries that were not identified during the primary survey are determined. This survey demands a rapid but organized and systematic approach. In addition, a high index of suspicion is required so that serious occult injuries (e.g., fractured spine, ruptured thoracic aorta, intraabdominal hemorrhage, ruptured urethra) are identified. Once again, priorities must be set. Although it is desirable to conduct a thorough evaluation, including use of radiologic and laboratory studies, the severity of the patient's injuries will determine the extent of the evaluation. It may be necessary to postpone certain studies, such as assessment of the genitourinary system, until more serious injuries have received definitive surgical therapy. No patient should ever be denied needed emergent surgery because of the desire to work up less serious injuries.

1. **History and physical examination.** Detailed information regarding the circumstances pertaining to the trauma and the patient's pertinent medical history should be obtained (to the extent possible). In addition, a rapid but thorough head-to-toe physical examination is performed; this examination entails inspecting, palpating, and, where appropriate, auscultating all body areas and performing a complete neurologic examination.

2. **Laboratory evaluation** depends on the nature and severity of the trauma. For potentially serious trauma, blood is obtained (usually when establishing IV lines) and sent for a complete blood count, type and cross-match, serum electrolytes and chemistries, coagulation indices, and, when indicated, toxicologic analysis. A voided or catheterized (unless contraindicated) urine specimen must be obtained for analysis. In addition, an arterial blood gas (ABG) and an electrocardiogram (ECG) generally are indicated. Laboratory results may indicate acute blood loss (e.g., an initial low-normal hematocrit that decreases with time, metabolic acidosis), pulmonary insufficiency, myocardial infarction or contusion, genitourinary tract injury (e.g., hematuria), or intraabdominal visceral injury (e.g., hyperamylasemia, leukocytosis).

3. Unless contraindicated, a **Foley catheter and nasogastric tube** should be inserted in serious trauma cases. Insertion of a Foley catheter enables obtaining a urine specimen for analysis and monitoring of the urinary output. A nasogastric tube allows detection of gastric blood (secondary to injury to the stomach or proximal gastrointestinal or pulmonary tracts) and effects gastric decompression (preventing aspiration). Contraindications to insertion of a Foley catheter and nasogastric tube include a suspected ruptured urethra (see Chap. 27) and fractured cribriform plate, respectively. In the former situation, a suprapubic cystostomy (see Chap. 38) may be performed if bladder drainage is required; in the latter situation, an orogastric tube should be passed in order to avoid possible intracranial intubation.

4. **Radiologic studies** depend on the nature and extent of the patient's suspected injuries, the patient's stability, and management priorities. Initial studies are directed at detecting potentially life-threatening injuries and those needing urgent therapy.

   a. **Plan roentgenograms**

      (1) In **penetrating trauma**, the location of entrance and exit wounds, if any, and suspected paths of penetrating missiles determines the x-rays to be obtained.

      (2) In potentially severe **blunt trauma**, the following x-rays usually are indicated, generally in the following order: cervical spine, chest, and pelvis.

         (a) **Cervical spine films.** Unless the patient is in respiratory distress, the first x-ray obtained is a lateral cervical spine. Since approximately 20% of serious injuries may be missed with the lateral view alone [33], anteroposterior (AP) and odontoid views also are required. The combination of all three views enables detection of about 95% of serious cervical spine injuries [35]. Later, when time permits, oblique views and tomograms may be obtained, as needed. For radiographic evaluation of the cervical spine to be complete, it is imperative that all seven cervical vertebrae be visualized, which may require either applying downward traction to the upper extremities to depress the victim's shoulders or obtaining a swimmer's view. If time does not permit undertaking these procedures, the cervical spine should be immobilized in a semirigid collar, and completion of the cervical spine series delayed until more severe injuries have been appropriately managed [11].

         (b) **Chest x-ray.** If the patient is in respiratory distress, the chest x-ray should precede the cervical spine series. If it is safe to do so, an upright chest x-ray should be obtained because it enables better identification of a pneumothorax or hemothorax and better delineation of the mediastinum.

(c) An **AP film of the pelvis** generally is dictated because of the potential seriousness of pelvic injuries.

(d) **Additional plain roentgenograms** are obtained as dictated by the apparent nature of the patient's injuries, the patient's clinical status, and management priorities. In particular, facial and extremity films are of low priority and should be obtained only when the clinical situation safely permits their being taken.

b. **Specialized radiologic procedures.** Once again, the patient's clinical status and management priorities will determine the timing of these radiologic tests. With a few exceptions (e.g., one-shot intravenous pyelogram [IVP]), these procedures are undertaken as indicated by the nature of the patient's injuries only when the patient has been stabilized and the information to be gained from the test is vital to the immediate management of the patient. In emergent situations, certain of these procedures (e.g., angiography, IVP) can be performed during surgery.

(1) **Computed tomography**

(a) **CT of the head** is now the preferred means of assessing intracranial pathology in trauma victims. It can rapidly and accurately diagnose intracranial hemorrhage, cerebral contusion, cerebral edema, radiodense foreign bodies, and skull fractures [13]. CT of the head is indicated in any patient with suspected head trauma and any sign or symptom suggestive of a structural intracranial injury, particularly a deteriorating level of consciousness or lateralizing signs.

(b) **CT of the abdomen.** Recent evidence indicates that an abdominal CT scan is accurate in detecting and quantifying intraperitoneal and retroperitoneal hematomas and in diagnosing the nature and extent of visceral injuries, particularly involving the liver, spleen, pancreas, and kidneys [14, 28]. If an abdominal CT scan is to be performed, peritoneal lavage should be avoided since it will interfere with the detection of hemoperitoneum. Because an abdominal CT scan is a rapid, noninvasive test with the ability to provide accurate and detailed information, it may be the preferred means of evaluating the abdomen in stable trauma victims.

(c) In addition, CT scanning is useful in assessing injuries to the spine, pelvis, maxillofacial area, neck, and chest [13].

(2) **IVP** is indicated in assessing the upper urinary tract in trauma victims with suspected renal or ureteral injuries. Indications for IVP include microscopic or gross hematuria; significant flank pain, tenderness, or hematoma; and gunshot wounds to the abdomen or corresponding back. Recent evidence, however, reveals that IVP may not be necessary for microscopic hematuria (with < 30 red blood cells [RBCs] per high-power field) alone [20]. In the emergent situation, a one-shot IVP may be obtained by injecting as a bolus 100–150 ml of an appropriate iodine contrast agent IV and obtaining an abdominal (kidneys, ureters, and bladder [KUB]) film 5 minutes after the injection.

(3) **Urethrography and cystography.** In stable trauma victims, these radiologic procedures are performed as indicated to assess the lower urinary tract.

(a) **Urethrography.** For a suspected urethral injury (e.g., inability to void, blood at the urethral meatus, evidence of perineal trauma, fractured pelvis, a boggy prostatic mass, a high-riding or absent prostate), a urethrogram is performed (prior to attempted insertion of a Foley catheter) by injecting 10–20 ml of an appropriate contrast agent via a Foley catheter inserted into the tip of the urethra and obtaining an x-ray.

(b) **Cystography.** If a bladder injury is suspected (e.g., inability to void, gross hematuria, fractured pelvis, absence of urine following bladder catheterization), a cystogram is performed (after the urethra has been cleared) by administering by gravity flow 200–400 ml of an appropriate contrast agent via a Foley catheter and obtaining AP and lateral radiographs pre- and postevacuation.

Table 17-1. Indications for arteriography following trauma

I. Neck injuries in relatively inaccessible regions (i.e., zones I and III)*
II. Thoracic trauma with suspected great-vessel injury (e.g., mediastinal widening, distortion or blurring of the aortic outline, penetrating mediastinal trauma)
III. Select abdominal injuries
    A. Nonvisualization of a kidney on IVP
    B. Pelvic fractures with excessive hemorrhage (for diagnostic and therapeutic purposes)
    C. Assessment of the abdomen when thoracic arteriography is required
IV. Extremity injuries with possibility of damage to major vessels
    A. Penetrating extremity wounds in proximity to major vessels
    B. Injuries (including fractures) with diminished or absent distal pulses, expanding hematoma, or evidence of major arterial bleeding
    C. Knee dislocations

*The neck is divided into three zones. Zone I is the area of the thoracic outlet extending to 1 cm above the clavicles; zone II extends from 1 cm above the clavicles to the angle of the mandible; and zone III is the area above the angle of the mandible.
Source: Adapted from A. J. Walt (ed.), *Early Care of the Injured Patient* (3rd ed.). Philadelphia: Saunders, 1982.

       (4) Radionuclide scans. A liver-spleen scan can reliably detect injuries to these organs [12]. In stable trauma victims, this test may be used to assess the integrity of the liver or spleen when isolated injury to one or both of these organs is suspected.
       (5) Gastrointestinal contrast studies with a water-soluble contrast agent may be useful in select, stable trauma victims to assess the integrity of the upper and lower gastrointestinal tracts (i.e., esophagus, stomach, duodenum, and colon).
       (6) Arteriography is a useful procedure in evaluating trauma victims. Indications for its use are given in Table 17-1.
    5. Peritoneal lavage is an accurate and sensitive means of rapidly assessing whether there is intraabdominal injury. It has consistently been shown to be superior to the physical examination in assessing the abdomen; its accuracy in diagnosing intraabdominal injury in blunt and penetrating trauma generally exceeds 98% and 90%, respectively [1, 15, 36–39]. For blunt trauma, use of peritoneal lavage has led to a decline in unnecessary laparotomies and reduced the mortality associated with abdominal trauma [15]. For penetrating trauma, the technique has resulted in a decline in unnecessary laparotomies and morbidity [37, 39]. In the absence of a contraindication (see Chap. 38), peritoneal lavage is indicated whenever there is uncertainty regarding the status of the abdomen, particularly when the patient has an altered mental status (secondary to a head injury or drug intoxication) or a spinal cord injury [40], and there is the need for rapid evaluation of the abdomen. The procedure is discussed in Chap. 38.
    6. Endoscopy. Laryngoscopy, bronchoscopy, esophagoscopy, and proctosigmoidoscopy may be used as indicated in stable patients to detect injuries to the larynx, trachea or bronchi, esophagus, and distal colon, respectively.
    7. Fracture care. Suspected fractures (and dislocations), based on the physical examination, should be immobilized pending radiologic evaluation and definitive care. Immobilization is required to minimize soft-tissue damage, reduce blood loss, prevent neurovascular damage, prevent conversion of a closed fracture to an open fracture, and relieve pain. Generally, suspected fractures are splinted without attempted realignment. For severely angulated fractures and fractures with distal vascular compromise, however, gentle application of axial traction and attempted correction of the deformity is indicated. Open fractures should not be reduced because of the risk of introducing debris and bacteria into the wound; such fractures should be covered with a sterile dressing soaked with povidone-iodine and splinted, pending irrigation, debridement, and reduction in the operating suite. A variety of immobilizing devices are available, including slings, prefabricated splints of various materials, plaster of paris, the MAST suit, and traction splints. Following splinting, cold should be applied to the

Table 17-2. Indications for urgent surgery*

I. Laparotomy
  A. Evidence of significant visceral injury
    1. Signs of peritoneal irritation
    2. Clinical evidence of intraabdominal hemorrhage (e.g., unexplained hypotension,
       expanding abdominal girth)
    3. Significant gastrointestinal bleeding
    4. Massive hematuria
    5. Positive peritoneal lavage
    6. Positive radiologic study
      a. Free intraperitoneal air or evidence of diaphragmatic rupture on plain radio-
         graphs
      b. Significant hemoperitoneum or organ injury demonstrated on CT scan
      c. Significant injury demonstrated on angiographic, contrast, or radionuclide
         study
  B. Gunshot wound with evidence of peritoneal penetration
  C. Significant fascial defect/evisceration
II. Thoracotomy
  A. Patient in extremis or in cardiac arrest (with recent signs of life) following
     thoracoabdominal trauma
  B. Cardiac tamponade
  C. Massive or persistent intrapleural hemorrhage
  D. Major intrathoracic vascular injury demonstrated on angiography (e.g., ruptured
     thoracic aorta)
  E. Evidence of tracheobronchial injury
  F. Evidence of esophageal injury
  G. Evidence of diaphragmatic injury
  H. Significant chest wall defect
  I. Large, clotted hemothorax
  J. Massive hemoptysis
  K. Gross contamination of the pleural space with foreign bodies
  L. Valvular or septal cardiac injuries with acute heart failure
III. CNS surgery
  A. Significantly depressed skull fracture
  B. Open skull fracture or cranial defect
  C. Penetrating skull injury
  D. Surgically correctable intracranial hematoma (e.g., epidural or subdural hematoma)
  E. Cerebral contusion acting as an expanding mass lesion
  F. Spinal cord compression that may benefit from decompression, or evidence of bone
     or foreign bodies in the spinal canal
IV. Other surgery
  A. Open fractures or joints
  B. Evidence of significant vascular injury
  C. Amputation or significant soft-tissue loss
  D. Compartment syndrome
  E. Neck trauma with signs suggestive of significant injury

*This table is only a guide. Other injuries may require urgent surgery depending on their nature and
extent. In addition, the timing of surgery will depend on the management priorities.
Source: Adapted from G. D. Zuidema, R. B. Rutherford, and W. F. Ballinger II (eds.), *The Management of
Trauma* (3rd ed.). Philadelphia: Saunders, 1979; and R. A. Cowley and C. M. Dunham (eds.), *Shock
Trauma/Critical Care Manual*. Baltimore: University Park Press, 1982.

> suspected fracture site, and, if possible, the injured part should be elevated to
> reduce swelling.
> 8. **Consultations** are requested by the team leader as needed to obtain advice and
>   guidance regarding the management of specific injuries. The consultants make
>   recommendations to the team leader regarding the evaluation and treatment of
>   injuries falling within their areas of expertise. The team leader weighs these
>   recommendations and establishes management priorities.
> 9. **Careful monitoring and frequent reassessment** of the patient's status are
>   vital components in the management of the trauma victim. For potentially
>   serious trauma, the following parameters require diligent monitoring: the vital

signs, cardiac rhythm, respiratory status (e.g., arterial blood gases [ABGs]), fluid status (e.g., hematocrit, intake and output, CVP), and neurologic status. Depending on the clinical situation, an arterial line may be established for accurate and continuous recording of the blood pressure, and a Swan-Ganz catheter inserted for measurement of left heart pressures and cardiac output. Any change in the patient's status must be conveyed immediately to the team leader for necessary corrective action and reassessment of management priorities.

E. **Definitive care** involves in-depth management of specific injuries, including any necessary surgical intervention. Refer to other sections of this book for definitive therapy of specific injuries.

1. **Adjunctive therapy**

   a. **Tetanus prophylaxis** (see Chap. 12) must be provided as indicated.

   b. Early administration of appropriate **antibiotics** is indicated in the following situations: suspected gastrointestinal perforation (gentamicin and clindamycin or cefoxitin for enteric organisms), open fractures (penicillinase-resistant penicillin or cephalosporin for gram-positive organisms), and obviously contaminated wounds (penicillinase-resistant penicillin or cephalosporin).

   c. **Narcotic analgesics** are withheld in patients who have head injury or are in shock; in addition, narcotics should be withheld until the nature and extent of the injuries have been determined, the treatment plan has been formulated, and consent for surgery has been obtained.

2. **Urgent surgery** (see Table 17-2) may be required, depending on the nature of the patient's injuries. Since many deaths from trauma tend to occur within 2 hours of injury (the second death peak), it is essential that trauma victims receive definitive surgical care within this time period, preferably within 1 hour of injury, in order to improve the chances for survival [42]. If the patient has sustained injury to more than one system, treatment priorities must be established. Initial surgical therapy must be directed at the patient's most life-threatening injury. In certain situations, surgery may be performed simultaneously on two or more systems (e.g., laparotomy and craniotomy). Generally, orthopedic injuries are of low priority.

3. **Disposition.** The disposition depends on the patient's condition, the nature and extent of the injuries, and the hospital's resources and available personnel. Hospital admission for observation or definitive care is indicated for all significantly injured patients. Following stabilization (if possible), transfer to another institution for definitive therapy is required if the hospital and available personnel are unable to provide the level of care necessary for the patient's injuries.

Bibliography

1. Alyono, D., and Perry, J. F. Value of quantitative cell count and amylase activity of peritoneal lavage fluid. *J. Trauma* 21:345, 1981.
2. Baker, C. C., Thomas, N. N., and Trunkey, D. D. The role of emergency room thoracotomy in trauma. *J. Trauma* 20:848, 1980.
3. Bivins, H. G., et al. Blood volume displacement with inflation of antishock trousers. *Ann. Emerg. Med.* 11:409, 1982.
4. Bodai, B. I., et al. Emergency thoracotomy in the management of trauma. A review. *J.A.M.A.* 249:1891, 1983.
5. Braakman, R., et al. Megadose steroids in severe head injury. Results of a prospective double-blind clinical trial. *J. Neurosurg.* 58:326, 1983.
6. Breaux, E. P., et al. Cardiac tamponade following penetrating mediastinal injuries: Improved survival with early pericardiocentesis. *J. Trauma* 19:461, 1979.
7. Callaham, M. Acute traumatic cardiac tamponade: Diagnosis and treatment. *J.A.C.E.P.* 7:306, 1978.
8. Callaham, M. Pericardiocentesis in traumatic and nontraumatic cardiac tamponade. *Ann. Emerg. Med.* 13:924, 1984.
9. Committee on Trauma. *Advanced Trauma Life Support Course.* American College of Surgeons, 1984.
10. Cooper, P. R., et al. Dexamethasone and severe head injury. A prospective double-blind study. *J. Neurosurg.* 51:307, 1979.
11. Cowley, R. A., and Dunham, C. M. (eds.). *Shock Trauma/Critical Care Manual.* Baltimore: University Park Press, 1982.

12. Danzl, D. F., and Berg, B. C., Jr. Peritoneal lavage and scintigraphic evaluation of blunt abdominal trauma. *J.A.C.E.P.* 6:397, 1977.
13. Federle, M. P. Comparative value of computed tomography in the evaluation of trauma. *Emerg. Med. Reports* 4:147, 1983.
14. Federle, M. P., et al. Computed tomography in blunt abdominal trauma. *Arch. Surg.* 117:645, 1982.
15. Fischer, R. P., et al. Diagnostic peritoneal lavage. Fourteen years and 2586 patients later. *Am. J. Surg.* 136:701, 1978.
16. Flint, L. M., Jr., et al. Definitive control of bleeding from severe pelvic fractures. *Ann. Surg.* 189:709, 1979.
17. Freeman, T., and Fischer, R. P. The inadequacy of peritoneal lavage in diagnosing acute diaphragmatic rupture. *J. Trauma* 16:538, 1976.
18. Gaffney, F. A., et al. Hemodynamic effects of medical anti-shock trousers (MAST garment). *J. Trauma* 21:931, 1981.
19. Gilliland, M. G., et al. Peritoneal lavage and angiography in the management of patients with pelvic fractures. *Am. J. Surg.* 144:744, 1982.
20. Guice, K., et al. Hematuria after blunt trauma. When is pyelography useful? *J. Trauma* 23:305, 1983.
21. Harnar, T. J., et al. Role of emergency thoracotomy in the resuscitation of moribund trauma victims. 100 consecutive cases. *Am. J. Surg.* 142:96, 1981.
22. Hubbard, S. G., et al. Diagnostic errors with peritoneal lavage in patients with pelvic fractures. *Arch. Surg.* 114:844, 1979.
23. Lowe, R. J., et al. Should laparotomy be mandatory or selective in gunshot wounds of the abdomen? *J. Trauma* 17:903, 1977.
24. Marshall, L. F., and Bowers, S. A. Rapid assessment and therapy of severe head injuries. *E.R. Reports* 1:13, 1980.
25. Mattox, K. L., Allen, M. K., and Feliciano, D. V. Laparotomy in the emergency department. *J.A.C.E.P.* 8:180, 1979.
26. May, H. L. The Critically Injured Patient. In H. L. May (ed.), *Emergency Medicine*. New York: Wiley, 1984.
27. McCabe, J. B., et al. New concepts concerning pneumatic antishock trousers. *Emerg. Med. Reports* 5:85, 1984.
28. Moon, K. L., and Federle, M. P. Computed tomography in hepatic trauma. *A.J.R.* 141:309, 1983.
29. Moore, J. B., et al. Diagnostic peritoneal lavage for abdominal trauma: Superiority of the open technique at the infraumbilical ring. *J. Trauma* 21:570, 1981.
30. Mueller, G. L., Burney, R. E., and Mackenzie, J. R. Sequential peritoneal lavage and early diagnosis of colon perforation. *Ann. Emerg. Med.* 10:131, 1981.
31. Niemann, J. T., et al. Hemodynamic effects of pneumatic external counterpressure in canine hemorrhagic shock. *Ann. Emerg. Med.* 12:661, 1983.
32. Pachter, H. L., and Hofstetter, S. R. Open and percutaneous paracentesis and lavage for abdominal trauma. A randomized prospective study. *Arch. Surg.* 116:318, 1981.
33. Shaffer, M. A., and Doris, P. E. Limitation of the cross table lateral view in dectecting cervical spine injuries: A retrospective analysis. *Ann. Emerg. Med.* 10:508, 1981.
34. Siemens, R., et al. Indications for thoracotomy following penetrating thoracic injury. *J. Trauma* 17:493, 1977.
35. Streitwieser, D. R., et al. Accuracy of standard radiographic views in detecting cervical spine fractures. *Ann. Emerg. Med.* 12:538, 1983.
36. Talbert, J., Gruenberg, J. C., and Brown, R. S. Peritoneal lavage in penetrating thoracic trauma. *J. Trauma* 20:979, 1980.
37. Thal, E. R. Evaluation of peritoneal lavage and local exploration in lower chest and abdominal stab wounds. *J. Trauma* 17:642, 1977.
38. Thal, E. R., May, R. A., and Beesinger, D. Peritoneal lavage. Its unreliability in gunshot wounds of the lower chest and abdomen. *Arch. Surg.* 115:430, 1980.
39. Thompson, J. S., et al. The evolution of abdominal stab wound management. *J. Trauma* 20:478, 1980.
40. Tibbs, P. A., et al. Diagnosis of acute abdominal injuries in patients with spinal shock: Value of diagnostic peritoneal lavage. *J. Trauma* 20:55, 1980.
41. Trunkey, D. D. (ed.). Symposium on trauma. *Surg. Clin. North Am.* 62:1, 1982.
42. Trunkey, D. D. The value of trauma centers. *Bull. Am. Coll. Surgeons* 67(10):5, 1982.
43. Vij, D., et al. The importance of the WBC count in peritoneal lavage. *J.A.M.A.* 249:636, 1983.
44. Walt, A. J. (ed.), *Early Care of the Injured Patient* (3rd ed.). Philadelphia: Saunders, 1982.

45. Ward, R. E., et al. Angiography and peritoneal lavage in blunt abdominal trauma. *J. Trauma* 21:848, 1981.
46. Wayne, M. A., Macdonald, S. C. Clinical evaluation of the antishock trousers: Retrospective analysis of five years of experience. *Ann. Emerg. Med.* 12:342, 1983.
47. Williams, G. O. Avoiding error with acute cervical spine injuries. *E.R. Reports* 3:9, 1982.
48. Young, G. P., and Purcell, T. B. Emergency autotransfusion. *Ann. Emerg. Med.* 12:180, 1983.

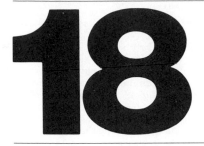

Cardiothoracic Emergencies

J. E. Martin, Jr., and
Jon F. Moran

Cardiothoracic injuries are present in nearly 50% of individuals dying as a result of trauma. In 25% of deaths from trauma, the thoracic injury is the actual cause of death. Isolated trauma to the chest has a mortality of approximately 5%. Cardiothoracic emergencies occur in every age group and range from blunt or penetrating trauma to spontaneously occurring intrathoracic catastrophies. Assessment and therapy of cardiothoracic emergencies requires a thorough knowledge of the anatomy of the thorax and a detailed understanding of cardiopulmonary physiology. This chapter presents the essentials for recognizing common cardiothoracic emergencies and expeditiously assessing their severity; in addition, the principles of initial stabilization and management are provided.

General Management Principles

Life-threatening cardiothoracic emergencies can be either traumatic or nontraumatic in etiology. Trauma to the chest may damage the chest wall, the lungs, the heart, the major airways, the esophagus, major intrathoracic blood vessels, or the diaphragm. The vast majority of penetrating trauma to the chest will be obvious by simple inspection. In contrast, blunt trauma may cause extensive intrathoracic damage with few, if any, external signs of injury. Other serious cardiothoracic emergencies arise without any preceding trauma and with no externally apparent evidence of the intrathoracic problem. Rapid, accurate assessment of cardiothoracic emergencies is critically important, since respiratory or circulatory embarrassment may be precipitated easily by many of these conditions.

I. **Assessment.** While assessing any cardiothoracic problem, it is essential that basic cardiopulmonary support be provided as needed. Frequently, basic maneuvers for maintenance of respiratory and cardiovascular stability will simultaneously help assess the extent of intrathoracic injury.

   A. **History.** The history can be critically important in reaching an expeditious diagnosis of nontraumatic or traumatic cardiothoracic emergencies. The presence or absence of chest pain (including its descriptive features), shortness of breath, and other associated features are important parameters in assessing both nontraumatic and traumatic disorders. Information regarding the forces involved (e.g., deceleration forces, penetrating trauma) and their magnitude (e.g., caliber of the injuring weapon, velocities of involved vehicles) is important in assessing the likelihood of various injuries. For example, involvement of deceleration forces suggests the possibility of a ruptured thoracic aorta or myocardial contusion.

   B. **Physical examination**

      1. **Airway.** The oral cavity is first examined for secretions, vomitus, or foreign bodies (e.g., avulsed teeth, dentures). Next, stability of the larynx is verified. The breathing pattern should be observed to assess the degree of respiratory distress, if any, and the breath sounds should be checked bilaterally.

      2. **Circulation.** The blood pressure and heart rate should be determined. While checking the apical heart rate, it is important to listen for a pericardial rub (suggestive of pericarditis), mediastinal crunch (suggestive of a pneumomediastinum), and cardiac murmurs. Any muffling of cardiac sounds (suggestive of a pericardial effusion) should be noted. Engorgement or collapse of neck veins provides a rapid qualitative measure of the right-sided cardiac filling pressure and the overall volume status. The carotid, brachial, and femoral pulses should be palpated, and any pulse deficits noted as possible indicators of a dissecting thoracic aneurysm or major intrathoracic vascular trauma. The presence or

absence of pulsus paradoxus (suggestive of cardiac tamponade) should be noted. Any sites of blood loss or accumulation should be identified.

  3. The **thorax** must be examined both anteriorly and posteriorly. Any areas of tenderness, contusion, open wounds, or chest asymmetry are noted.

  C. **Laboratory.** Appropriate radiologic examination, usually a portable chest x-ray but a standard upright posteroanterior (PA) and lateral chest x-ray whenever possible (for better delineation of the mediastinum and identification of a pneumo- or hemothorax), should be obtained as early as possible after presentation but should not delay any necessary therapeutic intervention (e.g., emergent tube thoracostomy). Arterial blood gases (ABGs) are useful in evaluating the respiratory status of the patient, and an electrocardiogram (ECG) helps assess possible cardiac involvement. A complete blood count (CBC), type and cross-match, and other laboratory tests are obtained as dictated by the clinical situation.

II. **Management**

  A. **Airway.** The posterior pharynx should be cleared of secretions, vomitus, and any foreign bodies. Supplemental oxygen is provided as needed. If necessary, the patient is ventilated via an endotracheal tube or face mask in order to achieve an adequate gas exchange.

  B. **Circulation.** Any external hemorrhage is controlled by application of direct pressure, and an appropriate volume of Ringer's lactate solution (and blood as needed) is infused. It may be necessary to immediately intervene operatively to control excessive blood loss.

  C. **Specific procedures**

   1. In trauma patients a **nasogastric tube** should be inserted initially to decompress the stomach, thereby lessening the likelihood of vomiting or aspiration. The position of the nasogastric tube on the initial chest x-ray can be helpful diagnostically, as deviation of the tube to the right suggests a transected thoracic aorta.

   2. An emergent **needle or tube thoracostomy** (see Chap. 38) is indicated (prior to obtaining a chest x-ray) if a tension pneumothorax is suspected.

   3. An emergent **pericardiocentesis** (see Chap. 38) is indicated in patients who have pericardial tamponade with hemodynamic compromise as a temporizing measure pending definitive surgical therapy.

   4. For patients in extremis or in cardiac arrest, an emergency **thoracotomy** may be indicated (see Chap. 38).

   5. Additional therapeutic measures will be guided by the specific clinical circumstances.

  D. Frequent or continuous **monitoring** of the vital signs, respiratory status, and ECG is required until the patient is stable.

III. The **disposition** will depend on the clinical situation. In particular, patients requiring a tube thoracostomy or suspected of having injury to the heart, a great vessel, lung, or esophagus require hospitalization.

Chest Wall Injuries

Most chest wall injuries occur secondary to blunt trauma to the thorax, resulting in rib fractures and interference with the bellows function of the chest wall. Occasionally, rib fractures are caused by malignant disease metastatic to bone or by vigorous coughing in elderly osteoporotic patients. Major penetrating trauma can also lead to instability of the thoracic cage.

I. **Soft-tissue wounds of the thorax** result from penetrating or blunt trauma. Those wounds that do not penetrate into the pleural space and do not expose any bony or cartilaginous portions of the chest wall are managed in a manner identical to soft-tissue wounds anywhere else in the body.

  A. **Treatment**

   1. As in any other soft-tissue wound, copious **irrigation** and meticulous **debridement** of any foreign material and all devitalized tissue should be performed as soon as possible. While irrigating and debriding these wounds, it is critically important to be certain that the thorax is not penetrated and that no damaged bone or cartilage is exposed at the base of the soft-tissue defect.

   2. **Closure** of simple, relatively clean lacerations that involve the soft tissue or muscles of the chest wall is undertaken following irrigation and debridement. Only rarely will such wounds become infected. However, if the traumatic soft-tissue defect is large or if the wound is heavily contaminated with foreign

material, the wound should be packed open with antiseptic-dampened gauze rolls after irrigation and debridement. These larger or more contaminated wounds may then be allowed to close by secondary intention or be closed by skin grafting or composite tissue grafting at a later time.

3. Adequate **analgesia** must be given to these patients to enable them to breathe deeply and cough despite their injuries. Analgesia is particularly important for those patients whose wounds will require repacking regularly.

4. **Antibiotics** are indicated for wounds that are contaminated, contain a significant amount of devitalized tissue, or are of major proportions.

5. **Tetanus prophylaxis** should be given as for any other soft-tissue wound.

B. **Complications.** A soft-tissue wound involving the chest wall that does not expose or penetrate the bony thorax may lead to two serious probems: (1) infection in the wound or (2) splinting of the chest wall with subsequent pulmonary infection.

1. **Wound infection** can develop in a soft-tissue wound of the chest wall. Because the muscular layers of the chest wall are particularly well vascularized, however, most soft-tissue wounds of the chest will not become infected if they are initially irrigated and debrided properly.

2. **Splinting of the chest wall** adjacent to a soft-tissue wound may significantly interfere with pulmonary toilet and ventilation. Splinting is probably the greatest source of morbidity from soft-tissue injuries of the thorax, since the splinting secondary to pain in the area of injury can rapidly lead to atelectasis, lobar collapse, and even pneumonia. Adequate analgesia that will allow the patient to cough and breathe deeply will help prevent this complication.

C. **Disposition.** Patients with major traumatic defects require hospitalization for operative debridement, IV antibiotics, dressing changes, and subsequent coverage or closure. Most patients with smaller wounds can be treated and released, with follow-up in 2–3 days.

II. **Chest wall fractures.** Usually chest wall fractures result from relatively major blunt trauma to the thorax; however, fractured ribs occasionally occur secondary to vigorous coughing or metastatic disease. The possibility of associated injury to intrathoracic vessels and organs must always be considered, and appropriate diagnostic studies undertaken as indicated. Chest wall fractures alone often seriously impair respiratory function by interfering with the normal bellows function of the thoracic cage. Simple rib fractures are associated with a 20% mortality in patients over the age of 80 years as a result of secondary pulmonary complications.

A. **Rib fractures** are a major cause of morbidity and mortality in patients sustaining blunt trauma to the chest. Severe pain often accompanies uncomplicated rib fractures, leading to marked splinting with decreased ventilation to the adjacent portions of the lung. Fractures of several ribs in two separate places interfere with expansion of the chest wall during inspiration, compounding the ventilatory disability from the pain and associated splinting.

1. **Simple rib fractures without paradoxical motion of the chest wall.** Ribs fractured at only one point along their course do not lead to paradoxical chest wall motion. In addition, fractures of one or two ribs, each at two points, rarely leads to a significant "flail," or inwardly moving, segment during inspiration because the chest wall musculature and overall chest wall integrity prevent paradoxical motion.

a. **Clinical features.** Chest pain is present; it is usually severe and pleuritic and can be localized to a particular site. Point tenderness can be elicited over the involved ribs, and a palpable click may occasionally be felt on deep inspiration or application of pressure.

b. **Diagnosis.** Chest- and rib-detail x-rays will usually confirm the diagnosis. However, fractures of the anterior portions of the ribs (particularly those involving the cartilage) can be very difficult to confirm radiographically.

c. **Associated injuries.** Significant intrathoracic injury (e.g., pneumothorax, hemothorax, pulmonary contusion, injury to the heart or great vessels) may accompany simple rib fractures. Appropriate diagnostic tests should be performed as indicated, based on the nature and magnitude of the thoracic trauma.

d. **Treatment.** In the absence of paradoxical chest wall motion, significant intrathoracic injury, or impaired gas exchange, treatment of rib fractures focuses on adequate pain relief to prevent splinting and resultant hypoventilation and atelectasis (and their adverse sequelae). Adequate analgesia may be obtained using either oral narcotics or regional block anesthesia. Although externally applied appliances (including strapping or taping of the chest wall) may give symptomatic relief by restricting movement of the fracture, they should not be used because splinting of the area occurs, leading to hypoventilation and atelectasis.

(1) **Oral analgesics,** including codeine, meperidine, or oxycodone, are prescribed for the pain caused by rib fractures. Side effects include mild depression of the respiratory drive, a diminished cough reflex, mild drowsiness, and constipation. Significant analgesic requirements generally continue for at least 3 weeks following most rib fractures.

(2) **Intercostal nerve blocks** using a relatively long-acting local anesthetic, such as 0.5% bupivacaine with epinephrine, provide an alternative method for relieving the pain caused by rib fractures. Four 5-ml doses of a local anesthetic are injected just below the lower border of each fractured rib several inches lateral to the spine; one extra rib above and below the fractured ribs should also be blocked to give nearly complete pain relief. The total dose of bupivacaine injected should not exceed 200 mg in an adult. Regional block anesthesia provides excellent pain relief without any depression of ventilatory drive or patient alertness. Unfortunately, regional blocks require considerable experience and usually afford only 4–6 hours of pain relief. Repeated blocks are not practical. The major complication of intercostal nerve blocks is a pneumothorax from insertion of the needle too far.

e. **Disposition.** Patients with complications of rib fractures (e.g., ventilatory impairment, pneumothorax, hemothorax, pneumonia) or at high risk for such complications (e.g., patients with chronic obstructive pulmonary disease [COPD] or multiple [three or more] rib fractures) generally should be admitted to the hospital. In addition, patients with severe or intractable pain may need to be hospitalized for pain control. Other patients require close follow-up for the possible development of complications. It is important to emphasize to these patients the pathophysiologic consequences of splinting secondary to chest wall pain, so that they will take adequate analgesics. These patients should also be warned about the signs and symptoms of potential complications.

2. **Multiple rib fractures with paradoxical motion of a significant portion of the chest wall.** If three or more ribs are fractured, each in two places or on both sides of the sternum laterally, an entire section of the chest wall may become unstable, allowing it to move inward as the diaphragm descends during inspiration. The anterior and lateral portions of the chest wall are most often involved, since the heavier musculature and scapulas help stabilize the posterior chest wall.

a. **Clinical features.** Considerable trauma is usually required to create a flail-chest segment. Typically, these injuries result from automobile accidents in which the chest strikes the steering wheel or the door of the car. Most patients present with a large area of contusion over the chest wall, severe pleuritic pain, and moderate respiratory distress.

b. The **diagnosis** is confirmed by observing the involved chest wall segment moving inward (paradoxically) with inspiration. Contraction of chest wall muscles surrounding the unstable area occasionally prevents the paradoxical motion initially. As these muscles tire and relax, however, the section will retract during inspiration, compromising the patient's ventilatory efforts.

c. **Associated injuries.** Because flail-chest segments usually result from relatively major blunt trauma, intrathoracic injury frequently coexists, and this possibility should be investigated thoroughly. A chest x-ray will document the number of fractured ribs and, simultaneously, the presence of any pneumothorax, hemothorax, widening of the mediastinum, or pulmonary parenchymal contusion. Practically every significant flail-chest injury is associated with an underlying pulmonary contusion, although the contused area may not be visible on an initial chest x-ray immediately following the injury.

d. **Management.** Maintenance of ventilation and avoidance of atelectasis are the goals of treatment. Since deterioration and decompensation can occur over a period of hours secondary to both the chest wall injury and the delayed effects of a pulmonary contusion, these patients require hospitalization and frequent monitoring of the vital signs and arterial blood gases. Fluid restriction is important in the presence of any concomitant lung contusion. Adequate relief of chest wall pain is essential.

(1) **Smaller flail segments** can be treated without ventilatory support by nerve blocks or careful titration of analgesics, fluid restriction, aggressive pulmonary toilet, and frequent respiratory monitoring. Treatment of flail-chest injuries without early intubation and ventilatory support, however, demands particularly close observation of these patients for later decompensation.

(2) **Larger flail segments or flail-chest injuries in patients with multiple-system injury**

(a) **Mechanical ventilation,** so-called internal pneumatic stabilization of the flail segment, is required. Following endotracheal intubation, moderate levels of positive end-expiratory pressure (PEEP) are applied to optimize the patient's arterial blood gases. Mechanical ventilation may be required for a period of 2–4 weeks in very severe flail-chest injuries.

(b) **Operative stabilization.** Pinning or mechanically realigning and stabilizing multiple rib fractures is rarely indicated. If a patient with blunt chest trauma is undergoing a thoracotomy for internal injuries, internal mechanical stabilization of the chest wall fractures can be accomplished simultaneously. Infrequently, a portion of the chest wall is depressed inwardly by trauma and requires operative realignment and fracture reduction.

B. **First rib or scapular fractures** rarely require reduction but serve as a hallmark of severe blunt trauma. The impact required to fracture a first rib or scapula is great because of the thickness of these bones. Thus, a relatively high incidence of intrathoracic injury can be expected in association with either of these fractures. First rib or scapular fractures alone are not indications for aortography, bronchoscopy, or other invasive diagnostic procedures. However, these injuries should serve as a warning that significant intrathoracic damage may be present, including a transected great vessel or bronchus. Patients with either of these fractures should be examined particularly closely for any evidence of such intrathoracic injuries. Generally, hospitalization is indicated for observation and further evaluation as appropriate.

C. **Sternal fractures** are associated with major blunt chest trauma. These fractures present with severe local pain, like other chest wall fractures, and are frequently associated with a myocardial contusion. Sternal fractures are usually seen easily on a lateral chest x-ray. If fractures of the costal cartilages occur bilaterally, fracture of the sternum can result in an unstable anterior chest wall with a flail segment and may even lead to respiratory failure. Rarely, the posteriorly displaced upper end of a fractured sternum will damage the innominate or left carotid artery, and such associated injuries should be ruled out. Analgesia is required, as for other chest wall fractures; however, operative reduction is rarely necessary. Patients with a sternal fracture should be hospitalized and evaluated for a myocardial contusion and other intrathoracic injuries.

D. **Clavicular fractures** (see Chap. 26) are generally not serious problems; however, possible damage to adjacent neurovascular structures must be evaluated. If the neurovascular examination of the arm on the side of the fracture is normal, clavicular fractures require only a figure-of-eight bandage or a similar clavicle splint for realignment. Stabilization in this manner reduces the pain and encourages callus formation with minimal deformity.

III. **Open chest wall defects.** Traumatic open chest wall defects occur infrequently, usually secondary to blast injuries from a shotgun.

A. **Pathophysiology.** Any significant full-thickness opening in the chest wall makes maintenance of negative pressure in the involved hemithorax impossible. This inability to maintain negative pressure results in a nearly complete pneumothorax on the injured side and enables the mediastinum to shift with inspiration and expiration, interfering with ventilation of the contralateral lung as well.

B. **Clinical features.** Patients with open chest wall defects manifest severe respiratory embarrassment and distress. The opening in the chest wall is obvious to inspection and frequently makes a "sucking" or "blowing" sound with each labored respiration.

C. **Treatment.** The opening in the chest wall should be sealed as soon as possible, using a sterile dressing. The dressing can be made nearly airtight by including an inner layer of petroleum jelly-impregnated gauze. Once the defect is sealed, the open pneumothorax has been converted to a closed pneumothorax and should be treated accordingly by prompt chest tube insertion (see Chap. 38). After complete evaluation, debridement and closure of the chest wall are performed in the operating room.

Pleural Space Disorders

A pneumothorax, pneumomediastinum, and subcutaneous emphysema are varied manifestations of a single underlying disorder. Most often, air enters the pleural space, mediastinum, or subcutaneous tissue through an abnormal opening along the tracheobronchial tree between the glottis and alveoli. Much less commonly, air is introduced directly through the skin or chest wall or through a ruptured upper gastrointestinal tract. Treatment of these disorders is dictated largely by the etiology of the individual case.

I. **Pneumothorax.** Any accumulation of air within the pleural space constitutes a pneumothorax.

   A. **Etiologies**

   1. **Trauma.** Penetrating trauma (either a laceration or a gunshot wound) commonly creates a pneumothorax as a result of direct penetration of the visceral pleura and the lung parenchyma. Blunt trauma can lead to a pneumothorax by several mechanisms. The sharp edges of a fractured rib can tear the underlying lung, or the force of the blunt trauma itself can rupture the lung tissue. Major blunt trauma occasionally tears the major bronchi or trachea as a result of shearing forces, creating a major air leak from the tracheobronchial tree into the pleural space.

   2. A **spontaneous pneumothorax** presents without a history of externally applied trauma. The leak from the tracheobronchial tree or pulmonary parenchyma into the pleural space in a spontaneous pneumothorax results either from elevated airway pressure rupturing a normal air-containing portion of the lung or from rupture of an abnormal area of lung parenchyma, such as an emphysematous bleb. A spontaneous pneumothorax is seen frequently in association with conditions predisposing to high airway pressures (e.g., asthma, cystic fibrosis, or other forms of obstructive lung disease). Any patient with emphysematous blebs in a lung is at increased risk for a spontaneous pneumothorax. Because asthenic individuals have an increased height of their lungs (i.e., length from diaphragm to apex), they have more dilated alveoli at the apices of their lungs compared with other individuals and as a result seem to be predisposed to a spontaneous pneumothorax.

   3. **Artificial ventilation** can cause a pneumothorax secondary to increased peak airway pressures.

   4. An **open pneumothorax** (see **Chest Wall Injuries**, sec. III) is associated with a chest wall defect.

   5. **Esophageal perforation** (see **Esophageal Disorders**) can lead to a pneumothorax.

   B. **Pathophysiology.** Any accumulation of air within the pleural space elevates the intrapleural pressure and impedes full inflation of the lung during inspiration. The more air that accumulates in the pleural space, the greater the collapse of the ipsilateral lung and the greater the impairment of respiratory function. If the source of air leak into the pleural space acts as a one-way valve, with air entering the pleural space during inspiration but not exiting on expiration, the pleural pressure may rise above atmospheric pressure, creating a "tension" pneumothorax. A tension pneumothorax may shift the mediastinum, compressing the opposite lung, and lead to cardiopulmonary collapse. The mechanism of cardiovascular collapse in a tension pneumothorax has been controversial but now appears to be a marked elevation of pulmonary vascular resistance secondary to compression and collapse of the lung, leading to acute right ventricular failure. Experimental studies have not supported earlier theories that a tension pneumothorax interferes with right heart filling by obstructing the venae cavae as a result of the mediastinal shift.

   C. **Clinical features**

   1. The **history** and **presenting symptoms** of a pneumothorax are highly variable, depending on the etiology.

      a. **Traumatic pneumothorax.** When the pneumothorax has resulted from penetrating or blunt chest trauma, there is usually an obvious chest wall injury

with pain in the area of the trauma. Most pneumothoraces secondary to chest trauma can be suspected from the nature of the injury.

   b. A **spontaneous pneumothorax** can present in either a subtle or a dramatic fashion, depending on the underlying pulmonary function in the individual affected. In the young, healthy individual, a spontaneous pneumothorax may cause only mild tachypnea and mild pleuritic chest pain. Conversely, in an individual with severe underlying lung disease, such as cystic fibrosis or obstructive pulmonary disease, a spontaneous pneumothorax may present with severe respiratory failure, extreme tachypnea, and cyanosis.

   2. The **physical examination** will reveal decreased or absent breath sounds on the side of the pneumothorax, with hyperresonance to percussion. Palpation of the trachea may reveal a shift of the trachea away from the side of the pneumothorax. Subcutaneous emphysema, although not always present, is a frequent physical finding, especially in traumatic pneumothoraces.

D. **Diagnosis.** Once the suspicion of a pneumothorax is raised by either the history or physical examination, the diagnosis is confirmed by x-ray examination of the chest, if time allows. Because of the separation between the visceral and parietal pleurae that is caused by the pneumothorax, an x-ray shows that lung markings do not extend all the way to the edges of the pleural space. This separation of the visceral and parietal pleurae with air just outside the visceral pleura allows the edge of the lung to be seen as a distinct line when a pneumothorax is present. Since a small pneumothorax can be difficult to discern on a supine x-ray examination, upright PA and lateral films of the chest should be obtained when possible. A chest x-ray obtained at end expiration will accentuate the relative size of a small pneumothorax and makes detection of a small pneumothorax easier.

E. **Treatment**
   1. **Traumatic pneumothorax.** Any pneumothorax, even a very small one, associated with a history of trauma or a rib fracture is an indication for insertion of a chest tube (see Chap. 38). Occasionally, a tube thoracostomy must be performed on an emergent basis before confirmation of the diagnosis with a chest x-ray. More frequently, however, it is possible to obtain a chest x-ray for confirmation of the diagnosis before inserting a chest tube.

   2. **Spontaneous pneumothorax**
      a. **Tube thoracostomy** (see Chap. 38). The majority of spontaneous pneumothoraces require a tube thoracostomy for treatment. After placement of a chest tube, a chest x-ray should be obtained to verify proper placement of the chest tube and full reexpansion of the lung.
      b. **Observation.** A small spontaneous pneumothorax (i.e., < 20%) can be followed with serial chest x-rays if the patient is relatively asymptomatic and reliable. If there is no ongoing air leak from the surface of the lung in a spontaneous pneumothorax, the air in the pleural space will gradually be resorbed. This resorption can be hastened by having the patient breathe a high concentration of oxygen continuously. Thus, a patient with a small spontaneous pneumothorax can be observed over a period of 24–48 hours in the hospital while being kept on 100% oxygen by face mask, and frequently the small pneumothorax will resolve over this time period. Any increase in the size of the pneumothorax, however, is an indication for a tube thoracostomy.
      c. **Needle aspiration** can be used in selected cases of small spontaneous pneumothoraces. However, the risks of needle aspiration usually outweigh its benefits.

F. **Disposition.** All patients with a traumatic pneumothorax require hospitalization. Most patients with a spontaneous pneumothorax should be hospitalized for 24–48 hours for observation, even if a tube thoracostomy is not performed.

II. A **pneumomediastinum** is defined as the presence of air within the mediastinum and outside the esophagus and tracheobronchial tree.

A. The most common **mechanism** whereby air reaches the mediastinum is rupture of a bronchiole or alveolus secondary to elevated intrapulmonary pressure, with dissection of air back along the small airways to the major bronchi and then into the mediastinum itself. Traumatic injuries to the esophagus or tracheobronchial tree may also lead to a pneumomediastinum without a pneumothorax. Direct introduction of air into the mediastinum by penetrating trauma is relatively unusual, with the exception of iatrogenic trauma to the esophagus.

B. **Clinical features.** The clinical signs of a pneumomediastinum range from minimal to catastrophic. A pneumomediastinum resulting from rupture of an alveolus with dissection of air back along the airways into the mediastinum generally will be asymptomatic. The patient may notice subcutaneous emphysema with swelling in the area of the neck, and the physical examination may reveal a "Hamman's crunch" that is characteristic of mediastinal emphysema. A pneumomediastinum resulting from perforation of the esophagus, on the other hand, will often have a dramatic clinical presentation with back pain, fever, and associated hypotension from mediastinal infection.

C. **Diagnosis.** The presence of subcutaneous emphysema without physical signs of a pneumothorax should suggest the presence of a pneumomediastinum. The diagnosis, however, is usually established by a chest x-ray.

D. **Treatment.** A pneumomediastinum by itself is not an indication for specific treatment. However, it should alert the clinician to consider a more serious underlying disorder, such as a bronchial or tracheal injury or rupture of the esophagus, which will require specific therapy.

E. **Disposition.** Patients with a pneumomediastinum generally require hospitalization for observation and further evaluation as appropriate.

III. **Hemothorax**

A. **Etiologies.** Hemorrhage into the pleural space occurs to some extent in almost every patient with a diagnosable chest injury, blunt or penetrating. In contrast, a nontraumatic hemothorax is very unusual. Bleeding from chest trauma can be from any intrathoracic structure, including the great vessels or heart; but most often it is from the lung parenchyma, an intercostal artery, or, in penetrating wounds, the internal mammary or subclavian vessels.

B. **Clinical features.** The blood in the pleural space may result in sufficient blood loss to cause hypovolemic shock or in sufficient lung compression to cause decreased ventilation and hypoxemia. If the hemothorax is small, the patient may be asymptomatic. If a large amount of blood loss has occurred, the patient may be in profound shock with respiratory distress. Other clinical signs include decreased breath sounds and dullness to percussion.

C. **Diagnosis.** A hemothorax is best diagnosed with an upright PA and lateral chest x-ray. A small hemothorax of only a few hundred milliliters may not be detectable on an upright chest x-ray, as 400–500 ml of fluid is required to cause discernible blunting of the costophrenic angle. A lateral decubitus film, however, usually will reveal layering of the blood. A large hemothorax of 1500–2000 ml will cause significant opacification of the hemithorax. However, a hemothorax of 800–1200 ml can easily be overlooked on x-rays obtained in supine patients. A history of an appropriate type of trauma combined with these x-ray findings is sufficient to make the diagnosis of a hemothorax, which is confirmed by a thoracentesis or tube thoracostomy.

D. **Treatment.** The goal in the treatment of any hemothorax is to expeditiously evacuate the blood from the pleural space. Evacuation of a hemothorax will allow full reexpansion of the underlying lung, which should improve pulmonary function. Full evacuation of a hemothorax will also prevent later complications, such as an empyema from superinfection of a retained hematoma or a fibrothorax from organization of the hematoma covering the visceral pleura.

1. **Tube thoracostomy.** For any detectable hemothorax, a tube thoracostomy (see Chap. 38) should be performed using a relatively large chest tube (e.g., 36 F). It is important to document evacuation of the hemothorax and full reexpansion of the lung by a chest x-ray after insertion of the chest tube. When the hemothorax is large, consideration should be given to autotransfusion (see Chap. 38) of the shed blood, if such equipment is available.

2. **Thoracotomy.** Between 80 and 90% of individuals with a traumatic hemothorax will require only chest tube placement for treatment of their hemothorax and not a thoracotomy. The amount of blood initially evacuated from the thorax is not a reliable indication for a thoracotomy. Much more important are the trend in blood loss from the chest tube and the relative stability of the patient. A thoracotomy is indicated when the chest tube drainage exceeds 200 ml/hour for 3–4 hours following chest tube insertion. In addition, a steady increase in the rate of chest tube drainage in the 2–3 hours after insertion is an indication for a thoracotomy. Inability to adequately drain the hemothorax with one or two large chest tubes and bleeding at a rate of 400 ml/hour or more

for 2 hours following chest tube insertion are additional indications for a thoracotomy.

E. Disposition. Patients with a hemothorax require hospitalization.

IV. A **hemopneumothorax** is defined as the presence of both blood and air within the pleural space. In the setting of blunt or penetrating trauma to the chest, a hemopneumothorax is the rule rather than the exception. This condition is generally treated by insertion of a large chest tube placed at about the sixth intercostal space in the midaxillary line and directed posteriorly and superiorly. However, it is sometimes helpful in patients with a hemopneumothorax to place both an anterior and a posterior chest tube, so that the anteriorly placed tube can effectively drain the air leak while the posterior tube drains the blood and fluid within the chest. The indications for an open thoracotomy are outlined in sec. **III.D.2.**

V. An **empyema** is defined as an infection of the pleural space.

A. Etiologies. Before the advent of modern antibiotic therapy, an empyema was seen as a complication in nearly 10% of all patients suffering from pneumonia. Now, an empyema is usually seen in debilitated or malnourished patients, in the setting of a partially treated pneumonia, or as a complication of penetrating chest trauma or pulmonary or esophageal surgery.

B. Clinical features. The presenting signs and symptoms of an empyema are a fever, pleuritic chest pain, tachypnea, and a tachycardia. X-ray examination of the chest reveals fluid that usually will layer out on lateral decubitus views.

C. Diagnosis. Given the proper history and a clinical setting consistent with infection, a diagnostic thoracentesis (see Chap. 38) is indicated to prove the presence of infected material within the pleural space. Even when the pleural fluid does not appear grossly infected, a pH of the pleural fluid of less than 7.20 is suggestive of infection.

D. Treatment. With the exception of a tuberculous empyema, treatment of an empyema should be prompt drainage of the pleural space. This drainage is accomplished in most cases by the placement of one or two large chest tubes, thereby effecting reexpansion of the underlying lung and, eventually, obliteration of the pleural space. If the pleural space can be obliterated in this way, the empyema will clear. However, treatment of an empyema with chest tubes involves prolonged drainage. When insertion of chest tubes and administration of appropriate antibiotics does not bring about both full reexpansion of the lung and dramatic improvement in the patient's clinical appearance, an open thoracotomy for decortication of the underlying lung and complete evacuation of any loculations of infected material is indicated.

Pulmonary Parenchymal Injuries

I. A **pulmonary contusion** can cause extensive parenchymal damage within the lung.

A. Etiologies. A pulmonary contusion is usually the result of blunt trauma to the chest wall, ranging from large flail segments to only minor chest wall abrasions. Penetrating trauma can also cause a significant pulmonary contusion.

B. Pathophysiology. Hemorrhage and interstitial edema result in both obliteration of the alveolar space and consolidation of areas of lung tissue. The consolidation of lung tissue allows large areas of the lung to become unventilated, resulting in pulmonary arteriovenous shunting and hypoxemia.

C. Clinical features. The patient with a pulmonary contusion usually exhibits mild respiratory distress initially. Chest wall abrasions or ecchymoses may or may not be present. Rib fractures are common but occasionally are absent. Because the physiologic derangements in a pulmonary contusion progressively worsen with administration of resuscitative IV fluids and passing time, a pulmonary contusion presenting initially with only mild respiratory distress and minimal changes on a chest x-ray often becomes obvious 1–2 hours later with marked respiratory decompensation. With a severe pulmonary contusion and extensive chest wall injuries, marked respiratory distress will be apparent initially.

D. Diagnosis. Given the history of blunt or penetrating trauma to the chest, a high index of suspicion should be maintained for a pulmonary contusion. The diagnosis is made by correlating the history of trauma to the chest with appropriate chest x-ray findings and respiratory insufficiency as shown by serial arterial blood gas determinations. The initial chest x-ray often shows a subtle, hazy infiltrate in the area of suspected contusion, and this infiltrate becomes steadily more apparent during the first 6–8 hours following injury. The chest x-ray also helps confirm the diagnosis by showing rib fractures, a hemothorax, or a pneumothorax on the side of the suspected contusion. Given the appropriate history, respiratory insufficiency (as evidenced by tachypnea or hypoxemia) out of proportion to the chest x-ray findings should suggest the probability of a significant pulmonary contusion.

E. **Treatment.** Once the diagosis of a significant pulmonary contusion is suspected, aggressive treatment should be directed toward optimizing pulmonary function.

1. **Fluid restriction.** Careful restriction of resuscitative IV fluids is particularly important in minimizing the edema and consolidation in the contused portions of the lung.

2. **Analgesia.** Since splinting of the traumatized chest wall compounds the ventilation-perfusion mismatches within the lung, measures should be taken to assure adequate pain relief either by giving small doses of a narcotic analgesic or by administering intercostal nerve blocks in the area of the contused chest wall. Relief of chest wall pain in this way will improve ventilation.

3. **Mechanical ventilation.** If there is an extensive flail segment or a particularly large pulmonary contusion, intubation and ventilation of the patient using PEEP is usually required.

4. **Monitoring.** Even after intubation and ventilation, a patient with a significant pulmonary contusion requires careful monitoring of ABGs, since marked hypoxemia frequently occurs several hours after the initial injury as more fluid accumulates in the area of the contusion.

II. A **pulmonary parenchymal laceration** can result from penetrating injuries (e.g., gunshot or stab wounds, fractured ribs) or blunt trauma. The laceration will usually manifest itself with a pneumothorax or hemothorax. A pneumothorax results from air leakage from the alveoli beneath the torn visceral pleura. Bleeding from the lung parenchyma itself causes a hemothorax. With significant lung lacerations, a tube thoracostomy will almost always be required. Rarely, if blood loss or an air leak cannot be controlled by a tube thoracostomy, a thoracotomy and suturing of the laceration may become necessary. A rare life-threatening complication of pulmonary parenchymal lacerations is a bronchopulmonary-venous fistula. With the development of this fistula, systemic air embolization can occur with acute cardiovascular or pulmonary deterioration. In this situation, an immediate thoracotomy is indicated to close the bronchial leak and thus prevent further systemic air embolization.

Injuries to the Major Airways

I. **Etiologies.** Injuries of the trachea and major bronchi can result from blunt or penetrating trauma and have been reported in increasing numbers in the past 10 years. Lesions that result from blunt trauma primarily occur within 2.5 cm of the carina. Penetrating trauma can injure the tracheobronchial tree at any level but is of special significance when the injury is proximal to the subsegmental bronchi.

II. **Pathophysiology.** Extensive trauma to the proximal airways can completely disrupt the continuity of the airway. Such an injury results in distal atelectasis and an extensive pneumothorax that is often refractory to tube thoracostomy. More commonly, despite traumatic disruption of the airway itself, continuity is maintained by the supporting tissues adjacent to the airway. In such cases a pneumothorax may be absent or minimal, but stenosis of the involved airway can develop subsequently.

III. **Clinical features.** Patients with tracheobronchial disruption may present with subcutaneous emphysema, a mild cough or respiratory distress, a pneumothorax, lobar atelectasis, or hemoptysis. When a pneumothorax occurs, it is frequently of a tension variety, and after tube thoracostomy there is usually failure of the lung to reexpand on repeat x-ray examination due to a major air leak.

IV. The **diagnosis** is usually made with bronchoscopy. This procedure almost always identifies the extent and location of the tracheal or bronchial tear.

V. **Management.** The first priority in the treatment of a patient with injury to the trachea or bronchial tree is to secure the airway and ventilate the patient. When a pneumothorax is present, a tube thoracostomy should be performed immediately; a very large air leak is an indication for bronchoscopy. If difficulty is encountered in ventilating the patient, the normal bronchus should be selectively intubated by passing a translaryngeal tube over a flexible bronchoscope. Small tears in the tracheobronchial tree can be managed conservatively if the lung can be reexpanded and the patient easily ventilated. However, if the patient requires ventilatory assistance, surgical repair usually is necessary to permit reexpansion of the distal lung, ventilate the patient, and prevent contamination of the pleural space and mediastinum.

Esophageal Disorders

I. Esophageal trauma

    A. Etiologies. Esophageal injuries can occur secondary to either blunt or penetrating trauma but are uncommon. The most frequent type of esophageal perforation is that resulting from endoscopic procedures. Since the esophagus is thin-walled and has no serosal covering, it is easily injured by intraluminal manipulations. Most endoscopic injuries should be recognized by the endoscopist.

    B. Clinical features. Clinical symptoms vary from no symptoms or minimal pain initially to fever, tachycardia, and cardiovascular collapse subsequently. Pain in the neck or chest, dysphagia, fever, and subcutaneous emphysema are common early symptoms of esophageal perforation. Occasionally, hypotension, sweating, or other findings of overwhelming sepsis may be the primary presentation.

    C. Diagnosis. X-ray examination of the cervical region and upper mediastinum usually shows air in the deep-tissue planes and widening of the retrotracheal space on a lateral view. A meglumine diatrizoate (Gastrografin) swallow (barium should be avoided if perforation is a possibility) may show extravasation at the site of the injury.

    D. Treatment. If the injury is minimal with little contamination and if antibiotics are started early, nonsurgical therapy of such an esophageal perforation can be attempted. Generally, however, immediate surgical management with operative drainage of the perforation and primary closure (when possible) should be undertaken. The potentially lethal course of mediastinitis places the emphasis on early surgical drainage as the procedure of choice.

II. Spontaneous or postemetic rupture of the esophagus (Boerhaave's syndrome) is an uncommon but frequently fatal condition. Rupture of the esophagus following emesis or attempted emesis usually occurs several centimeters above the diaphragm, with the perforation usually on the left lateral side communicating with the mediastinum and left pleural space. Rupture can occur at other levels with emesis, however, and the perforation may be into the right pleural space. The level of the perforation may be modified by previous disease in or around the esophagus, such as reflux strictures or an inflammatory reaction from previous esophageal procedures.

    A. Clinical features. Patients suffering from Boerhaave's syndrome usually present with pain and fever following an episode of violent vomiting. The pain tends to be severe and substernal or interscapular in location. The mediastinitis that results from perforation of the esophagus usually leads to rapid clinical deterioration over a period of 24–48 hours, if untreated.

    B. The **diagnosis** is usually established by x-ray examinations. A chest x-ray often shows widening of the mediastinal shadow, mediastinal air, air in the cervical tissue planes, and a pleural effusion on one or both sides. The diagnosis is most easily confirmed by a contrast examination (using meglumine diatrizoate) of the esophagus, since the tear in the esophagus is usually large enough to be seen at the time of fluoroscopy.

    C. Treatment. Once the diagnosis is established, a thoracotomy with closure of the perforation, mediastinal and pleural irrigation, and pleural drainage should be performed immediately. Early repair, drainage, intensive antibiotic therapy, and nutritional support can achieve a high survival rate. However, a delay in diagnosis or operative treatment will lead to an unnecessarily high morbidity and mortality in this setting.

III. Retained foreign body. A foreign body tends to lodge at one of three sites in the esophagus: (1) in the cervical area at or just below the cricopharyngeal sphincter, (2) at the level of the aortic arch, and (3) at the esophagogastric junction. These sites are the three normal areas of narrowing within the esophagus. If not removed, a retained foreign body within the esophagus tends to penetrate or erode through the esophageal wall.

    A. Clinical features. Some patients realize immediately that a foreign body has lodged in their esophagus during attempted swallowing. Other patients with a retained foreign body present with pain in the neck or dysphagia.

    B. The **diagnosis** can usually be made by taking a careful history and is confirmed with a contrast (barium) x-ray examination of the esophagus.

C. **Treatment.** Glucagon, 1 mg IV, may help cause passage of the retained foreign body. If not, early endoscopic removal under general anesthesia by a skilled endoscopist is required.

Diaphragmatic Injuries

I. **Etiologies.** Penetrating injuries usually cause relatively minimal injury to the diaphragm; however, there may be associated damage to vital intraabdominal or intrathoracic structures. The majority of diaphragmatic injuries secondary to blunt trauma occur on the left side.

II. **Clinical features.** Patients with diaphragmatic injuries are frequently asymptomatic; however, they may be in respiratory distress or shock from associated injuries. Bowel obstruction or strangulation with perforation may appear after a variable period of time if the lesion is not identified and repaired after injury.

III. The **diagnosis** is usually made by x-ray examination. The chest x-ray may reveal an elevated left hemidiaphragm or visceral herniation into the thorax. Visceral herniation can be confirmed by x-ray examination using contrast.

IV. **Treatment.** Once the diagnosis of diaphragmatic injury has been confirmed, immediate operative repair is indicated.

Cardiac Injuries

I. **Penetrating injuries of the heart.** The incidence of penetrating wounds of the heart is increasing, and the number of patients reaching the hospital alive after such injuries is also increasing due to improved prehospital emergency care. Approximately 50% of patients with penetrating cardiac injuries arrive in the emergency department alive.

A. **Pathologic features.** Stab wounds of the heart are more likely to seal and result in pericardial tamponade without major hemorrhage, whereas gunshot wounds are frequently associated with major hemorrhage into the chest. The most common site of cardiac injury is the right ventricle, since the anterior surface of the heart is most accessible to penetrating injury. The second most common site is the left ventricle.

B. **Clinical features.** Patient with penetrating injuries to the heart have external evidence of trauma. They may be in shock from pericardial tamponade or from hemorrhage into the chest (hemothorax). A pneumothorax may be a concomitant finding.

1. **Pericardial tamponade** (see Chap. 5). Early signs of pericardial tamponade include tachycardia and hypotension; the latter cannot be explained by apparent blood loss or other factors (e.g., a tension pneumothorax). Because of the hemopericardium, there is poor cardiac filling and diminished cardiac output. The central venous pressure is elevated, and clinically the patient's neck veins in the supine position are distended (unless there is concomitant hypovolemia). The heart sounds may be distant, and classically there is a pulsus paradoxus of greater than 10 mm Hg during spontaneous inspiration. With the noise and high activity level in the emergency center, however, cardiac auscultation may be difficult. Arrhythmias and even sudden cardiac asystole can also occur. Agitation and restlessness to the point of requiring restraint are common.

2. A **hemothorax** (see **Pleural Space Disorders,** sec. **III**) with associated hypotension may be present if there is hemorrhage into the pleural space.

C. **Evaluation**

1. **Central venous pressure measurement.** All patients with a penetrating injury to the chest should have a central venous pressure line placed. If injury to the heart is suspected and if the central venous pressure is greater than 15 mm Hg, the diagnosis of tamponade is very likely.

2. A **chest x-ray** should be obtained if time permits. Generally, the chest film will not be helpful in evaluating for pericardial tamponade, as the pericardium is unable to distend rapidly; however, a chest x-ray may identify a hemothorax or pneumothorax.

3. An **electrocardiogram** may reveal evidence of a pericardial tamponade (e.g., low voltage, electrical alternans), myocardial injury (e.g., arrhythmias, conduction disturbances, ST–T changes), or ischemia due to hypotension or coronary artery injury.

4. If the patient is stable, **echocardiography,** if immediately available, may demonstrate fluid within the pericardium.

D. Treatment. Standard resuscitative measures (i.e., airway, ventilation, circulation) should be initiated as needed.

    1. If **cardiac tamponade** is suspected in an appropriate clinical setting, the patient should be transferred immediately to the operating suite for exploration, rather than delaying while further diagnostic procedures are performed. However, if the patient is hemodynamically compromised and cannot be stabilized or is deteriorating, pericardiocentesis (see Chap. 38) is indicated as a temporizing measure; the subxiphoid approach is preferred to reduce the chance of either injury to the coronary arteries or a pneumothorax. The patient should then be moved immediately to the operating suite for a thoracotomy and repair of the penetrating cardiac injury. It is important to remember that failure to obtain blood from the pericardium does not exclude a hemopericardium because of clotting of intrapericardial blood.

    2. A **hemothorax** or pneumothorax (or both) is treated initially with a tube thoracostomy (see Chap. 38). Major or persistent hemorrhage, as might be seen with a penetrating cardiac injury, is an indication for a thoracotomy and definitive surgical repair.

II. Blunt injuries of the heart usually occur in vehicular accidents when the steering wheel forcefully compresses the heart between the sternum and the vertebral column, resulting in a wide variety of injuries.

  A. Pathologic features

    1. The most common injury is a **myocardial contusion,** which may vary from superficial epicardial petechiae to a complete transmural infarction.

    2. **Rupture of an atrial or ventricular chamber** due to blunt trauma is uncommon but does occur. Most patients suffering rupture of a cardiac chamber do not reach a medical facility alive; however, if the pericardium is intact, the patient may reach the emergency department with signs and symptoms of pericardial tamponade.

    3. Occasionally, a severe cardiac contusion will result in a **ventricular septal defect** 3–14 days postinjury when the contused, infarcted area breaks down.

    4. Rarely, blunt injury to the heart can cause **valvular injury.**

  B. Diagnosis. Clinical findings in blunt injuries to the heart may include obvious trauma to the anterior chest wall, such as a sternal fracture or an anterior chest wall flail segment. Hypotension that does not respond to fluid administration suggests a cardiac tamponade or myocardial contusion. A pericardial friction rub or any new electrocardiographic findings in the appropriate clinical setting should raise the suspicion of a myocardial contusion. However, the electrocardiographic abnormalities most frequently attributable to a myocardial contusion (i.e., a sinus tachycardia and ST and T-wave alterations) are nonspecific and may be secondary to hypotension or associated injuries; furthermore, a normal ECG does not rule out the diagnosis of a cardiac contusion. Given the appropriate clinical setting, the existence of a cardiac contusion should be assumed and the patient managed accordingly. Further studies that may be helpful in diagnosing a myocardial contusion include laboratory evaluation of the total creatine kinase (CK) and the MB fraction of this enzyme. Radionuclide scanning may also be helpful in demonstrating wall-motion abnormalities and a decreased ejection fraction. Echocardiography may demonstrate both functional and anatomic abnormalities secondary to a cardiac contusion.

  C. Treatment of blunt cardiac injuries is variable, depending on the severity and nature of the injury. All patients with a history of significant blunt trauma to the chest should have continuous cardiac monitoring for at least 1–2 days. Cardiac isoenzyme determinations should be followed closely over the first 24–48 hours, and serial ECGs should be obtained. In most respects, treatment of a myocardial contusion is similar to that of an acute myocardial infarction (see Chap. 5). Other injuries, such as rupture of a cardiac chamber or intracardiac anatomic defects, should be treated individually.

Great-Vessel Injuries

I. Penetrating injuries to the great vessels. The aorta, its arch branches, and the pulmonary hilar vessels may be injured in penetrating trauma. Massive hemorrhage with a hemothorax and hypotension usually results from penetrating trauma to any of these structures. Injury is usually from a gunshot or stab wound to the neck or chest. These injuries are often fatal before the patient reaches medical attention.

  A. Clinical features. Patients with penetrating injuries of the great vessels usually present with hemorrhage and hypotension. However, pericardial tamponade can occur if an intrapericardial portion of a vessel has been injured. Any entry wound in the chest or neck should be assumed to have penetrated the mediastinal structures until proved otherwise because of the extremely grave implications of penetrating injuries to these structures, such as the heart or great vessels. As a result of hypotension and direct damage to the vessels themselves, the carotid or brachial pulses may be diminished. These patients often have an altered mental status and may have significant cervical or supraclavicular hematomas that compromise the airway.

B. Diagnosis. If the patient is stable, a chest x-ray should be taken immediately. Radiographic findings in injury to the great vessels are not entirely specific, but either widening of the mediastinal shadow or a definite hemothorax will usually be seen. In a patient who remains hypotensive despite attempted volume replacement, an emergency thoracotomy (see Chap. 38) may be necessary to control the hemorrhage. However, if the patient can be stabilized, aortography can be useful to establish the diagnosis and identify the location of a great-vessel injury.

C. Treatment. When a patient sustains injury to a great vessel, an emergency thoracotomy (see Chap. 38) may be necessary as part of the resuscitation, as the patient usually exsanguinates quickly if control of hemorrhage is not obtained. A patient presenting in extremis from injury to a great vessel should be immediately intubated for control of the airway, and mechanical ventilation instituted. Vascular access should be obtained with numerous large-bore IV catheters, including at least one large-bore IV catheter below the diaphragm. The patient should then be moved immediately to the operating suite for operative control of hemorrhage and further resuscitation.

II. Blunt injuries of the great vessels occur secondary to chest compression or deceleration accidents, such as automobile or motorcycle accidents, auto-pedestrian accidents, or falls from heights. Patients sustaining **blunt injury to the aorta** usually die at the scene; however, approximately 15% will survive to reach the hospital. Of these survivors, the majority will die within 1 week if the aortic injury is not recognized and repaired. These statistics mandate early and aggressive diagnosis and surgical treatment.

A. Pathologic features. The exact mechanism of injury is not fully understood, but the aorta or, uncommonly, one of its major branches tears at a point of fixation of the vessel. The most common site of injury to the thoracic aorta is at the ligamentum arteriosum (i.e., just distal to the left subclavian artery). The tear is generally transverse and involves a variable portion of the circumference of the vessel. The tear may extend through the intima only or through all layers of the vessel wall, bringing about a complete disruption.

B. Clinical features. There is usually a history of deceleration or compression trauma. External evidence of chest trauma may or may not be present; however, extrathoracic injuries are relatively common. The most common symptom (in conscious patients) is retrosternal or interscapular pain. Other symptoms that may be present include dyspnea from tracheal compression, hoarseness secondary to compression of the recurrent laryngeal nerve, or dysphagia from esophageal compression. Physical findings may include a harsh systolic murmur over the precordium or interscapular area, relative upper-extremity hypertension, pulse deficits (particularly from injury to aortic arch vessels), or a cervical or supraclavicular hematoma.

C. Diagnosis. All patients with a history of deceleration trauma should be examined for aortic rupture (or injury to aortic arch vessels). The diagnosis is usually suggested from careful examination of a chest roentgenogram (preferably an upright PA film, if possible) revealing a superior mediastinal hematoma, which is evidenced by an ill-defined aortic knob, superior mediastinal widening (i.e., > 8 cm), depression of the left main stem bronchus, obliteration of the aortopulmonary window, deviation of the trachea or esophagus (i.e., a nasogastric tube) to the right, or the presence of a left apical "cap" or left pleural effusion (hemothorax). Patients in whom the diagnosis of an aortic (or other great vessel) injury is suspected should undergo an immediate, appropriate radiologic study (e.g., aortography, digital subtraction angiography, contrast-enhanced computed tomography) to confirm the diagnosis and identify the site of rupture (unless rapid deterioration of the patient precludes the study).

D. Treatment. Once the diagnosis is made, surgical repair should be performed immediately because of the risk of fatal hemorrhage at any moment.

III. Dissecting aneurysm of the thoracic aorta. See Chap. 5.

Bibliography

1. Ayella, R. J., et al. Ruptured thoracic aorta due to blunt trauma. *J. Trauma* 17:199, 1977.
2. Beel, T., and Harwood, A. L. Traumatic rupture of the thoracic aorta. *Ann. Emerg. Med.* 9:483, 1980.
3. Callaham, M. Acute traumatic cardiac tamponade: Diagnosis and treatment. *J.A.C.E.P.* 7:306, 1978.
4. Callaham, M. Pericardiocentesis in traumatic and nontraumatic cardiac tamponade. *Ann. Emerg. Med.* 13:924, 1984.
5. Cowley, R. A., and Dunham, C. M. (eds.). *Shock Trauma/Cricital Care Manual.* Baltimore: University Park Press, 1982.
6. Curci, J. J., and Horman, M. J. Boerhaave's syndrome: The importance of early diagnosis and treatment. *Ann. Surg.* 183:401, 1976.
7. DeLuca, S. A., Rhea, J. T., and O'Malley, T. Radiographic evaluation of rib fractures. *A.J.R.* 138:91, 1982.
8. Feliciano, D. V., et al. Civilian trauma in the 1980's. *Ann. Surg.* 199:717, 1984.
9. Graham, J. M., Mattox, K. L., and Beall, A. C. Penetrating trauma of the lung. *J. Trauma* 19:665, 1979.
10. Marshall, W. G., Jr., Bell, J. L., and Kouchoukos, N. T. Penetrating cardiac trauma. *J. Trauma* 24:147, 1984.
11. Martin, T. D., et al. Blunt cardiac rupture. *J. Trauma* 24:287, 1984.
12. Mattox, K. L. Suspecting thoracic aortic transection. *J.A.C.E.P.* 7:12, 1978.
13. Mattox, K. L., and Allen, M. K. Emergency department treatment of chest injuries. *Emerg. Med. Clin. North Am.* 2:783, 1984.
14. Nowak, R. M., and Tomlanovich, M. C. Subcutaneous emphysema. *J.A.C.E.P.* 6:269, 1977.
15. Oparah, S. S., and Mandal, A. K. Penetrating stab wounds of the chest: Experience with 200 consecutive cases. *J. Trauma* 16:868, 1976.
16. Rothstein, R. J. Myocardial contusion. *J.A.M.A.* 250:2189, 1983.
17. Shaffer, K. R., and Franaszek, J. B. Emergency diagnosis, resuscitation, and treatment of acute penetrating cardiac trauma. *Ann. Emerg. Med.* 11:504, 1982.
18. Sherman, M. M. Management of penetrating heart wounds. *Am. J. Surg.* 135:553, 1978.
19. Sturm, J. T., Marsh, D. G., and Bodily, K. C. Ruptured thoracic aorta: Evolving radiologic concepts. *Surgery* 85:363, 1979.
20. Sturm, J. T., Olson, F. R., and Cicero, J. J. Chest roentgenographic findings in 26 patients with traumatic rupture of the thoracic aorta. *Ann. Emerg. Med.* 12:598, 1983.
21. Symbas, P. N. Cardiac trauma. *Am. Heart J.* 92:387, 1976.
22. Symbas, P. N. Great vessel injury. *Am. Heart J.* 93:518, 1977.
23. Symbas, P. N., Hatcher, C. R., and Harlaftis, M. Spontaneous rupture of the esophagus. *Ann. Surg.* 187:634, 1978.
24. Tenzer, M. L. The spectrum of myocardial contusion: A review. *J. Trauma* 25:620, 1985.
25. Trinkle, J. K., et al. Management of flail chest without mechanical ventilation. *Ann. Thorac. Surg.* 19:355, 1975.
26. Waldschmidt, M. L., and Laws, H. L. Injuries of the diaphragm. *J. Trauma* 20:587, 1980.
27. Weil, P. H., and Margolis, I. B. Systemic approach to traumatic hemothorax. *Am. J. Surg.* 142:692, 1981.
28. Wilson, R. F., Murray, C., and Antoneko, D. R. Nonpenetrating thoracic injuries. *Surg. Clin. North Am.* 57:17, 1977.
29. Wilson, J. M., et al. Severe chest trauma. Morbidity implication of first and second rib fractures in 120 patients. *Arch. Surg.* 113:846, 1978.
30. Woodring, J. H., and Dillon, M. L. Radiographic manifestations of mediastinal hemorrhage from blunt chest trauma. *Ann. Thorac. Surg.* 37:171, 1984.
31. Woodring, J. H., et al. Fractures of first and second ribs: Predictive value for arterial and bronchial injury. *A.J.R.* 138:211, 1982.

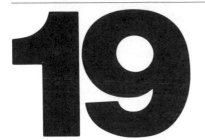

Abdominal Emergencies

Michael B. Freeman and
Charles B. Anderson

Abdominal Pain

In most cases of acute abdominal disease, pain is the primary presenting symptom. The etiology of the pain usually can be ascertained by means of a careful history and complete physical examination supplemented by a few laboratory tests. It is important to exercise careful judgment in order to arrive at a prompt and accurate diagnosis, so that appropriate treatment can be instituted expeditiously.

I. **Anatomic considerations.** To accurately evaluate the etiology of abdominal pain, the basic neuroanatomy of abdominal pain fibers must be understood. There are three distinct types of abdominal pain: visceral, somatic, and referred.

A. **Visceral pain** is mediated by the autonomic nervous system. These pain fibers are stimulated by stretch or distention of a viscus structure. Visceral pain is usually characterized as diffuse, poorly localized, crampy abdominal pain with a high threshold. The area of general localization is influenced by the embryologic derivation of the involved viscus; pain from structures originating from the foregut, midgut, and hindgut is generally felt in the midepigastrium, periumbilical region, and hypogastrium, respectively. Also mediated through the autonomic nervous system are reflexes associated with severe pain; these reflexes are manifested as nausea, tachycardia, bradycardia, and muscular rigidity.

B. **Somatic pain** results from stimulation of the parietal peritoneum, root of the mesentery, and the diaphragm. Compared with visceral pain, somatic pain generally is sharper and more well defined. In several abdominal diseases, visceral and somatic pain fibers may be stimulated; however, it is the somatic component that generally is manifested. For example, in acute appendicitis, the patient initially has dull periumbilical pain (visceral pain) that subsequently localizes in the right lower quadrant (somatic pain) once the parietal peritoneum becomes involved in the inflammatory process.

C. **Referred pain** is felt in the areas supplied by the same neurologic segment as a diseased organ and is due to the existence of a shared central pathway for afferent neurons from different sites. Thus, pain can be perceived in a part of the body that is a considerable distance from the tissue causing the pain.

II. **Evaluation**

A. **History of pain.** A careful history is essential in ascertaining the etiology of abdominal pain. The pain must be analyzed with regard to its onset, location, character, and associated symptoms.

1. **Onset of pain.** The examiner should determine the exact time and severity of pain at its onset. Certain clues about the onset of pain aid in the diagnosis. Severe pain at the time of onset and pain that awakens the patient from sleep are of a serious nature. Pain related to meals suggests the possibility of peptic ulcer or gallbladder disease. Sudden pain in which a previously well patient can recall the exact time of onset is classic for a perforated viscus or an intraabdominal vascular accident.

2. **Location.** The location of pain should include a description of its original location and any shifting or radiation of the pain. The initial location may better define the viscera involved, since once peritonitis occurs, the pain becomes diffuse. Table 19-1 shows the characteristic location of abdominal pain associated with various diseases. Change in location of pain, as in appendicitis, can be an important clue to the etiology of the pain. In addition, referral of pain may be diagnostic in that certain disorders are associated with a typical pattern of radiation (e.g., radiation of pancreatic pain to the back and of ureteral pain to the groin).

Table 19.1 Location of abdominal pain associated with various diseases

I. *Right upper quadrant*
   Gallbladder/biliary disease
   Hepatitis
   Peptic ulcer
   Pancreatitis
   Renal pain
   Appendicitis
   Myocardial infarction
   Pneumonia/empyema

II. *Right lower quadrant*
   Appendicitis
   Meckel's diverticulitis
   Regional enteritis
   Mesenteric lymphadenitis
   Diverticulitis
   Cholecystitis
   Renal pain
   Ureteral calculi
   Salpingitis
   Ectopic pregnancy
   Ovarian disorders
   Ruptured aneurysm

III. *Left upper quadrant*
   Pancreatitis
   Gastritis
   Splenic rupture/infarction
   Renal pain
   Myocardial infarction
   Pneumonia/empyema

IV. *Left lower quadrant*
   Diverticulitis
   Appendicitis
   Ectopic pregnancy
   Ovarian disorders
   Salpingitis
   Renal pain
   Ureteral calculi
   Ruptured aneurysm

3. **Character of pain.** The examiner must determine the exact character of the abdominal pain.
   a. **Excruciating pain unrelieved by narcotics** indicates a vascular lesion, such as intestinal infarction or rupture of an abdominal aortic aneurysm.
   b. **Very severe pain relieved by narcotics** is typical of acute pancreatitis or peritonitis associated with a ruptured viscus. Other examples include appendicitis, incarcerated small bowel, and biliary and renal colic.
   c. **Dull, vague, poorly localized pain** that is usually gradual in onset suggests an inflammatory process or low-grade infection.
   d. **Colicky pain** suggests gastroenteritis or obstruction of a hollow viscus (e.g., mechanical intestinal obstruction, ureteral or biliary obstruction).
4. **Symptoms associated with pain**
   a. **Nausea/vomiting.** Vomiting is an indication of a viral illness, severe irritation of the peritoneum, stretching of the mesentry, obstruction, or the presence of local or absorbed toxins. The character of the vomitus should be determined with regard to its color, volume, and frequency. Feculent vomitus is indicative of bowel obstruction. Hematemesis of a massive nature is suggestive of bleeding esophageal varices or peptic ulcer disease. Coffee ground vomitus is found in any number of pathologic states with upper gastrointestinal hemorrhage, including duodenal ulcer, gastritis, and gastric ulcer. Frequent bilious vomiting suggests a high intestinal obstruction. It is of diagnostic importance to elicit whether the abdominal pain occurred before or after the onset of vomiting. Upper abdominal pain occurring after severe vomiting and retching suggests the possibility of esophageal perforation (Boerhaave's syndrome).
   b. **Bowel habits.** Evaluation of bowel habits with regard to diarrhea, constipation, or obstipation is particularly pertinent in patients presenting with abdominal pain. In general, if a patient has not passed flatus in 24 hours, there is a profound paralytic ileus or intestinal obstruction. Although diarrhea may suggest colitis or gastroenteritis, it can be found in association with any number of intraabdominal diseases, including partial bowel obstruction and inflammatory processes such as appendicitis. The color of the stool and the presence of blood should also be noted, since these characteristics often provide important diagnostic clues.
   c. **Chills/fever.** High fevers and chills are usually associated with renal, biliary, or pelvic inflammatory disease. In contrast, appendicitis is rarely associ-

ated with a high fever; if it occurs, perforation or pyelophlebitis should be suspected.

   d. **Urinary symptoms.** Hematuria or dysuria are indicative of urinary tract disease. It should be emphasized that a distended bladder can produce abdominal pain; therefore, the frequency of voiding and the volumes of urine should be ascertained.

5. **Gynecologic history.** A gynecologic history including a menstrual history and the presence or absence of vaginal discharge or bleeding should be determined. Pain in association with ovulation characteristically occurs at midcycle. Severe lower abdominal pain and purulent vaginal discharge are characteristic of pelvic inflammatory disease. If the patient has lower abdominal pain and a history of missed menses, an ectopic pregnancy should be suspected.

6. **Cardiopulmonary history.** Disease processes involving the cardiopulmonary system may produce abdominal pain. Symptoms such as chest pain, shortness of breath, productive cough, or irregular heart beat should be ascertained. Pneumonia sometimes produces a paralytic ileus and abdominal pain. Atrial fibrillation may lead to embolic disease affecting the mesenteric vasculature. Other conditions of the cardiorespiratory system that may produce abdominal pain include myocardial infarction, empyema, and pneumothorax.

7. **Past medical history.** It is important to ascertain whether the patient has had any previous episodes of pain. In addition, it is important to determine whether the patient has any underlying medical illnesses or has had any hospitalizations or surgery. Also important are the patient's use of medications, alcoholic beverages, or drugs.

B. **Physical examination.** A complete physical examination, with special emphasis on the abdominal examination, should be performed on all patients with abdominal pain. The appearance and position of the patient will often given clues as to the severity of the illness. Restricted motion in bed suggests peritonitis, whereas writhing suggests biliary or renal colic. Vital signs should be obtained, with special note made of the character and rate of respirations. Patients with peritonitis often have frequent shallow respiratory efforts. The abdominal examination itself should include inspection, auscultation, percussion, and palpation in addition to careful gynecologic and rectal examinations.

1. **Inspection.** The abdomen should be noted for distention and restricted motion of the abdominal wall during respiration, which suggests peritonitis. Maintenance of the hip in a position of flexion is suggestive of inflammation involving the psoas muscle, which can occur in appendicitis or pelvic abscess.

2. **Palpation** is the most important facet of the physical examination. It should be done in a gentle manner, beginning in an area remote from the indicated site of maximal discomfort. When palpation is begun, the degree of muscular rigidity should be assessed. The presence or absence of either organomegaly or intraabdominal masses should be ascertained. Rebound tenderness should be sought, and when present, signifies peritoneal inflammation; rebound tenderness is elicited by the sudden removal of the palpating hand from the abdomen and should be done without warning. Potential sites of hernia, including both groins and previous surgical scars, should be examined.

3. **Percussion** may be helpful in determining the etiology of abdominal distention. Tympany suggests a gas-filled bowel; shifting dullness, ascites; and suprapubic dullness, urinary retention.

4. **Auscultation** is an essential part of the abdominal examination and can often narrow the differential diagnosis. Absence of audible peristalsis usually signifies peritonitis or a severe ileus. The examiner may, however, need to listen for 3 minutes to verify the absence of peristalsis. Conversely, in patients with intestinal obstruction, the bowel sounds are increased in frequency and are high-pitched. It should be pointed out that although certain generalities exist among disease processes, the presence or absence of bowel sounds does not necessarily confirm or rule out the diagnosis. Severe catastrophies such as a strangulated small-intestinal obstruction can occur in the presence of normal peristalsis.

5. **Rectal examination** should be performed, noting the stool color and result of test with guaiac as well as the presence or absence of pelvic masses or tenderness. Acholic stools are virtually diagnostic of biliary obstruction. The combination of guaiac-positive stools and intestinal obstruction is suggestive of strangulated bowel or possibly an obstructing carcinoma.

6. **Gynecologic examination.** A thorough pelvic examination should be performed, including speculum and bimanual examination. Any vaginal discharge should be cultured. On bimanual examination, every effort should be made to determine the size of the uterus and the presence or absence of adnexal masses; in addition, any abnormal tenderness should be noted.

7. **Supplemental physical findings**
   a. The **iliopsoas sign** tests for an inflammatory process in contact with the psoas muscles. This test is performed by having the patient lie in the supine position with the legs fully extended. The patient is then requested to elevate each leg. Pain is experienced if the inflammatory process involves the psoas muscle.
   b. The **obturator sign** tests for an inflammatory process in contact with the obturator internus muscle. This test is performed by placing the patient in a supine position, with the thigh flexed at a right angle. The leg is then rotated internally and externally. Pain on rotation is considered a positive test. This test may be positive with pelvic abscesses, acute appendicitis in which the appendix extends into the pelvis, or a strangulated obturator hernia.
   c. **Murphy's sign** is associated with acute cholecystitis and gonococcal perihepatitis (Fitz-Hugh–Curtis syndrome). The examiner exerts pressure against the abdominal wall in the right upper quadrant and asks the patient to breathe deeply. With descent of the diaphragm, an acutely inflamed gallbladder or liver capsule will come in contact with the examining fingers, causing accentuation of pain and arrest of the inspiratory effort.
   d. **Cullen's sign** is a bluish or purplish discoloration in the region of the umbilicus associated with blood in the retroperitoneum.

C. **Laboratory evaluation.** The two most important laboratory tests in evaluating abdominal pain are a complete blood count and urinalysis. Other tests may be of benefit, but unnecessary tests can delay treatment of patients with acute abdominal illnesses.

1. **Complete blood count.** This test should include a white blood cell (WBC) count, hematocrit, red cell count, and differential count. The hematocrit can reflect changes in plasma volume and red cell mass (e.g., hemoconcentration and anemia). An elevated WBC count suggests an inflammatory process, as does a shift to the left on the peripheral smear; however, normal or even low counts may be associated with peritonitis. A low blood count with lymphocytosis usually signifies a viral illness or gastroenteritis.

2. **Urinalysis** may aid in the diagnosis of primary renal disease, dehydration, and other systemic and intraabdominal diseases. A urinalysis should include the specific gravity; pH; tests for albumin, blood, and urobilinogen; and a careful microscopic examination.

3. **Amylase.** An elevated serum amylase is usually indicative of primary pancreatic disease. However, an elevated amylase may also be found in mesenteric ischemia, intestinal obstruction, perforated ulcer, or ectopic pregnancy. In addition, it should be noted that acute pancreatitis may be associated with a normal serum amylase. Urinary amylase excretion may be measured and, when expressed as a ratio of amylase to creatinine clearance, can be diagnostic of pancreatitis if greater than 5:1.

4. **Serum chemistries.** Standard serum electrolytes (Na^+, K^+, Cl^-, CO_2), blood urea nitrogen (BUN), creatinine, and glucose should be obtained, especially in those with protracted symptoms of vomiting and diarrhea. A hypokalemic metabolic alkalosis is encountered frequently in patients with prolonged vomiting, whereas those with protracted diarrhea will develop a hypokalemic metabolic acidosis. The BUN and creatinine levels often give an estimate of the amount of dehydration and help determine the presence of renal insufficiency. Diabetics with pathologic intraabdominal conditions often have a marked hyperglycemia.

D. **Radiologic evaluation.** There should be specific indications for requesting radiologic studies. In some instances, a trip to the radiology suite will unnecessarily delay needed surgery and constitute a hazard to the patient. In addition, there seems little reason to obtain films of the abdomen when the diagnosis can be made on clinical grounds (e.g., appendicitis). If the diagnosis is obscure in patients presenting with significant abdominal pain, supine and upright abdominal films and an upright chest x-ray should be obtained.

1. **Chest x-ray.** An upright chest x-ray is the best radiologic study to demonstrate

free air in the abdomen. The patient should remain in the upright position for 5 minutes before taking the chest x-ray to completely rule out free air. The chest radiograph also allows for evaluation of pulmonary disease, mediastinal air, and the possibility of air-filled viscera in the chest.

2. **Supine and upright abdominal films.** These studies should be examined for the gas pattern, abnormal calcifications, outline of viscera, and obliteration of the psoas shadows.

   a. **Abnormal gas patterns.** Small amounts of air are normally seen in the stomach, small intestine, and colon. Obstruction of the bowel has characteristic patterns depending on the location of the blockage. A large-bowel obstruction shows a markedly dilated proximal colon, with or without air-fluid levels in the small bowel. Depending on the location, a small-bowel obstruction may show multiple distended loops of small bowel with air-fluid levels without large-bowel gas. It should be remembered that a high-intestinal obstruction may not be associated with dilated loops of small bowel and that in certain instances when the small bowel is completely filled with fluid, the abdominal film will fail to demonstrate air-fluid levels. Other abnormal gas patterns include air in the biliary tree or bowel wall and outlining viscera.

   b. **Abnormal calcifications** include gallstones, renal calculi, uterine fibromas, pancreatic calcifications, and vascular calcifications (e.g., in the wall of an abdominal aortic aneurysm).

   c. **Viscera.** It is important to note the location and size of the various intraabdominal viscera. It may be possible to identify enlargement of the liver and spleen, as well as a distended bladder or cecal volvulus.

   d. **Psoas shadow.** An obscured psoas shadow suggests retroperitoneal disease.

3. **Lateral decubitus abdominal radiograph.** In those instances where upright films cannot be obtained, a left lateral decubitus film of the abdomen is useful in demonstrating free air (over the dome of the liver) and air-fluid levels.

4. **Other radiologic studies.** With the aid of clinical evaluation, laboratory examination, and plain radiographs, the etiology of abdominal pain usually can be determined. However, it is occasionally necessary to obtain other radiologic studies to establish the diagnosis. These studies include intravenous pyelography (IVP), an upper gastrointestinal series, barium enema, oral cholecystogram, isotopic cholescintigraphy (with technetium 99m[^{99m}Tc]-labeled derivative of acetanilide iminodiacetic acid [IDA]), ultrasonography, computed tomography (CT), and angiography.

III. **Differential diagnosis.** When a specific diagnosis cannot be made, several disease processes must be considered in the differential diagnosis. Although abdominal pain is usually the result of an intraabdominal disease process, the pain may be secondary to an extraabdominal disorder.

A. **Myocardial infarction.** An acute myocardial infarction can mimic the pain pattern of a perforated ulcer or acute cholecystitis. Examination of the abdomen fails to reveal muscular rigidity or absent peristalsis. A careful history and an electrocardiogram (ECG) generally will lead to the diagnosis.

B. **Pneumonia/pleurisy/empyema.** These entities can produce upper abdominal pain and an intestinal ileus. A careful history, physical examination, and chest x-ray usually will clarify the diagnosis. Occasionally, pneumonia may not be radiographically apparent until the hypovolemic patient is rehydrated.

C. **Spontaneous pneumothorax** may present with pain similar to that of acute cholecystitis. The chest x-ray is diagnostic.

D. **Acute hepatitis** may be easily confused with biliary tract disease, since both are associated with right upper quadrant pain, jaundice, and fever. Tenderness diffusely over the liver may provide the clue that hepatitis is the etiology.

E. **Acute porphyria.** Severe abdominal pain is often a classic presentation for acute porphyria. These patients often have multiple surgical scars from previous negative laparotomies. The diagnosis can be made by examination of the urine for porphobilinogens (Watson-Schwartz test).

F. **Lesions of the spine.** Acute lumbar disk disease, as well as thoracic spine compression, may present with abdominal pain, profound ileus, and involuntary guarding. The abdominal pain is often atypical. With physical examination and appropriate radiologic studies, a diagnosis can usually be made.

G. **Other unusual causes** of abdominal pain include hyperparathyroidism, lead intoxication, herpes zoster, tabes dorsalis, epilepsy, spider bites, infectious mononucleosis, diabetic ketosis, and diseases of the hip joint.

IV. General management principles. Once an extensive evaluation of the patient has been completed, a specific diagnosis or at least a differential diagnosis can be reached. If a pathologic process is identified, appropriate treatment should be instituted; however, in those in whom the diagnosis is obscure, a period of observation may be appropriate. Certain principles apply during this observation period.

    A. Reevaluation. Frequent reevaluation for progression of signs and symptoms is essential and should include frequent examination of the abdomen, preferably by the same observer, and follow-up of appropriate laboratory tests.

    B. Antibiotics should be withheld until the diagnosis is established, since their use can mask progression of the disease process.

    C. Pain medications should be used judiciously, if at all. However, analgesia may be of benefit for severe pain in that diffuse tenderness may become more localized and examination for masses facilitated.

    D. Exploratory laparotomy. Progression of signs, particularly development of peritoneal signs, generally signifies the need for exploratory laparotomy. Such patients should be prepared for the operating room. This preparation may require (1) fluid hydration, (2) nasogastric suction, and (3) administration of intravenous antibiotics.

V. Specific entities

    A. Appendicitis. Acute appendicitis is the most common acute surgical condition of the abdomen. It has been estimated that 6% of the population will develop acute appendicitis during their lifetime [6]. The condition most commonly occurs in the young; its maximum incidence is in the first and second decades of life. The etiology is almost always due to obstruction of the lumen by lymphoid tissue or a fecalith. Obstruction of the lumen ultimately leads to distention, bacterial overgrowth and suppuration, venous thrombosis, arterial ischemia, and, ultimately, perforation.

        1. Clinical features

            a. History. The classic sequence of symptoms in a patient with appendicitis is that of initial periumbilical pain associated with anorexia and nausea that subsequently becomes more localized in the right lower quadrant. This presentation is found in 55% of patients with appendicitis [3]. Atypical pain, however, can occur with various locations of the appendix. For example, a retrocecal appendix may present with flank pain and urinary symptoms due to its proximity to the ureter; a pelvic appendix may produce either urinary symptoms when adjacent to the bladder or diarrhea, tenesmus, and rectal pain when adjacent to the sigmoid colon; and a high cecum may place the appendix near the gallbladder and therefore mimic cholecystitis. When vomiting is present, it occurs after the onset of pain and usually is not persistent or prolonged; if vomiting precedes the pain, the diagnosis of appendicitis should be questioned. Bowel function is of little benefit since the patient may have either diarrhea or constipation.

            b. Physical examination. The traditional sign of appendicitis is right lower quadrant tenderness with rebound and muscle guarding. Other findings include a positive Rovsing (pain in right lower quadrant produced by palpation in left lower quadrant), obturator, or psoas sign as well as a tender rectal examination. Fever, when present, is usually mild; when markedly elevated, it suggests perforation or another intraabdominal inflammatory condition. It should be remembered that the signs and symptoms of appendicitis may be diminished in both infants and the elderly. Although it is unusual for these age groups to present with appendicitis, this diagnosis must be kept in mind to prevent the increased morbidity and mortality commonly associated with appendicitis in these age groups.

            c. Laboratory findings. Although laboratory tests may help in confirming the diagnosis of acute appendicitis, this diagnosis can never be ruled out on the basis of normal laboratory work. The WBC count and differential are usually abnormal, showing a mild leukocytosis with shift to the left; however, 5% of patients with acute appendicitis have both a normal leukocyte count and a normal differential count [1].

            d. Radiologic evaluation. Abdominal films usually demonstrate nonspecific findings in acute appendicitis. A barium enema can be of diagnostic aid if the diagnosis is obscure after a period of observation; positive findings suggestive of appendicitis include nonfilling or partial filling of the appendix and a mass effect compressing the cecum. It has been reported, however, that the false-negative rate of barium enemas in selected patients with appendicitis is approximately 12% [5].

2. The **differential diagnosis** in patients suspected of having appendicitis includes almost any intraabdominal inflammatory condition, e.g., mesenteric lymphadenitis, acute gastroenteritis, urinary tract infection, Meckel's diverticulitis, intussusception, regional enteritis, primary peritonitis, Henoch-Schönlein purpura, pelvic inflammatory disease, ectopic pregnancy, ruptured graafian follicle, epididymitis, perforated peptic ulcer, diverticulitis, and ureteral calculi.

3. The **treatment** of acute appendicitis is appendectomy. Preoperative preparation should begin as soon as possible and includes IV hydration, nasogastric suction, and antibiotic administration. A broad-spectrum, third-generation cephalosporin is recommended unless there is evidence that the appendix has ruptured; in this instance, an aminoglycoside and ampicillin along with either clindamycin or metronidazole are given.

B. **Diverticulitis.** Diverticular disease is a malady of Western culture thought to be secondary to low-residue diets and stress. There are two types of diverticula: (1) congenital, consisting of all layers of the bowel wall, and (2) acquired, consisting of mucosa covered with serosa. Diverticula are most commonly found in the sigmoid colon. The incidence of diverticulosis in the population rises precipitously from age 35, where the incidence is almost zero, to age 80, where the incidence is 65% [2]. Although most patients with diverticulosis remain asymptomatic, if the orifice of a diverticulum becomes obstructed, the diverticulum can perforate with resultant surrounding inflammatory reaction. An acute peridiverticulitis may heal spontaneously, or an abscess, free perforation with spreading peritonitis, fistula formation, or obstruction may develop.

1. **Clinical features.** The classic presentation of a patient with diverticulitis is that of fever, usually left lower abdominal pain associated with constipation, mild abdominal distention, and leukocytosis. The clinical picture of sigmoid diverticulitis has often been called left-sided appendicitis since the clinical picture is almost identical. The pain is usually characterized as constant and dull; however, it can be intermittent and crampy. Although constipation is the most common associated change in bowel habit, diarrhea may also be found. If the patient has either a redundant sigmoid colon that lies in the right lower quadrant or congenital diverticular disease affecting the right colon, the diverticulitis may mimic appendicitis. A mass palpated in the left lower quadrant suggests possible abscess formation.

2. The **diagnosis** of acute diverticulitis can usually be made by a careful history and physical examination. If there is doubt as to the disease process involved, a sodium diatrizoate (Hypaque) enema can be obtained. This enema may demonstrate perforation or show an extrinsic mass effect on the colon. If possible, the contrast enema should be delayed until after the acute stage, since there is always the risk of turning a sealed perforation into a free perforation. If an abscess is suspected, it can be confirmed by ultrasonography or CT scanning. Sigmoidoscopy can also be performed and may be characterized by an inability to introduce the scope beyond 15 cm because of immobility of the bowel and fixed angulation at that point.

3. The **differential diagnosis** of patients presenting with diverticulitis includes pelvic inflammatory disease, colon carcinoma, ovarian diseases, colitis (granulomatous, ulcerative, ischemic), and appendicitis.

4. **Treatment** of uncomplicated diverticulitis should be conservative with bowel rest and administration of antibiotics. Mild cases can be treated with oral antibiotics and a liquid diet. In all other cases, broad-spectrum IV antibiotics should be used, consisting of ampicillin, a wide-spectrum cephalosporin, or a combination of an aminoglycoside and either clindamycin or metronidazole. These patients usually do not require nasogastric suction; however, it should be employed if an adynamic ileus develops. If the patient either fails to improve on medical management or develops one of the complications of diverticulitis (i.e., abscess formation, perforation, fistula formation, or intestinal obstruction), surgical intervention should not be delayed.

C. **Intestinal obstruction** refers to the interference of normal transit of intestinal contents.

1. **Etiologies.** Intestinal obstruction can be produced by mechanical obstruction or by paralysis of intestinal motility.

a. By definition, an **ileus** refers to all intestinal obstructive processes; however, it has come to be associated with an adynamic or paralytic state of the intestinal musculature. An adynamic ileus occurs most commonly after trauma or laparotomy; however, it may be due to serum electrolyte abnormalities, associated intraabdominal inflammatory processes, or chemical irritation from blood, bile, or bacteria.

b. **Mechanical obstruction** can result from encroachment of the lumen by intrinsic disease or extrinsic bowel lesions. The most common causes of intestinal obstruction (in decreasing order of frequency) are adhesions, hernias, and neoplasm. The order of frequency, however, varies with age, with hernias being more common in the young and neoplasms playing a more prominent role in the elderly.

Mechanical intestinal obstruction can be further subclassified according to the physiologic process involved. In simple mechanical obstruction, there is lumenal obstruction but no vascular abnormality. In strangulated obstruction, there is compromise of both the lumen and the vascular supply. Closed obstruction occurs when both limbs of the loop are obstructed; if left untreated, closed loop obstruction will lead to strangulation, since the marked increase in pressure will compromise the bowel wall vascularity.

2. **Pathophysiology.** Intestinal obstruction results in proximal bowel distention from accumulation of fluid and gas. Due to loss of fluid and electrolytes into the bowel lumen, bowel wall, and free peritoneal cavity, as well as losses incurred with vomiting or nasogastric suction, the extracellular fluid space may become contracted. Contraction of this space is manifested by hypovolemia, hemoconcentration, renal insufficiency, shock, and death if left untreated. To overcome the obstruction, the usual peristalsis is replaced by recurring bursts of peristaltic activity with interspersed quiescent periods. The bowel distal to the obstruction will be evacuated and will collapse. In contrast to small-bowel obstruction, colonic obstruction is often not so dramatic. In particular, fluid and electrolyte losses are not as marked. If the ileocecal valve is competent, a closed-loop obstruction will result between the valve and the point of obstruction. When the colon becomes distended, it may perforate; perforation usually occurs in the cecum, because it is the segment of colon with the largest diameter (Laplace's law) and a relatively thin wall.

3. **Clinical features**

a. The initial **symptoms and signs** of intestinal obstruction include crampy abdominal pain, vomiting, abdominal distention, and failure to pass flatus. Severity of each of these symptoms and signs depends on the site, degree, and duration of the obstruction. Initially, the pain may be unrelenting; however, this type of pain usually gives way to the more characteristic crampy abdominal pain. Patients with a high-intestinal obstruction usually have cramps that occur every 4–5 mintues; in contrast, with distal obstruction, the cramps are less frequent. Severe, constant pain suggests strangulation. In those patients in which the obstruction becomes chronic and in those patients with an adynamic ileus, the pain is characterized as a constant, dull, generalized abdominal discomfort. The amount of distention and vomiting vary according to the site of obstruction. A high-intestinal obstruction is usually characterized by frequent vomiting in the absence of distention; in contrast, more distal lesions characteristically produce marked distention but fewer episodes of vomiting.

b. **Physical examination.** Tenderness is a frequent finding; however, if peritoneal signs develop, strangulation or perforation should be considered. On auscultation, characteristic peristaltic rushes may be found. Signs of dehydration are often present, including lethargy, tachycardia, orthostatic changes, and dry mucous membranes.

c. **Laboratory findings.** Although there are marked shifts of fluid and electrolytes in intestinal obstruction, these patients' serum electrolytes are normal early in the disease. The only demonstrable abnormality may be an increased hematocrit secondary to dehydration; since the body responds to dehydration by antidiuresis, the urine specific gravity frequently approaches 1.030. If these patients are not treated, they will develop further dehydration, metabolic acidosis, hyponatremia, hypochloremia, and hypokalemia. If a metabolic alkalosis occurs, it is usually due to a high-intestinal obstruction with marked vomiting and the loss of a large volume of gastric juices. The

WBC count may be normal or mildly elevated up to 15,000/mm^3; a count greater than 15,000/µl suggests strangulation or mesenteric infarction. The serum amylase may also be elevated in obstruction and is suggestive of ischemic bowel.

    d. Radiologic evaluation. The most important radiographs in intestinal obstruction are the upright chest x-ray and supine and upright abdominal films. If the patient is unable to stand or assume an upright position, a left lateral decubitus film can be substituted. Air-fluid levels may be seen in the upright or lateral films; however, they may also be present in an ileus, gastroenteritis, and severe constipation. Supine films often demonstrate the amount of bowel distention. If complete obstruction is present, there will be no gas distal to the point of obstruction. Additional radiographs, such as a barium enema and upper GI series with small-bowel follow-through, are occasionally indicated. A barium enema should always be obtained first if colonic obstruction cannot be ruled out. A barium or water-soluble contrast can be given orally and is often helpful in determining whether a partial obstruction or ileus is present. The barium enema is indicated to define colonic obstruction or to differentiate dilated loops of bowel as either small bowel or colon. A barium enema may also be therapeutic in children in helping to reduce an intussusception. The risks of a barium enema are the possibility of perforation of an inflammatory lesion and the possible changing of a partial colonic obstruction to a complete colonic obstruction, since barium may become inspissated proximal to the obstruction.

   4. Treatment. The principles in the management of intestinal obstruction are fluid and electrolyte replacement, bowel decompression, and operative intervention.

    a. Isotonic fluid should be administered to achieve and maintain an adequate urine output, at which time potassium chloride may then be added to the IV fluids.

    b. Nasogastric suction should be initiated to decompress the proximal bowel, prevent further distention, and prevent pulmonary aspiration of vomitus. Some surgeons prefer intubation with long intestinal tubes; however, this procedure may be time-consuming unless placed under fluoroscopic control.

    c. Timely **surgical intervention** is indicated in **complete mechanical obstruction** since there is no infallible means of determining whether strangulation has occurred. An exception to this rule includes those patients with a sigmoid volvulus who may have endoscopic relief of the obstruction and later undergo elective resection of the sigmoid colon. Surgery may be delayed until the patient receives the necessary preoperative preparation to correct any hemodynamic and electrolyte abnormalities.

    d. Should an **ileus or partial obstruction** be diagnosed, these patients may be treated conservatively with IV fluids, nasogastric suction or decompression with a long intestinal tube, and close observation. If an ileus is diagnosed, the underlying cause should be determined and treated appropriately.

  D. Perforated peptic ulcer can involve the duodenum or stomach. Men are more commonly affected than women, and the peak incidence occurs between the ages of 25 and 45 years.

   1. Clinical features

    a. History. Free perforation into the peritoneal cavity is usually quite dramatic; the patient develops sudden, severe midepigastric pain that subsequently spreads to involve the entire abdomen. The patient can often recall the exact moment the pain occurred. Most patients present to the hospital within several hours of the initiating event. On close questioning, previous symptoms of ulcer disease may occasionally be elicited, with exacerbation occurring several days prior to perforation. The pain can be so severe that the patient suffers a syncopal episode at the time of perforation. Vomiting is not a prominent feature of perforated peptic ulcer. Patients on immunosuppressive drugs and elderly patients may have less dramatic symptoms, with the presentation being more slow and insidious.

    b. Physical examination. These patients characteristically present with a rigid, "boardlike" abdomen. Fever is usually absent early in the course of the disease but develops subsequently. The patient frequently appears ill and in marked distress with a moderate tachycardia and shallow respirations. Bowel sounds are typically absent; however, this finding is variable.

    c. Laboratory findings include a mild leukocytosis to 15,000/mm^3 within several hours of perforation. Hemoconcentration may be demonstrated due to the large shift of plasma into the peritoneal cavity. An elevated amylase level may be present also. An upright chest or abdominal radiograph will usually demonstrate free air beneath the diaphragm; however, 20% of patients with a perforated ulcer will fail to demonstrate free air on the appropriate radiographs. It may be necessary to leave the patient in the upright position for 5 minutes before taking the radiograph. For those patients unable to assume an upright position, a left lateral decubitus film can be obtained. When the diagnosis remains in doubt, water-soluble contrast material can be administered orally or via a nasogastric tube to demonstrate the perforation.

  2. The **differential diagnosis** includes acute pancreatitis, acute cholecystitis, appendicitis, and a ruptured abdominal aortic aneurysm.

  3. Treatment. Although there have been proponents for nonoperative therapy in patients with a perforated peptic ulcer, this therapy has been associated with a high rate of complications, including intraabdominal sepsis. Thus, operative therapy is the treatment of choice and should be delayed only in allowing preoperative preparation of the patient. Preoperative preparation includes use of nasogastric suction, fluid and electrolyte replacement, and administration of appropriate antibiotics.

E. Biliary tract disease. Acute cholecystitis is a common complication of chronic gallbladder disease. It is associated with cholelithiasis in 95% of instances; however, only 25% of patients with cholelithiasis develop acute inflammation of the gallbladder. This disease is more common in women than men, reflecting the incidence of gallstones. Although acalculous cholecystitis can occur, the factor most commonly responsible for development of acute cholecystitis is obstruction of the cystic duct by a calculus, leading to gallbladder distention and subsequent wall ischemia. Chemical injury and bacterial invasion of the gallbladder wall then ensue, resulting in the characteristic findings of acute cholecystitis. Although the acute inflammation may resolve spontaneously or with appropriate antibiotics, if left untreated, complications can develop, including gangrene, empyema, and perforation of the gallbladder.

  1. Clinical features

    a. History and physical findings. Patients presenting with biliary tract disease frequently have a history of previous biliary colic consistent with chronic gallbladder disease. It is necessary to distinguish the symptoms of biliary colic, acute cholecystitis, and complicated cholecystitis in order to determine the best treatment for the patient.

      (1) Biliary colic occurs when there is obstruction of the cystic duct and is characterized by a steady right upper quadrant pain that is abrupt in onset and colicky in nature. These episodes are not associated with acute inflammation, and usually the pain subsides within 4 hours. Although these patients may be restless, physical findings are minimal with only occasional right upper quadrant tenderness elicited.

      (2) Acute cholecystitis. The onset of symptoms in patients with acute cholecystitis can appear similar to previous attacks of biliary colic. The pain, however, does not subside and becomes more localized in the right subcostal area, with occasional radiation to the right scapula. Nausea and vomiting are frequent associated symptoms; however, if they are marked, the presence of choledocholithiasis, acute pancreatitis, or bowel obstruction is suggested. On physical examination, patients with acute cholecystitis frequently are mildly febrile (up to 100°F) and have localized tenderness and guarding in the right upper quadrant. Murphy's sign (see sec. **II.B.7.c**) may be elicited. One-third of patients will have a palpable gallbladder on physical examination. In contradistinction to patients with biliary colic, those with acute cholecystitis generally appear toxic and often remain quiet since movement exacerbates the pain. Although mild icterus may be present, this finding should suggest the possibility of associated choledocholithiasis.

      (3) Patients who present with **suppurative complications** of acute cholecystitis may have the same symptoms and physical findings as those with acute cholecystitis. These patients almost always have marked right upper quadrant tenderness with rebound. Temperature elevations greater than 101°F are quite common. Such complications should be suspected in elderly and diabetic patients who present with symptoms of acute cholecystitis.

b. Laboratory findings. Patients with biliary colic characteristically present with a normal WBC count; however, those with acute cholecystitis generally have a mild leukocytosis, and counts greater than $15,000/mm^3$ are suggestive of the development of suppurative complications. Whereas mild hyperbilirubinemia occurs in 25% of patients with acute cholecystitis, hyperbilirubinemia greater than 3 mg/dl is suggestive of choledocholithiasis. Mild elevations in the alkaline phosphatase, serum aspartate aminotransferase (AST), and serum alanine aminotransferase (ALT) can also be encountered in acute cholecystitis and usually resolve within 24–48 hours; with viral hepatitis, however, these enzymes continue to increase. The serum amylase is abnormal in 15% of patients with acute cholecystitis and may approach 1000 Somogyi units.

c. Radiologic studies. The mainstays for diagnosing gallbladder disease are oral cholecystography and ultrasonography. Recently, radionuclide cholescintigraphy has also been used with good results. More invasive procedures include IV cholangiography, percutaneous transhepatic cholangiography, and endoscopic retrograde cholangiopancreatography. Less than 20% of gallstones are radiopaque.

(1) Oral cholecystography (OCG). With the use of iodinated organic compounds administered orally and concentrated by the gallbladder, it is possible to demonstrate the shadows of calculi, if present. Failure of visualization of the gallbladder usually indicates obstruction of the bile ducts or inability of the gallbladder to concentrate the dye. Other causes of failure include inadequate doses of the dye, failure of intestinal absorption, or inadequate hepatic excretion due to primary liver disease. Oral cholecystography has been reported to be 95% accurate.

(2) Ultrasonography is a noninvasive method of visualizing the gallbladder and demonstrating calculi. The accuracy of this test approaches that of oral cholecystography. Ultrasonography allows visualization not only of the gallbladder but also the liver, common bile duct, and pancreas. Since this study does not require ingestion of contrast material, it is useful in patients who have associated nausea and vomiting. It is also advantageous in pregnant patients (since no radiographs are required) and in patients who are jaundiced (since oral cholecystography is inaccurate when the bilirubin exceeds 3 mg/dl).

(3) Radionuclide cholescintigraphy. The use of technetium-labeled iminodiacetic compounds usually delineates the common bile duct, gallbladder, and duodenum 10–20 minutes after injection. If the cystic duct is obstructed, the isotope cannot enter the gallbladder, and thus an image of the gallbladder will not be seen. In acute obstruction of the cystic duct, this test is 95% accurate. However, it will not demonstrate calculi that are present within the gallbladder if they are not obstructing the duct. In addition, radionuclide cholescintigraphy is an unreliable indicator of common bile duct obstruction.

2. The **differential diagnosis** of patients with acute cholecystitis includes hepatitis, acute pancreatitis, a perforated ulcer, pyelonephritis, gonococcal perihepatitis, myocardial infarction, pneumonia, and herpes zoster.

3. Treatment

a. Patients who present with **symptomatic cholelithiasis** should be treated with cholecystectomy. Uncomplicated biliary colic is treated with an analgesic, and an elective cholecystectomy may be arranged.

b. Patients with **acute cholecystitis** should be hospitalized and placed on an appropriate antibiotic (e.g., ampicillin, cephalosporin, or an aminoglycoside); however, controversy exists over the timing of surgery. Some physicians prefer operative intervention within 72 hours of the onset of the acute process; however, others like to delay operative management until the acute inflammation has subsided.

c. Patients with suspected **complications** of acute cholecystitis should undergo emergency cholecystectomy.

F. Hernia. The term *hernia* is defined as any protrusion of tissue through an abnormal opening in a body cavity. Hernias of the abdominal wall most commonly occur at the groin and umbilicus.

1. **Clinical features.** Although hernias frequently are asymptomatic and easily reducible, the bowel may become incarcerated within the hernial sac. The size of the hernia defect often determines the symptomatology and potential for incarceration. In general, smaller fascial defects lead to more pronounced symptoms and are associated with a higher incidence of incarceration. Most hernias, when symptomatic, present with pain in the area of the fascial defect. If bowel becomes incarcerated within the hernial sac, obstructive symptoms, including nausea, vomiting, and abdominal distention, will result. If this condition is left untreated, strangulation will occur with subsequent intestinal gangrene. Should strangulation ensue with subsequent gangrene, there will be surrounding erythema as well as fever and possible signs and symptoms of sepsis. When obstructive symptoms are absent in an incarcerated hernia, the contents of the hernial sac may contain omentum, ovary, or other nongastrointestinal viscera. Richter's hernia occurs when only the nonmesenteric portion of the bowel wall becomes incarcerated within the fascial defect and may subsequently strangulate without signs of intestinal obstruction.

2. **Differential diagnosis.** Although the diagnosis of an incarcerated hernia is usually not difficult, several entities can mimic this condition. In the inguinal region, the differential diagnosis includes a hydrocele, groin hematoma, femoral lymphadenopathy, and femoral artery aneurysm. When the diagnosis of a Spigelian hernia is entertained, hematoma of the rectus sheath should be ruled out.

3. **Treatment**

   a. Patients presenting with a relatively **asymptomatic and easily reducible hernias** should be referred for operative repair. Patients who are considered not to be candidates for surgical management can be fitted with a truss, but these devices are cumbersome.

   b. Patients who present with an **incarcerated hernia** of less than 4–6 hours' duration without signs of strangulation should have the hernia carefully reduced by gentle but firm pressure. This procedure is often facilitated by placing the patient in the Trendelenburg position and administering a parenteral narcotic. Following successful reduction of the hernia, patients generally should be hospitalized for observation and definitive hernia repair. The advantage of reducing an incarcerated hernia is that the repair can be done 2–3 days later when edema of the surrounding tissues is reduced, and, if necessary, the patient's general medical condition is improved through appropriate therapy. Inability to reduce an incarcerated hernia, however, is an indication for emergent surgical reduction and repair.

   c. Should there be any question of possible **strangulation** (as evidenced by prolonged incarceration, fever, leukocytosis, elevated amylase, guaiac-positive stools, or peritonitis), immediate operative repair should be performed to determine whether irreversible intestinal ischemia has occurred. It should be noted that the fatality rate for elective hernia repair averages approximately 0.2%, whereas that for repair of strangulated hernias is 8–10% [10].

Abdominal Trauma

Abdominal trauma can be classified as penetrating, nonpenetrating, or iatrogenic. The emergency department physician is most often called on for the initial evaluation and management of penetrating and nonpenetrating trauma, which involves a rapid assessment, resuscitation, diagnosis, and disposition.

I. **Assessment**

A. **History.** An accurate history is essential in assessing abdominal trauma. Information should be obtained regarding the time of the injury, the circumstances pertaining to the injury, the strength of the forces involved (or the seriousness of the accident), the status of the patient at the scene of the accident and en route to the hospital, the patient's complaints of pain, history of previous illnesses, the patient's allergies and use of medications, and the time of the patient's last meal. Such information should be sought, when appropriate, from the patient, relatives, friends, bystanders, and the emergency medical technicians (EMTs). Depending on the urgency of the situation, it may be necessary to gather information to the extent possible during the resuscitation of the patient.

B. The **physical examination** should be rapid but thorough, and basic rules should be followed in assessing the patient. Assessment of the patient's airway is top priority, followed by assessment of the cardiovascular system, central nervous system, abdomen, and extremities, respectively. Depending on the clinical circumstances, the initial examination may need to be performed simultaneously with the resuscitation of the patient. Following stabilization of the patient, which takes precedence, a more thorough head-to-toe examination can be performed.

   1. **Inspection.** Examination of the abdomen should begin with an inspection. In addition, the back, flank, buttocks, and posterior thighs should be inspected when first seen, since after insertion of multiple catheters, the examination may be hindered. The location of any entrance and exit wounds as well as the angle of the trajectory should be noted. For any wounds below the level of the nipples, consideration should be given to the possibility of intraabdominal injury. Distention of the abdomen with evidence of hypovolemia strongly suggests significant internal injury.

   2. **Palpation** of the abdomen should begin gently, away from the site of possible injury. The findings on examination may be quite variable since more than one organ system may be involved. In addition, the abdomen can be difficult to assess in patients with a depressed level of consciousness. Rigidity when present is usually an indication for laparotomy; however, it may merely reflect injury to the abdominal wall and not visceral damage. Voluntary guarding may be present with lower rib fractures, which makes the abdominal examination difficult to interpret. Abdominal masses when discovered can be assumed to represent a contained or semicontained collection of blood, as would occur with a subcapsular hematoma of the spleen. Subcutaneous emphysema of the abdominal wall is most likely from intrathoracic injury; however, rupture of an air-filled abdominal viscus can also produce this finding.

   3. **Auscultation** of the abdomen for bowel sounds in trauma is unreliable. The presence of peristaltic sounds may be heard in spite of active intraperitoneal hemorrhage or following hollow visceral rupture.

   4. **Rectal and pelvic examinations** should not be omitted. A stool guaiac should be obtained, and the presence of any masses (e.g., hematoma) or tears in the mucosa noted. In addition, in males the position and integrity of the prostate gland should be assessed; displacement of the gland suggests a urethral injury. In women, culdocentesis may demonstrate the presence of blood in the peritoneal cavity.

C. **Laboratory evaluation.** In the acutely injured patient, blood for type and crossmatch and a complete blood count (CBC) should be sent within minutes of the patient's arrival. In addition, a urinalysis should be performed. Other useful diagnostic tests include arterial blood gases; serum electrolytes, glucose, and creatinine; serum amylase; blood alcohol; and a toxicology screen.

D. **Radiologic evaluation.** Radiologic studies are helpful in assessing patients with traumatic injuries. It must be stressed, however, that time is often of the essence in these critically injured patients and time spent in the radiologic suite obtaining x-rays may be detrimental. A patient with obvious indications for an exploratory laparotomy should undergo only absolutely essential studies in order to expedite getting the patient to the operative suite. Useful radiologic studies are as follows:

   1. A **chest x-ray** is an integral part of the evaluation of any patient with traumatic injuries. These patients often have associated thoracic injuries, and even if the chest x-ray is negative, it will provide a valuable baseline study.

   2. **Supine and, if possible, upright abdominal x-rays** should be obtained in patients who have suspected abdominal injuries, if time allows. These x-rays allow for inspection of bony injuries, foreign bodies, free intraperitoneal air, and retroperitoneal injury; the last is suggested either by obliteration of the psoas shadow or by stippling of the retroperitoneum.

   3. **Pelvis radiograph.** Because of the relatively high frequency and potential seriousness of pelvic fractures in blunt trauma victims, a radiograph of the pelvis generally should be obtained in such patients.

   4. **IVP/cystourethrogram.** These studies are used to assess the integrity of the urinary tract. Detailed discussion of these tests is covered in Chaps. 17 and 27.

   5. **CT scanning.** Use of CT scanning has been one of the most important recent advances in the evaluation of the patient with blunt abdominal trauma. Scan-

ning can usually be accomplished within 30 minutes, and when combined with PO and IV contrast, provides an accurate, noninvasive diagnostic test for intraabdominal injuries. Several institutions report a less than 1% incidence of false-negative or -positive studies with the use of CT scanning in the evaluation of patients with blunt abdominal trauma [4]. Patients best suited for evaluation by CT include stable patients in whom the abdominal examination is unreliable, such as those with neurologic injuries or alcohol or drug intoxication.

6. **Hypaque studies.** The use of sodium diatrizoate (Hypaque) allows for evaluation of the esophagus, stomach, and duodenum, as well as the colon and rectum.

7. **Ultrasound.** This noninvasive study can provide information regarding pancreatic or renal injury; however, examination may be hindered by overlying intestinal gas, abdominal wounds, and obesity.

8. **Radionuclide scans.** With the advent of nuclear medicine scanning, it is possible to evaluate the spleen, liver, and kidneys by noninvasive techniques without the risk of administering intravenous contrast. Technetium sulfur colloid scans may demonstrate splenic and liver injuries. This study is most helpful in the individual with blunt trauma who is otherwise stable and can be treated nonoperatively. The renal scan, although not providing the detail of an IVP, can be useful in indicating parenchymal injuries.

9. **Arteriography.** Although arteriography is useful in assessing abdominal trauma, other less invasive studies are usually employed. Arteriography, however, is useful in patients with puzzling diagnostic problems, pelvic fractures with massive hemorrhage (for diagnostic or therapeutic purposes), or suspected aortic injuries.

10. **Sinograms.** Although there had been proponents for this technique in the past, it has been abandoned because of a high rate of unnecessary laparotomies and the availability of more reliable techniques.

E. **Diagnostic procedures**

1. **Peritoneal lavage.** Since its introduction in 1964, peritoneal lavage has gained wide acceptance as the best diagnostic tool to determine significant intraabdominal injury. Its diagnostic accuracy has been reported in one large series to approach 95%, with few false-negatives and -positives [8]. When employed, it may help in reducing unnecessary laparotomies. Peritoneal lavage is of greatest value both in patients in whom the abdomen is difficult to evaluate (e.g., secondary to an altered mental status or spinal cord injury) and in patients with unexplained hypotension. When the open technique (see Chap. 38) is used, the complication rate approaches zero. Findings indicative of a positive lavage include free aspiration of blood from the catheter on insertion or a lavage fluid with greater than 100,000 RBC/mm^3, 500 WBC/mm^3, or 175 IU amylase/dl.

2. **Endoscopy** is most frequently used in the removal of foreign bodies from the esophagus and stomach and in the evaluation of the esophagus and stomach following ingestion of alkalies or acids. This study is rarely used in patients with traumatic injuries. Proctosigmoidoscopy, however, may be useful in evaluating the integrity of the rectum and sigmoid colon (e.g., when there is penetrating trauma in proximity to those structures).

3. **Paracentesis** can be utilized to help determine the presence of intraabdominal injuries. It has been reported to have up to a 90% diagnostic accuracy when positive [11]. A negative abdominal tap, however, has no diagnostic significance. If negative, it may be necessary to repeat the paracentesis at a later time. This procedure is most advantageous in that it can often provide a quick diagnosis that will expeditiously lead to laparotomy. Paracentesis is performed as follows.

   a. It is mandatory to have the patient void or have the bladder emptied by catheterization before needle aspiration.

   b. The four quadrant approach should be used. The sites of penetration should be away from any surgical scars and lateral to the rectus sheath to avoid complications (e.g., bowel perforation, hematoma formation). The tap is contraindicated in the presence of extensive adhesions.

   c. A local anesthetic should be injected into the skin to create a "wheal."

   d. Using an 18- or 20-gauge spinal needle on a 10-ml syringe, the needle should be inserted through the abdominal wall into the peritoneal cavity; the peritoneum is entered when there is minimal resistance followed by a slight give.

   e. Intraabdominal injuries are suggested by a bile-colored aspirate or the return of nonclotting blood. Any nonbloody fluid obtained should be cultured and smeared for bacteria immediately.

4. **Laparoscopy.** Although there are proponents for the use of laparoscopy in abdominal trauma, this procedure has limited application because of the inability to carefully inspect the entire abdomen.

II. Treatment

A. Penetrating abdominal injuries

1. **Gunshot wounds.** Although there are some proponents for selective observation of gunshot wounds of the abdomen, most would agree that these patients are best treated with exploration if there is evidence of peritoneal penetration. Tangential bullet wounds that miss the peritoneal cavity, however, can cause visceral injury from a blast effect, particularly if a large-caliber or high-velocity missile is involved; evidence of visceral injury is an indication for exploratory laparotomy. The examiner should always search for an exit wound and determine the path of the bullet. If there is no exit wound, the bullet location must be accounted for by radiographs. Many shotgun injuries can be observed if the patient was shot from a long distance, since the pellets are often imbedded in the abdominal wall and uncommonly cause significant damage. It should be stressed that although the gunshot wound may appear to involve only the thoracic cavity, if the bullet traverses a path below the level of the nipples, intraabdominal injury should be suspected.

2. **Stab wounds.** Controversy exists regarding the use of selective management versus routine laparotomy in the treatment of abdominal stab wounds. Selective management involves frequent observations (usually hourly by a qualified surgeon) and the use of ancillary laboratory (e.g., CBCs) and radiologic tests. Reports have shown that the use of laparotomy for all penetrating injuries has an associated 25–75% incidence of negative laparotomies. Proponents of selective management have reported a lower morbidity and equal mortality with their approach.

   a. **Absolute indications for surgery** in patients with stab wounds to the abdomen include shock, signs of peritoneal inflammation, evidence of gastrointestinal bleeding, free air within the peritoneal cavity, evisceration, or massive hematuria.

   b. **Selective management.** If a patient does not have a mandatory indication for laparotomy, selective management can be employed. A useful approach is as follows:

      (1) A patient without a mandatory indication for laparotomy who presents with a stab wound less than 6 hours old undergoes exploration of the stab wound under local anesthesia. If penetration of the peritoneal cavity is confirmed, laparotomy is performed.

      (2) If a patient presents after 6 hours and is stable without an indication for laparotomy, the patient is observed. However, if abdominal findings are questionable or if the patient has a depressed state of consciousness, the wound is explored. Should peritoneal injury be confirmed with local wound exploration, peritoneal lavage is then performed. Laparotomy is carried out if the RBC count in the lavage fluid is greater than 100,000/mm^3, if the WBC is greater than 500/mm^3, or if the amylase level is elevated.

B. Nonpenetrating abdominal trauma presents the most difficult problem in assessing for intraabdominal injury. If the patient is alert and cooperative, the physical examination is usually quite reliable; however, contusions of the abdominal wall and depressed states of consciousness make it less accurate. Each patient must be individualized with regard to management, although certain generalities exist.

1. **Immediate laparotomy** is indicated if (1) there are unequivocal signs of peritoneal irritation, (2) free air is demonstrated in the peritoneal cavity, (3) hypotension is present in the absence of other causes, or (4) there is evidence of gastrointestinal hemorrhage.

2. **Peritoneal lavage** is indicated if there are equivocal abdominal findings or if the physical examination is unreliable. **CT scanning** can also be used in these patients who are stable.

3. **Radionuclide scans** are warranted if the patient is stable and there is no indication for laparotomy but the injury is suggestive of specific organ injury.

4. **Observation.** Stable patients not falling into the above categories may be observed. All patients observed must be followed closely.

C. **General measures.** Once the decision has been made to proceed with laparotomy, the patient should be prepared for the operating suite. General measures include the following:

1. A **patent airway** must be secured. It is occasionally necessary to perform a cricothyrotomy or tracheostomy in patients with unstable neck injuries.

2. The **intravascular volume** must be repleted through infusion of Ringer's lactate solution and blood as needed. Diuretics are contraindicated in trauma patients except when adequate replacement therapy has been achieved.

3. The **antishock trousers** (see Chap. 38) can be utilized to control intractable abdominal bleeding by external counterpressure. There has been some controversy regarding their use; however, proponents point out that the antishock trousers will often support a patient in hemorrhagic shock until operative correction of the internal bleeding can be performed. Circumferential pneumatic compression has been used to control hemorrhage from pelvic fractures, retroperitoneal hematomas, and disseminated intravascular coagulation and following penetrating abdominal injuries and blunt abdominal trauma. Pressures of 20–25 mm Hg are usually sufficient to stop hemorrhage; higher pressures can be used if needed. Prior to deflation of the suit, it is essential that the blood volume be restored. The antishock trousers usually should not be deflated until the patient is under anesthesia in the operating suite.

4. Patients with multiple rib fractures or penetrating wounds of the thorax need insertion of a chest tube (although the chest x-ray may be without evidence of a pneumothorax or hemothorax), because these patients are at risk of developing a tension pneumothorax when placed on positive pressure ventilation during anesthesia.

5. A **nasogastric tube** and **Foley catheter** should be inserted unless contraindicated (see Chap. 17).

6. **Blood** should be made available to the emergency departments and operating suite.

7. **Fractures** should be stabilized.

8. **Prophylactic antibiotics** should be administered before proceeding with laparotomy. The choice of antibiotics is often the surgeon's preference and can be either a cephalosporin or, if colonic injury is suspected, an aminoglycoside plus clindamycin or metronidazole.

9. The patient's cardiac rhythm, blood pressure, pulse pressure, and urine output should be monitored while the operating suite is being prepared. The CVP is also a useful parameter to follow.

III. **Specific entities**

A. **Abdominal wall injuries.** Injuries to the abdominal wall alone can produce signs and symptoms that suggest significant intraabdominal injury. Pain, nausea, vomiting, guarding, and rigidity can all be associated with abdominal wall injuries.

1. A **hematoma,** when present, is usually found within the rectus sheath and represents rupture of the muscle or a tear in an epigastric vessel. It may simulate an intraabdominal mass but can be differentiated by having the patient tense the abdominal muscles. If the mass disappears, it is intraabdominal; however, if it is persistent and cannot be moved from side to side, a hematoma is most likely. A hematoma by itself usually does not require operative intervention. However, if it is associated with a significant intraabdominal injury that requires laparotomy, it should be evacuated and the bleeding site controlled at the time of surgery.

2. **Abdominal wall defects** may be encountered with large-caliber gunshot wounds and close-range shotgun injuries. These patients require exploratory laparotomy and repair of any intraabdominal injuries and the defect in the abdominal wall, which may require the use of flaps or synthetic mesh. As with any patient with an evisceration, these wounds should be covered with moistened sponges until the patient can reach the operating suite.

B. **Splenic trauma.** Although the spleen is protected by the lower rib cage, it is the intraabdominal organ most frequently injured in blunt trauma. Penetrating trauma can also injure this highly vascular organ. Resulting hemorrhage can be massive even when the injury seems minimal, and multiple organ injuries often occur when the spleen is ruptured. The mortality for splenic trauma is 11% but is higher when there are associated organ injuries. In the past, splenectomy was the treatment of choice; however, now the trend is toward nonoperative management to prevent postsplenectomy sepsis.

1. Clinical features
  a. Signs and symptoms. The clinical spectrum in splenic trauma varies from minimal or no symptoms to hypovolemic shock. In general, the findings are related to the extent of hemorrhage, presence of other organ system injuries, and the time since the injury occurred. Patients who develop a subcapsular hematoma that goes unrecognized may present several weeks after the event with rupture and internal hemorrhage. In general, patients with splenic injury present with a history of trauma and left upper quadrant pain and tenderness. Left shoulder pain **(Kehr's sign),** when manifested, is due to blood irritating the left hemidiaphragm; this pain can be made more pronounced by placing the patient in the Trendelenburg position and applying pressure in the left upper quadrant. **Ballance's sign,** which refers to an area of fixed dullness to percussion in the left flank, is found with large extra- or subcapsular hematomas.
  b. The most useful **laboratory tests** include the leukocyte count and hematocrit. Leukocytosis is generally present and may range from 12,000–30,000/mm^3. The hematocrit is usually low, although it may be normal initially.
  c. Radiologic evaluation is often helpful in confirming a suspected splenic injury. The chest x-ray may demonstrate fractures of the lower left ribs, which should arouse suspicion of a possible splenic injury. Abdominal x-rays in patients with a splenic injury may show an increased splenic shadow or loss of outline of the spleen, left kidney, or left psoas muscle; in addition, the greater curvature of the stomach may be serrated due to blood dissecting into the gastrosplenic ligament, the stomach may be shifted medially, and the transverse colon may be depressed. A technetium sulfur colloid scan may demonstrate splenic enlargement and intraparenchymal hematomas. CT is the best noninvasive diagnostic tool for splenic injuries and has a reported accuracy of 95%.
2. Treatment. At present, controversy exists regarding the management of splenic injury. Patients who are unstable should undergo immediate laparotomy with splenectomy. Immediate laparotomy is indicated in patients with penetrating trauma, continued hemorrhage, associated gastrointestinal injuries, or a scan demonstrating devascularization or severe fragmentation. Splenectomy is indicated if there is severe injury to the spleen or severe or persistent hemorrhage from the spleen; otherwise, an attempt should be made at splenic salvage. In stable patients without associated injuries, laparotomy can be performed in an attempt at splenic salvage; however, if bleeding persists despite splenorrhaphy, splenectomy should be performed. A more conservative approach with nonoperative management has recently been proposed in the stable patient and has been successfully employed, particularly in children. Approximately 50% of the children with radionuclide-proved splenic injuries can be managed conservatively. It should be pointed out, however, that up to 48% of those with splenic injuries will have associated visceral injuries requiring surgery. When the conservative approach is utilized, frequent reexamination is necessary, including following serial hematocrits. If there is deterioration in the patient's status or evidence of continued hemorrhage, associated injuries, or severe injury to the spleen on scan, laparotomy is indicated. If the conservative approach is followed and the patient remains stable, he or she is hospitalized for 1–2 weeks. On discharge from the hospital, the patient is instructed to avoid strenuous physical activity for 2 months and contact sports for 6 months.
C. Liver injuries. The liver is the second most frequently injured organ following blunt or penetrating trauma. The liver size, weight, consistency, location, and attachments make the organ particularly susceptible to blunt trauma. Although stab wounds previously were the most frequent initiating factor, blunt trauma and gunshot wounds have been more common in recent years. These injuries vary from superficial lacerations to massive parenchymal destruction. The mortality of liver trauma has been estimated at 10–20%. As with splenic injury, there is often other organ system involvement.
  1. Clinical features
    a. The **signs and symptoms** of liver injury are similar to those of the spleen, except that the right side is usually affected. The patients typically complain of right-sided to midabdominal pain and have right upper quadrant tenderness; they may also have associated right shoulder pain.

   b. Laboratory evaluation may demonstrate, as with splenic injuries, a leukocytosis and decreased hematocrit.
   c. Radiologic evaluation of patients with hepatic injury may reveal abnormalities on the chest x-ray and abdominal x-ray. These findings may include right lower rib fractures, a right hemothorax, loss of the liver shadow, and evidence of blood or fluid in the abdomen. A technetium sulfur colloid scan may demonstrate liver injury and is useful in following a subcapsular hematoma in stable patients. A CT scan, however, is the best diagnostic test for evaluating liver injury. It provides a better view of hepatic parenchymal injuries compared with the technetium sulfur colloid scan and is capable of demonstrating significant hemoperitoneum or associated organ injuries that would necessitate laparotomy. Arteriography may be utilized both to demonstrate active bleeding within the liver and to control hemorrhage by embolization.

2. **Treatment**
   a. The treatment of all **penetrating liver injuries** and blunt trauma resulting in **significant liver parenchymal injuries** involves laparotomy. The primary goals of management are control and prevention of bleeding and bile drainage, removal of all severely damaged nonviable liver tissue, and adequate wound drainage.
   b. Patients with an isolated **subcapsular hematoma** who are stable can be treated with observation. Although the hematoma usually will resolve spontaneously, it eventually may expand and rupture, develop into a hepatic abscess, or decompress into the biliary tree with subsequent hemobilia. The risk of operation is considerable because, if the hematoma is unroofed, troublesome bleeding is usually encountered. If observation is employed, the injury should be documented with either a liver scan or a CT scan. CT is preferable, since it better delineates the extent of parenchymal damage and allows for evaluation of other possible visceral injuries. As with splenic injury, if the patient being observed develops signs or symptoms of associated gastrointestinal injuries, an enlarging hematoma, or complications, the patient should undergo laparotomy. If the patient has an isolated liver injury with hemorrhage, the bleeding may be controlled with embolization by arteriography.

D. **Pancreatic injuries** account for 1–2% of all abdominal trauma, with penetrating trauma accounting for two-thirds of the injuries. The mortality varies with the etiology of the injury: stab wound, 8%; gunshot wound, 25%; and shotgun or blunt injury, 50% [7]. Major complications of pancreatic injury include pancreatic fistula, pancreatic abscess, hemorrhage, and pancreatitis.
   1. **Clinical features.** The diagnosis of pancreatic injury is often difficult to make, since the signs and symptoms are often slow to appear after injury. The history and a high index of suspicion are the best aids in making the diagnosis. Generally, these patients present with midabdominal pain and tenderness, but patients with blunt pancreatic injury may remain asymptomatic for days to years and then suddenly manifest one of the complications of pancreatic injury. Ninety percent of patients presenting with blunt abdominal trauma have mildly elevated amylase levels, which may only be secondary to a transient delay in secretory excretion; marked elevation, however, is suggestive of pancreatic or duodenal injury. Serial values are useful in that persistent elevation for 6 days may signal pseudocyst formation. When employing peritoneal lavage, an elevated amylase level may be obtained on the lavage effluent. A normal amylase level, however, does not rule out pancreatic injury since this organ sits in a retroperitoneal location. CT examination is of benefit in determining pancreatic injury in patients in whom there is suspicion of such injury.
   2. **Treatment** of pancreatic trauma is usually observation when blunt injury has been sustained. In contrast, in penetrating injuries to the abdomen involving the pancreas, surgery is usually required because of the high incidence of associated visceral injury. When observation is employed, the pancreas may be studied using CT or ultrasonography. Endoscopic retrograde cholangiopancreatography (ERCP) may be used to demonstrate significant ductal injury if this is suspected.

E. **Gallbladder/biliary tract trauma.** Injury to the extrahepatic biliary system most often results from penetrating injuries or, in more rare circumstances, from blunt trauma. There are no characteristic signs or symptoms. These injuries can be identified by the return of bile-stained peritoneal lavage fluid, but most such injuries usually are identified at the time of surgery by evidence of bile leakage from lacerated ductal structures. Development of hematobilia is unusual in injuries limited to the bile ducts unless there is associated vascular injury to the portal vein or hepatic artery. Injuries to the gallbladder are usually best treated with cholecystectomy; however, in simple stab wounds, the gallbladder wall may be repaired primarily. Injuries to the common bile duct are best treated by either primary repair or Roux-en-Y jejunal anastomosis.

F. **Gastric injuries** are almost always due to penetrating trauma. Due to its protected location and mobility, the stomach is rarely injured in blunt trauma. Injury can often be suspected by the trajectory of the penetrating object. As in perforated ulcers, the caustic nature of the stomach contents generally leads to severe abdominal pain with marked peritoneal signs when leakage occurs. Gastric injury may also be suspected by a bloody nasogastric aspirate. Abdominal x-rays will usually demonstrate free air; if necessary, a sodium diatrizoate study may be obtained to demonstrate the gastric injury. Treatment of gastric trauma is laparotomy with repair of the injury.

G. **Duodenal injuries** range from simple stab wounds to blast or crush trauma. The mortality following duodenal trauma depends on the time of presentation since injury and the extent of associated visceral injuries. Due to its retroperitoneal location and its contents being relatively sterile with a neutral pH, the injury may go unrecognized at the initial presentation. A delay of 24 hours prior to surgical intervention in an isolated duodenal injury is associated with a 65% mortality; however, if surgical intervention occurs within 24 hours, the mortality is only 5% [9]. Associated injuries to the pancreas, liver, and biliary system present complex management problems and are associated with the highest morbidity and mortality.

1. **Blunt injuries** to the duodenum most commonly occur in the second and third portion. These injuries can take the form of intestinal rupture or intramural hematoma.

   a. **Rupture** has been postulated to be due to a rapid increase in the intraluminal pressure of a loop of duodenum closed between the pylorus and ligament of Treitz. The patient may go on to develop fever, jaundice, and signs of high-intestinal obstruction if the injury is not recognized. Since the duodenum is in a retroperitoneal location, peritoneal lavage may be unremarkable in this instance. Elevated amylases are often present in blunt duodenal injuries, and abdominal x-rays may demonstrate retroperitoneal air. The diagnosis can be confirmed by duodenography with sodium diatrizoate. Treatment of duodenal rupture is always operative intervention.

   b. **Intramural hematomas** are the result of nonpenetrating trauma. These patients commonly present with signs and symptoms of upper intestinal obstruction. The diagnosis can be made by an upper GI series that shows the characteristic "coiled spring" appearance. If a hematoma is found during laparotomy, it should be decompressed. If this injury occurs alone without other evidence of visceral injury, treatment can be conservative. The patient is placed on nasogastric suction and total parenteral nutrition. If after a period of 10–14 days of conservative therapy the hematoma persists, operative decompression should be considered.

2. **Penetrating injuries** involving the duodenum usually involve other visceral structures. Operative intervention is required.

H. **Small-bowel injuries.** Of all intestinal trauma, the small bowel is most frequently involved. Eighty percent of bowel injuries occur between the ligament of Treitz and distal ileum, with 10% involving the duodenum and 10% the colon. In blunt trauma, the usual mechanism of injury to the small bowel is crushing of the small bowel against the vertebral column; however, shearing and tearing forces or acute increase in intraluminal pressure may also play an important role. Injuries to the mesentery may compromise the vascular supply to the bowel and lead to mesenteric ischemia. The diagnosis is usually made from the clinical findings of abdominal tenderness (progressing to rebound), fever, and leukocytosis. Treatment of small-bowel injuries is laparotomy with repair or resection of the involved bowel.

I. **Colonic injuries.** The morbidity and mortality of colonic injuries has declined over the past 50 years from 60% to 10%, due mostly to a more aggressive surgical approach. In blunt trauma, the mechanism of injury is similar to that of the small intestine. Due to the high bacterial content of the colon, untreated colonic injuries can develop diffuse peritonitis quite rapidly. Stab injuries to the flank may perforate the colon in a retroperitoneal location; if left untreated, these patients develop abscesses. The diagnosis can be confirmed by a sodium diatrizoate enema, which is also helpful in suspected rectal injuries. The treatment of colonic injuries is always surgical.

J. Vascular injuries (see Chap. 20). Penetrating wounds account for the vast majority of injuries to the abdominal aorta and inferior vena cava. These patients often present to the emergency department in a moribund condition. They require immediate laparotomy if there is any chance for survival. When dealing with vascular injuries, any bullets not accounted for must be sought with appropriate plain radiographs to rule out peripheral or central embolization. It should be noted also that combined arteriovenous injuries may occur with subsequent fistula formation. Any time a retroperitoneal hematoma is encountered, consideration should be given to performing arteriography to search for a major vascular injury.

Bibliography

1. Bolton, J. P., et al. An assessment of the value of the white blood cell count in the management of suspected acute appendicitis. *Br. J. Surg.* 62:906, 1975.
2. Cohn, I., Jr., and Nance, F. C. Mechanical, Inflammatory, Vascular, and Miscellaneous Benign Lesions. In D. C. Sabiston, Jr. (ed.), *Davis-Christopher Textbook of Surgery* (12th ed.). Philadelphia: Saunders, 1981. Pp. 1077–1085.
3. Condon, R. E. Appendicitis. In D. C. Sabiston, Jr. (ed.), *Davis-Christopher Textbook of Surgery* (12th ed.). Philadelphia: Saunders, 1981. Pp. 1048–1064.
4. Federle, M. D., et al. Computerized tomography in blunt abdominal trauma. *Arch. Surg.* 117:645, 1982.
5. Fee, H. J., et al. Radiologic diagnosis of appendicitis. *Arch. Surg.* 112:742, 1977.
6. Ludbrook, J., and Spears, G. F. S. The risk of developing appendicitis. *Br. J. Surg.* 52:856, 1965.
7. Northrup, W. R., III, and Simmons, R. L. Pancreatic trauma: A review. *Surgery* 71:27, 1972.
8. Powell, D. C., Bivins, B. A., and Bell, R. M. Diagnostic peritoneal lavage. *Surg. Gynecol. Obstet.* 155:259, 1982.
9. Roman, E., Silva, Y. J., and Lucas, C. Management of blunt duodenal injury. *Surg. Gynecol. Obstet.* 132:7, 1971.
10. Rydell, W. B., Jr. Inguinal and femoral hernia. *Arch. Surg.* 87:493, 1963.
11. Yurko, A. A., and Williams, R. D. Needle paracentesis in blunt abdominal trauma: A critical analysis. *J. Trauma* 6:194, 1966.

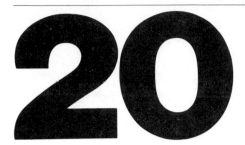

Vascular Disorders

Gregorio A. Sicard,
John C. Vander Woude, and
Timothy I. Shoen

Arterial Disorders

I. **Peripheral arterial occlusive disease**
   A. **Acute peripheral arterial occlusive disease.** Since acute arterial occlusion can lead to irreversible ischemic necrosis of striated muscles in 4–8 hours following the onset of symptoms, acute arterial occlusive disease is a surgical emergency requiring prompt diagnosis and treatment.
   1. **Etiology.** The usual causes of acute arterial insufficiency are emboli, acute arterial thrombosis, and trauma.
      a. **Emboli** can be cardioarterial or arterioarterial. They usually lodge where vessels bifurcate or taper. Between 70 and 90% of surgically treatable emboli affect the lower extremities, most frequently lodging in the femoral, popliteal, or iliac arteries. In the upper extremity, the brachial artery is most commonly involved, but emboli can also obstruct the subclavian or axillary artery.
         (1) **Cardioarterial emboli** account for 90% of acute emboli; embolization may be the first clinical sign of underlying heart disease, such as atrial fibrillation, mitral stenosis, or a myocardial infarction. Less common sources include debris from bacterial endocarditis or an atrial myxoma and paradoxical emboli that pass right to left through septal defects.
         (2) **Arterioarterial emboli** occur in patients with arterial aneurysms or severe atherosclerotic disease, with embolization distally. Microscopic debris from these arterial lesions can result in repetitive occlusion of small end arteries. The "blue-toe" syndrome, i.e., severe ischemia of both feet with palpable pulses, results from embolic debris from the distal aorta.
      b. **Acute arterial thrombosis** occurs where vessels are very stenotic, usually from atherosclerotic disease. Thrombosis generally occurs in conjunction with low-flow syndromes, such as congestive heart failure (CHF), shock states, or blood dyscrasias. Acute thrombosis can also be an iatrogenic event following percutaneous catheterization procedures, such as angiography. Other unusual causes include intraarterial drug injections, compression from cervical ribs, and occupational trauma (such as that seen in workers using pneumatic tools).
      c. **Trauma** (see **Vascular Injuries**). Penetrating or blunt trauma can cause intimal damage and subsequent thrombotic occlusion of the vessel.
   2. **Pathophysiology.** Ischemia can occur distal to the occlusion, depending on the extent of collateral circulation. Peripheral nerves are most sensitive to anoxia, with an early onset of paresthesias and paralysis. Persistent ischemia can result in muscle necrosis in 4–8 hours; however, some patients may tolerate ischemia for a longer period without irreversible necrosis due to their collateral circulation. Sluggish arterial blood flow at the site of occlusion allows extension of the clot both proximally and distally, which may occlude collateral vessels. If stasis results in venous thrombosis, embolectomy or thrombectomy will not restore blood flow.
   3. **Clinical manifestations** result from an acute ischemic event that may or may not be superimposed on chronic arterial insufficiency.
      a. **History.** In 80% of patients, there is a sudden onset of severe unremitting pain, followed by paralysis and paresthesias; these neurologic symptoms signify severe ischemia and portend the development of gangrene. A history of heart disease or an aneurysm suggests an embolic phenomenon; in con-

trast, a history of claudication without significant heart disease favors a thrombotic event.

  b. The **physical examination** reveals pallor and pulselessness in a cold extremity with collapsed peripheral veins. Examination of the skin temperature demonstrates a definite line of change that is somewhat below the true level of occlusion. Pulsations proximal to the obstruction usually are prominent. With prolonged ischemia, involved muscles become edematous and necrotic and progress to the very stiff muscular state of rigor mortis. Examination may reveal signs of chronic arterial insufficiency (e.g., trophic changes of the skin and nails, hairlessness) suggestive of a thrombotic event or signs of cardiac disease (e.g., atrial fibrillation) or an aneurysm that could be the source of emboli.

  c. **Laboratory.** An electrocardiogram (ECG), chest x-ray, complete blood count (CBC), muscle enzyme determinations, serum electrolytes and creatinine, coagulation studies, arterial blood gas, type and cross-match, and a urinalysis should be obtained in the emergency department.

4. The **diagnosis** of acute arterial occlusion is a clinical diagnosis that can be made from the characteristic findings described by the 5 Ps: pain, pallor, paresthesias, paralysis, and pulselessness. Doppler ultrasonography is useful in demonstrating pulselessness and may be helpful in localizing the site of occlusion. The diagnosis can be confirmed, if time permits, by **arteriography.** Arteriography will demonstrate the site of an arterial occlusion as well as distinguish between an embolus and thrombosis; coexistent atherosclerotic disease is also revealed. However, surgical therapy should not be delayed for arteriography if gangrene is imminent.

5. **Management.** All patients with evidence of significant acute arterial occlusion warrant hospitalization and urgent surgical care.

  a. **Anticoagulation.** Pending surgical intervention, the patient should receive anticoagulant therapy to prevent propagation of the embolus or thrombus. Heparin, 5000–10,000 units, is given IV and is followed by a continuous infusion of 1000–2000 units/hour or by repeat boluses at 4- to 6-hour intervals while monitoring the partial thromboplastin time (PTT).

  b. **Surgery** is most successful if performed within 4–8 hours of the onset of symptoms. The goal of surgery is to restore blood flow before irreversible changes occur. Depending on the clinical situation, this goal may be accomplished by embolectomy, thrombectomy, or graft interposition.

B. **Chronic peripheral arterial occlusive disease** is usually secondary to atherosclerosis. Other conditions, such as collagen vascular disease or hematologic abnormalities, are occasionally responsible for both occlusion of extremity vessels and manifestations of extremity ischemia. In general, this section discusses atherosclerotic chronic peripheral arterial occlusive disease.

  1. **Pathophysiology.** Atherosclerosis predominantly involves the arterial intima, with extension into the media, but usually spares the outer media and adventitia. Initially, there is focal accumulation of platelets and cholesterol, particularly in association with deposition of proteoglycan in the vessel wall. Accumulation of thrombus or the development of fibrosis leads to plaque formation and lumenal encroachment, which may progress to total occlusion of the vessel lumen. Progressive narrowing of the arterial lumen at any site stimulates the development of collateral circulation about the obstructed segment. When stenosis exceeds 50% of the lumen, the arterial pressure is usually reduced beyond the stenotic zone. As the stenosis approaches total occlusion, the sharply reduced blood flow usually leads to thrombosis. A clot may then propagate in the stagnant column of blood both proximally and distally. If blood flow through the collateral channels is not enough to meet the metabolic demands of the extremity, the patient may develop symptoms of ischemia in the muscle group supplied by the obstructed vessel.

  2. **Pathologic features**

  a. **Incidence and course.** Atherosclerotic peripheral arterial occlusive disease is chiefly a disease of the elderly, with a 10:1 predominance of males over females. The course of the disease is usually gradual and progressive, but it may be accelerated by acute episodes due to segmental arterial thrombosis or traumatic injuries to the digits, resulting in peripheral gangrene. Furthermore, the incidence and progression of atherosclerotic peripheral arterial occlusive disease are clearly accelerated by diabetes mellitus, hypertension, lipoprotein abnormalities, and the chronic use of nicotine-containing substances such as tobacco.

   b. Involvement. Atherosclerotic peripheral arterial disease is predominantly a disease of the lower extremities. Obstructive lesions are usually found from the infrarenal aorta to the tibial vessels, with diabetic patients tending to have more distal arterial involvement of the popliteal and tibial arteries. Obliterative lesions occur preferentially in areas of high turbulent flow, as seen at arterial bifurcations. Sites that exhibit a predilection for atherosclerotic involvement include the common iliac bifurcation, the superficial femoral artery, the midpopliteal artery opposite the knee joint, and the popliteal trifurcation just distal to the knee. In cases of upper-extremity atherosclerotic peripheral vascular disease, arterial lesions are usually confined to the axillary and subclavian arteries.

3. **Clinical manifestations** of peripheral arterial occlusive disease are related to a decrease in perfusion and the resultant ischemia.

   a. Claudication is a highly specific symptom virtually diagnostic of chronic arterial insufficiency. It is characterized by muscular pain or fatigue of the lower extremity caused by walking and relieved by bed rest. The pain is a deep ache that generally progresses to halt further activity and is completely relieved after 2–5 minutes of inactivity. The distance such a patient can walk varies with the rate of walking, degree of incline, and extent of arterial obstruction. Since claudication involves the muscle groups distal to the occlusion, a patient with calf pain has distal disease, whereas a patient with thigh or buttock claudication has occlusion in the iliac system; aortoiliac occlusion usually presents with hip or thigh claudication. Claudication is distinguishable from other forms of pain in that some exertion is always required before it appears, it does not occur at rest, and it is relieved by standing. **Pseudoclaudication** is a symptom, usually neurogenic in origin, that can be worsened by exercise but commonly lasts longer than 30 minutes and is relieved frequently only by lying down.

   b. Impotence in males can occur as a manifestation of chronic peripheral arterial occlusive disease involving the aortoiliac vessels. In partial obstruction, the presenting symptom may be an inability to sustain an erection, rather than complete impotence.

   c. Diminished pulses and **bruits** of affected vessels are often found.

   d. Pallor of the foot on elevation of the extremity may occur as arterial insufficiency progresses.

   e. Dependent rubor is usually found in more advanced stages of arterial insufficiency, with the foot displaying a marked cyanosis on dependency. With arterial occlusion, the blood in the capillary network of the foot is stagnant with a high oxygen extraction. Thus, the capillary blood in the foot becomes the color of that found in the venous circulation; and the concurrent vasodilation due to ischemia causes blood to suffuse the skin, imparting this livid appearance to the ischemic foot.

   f. Temperature. With chronic ischemia, the temperature of the extremity usually approaches that of its surroundings; thus, the ischemic extremity is usually cool.

   g. Trophic changes. Skin and muscular atrophy, decreased skin turgor and thickness, loss of hair, and brittle nails can be found in patients with chronic ischemia.

   h. Paresthesias. Patients may report numbness in the extremity; however, sensory abnormalities are generally not present on examination if the patient does not have diabetes mellitus. If decreased sensation is found in the foot, a peripheral neuropathy from diabetes mellitus or alcohol abuse should be considered, if the extremity is otherwise viable.

   i. Rest pain. Severe peripheral vascular insufficiency is characterized by rest pain, which is a constant discomfort occurring without exercise in the area of the metatarsal heads or ankle. Exacerbation of pain may occur in a recumbent position, leading the patient to place the leg in a dependent position to obtain relief. The recognition and treatment of ischemic rest pain is important, since this type of pain precedes gangrene and limb loss.

   j. Tissue necrosis is the final and most advanced sign of peripheral vascular disease. Every effort should be made to limit the extent of tissue loss by revascularization, when possible.

k. Peripheral arterial insufficiency is accompanied by a marked susceptibility of the patient to **long-term sequelae from trivial trauma** to the involved extremity. Foot and toe ulcerations, infection, or gangrene may result from minor trauma (e.g., from wearing improper shoes or trimming calluses, corns, or toe nails).

4. Evaluation. Patients with evidence of chronic peripheral vascular disease deserve a thorough medical workup in search of significant cardiac, renal, or pulmonary disease, since atherosclerotic cardiovascular and cerebrovascular disease, as well as chronic pulmonary insufficiency, are often present. Thus, any patient being considered for vascular reconstruction should generally receive a 12-lead ECG with a rhythm strip, pulmonary function tests with an arterial blood gas, a serum creatinine, and, if time permits, a radionuclide-gated blood-pool scan to assess the left ventricular ejection fraction. In particular, a careful history for symptoms of coronary artery disease is essential, as a thallium stress test, cardiac catheterization, and possibly coronary artery bypass surgery may be indicated prior to a peripheral revascularization procedure.

5. Diagnosis

a. Doppler blood flow meter. Segmental Doppler pressures can be obtained with a Doppler blood flow meter. Pressures can be measured high in the thigh, above the knee, below the knee, and at the ankle and can be compared with the blood pressure in the brachial artery. The **ankle-brachial index (ABI)** compares the Doppler systolic blood pressure at the ankle with the blood pressure in the brachial artery; normally the ratio should be greater than or equal to one. An ABI of 0.5–0.8 is compatible with claudication. Rest pain usually occurs when the ABI is between 0.1 and 0.5. An ABI of 0.2 or less is usually seen in patients with impending gangrene or ulceration.

b. Plain radiographs of the extremity may reveal calcification in the walls of atherosclerotic arteries. In particular, patients with diabetes mellitus can have diffuse medial calcification **(Mönckeberg's calcification)** involving the arteries of the upper and lower extremities, including the digital arteries.

c. Arteriography. Determination of the severity of chronic arterial occlusion ultimately requires arteriography. This procedure is useful in determining the location and anatomic extent of the lesion(s) and the status of the collateral circulation; in addition, it is extremely helpful in planning the operative approach. However, only those patients who are candidates for surgical treatment of their peripheral vascular disease should undergo arteriography. Prior to arteriography patients should have a determination of their serum creatinine to be sure that coincident renal insufficiency is not present. In addition, all patients undergoing arteriography should receive IV hydration (for at least 6 hours if possible) prior to the procedure. Recent studies have shown that the infusion of 12.5–25.0 gm of mannitol immediately prior to arteriography, along with intravenous hydration, decreases the incidence of postarteriography renal insufficiency.

6. Prognosis. Complications of atherosclerotic disease remain the most common cause of death and significant morbidity in the United States. The 5-year mortality of atherosclerotic disease is approximately 40–50%, with most deaths being related to cardiac or cerebrovascular disease. Patients with ischemic ulcerations, rest pain, advanced limb infections, or gangrene have an increased incidence of amputations, with immediate amputation needed in approximately 20% of cases. In contrast, patients with intermittent claudication can expect their symptoms to remain stable, with a risk of gangrene of under 5% when followed for 5 years. Untreated symptomatic superficial femoral artery obstruction also has a relatively benign course, with approximately 10% of patients requiring amputation within 10 years after the onset of symptoms. However, the presence and control of associated risk factors significantly influence the natural history of atherosclerosis. Those patients who continue to smoke, do not control their diet, have uncontrolled hypertension, or do not exercise have a much higher amputation rate. Similarly, patients with diabetes mellitus have a higher incidence (compared with nondiabetics) of lower-extremity vascular problems leading to amputation.

7. Treatment. The objectives of treatment of patients with chronic peripheral vascular disease are relief of symptoms and prevention of limb loss, with the ultimate goal being to maintain bipedal gait.

a. Progression of chronic peripheral vascular disease can generally be greatly reduced by (1) abstinence from tobacco, (2) regular exercise, and (3) control of any associated medical condition (e.g., diabetes mellitus, hypertension).

b. Infection. Treatment of soft-tissue infection of extremities with peripheral vascular disease involves (1) debridement of all necrotic tissue and (2) administration of an appropriate antibiotic. A basic guideline is that all necrotic tissue must be completely debrided if the limb and patient are to be salvaged. When infection is the dominant process without extensive tissue necrosis, intensive antibiotic therapy along with debridement will often suffice. However, if the patient presents with a rampant, uncontrolled infection of a lower extremity, an emergent guillotine amputation may be necessary to prevent a septic death.

c. Ischemic necrosis (gangrene). If tissue necrosis is not complicated by infection **(dry gangrene),** a conservative approach can be taken, in contrast to the urgency required when the patient has a necrotizing infection **(wet gangrene).** Dry gangrene is best treated by allowing the involved part to autoamputate over a period of weeks. On the other hand, wet gangrene requires aggressive measures (see **b**).

d. Ulcers of the digits overlying the metatarsal heads or involving the tips of the toes, but without osteomyelitis, can often be managed by local care, protection from trauma, and immobilization. Ulcers with superimposed infection require antibiotics and local debridement. In addition, particularly in diabetic patients in whom ulcers are the result of tissue breakdown at pressure points in an insensate foot, adequate footwear by an orthotist is mandatory in order to avoid recurrence of the ulceration.

e. Operative therapy (e.g., revascularization, amputation) is usually reserved for patients with rest pain, impending tissue loss, gangrene, or incapacitating claudication.

8. Disposition. Patients with chronic occlusive peripheral vascular disease and associated lower-extremity infection, gangrene, advanced ulcers, or rest pain generally need hospitalization for further evaluation and therapy.

II. Arterial aneurysms
A. Abdominal aortic aneurysm

1. Etiology. The abdominal aorta is a common site for atherosclerosis, with the infrarenal portion of the aorta most commonly involved. The vast majority of abdominal aortic aneurysms (AAAs) are a manifestation of atherosclerotic disease. Rarely, syphilis, trauma, or cystic medial necrosis has been reported as causing an AAA, but these conditions are more commonly associated with thoracic aortic aneurysm formation.

2. Pathology. Although atherosclerosis is a disease of the arterial intima, with atheromatous plaques, ulceration, and thrombus formation involving the damaged intima, severe disease can penetrate to the arterial media. When the media is damaged, a fusiform or saccular aneurysm may result as the weakened arterial wall dilates. Consistent with the incidence of atherosclerosis, 80–85% of aortic aneurysms occur in the infrarenal portion of the aorta. Males are affected 10 times more often than females, and the incidence peaks in the sixth and seventh decades.

3. Clinical features. AAAs may be asymptomatic and incidentally discovered on physical examination or when calcification outlining the aneurysm is noted on an abdominal x-ray taken for another reason. Rarely, emboli from an asymptomatic aneurysm may present as acute peripheral arterial occlusion. Abdominal or back pain results from expansion of an aneurysm or from bleeding into the arterial wall or the retroperitoneal space. With rupture of an AAA, which can occur without prodromal symptoms, the patient experiences sudden, severe abdominal pain radiating to the back or groin or both; syncope can occur, and the patient usually presents with hypotension or shock. Rupture of an AAA may also be associated with abdominal or flank ecchymosis or with femoral, obturator, or sciatic nerve neuropathy. Rarely, a primary aortoenteric fistula may develop and present as a gastrointestinal hemorrhage.

4. Differential diagnosis. Symptomatic AAAs may mimic a variety of conditions. Lumbar back pain or pain radiating to the left flank or groin may give the impression of a spine problem or nephrolithiasis, respectively. Pain referred to the epigastric or periumbilical area may be erroneously diagnosed as pancreatitis, peptic ulcer disease, or a myocardial infarction.

5. The **diagnosis** of an AAA frequently can be made on clinical grounds. Patients with a suspected expanding or ruptured aneurysm (e.g., tender, pulsatile abdominal mass; abdominal or back pain plus hypotension should forgo diagnostic tests and be prepared for emergent repair of the aneurysm, as any delay may lead to the patient's demise. Use of diagnostic tests to establish or delineate the extent of an AAA should be reserved either for patients with a nonexpanding or nonruptured aneurysm or for stable patients in whom the diagnosis is in doubt.

   a. **Physical examination.** AAAs greater than 5 cm in size can usually be detected by palpating the abdomen. A ruptured aneurysm typically presents as a tender, pulsatile mass in the epigastrium in a hypotensive patient with severe back pain and occasionally left lower quadrant pain.

   b. **Plain radiographs** (anteroposterior [AP] and cross-table lateral) of the abdomen may reveal the presence of a calcified wall of an AAA. However, abdominal plain films may overestimate the size of an aneurysm by as much as 1.0–1.5 cm.

   c. **Ultrasound examination** of the aorta accurately detects AAAs and determines aneurysmal size within 2–4 mm of intraoperative measurement of aneurysmal size. Although ultrasonography is not sensitive in detecting bleeds, it will detect large hematomas.

   d. **Arteriography** is useful in planning elective surgical repair of an AAA, because it may detail the extent of the aneurysm and determine whether other vessels (e.g., renal or iliac arteries) are involved with the process. In contrast, arteriography is of limited usefulness in the acute setting, because it may miss the diagnosis in the presence of an intralumenal clot and will not detect hemorrhage that has been tamponaded; furthermore, it will delay surgical intervention.

   e. An **abdominal computed tomographic (CT) scan** with contrast accurately evaluates AAAs and may detect other causes of abdominal or back pain, such as cholelithiasis, hydronephrosis, and intraabdominal tumors. The CT scan can also detect dissection of blood between a laminated clot and the aneurysm wall (indicating expansion of the aneurysm) and any retroperitoneal or intraperitoneal hematoma. The CT scan is particularly useful when a stable patient presents with back or abdominal pain and a question exists as to whether an aneurysm is causing the symptoms; however, if it is apparent clinically that the patient's symptoms are attributable to an aneurysm (e.g., by the presence of a tender, pulsatile abdominal mass), time must not be lost to obtain radiographic confirmation.

6. **Prognosis.** For untreated AAAs, there is about a 50% risk of rupture within 5 years. The mortality associated with intraperitoneal rupture of an AAA is 70–90%, while retroperitoneal rupture has a slightly lower mortality (40–60%). In contrast, elective resection of an AAA has a mortality of 2–5%.

7. **Management**

   a. **Asymptomatic patients** who present to the emergency department for evaluation of other medical or surgical problems and are found to have an incidental AAA should be referred to a general or vascular surgeon for evaluation. Generally, patients who have no medical contraindications to an aneurysmectomy should have any aneurysm larger than 4 cm by ultrasound electively repaired. For patients with significant cardiac or pulmonary insufficiency, biannual follow-up sonographic evaluation of the aneurysm is recommended; if the aneurysm increases in size by more than 0.5 cm in a 6-month period, surgical therapy should be considered.

   b. **Symptomatic patients.** Once the diagnosis of an expanding or ruptured AAA is suspected, prompt surgical consultation should be obtained.

      (1) **Supportive care. Volume repletion** with Ringer's lactate solution and blood (as needed) should be administered commensurate with the clinical situation. In markedly hypotensive patients, type-specific or O-negative blood should be infused immediately (prior to anesthesia induction) to avoid circulatory collapse. The military antishock trousers (MAST) suit (see Chap. 38) is a useful device in tamponading bleeding and raising the blood pressure.

      (2) **Surgery.** Once the diagnosis of a ruptured AAA is made, the patient should be promptly transferred to the operating suite for control of bleeding and surgical repair of the aneurysm. In such a situation, there should be no significant delay in transfer to the operating suite (e.g., to

obtain radiographic studies), as proximal control of the ruptured aorta is a lifesaving maneuver. Although the signs and symptoms of impending rupture of an AAA are not specific, the presence of back pain or abdominal tenderness in a stable patient with an AAA should be regarded as an ominous sign, and prompt surgical therapy considered because of the very high mortality associated with surgery after the patient's hemodynamic status has deteriorated.

B. Uncommon intraabdominal aneurysms

1. **Iliac artery aneurysms** are extremely rare and are usually associated with an abdominal aortic aneurysm. An internal iliac artery aneurysm can present with rectal pain and may be palpable on rectal or pelvic examination. Rupture of these aneurysms causes pain similar to that of renal colic, with pain radiating into the scrotum, inner thigh, or perirectal region. In stable patients, the diagnosis can be established by CT scanning, ultrasonography, or arteriography. Symptomatic patients with an iliac artery aneurysm require emergent surgery.

2. Other **unusual types of intraabdominal aneurysms** include splenic, renal, celiac axis, hepatic, superior mesenteric, and inferior mesenteric artery aneurysms. Rupture of any of these rare aneurysms can present as an intraabdominal catastrophe requiring an emergency operation; however, surgery is usually delayed because the preoperative diagnosis is rarely made. In stable patients, CT scanning, arteriography, or ultrasonography can be used to establish the diagnosis.

C. Peripheral arterial aneurysms

1. **Types. Popliteal artery aneurysms** account for approximately 70% of peripheral aneurysms. Popliteal aneurysms usually are atherosclerotic in origin, although traumatic false aneurysms can occur occasionally. Various series have reported an amputation rate of 20–30% in patients who have thrombosis or significant embolization secondary to a popliteal artery aneurysm. Femoral artery aneurysms, which are not associated with a significant amputation rate, are less common peripheral aneurysms; and aneurysms of the carotid and subclavian arteries occur very rarely.

2. **Clinical manifestations.** Approximately 50–70% of patients with a popliteal aneurysm also have an aneurysm of the aorta, iliac, or femoral artery; and two-thirds of patients have bilateral popliteal aneurysms. Since 50–70% of patients with a popliteal aneurysm present with acute arterial occlusion from thrombosis or emboli, the diagnosis should be considered in any patient presenting with an acute unilateral infrapopliteal vascular occlusion. Less than 10% of patients with a popliteal aneurysm present with acute rupture of the aneurysm. A small percentage of patients will have either edema of the lower extremity secondary to popliteal vein obstruction or motor and sensory changes secondary to nerve compression.

3. **Diagnosis.** Physical examination will often reveal the aneurysm as a pulsatile mass, but small or thrombosed aneurysms may be difficult to detect on examination. Ultrasonography can be diagnostic. Arteriography can also confirm the diagnosis. Because of the high incidence of multiple aneurysms in patients with a popliteal artery aneurysm, these patients should have popliteal, femoral, and iliac arteries, as well as the abdominal aorta, evaluated by sonography.

4. **Management.** Patients with a peripheral artery aneurysm detected on examination should be referred to a vascular or general surgeon. Elective repair should be considered in patients with a peripheral artery aneurysm (e.g., popliteal artery aneurysm) before complications occur. Patients who present with acute arterial occlusion of a lower extremity secondary to embolism from a popliteal artery aneurysm should receive prompt evaluation and treatment by a vascular surgeon. A ruptured aneurysm requires immediate surgical intervention.

Venous Disorders

I. **Varicose veins** represent dilated and tortuous branches of the lesser and greater saphenous systems.

  A. **Etiology.** The main abnormality responsible for varicose veins is valvular incompetence. Many causes of varicose veins have been described.

   1. **Familial varicosities** are common and can affect both males and females.

   2. **Pregnancy** is associated with an increased incidence of varicose veins and may

be the result of various factors, such as hormonal factors or the mechanical effect of the gravid uterus.

   3. **Congenital** or **acquired arteriovenous (AV) malformations** are a rare cause of varicose veins. The congenital form is present at an early age, whereas the acquired form usually results from trauma.

B. **Clinical features.** Patients with varicose veins seek medical attention because of the undesirable cosmetic appearance of the dilated veins or, less commonly, because of manifestations of venous insufficiency (see sec. II).

C. **Complications**

   1. **Hemorrhage,** sometimes of serious magnitude, can result from traumatic rupture of a varix or can be spontaneous. If the bleeding is readily controlled by direct compression and elevation of the leg, a compression dressing and instructions to keep the leg elevated for 24–48 hours are all that is necessary. For bleeding that is recurrent or not easily controlled, suture ligation of the bleeding vessel is indicated.

   2. Other complications associated with varicose veins include thrombosis (see sec. III) and venous insufficiency (see sec. II).

D. **Treatment**

   1. **Conservative management** is indicated for patients with mild varicosities, elderly patients, and patients who refuse surgery. This therapy consists of elastic support in combination with periodic leg elevation and exercise. Prolonged standing or sitting should be avoided.

   2. **Sclerotherapy** with 3% sodium tetradecyl sulfate in benzyl alcohol is indicated for small unsightly veins, dilated superficial veins, lower leg perforators, and recurrent or persistent veins after operation.

   3. **Surgical therapy** (i.e., vein stripping) is indicated for patients with (1) severe symptoms, (2) very large varices, (3) recurrent attacks of superficial phlebitis or bleeding, or (4) ulceration from venous stasis. Surgery can also be performed for cosmetic reasons.

II. **Chronic venous insufficiency** results from obstruction or valvular incompetence (or both) of the deep, communicating (perforating), or superficial veins.

A. **Etiology.** The most common cause of chronic venous insufficiency is previous deep vein thrombosis (i.e., postphlebitic syndrome). Other causes include varicose veins, venous trauma, and incompetent perforators. Uncommonly, nonthrombotic venous obstruction can occur secondary to an extrinsic mass lesion (e.g., abdominal aneurysm, pelvic cyst or benign tumor, pregnancy, malignant neoplasm).

B. **Clinical manifestations** involving the affected extremity include aching pain, edema, and, occasionally, night cramps. The aching pain and edema are worse toward the end of the day and are usually relieved by elevation of the affected limb. Night cramps usually present while the patient is asleep and require massage of the affected muscle group and ambulation for relief. Stasis dermatitis, brown pigmentation, chronic induration, and ulcerations of the affected extremity are also common manifestations of chronic venous insufficiency. The brown pigmentation is secondary to hemosiderin deposition in the subcutaneous tissue, thought to be derived from the breakdown of extravasated blood. Ulcerations usually involve the lower third of the affected extremity, with ulcers most commonly found posterior and superior to the medial malleolus and, less commonly, in relation to the lateral malleolus. These ulcers are usually shallow in nature and can appear following minimal trauma. Occasionally, the dermatitis is very severe, related either to a secondary infection with cellulitis or a superimposed allergic reaction from medication used by the patient. Patients with chronic venous insufficiency are at an increased risk for developing acute thrombosis of the deep system (see sec. III).

C. **Evaluation**

   1. **Noninvasive tests.** The standard test is Doppler ultrasonography, with venous insufficiency demonstrating incompetence of the valves at different sites. Other noninvasive tests include photoplethysmography, calf-volume plethysmography, and impedance plethysmography.

   2. **Invasive tests** include ambulatory venous pressure measurements and contrast phlebography.

D. **Treatment**

   1. **Conservative therapy** is directed toward decreasing the amount of stasis in the lower-extremity veins and decreasing the pressure in the superficial venous system. The patient should attempt to elevate the involved leg as much as possible during the day as well as during the night. Active exercise to maintain

an adequate blood flow and diminish the stasis is recommended. Elastic compression, preferably custom fit, will diminish the swelling of the leg and will usually relieve the symptoms of venous claudication.

2. **Stasis ulcers** are treated by rest, elevation of the extremity, and good general foot care. A gelatinized pressure dressing (e.g., Unna Boot) is also beneficial in selected cases. Appropriate antibiotics should be used if there is evidence of superimposed infection. Skin grafting may be necessary in severe cases.

3. **Surgical treatment.** Patients who have severe varicosities and a patent deep venous system can benefit from ligation and stripping of the greater or lesser saphenous veins (or both), as well as ligation of incompetent perforators.

E. **Disposition.** Most patients with chronic venous insufficiency can be discharged from the emergency department. However, admission to the hospital is generally recommended for patients with (1) severe symptoms, (2) severe ulcerations requiring skin grafting, or (3) cellulitis complicating ulcers or a stasis dermatitis.

III. **Venous thrombosis** can be associated with venous inflammation **(thrombophlebitis)** or unassociated with venous inflammation **(phlebothrombosis)**. Both entities are variants of the same process, and both are potentially lethal conditions. The development of venous thrombosis is related to three factors **(Virchow's triad)**: (1) abnormalities of the vein wall (e.g., from trauma, previous thrombophlebitis, perivenous inflammation, venous disease, or injection of irritant solutions), (2) venous stasis (e.g., secondary to prolonged bed rest, sitting, or standing; congestive heart failure; low cardiac output states; immobilization of an extremity; venous insufficiency; extrinsic venous compression; age over 40 years; or obesity), and (3) hypercoagulability of the blood (e.g., from trauma, hyperviscosity, malignancy, use of oral contraceptives, inherent antithrombin III deficiency, pregnancy, diabetes mellitus, smoking, or liver disease).

A. **Superficial thrombophlebitis**

1. **Uncomplicated superficial thrombophlebitis**

a. **Clinical manifestations** include pain, swelling, warmth, erythema, tenderness, and induration along the course of a superficial vein. Generally, there is an absence of significant extremity swelling with uncomplicated superficial thrombophlebitis. Superficial thrombophlebitis rarely embolizes, because inflammation produces firm adherence of the thrombus to the vein wall. However, pulmonary emboli can occur in association with this condition as a result of propagation of the superficial thrombus into the deep vein system or because of the increased incidence of concomitant deep vein thrombosis.

b. **Diagnosis.** Doppler examination can confirm the occlusion of the affected superficial vein and is useful in excluding the diagnosis of deep vein thrombosis. In patients with suspicion of an associated deep vein thrombosis and equivocal noninvasive studies, a venogram may be required.

c. **Treatment.** For a superficial thrombophlebitis that is localized and mildly tender, treatment with a mild anti-inflammatory agent (e.g., aspirin), local heat, and an elastic compression bandage is recommended. For more severe superficial thrombophlebitis, bed rest with elevation of the affected extremity and a more potent nonsteroidal anti-inflammatory agent (e.g., ibuprofen, indomethacin) may be required. Rarely, a high saphenous vein thrombophlebitis, with evidence of propagation toward the saphenofemoral junction, requires ligation and stripping of the greater saphenous vein.

d. **Disposition.** Most patients with superficial thrombophlebitis can be treated on an outpatient basis. However, admission is recommended for patients with (1) extensive superficial venous involvement, (2) superficial thrombophlebitis occurring in close proximity to the deep venous system (e.g., at the saphenofemoral, saphenopopliteal, or cephaloaxillary junction), (3) progression of the process despite adequate therapy, or (4) a severe inflammatory reaction.

2. **Superficial septic thrombophlebitis** can occur as a result of an indwelling intravenous catheter, parenteral drug abuse, an infected venipuncture site, or adjacent soft-tissue infection.

a. **Etiologic agents.** Although *Staphylococcus aureus* has been the most common organism responsible for septic thrombophlebitis in the past, infection with a wide variety of organisms, including the Enterobacteriaceae, *Pseudomonas, Bacterioides,* and *Candida,* is becoming more common as a result of parenteral drug abuse and the use of broad-spectrum antimicrobial agents in hospitalized patients for prolonged periods.

   b. Clinical manifestations are the same as those associated with uncomplicated superficial thrombophlebitis plus evidence of an infectious process (e.g., fever, chills, leukocytosis, positive blood cultures). Purulent drainage may be expressed from the vein, and abscesses may occur along the course of the affected vein. Septic embolization may complicate septic thrombophlebitis.

   c. Management consists of hospitalization, appropriate intravenous antibiotic therapy, and excision of the infected vein.

   3. Migratory thrombophlebitis. Recurrent superficial thrombophlebitis occurring at different sites may indicate the presence of a systemic disease such as Buerger's disease, a malignant neoplasm (especially bronchial or pancreatic), systemic lupus erythematosus, or ulcerative colitis. Migratory thrombophlebitis is an indication for a workup for such disease entities.

B. Deep vein thrombosis is a medical emergency due to the risk of embolization into the pulmonary circulation.

   1. Lower-extremity deep vein thrombosis is the source of pulmonary emboli in about 85% of patients [14]. Although the soleus plexus of veins in the calf is the most common location for deep vein thrombosis, thrombosis limited to the calf is rarely life-threatening because of the small risk of embolization from calf-vein thrombi [6] and the fact that emboli originating from the smaller veins of the calf seldom cause serious clinical manifestations [16]. However, calf-vein thrombosis can cause postthrombotic sequelae, and about 20% of these thrombi propagate proximally into the popliteal vein where the risk of major embolization is significant [6].

   a. Clinical manifestations include an aching pain in the involved calf or thigh muscles that is aggravated by muscular activity, systemic signs of inflammation (e.g., fever, chills, tachycardia, leukocytosis, anxiety), edema of the affected extremity, increased skin warmth and erythema in the affected extremity, a positive Homans' sign (i.e., calf pain with dorsiflexion of the foot), dilatation of superficial veins, deep induration of calf muscles, and tenderness in the calf, thigh, popliteal fossa, adductor canal, or groin (depending on the site of the thrombosis). Unilateral extremity swelling (i.e., a difference in calf circumferences of greater than 1.5 cm) is the most valuable clinical manifestation in the diagnosis of deep vein thrombosis. Iliofemoral thrombosis may present with severe pain, massive swelling, marked elevation in the venous pressure, and a bluish discoloration of the affected extremity. A severe form of this entity is called **phlegmasia cerulea dolens** (blue leg); another variant is **phlegmasia alba dolens** (milk leg), characterized by arterial spasm and a pale cool leg with diminished pulses. These entities are rare, but they can progress to massive thrombosis of the venous system and gangrene of the affected extremity. Except in extreme cases, clinical manifestations are notoriously inaccurate in predicting deep vein thrombosis, with studies indicating an equal frequency of positive clinical findings in patients with and without this condition [2], as well as no clinical evidence of this type of thrombosis in 50% of patients dying of pulmonary emboli from deep vein thrombosis [15].

   b. Differential diagnosis. Conditions that may mimic deep vein thrombosis include superficial thrombophlebitis; venous insufficiency; varicose veins; arterial insufficiency; infection (e.g., lymphangitis, cellulitis); extremity swelling (e.g., secondary to venous compression by an extrinsic mass, congestive heart failure, renal insufficiency, pregnancy, or a paralyzed limb); lymphedema (e.g., from lymphatic obstruction by a tumor); arthritis; ruptured Baker's cyst; and traumatic injuries to an extremity resulting in a contusion, subfascial hematoma, or a ruptured muscle or tendon (e.g., involving the gastrocnemius or soleus muscle).

   c. Diagnosis

   (1) Contrast phlebography is the most accurate test for diagnosing deep vein thrombosis. However, this procedure is invasive, may be technically difficult to perform in a swollen extremity, and has been implicated in the generation of venous thrombi.

   (2) Doppler ultrasonography is the most sensitive noninvasive test for detecting calf vein thrombosis; it is also accurate in detecting proximal vein thrombosis. The accuracy, sensitivity, and specificity of the technique are directly related to the experience of the technician performing the test, with an accuracy approaching 95% in proper hands.

(3) Impedance plethysmography is the most accurate noninvasive test for diagnosing proximal vein thrombosis. However, this test is not accurate in detecting thrombi distal to the popliteal vein.

(4) I^{125}-labeled fibrinogen test is extremely sensitive and can identify small areas of thrombosis. The clinical usefulness of this test is limited, however, because of its cost and the fact that it may identify areas that are of questionable clinical significance.

(5) Recommendation. It is recommended that Doppler ultrasonography be performed for suspected deep vein thrombosis distal to the popliteal vein, and that Doppler ultrasonography in combination with impedance plethysmography be performed for suspected proximal thrombi. If the results of these noninvasive studies are unequivocal, additional tests are unnecessary. However, if these noninvasive studies yield equivocal results or if there is a discrepancy between the clinical impression and the test results, contrast phlebography is required.

d. Treatment

(1) Supportive care includes bed rest, elevation of the affected extremity to 15–20 degrees, and application of warm, moist dressings to the affected extremity.

(2) Anticoagulation, unless specifically contraindicated, should be instituted for all patients with deep vein thrombosis. Anticoagulation prevents propagation of the original thrombus, averts the development of new thrombi, prevents pulmonary embolization of the thrombus, and hastens dissolution of the thrombus by allowing natural fibrinolysis to operate unopposed. Following initiation of anticoagulation therapy, patients remain at risk for embolization until normal physiologic mechanisms dissolve the existing thrombus (in 3–7 days). Due to the unreliability of clinical findings and the significant risk of anticoagulant therapy, deep vein thrombosis should be confirmed by noninvasive or invasive tests (or both) either prior to or shortly after instituting anticoagulant therapy, depending on the clinical suspicion and availability of the tests.

(a) Heparin therapy is initiated with an IV bolus of 5000–10,000 units as a loading dose, followed by 1000–2000 units/hour via a mechanical infusion pump. The dosage is then adjusted to maintain the PTT at 1.5–2.5 times the control.

(b) Warfarin therapy is initiated when patients show evidence of stabilization or resolution of clinical manifestations (i.e., 2–3 days following initiation of heparin therapy). After anticoagulation is achieved with warfarin, heparin is discontinued. The warfarin is then continued for 3 months.

(c) Fibrinolytic therapy (e.g., with streptokinase or urokinase) may reduce the incidence of postphlebitic complications but apparently does not affect the incidence of pulmonary embolism [3]. Fibrinolytic therapy is recommended only in specific circumstances and should be given by a physician familiar with its usage.

(3) Surgery. Venous interruption by a transvenous umbrella filter or surgically placed clips on the involved vessel is indicated for patients who continue to embolize despite adequate anticoagulation or for patients in whom anticoagulant therapy is contraindicated (e.g., because of recent active bleeding). Rarely, venous thrombectomy may be required for severe iliofemoral thrombosis with impending gangrene.

2. Upper-extremity thrombosis involving the axillary or subclavian vein can occur as a result of an indwelling venous catheter, external trauma, or repetitive or unusual muscular activity of the affected upper extremity **(effort thrombosis).**

a. Clinical manifestations include pain and swelling of the involved extremity, a prominent collateral pattern over the anterior chest and shoulder, cyanosis of the involved extremity, and a palpable axillary cord.

b. The **diagnosis** of upper-extremity thrombosis can be established with Doppler ultrasonography or venography.

c. The **treatment** is the same as that of lower-extremity deep vein thrombosis (see **1.d**).

IV. Venous trauma. See **Vascular Injuries,** sec. **III.**

Acute Mesenteric Ischemia

Acute mesenteric ischemia is the presenting diagnosis at least once per every 1000 admissions at major medical centers. Therapeutic modalities for this entity have yielded poor results, with mortality in most reported series ranging from 60 to 100%. Since 30 minutes of ischemia can result in extensive damage to the intestinal wall, a delay in diagnosis is at least partly responsible for the high mortality.

I. Etiology. Embolic occlusion of a mesenteric artery is currently the most common cause of acute mesenteric ischemia. One-half of cases are due to acute arterial occlusion, one-fourth to nonocclusive mesenteric infarction, and the remainder to mesenteric venous thrombosis.

A. Embolic occlusion. Sudden complete occlusion of a mesenteric artery is due more often to an embolus than to thrombosis. The superior mesenteric artery (SMA) is the mesenteric artery most susceptible to embolic occlusion because it leaves the aorta at an acute angle and parallels it. Emboli tend to lodge at points of anatomic narrowing, usually just distal to the origin of a major arterial branch, such as the inferior pancreaticoduodenal or middle colic artery. Most emboli originate in the heart, either from a mural thrombus following a myocardial infarction or from an atrial thrombus in patients with atrial fibrillation. Less frequently, emboli arise from vegetative endocarditis or from atheromatous plaques within the aorta. A large number of patients will have a history of peripheral arterial embolism, and approximately 20% can be expected to have synchronous emboli to other arteries.

B. Thrombotic occlusion. Acute thrombosis of a mesenteric artery usually occurs where there is significant atherosclerotic disease. The extent of the intestinal ischemia or infarction is dependent on the site of thrombosis and the status of collateral channels. Sudden thrombosis of the main stem SMA usually results in infarction of the entire small intestine and right colon, whereas distal thrombosis of a segmental artery results in segmental bowel infarction. Slowly developing stenosis, on the other hand, may allow for the development of a collateral circulation so that bowel viability is preserved when complete occlusion occurs. The final thrombotic event is usually precipitated by a sudden decrease in cardiac output, such as occurs in acute CHF or an acute myocardial infarction, that results in a sluggish arterial blood flow and subsequent thrombus formation in the stenotic vessel.

C. Nonocclusive mesenteric infarction. This entity is thought to be caused by enteric small-vessel vasoconstriction occurring in response to a decrease in cardiac output, severe dehydration, use of vasopressor agents, or prolonged hypotension. Predisposing conditions include an acute myocardial infarction, CHF, aortic insufficiency, and major abdominal or cardiac surgery; digitalis and diuretic therapy have also been implicated as predisposing factors.

D. Mesenteric vein occlusion. Mesenteric vein thrombosis was cited as the most frequent cause of intestinal infarction 50 years ago but is relatively uncommon today. Mesenteric vein occlusion can be primary (agnogenic) or secondary to a variety of conditions. Predisposing factors to secondary mesenteric vein thrombosis are (1) infection, usually secondary to appendicitis, diverticulitis, or a pelvic abscess; (2) local vein congestion, as occurs with hepatic cirrhosis and portal hypertension; (3) accidental operative trauma to mesenteric veins, particularly during portocaval shunting procedures; and (4) hematologic conditions, such as polycythemia vera, hypercoagulability associated with oral contraceptives, and antithrombin III deficiency.

II. Pathophysiology. Although there are different causes of mesenteric ischemia, the final pathway leading to irreversible intestinal infarction is essentially the same for each cause. The mucosa and submucosa are most sensitive to ischemia and respond with edema, hemorrhage, and sloughing. Initial spasm in the muscularis is followed by atonia. The bowel wall becomes edematous and infiltrated with blood; and wall perforation, leading to bacterial peritonitis, ensues. As necrosis of the intestine progresses, massive plasma losses into the bowel lumen and peritoneal cavity occur. Since the alimentary tract contains 95% of the vasoactive serotonin in the body, intestinal cell necrosis results in liberation of this agent; serotonin promotes platelet aggregation and peripheral platelet clumping, and contributes to disseminated intravascular coagulation and failure of organ perfusion. The end result is sepsis and multiple organ system failure, culminating in death.

III. The **clinical features** of mesenteric ischemia are the same whether occlusion is from thrombosis or an embolus.

    A. **Historic features.** Patients with mesenteric ischemia are usually over 50 years of age, and there is often a history of longstanding CHF, cardiac arrhythmias (particularly atrial fibrillation), or a recent myocardial infarction. A history of crampy postprandial abdominal pain may be present in one-third of these patients. Patients with hypovolemia and hypotension, such as occurs in burns and pancreatitis, may develop nonocclusive intestinal ischemia. There may be a prior history of embolization or a familial tendency for diffuse clotting disorders or thrombotic events.

    B. **Physical features.** Severe abdominal pain is present in 75–98% of these patients. The pain is continuous or colicky in nature; it is unresponsive to narcotics and, in the early phases, is out of proportion to the abdominal findings, which initially may be minimal. Abdominal distention and lack of audible peristalsis are common. Hematemesis or bloody diarrhea may occur. As intestinal infarction progresses, perforation occurs, and peritonitis develops with the physical findings of rebound tenderness and rigidity. Sepsis, hypotension, and multiple organ system failure ensue, culminating in death.

    C. **Laboratory features.** A leukocytosis (i.e., $> 15,000/mm^3$) occurs in 75% of patients with acute mesenteric ischemia. Hemoconcentration develops and reflects plasma loss into the peritoneal cavity. Moderate elevation of the serum amylase can be found in half of the patients but is not diagnostic. Late in the course of mesenteric infarction, the serum levels of lactic dehydrogenase (LDH), aspartate aminotransaminase (AST), and alanine aminotransaminase (ALT) rise significantly. A progressive metabolic acidosis ensues as necrosis of the intestine progresses.

    D. **Radiographic studies.** Signs of acute ischemia on plain radiographs tend to be nonspecific and usually do not occur until late, when bowel infarction and perforation are present. Mesenteric arteriography can be helpful when the diagnosis is questionable but should be undertaken only if it can be performed expeditiously. Arteriography can determine the type of obstruction and identify the site of obstruction. However, in patients with severe acidosis or peritonitis, the procedure should not delay emergent surgical intervention.

IV. **Diagnosis.** The clinical diagnosis of intestinal ischemia can be difficult unless a high degree of suspicion is present. Identification of acute mesenteric ischemia depends on recognition of patients at risk (see sec. III.A). In particular, any patient with abdominal pain out of proportion to the physical findings, a leukocytosis, and a marked metabolic acidosis should be suspected of having a mesenteric infarction. The diagnosis can be confirmed by mesenteric arteriography, but only if time allows.

V. **Management.** Patients with mesenteric ischemia require immediate surgical consultation.

    A. **Supportive care.** IV fluids are administered to replace third-space fluid losses, and sodium bicarbonate is used to ameliorate a metabolic acidosis. Cardiac arrhythmias and CHF require appropriate therapy. Hypotension unresponsive to volume infusion requires administration of a vasopressor.

    B. **Vasodilator therapy.** If arteriography demonstrates mesenteric vasoconstriction, the procedure may be therapeutic, as an infusion of a vasodilator (e.g., papaverine, isoproterenol, tolazoline) can be delivered directly into the involved artery. Papaverine is the most commonly used agent; it is usually infused at a rate of 30–60 mg/hour via an arterial infusion pump. Occasionally, this form of therapy may be successful, and abdominal pain will subside.

    C. **Surgery.** The essential treatment of acute mesenteric ischemia is prompt surgical intervention to restore perfusion before gangrene and perforation occur. Patients with a severe acidosis or peritonitis also require emergent surgery for resection of infarcted bowel.

Vascular Injuries

Vascular trauma poses a significant challenge to the emergency physician and surgeon. Experience gained in wartime with the management of vascular injuries led to the advances that have resulted in a higher limb salvage rate for civilians. Amputation rates for major-extremity arterial injuries in World War II approached 50% but fell to about 13% in the Korean conflict. Successful limb salvage depends on prompt diagnosis, accurate resuscitation, and early revascularization.

I. **Pathophysiology.** Vascular injury can result from either penetrating or blunt trauma to a vessel.

  A. **Penetrating injuries** can result from knife or gunshot wounds and are characterized by puncture, laceration, or transection of vessels. A loss of arterial substance, false aneurysm formation (presenting as a pulsating hematoma), AV fistula formation, vessel contusion, or missile embolism may occur.

   1. **Knife wounds** can cause direct injury to vessels in their path.

   2. **Gunshot injuries.** Some knowledge of missile ballistics is important in the evaluation of vessels following a gunshot wound. Basic physics relates that kinetic energy is equal to one-half the mass of a missile times the square of its velocity. Thus, velocity is the critical variable in the production of kinetic energy and, subsequently, in determining the extent of tissue damage.

      a. **Low-velocity injuries,** i.e., associated with velocities less than 1000 feet/second, generally result from handguns used by civilians. These missile wounds may cause direct vascular injury but usually do not result in extensive soft-tissue damage.

      b. **High-velocity missiles** have velocities greater than 2000 feet/second and are usually associated with war wounds and the use of high-powered hunting rifles. A large amount of kinetic energy is dissipated by such missiles, creating a cavity in their wake, with the size of the cavity being directly proportional to the projectile's velocity. This cavitation can have an explosive effect that, even at a distance removed from the tract of the missile, disrupts tissue, ruptures blood vessels and nerves, and even fractures bones. The external appearance of high-velocity wounds, therefore, may be misleading, and the possibility of distant vascular injuries must be suspected.

  B. **Blunt trauma** can damage the intima of blood vessels (leading to thrombosis), cause spasm, or produce complete or incomplete division of vessels (the latter occurs when all layers except the adventitia have been separated).

II. **Arterial trauma**

  A. **Clinical manifestations.** The history and physical examination are the basis for suspecting arterial injury in the emergency department. Arterial injury must always be considered in the presence of brisk bleeding, an expanding hematoma, or obvious major blood loss. In an extremity, the most prominent features of a major arterial injury may be signs of ischemia (e.g., pulselessness, pallor, paresthesias). Palpation of a pulsating hematoma may indicate the presence of a pseudoaneurysm, while auscultation along the trajectory of the injury may reveal a bruit indicative of an AV fistula. The presence of a distal circulatory deficit, an auscultated bruit, a pulsatile hematoma, or bright-red spirting bleeding is pathognomonic of an underlying arterial injury and must be treated as such. An important observation is that the presence of a pulse does not preclude the presence of a proximal arterial injury.

  B. **Diagnosis.** Arteriography is the most important diagnostic study in suspected arterial injuries. This study is sensitive enough to detect or exclude the presence of an arterial injury in patients with equivocal clinical signs. If there are soft signs of arterial injury on physical examination, such as the presence of a nonexpanding hematoma, an adjacent neurologic deficit, or injury in proximity to a major vascular structure, an arteriogram can confirm or exclude the presence of arterial injury. On arteriography, obstruction to the column of dye, extravasation of dye into the surrounding soft tissues, early venous filling, an irregular wall defect, or the presence of a false aneurysm is indicative of vascular injury. With evidence of distal ischemia or significant hemorrhage, injury localization can be obtained (if necessary) in the operating suite with a single film arteriogram. Otherwise, stable patients with equivocal or definite signs of vascular injury can be managed expectantly and brought to the arteriography suite for evaluation.

  C. **Management.** Patients presenting to the emergency department with a potential vascular injury are managed selectively on the basis of their physical examination. Consultation with a vascular or general surgeon is indicated.

   1. **Hemorrhage** is controlled by packing the wound with gauze and applying pressure; however, a tourniquet should be avoided. Since clamping of vessels may further damage the vessel and can damage adjacent structures (e.g., nerves), it should also be avoided.

   2. **Shock,** which is present in 50–60% of patients with significant arterial injury, is treated with rapid infusion of Ringer's lactate solution and, if needed, blood

via multiple large-bore IV catheters (see Chap. 17). The MAST suit (see Chap. 38) is a useful adjunct in shock resuscitation because it raises the blood pressure and tamponades bleeding beneath the device.

3. **Prophylactic antibiotics** are given as soon after the injury as possible. For an extremity injury, an agent effective against gram-positive skin organisms, including *S. aureus,* is used. With abdominal injuries in which enteric contamination is possible, agents effective against gram-positive bacteria and enteric aerobes and anaerobes are administered.

4. **Tetanus prophylaxis.** Since penetrating wounds are tetanus-prone, appropriate tetanus prophylaxis with toxoid and human immune globulin, depending on the patient's status, is indicated.

5. **Associated injuries.** Since patients with fractures or dislocations can have associated vascular injuries, precise and complete assessment of the vascular status is imperative. Stabilization of fractures is necessary to prevent further damage to surrounding vascular structures. If there is any question regarding possible injury to an adjacent major artery, an arteriogram should be performed.

6. **Surgery.** Arterial injuries generally should be repaired, with the possible exception of distal or minor vessels that can be sacrificed (ligated) without risk of circulatory insufficiency (e.g., radial artery in the presence of a patent ulnar artery). Injuries resulting in distal ischemia require urgent operation (i.e., within 4–6 hours of injury) to prevent irreversible muscle and nerve damage.

D. **Disposition.** With the exception of an isolated injury to a distal artery with good collateral circulation (e.g., radial artery) that can be treated with ligation, patients with a suspected arterial injury require hospitalization.

E. **Special anatomic considerations**
  1. **Injuries to the neck**
    a. **Penetrating injuries to the neck** (extending below the platysma muscle) require surgical consultation.
      (1) **Symptomatic wounds.** Patients with clinical findings of arterial injury (e.g., brisk bleeding, expanding hematoma) require urgent operative treatment. Preoperative or intraoperative arteriography is indicated, if time permits, for wounds at the base of the neck (zone 1) or above the angle of the mandible (zone III). Special attention should be paid to clinical findings of dysphagia, hoarseness, hemoptysis, or subcutaneous emphysema suggestive of esophageal or tracheal injury coincident with the vascular injury; esophagoscopy or bronchoscopy (or both) is indicated for these clinical findings.
      (2) **Asymptomatic wounds.** Controversy exists regarding the proper management of patients with asymptomatic wounds to the neck. Recommendations vary from mandatory operation to observation supplemented by diagnostic tests (e.g., arteriography, esophagoscopy, bronchoscopy). In general, arteriography is mandated for wounds at the base of the neck (zone I) and for wounds above the angle of the mandible (zone III); however, since wounds between the mandible and 1 cm above the clavicles (zone II) are accessible for observation or exploration, arteriography is less important in their management.
      The risks associated with **penetrating trauma to the base of the neck** are related to the possibility of exsanguination into the pleural cavities and the possibility of other injuries such as a hemopneumothorax, tracheal disruption, or esophageal perforation. These patients may appear well at first, but bleeding can occur spontaneously, oftentimes aggravated by changes in the intrathoracic pressure. Therefore, treatment modalities that may increase the intrapleural pressure, including tracheal intubation and nasogastric intubation, should be avoided if possible. No wound involving the base of the neck should be probed in the emergency department, since dislodgement of a clot tamponading a proximal carotid or subclavian artery injury can lead to massive hemorrhage and even death, particularly if the hemorrhage occurs intrapleurally; in addition, a pneumothorax can be created.
    b. **Blunt trauma to the neck** can cause vascular injury. In the presence of neurologic signs (e.g., syncope, hemiparesis) or signs suggestive of an arterial injury (e.g., bruit, expanding hematoma), arteriography or exploration or both are indicated.

2. **Upper-extremity vascular injuries** constitute about 40% of vascular injuries presenting to the emergency department.
   a. **Types of injuries**
      (1) The **brachial artery** is the most commonly injured artery in the upper extremity. Injury to this vessel usually results from penetrating trauma but can occur with either supracondylar fractures of the humerus or posterior dislocation of the elbow. Since the median nerve travels in the neurovascular sheath of the brachial artery, a neurologic deficit in the median nerve distribution is often associated with injury to the brachial artery.
      (2) Injury to the **axillary artery** can occur from penetrating trauma or secondary to a shoulder injury. However, since there is an extensive collateral system of vessels about the shoulder, distal perfusion may be maintained even with axillary artery damage.
      (3) Injuries to the **radial and ulnar arteries** are common civilian vascular injuries, usually from penetrating trauma. Ultimate amputation secondary to the loss of either of the arteries is rare, but the probability increases if both arteries are transected.
   b. **Management.** With the possible exception of an isolated radial or ulnar artery injury at the wrist with good collateral circulation, arterial injuries of the upper extremity require repair. Arteriography is useful in assessing for injury to the axillary or brachial artery if there is any suspicion of injury to those vessels.
3. **Lower-extremity vascular injury** is usually the result of penetrating trauma; distal to the common femoral artery, however, injury occurs with some frequency from blunt trauma. Repair of most lower-extremity arteries, including the common femoral, superficial femoral, and popliteal arteries, is mandatory, as amputation can be expected in 50% of limbs in which one of these vessels is ligated. The patient presenting with a lower-extremity fracture and signs of arterial compromise warrants arteriography in spite of any improvement noted in the limb after the bone is realigned.
   a. **Popliteal artery trauma** results in amputation more frequently than any other lower-extremity vascular injury, with unrecognized injury to the popliteal artery resulting in limb loss in approximately 75% of cases. This injury should be suspected with knee joint dislocation or tibial plateau fractures. Arteriography is recommended to assess for blunt arterial injury in patients with a posterior knee dislocation, knee instability after blunt trauma, displaced fractures near the knee, or severe compression injuries involving the knee.
   b. With **vascular injuries distal to the trifurcation of the popliteal artery,** the guideline to treatment is to ensure revascularization and patency of at least one of two vessels (posterior tibial or anterior tibial artery) forming the plantar arch.
4. **A traumatic AV fistula** can develop anywhere a penetrating injury causes a communication between an artery and an adjacent vein; however, these fistulas tend to occur more commonly in the lower extremity. The bruit (i.e., machinery murmur) characteristic of an AV fistula should be sought whenever there is any suspicion of an arteriovenous injury, but it is usually not audible until weeks or months after the injury. **Branham's sign,** which is the slowing of the patient's pulse when the artery is compressed proximal to the fistula, is present rarely in large AV fistulas. The diagnosis is established with arteriography, and the treatment is surgical repair unless the fistula is extremely small. The long-term sequelae of an untreated AV fistula include left ventricular enlargement, left ventricular failure, subacute bacterial endocarditis, and aneurysm formation.
III. **Venous trauma** can result in venous thrombosis, venous laceration, or an AV fistula. Venous injuries occur concomitantly with approximately 40% of arterial injuries.
   A. **Clinical manifestations** associated with major venous injury include extremity edema and venous engorgement distal to the site of injury, brisk bleeding from a wound in proximity to a major vein, an expanding hematoma, a hemothorax or hemoperitoneum, and hemorrhagic shock.
   B. The **diagnosis** can be confirmed, if necessary, by venography.
   C. **Treatment**
      1. **Bleeding** is usually controlled by direct pressure.
      2. **Injury to a major vein** (e.g., vena cava; portal, jugular, axillary, subclavian,

iliac, or femoral vein) warrants operative intervention to control bleeding or to avert chronic edema (or both).

3. **Injured extremity veins.** With the exception of the axillary vein, injured veins in the upper extremity can be ligated without increasing morbidity. In contrast, the major lower-extremity deep veins (e.g., superficial femoral vein, popliteal vein) should be surgically repaired, since ligation increases the incidence of venous stasis disease, including edema and thrombosis; consideration should be given to anticoagulation postoperatively and, with massive swelling, fasciotomy. Veins comprising the superficial system can be ligated with impunity.

Bibliography

1. Baker, C. C., Peterson, J. K., and Sheldon, G. F. Septic phlebitis: A neglected disease. *Am. J. Surg.* 138:97, 1979.
2. Cranley, J. J., Canos, A. J., and Sull, W. J. The diagnosis of deep vein thrombosis. Fallibility of clinical symptoms and signs. *Arch. Surg.* 111:34, 1976.
3. Elliot, M. S., et al. A comparative randomized trial of heparin versus streptokinase in the treatment of acute proximal venous thrombosis: An interim report of a prospective trial. *Br. J. Surg.* 66:838, 1979.
4. Hardy, J. D. *Critical Surgical Illness* (2nd ed.). Philadelphia: Saunders, 1980. Pp. 177–190.
5. Hardy, J. D. *Hardy's Textbook of Surgery.* Philadelphia: Lippincott, 1983. Pp. 936–952.
6. Kakkar, V. V. The diagnosis of deep vein thrombosis using the I^{125} fibrinogen test. *Arch. Surg.* 104:152, 1972.
7. Karl, R., et al. Surgical implications of antithrombin III deficiency. *Surgery* 89:429, 1981.
8. Moser, K. M., and LeMoine, J. R. Is embolic risk conditioned by location of deep venous thrombosis? *Ann. Intern. Med.* 94:439, 1981.
9. O'Gorman, R. B., et al. Emergency center arteriography in the evaluation of suspected peripheral vascular injuries. *Arch. Surg.* 119:568, 1984.
10. Ross, S. E., Ransom, K. J., and Shatney, C. H. The management of venous injuries in blunt extremity trauma. *J. Trauma* 25:150, 1985.
11. Rutherford, R. B. *Vascular Surgery* (2nd ed.). Philadelphia: Saunders, 1984. Pp. 440–572.
12. Sachs, S. M., Morton, J. W., and Schwartz, S. I. Acute mesenteric ischemia. *Surgery* 92:646, 1982.
13. Schwartz, G. R., et al. *Principles and Practice of Emergency Medicine* (2nd ed.). Philadelphia: Saunders, 1986.
14. Schwartz, S. I. *Principles of Surgery* (4th ed.). New York: McGraw-Hill, 1984.
15. Sevitt, S., and Gallagher, N. G. Venous thrombosis and pulmonary embolism. A clinicopathological study in injured and burned patients. *Br. J. Surg.* 48:475, 1961.
16. Way, W. W. (ed.). *Current Surgical Diagnosis and Treatment* (6th ed.). Los Altos, Calif.: Lange, 1983.

21

Thermal Injuries

William W. Monafo, Jr.

The American Burn Association has categorized burn injuries according to severity and has provided recommendations for their optimal triage (Table 21-1) and method of treatment. These recommendations, which are purposely broad so as to allow for unique circumstances, are based primarily on the extent of the body surface area involved, the depth and location of injury, age and general fitness of the patient, the presence of associated injuries, and the capabilities (personnel and equipment) of the in- and outpatient facilities of the institution in question. Accurate initial evaluation and management, coupled with appropriate triage by the emergency department physician, will improve both morbidity and mortality. In addition, optimal care of the severely burn-injured patient requires an organized and properly trained professional team along with the facilities and equipment that comprise a burn center.

I. **Assessment.** A brief but pertinent **history** is essential. The circumstances under which the injury was sustained should be elicited in detail. First aid measures that have been applied in the field, either by onlookers or ambulance attendants, should be noted and clearly recorded. A properly obtained history will alert the emergency department physician to the possibility of associated injuries that might otherwise be overlooked; in addition, the probable depth of the injury (see **B**) can usually be predicted with a fair degree of accuracy. For example, a person involved in a closed-space fire or explosion may have sustained an inhalation injury; and a patient whose clothing ignited generally will have deeper burns compared with someone who had only momentary contact with a moderately hot liquid or object. A careful **physical examination** is of paramount importance to determine not only the extent and probable depth of the burn injury but also the nature and severity of any associated injuries.

A. **Burn extent.** The simple and convenient rule of nines (see Table 21-2) is suitable for initial assessment, provided that the proportionally greater contributions of the head and neck in infants are taken into account. Burn injury of the head and neck in an infant involves approximately 20% of the body surface area (BSA) compared with about 9% in an adult. A helpful supplement to the rule of nines, particularly if the burns are patchy or discontinuous, is to remember that the palm of the subject's hand encompasses approximately 1% of the skin surface area.

B. **Depth of injury**

1. **First-degree (epidermal) burns** are confined to the epidermis. The involved area is hypersensitive to pinprick and air currents. There are no blisters initially, although delayed vesicle formation and desquamation can occur during the subsequent few days. Edema in the dermis is variable but may be especially pronounced about the burned face and eyes. The surface is warm and red, and capillary filling is brisk. Although these injuries are painful, they impose no subsequent physiologic burden, and there is little risk of secondary infection. Epidermal burns are not included in area estimates of injury because their ill effects are short-lived.

2. **Second-degree (intradermal) burns** are subdivided into two major categories because of important differences in prognosis and management.

   a. **Superficial second-degree burns** extend into but not deeper than the superficial papillary layer of the dermis; this layer contains numerous epithelial-lined skin appendages from which spontaneous reepithelialization will result in wound resurfacing within approximately 14 days, provided that secondary infection does not occur and histotoxic substances that impede reepithelialization are not applied to the wound. In these burns, blisters or blebs are present, and there is moderate spontaneous local swelling. Dermal capillary filling and sensitivity to pinprick are retained. Deep intradermal and third-degree burns typically lie centrally, surrounded by a shal-

411

Table 21-1. Guidelines for appropriate triage of burn victims

Burn severity		Optimal place of treatment
Major		Burn center
Second degree:	> 25% (20% child)	
or		
Third degree:	> 10%	
or		
Special burn areas*:	Severe involvement	
or		
Complicating factors:	Inhalation injury, fractures, electrical injury, or poor risk	
Moderate		General hospital (some special expertise in burn management is preferable)
Second degree:	15–25% (10–20% child)	
or		
Third degree:	2–10%	
or		
Special burn areas*:	Significant involvement	
or		
Complicating factors:	None	
Minor		Outpatient treatment
Second degree:	< 15% (10% child)	
or		
Third degree:	< 2%	
or		
Special burn areas*:	Little or no involvement	
or		
Complicating factors:	None	

*Special burn areas include the face, hands, feet, and perineum.
Source: Adapted from American Burn Association, Guidelines for service standards and severity classifications in the treatment of burn injury. *Bull. Am. Coll. Surgeons* 69(10):24, 1984.

lower zone of superficial second-degree injury at the periphery where the distance from the heat source is greater; thus, a variable width of superficial second-degree injury surrounds most deep burns. After reepithelialization has occurred, dermal hyperemia persists for a variable period of weeks to months, but this condition eventually resolves, leaving (at most) minor hypopigmentation but little or no raised hypertrophic scar. Spontaneous wound contraction is minimal; thus, the final cosmetic and functional results are excellent.

    b. **Deep second-degree burns** extend into the lower reticular layer of the dermis, where skin appendages are relatively sparse. Clinically, blebs or blisters may be present as in superficial dermal burns; however, dermal capillary refilling is sluggish or absent ("zone of stasis") and, if present initially, ceases within 24 hours. Pinprick sensation is absent, although that of light touch or pressure usually is retained. There is a varying degree of spontaneous wound edema. The color may be ivory or red, the latter being due to punctate or confluent interstitial hemorrhage (or both) that is always present microscopically. Although burns of this depth eventually reepithelialize spontaneously, healing requires at least 21 days and may take 60 days or longer. An outermost layer of devitalized papillary dermis, which is gray or brown in color, demarcates during the first week or two following injury and slowly separates spontaneously as epithelial ingrowth occurs beneath it. Wound contraction is significant in injuries of this depth, with hypertrophic scar formation being the rule.

  3. **Third-degree (subdermal) burns.** In this injury all the layers of the skin are destroyed. Blebs or blisters may be present. Since the circulation is obliterated, there is no dermal capillary refilling, although these wounds may also be red in color due to extensive interstitial hemorrhage. The denatured dermal collagen

Table 21-2. Rule of nines estimation of burn extent*

Body part	Surface area (%)
Head and neck	9
Anterior torso	18
Posterior torso	18
Lower limb	18 each
Upper limb	9 each
Genitalia and perineum	1
Total	100

*The Rule of Nines accurately estimates burn extent in adults. In infants, however, the head and neck comprise nearly 20% of the body surface area. It is also helpful to remember that the patient's palm comprises about 1% of the body surface area.

loses its elasticity, has a leathery feel, and tends to wrinkle over joints and bony prominences. Thrombosed subcutaneous veins may be visible through the dermis, which may be translucent. This type of injury can extend to the subcutaneous fat or through it to the investing muscle fascia and bone, depending on the heat source and duration of exposure. Thus, shriveled, desiccated soft tissue involving the digits, hands, feet, and other areas where there is little soft tissue intervening between skin, fascia, and bone is relatively common. In this injury healing can occur only from the wound margins (with resultant scar formation).

C. **Associated injuries**
1. **Carbon monoxide poisoning** can accompany burn injuries, particularly in patients involved in a closed-space fire or explosion or in patients with a history of coma or confusion. In such situations an arterial blood carbon monoxide determination is indicated. See Chap. 16 for a discussion of carbon monoxide poisoning.
2. **Inhalation injury.** Although respiratory tract injuries can occur without any cutaneous injury, patients with burns involving the head and neck or with extensive flame burns (i.e., > 50% BSA) commonly have associated respiratory tract lesions. The circumstances of the accident are relevant. Fires or explosions in closed spaces or, less commonly, exposure to steam are the usual historic findings. Asphyxia, with severe obtundation or transient apnea and loss of consciousness, may result from depletion of atmospheric oxygen by the burning fire or from accumulation of carbon monoxide in the blood and tissues. Asphyxia syndromes aside, it is convenient to subdivide inhalation injuries into two types: (1) **upper airway injury,** in which the injury extends only to the level of the glottis, and (2) **lower airway injury,** in which there is also subglottic involvement that may extend to the pulmonary parenchyma.
   a. **Upper airway injury** can be thermal or chemical or both. Cutaneous burns, if present, usually involve the perioral or perinasal area, with singeing of the nasal hairs. Carbon is often present within the pharynx, inspection of which discloses erythema, ulceration, and edema in various combinations. Progressive glottic swelling during the first 24 hours after injury can produce hoarseness, which, especially if progressive, may be a significant clinical sign portending abrupt airway closure. Laryngoscopy, usually done with a fiberoptic instrument, discloses findings in the glottis similar to those in the pharynx. Elective endotracheal intubation is indicated if there is appreciable narrowing of the airway at the glottis.
   b. **Lower airway injury**
      (1) **Pathophysiology.** Lower airway injury is nearly always chemical in origin. The specific toxic gaseous products responsible depend on the fuel source combusted. In severe cases the injury may extend distally to the alveolus. Loss of ciliary action, progressive inflammation, and edema are followed by intraluminal slough of mucosal fragments. These fragments usually are conglutinated with carbon particles and tenacious secretions and often are subsequently aspirated distally. This sequence of events leads to atelectasis.

(2) **Clinical features.** The clinical progression is typically gradual. Arterial blood gases are often normal, although in severe cases there may be hypoxemia initially. The FiO_2/PaO_2 ratio characteristically increases during the first 12–24 hours, after which the chest radiograph, which is also usually normal initially, begins to show evidence of edema. Secondary bacterial infection tends to supervene during the succeeding days with a rapidity that depends on many other variables, the most important of which appears to be the extent of the cutaneous burn. In the absence of extensive burns, the prognosis is excellent; however, if extensive burns are present, the mortality (which usually is secondary to sepsis) is considerable. If the cutaneous burns exceed 50% BSA and if the inhalation injury is severe, less than 25% of these patients will survive.

(3) **Diagnosis.** Visual inspection of the airways with a fiberoptic bronchoscope should be carried out in all patients in whom the diagnosis is in doubt. However, this procedure should be deferred until fluid resuscitation (see sec. **II.A.2**) has resulted in hemodynamic stability because the diagnostic tracheobronchial inflammatory changes may be less prominent or even absent if the patient is in shock, and a false-negative examination may result. The diagnostic accuracy of endoscopy, when performed at the proper time, is better than 90%. The 133-xenon lung scan is also a highly accurate method of diagnosing lower airway injury but has been less widely used than bronchoscopy because of logistic considerations [12, 15].

3. **Other associated injuries.** Burns resulting from motor vehicle accidents, explosions, and high-voltage electrical injuries may be associated with visceral or skeletal trauma that is easily overlooked if pertinent historic details, careful clinical examination of the skeleton, and appropriate confirmatory radiographs are not performed.

II. **Management**

A. **Major and moderate burn injuries** (see Table 21-1). The conventional treatment priorities pertain to the burn patient, i.e., airway patency and circulatory and ventilatory adequacy.

1. **Respiratory care**

   a. **Oxygen.** Patients with major burns or suspected carbon monoxide poisoning should be given 100% oxygen to breathe.

   b. **Airway.** If there is significant upper airway (including pharyngeal) edema or if its development appears probable, based on the severity of the burns of the head and neck or on evidence of mucosal injury, elective endotracheal intubation should be carried out, preferably by the nasal route. If, at the initial assessment, there is any doubt about the security of the upper airway in the succeeding hours when fluid resuscitation will exacerbate wound edema accumulation, prophylactic intubation is indicated. There should be no hesitancy in performing intubation, as the edema and inflammation will rapidly subside and the mucosal lesions will heal within a few days. Tracheostomy or cricothyrotomy (see Chap. 38) for upper airway edema or massive facial burns, however, is an obsolete procedure that is indicated only if nasotracheal or orotracheal intubation is technically impossible.

   c. The necessity for instituting **mechanical ventilation** is based on the same criteria utilized in nonburned subjects (see Chap. 7).

   d. **Ancillary measures.** Many cases of smoke inhalation without significant upper airway edema can be satisfactorily managed by humidification of the inspired air and vigorous pulmonary toilet, which should include chest physiotherapy. Bronchodilators should be used as needed.

   e. **Corticosteroids.** There is no clinical evidence that corticosteroids, either systemically or tracheally administered, are of benefit. Moreover, in severely burned patients with smoke inhalation, their use significantly increases the septic death rate [15]. Corticosteroids should not be used.

2. **Fluid resuscitation.** IV fluid therapy is necessary to prevent or treat hypovolemic shock in the following circumstances: (1) a total burn area of 20% or more in adults, (2) full-thickness burns exceeding 10% BSA, or (3) burn injuries of somewhat less severity in the elderly or very young. Since burn shock results from shifts and losses of fluid similar in composition to the interstitial fluid and since these events occur most rapidly during the first 8–12 hours following

injury, the most critical component of fluid therapy is a sodium salt crystalloid solution administered promptly and in sufficient quantity. **Ringer's lactate solution** is the most satisfactory crystalloid with which to initiate fluid therapy. Plasma, human albumin, blood, or another macromolecular solution is not routinely necessary initially, if at all; moreover, the timing and specific indications for their use remains controversial.

   a. Venous access. At least one secure **large-bore IV line** should be inserted as soon as airway patency and ventilatory support, if necessary, have been instituted. The line should be inserted through unburned skin, if possible, even if it means achieving venous access in a lower extremity. A central venous line is not necessary initially in most instances. If the skin overlying all venous access sites is deeply burned, an open surgical cutdown may be necessary.

   b. Fluid requirements. Although the fluid requirement is variable and tends to be larger in the elderly and when there is associated inhalation injury, most patients require between 2 and 4 ml of Ringer's lactate solution per percent of burn and kilogram of body weight during the first 24 hours. This range of fluid requirement, which is easily and quickly calculated, should be used to set the initial hourly rate of fluid administration once the burn extent has been determined. For example, a 70-kg patient with a 50% BSA burn will require a fluid volume of 7000 ($2 \times 50 \times 70$) to 14,000 ($4 \times 50 \times 70$) ml in the first 24 hours postinjury. About one-half of the total requirement is usually necessary during the first 8 hours. If considerable time has elapsed between the time of injury and the initiation of fluid therapy, any estimated preexistent fluid deficit should be corrected rapidly. Although crystalloid infusion rates greater than 2 liters/hour in adults are rarely necessary, rates of 500–1500 ml/hour, particularly during the first 8–12 hours, are not unusual in severe injury.

   c. Monitoring fluid resuscitation. The urine flow rate is the best and simplest single criterion of the adequacy of fluid therapy. Thus, a Foley catheter should be inserted, the bladder emptied, and hourly measurements of urine flow rates initiated; penile burns are not a contraindication for transurethral bladder catheterization. Flow rates between 0.5 and 1.0 ml/kg body weight/hour are sufficient (the higher value being used for patients who weigh less than 20 kg), provided the arterial blood pressure, which can be measured even on circumferentially burned limbs using a Doppler probe, is not low. Thus, the rate of lactated Ringer's administration should be adjusted according to the urine output. Persistent oliguria, hypotension, obtundation, metabolic acidosis, or other clinical or laboratory indices of refractory or deepening shock in most instances signal the need for a trial of a more rapid rate of fluid administration, even if the estimated fluid requirement has already been exceeded. Congestive heart failure is uncommon during the early shock phase, even in the elderly. In those with seriously impaired cardiopulmonary function, a pulmonary artery catheter is helpful in guiding fluid therapy but is unnecessary in most patients and should never be used routinely.

   d. Special considerations. If gross **pigmenturia** is present, as occurs in extensive full-thickness thermal burns and in high-voltage electrical injury, urine flow rates should be titrated with crystalloid infusion to a range of 1–2 ml/kg/hour for several hours until there is gross clearing of the urine. If pigmenturia is severe or persistent (i.e., > 4 hours), mannitol, 12.5 gm/liter of crystalloid, is useful to augment diuresis. Systemic acidosis should also be rapidly corrected, using supplemental IV sodium bicarbonate as needed, since tubular precipitation is favored by acidosis as well as by a decreased renal blood flow. However, vigorous fluid resuscitation alone often results in rapid correction of acidemia.

3. Surgical release (i.e., escharotomy/fasciotomy)

   a. Indications. Circumferential or near-circumferential burns of the limbs may lead to inadequate perfusion due to a combination of heat-induced shortening of the dermal collagen and edema accumulation, and thus require early surgical release. If the distal parts are unburned, cutaneous capillary filling, sensation, temperature, and color, combined with palpatory assessment of the pulses and wound turgor, can be used to judge the need for surgical release. Unfortunately, the distal parts frequently are confluently burned; in this situation, auscultation of the distal pulses with the Doppler probe may

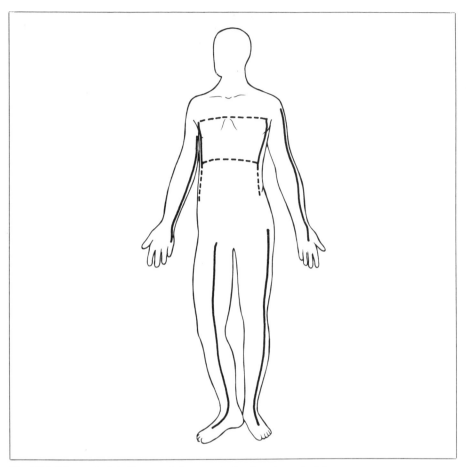

Fig. 21-1. Figure depicts the usual placement of escharotomy incisions.

be necessary to determine the adequacy of distal blood flow in the injured part. Absence or disappearance of distal pulses is an absolute indication for surgical release. Confluent burns of the torso may significantly impair the excursions of the thoracic cage and diaphragm and result in an inadequate tidal volume. If such is the case, as evidenced by clinical observation or by direct measurement of the tidal volume, escharotomy is indicated.

  b. Method (Fig. 21-1). On the limbs, escharotomy is always performed initially in the long axis using aseptic technique. Local infiltration of anesthesia occasionally is necessary, but the burns are typically deep and insensate. The depth of the skin incision should be palpated to ensure that all constrictive subcutaneous collagenous bands have been divided. The underlying muscle fascia should also be incised unless escharotomy alone results in a clear-cut and dramatic improvement, with return of previously absent pulses and an obvious decrease in wound turgor; supplemental fasciotomy is often necessary in high-voltage electrical injury but is uncommonly required in thermal burns. Thoracic escharotomy is usually performed initially in the anterior axillary lines bilaterally. These incisions can be connected, if necessary, in severe cases by supplementary transverse subclavicular or subcostal incisions (or both).

4. Nasogastric intubation. Since adynamic ileus, at times accompanied by acute gastric dilatation, occurs in all major and many moderate burn injuries, an 18 F nasogastric tube with a sump port should be inserted, the stomach emptied of its contents, and continuous drainage instituted. Aspiration of gastric contents is a serious hazard, particularly in the obtunded patient and during transport or transfer. Antacids should be administered hourly through the tube as needed to maintain the pH of the gastric aspirate above 4.5. Cimetidine is not routinely administered.

5. Wound management

a. Emergency department care. Since patients with burn injuries of major or moderate severity require hospitalization, they should not be unduly detained in the emergency department with their wounds exposed and subject to environmental contamination. The burns should be covered with dry sterile sheets, preferably water-repellent ones. Alternatively, if the patient is to be transported to another hospital for definitive treatment, temporary dressings can be applied to minimize the risk of contamination during transport. Nonconstrictive, dry gauze dressings of thickness sufficient to absorb the wound secretions are best. Wet dressings should be avoided. It is advisable to consult with the responsible physician at the accepting institution regarding other details of emergent wound management.

b. Subsequent early wound care involves atraumatic cleaning with saline or a bland soap, removal of detritus and loose skin fragments, and the application of a topical ointment such as 1% silver sulfadiazine. The burns are then covered with overlie dressings, and the dependent parts are elevated to minimize edema accumulation.

6. Antibiotic prophylaxis. Beta-hemolytic streptococcal infections occur with some regularity during the first 5–7 days after burn injury. Prophylactically administered penicillin, 250,000 units IV q6h, essentially eliminates the hazard of this infection, which can be fulminating. Erythromycin, 250 mg IV q6h, can be substituted if the patient is allergic to penicillin. Other antibiotic therapy is not routinely necessary or desirable.

7. Tetanus prophylaxis (see Table 12-6). Since the ischemic burn wound is tetanus-prone, a booster injection of tetanus toxoid should be administered IM to patients who have previously been actively immunized but have not received a booster injection within the past 5 years. In patients who have not been actively immunized, antitetanus globulin, 250–500 units IM, depending on injury severity, should be administered in addition to tetanus toxoid using a separate syringe and injection site.

8. Analgesia. A narcotic should be administered only if the patient is complaining of pain, which is often absent in deep second- or third-degree burns. If a narcotic is required, it is always administered intravenously in small increments (e.g., 2–3 mg of morphine sulfate in adults) until analgesia is achieved. The absorption of narcotics from subcutaneous or intramuscular sites is unreliable in severely burned patients; in addition, repetitive injections in an attempt to achieve analgesia can result in respiratory arrest due to rapid drug absorption after fluid resuscitation has restored blood flow to those tissues.

9. Disposition. Major and moderate burn injuries require hospitalization, the former preferably at a burn center (see Table 21-1). If transfer to a burn center is indicated, telephone contact with a responsible physician at the institution to which transfer is contemplated should be carried out as soon as the initial assessment has been completed and the necessary resuscitative and supportive measures are underway. Prior to transfer, the airway should be secure, fluid resuscitation at an appropriate rate in progress, and the patient sufficiently stabilized. The wounds should be managed as described in **5.a,** and both the stomach and urinary bladder should be intubated and draining.

B. Minor burn injuries (see Table 21-1)

1. First-degree burns. Systemic or topical analgesics (or both) may be used as necessary, bearing in mind that if extensive areas are involved, topically applied agents that are absorbed percutaneously may cause systemic toxicity. Local cooling with ice water of limited areas of involvement (i.e., < 15% BSA) provides effective analgesia; however, in patients with more extensive burn injuries, use of ice water generally should be avoided because of the risk of inducing corporal hypothermia, which can be lethal. Tetanus prophylaxis should be administered as needed.

2. Second-degree burns

a. Superficial second-degree burns

(1) Analgesia. Since these burns are painful and there is typically anxiety and fear of disfigurement that magnify the discomfort, analgesia generally is required. Application of ice water (see **1**) is effective for superficial dermal burns of less than 15% BSA, or simply covering the wound with a sterile towel (while the history is being obtained) provides some relief of pain by eliminating convection currents from the sensitive wound surface. In addition, intramuscular analgesics such as codeine or meperidine, in appropriate doses have beneficial pharmacologic and psychologic effects; they should be given prior to any manipulation of the wound.

(2) Wound care
  (a) Wound cleansing and debridement. Gentle sterile saline cleansing is sufficient unless the burn is grossly contaminated, in which case a mild soap should be used. Thick, unruptured blisters, such as occur typically on the palms, can safely be left intact until healing has occurred, a maneuver that essentially eliminates pain. In contrast, thin blisters generally are debrided, since they usually will rupture spontaneously, and loose skin is trimmed after the wound has been cleansed.
  (b) Topical therapy and dressings. A sterile occlusive dressing provides comfort, insulates the wound from the (small) risk of bacterial contamination, and, by helping splint the part, further relieves pain. The dressing should be nonconstrictive and should allow for subsequent edema formation. It is also important that the dressing be of sufficient thickness so that the wound secretions, which may be considerable, do not wet its outer layer. An inner layer of petrolatum gauze will prevent unnecessary pain from the adherence of dry gauze in the subsequent dressing change. Alternatively, or if the burn depth is uncertain, a topical antibacterial agent, such as 1% silver sulfadiazine cream, may be used. The dressing is removed daily, the wound cleansed, and the topical agent and dressing reapplied. However, if the burn is unequivocally superficial dermal, a topical antiseptic is not necessary and adds expense. Superficial second-degree burns of the face and perineum are difficult to dress effectively. They can be treated by exposure (with daily or twice-daily rinsing with soap and water) and usually the application of a topical antibacterial, such as silver sulfadiazine cream or polymyxin B-bacitracin (Polysporin) ointment, which is replaced as necessary. The somewhat greater propensity for staphylococcal colonization of burns in these areas justifies the use of an antibacterial agent.
(3) Tetanus prophylaxis should be carried out as described in **A.7.**
(4) Oral **penicillin** for streptococcal prophylaxis is often administered for 5 days but probably is not essential.
(5) Disposition. Patients with minor superficial second-degree burns are appropriately managed on an outpatient basis. They should be followed up in 4 days, or sooner if there is concern regarding the quality of home care.
b. Deep second-degree burns are more likely to become infected than superficial second-degree burns because the eschar that forms provides a pabulum for bacterial growth and because they take twice as long (or more) to heal spontaneously. Thus, silver sulfadiazine cream or some other topical antibacterial agent should be used prophylactically. Oral penicillin may be prescribed, and tetanus prophylaxis is administered as needed. Although initial outpatient management is safe and appropriate, these patients should be seen by a surgeon within the first few days, since many of them are best treated by early excision and split-skin grafting within the first week, particularly if the burns involve functionally or cosmetically important areas (e.g., face, hands).
3. Full-thickness burns. In minor injuries, these burns are of limited extent. Burns of this depth that are less than 2% BSA can be managed in the same manner as deep second-degree burns (see **2.b**) on an ambulatory basis. However, unless the burns are of such small size that they can be expected to heal by contracture without significant residual deformity, early or immediate excision and primary closure with a skin graft using local anesthesia is often preferable to expectant treatment in order to shorten convalescence, avoid secondary infec-

tion, and lessen functional and cosmetic deformity. Thus, these patients should be seen by a surgeon within a few days after injury.

III. Special considerations

A. Electrical injury

1. Pathophysiology

a. There are three mechanisms of **heat injury** to the skin and soft tissues associated with electrical and lightning accidents.

(1) If an electrical current traverses the body, some of its energy is converted to heat with resultant tissue injury along its path to the ground. Since the current is collected at the points of entrance and exit, tissue damage tends to be more severe in these areas, with variable injury severity along the current path.

(2) Arcing from an electrical source can occur, producing transient ionization and extreme heating of the surrounding air with resultant thermal injury.

(3) Clothing can ignite from either of the above mechanisms, superimposing flame burns of variable extent and depth.

b. Other effects, which are more frequent in high-voltage accidents, include transient or permanent dysfunction or injury of various organs, principally the heart and nervous system.

2. Classification

a. Low-voltage electrical injury (i.e., < 1000 volts). Significant tissue damage from household current sources is generally confined to the points of entrance and exit. These soft-tissue injuries, although deep, are usually minor in extent. A common example is the oral burn sustained by toddlers who have inserted a live current source into their mouth. Although ventricular fibrillation or other arrhythmias can occur, which must be dealt with individually, the soft-tissue injuries (including those of the mouth and oral commissure) are usually managed on an outpatient basis (see sec. **II.B**), provided the evaluations of neurologic and cardiac function are normal. Delayed hemorrhage from orolabial electrical burns is not infrequent. Patients or parents should be informed of this possibility and instructed to use firm manual compression should it occur.

b. High-voltage electrical injury (i.e., > 1000 volts). If the electrical source exceeds 1000 volts, skin and soft-tissue damage can be much more extensive. The major amputation rate approximates 20% in high-voltage electrical injuries due to the destruction of muscle in the path of the current, which typically traverses the limb. In addition, depending on the current path, the heart, brain, and spinal cord can be injured. Urgent fasciotomy and escharotomy commonly are necessary in these injuries and should not be delayed for more than a few hours because the unrelieved ischemia will result in additional tissue necrosis. After careful evaluation, monitoring of cardiac and neurologic function should begin promptly. Pigmenturia is common and requires prompt fluid therapy and correction of systemic acidosis (see sec. **II.A.2.d**). Fluid resuscitation requirements tend to be 2–3 times larger than estimates based on the skin surface area burns because of the volume of deeper tissue also involved. In addition, tetanic contractions induced by an alternating current can result in fracture-dislocations. These accidents often result in falls with accompanying significant blunt visceral or skeletal trauma that requires appropriate evaluation and treatment. Hospitalization generally is indicated.

B. Lightning stroke

1. The **spectrum of injury** varies widely. Most of the electrical energy ordinarily does not traverse the body but flows around it ("flashover"), sometimes vaporizing cutaneous sweat droplets and disrupting clothing and shoes, due to the transient shock wave produced by the mutual repellance of accumulated like charges. The violence of the shock wave, the so-called sledge hammer blow, should not be underestimated. Fractures of the skull, which can easily be overlooked, are common. Long bone fractures, dislocations, and associated visceral injuries have also been reported frequently. Due to the flashover phenomenon, cutaneous electrical injuries are surprisingly limited in extent in most cases compared with those seen after contact with man-made high-voltage sources. Cardiorespiratory arrest at the scene is often due to ventricular standstill, although fibrillation and other arrhythmias can occur. Apnea, presumably due to current flow through the brain, may be prolonged. Transient, spidery skin lesions that follow the course of the cutaneous vasculature, the so-called Lichtenberg's flowers, are said to be pathognomonic. Paresthesias or paralysis, both of which are usually temporary, are present in 70% or more of patients. Cerebral concussion is not uncommon.

2. **Treatment.** Cardiopulmonary resuscitation should be aggressive and prolonged, as recovery of neurologic function after lengthy apneic periods due to lightning stroke has been reported; this phenomenon may be due to some unique protective effect of lightning on the cellular metabolism of neural tissue. Otherwise, the usual fluid resuscitative measures should be carried out as necessary, depending on the extent of associated injuries and burns. Fasciotomy is occasionally necessary, usually in the lower limbs, because of swelling. Associated electrical or thermal burns are treated as previously described.

3. **Disposition.** Hospitalization is warranted if there are major or moderate burns, significant cardiac or neurologic abnormalities, or serious associated injuries.

C. **Asphalt and tar burns.** These materials adhere tenaciously to the skin. Removal is greatly facilitated by the application of solvents such as household shortening, Goup, or polymyxin B-bacitracin (Polysporin) ointment, the ointment base of which contains an effective solvent. Additional tissue trauma imposed by ill-advised attempts to mechanically remove asphalt or tar without the aid of such solvents should be avoided. The depth of burn injury varies, depending on the temperature of these materials at the time of contact with the skin and the duration of exposure. Deep dermal and full-thickness burns are not uncommon. The methods of wound management and the criteria for hospital admission are the same as for any other type of thermal injury.

D. **Chemical burns**
   1. **General principles.** A variety of chemicals and caustic substances can produce cutaneous burns [9]. The burn depth will vary with the agent involved, its concentration, the exposure time, and the mechanism of action of the agent. In general, concentrated alkalis are more destructive than acids. Consideration should be given both to the systemic effects, if the offending agent is known to be absorbed readily through the skin (e.g., phenol), and to local wound care. The regional poison control center or toxicology texts should be consulted for specific therapeutic measures. Emergency treatment consists of removing all garments and solid materials, followed by copious water irrigation of the involved areas. Although chemical neutralization with an appropriate antidote (if one exists) is preferred, this approach is usually not practical. Water irrigation is always immediately available in the emergency department, and the benefits of prompt irrigation more than counterbalance the delay inherent in procuring a specific antidote; minimizing exposure time is by far the most critical factor in the prevention of additional tissue necrosis. Specific therapeutic measures and standard burn therapy should follow.
   2. **Hydrofluoric acid.** This common chemical burn results in the transcutaneous absorption of fluoride ions into the subcutaneous tissues where it binds with calcium and may produce severe burning pain. Copious water lavage and the application of magnesium hydroxide paste to bind the fluoride are appropriate. Injection of calcium gluconate into the subcutaneous tissue may be beneficial if there is persistent burning pain after surface lavage and neutralization have been carried out. Care should be taken, however, not to overdistend the soft tissue with the calcium injection, since overdistention can result in additional tissue loss from pressure necrosis.

E. **Lacerations of burned skin.** Approximation of the dermal edges of deep lacerations of the face or hands that are situated within superficial second-degree burns, using subcuticular absorbable sutures, may minimize late deformity, but careful follow-up is necessary. Superficial second-degree burns in other areas of the body and lacerations in deep dermal burns in any location, however, are best left unsutured initially. It is pointless to attempt to suture lacerations that lie within areas of third-degree burns, since dead tissue cannot heal.

Bibliography

1. American Burn Association. Guildlines for service standards and severity classifications in the treatment of burn injury. *Bull. Am. College Surgeons* 69(10):24, 1984.

2. Butler, E. D., and Gant, T. D. Electrical injuries, with special reference to upper extremities. A review of 182 cases. *Am. J. Surg.* 134:95, 1977.
3. Cahalane, M., and Demling, R. H. Early respiratory abnormalities from smoke inhalation. *J.A.M.A.* 251:771, 1984.
4. Cooper, M. A. Lightning injuries: Prognostic signs for death. *Ann. Emerg. Med.* 9:134, 1980.
5. Crapo, R. O. Smoke-inhalation injuries. *J.A.M.A.* 246:1694, 1981.
6. Demling, R. H. Burns. *N. Engl. J. Med.* 313:1389, 1985.
7. Demling, R. H., Buerstatte, W. R., and Perea, A. Management of hot tar burns. *J. Trauma* 20:242, 1980.
8. Edlich, R. F., et al. Emergency department treatment, triage and transfer protocols for the burn patient. *J.A.C.E.P.* 7:152, 1978.
9. Jelenko, C., III. Chemicals that "burn." *J. Trauma* 14:65, 1974.
10. Moncrief, J. A. Burns. Parts I and II. *J.A.M.A.* 242:72, 179, 1979.
11. Moylan, J. A., and Chin-Keung, C. Inhalation injury—An increasing problem. *Ann. Surg.* 188:34, 1978.
12. Petroff, P. A., and Pruitt, B. A., Jr. Pulmonary Disease in the Burn Patient. In C. P. Artz, J. A. Moncrief, and B. A. Pruitt, Jr. (eds.), *Burns. A Team Approach.* Philadelphia: Saunders, 1979.
13. Proceedings of the NIH Conference. Frontiers in understanding burn injury. *J. Trauma* 24(9 Suppl.):S1, 1984.
14. Proceedings of the NIH Conference. Second conference on supportive therapy in burn care. *J. Trauma* 21(8 Suppl.):665, 1981.
15. Proceedings of the NIH Consensus Development Conference. Supportive therapy in burn care. *J. Trauma* 19(11 Suppl.):855, 1979.
16. Pruitt, B. A., Jr., and Edlich, R. F. Treatment of bitumen burns. *Ann. Emerg. Med.* 11:697, 1982.
17. Rouse, R. G., and Dimick, A. R. The treatment of electrical injury compared to burn injury: A review of pathophysiology and comparison of patient management protocols. *J. Trauma* 18:43, 1978.
18. Sances, A., Jr., et al. Electrical injuries. *Surg. Gynecol. Obstet.* 149:97, 1979.
19. Sevitt, S. A review of the complications of burns, their origin and importance for illness and death. *J. Trauma* 19:358, 1979.
20. Tintinalli, J. E. Hydrofluoric acid burns. *J.A.C.E.P.* 7:24, 1978.
21. Trunkey, D. D. Inhalation injury. *Surg. Clin. North Am.* 58:1133, 1978.
22. Wilkinson, C., and Wood, M. High-voltage electrical injury. *Am. J. Surg.* 136:693, 1978.

22

Soft-Tissue Disorders

Barbel Holtmann

Soft-Tissue Injuries

Tissue injury produces local and systemic responses that ultimately result in wound healing, the fundamental elements of which are epithelialization, collagen synthesis, and contraction.

I. **Management principles.** Healing at maximal speed with minimal scar formation is the objective of wound management and is influenced by the local state of the wound and by the general state of the patient. Healing is impaired by necrotic tissue, foreign bodies, bacteria, hematoma, edema, decreased vascularity, wound tension, and alteration in the patient's capacity to respond to injury (e.g., diabetes mellitus, malnutrition, endogenous or exogenous immunosuppression). The treating physician's initial wound management has perhaps the single most decisive influence on healing.

A. **Wound assessment** includes evaluation of the mechanism, site, and type of injury; the extent of tissue damage; and the presence of foreign bodies or other contaminants. This evaluation requires adequate lighting and instruments, use of sterile technique, and gentle tissue handling to avoid additional wound contamination and tissue damage. Proper wound evaluation may require anesthesia, but motor function and sensation in the immediate wound area or of distant points potentially affected by the area of injury must be evaluated before any type of anesthetic is administered. By testing for their appropriate function, the diagnosis of tendon or nerve laceration (or both) can almost always be made without probing the wound (and inflicting further damage). In addition to consideration of the patient's overall status, the plan for wound management is formulated on proper diagnosis of the extent of tissue damage and injury to specific structures.

1. **Tidy wounds** produced by sharp objects usually have minimal tissue injury or contamination and can usually be managed in the emergency department.

2. **Untidy wounds** characterized by extensive soft-tissue injury with or without contamination usually require major intervention to convert them into tidy wounds; they may or may not be amenable to emergency department treatment. As a general rule, extensive wounds and minor wounds involving major structures are best managed in the operating room. Wounds not amenable to emergency department management should be covered with a sterile, bulky, moist dressing and the injured part elevated, if possible, to reduce edema formation until definitive treatment is undertaken.

B. **Anesthesia** is required for proper wound management in most instances. **A motor and sensory examination must be performed prior to administration of any anesthetic.**

1. **Local infiltration anesthesia.** A premixed solution of 0.5 or 1.0 percent lidocaine with 1:200,000 epinephrine is the anesthetic of choice for most emergency procedures. However, epinephrine should not be used around end arteries (i.e., fingers and toes), and its systemic effects should be considered in patients with cardiovascular disease. Multiple injections are administered via a 25- or 27-gauge needle through intact skin adjacent to the wound edges or directly into the wound margins.

2. **Regional nerve block anesthesia** is indicated for some emergency department procedures if the procedure site is localized to an area supplied by discrete peripheral sensory nerves (see Chap. 38).

3. **Topical anesthesia** with freezing agents such as ethyl chloride is very superficial, short in duration, and generally unreliable. Lidocaine produces very superficial anesthesia when applied topically to mucous membranes, but has little or no effect when applied topically to skin.

4. **General and intravenous regional anesthesia** are used in properly equipped facilities.

C. **Wound preparation**

1. **Wound cleansing** with a soap solution, saline wash, and an iodinated disinfectant is adequate preparation for most simple wounds. Soaps, detergents, and skin disinfectants, however, should not be instilled directly into the open wound because they may cause tissue injury. Petroleum products, such as grease or motor oil, present on the skin can be effectively removed with Goop hand cleaner (available in hardware and grocery stores). Shaving of hair around wound edges should be avoided, since it may increase bacterial proliferation or may destroy critical landmarks necessary for accurate wound edge alignment. In particular, the eyebrows should never be shaved. Hair may be clipped a few millimeters above skin level in a limited area to facilitate scalp wound management.

2. **Irrigation** with a physiologic solution (e.g., normal saline, Ringer's lactate) is indicated for extensive or contaminated wounds. Dilution of the bacterial inoculum and removal of foreign matter, blood clots, and tissue debris are dependent on the irrigant volume and stream force. Untidy wounds with extensive tissue damage or gross contamination are best irrigated with several liters of solution delivered as a pulsating jet stream (Teledyne Waterpik, Stryker Surgilav). Irrigation with antibiotic solutions is of no benefit unless the wound is known to be contaminated with specific bacteria.

3. **Draping** around the wound with sterile cloth towels, sheets, or self-adherent plastic drapes is done to prevent contamination of instruments, sutures, and gloves by surrounding skin, hair, or clothing. The drapes are arranged to expose the entire wound plus enough surrounding area to avoid distortion of adjacent anatomic landmarks. In facial wounds, the skin of the entire face is cleansed; and drapes are placed to expose the eyes, nose, and mouth to preserve symmetry of anatomic structures and to prevent patient discomfort from inability to breathe beneath drapes.

4. **Debridement** is limited to removal of foreign matter, excision of devitalized or contaminated tissue, and excision of wound margins so irregular as to make wound closure impractical. Caution must be exercised in excising irregular wound margins since it may produce significant tension on wound closure or limit tissues available for later use in scar revision. Some irregular scars are ultimately less noticeable than straight-line scars.

5. **Hemostasis** is necessary for proper visualization of injured structures in the wound and prevention of hematoma formation.

   a. **Continuous pressure** is applied for a minimum of 5–10 minutes.

   b. **Vasoconstrictors,** such as epinephrine 1:200,000, are injected together with the local anesthetic or applied topically in conjunction with light pressure (taking the wound location and the patient's cardiovascular status into account). At least 5 minutes must elapse from the time of injection or topical application for the vasoconstrictive effect of epinephrine to be apparent.

   c. **Ligation** of specific blood vessels with sutures is the most reliable method of hemostasis, but the procedure introduces foreign bodies into the wound. Vessels are clamped under adequate visualization (which may require suction equipment and an assistant) to avoid injury to structures, such as nerves, particularly in facial and hand wounds. A suture is tied around the vessel distal to the tip of the hemostat or is first passed through tissue adjacent to the hemostat tip before being tied.

   d. **Electrocautery** generates heat, resulting in coagulation of blood vessel ends. Pinpoint accuracy is important to avoid leaving unnecessary charred tissue in the wound, and a dry field is required for an effective electrical current to pass into the tissues. Monopolar cautery causes approximately three times as much tissue necrosis as bipolar cautery. Self-contained, sterile, disposable, hand-held, battery-powered ophthalmic cautery units are useful for coagulating small vessels, particularly along skin edges.

   e. **Topical agents** such as Gelfoam, Surgicel, and Avitene promote coagulation but introduce a foreign body into the wound, some remnants of which may persist if left in place.

   f. The **pneumatic tourniquet** can be helpful in extremity wounds but requires proper maintenance and routine calibration; ordinary blood pressure cuffs should not be used for this purpose.

6. **Undermining** of tissues at the wound margin can decrease tension on wound closure. It is indicated in wounds where actual tissue loss has occurred or in areas of scant tissue laxity (e.g., trunk, extremities). Blunt undermining is done with the fingertip or dissecting scissors, using a spreading technique. Sharp undermining is performed with a scalpel blade or the dissecting scissors, using a cutting motion. The wound edge being undermined should be held with a forceps or skin hook, exerting mild tension on the tissue. The level of undermining depends on the wound depth (e.g., at the fascial level in wounds that extend to that depth, or just beneath the dermis in more superficial wounds), taking care not to devascularize the overlying skin. Undermining must extend from one end of the wound to the other to be effective.

D. **Suture materials** vary in their degree of tensile strength, tissue reactivity, and ease of handling.

1. **Absorbable sutures** are biodegradable. Gut is digested by proteolytic enzymes in the wound; synthetic sutures are hydrolyzed. Gut is degraded more rapidly in the presence of infection, whereas the synthetics are not affected by infection. The synthetics are used most commonly for vascular ligation and dermal closure. All absorbable sutures lose tensile strength more rapidly and incite a more intense inflammatory response than nonabsorbables. Their use is therefore restricted primarily to subcutaneous locations, since skin placement results in additional visible scarring from the tissue reaction they produce. Exceptions to this restriction include skin closures of the palm and plantar surface of the foot, where suture marks are less obvious. Absorbable sutures can also be used for mucous membrane closures, but their staying power is unreliable.

   a. **Catgut** is made from sheep and cattle small intestine; it is the most rapidly absorbed suture (3–10 days) and produces the most intense inflammatory response.

   b. **Chromic catgut** is catgut treated with chromium salts to retard absorption and reduce the inflammatory response. The absorption rate varies with the location (being faster in mucous membranes than in muscle), extending from 14 days to 6 months.

   c. **Dexon** is a synthetic suture made of polyglycolic acid. It is stronger than catgut of comparable size, has greater knot security, and produces less inflammation. The absorption rate varies with the location, extending from 14–34 days in skin to up to 80 days in muscle. Fifty percent of its tensile strength is lost in 20–30 days.

   d. **Vicryl** is a synthetic suture made of polyglactin, with properties similar to Dexon, except for a slightly slower absorption rate (up to 120 days).

2. **Nonabsorbable sutures** are classified as organics, synthetics, and metallics. They produce less tissue reaction than absorbable sutures and are therefore indicated for most skin closures. They are also used in subcutaneous locations where motion or tension is present with tissue approximation (e.g., tendon repair) or when suture absorption is undesirable (e.g., ligation of major blood vessels). They do, however, introduce a permanent foreign body into the wound when placed deep to the skin.

   a. **Silk** is a braided organic suture and is the easiest suture material to handle. It has excellent knot security and pliability but is considerably more reactive than synthetic and metallic nonabsorbables.

   b. **Nylon** is a synthetic suture available in monofilament or braided form. Monofilament nylon is the suture of choice for most skin closures because of its minimal tissue reactivity, excellent tensile strength, and low friction coefficient. However, it is more difficult to handle than silk because of its stiffness and lesser knot security (requiring at least five throws for each knot).

   c. **Prolene** is a synthetic suture similar to nylon but with greater tensile strength, lower friction coefficient, and less elasticity. These properties make it the suture of choice for pull-out running subcuticular closures, but they also make it stiffer and decrease knot security.

   d. **Polyester fiber** sutures such as Mersilene are braided synthetics that are easy to handle and may be used for skin closure. They are not quite as pliable and have less knot security than silk. Application of a Teflon coating (Ethibond, Tevdek) increases smoothness and decreases suture fraying but does not alter tissue reactivity.

   e. **Stainless steel** is a metallic suture available in monofilament or braided form. It is more difficult to handle than other suture materials and is of limited value for emergency department use.

3. **Monofilament sutures** produce less tissue reaction and less tissue injury caused by friction and have a decreased surface area for harboring bacteria, compared with multifilament sutures. They are, however, stiffer and have less knot security. They are the suture material of choice for most skin closures (nylon) and for pull-out running subcuticular closures (Prolene).

4. **Multifilament (braided) sutures** are easier to handle, more pliable and have greater knot security than monofilament sutures. However, they cause more tissue reaction and more tissue damage due to their high friction coefficient, and their interstices are more likely to harbor bacteria that can produce a pustule or discharging sinus where they penetrate skin. Nonabsorbable braided sutures are ideal for mucous membrane closures and skin closures adjacent to the eye because the pliable suture ends lie flat after the knot is tied. All absorbable sutures are braided, and most nonabsorbables are available in braided form (except Prolene).

5. **Other considerations.** Suture material is most frequently used with a needle swaged onto one end. The needle size and suture thickness, or caliber, are not factors in the production of skin suture marks, but some judgment should be exercised regarding their use.

   a. **Needles** are cutting or noncutting (taper). Their use varies with the consistency of the tissue they must penetrate. Cutting needles are always used for placing sutures in skin and dermis because these tissues are relatively tough and penetration with a cutting needle is less traumatic. Taper needles are used in soft, easily penetrated tissues, i.e., most layers beneath the dermis, although cutting needles can be used there also.

   b. The **suture caliber** affects tensile strength and tissue reactivity, i.e., the larger the suture, the greater the tensile strength and tissue reaction. As a general rule, the smallest suture caliber that will hold securely should be used; 6-0 caliber suture is usually used for skin closure on the face, 5-0 on the hand, and 4-0 or 5-0 on the trunk and extremities. Smooth-jawed needleholders are necessary to adequately grasp fine-caliber sutures.

E. **Wound closure** restores function and appearance to the injured area.

   1. **Indications and contraindications** for wound closure rarely can be stated in absolute rules. Bacterial contamination and blood supply to the wound are the two interrelated factors that must be considered in determining whether or not to close a wound. Ischemic wounds heal poorly and frequently become infected, whereas well-vascularized tissues heal well and are markedly resistant to bacterial invasion. Infection usually results if the number of bacteria in the wound exceeds 10^5 per gram of tissue at the time of closure, but this number is markedly less in the presence of a foreign body, necrotic tissue, or diminished local blood supply. Trunk and extremity wounds have less blood supply than facial and scalp wounds. Wounds produced by blunt, crushing forces are more likely to have areas of decreased tissue vascularity than wounds produced by sharp objects. Under ideal circumstances, quantification of wound bacteria should determine whether closure is indicated or not, but practical methods for this analysis are lacking in most emergency department settings. Therefore, the decision regarding wound closure rests on the judgment of the treating physician.

      a. The **time interval** between injury and wound closure is not critical, except that a longer interval makes infection more likely due to bacterial proliferation in the open wound and makes repair more difficult because retracted, edematous tissues are stiff, do not hold sutures well, and obscure landmarks necessary for precise tissue alignment. Most clean wounds can be closed as late as 18 to 24 hours after injury if tissue pliability remains adequate.

      b. **Heavily contaminated wounds,** including **bites** (see **Bites and Stings**) can be closed in well-vascularized areas (e.g., the face) after copious irrigation and adequate debridement, using as few sutures as possible (with none in buried locations) and sometimes a drain. Wounds of this nature on the trunk and extremities, however, are best left open. Human bite wounds are usually left open.

      c. The presence of **inflammation** (i.e., erythema, edema, and tenderness) around a wound is a contraindication to closure.

      d. When significant **edema** is present or anticipated in the postoperative period (e.g., after crushing injuries), wound closure may be contraindicated to prevent underlying tissue ischemia and necrosis.

e. Wounds with **missing tissue** that require a skin graft or flap repair are referred to a specialist.

2. **Repair of tissue layers.** Repair of tissue layers deep to the skin is indicated when gaps exist between the wound edges in order to reduce tension on skin approximation and restore function. A gap between tissue layers at any level of a closed wound is **dead space.** Dead space permits accumulation of blood or serum, which may produce wound dehiscence, act as a culture medium for bacteria, or produce a bulky mass of irregular scar tissue or an area of depression beneath the skin. In addition to the length of time sutures are left in place (see Chap. 38, **Wound Closure Techniques**), the factor most responsible for producing skin suture marks is **tension.** A layered wound repair facilitates healing by obliterating the dead space and reducing tension on skin closure. Wounds with buried sutures, however, have a higher infection rate than those with skin sutures only. Tissue surfaces that fall together do not require sutures unless tension or motion is anticipated during the healing period. As a general rule, hand and foot wounds can be repaired effectively with a single-layer skin closure. This type of closure is also effective for most scalp and facial wounds. Repair of major structures (e.g., tendons, nerves, blood vessels) is not an emergency department procedure; patients with these injuries should be referred to a specialist.

a. **Periosteum** and **perichondrium** are repaired with interrupted or continuous absorbable sutures when possible, but these tissues are inelastic and hold sutures poorly. The suture caliber depends on the location (e.g., 3-0 or 4-0 for long bone periosteum, 5-0 or 6-0 for ear perichondrium and short bone periosteum [phalanges]). **Joint capsules** are repaired with interrupted or continuous absorbable or nonabsorbable sutures of caliber appropriate for the joint size and location.

b. **Muscle** holds sutures poorly, so suture bites should include muscle fascia. Interrupted 3-0 or 4-0 absorbable or nonabsorbable sutures are used, depending on the amount of tension present.

c. **Fascia,** when present as a distinct subcutaneous tissue layer (other than muscle fascia), should be repaired with 4-0 or 5-0 absorbable or nonabsorbable interrupted sutures.

d. **Subcutaneous fatty tissue** may be repaired with interrupted 4-0 or 5-0 absorbable sutures, with buried knots to obliterate dead space and help evert the skin edges. Since this layer holds sutures poorly, it may be necessary to include a portion of fibrous dermal tissue with each bite for the suture to hold. It may also be possible to obliterate dead space in this layer with skin sutures that are placed deeply (see Chap. 38). Since subcutaneous fat is relatively avascular, sutures placed in this layer tend to devitalize tissue (when tied tightly) and increase the inflammatory response.

e. **Dermis** repair **(subcuticular closure)** with interrupted, inverted 4-0 or 5-0 synthetic absorbable sutures is very useful in relieving tension on skin closure. Properly placed subcuticular sutures are superficial enough to hold the skin edges in close approximation but deep enough so that a healthy layer of epithelium will cover them. The disadvantages of dermal sutures are tissue reaction near the skin surface and possible suture extrusion through the skin before absorption is complete. A continuous pull-out dermal suture technique using 3-0, 4-0, or 5-0 Prolene can also be used for dermal repair (see Chap. 38).

f. **Epidermis**

(1) **Epidermis approximation** in wound repair is the step most responsible for minimizing the skin scar. Epidermal healing occurs by migration and proliferation of epithelial cells originating in the wound margin. Eversion of skin edges without an intervening gap produces the most favorable skin scar. Inverted skin edges require epithelial cells to travel a greater distance from each skin edge before meeting, resulting in a wider skin scar that usually persists as a valley trapping shadows as light is cast across its surface, thus making it more noticeable. When the wound edges are of unequal thickness, the two sides must be equalized to minimize the distance over which epithelial cell migration has to occur. Thus, exact and accurate approximation of epidermal edges is

necessary to produce a favorable skin scar. Various suture and nonsuture techniques for skin edge approximation are described in Chap. 38.

(2) Suture marks. Scars from the permanent imprints of suture material on the skin surface are dependent on the length of time skin sutures are left in place (see Chap. 38), their tension, the relationship of the sutures to the wound edge, the region of the body, and the presence or absence of infection. Tension from sutures tied too tightly or from the lateral pull on the wound margins (due to little or no skin laxity, tissue loss, tissue edema, or underlying muscle pull at right angles to the wound) produces suture marks. In addition, tissue encircled by a suture becomes ischemic and may become frankly necrotic. It is therefore important to reduce lateral pull on skin edges with a judiciously layered wound closure and to tie sutures just tight enough to coapt the skin edges, but no tighter. Large bites of tissue can result in larger amounts of tissue strangulation and larger suture marks (e.g., railroad track scars); thus, skin sutures must be placed close to the wound edge. Because natural tissue tension exerts greater lateral pull on wound margins of the trunk and extremities, suture marks are more likely to occur in those areas than on the face. Infection around a skin suture producing a pustule or draining sinus can also lead to suture marks.

3. Drains are indicated in contaminated wounds that are likely to become infected and in wounds with actual or potential dead space that cannot be obliterated with sutures and in which there is an increased likelihood of serum accumulation that could result in a seroma (e.g., large raw surfaces beneath traumatically elevated flaps). Drains are effective in evacuating serum, pus, and necrotic exudates. They do not, however, drain blood or prevent hematomas and should never be used as a substitute for adequate hemostasis. Drains can be brought out between the wound edges (preferably at one end of the wound), with the disadvantage of producing a less satisfactory scar at the drain exit site, or through a separate small incision near the wound, with the disadvantage of adding an additional scar. Drains should be secured to the skin with a suture if there is any possibility of their becoming dislodged or retracted into the wound. Since drains act as conduits for bacterial entry into the wound, they must be cared for with aseptic technique and removed promptly when the volume of drainage decreases significantly.

a. Passive drains, such as latex and rubber band drains, act as wicks for egress of minor amounts of wound fluid.

b. Active (suction) drains, such as Hemovac and Jackson-Pratt drains, require a closed system to suction fluid from the wound into a vacuum reservoir via perforated plastic tubing. A convenient suction drain for small wounds is the plastic tubing of a butterfly needle (with the connector cut off); this tubing is perforated and placed into the wound, while the needle at the other end of the tubing is inserted into a blood-collecting vacuum test tube.

F. Tetanus prophylaxis (see Chap. 12) must be considered for any wound involving a break in the skin or mucous membrane. Tetanus is caused by *Clostridium tetani*, an anaerobe, and its exotoxin, which produces skeletal muscle spasms that can lead to respiratory arrest and death. The organism is present in soil as well as in the intestine of humans and animals, thus assuring its contamination potential in a variety of wounds. Adequate wound debridement and provision of wound conditions favoring a high oxygen tension discourage colonization of *C. tetani*. Antibiotic therapy with penicillin (or tetracycline or chloramphenicol) may also be considered in tetanus-prone wounds but is unreliable as adequate prophylactic therapy. In addition to adequate wound debridement, immunization remains the standard of care in preventing tetanus.

1. Active tetanus immunization in adults consists of IM administration of tetanus and diphtheria toxoid, adult type (Td), 0.5 ml, repeated 4–6 weeks later and again in 6–12 months. In children age 6 or younger, immunization is achieved by administering diphtheria, tetanus, and pertussis (DTP) vaccine at approximately 2, 4, 6, and 18 months of age, with a booster given at 5 years of age. With completion of this basic series of injections, a booster dose of Td, 0.5 ml, is required approximately every 10 years to maintain active immunity. In previously immunized patients with tetanus-prone wounds (e.g., wounds > 6 hours old, contaminated wounds, penetrating wounds, presence of devitalized tissue), tetanus toxoid is usually given if at least 5 years have elapsed since the last dose (see Table 12-6). In patients with a history of an allergic reaction to previous Td (as evidenced by localized erythema, induration, and tenderness at the injection site), the booster dose can be administered as tetanus toxoid (T).

2. **Passive tetanus immunization** (see Table 12-6) consists of IM injection of human tetanus globulin (Hypertct), 250 500 units, depending on the patient immunization history and wound conditions. Hypertet is indicated in patients with a tetanus-prone wound and not previously immunized or only partially immunized. Tetanus toxoid is always administered concurrently at a separate site as a booster dose or to initiate active immunization.

G. **Wound aftercare** consists of providing an ideal environment for wound healing. A dressing should be applied, when feasible, for purposes of protection, immobilization, compression, absorption, and cosmesis. An attempt should be made to limit postoperative edema, because excess wound tissue fluid causes delay in the stages of healing and increases fibrous tissue proliferation (scar). Edema control is achieved by elevating the wound above heart level or by applying judicious compression or immobilization when wound elevation is impractical. Suture care and removal are discussed in Chap. 38.

II. **Specific injuries**

A. **Contusions** (bruises) are injuries without a break in the skin or mucous membrane, usually produced by blunt trauma. They frequently are accompanied by erythema, ecchymosis, edema, pain, and hyperesthesia or hypoesthesia of the overlying skin. A thorough examination of contused areas, including x-rays when indicated, is necessary to rule out underlying fractures and injury to specific structures (e.g., ocular globe; intracranial, intrathoracic, or intraabdominal organs; major vessels). A contusion alone requires only symptomatic treatment, including iced compresses, elevation when possible, and analgesics. Follow-up may be necessary to check for subsequent hematoma formation.

B. **Abrasions** are friction wounds of variable depth that result from scraping or rubbing trauma to the skin. Skin loss is an inherent feature of all abrasions and may be partial or full thickness (similar to burn wounds), depending on the depth of skin loss. Findings include bleeding, serous drainage (weeping), burning pain, loss of epidermis with exposure of dermis, loss of dermis with exposure of subcutaneous fat, or embedded foreign material. Treatment depends on the wound depth and whether foreign material is present or not.

1. **Partial-thickness abrasions** involve loss of the epidermis and upper dermis. These wounds heal by reepithelialization from the remaining dermal elements and skin appendages (i.e., hair follicles and sweat and sebaceous glands). **Treatment** is directed toward local wound care, prevention of infection, removal of embedded foreign bodies, and tetanus prophylaxis. Infection can convert a partial-thickness wound into a full-thickness one. To prevent this conversion, the wound is cleansed under adequate anesthesia and any foreign material is removed; a topical antibacterial ointment or cream is applied; and, depending on the wound location, a dressing is usually applied. Aftercare is most often performed by the patient; instructions for this care should be simple, keeping the patient's comfort and prevention of infection in mind. Twice-daily gentle washings of the abraded wound with mild soap and water, followed by patting the area dry and applying an antibacterial ointment or cream with or without a dressing, usually satisfy these requirements. In some instances, particularly abraded wounds in children, the dressing applied in the emergency department can be left in place for 7–10 days, at which time it is removed by a physician; however, if any evidence of wound infection (e.g., excessive pain, fever, foul-smelling drainage) intervenes, the dressing should be removed sooner. Most superficial abrasions heal in 7–14 days. Depending on the wound depth, some degree of scarring may result from an abrasion. Patients should be told to avoid sun exposure to healed abrasion sites for approximately 6 months to minimize permanent pigmentation changes in abrasion scars.

2. **Full-thickness abrasions** involve loss of the epidermis, dermis, and skin appendages, so that subcutaneous fat is visible in the wound. Full-thickness wounds 1 cm or less in diameter may heal within 2–4 weeks by reepithelialization from the wound edges. Healing in larger full-thickness wounds (and some small ones) is facilitated by a local tissue transfer or application of a skin graft; referral to a specialist is indicated for these patients. Linear full-thickness abrasions may be amenable to treatment by elliptical wound excision and primary closure with sutures.

3. **Traumatic tattooing** occurs when pigmented particles are embedded in the dermis of an abraded wound. Carbon from blacktop roads is the most common material found in such tattoos; it results in a black or dark blue discoloration in the skin if left in place. Once the particles are embedded, removal without scarring becomes difficult. However, this problem can be obviated by treatment immediately following the injury, and every effort should be made to remove these pigmented particles. Removal may require the use of magnifying loupes and a scrub brush in addition to standard wound cleansing, irrigation, and extraction of particles with a forceps under adequate anesthesia. Extensive wounds with foreign body tattooing and deeply embedded particles, such as from gunpowder or other explosive sources, may require general anesthesia for removal by means of dermabrasion or multiple excisions. Patients with these wounds should be referred to a specialist.

C. **Lacerations** are breaks in the continuity of the skin (or other organ) surface. The risk of infection in cleanly lacerated wounds is low, and the general demands for wound healing are easily satisfied. Skin lacerations can be very superficial, extending through the epidermis and upper dermis only, or they can extend through all layers of the skin and include the underlying deep tissues and structures.

1. **Management principles** for the treatment of lacerations are outlined in sec. I.; specific suture techniques are described in Chap. 38. In addition, the following general rules apply to the treatment of most lacerations in the emergency department.

    a. **Lacerations without obvious contamination** can be closed up to 24 hours after injury; with some exceptions (see **Bites and Stings**, sec. I), contaminated wounds are usually left open.

    b. Regardless of the depth, any **skin laceration with gaping wound edges** should be repaired.

    c. Debridement of skin edges should be kept to a minimum. Obviously devitalized tissue should be removed, and beveled wound edges should be excised to create sharp, right-angled margins for wound approximation.

    d. **Lacerations within abrasions** should be sutured.

    e. **Stellate and other complex lacerations** are accurately repaired by fitting together the pieces of what appears to be a jigsaw puzzle; in applying this principle, "missing tissue" is usually found.

    f. The smallest suture caliber that will hold securely in a given location (i.e., 6-0 for skin closure on the face, 5-0 on the hands, and 4-0 or 5-0 on the trunk and extremities) should be used.

    g. The least amount of suture material necessary to effect accurate wound edge approximation should be used; in many lacerations, a single-layer skin closure suffices.

2. **Problem areas**

    a. **Scalp** lacerations have a significant incidence of hematoma formation with or without infection subsequent to repair. They are best managed with careful hemostasis, copious irrigation to remove blood clots, and a single-layer skin closure with interrupted simple or mattress nonabsorbable sutures.

    b. Full-thickness **ear** lacerations are repaired in two layers, using 5-0 or 6-0 absorbable sutures placed through the perichondrium to approximate the cartilage and 5-0 or 6-0 nonabsorbable sutures to approximate the skin. Sutures aligning the helical rim should be placed first to prevent notching deformities.

    c. **Eyelid** lacerations that do not involve the ciliary margin are usually repaired with 6-0 nonabsorbable skin sutures, which are removed 4–5 days later to prevent milia. Full-thickness lacerations involving the ciliary margin require careful alignment of the ciliary border with placement of the first suture, the ends of which can be left long for use as a traction suture. The conjunctival surface and edges of the tarsal plate are repaired with the same 6-0 absorbable sutures that catch both layers; the knots should be buried to prevent corneal irritation. Skin closure is with 6-0 nonabsorbable sutures; braided suture material is preferred because the suture ends are less stiff and less likely to irritate the globe.

    d. Full-thickness **nose** lacerations extending through the nostril rim are repaired by placing the initial suture at the free nostril border to prevent notching or malalignment of this border.

    e. **Lip** lacerations extending through the vermilion must be carefully approximated to prevent a step-off deformity. The first suture placed should always be that which aligns the vermilion-skin border ("white roll") immediately adjacent to the vermilion edge; a layered closure (involving muscle, mucosa, and skin) follows as necessary.

   f. Lacerations **perpendicular to skin flexion creases** (e.g., upper eyelid, palmar surface of the hands and fingers) frequently heal with scar contracture unless a primary z-plasty is incorporated into the repair. These lacerations should be referred to a specialist for management.

D. Avulsions result from tensile forces that forcibly separate or tear tissues. The area of energy absorption in the soft tissue is much greater than that seen in simple lacerations. Consequently, the extent of tissue injury may be much greater and more deceptive. Avulsion injuries can produce intimal blood vessel damage with subsequent thrombosis and alteration in blood flow to injured parts. In addition, nerves, muscles, and ligaments may suffer disruption of their structural integrity. The viability of all portions of these wounds must be carefully evaluated and the integrity of underlying structures assessed.

   1. Incomplete avulsions maintain an intact blood supply to the avulsed tissue and are managed as lacerations or flaps, depending on the degree of tissue separation.

   2. Complete avulsions are tissues completely separated from underlying and adjacent structures and from their blood supply. Small segments of completely avulsed tissue can be discarded and the remaining wound edges approximated after appropriate debridement and undermining. If the avulsed segment is too large to permit approximation of the remaining wound edges, wound closure by other methods is indicated; such methods include a skin graft taken from the avulsed segment or a distant site, use of a local or distant flap, or, in some instances, microvascular reattachment of the avulsed segment (e.g., scalp avulsions, digital degloving injuries). These patients are referred to a specialist for treatment (see J for care of the wound and avulsed tissue segment).

E. Flaps are three-sided tongues of tissue with an intact vascular pedicle or attachment to the body along the fourth side that maintains nourishment to the tissues within the flap. Flap lacerations are traumatically elevated flaps that result from sharp or blunt avulsion injuries. Flaps with a direct cutaneous artery and vein coursing along their longitudinal axis are **axial pattern** flaps, while those without large direct blood vessels are **random pattern** flaps. Skin flaps contain only skin and subcutaneous tissue, while composite flaps incorporate various other tissue layers. A vast majority of traumatically elevated flaps are random pattern skin flaps. Management principles for treatment of flap lacerations include the following:

   1. Evaluation of the wound for missing tissue. Flap tissues frequently retract or curl up, giving the appearance that tissue has been lost. Unfurling of flap tissues usually results in the discovery that no tissue has been lost and that wound edge approximation is possible, although with some degree of tension.

   2. Careful assessment of flap tissues for viability, particularly at the tip of the flap (the portion farthest from the base and thus farthest from the blood supply in a random pattern flap), is essential. This assessment includes observation of skin color, capillary refill, and bleeding (particularly dermal) from the flap wound edges. In general, flaps located in the head and neck area have excellent vascularity and survive under most circumstances. In contrast, distally based flaps on extremities have a poor blood supply and tend to necrose, particularly if sutured under tension. Portions of flaps felt to be nonviable should be excised. If excision results in a wound that cannot be closed primarily, referral to a specialist is indicated.

   3. Removal of blood clots and other debris from beneath the flap, both from the undersurface of the flap and the wound bed, is usually best accomplished with copious wound irrigation.

   4. Careful wound hemostasis of both the undersurface of the flap and the wound bed to prevent hematoma formation, which can be particularly deleterious to flap wound healing (see H), is essential.

   5. Drains are useful in large flap lacerations to eliminate dead space (see sec. I.E.3).

   6. Closure of the wound is performed by carefully approximating tissue layers (see sec. I.E.2). This technique may help prevent trapdoor scar formation, a not infrequent consequence of flap laceration healing. Since these scars may require later scar revision, it is important to preserve as much tissue as possible at the time of injury. The interrupted half-buried horizontal mattress suture technique (see Chap. 38) is useful for skin closure of flap lacerations.

F. **Crush injury** results from compression of soft tissue between two opposing forces, frequently with more tissue damage than any other type of injury.

1. **Clinical features.** Hemorrhage into soft tissues is common, leading to ecchymosis and hematoma formation. Edema is often significant, not only prolonging the normal process of wound healing but also potentially leading to vascular occlusion and nerve compression, particularly in crush injuries of the extremities. Crush injuries may or may not have associated skin abrasions, lacerations, avulsions, or friction burns. Crush injuries resulting from industrial or farm machinery are frequently accompanied by severe skin damage as well as direct injury to underlying muscles, nerves, blood vessels, bones, and joints. Wringer injuries may display minor skin lacerations or friction burns with infrequent fractures of underlying bones. A compartment syndrome (see Chap. 26) must be suspected in any extremity crush injury, including the comatose drug addict whose body has compressed an extremity for several hours. In a compartment syndrome, swelling of the limb may not be seen early but develops subsequently. An early, reliable sign of impending muscle damage is increased turgor involving a muscle compartment, with pain on passive muscle stretch. Nerve compression is indicated by loss of sensory and motor function. Peripheral pulses, however, may be normal to palpation and Doppler examination. Unrecognized and untreated, an extremity compartment syndrome can lead to Volkmann's ischemic contracture with varying degrees of nerve and muscle damage.

2. **Evaluation** of crush injuries includes the following: (1) examination of the skin and any obvious wounds, (2) determination of the presence or absence of edema, (3) assessment of sensation and motor nerve function at the site of injury and distal to it, (4) assessment of muscle turgor at the site of injury and passive stretching of muscles in that compartment, (5) evaluation of vascularity at the site of injury and distally (e.g., assessment of capillary refill and distal pulses), and (6) testing for myoglobinemia and myoglobinuria when extensive muscle necrosis is suspected.

3. **Management** of crush injuries involves (1) debridement of nonviable tissues, (2) primary closure of small lacerations if contamination or a compartment syndrome is not suspected, and (3) immediate referral to a specialist and hospitalization for extensive crush injuries with damage to multiple tissues.

   a. If **myoglobinemia** or **myoglobinuria** is present, hydration of the patient is instituted in the emergency department and continued after hospital admission.

   b. If a **compartment syndrome** is possible, the extremity is immobilized in a soft, compressive dressing and elevated to prevent additional edema formation, and the patient is admitted to the hospital. Fasciotomies may be necessary to reduce compartmental pressure and prevent further ischemic injury.

G. **Puncture wounds** are produced by sharp objects that may drive foreign-body debris deeply through a small skin entrance wound. Graphite fragments from lead pencils, paint chips, rust particles, and wood splinters are the more common foreign bodies implanted by puncture. Tissue destruction, bleeding, and contamination may be present deep in the wound and covered by relatively normal-appearing tissues. X-rays are usually indicated. **Treatment** consists of debridement or excision of a small area of skin and subcutaneous tissue at the entrance site, removal of obvious foreign material, copious irrigation, and careful hemostasis. Because puncture wounds provide a particularly favorable environment (i.e., low oxygen tension) for growth of *Clostridium tetani*, most puncture wounds are treated open and allowed to heal by secondary intention. Antibiotics are used when there is evidence of contamination of the wound.

H. A **hematoma** is an abnormal, ectopic collection of blood characterized by swelling, ecchymosis, blanching, pain, and distortion of normal anatomy. Hematomas can act as a culture medium for bacterial growth, produce ischemia and necrosis of overlying skin (by pressure injury and a direct toxic effect), and produce an additional mass of scar tissue in the depth of the wound. **Treatment** varies with the location, size of the collection, and whether the collection is observed early or late. Early hematomas that are small, not expanding, not painful, and show no compromise of the overlying skin may be treated conservatively with a pressure dressing, immobilization, and elevation (if possible). Some hematomas will resorb spontaneously while others will require evacuation, particularly if they liquefy and become fluctuant. Larger hematomas, expanding hematomas, liquefied hematomas, and those in danger of producing pressure necrosis of underlying structures or overlying skin are treated by evacuation, i.e., incision with a scalpel blade and drainage or aspiration with a large-bore needle. A pressure dressing is usually necessary to prevent reaccumulation of the hematoma.

1. An **external ear hematoma** (see Chap. 24) commonly results from contact sports and can ultimately lead to a "cauliflower ear" deformity unless treated aggressively. Treatment consists of evacuation or aspiration of the hematoma and placement of through-and-through interrupted horizontal mattress sutures (see Chap. 38) tied over gauze bolsters on both surfaces of the ear to hold the elevated skin in place over the cartilage and prevent reaccumulation of blood or serum. These sutures are left in place 7–10 days.

2. A **nasal septal hematoma** (see Chap. 24) is relatively rare but should be ruled out in any patient with a history of nasal trauma, whether a fracture is present or not. An untreated septal hematoma may result in septal perforation by pressure necrosis or from infection of the hematoma. The septum is examined with a nasal speculum. A hematoma is evacuated by incision or aspiration on one or both sides of the septum, and nasal packing or septal stents are placed on one or both sides for 5–7 days.

3. A **subungual hematoma** (see Chap. 23) accompanies a fingertip crush injury and is often quite painful. X-rays are usually indicated to assess for fracture of the distal phalanx. **Treatment** consists of making a hole through the nail plate using the tip of a heated paper clip, the hot tip of a Concept disposable cautery, or the pointed tip of an 18- or 20-gauge needle. This treatment usually produces dramatic pain relief.

4. **Wound hematomas** should be evacuated by removing one or more sutures, separating the coapted wound edges with a hemostat directly over the collection, and rolling or pressing the clotted blood out. The skin edges may be reapproximated with Steri-Strips or left open to permit further drainage of blood or serum. A pressure dressing should be applied, if possible.

I. **Foreign body** contamination of wounds can (1) introduce large numbers of microorganisms into the wound, increasing the likelihood of infection; (2) elicit a more intense local inflammatory reaction, which ultimately results in more scar tissue; (3) leave permanent visible evidence of the foreign material by discoloring the scar or skin (e.g., pencil lead); or (4) produce prolonged or permanent discomfort from the physical presence of the foreign body. Therefore, foreign bodies should always be removed unless removal would produce additional injury to a critical structure. In addition to visual wound inspection and palpation, x-rays are obtained when a foreign body is suspected. If the foreign body is visible on x-ray, posteroanterior (PA), lateral, and oblique views with a small lead marker directly on the skin wound are obtained so that the foreign body can be located accurately in relation to the skin marker. The physician removing a foreign body must know the exact position of the skin marker when attempting to retrieve the foreign body. Fluoroscopy or an image intensifier, if available, may be used to remove foreign bodies. Patients either with multiple foreign bodies or with a foreign body located in deep tissues or a critical area where injury to structures such as nerves, tendons, or blood vessels is possible during attempted removal should be referred to a specialist for treatment under optimal conditions in the operating suite. Following removal of a foreign body, the wound can be closed unless there is concern about significant bacterial contamination. Antibiotics are not necessary in the absence of signs of infection or gross contamination.

1. A **fishhook** embedded in tissue is most easily removed by passing the point and barb out through the skin as if completing the passage of a curved needle through tissue. After the point and barb have penetrated out through the skin, they are grasped with a needle-holder or hemostat. Once the point and barb have been secured, the eye of the hook is cut off with an appropriate instrument (e.g., wire cutter, pliers, scissors), and the remainder of the hook is withdrawn with the instrument securing the point and barb.

2. **Foreign body tattooing** is discussed in **B.3.**

J. **Traumatic amputations** (see Chap. 23) should be considered as potentially replantable severed tissues that can be reattached utilizing techniques of microvascular surgery. Although the majority of traumatic amputations involve digits or limbs, other severed body parts (e.g., ear, penis, scalp, degloving ring avulsions) are also potentially replantable.

1. **Contraindications** to replantation that can be determined by the emergency department physician include (1) the presence of significant associated injuries that may be life-threatening, (2) a major systemic disease of sufficient magnitude to make transportation or prolonged surgery hazardous, (3) inability to retrieve the amputated part, and (4) a prolonged ischemia time (the maximum warm ischemia time is approximately 6 hours, but immediate cooling of the amputated part extends the tolerable ischemia time to 12–24 hours). Other contraindications to replantation, such as extent of injury to the amputated part, are determined by the replant surgeon.

2. Emergency department **management** of traumatic amputations includes the following: (1) evaluation of the patient's overall status, including assessment of other injuries; (2) control of hemorrhage from the stump with direct pressure; (3) fluid resuscitation and, if necessary, blood transfusion to restore an adequate blood volume; (4) administration of antibiotics and tetanus prophylaxis (if needed); (5) saline lavage of the stump and application of a stump dressing with moderate pressure for additional hemostasis; (6) after gentle saline lavage to remove only gross debris, wrapping the amputated part in a sterile, saline-moistened gauze and then placing it in a dry plastic bag that is sealed and placed on regular crushed ice; (7) x-rays of the stump and amputated part; and (8) transport of the stabilized patient, amputated part, and any x-rays with appropriate personnel via appropriate means (e.g., ambulance, helicopter) to a replant facility that has been notified of the patient's arrival. Incompletely amputated parts should be immobilized or splinted to minimize further vascular injury.

Soft-Tissue Infections

I. **General principles.** Infection results from invasion of a vulnerable host by pathogenic microorganisms that produce tissue injury characterized by inflammation, suppuration, and necrosis.

A. **Host factors** that influence the proliferation and invasive capacity of microorganisms include tissue integrity and viability, local circulation, and immune competence. Dehydration, shock, malnutrition, obesity, diabetes mellitus, or adrenal insufficiency may decrease host resistance enough to allow microbial invasion in wounds that would ordinarily be resistant to infection. Drug therapy with steroids, cytotoxic agents, immunosuppressive agents, or antimicrobials may render the host more susceptible to infection. A majority of soft-tissue infections are associated with an obvious break in the protective skin or mucous membrane barrier (i.e., acute or chronic wounds) that permits entry of a bacterial inoculum. When soft-tissue infection occurs in the presence of intact skin or mucous membrane, a source for bacterial seeding of a vulnerable body part must be sought elsewhere (e.g., infection in an area of decreased blood supply or otherwise compromised tissue from seeding from a dental abscess, recent dental manipulation, or urinary tract infection).

B. **Microbial factors** that influence the development of infection include an inoculum of sufficient density (usually 10^5 or more organisms/gram of tissue) and virulence to produce tissue damage and disease in the host. Microorganisms cause disease by invading tissues, producing toxins, or both. Bacterial invasion leads to demonstrable damage of host cells and tissues in the vicinity of the invasion, whereas bacterial toxins are transported via the blood and lymph to produce cytotoxic effects at distant sites.

C. The classic **signs and symptoms** of soft-tissue infection are redness, swelling, heat, and pain. Pain is the most reliable symptom of infection and is accompanied by tenderness to palpation, greatest over the area of maximal involvement, and by loss of function resulting from patient immobilization of the painful part in the most comfortable position. Fever, tachycardia, and leukocytosis are nonspecific signs that frequently accompany infection. Gram's stain of wound exudate or material obtained by needle aspiration of subcutaneous infections may confirm the presence of bacteria.

D. **Treatment** of infections involves local measures and antibiotic therapy as appropriate.

1. **Local therapy** consists, where appropriate, of adequate debridement of necrotic

or injured tissue, removal of foreign bodies, and establishment of adequate drainage.

2. **Antibiotic therapy**
   a. **Systemic antibiotics** are primary treatment for acute spreading infections (e.g., cellulitis, lymphangitis, septicemia, peritonitis). Antibiotics are adjuvant therapy for all other infections where local therapy (see 1) takes precedence. The use of antibiotics in the treatment of infections depends on an adequate blood supply to the infected area. The selection of appropriate systemic antibiotic therapy is based on clinical judgment. Clinical judgment is aided by microscopic examination of the Gram stain of any exudate or pus and by familiarity with the more common infecting organisms. The mechanism of injury, wound type and location, source of bacterial contamination or seeding, and history of recent antibiotic therapy all provide clues to the identity of the infecting organism.
      (1) A majority of skin and subcutaneous infections are caused by staphylococci or streptococci. Staphylococcal infections are treated with a semisynthetic pencillin or first-generation cephalosporin; either medication usually is effective against even penicillin-resistant *Staphylococcus aureus* and *Staphylococcus epidermidis*. Penicillin is the antibiotic of choice for treatment of hemolytic streptococcal infections.
      (2) **Gram-negative bacterial infection** should be suspected in wounds produced by farm machinery or when the source of bacterial contamination or seeding is likely to be the gastrointestinal or genitourinary tract. Gram-negative infections are treated with an aminoglycoside, some of the newer semisynthetic penicillins, or a second- or third-generation cephalosporin.
      (3) **Anaerobic infections** occur infrequently; when they do, they are usually seen in patients with a chronic systemic illness. Penicillin G is the drug of choice for most anaerobes except for *Bacteroides fragilis,* which requires chloramphenicol or clindamycin.
   b. **Topical antibiotic therapy** to wounds other than burns or abrasions is seldom indicated.

II. **Specific infections**
   A. **Cellulitis and lymphangitis. Cellulitis** is a nonsuppurative inflammation of the subcutaneous tissues extending along connective tissue planes and across intercellular spaces; it is characterized by widespread swelling, redness, heat, and pain without definite localization. **Lymphangitis** is an inflammation of lymphatic pathways; it is characterized by visible erythematous streaking of the skin. These infections are discussed in Chap. 31.
   B. **Cutaneous abscesses.** An **abscess** is a localized, walled-off collection of purulent material (i.e., white blood cells and cellular debris) surrounded by an area of inflamed tissue (cellulitis) in which hyperemia and infiltration of leukocytes is marked. Cutaneous abscesses can arise in a sweat gland or hair follicle (furuncle or boil), in a preexisting keratinous cyst, in areas of trauma or surgical wounds, or apparently de novo. A carbuncle is a multilocular suppurative extension of a cutaneous abscess into subcutaneous tissues. Individual compartments in a carbuncle are maintained via persistent fascial attachments to skin. When individual loculations rupture through the skin, fistulas may appear.
      1. **Etiologic agents.** Most cutaneous abscesses are caused by staphylococci. However, gram-negative bacilli or streptococci may be involved.
      2. **Management**
         a. **Incision and drainage** are the essence of treatment for any abscess. An abscess is ready for drainage when the infection has localized, i.e., when an area of softness or fluctuance appears, usually near the center of the area of inflammation. To encourage the process of localization from a state of diffuse induration, continuous warm soaks may first be applied to the area for 24–48 hours. No effort should be made to completely excise an abscess since (1) its boundaries are ill-defined, (2) the resulting tissue defect may be much larger than necessary, and (3) the secondary wound is likely to become infected, producing additional tissue damage. Drainage is performed as follows:
            (1) **Aseptic technique** is used for the procedure.
            (2) Local infiltration **anesthesia** is injected into the skin over the fluctuant area. No effort is made to infiltrate the subcutaneous tissues since pas-

sage of the needle into the surrounding tissues may seed bacteria and since the low pH in areas of infection generally negates the action of local anesthetics. Regional nerve block anesthesia (see Chap. 38) can be used in suitable anatomic regions if there is no danger of seeding bacteria to the area of injection.

   (3) **Incision.** The skin over the area of fluctuance is incised with a No. 11 or 15 scalpel blade. The incision is made deep enough to enter the abscess cavity and long enough to establish adequate drainage.

   (4) Material for **Gram's stain** and **culture** is obtained immediately on entering the abscess cavity.

   (5) **Drainage.** The abscess cavity is drained passively. Tissue septae between loculations are broken down with a hemostat.

   (6) **Irrigation.** The cavity is then irrigated with saline.

   (7) A small latex **drain** or gauze **wick** is placed between the skin edges and is secured to one skin edge with a suture if there is any possibility of the drain or wick becoming dislodged prematurely. Packing of the abscess cavity is less satisfactory, since it may impair continued wound drainage.

   (8) An **absorbent dressing** is then applied.

   b. **Wound care** involves (1) application of warm soaks to the wound 3 or 4 times daily or continuously until pain is no longer present, (2) elevation of the part, and (3) immobilization of the part. The drain or gauze wick should be removed by the patient or physician in 1–3 days. The wound should then be washed with soap and water 2–4 times daily; when conditions permit, cleansing is best accomplished by washing the wound under running water (e.g., in the shower). The patient should gently pry the wound edges apart during washings to prevent recurrence of the abscess, which can occur when the skin heals prematurely.

   3. **Antibiotics** are indicated as adjunctive therapy when there is significant concurrent cellulitis or lymphangitis or complicating factors (e.g., the presence of diabetes mellitus or immunosuppression).

   4. **Disposition.** Most cutaneous abscesses can be drained in the emergency department and followed up on an outpatient basis. However, hospitalization is indicated for patients with extensive abscesses requiring drainage in the operating suite or for patients with extensive surrounding cellulitis or lymphangitis or coexisting illness (e.g., impaired circulation or immune competence) mandating the use of parenteral antibiotics.

C. **Gas gangrene** (myonecrosis) is a rapidly progressive, rarely pure culture infection.

   1. **Etiologies.** The most important causative microorganism is *Clostridium perfringens,* which produces a lethal, necrotizing, hemolytic exotoxin. This anaerobic infection **(clostridial myonecrosis)** is most likely to occur in extensive wounds with devitalized muscle (e.g., injuries from high-velocity missiles), wounds with an impaired blood supply, wounds with gross foreign body contamination, and wounds in which there was incomplete initial debridement. It may also follow clean elective surgical procedures or may appear suddenly in chronic wounds, such as pressure sores. The average incubation period for clostridial myonecrosis is 48 hours, but the infection can appear as early as 6 hours after injury, particularly in wounds with grossly devitalized and contaminated muscle. Anaerobic streptococci can also cause gas gangrene; streptococcal myonecrosis resembles subacute clostridial gas gangrene.

   2. **Clinical features.** Pain due to the rapid infiltration of infected muscle by edema and gas is the earliest and most important symptom. A rapid, feeble pulse, characteristically out of proportion to the temperature elevation, usually follows the onset of pain. The blood pressure is normal or slightly elevated early in the course of infection; however, hypotension may ensue. Fever is an unreliable index of the severity and extent of infection, since the temperature may be elevated or subnormal. The patient usually is pale, weak, diaphoretic, and apathetic. Crepitus may or may not be present. A dirty-brown watery fluid with a peculiar foul odor is usually present in the wound; the Gram stain shows characteristic bacteria. Radiographs taken at 2- to 4-hour intervals reveal a visible increase in the amount of wound gas or a linear spread of gas along muscle and fascial planes.

   3. **Treatment**

   a. **Surgical decompression and debridement.** Immediate and radical surgical decompression of the involved fascial compartments by extensive longitudinal incisions (fasciotomies) and excision of infected and devitalized muscle are the most effective means of treating clostridial myonecrosis. Open guillotine amputation may be necessary for advanced gangrenous changes. These procedures are performed in the operating suite under general anesthesia.

   b. IV **antibiotics** (i.e., penicillin G, cephalothin, or clindamycin, in that order, or chloramphenicol) using maximum doses (e.g., penicillin G, 3 million units q3h) should be started in the emergency department after obtaining aerobic and anaerobic wound cultures.

   c. Fluid resuscitation, including blood transfusions, if indicated, with maintenance of fluid and electrolyte balance is important.

   d. Analgesics should be administered as necessary, and the infected injured part immobilized.

   e. Hyperbaric oxygen, if available, may be used to combat the anaerobic infection.

   4. Disposition. Hospitalization is always necessary, with referral to a specialist for surgical decompression and debridement.

D. Necrotizing fasciitis. This relatively rare, life-threatening infection is characterized by extensive necrosis of the superficial fascia, with resultant widespread undermining of the surrounding tissue and extreme toxicity. In contrast to gas gangrene, muscle is not involved. The disease appears to be a clinical entity and not a specific bacterial infection.

   1. Etiologies. The bacteria involved in 90 percent of cases are beta-hemolytic streptococci or coagulase-positive staphylococci or both. Gram-negative enteric pathogens are involved in 10 percent of cases. Anaerobic or microaerophilic streptococci or synergistic microorganisms (i.e., peptostreptococci, aerobic gram-negative rods, and frequently bacteroides) are sometimes involved in necrotizing fasciitis. A majority of cases follow minor trauma, especially in extremities of individuals with diabetes mellitus or peripheral vascular disease. Necrotizing fasciitis may also develop after clean surgical procedures or in chronic wounds.

   2. Clinical features. The patient exhibits signs and symptoms of systemic toxicity. A serosanguineous wound exudate is usually present. The fascia is swollen, stringy, dull-gray, and necrotic with extensive undermining. In an open wound, the extent of undermining can be determined by passing a sterile hemostat along the plane just superficial to the deep fascia; in contrast, in simple cellulitis or erysipelas, the hemostat cannot be passed. Crepitus may or may not be present. Radiographs may show linear streaking of gas along fascial planes. A Gram-stained smear of the wound exudate shows one or more of the above bacteria (see **1**).

   3. Treatment

   a. Resuscitation with **IV fluids** should be started immediately.

   b. IV **antibiotics** (i.e., aqueous penicillin and a broad-spectrum antibiotic that covers coagulase-positive staphylococci as well as gram-negative bacteria) should be initiated as soon as appropriate cultures have been obtained.

   c. To effect **decompression and drainage,** multiple linear incisions are made over the affected area in the operating suite after referral to a specialist.

   4. Disposition. Hospitalization is always necessary.

E. Foot infection. Infection in the foot occurs with relative frequency because minor trauma is often ignored and because the local blood supply is poorer than in other body parts. Individuals with diabetes or peripheral vascular disease are especially prone to developing foot infections.

   1. Preventive measures. To prevent foot infections, even apparently minor wounds should be evaluated carefully and treated aggressively. Radiographs to assess for foreign bodies, debridement of puncture wounds, leaving potentially contaminated wounds open to heal by secondary intention, use of adjunctive antibiotics when there is evidence of contamination, elevation and immobilization, and meticulous wound aftercare should all be considered in the treatment of foot wounds.

   2. Evaluation. Established foot infections are carefully evaluated for signs and symptoms of tenosynovitis (i.e., swelling, tenderness, and erythema along the course of the involved tendon, plus pain on passive stretch of the tendon). X-rays are obtained to assess for foreign bodies and osteomyelitis. A Gram stain and culture of wound exudate for aerobes, anaerobes, fungi, and mycobacteria (as indicated) are obtained.

3. **Management** includes local wound debridement and drainage, administration of antibiotics, elevation, immobilization, and dressing changes. Except when the infection is very superficial and localized, patients should be referred to a specialist for wound debridement and drainage in the operating suite to achieve adequate debridement and drainage and avoid possible damage to tendons, vessels, and nerves.

4. **Disposition.** Unless the infection is obviously minor and superficial, hospitalization is indicated to effect appropriate management of the infection and any coexisting systemic illness.

F. **Wound infection.** Infection can occur in any wound, but is more likely to occur following trauma. Hemolytic streptococci and staphylococci are the most common pathogens in wound infections. Other microorganisms may be involved, depending on the source of wound contamination, mechanism of injury, and various host factors.

1. **Diagnosis.** Wound infection must be differentiated from normal wound inflammation and suture reaction, which are characterized by localized, nonprogressive erythema of the wound margins or around sutures and resolve as swelling regresses and sutures are removed. Wound infection is an abscess, often with surrounding cellulitis, induration, lymphangitis, and possibly tissue necrosis. Characteristic features include excessive pain (frequently throbbing in nature), persistent swelling, redness, localized warmth, and possibly exudate at the wound site. Fever, chills, or leukocytosis may or may not be present.

2. **Management** includes the following: (1) adequate drainage by removing some or all sutures and evacuating pus and necrotic debris, (2) obtaining aerobic and anaerobic cultures as well as a Gram stain of the wound exudate, (3) insertion of a gauze wick or drain to prevent premature skin edge closure and reaccumulation of pus, (4) application of an absorbent dressing, (5) elevation of the part (when possible) to reduce swelling, (6) intermittent or continuous warm moist soaks or compresses (with care to avoid burning of skin), (7) dressing changes 2–4 times daily, accompanied by washing the wound under running water (e.g., a shower) when possible, and (8) adjunctive antibiotic therapy, especially in the presence of surrounding cellulitis, lymphangitis, or induration. The choice of an antibiotic is based on the Gram stain until the culture report is available.

3. **Disposition.** Hospitalization is sometimes necessary, depending on the severity of the wound infection, patient reliability, and the ability of the patient to care for the wound.

Bites and Stings

Animal bites and stings inflict damage via a variety of mechanisms: direct tissue destruction, microbial tissue contamination, venom or toxin injection, or foreign body reaction to retained portions of the biting or stinging animal.

I. **Animal bites** cause direct tissue destruction or wound contamination with oral microbial flora (or both). In addition, animals infected with rabies can transmit the virus via direct contact of the animal's saliva with an open wound or mucous membranes.

A. **Dog bites** (see Chap. 23) are managed as follows:

1. Copious **wound cleansing**, vigorous wound irrigation, and careful debridement of crushed and contaminated tissue are essential to avoid subsequent infection.

2. **Primary wound closure** without buried sutures is permissible, particularly if the wound is located on the face or neck. Wounds on the extremities have a higher infection rate, however, and consideration should be given to treating them open initially, with referral to a specialist for delayed primary closure or management during healing by secondary intention. Bites from dogs suspected to be rabid should be left open.

3. An **antibiotic** should be administered whether the wound is closed or left open. Penicillin is the antibiotic of choice, since the bacteria found in most infected dog bites are streptococci, *S. aureus*, or *Pasteurella multocida*. Alternative antibiotics are erythromycin or a cephalosporin.

4. Wound **elevation** (if possible) and **immobilization** are instituted.

5. **Tetanus prophylaxis** is given, if needed.

6. **Rabies prophylaxis** (see Chap. 12) is initiated, if indicated.

7. Close **follow-up** is essential.

B. **Cat bites and scratches** are treated the same as dog bites (see Chap. 23).

C. **Wild animal bites,** including those from skunks, bats, raccoons, foxes, coyotes, bobcats, and other carnivores, should be washed immediately and thoroughly with soap and water and followed by copious irrigation with saline and a germicide. The wound is debrided and usually left open, especially if rabies exposure is a concern. Tetanus prophylaxis (if needed) and an antibiotic are administered. Public health officials should be contacted regarding the need for rabies prophylaxis.

D. **Other animal bites,** including those from livestock, rodents, squirrels, hamsters, guinea pigs, gerbils, chipmunks, rabbits, and hares, are treated with thorough cleansing, irrigation, and debridement. They can be closed primarily or left open, depending on the wound location and extent of injury. Bites from these animals almost never require antirabies prophylaxis, but local and state public health officials can be consulted for individual cases.

II. **Human bites** (see Chap. 23). Any break in the skin or mucous membrane caused by human teeth or contaminated by human oral flora constitutes a human bite injury.

A. **Clinical features.** Human bite wounds are more likely to become infected than animal bite wounds because of the mixed bacterial flora present in the human mouth (i.e., streptococci, staphylococci, *Micrococcus, Eikenella corrodens, Bacteroides,* and anaerobes) and because they are often neglected. Human bites occur most commonly on the hand as a result of a fist striking a mouth. Other common locations are the genitalia, breast, buttock, and earlobe. Because of the mechanism of injury, these wounds are frequently minimized or overlooked until infection becomes well established.

B. **Treatment** of human bites is as follows:

1. Copious **wound cleansing,** vigorous wound irrigation, and careful debridement of crushed and contaminated tissue are essential; provision should be made for adequate drainage of puncture wounds by enlarging skin openings, if necessary.

2. **Open wound treatment,** rather than wound closure, is indicated. The wound may be packed loosely with gauze, and the patient instructed regarding dressing changes 2–4 times daily, with wound washing under running water with each dressing change.

3. **Tetanus prophylaxis** should be administered, if needed.

4. An **antibiotic** (i.e., a semisynthetic penicillin or, alternatively, erythromycin, a cephalosporin, or clindamycin) should be administered.

C. **Disposition.** Patients with human bite injuries require close follow-up; referral to a specialist is indicated if wound healing will require a skin graft or if scar revision is likely. Established human bite wound infections with cellulitis or lymphangitis require hospitalization for vigorous local wound care and parenteral antibiotics.

III. **Reptile bites** injure by direct tissue destruction or by local and systemic effects of venom injection.

A. **Venomous snake bites.** Snake venoms are highly complex mixtures of proteins and peptides, including some enzymes, that can cause local effects such as inflammation, damage to vascular endothelium, and tissue necrosis. Venoms can also cause neurotoxicity and interfere with blood clotting.

1. **Pit vipers** in the United States include rattlesnakes, cottonmouths (water moccasins), and copperheads. They have deep pits lined with heat receptors in their cheeks between the eyes and nostrils; these receptors are thought to detect the presence of prey and guide the direction of the strike. About 20% of bites by pit vipers are "dry" with no venom injected. Pit viper venom contains hematologic, neurologic, and other systemic toxins.

a. **Clinical manifestations** of pit viper envenomation vary with the type of snake and degree of envenomation. The following may be encountered: (1) immediate local pain at the site of visible fang marks, followed within 1–2 hours by swelling, erythema, and ecchymosis and subsequent bleb formation; (2) edema and ecchymosis of an entire limb (if the limb was bitten) along with lymphadenopathy; and (3) systemic signs and symptoms including weakness, sweating, chills, perioral numbness and paresthesias, nausea and vomiting, muscle fasciculations, bleeding, hypotension, seizures, respiratory depression, and renal failure.

b. **Laboratory data** may reveal hematuria, glycosuria, and proteinuria; anemia; thrombocytopenia; or abnormal clotting studies.

c. **Treatment** remains controversial in regard to wound incision and suction, use of tourniquets, application of ice packs, surgical excision of the bite wound, and administration of corticosteroids, because these measures may increase tissue damage or have not been shown to be of definite benefit.

(1) **First aid** should be limited to immediate application of a broad, firm,

constrictive bandage over the bitten area and immobilization of the part, if possible.

(2) Antivenin specific for North American pit vipers (antivenin Crotalidac polyvalent) is recommended to be given if there are signs of envenomation. However, the potential benefits from administering antivenin must be weighed against the risks. Since antivenin is made from horse serum, it frequently causes hypersensitivity reactions; anaphylaxis (see Chap. 31) can occur, and the incidence of posttreatment serum sickness is 30–75%, depending on the dose. Skin testing is performed routinely, but regardless of the result, patients with severe envenomation must be given antivenin. For best results, antivenin must be administered early, preferably within 4 hours of the bite. Antivenin is administered by slow IV infusion. Dosages vary depending on the type of snake, severity of envenomation, and the age and size of the patient. Doses of two to four vials may be adequate for patients with minimal envenomation, whereas patients with severe envenomation may require 10–15 vials or more. Hypersensitivity reactions can be managed by slowing or stopping the infusion as appropriate and giving an antihistamine (e.g., diphenhydramine, 50 mg IV) or epinephrine (or both); the former can also be given prophylactically before infusing antivenin. Specific guidelines regarding the use of antivenin are presented in the *Physicians' Desk Reference.*

(3) Tetanus prophylaxis is administered, if needed.

(4) Other measures, including supportive measures for shock, respiratory depression, and renal failure, may be necessary for severe envenomation. Bleeding secondary to envenomation responds to antivenin, not heparin; blood components may·be helpful. Antibiotics are recommended only for specific bacterial infection as determined by cultures; prophylactic antibiotics are not recommended.

2. Coral snakes

a. Clinical manifestations may include the following: (1) minor local bite wound pain and minimal swelling, with hard-to-detect fang marks; (2) occasional regional numbness or weakness of a bitten extremity; and (3) systemic signs and symptoms that are primarily neurotoxic and may be delayed for many hours, including drowsiness, weakness, nausea, vomiting, bulbar signs (such as tongue fasciculations, dysphagia, and extraocular muscle paresis), late paresis of limbs, a weak irregular pulse, and occasionally hypotension. Death may result from respiratory or cardiac failure.

b. Treatment is the same as for pit viper envenomation, except that antivenin *(Micrurus fulvius)* specific for the eastern coral snake is used.

B. Other reptiles

1. Gila monsters hang on tenaciously when biting; they can be detached by introducing a hemostat, stick, or spoon between the jaws posteriorly to pry them apart. Gila monster venom is primarily neurotoxic, producing pain, edema, and mostly a local reaction. There is no known antivenom. Management consists of supportive measures, tetanus prophylaxis (if needed), and pain relief.

2. Alligator bites are crushing in nature and cause severe tissue destruction. Management consists of appropriate resuscitation and surgical wound repair.

IV. Insect and spider bites (see Chap. 31)

A. Brown recluse spider bites. The brown recluse spider (*Loxosceles reclusa*), which has a distinguishing violin-shaped mark on its dorsal cephalothorax, most often produces trivial bite wounds, but envenomation may produce significant local or systemic reactions (or both).

1. Clinical manifestations. The initial bite frequently goes unnoticed but in a few hours may become painful, with formation of a cyanotic bleb at the bite site with a white ischemic periphery surrounded in turn by an erythematous, often indurated, halo. This reaction may progress to eschar formation and ulceration several days later, producing an indolent wound that may take weeks or months to heal but rarely becomes secondarily infected. Systemic symptoms include fever, chills, malaise, weakness, nausea, vomiting, arthralgias, petechiae, and seizures. Rarely, hemolysis may occur with subsequent hemoglobinuria, renal failure, and death. Thrombocytopenia and disseminated intravascular coagulation have also been reported. Significant systemic reactions are more likely in children.

2. **Evaluation.** Laboratory tests of renal function, a urinalysis, complete blood count (CBC), platelet count, prothrombin time, and partial thromboplastin time should be obtained if systemic symptoms are present.

3. **Treatment**

   a. **Conservative management** of the early bite wound with bandaging and immobilization to prevent further trauma to the area is appropriate. Most small lesions regress without treatment. Overzealous treatment (including early excision and local steroid injection) may produce more harm than good, resulting in increased scarring or cutaneous atrophy.

   b. **Tetanus prophylaxis** should be provided, if needed.

   c. **Analgesics** should be administered as necessary.

   d. **Antihistamines** are useful if itching is a symptom.

   e. **Antibiotics** are indicated only if secondary bacterial infection is demonstrated by cultures.

   f. **Dapsone** in low doses (i.e., 50–100 mg per day) may be beneficial in the treatment of large cutaneous lesions of loxoscelism.

   g. High-dose systemic **steroids** (i.e., the equivalent of 100 mg of prednisone/day) are administered when there is evidence of hemolysis or renal failure.

   h. Dialysis may be necessary to manage renal failure.

4. **Disposition.** Close patient follow-up is important; patients should be referred to a specialist if an indolent ulcer develops. Hospitalization is indicated for patients with systemic loxoscelism to provide adequate hydration and other supportive measures.

B. **Black widow spider bites** are produced by *Latrodectus mactans,* a globular black spider with a red hourglass mark on its ventral surface. Envenomation usually produces only minor discomfort at the bite site, but the neurotoxic venom may produce significant systemic symptoms.

   1. **Clinical manifestations.** The initial bite may go unnoticed; even with significant systemic symptoms, local bite wound manifestations may remain mild with minor discomfort, edema, and erythema surrounding punctate fang marks. Within one or more hours, severe cramps, fasciculations, muscle spasms, rigidity, pain, and ascending paralysis may ensue with progressive involvement of the more proximal muscle groups (i.e., abdominal, shoulder, chest, and back muscles). Rigidity and spasms are continuous and eventually involve all skeletal muscle groups. These symptoms may mimic peritonitis, acute myocardial infarction, or pneumonia. Other systemic symptoms may include fever, diaphoresis, nausea, vomiting, dyspnea, paresthesias, extreme restlessness, seizures, shock, cyanosis, and hyperreflexia.

   2. **Laboratory tests** may show a leukocytosis, albuminuria, or hematuria.

   3. **Treatment**

      a. For bite wound discomfort, **cold compresses** and a **steroid ointment** may be helpful.

      b. **Tetanus prophylaxis** should be provided, if needed.

      c. **Calcium gluconate,** 10 ml of a 10% solution, is slowly infused intravenously for muscle spasms, rigidity, and pain. It is both diagnostic and therapeutic and may be repeated at 4-hour intervals.

      d. **Diazepam** by slow IV infusion in doses of 1–5 mg for infants and toddlers, and up to 10 mg for older children and adults, may be used to treat apprehension, nausea, and muscle spasms.

      e. **Methocarbamol** (Robaxin), 10 ml, may be given by slow IV infusion for continuous and severe muscle spasms.

      f. An **analgesic** should be administered as needed for pain relief, with cautious use of narcotics to avoid respiratory depression.

      g. Specific **antivenin** (made from horse serum) is reserved for critical envenomation. Administration of antivenin must be preceded by skin testing; the usual dose is 2.5 ml IV (or IM). The need for antivenin, however, is rare.

   4. **Disposition.** Hospitalization is required for patients with systemic manifestations of latrodectism.

C. **Scorpion stings** produced by most species are of little significance, causing only local pain and edema that lasts up to several hours. Envenomation by *Centruroides sculpturatus,* endemic to the Southwest, however, can be serious. Immediate excruciating local pain and itching can be relieved with application of cold compresses, household ammonia, or a steroid ointment. IV diazepam (up to 5 mg for infants and 5–10 mg for adults), methocarbamol (10 ml), and/or calcium gluconate (10 ml of a

10% solution) may be infused to counteract apprehension, fasciculations, and seizures. Atropine sulfate in IM doses of 0.3 mg may be used to reduce hypersalivation. However, epinephrine and narcotics are contraindicated, since they may potentiate the effects of the venom.

D. Tick bites may be problematic because various diseases can be transmitted to humans via tick vectors. The local bite wound may display signs of inflammation for several days; symptomatic treatment with an anti-inflammatory ointment and antihistamines may be helpful. For bite wounds with persistent inflammation beyond 2 weeks, excision is recommended since this inflammation may represent foreign body reaction to retained fragments of the tick's head.

E. Hymenoptera stings are produced by bees, wasps, hornets, yellow jackets, ants, and membranous-winged insects. Over 25% of the world's inhabitants are hypersensitive to Hymenoptera venoms. The effects of envenomation vary, depending on the venom components, volume injected, patient hypersensitivity, and site of the sting.

  1. Clinical manifestations. Local findings may be limited to itching, burning pain, swelling, and urticaria. Systemic symptoms include nausea, vomiting, anxiety, and a heavy feeling in the chest; fatal anaphylactic reactions can occur.

  2. Treatment

   a. Immediate **removal of the stinger,** if present in the wound, is indicated. The stinger is retrieved with a No. 11 scalpel blade or needle. Squeezing or tweezing to remove the stinger is contraindicated, since this may cause additional venom injection.

   b. Local pain is relieved by application of cold compresses and elevation. Lidocaine 0.5 or 1.0% with epinephrine 1:100,000 can be injected into the affected area.

   c. An analgesic, antihistamine, and/or steroid ointment or calamine lotion may be used to relieve **local wound discomfort.**

   d. Tetanus prophylaxis should be given, if needed.

   e. Treatment of **significant local manifestations** includes diphenhydramine hydrochloride, 25–50 mg PO qid for several days, and/or prednisone, 20–40 mg PO once daily for several days, followed by rapid tapering of the dose.

   f. Generalized **urticaria** (see Chap. 31) can be treated with epinephrine (0.3–0.5 ml, or 0.01 ml/kg in children, of a 1:1000 solution), injected subcutaneously and repeated in 30 minutes if necessary, unless contraindicated. Diphenhydramine, corticosteroids, and/or baking soda baths may also be helpful.

   g. Bronchospasm not relieved by epinephrine is treated with IV aminophylline, 6 mg/kg given over 20–30 minutes. Oxygen should be administered; assisted ventilation may be required.

   h. Hypotension is treated aggressively with IV fluids, epinephrine SC or IV (depending on the patient's condition), and other standard life-support measures.

   i. Preventive care (e.g., avoidance of areas infested with stinging insects, brightly colored clothing, and perfumes) is advised. Commercial kits with preloaded syringes containing epinephrine and antihistamine tablets are available for patients prone to anaphylaxis.

  3. Disposition. Patients with acute urticaria should be observed for at least 2 hours. Hospitalization is indicated for patients with hypotension, upper airway obstruction, or persistent bronchospasm. Other patients may be referred to an allergist for hyposensitization.

V. Marine fauna bites

A. Marine animal stings are produced by coelenterates, including **jellyfish, Portuguese man-of-war, sea anemones, hydras, and corals,** whose dominant characteristic is the presence of tentacles equipped with venom-containing nematocysts that are activated by contact (see Chap. 31).

  1. Clinical features. Injurious effects resulting from nematocysts embedded on and in the skin range from a mild dermatitis to instant death. Intense local pain may be present, extending proximally along the affected limb, similar to an electric shock. Generalized symptoms such as headache, urticaria, shock, muscle cramps, nausea, and vomiting may also occur.

  2. Treatment consists of pulling off any adherent tentacles, inactivating the nematocysts by flushing the involved skin with alcohol followed by household ammonia, and applying a paste of baking soda or flour, which removes the remaining nematocysts when moistened with water and scraped off about 1 hour later. Tetanus prophylaxis is administered, as indicated. Allergic reactions are treated with an antihistamine or corticosteroids or both. Severe systemic reactions are treated with the usual supportive measures. Muscle spasms and rigidity may be treated with 10% calcium gluconate, given by slow IV infusion.

B. Aquatic puncture wounds are produced by marine animals with spines, such as **segmental worms, sea urchins, conus shells, stingrays, catfish, and spiny fish.** Slime and debris can be introduced into puncture wounds produced by spines, some of which also contain venom apparatuses. **Treatment** consists of debridement of the puncture wound, exploration to remove any foreign body (including spine), and irrigation to remove venom. Hot-water immersion of the injured area for at least 60 minutes is recommended for stingray injuries to deactivate its heat-labile venom. Tetanus prophylaxis (as indicated), broad-spectrum antibiotic coverage, and an analgesic (if necessary) are provided. Patients with systemic symptoms should be hospitalized, and supportive therapy instituted. Wounds that remain painful, swollen, and infected days after the initial injury must be explored for a possible retained foreign body.

Miscellaneous Disorders

I. Ingrown toenail. When the edge of the nail plate cuts into the adjacent soft tissue of the lateral nailfold (eponychium), an ingrowing nail develops.

A. Characteristic features include episodic pain, erythema, and swelling as injury to the eponychium occurs. Although this process may involve fingernails, toenails are affected much more commonly. Factors predisposing to the development of an ingrowing toenail are an abnormal lateral nail plate curvature, pressure from shoes on the soft tissues about the nail plate margin, and any process (e.g., trauma, infection) that alters the normal anatomy of the nail plate, sterile matrix, and/or adjacent soft tissues. Bacterial infection of the eponychium injured by an ingrowing toenail can occur at any time but achieves clinical significance primarily in patients with diabetes mellitus or peripheral vascular disease. With decreased circulation to the toe, infection becomes more difficult to treat, and gangrene may ensue. Thus, an ingrown toenail in the presence of a decreased blood supply may herald the first stage of a pathologic process that ultimately ends in amputation.

B. Treatment

1. **Removal of the involved lateral edge of the nail plate** is performed under digital block anesthesia. When the toe is numb, the portion of the nail plate to be removed can be detached from the sterile matrix by inserting a straight scissors or a straight hemostat beneath it and employing a spreading motion. The nail plate is then cut longitudinally with a scissors or scalpel blade to just beneath the proximal nail fold, and the lateral portion of the nail plate is removed (with some tugging or pulling). Hemostasis is achieved with local pressure; if chronic granulation tissue is present, it is cauterized. The wound is Gram stained and cultured. The wound is then packed with petrolatum gauze or dry gauze impregnated with povidone-iodine (Betadine) ointment, and a larger, dry gauze dressing is applied.

2. **Tetanus prophylaxis** is administered, as indicated.

3. An **antibiotic** is prescribed, based on the Gram stain of the wound, if infection is suspected.

4. An **analgesic** is prescribed, as necessary.

5. The patient is instructed regarding leg elevation, minimal ambulation for several days, and dressing changes 2–4 times daily. Adherent dressings may be soaked off, and the wound washed under running warm water with each dressing change. If the packing falls out, it should be replaced with lubricated gauze until the eponychium becomes adherent laterally. Dressing changes are discontinued when the open wound has healed.

6. As the lateral nail plate regrows, the eponychium may periodically have to be pushed laterally to prevent recurrent ingrowing of the nail plate until it has grown past the distal skin margin of the toe.

7. The patient is instructed both in trimming the nail plate straight across when regrowth is complete and in avoiding recurrent pressure from shoes or other obvious sources of trauma to the area.

C. Disposition. Patient follow-up is necessary until nail plate regrowth is complete (i.e., 6 months). Patients with associated disease (e.g., diabetes mellitus, peripheral vascular disease) should be referred to a specialist immediately. Patients with recurrent infected ingrowing toenails are referred to a specialist for extirpation of the involved germinal matrix.

II. **Cutaneous ulcers.** Skin loss resulting from vascular disease (see Chap. 20), trauma, or prolonged pressure produces cutaneous ulcers that occur on any part of the body but are found most commonly on the lower extremities. Cutaneous ulcers are frequently painful, almost always contaminated by bacteria, and at constant risk for invasive infection; underlying systemic disease often retards healing. Longstanding lesions are also at risk of undergoing neoplastic change (e.g., epidermoid carcinoma).

A. **Ischemic ulcers** are caused by chronic arterial insufficiency, i.e., large- or small-vessel occlusive disease.

1. **Clinical manifestations.** Ischemic ulcers are usually located on the toes and feet, but are occasionally found on the lower leg or ankle without foot involvement. One or more of the following signs and symptoms of large-vessel occlusive disease are present: hair loss from the toes; brittle, opaque nails; atrophic, shiny skin; atrophy of foot muscles; dependent rubor; pallor with extremity elevation; decreased skin temperature; decreased or absent distal pulses; bruits over proximal limb arteries; prolonged venous filling time; significant pain, often relieved by holding the extremity in a dependent position; and a history of intermittent claudication.

2. **Evaluation** should include a wound culture and x-rays to rule out osteomyelitis.

3. **Treatment**
   a. A **dry dressing** should be applied to prevent further trauma and contamination to the area; a topical antibiotic ointment may be applied, but in small quantities to prevent adjacent skin maceration.
   b. **Tetanus prophylaxis** should be provided, if needed.
   c. **Systemic antibiotics** are of little benefit because of the decreased local blood supply; they are indicated only if frank signs of cellulitis or lymphangitis are present.

4. **Disposition.** These patients should be referred to a specialist for management and evaluation for arterial revascularization of the extremity, which may be the primary treatment for some ischemic ulcers.

B. **Venous stasis ulcers** are caused by chronic venous insufficiency resulting from varicose veins, incompetent perforators, or deep vein thrombosis. The common abnormality is reflux of blood from deficient or incompetent venous valves.

1. **Clinical features** include one or more of the following: (1) an ulcer usually located posterior to the medial or lateral malleolus; (2) chronic stasis changes around the ulcer (e.g., brownish skin discoloration and brawny induration); (3) a surrounding dermatitis (e.g., dry, scaling, pruritic skin; allergic dermatitis secondary to local medications); (4) chronic pitting edema, often progressive throughout the day, especially with prolonged standing and sitting; (5) symptoms of aching, tenderness, or heaviness in the involved lower extremity, usually related to edema; (6) superficial varicosities; (7) normal peripheral pulses; (8) pain at the site of ulceration, usually worse in the presence of infection; and (9) a history of deep vein thrombosis or thrombophlebitis.

2. **Evaluation** should include a wound Gram stain and culture and x-rays to assess for osteomyelitis.

3. **Treatment**
   a. **Debridement** of fibrotic, indolent granulation tissue is indicated if adequate local anesthesia can be obtained. Slow debridement can be achieved with wet-to-dry dressing changes, i.e., coarse mesh gauze saturated with saline or tap water and wrung out (to avoid skin maceration), applied to the ulcer 2–4 times daily, and removed dry to remove superficial debris.
   b. **Tetanus prophylaxis** is administered, if necessary.
   c. Systemic **antibiotics** are indicated only for an associated cellulitis or lymphangitis. Topical antibiotics should be avoided to prevent additional problems from an allergic dermatitis.
   d. **Leg elevation** above heart level and avoidance of standing and sitting (except with leg elevation) are important therapeutic measures. However, walking is permitted since muscle contractions help venous return.
   e. **Compression therapy** (e.g., with an ace bandage or Jobst pressure-gradient stocking) is almost always helpful but may be too uncomfortable during the acute treatment phase.

4. **Disposition.** Patients should be referred to a specialist for follow-up of this long-term, often recurrent problem and for possible surgical treatment.

C. **Diabetic ulcers** are usually caused by small-vessel occlusive disease. Since diabetic ulcers often occur in areas of excessive callus formation on the toes and plantar surface of the foot, particularly over the metatarsal heads, skin anesthesia from the peripheral neuropathy of diabetes combined with local pressure is another presumed etiologic factor. In addition, there may be signs and symptoms of large-vessel occlusive disease or chronic venous insufficiency or both. Patients must be carefully evaluated for ulcer etiology, diabetes control, and evidence of infection. Standard **management** includes obtaining a wound culture and x-rays, tetanus prophylaxis, and application of a dressing (preferably dry). Specialist referral for possible surgical intervention or diabetes management (or both) is indicated.

D. **Vasculitic ulcers** are painful, small, round, punched-out ulcerations seen in the lower extremities of patients with collagen vascular disease. The diagnosis is established by a biopsy of the ulcer. These ulcers require standard local wound evaluation and management, plus referral to a specialist, since the onset of vasculitic ulcers is usually associated with exacerbation of the collagen vascular disease. Healing is prolonged and usually best accomplished by the slow process of wound contraction and epithelialization.

E. **Traumatic ulcers** are due to acute injuries with prolonged healing of the skin and soft tissues. Although they may be associated with underlying vascular occlusive disease, chronic venous insufficiency, diabetes mellitus, or other systemic factors that retard wound healing, they also occur in otherwise healthy, young individuals because of altered local vasculature (arterial or venous), infection, envenomation with dermonecrotoxins (brown recluse spider bites), retained foreign bodies, and/or tissue loss. Management consists of standard patient and wound evaluation, local wound care, and referral to a specialist for treatment of any associated systemic disease or for reconstruction of lost tissues.

F. **Pressure sores** result from excessively long compression of soft tissues between a bony prominence and an external object. The discomfort from ischemic changes that cause the average individual to change position under these circumstances is not felt by the patient with skin anesthesia (e.g., paraplegic), or the patient may be too ill or weak to change position. Contributing factors are friction, contusion, spasticity, and malnutrition. Prolonged pressure causes tissue anoxia and small-vessel thrombosis with subsequent necrosis. When the necrotic tissue sloughs or is debrided, an ulcer is left. The most common sites for pressure sores are over the sacrum, greater trochanter, and ischial tuberosity.

1. **Clinical manifestations** may include the following: (1) presence of skin erythema over a bony prominence with or without underlying induration, superficial skin blistering, or excoriation; (2) presence of a dry, black eschar over a bony prominence; (3) presence of a draining, foul-smelling necrotic ulcer over a bony prominence (the underlying bone may be visible or palpable at the base of the ulcer, and the surrounding skin may or may not be erythematous); and (4) evidence of a systemic illness, ranging from simple fever to sepsis and shock associated with an infected pressure sore.

2. **Evaluation.** Radiographs should be obtained to assess for osteomyelitis or gas in the soft tissues. A urinalysis, urine culture, and chest x-ray are obtained in patients with systemic symptoms (a necrotic pressure sore should be assumed to be the etiology of a systemic illness until proved otherwise).

3. **Management**
   a. **Early pressure changes** (e.g., skin erythema with superficial skin loss only and absence of systemic symptoms) may be managed by avoidance of pressure on the area and use of drying agents or procedures (e.g., exposure to air, application of thimerosal [Merthiolate], use of a hair dryer on a "cool" setting).
   b. **Dry eschars** can be treated conservatively but require close follow-up.
   c. All **other pressure sores** require a Gram stain and culture and excision of all necrotic tissues with appropriate hemostasis; the wound is packed loosely with gauze moistened with a saline or povidone-iodine solution. Tetanus prophylaxis is administered, if necessary. Systemic antibiotics are administered (based on the Gram stain or to provide broad-spectrum coverage) if there are signs of infection. These patients usually require hospitalization and are referred to a specialist for surgical treatment (i.e., excision of the ulcer and underlying bony prominence and flap tissue coverage).

G. **Miscellaneous ulcers** include those caused by sickle cell disease (which usually occur on the lower extremities), Buerger's and Raynaud's disease (which usually involve the digits of the upper extremities), and those of mixed arterial and venous etiology occurring in the lower extremities. Fictitious ulcerations must also be considered. Standard principles of patient and wound evaluation, local wound management, treatment of underlying disease, and referral to a specialist apply.

III. **Gangrene.** Acute or chronic loss of arterial blood supply to any portion of the body produces tissue death, i.e., gangrene. Gangrene occurs most commonly in the toes and feet but, depending on the etiology and mechanism of vascular occlusion, can occur elsewhere as well. Vascular occlusion may be secondary to emboli, thrombi, atherosclerotic plaques, increased blood viscosity with sludging, intense vasoconstriction, or vasospasm. The process may involve large or small vessels or both. Gangrene is most common in patients with atherosclerotic peripheral vascular disease or diabetes mellitus. It also occurs in patients with vasospastic disease (i.e., Raynaud's or Buerger's disease), following frostbite injuries, or with certain types of necrotizing infections (e.g., gas gangrene). Ischemic ulcers and pressure sores are preceded by localized areas of gangrene.

A. **Dry gangrene** refers to tissue necrosis in the absence of infection. The characteristic lesion of dry gangrene is a black crust surrounded by a zone of erythematous skin, the zone of demarcation. Skin erythema in areas of chronic arterial insufficiency (including chronic localized pressure) may precede frankly gangrenous changes. It is often difficult to judge the depth of tissue necrosis and how much tissue in the zone of demarcation will ultimately remain viable. When gangrene involves a digit, the full thickness of a part or the whole length of the toe or finger is usually black and mummified with a proximal zone of demarcation. Dry gangrene is frequently painless and may heal spontaneously, with the development of collateral circulation and separation of the black eschar as epithelialization occurs beneath it over a period of time (i.e., autoamputation).

1. **Evaluation.** Careful patient evaluation is important to determine the etiology of the lesion and the nature and extent of underlying disease. Careful wound evaluation is essential to rule out infection. X-rays are necessary to assess for osteomyelitis.

2. **Treatment** of dry gangrene is directed toward conserving as much tissue as possible by preventing progression of tissue necrosis and secondary bacterial infection.

   a. **Application of a dry dressing** is indicated to prevent skin maceration, bacterial contamination, and further trauma.

   b. If infection is absent, the eschar is not debrided.

   c. **Tetanus prophylaxis** is administered, if needed.

   d. **Analgesics** are administered as necessary.

   e. **Patient instructions** include keeping the area dry and meticulously clean and preventing further trauma.

   f. **Intraarterial reserpine** may be indicated for gangrene due to vasospastic disease to prevent progressive ischemia and necrosis.

3. **Disposition.** These patients should be referred to a specialist for consideration for arterial reconstruction or amputation and treatment of associated systemic disease. Close patient follow-up is essential.

B. **Wet gangrene** occurs when there is bacterial invasion of necrotic tissue, producing a moist, draining, often painful, malodorous black eschar or ulcer. Cellulitis and edema may be superimposed on the zone of demarcation.

1. **Evaluation** involves a wound Gram stain and culture and x-rays to assess for osteomyelitis and soft-tissue gas.

2. **Treatment** is directed toward control of the infection to prevent additional tissue necrosis.

   a. **Debridement** of all necrotic and infected tissues is indicated.

   b. Dry **dressings** or dressings moistened with povidone-iodine solution are applied to the gangrenous area and changed 2–4 times daily. The purpose of dressings is to debride superficial wound debris, prevent further bacterial contamination and trauma, and absorb wound drainage, while preventing skin maceration.

   c. Systemic **antibiotics** are administered, based on the Gram stain (or to provide broad-spectrum coverage).

   d. **Tetanus prophylaxis** is administered, if needed.

   e. **Analgesics** are given as needed.

3. **Disposition.** Hospitalization is generally indicated, with referral to a specialist for arterial reconstruction or amputation and treatment of associated systemic disease.

IV. **Cysts and tumors.** A large variety of skin and subcutaneous lesions present as cysts or tumors, which generally are best treated by specialists under nonemergent conditions.
- A. **Keratinous cysts,** epidermal or pilar type, are round, moderately firm subcutaneous lesions that can occur on any part of the body. The etiology of keratinous cysts is unknown; they usually occur in adults but can also occur in children. The material within the cyst is keratin (the term **sebaceous cyst** is a misnomer), which presumably accumulates because there is no avenue of escape from beneath the skin surface.
  1. **Clinical features.** Keratinous cysts range from a few millimeters to several centimeters in size and may slowly enlarge. A dark skin punctum is sometimes present over the subcutaneous mass, which is usually attached at some point to the overlying skin. There may be an antecedent history of trauma (with trapping of epithelium subcutaneously); a history of drainage of thick, white, cheesy material from the punctum; or a history of previous inflammation involving the lesion. Keratinous cysts sometimes rupture, producing an intense inflammatory response to keratin in the subcutaneous tissues; in this situation, patients present to the emergency department with a swollen, red, painful area where they previously noted a subcutaneous lump. *S. epidermidis* is the most frequent organism cultured; however, the lesion may be sterile. Occasionally, the inflammatory process associated with rupture will destroy the entire cyst wall, and the lesion will resolve. Several weeks or months must elapse following acute rupture to distinguish the difference between indurated scar tissue and residual cyst.
  2. Adequate **treatment** of keratinous cysts consists of total excision, including all portions of the cyst wall, to prevent recurrence. If there is inflammation, however, incision and drainage and other steps of cutaneous abscess management (see **Soft-Tissue Infections**, sec. II.B) are indicated; adjunctive antibiotics may or may not be used. Because of the intense inflammatory reaction, it is difficult to adequately anesthetize the area and also impossible to identify the wall of the cyst when acute rupture has occurred. Excision of the entire lesion is thus delayed for several weeks or months, or at least until all evidence of inflammation has subsided.
- B. **Capillary (strawberry) hemangiomas** usually appear shortly after birth and may enlarge progressively up to the age of 12 months. They can be found on any part of the body. Capillary hemangiomas consist of bright red, sometimes bluish-red, raised lesions of the skin surface and may have a subcutaneous component that is soft and compressible. Over 95 percent of capillary hemangiomas undergo spontaneous involution by 8 years of age or earlier with minimal or no scarring. The onset of spontaneous involution is marked by the appearance of white or gray areas (herald spots) in the center of the lesion. These areas gradually enlarge and are accompanied by flattening of the lesion. Ulceration of capillary hemangiomas sometimes occurs, especially in the diaper area. Significant bleeding from areas of ulceration is rare but can be of concern to parents. Ulcerated hemangiomas are treated with air drying (which is difficult in infants) or wound care consisting of appropriate cleansing to prevent bacterial infection and application of dressings lubricated with povidone-iodine ointment (to prevent recurrent trauma with each dressing change). When applicable, a moderate pressure dressing technique is employed, since pressure may hasten the normal involution process. Parental reassurance regarding spontaneous involution of most capillary hemangiomas is indicated, pointing out that scarring from involution is almost always less than that produced by surgical treatment. Referral to a specialist is indicated for lesions involving eyelids or any orifice, ulcerated lesions or lesions that continue to enlarge after 12 months of age, or if help with parental reassurance is needed.
- C. **Cavernous hemangiomas and lymphangiomas** (cystic hygromas) occurring in the neck of children sometimes enlarge suddenly, prompting an emergency department visit. The patient's airway must be carefully evaluated; if airway compromise is imminent, immediate control of the airway and referral to a specialist are indicated.
- D. **Pyogenic granulomas** are rapidly enlarging, vascular, papular lesions that bleed readily with slight trauma. They are round, red, often sessile lesions that frequently occur following minor trauma. They presumably represent exuberant granulation tissue. **Treatment** consists of excision and wound closure or electrocautery of the base of the lesion. The tissue removed must be sent to pathology for histologic examination to confirm the diagnosis and exclude a neoplastic process. Pyogenic granulomas sometimes recur following treatment.

Bibliography

1. Anderson, P. C. Necrotizing spider bites. *Pract. Ther.* 26:198, 1982.
2. Converse, J. M. (ed.). *Reconstructive Plastic Surgery* (2nd ed.). Philadelphia: Saunders, 1977.
3. Grabb, W. C., and Smith, J. W. (eds.). *Plastic Surgery* (3rd ed.). Boston: Little, Brown, 1979.
4. Grossman, J. A. *Minor Injuries and Disorders: Surgical and Medical Care.* Philadelphia: Saunders, 1982.
5. Haddad, L. M., and Winchester, J. F. (eds.). *Clinical Management of Poisoning and Drug Overdose.* Philadelphia: Saunders, 1983.
6. King, L. E., Jr., and Rees, R. S. Dapsone treatment of a brown recluse bite. *J.A.M.A.* 250:646, 1983.
7. Medical Letter. Treatment of snakebite in the USA. *Med. Lett. Drugs Ther.* 24:87, 1982.
8. Peacock, E. E., Jr. *Wound Repair* (3rd ed.). Philadelphia: Saunders, 1984.
9. Walt, A. J. (ed.). *Early Care of the Injured Patient* (3rd ed.). Philadelphia: Saunders, 1982.
10. Wray, R. C., Holtmann, B., and Weeks, P. M. Factors in the production of inconspicuous scars. *Plast. Reconstr. Surg.* 56:86, 1975.

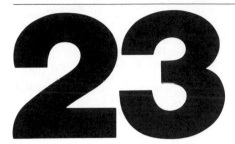

Hand Injuries and Infections

V. Leroy Young

Hand Examination

I. **Anatomy.** The hand and digits have dorsal and volar surfaces and radial and ulnar borders. The palm is divided into the thenar, hypothenar, and midpalmar areas. The digits should be referred to as the thumb and index, long, ring, and little fingers. The thenar mass corresponds to that muscular area on the palmar surface overlying the thumb metacarpal; the hypothenar area corresponds to the muscle mass on the palmar surface overlying the little finger metacarpal. Each finger has three joints: the metacarpophalangeal (MCP) joint, the proximal interphalangeal (PIP) joint, and the distal interphalangeal (DIP) joint. In contrast, the thumb has only an MCP and an interphalangeal (IP) joint. There are proximal, middle, and distal phalanges in the fingers and a proximal and distal phalanx in the thumb. The proximal part of each metacarpal and phalanx is referred to as the base, and the distal aspect as the head.

There are eight carpal bones divided into two rows. In the proximal carpal row beginning on the radial side are the scaphoid, lunate, triquetrum, and pisiform. Bones in the distal carpal row are the trapezium, trapezoid, capitate, and hamate.

II. **History.** Prior to any hand examination, a detailed history of the present problem should be obtained. This history should include the patient's age, occupation, pursuits, and the dominant hand. Any previous hand impairment or injury should also be documented. In the case of injuries, the following should always be sought: (1) the time when the injury occurred, (2) the place (e.g., at work, home, or play) and under what conditions (e.g., clean versus dirty environment) it occurred, (3) the mechanism (e.g., crushing force, laceration) of the injury, (4) the status of the wound (e.g., clean versus contaminated) and the extent of blood loss, (5) the posture of the hand at the time of injury, and (6) the nature of any treatment that may have been rendered prior to examination. For nontraumatic problems, emphasis should be placed on (1) the timing and sequence of signs and symptoms, including pain, sensory changes, and swelling; (2) any functional impairment, particularly with respect to the patient's occupation or hobbies; (3) any involvement of joints or tendons; (4) any activities that make the symptoms worse; and (5) any history of prior problems.

III. **Physical examination.** The entire upper extremity should be exposed when the hand is examined. Active and passive shoulder and elbow motion and pronation and supination of the forearm should be determined, since abnormalities at these joints or in the arm or forearm can significantly affect hand function. Both the radial and ulnar pulses should be palpated and the hand inspected for color and capillary refill as measures of the circulation. The hand posture and any swelling or edema (which is an important cause of limited function of the hand) should be noted. Localized tenderness is one of the most important diagnostic signs in the hand evaluation and, if present, should be accurately localized and described in the physical examination. Likewise, skin sensibility is the most accurate means of assessing sensory nerve function and should be objectively measured (including determination of two-point discrimination) and recorded. Skin moisture can also be a helpful method of evaluating innervation, since it does not require the cooperation of the patient. Passive and active motion should be noted for the wrist, MCP, and IP joints of all digits. The range of motion can be simply and accurately measured with a small, pocket-sized goniometer, which should be available wherever hand examinations are routinely performed. Muscle strength should be tested against resistance. The ability to perform simple functions such as writing or identifying objects such as coins also should be tested. Just as important as an accurate examination is the accurate recording of the findings of the examination. Often, this record can be best portrayed by a simple diagram noting the location and extent of injuries, including any altered sensation, lacerations, fractures, or tendon injuries. This diagram provides a readily and easily interpretable record of the examination and the extent of the problem.

A. Skin. The general appearance of the skin of the hand should be noted, as should the presence or absence of edema, moisture, scars, calluses, skin lesions, or surface irregularities. Swelling is most often manifested on the dorsum of the hand, whereas the circulation is most easily evaluated on the palmar surface of the hand or in the nail beds. Absence of moisture indicates loss of sympathetic innervation.

B. Muscles. Intrinsic and extrinsic muscles provide the power that moves the hand. Systematic testing of these muscles for function and strength is essential.

  1. The **extrinsic muscles** have their origin in the forearm and their tendinous insertions in the hand. The flexor muscles are on the volar surface of the forearm and flex the wrist and the digits. The extensor muscles are on the dorsum of the forearm and extend the wrist and digits.

    a. Extrinsic flexor muscles

      (1) The **flexor pollicis longus muscle** has its tendinous insertion on the volar base of the distal phalanx of the thumb. It is evaluated by having the patient bend the tip of the thumb.

      (2) The **flexor digitorum profundus muscles** insert on the volar base of each distal phalanx. They are evaluated by having the patient bend the tip of each finger while the PIP joint is stabilized in extension.

      (3) The **flexor digitorum superficialis muscles** insert on the volar surface of the middle phalanges. They are individually tested by having the patient flex the specific finger at the PIP joint while the other fingers are stabilized in extension to block flexion produced by the flexor digitorum profundus.

      (4) The **flexor carpi ulnaris, flexor carpi radialis,** and **palmaris longus muscles** insert into the pisiform, the volar aspect of the index metacarpal, and the palmar fascia of the hand, respectively; the pulmaris longus muscle unit is absent in approximately 10% of patients. These muscles are evaluated by having the patient flex the wrist while the examiner palpates the tendons.

    b. The **extrinsic extensor muscles** lie on the dorsum of the forearm. Their tendons pass through six tendinous compartments of the dorsum of the wrist and insert in the hand. The tendons passing through each compartment should be systematically examined.

      (1) The **first dorsal wrist compartment** contains the tendons of the **abductor pollicis longus** and the **extensor pollicis brevis.** The abductor pollicis longus inserts on the dorsal base of the thumb metacarpal, and the extensor pollicis brevis inserts at the base of the proximal phalanx of the thumb. These tendons are evaluated by having the patient extend and radially deviate the thumb while the examiner palpates the tendons on the radial side of the wrist.

      (2) The **second dorsal wrist compartment** contains the **extensor carpi radialis longus** and **extensor carpi radialis brevis** tendons. These tendons insert at the base of the index and middle finger metacarpals, respectively. They are evaluated by having the patient make a fist and extend the wrist while the tendons are palpated over the dorsal and radial aspects of the wrist.

      (3) The **third dorsal wrist compartment** contains the **extensor pollicis longus** tendon as it passes around Lister's tubercle on the radius to insert at the dorsal base of the distal phalanx of the thumb. This muscle tendon unit is evaluated by having the patient extend the distal phalanx of the thumb.

      (4) The **fourth dorsal wrist compartment** contains the **extensor digitorum communis** tendons and the **extensor indicis proprius** tendon. These tendons insert on the base of the proximal and middle phalanges and are responsible for extension at the MCP and PIP joints. They are evaluated by having the patient actively extend the MCP and PIP joints. The extensor indicis proprius can be independently examined by having the patient extend the index finger while the other fingers are held in flexion.

      (5) The **fifth dorsal wrist compartment** contains the **extensor digiti minimi** tendon, which inserts through the tendon of the extensor digitorum on the dorsum of the little finger. This muscle-tendon unit is evaluated by having the patient actively extend the little finger (at the MCP joint) while the other fingers are held in flexion.

(6) The **sixth dorsal compartment** contains the tendon of the **extensor carpi ulnaris,** which inserts at the dorsal base of the little finger metacarpel. This muscle-tendon unit is evaluated by having the patient extend and ulnarly deviate the hand while the tendon is palpated at the ulnar side of the wrist just distal to the head of the ulna.

2. The **intrinsic muscles** of the hand have their origins and insertions within the hand. The specific muscles are the thenar muscle group, the adductor pollicis, the lumbricals, the interosseous muscles, and the hypothenar muscle group.

   a. The **thenar muscles,** which usually are innervated by the motor branch of the median nerve but occasionally partially or totally by the ulnar nerve, overlie the thumb metacarpal. Included in this group are the **abductor pollicis brevis, opponens pollicis,** and **flexor pollicis brevis.** These muscles pronate or oppose the thumb and are evaluated by having the patient touch the thumb and the little fingertip together. Another test for thenar muscle function is to have the patient place the dorsum of the hand flat on a table and raise the thumb so that it forms a 90-degree angle with the palm while the examiner palpates the thenar muscles for strength of contraction. It is important to compare thenar muscle function in both hands for any difference in muscle mass and function.

   b. The **adductor pollicis muscle,** which is innervated by the ulnar nerve, adducts the thumb. It is tested by having the patient forcibly hold a piece of paper between the thumb and the radial side of the proximal phalanx of the index finger. If this muscle is weak or nonfunctioning, the patient will pinch against the index proximal phalanx by flexing the IP joint of the thumb. Again, the function in both hands should be compared to detect subtle differences.

   c. The **interosseous and lumbrical muscles** flex the MCP joints of the fingers and extend the IP joints. The interosseous muscles, which lie on either side of the finger metacarpals, are innervated by the ulnar nerve; they also adduct and abduct the fingers. The function of these muscles is tested by having the patient spread the fingers apart while the examiner palpates the first dorsal interosseous on the radial side of the index finger metacarpal for the strength of contraction. Another test of interosseous muscle function involves having the patient hyperextend the middle finger at the MCP joint (with the IP joint held in extension to eliminate the function of the extrinsic extensor muscles) and ulnarly and radially deviate it. The two ulnarmost lumbrical muscles are innervated by the ulnar nerve, and the two radial lumbrical muscles are innervated by the median nerve. All four participate in extension of the IP joints.

   d. The **hypothenar muscles,** which are innervated by the ulnar nerve, consist of the **abductor digiti minimi, flexor digiti minimi,** and **opponens digiti minimi.** These muscles are evaluated as a group by palpating the muscle mass while the little finger is forcefully abducted away from the other digits.

C. **Nerves.** The median, ulnar, and radial nerves all are involved in the innervation and function of the hand. These nerves are evaluated by assessing the motor function of the muscles they innervate (see sec. **B**) and determining sensibility in the hand. The latter is evaluated by assessing light touch and two-point discrimination and noting whether sweating (moisture) is present or absent. Light touch is evaluated by having the patient either close the eyes or look away from the hand while the examiner strokes the pulp of the thumb or finger with a wisp of cotton; if the patient is able to feel this, light touch is intact or present. Two-point discrimination is evaluated by taking a paper clip, initially setting the points at 4–5 mm apart, and then, with the patient closing the eyes or looking away, touching the radial or ulnar aspect of the finger pulp with the tips of the clip oriented in a longitudinal direction; the amount of two-point discrimination present is recorded in millimeters. Normal two-point discrimination is less than 6 mm at the tips of the fingers. The presence or absence of sweating (moisture) can be assessed by looking at the pulp of the finger with an ophthalmoscope or magnifying lens. Absence of sweating signifies loss of sympathetic innervation to the skin.

1. The **median nerve** courses through the arm with the brachial artery and enters the forearm by passing through the pronator teres muscle. In the proximal

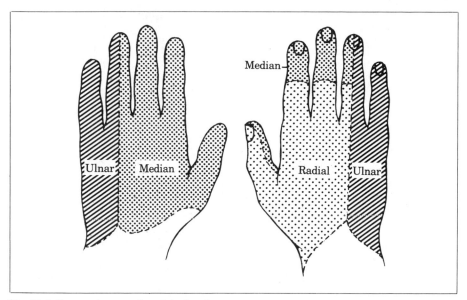

Fig. 23-1. Sensory innervation of the hand.

forearm, the median nerve innervates the flexor pronator muscles, which consist of the pronator teres, flexor carpi radialis, and palmaris longus. In the proximal forearm the anterior interosseous nerve branches from the main nerve trunk and innervates the flexor pollicis longus, flexor digitorum superficialis, radial half of the flexor digitorum profundus, and the pronator quadratus. The remainder of the main median nerve trunk passes through the volar aspect of the forearm, entering the hand through the carpal tunnel. Just distal to the transverse carpal ligament, the motor (recurrent) branch to the thenar muscles (i.e., abductor pollicis brevis, flexor pollicis brevis, opponens pollicis) separates from the sensory branches. In addition, the median nerve innervates the index and long finger lumbrical muscles. The sensory branches continue on to provide sensation to the thumb, index, long, and radial half of the ring fingers (Fig. 23-1).

2. The **ulnar nerve** passes from the arm into the forearm posterior to the medial epicondyle of the humerus. It enters the forearm between the two heads of the flexor carpi ulnaris muscle, innervating that muscle. Distally it innervates the flexor digitorum profundus muscle to the ring and little fingers. It then passes along the ulnar volar aspect of the forearm and gives off a dorsal sensory branch at the level of the ulnar styloid, which provides sensation to the dorsum of the ulnar side of the hand (see Fig. 23-1). The ulnar nerve then passes from the forearm into the hand through Guyon's canal, where it divides into motor and palmar sensory branches. The motor branches innervate all the interosseous muscles and the lumbrical muscles to the ring and little fingers. In addition, there are motor branches to the palmaris brevis, adductor pollicis, the hypothenar (digiti minimi) muscles, and all or part of the flexor pollicis brevis. The palmar sensory branches continue into the hand to provide sensation to the little finger and ulnar half of the ring finger (Fig. 23-1).

3. The **radial nerve** innervates the triceps, anconeus, brachioradialis, extensor carpi radialis longus and extensor carpi radialis brevis proximal to the elbow. At the elbow, the nerve divides into motor and sensory components. The sensory branch provides sensation to the radial side of the dorsum of the hand and the thumb (see Fig. 23-1). The motor branch, the posterior interosseous nerve, passes between the two heads of the supinator muscle, innervating it in its course. After exiting from the supinator, it continues dorsally and laterally, innervating the wrist and finger extensors, i.e., extensor digitorum communis, extensor digiti minimi, extensor carpi ulnaris, extensor pollicis longus, extensor

pollicis brevis, extensor indicis proprius, and abductor pollicis longus. The radial nerve does not innervate any of the intrinsic hand muscles.

D. **Circulation.** The blood supply to the hand comes from the radial and ulnar arteries through the superficial and deep palmar arches. Circulation in the hand is evaluated by observing skin color and capillary refill in the pulp and nail beds of the fingers. Capillary circulation within the nail bed is tested by compressing the nail bed and observing the time it takes for blanching to be replaced by a pink flush; normally, this is less than 2 seconds. The Allen test is useful in determining the patency of the radial and ulnar arteries. It is performed by compressing both arteries at the wrist and having the patient make a tight fist several times in succession to express blood from the fingers. The fingers are then extended and one artery is released; the hand is observed for extent and rate of capillary refill. The Allen test can also be performed on a single digit by expressing the blood from the digit, occluding both digital arteries, subsequently releasing one digital artery, and noting the capillary refill. The test is repeated, and this time the opposite artery is released. If there is a prompt flush in the hand or digit on release of the artery, the artery is patent. The Allen test can also be performed using a Doppler device. The Doppler is also useful in evaluating arterial flow in the fingers; this test is performed by placing the Doppler along the digital artery on the volar surface of the finger and tracing it distally as far as there is pulsatile flow. This procedure is very useful in detecting occlusions of digital arteries.

IV. **X-rays** are an integral component in the evaluation of hand injuries, infections, and suspected foreign bodies and should always be obtained when evaluating these problems. X-rays of the hand should include anteroposterior (AP), lateral, and oblique views. Any time a single digit is x-rayed, both an AP and lateral view should be obtained. The presence or absence of soft-tissue swelling, fractures, dislocations, subluxations, and foreign bodies should be noted. With regard to foreign bodies, most glass is radiopaque and hence may be demonstrated on x-rays.

Lacerations

I. **General management principles.** A systematic approach should be used in evaluating and examining patients with lacerations involving the forearm, wrist, or hand. Such an approach will prevent missing injuries, particularly tendon and nerve injuries.

A. **Control of bleeding.** Patients who present with bleeding following an injury should be made comfortable in a recumbent position, with the hand elevated and a sterile dressing applied. If bleeding continues, direct gentle pressure should be applied; this procedure will almost always control the bleeding. Clamping and tying of vessels in the hand should be avoided in order to prevent inadvertent and permanent damage to vital structures such as nerves and tendons.

B. **Examination.** Essentially all necessary information following an injury to the hand can be gained by a thorough and systematic examination of the forearm and hand (see **Hand Examination,** sec. III); the tendency to explore wounds to inspect for injured structures should be avoided initially. Furthermore, local anesthetics should not be injected until a thorough examination has been completed and recorded.

C. **Wound care.** Wounds should be copiously irrigated with saline. To avoid further tissue damage, antiseptic solutions should not be placed directly in the wound. Debridement should be kept to a minimum, as the hand is devoid of excess tissue. In repairing hand lacerations, it is best to avoid placing deep sutures. Tetanus prophylaxis should be administered if needed. However, antibiotics are not indicated unless there is evidence of contamination.

D. **Consultation.** If any questions exist regarding the evaluation and treatment of hand lacerations, consultation with a hand surgeon should be sought. In particular, suspected injury to vital structures, significant tissue loss, or gross contamination generally warrants consultation.

II. **Specific injuries**

A. **Fingertip injuries**

1. **Loss of skin and pulp only.** Amputations of the tips of the fingers or thumb without loss of bone can be treated by (1) allowing the area to heal by secondary intention, (2) skin grafting with split- or full-thickness skin grafts, or (3) local flaps.

a. **Healing by secondary intention.** In young children below the age of 13, the results of allowing the wound to heal by secondary intention are superior to those of any of the other techniques. Healing by secondary intention is also an excellent choice in other age groups for transverse amputations or amputations in which there is a relative excess of tissue on the volar surface following the amputation. This technique consists of dressing the amputated digit with Xeroform and gauze and changing the dressing daily. The patient should be followed closely by a surgeon who specializes in hand surgery. Healing will occur in 14–21 days, and the patient is often able to return to work within 1 month. Complications include cold intolerance, hypersensitivity in the area of the scar, and a volar curving of the nail at the amputation site.

  b. Treatment with skin grafts. Either full- or split-thickness skin grafts can be used for amputations of digits in which there is no exposed bone. If there is a small area of exposed bone, this approach may still be reasonable if sufficient bone can be removed with a rongeur to allow soft-tissue closure over the bone. There is controversy as to whether split-thickness or full-thickness skin grafts are better. Full-thickness skin grafts have the advantage that they contract minimally and the donor site can be placed in a concealed area and closed primarily. Split-thickness skin grafts have the advantage of being easy to obtain, but the disadvantage that the donor site is usually visible and cannot be closed primarily. Results following closure with skin grafts are usually excellent, although there is always altered sensation in the area of the skin graft. Wound healing is usually by primary intention, and there are few complications. These patients usually can return to work within 3–4 weeks.

  c. Local flaps. It is unusual to have to use local flaps when there is no exposed bone. Occasionally, local flaps will be necessary, and this decision should be made by an experienced hand surgeon.

2. Digital amputation with exposed bone

  a. Exposed bone in which soft-tissue closure is possible. Occasionally amputations with exposed bone can be closed primarily when the exposed bone can be eliminated with a rongeur. Closure either by direct suturing or by skin grafting may be used. The result following either of these techniques is good. Management and follow-up of these patients should be by an experienced hand surgeon.

  b. Exposed bone requiring closure by local flap techniques. Local flap techniques can be used to cover exposed bone when skin grafting or primary closure is not possible. The most useful of these techniques is the **volar VY advancement flap** described by Atasoy [2]. This procedure can be performed in the emergency department under digital block anesthesia; however, it should be performed by someone with experience in the management of hand problems. Follow-up should be by a hand surgeon.

3. Amputations of the tip of the thumb. Thumb tip amputations are unique in that they should be managed with the goal of maintaining normal sensation and length in the thumb. Generally, either primary closure or VY advancement flaps are perferred. If there is an amputation of the pulp or skin only, healing by secondary intention is still applicable. These patients should always be managed by a physician experienced in hand surgery.

4. Nail bed injuries

  a. Avulsion of the nail. Nail avulsions are extremely painful. Unless associated with lacerations of the nail bed or with avulsion of a portion of the nail bed, they rarely produce permanent disability or deformity. If the nail remains partially attached to the nail bed, it should be elevated under digital block anesthesia with a tourniquet and the nail bed examined to be certain there are no lacerations. If there are no lacerations and the nail is available, it should be cleansed and any soft tissue remaining on the volar surface removed. The nail is then replaced beneath the nail fold and sutured in place with 5-0 or 6-0 nylon sutures. The nail functions as both a splint and a protective covering for the nail bed until a new nail regrows. It takes approximately 6 months to complete regrowth of a new nail. If the nail is not available, Silastic sheeting should be placed beneath the nailfold and over the nail bed and anchored in place with 5-0 or 6-0 nylon sutures. When either Silastic sheeting or the nail is used to cover the nail bed, a hole should be drilled in the surface to allow drainage and prevent the occurrence of a subungual hematoma. Failure to place either the nail or Silastic sheeting beneath the nail fold can result in adherence of the nail fold to the nail bed, with subsequent deformity of the regrowing nail. These injuries are best managed by hand surgeons.

b. **Subungual hematomas** result from disruption of blood vessels in the nail bed. They are extremely painful, and the pain is of a throbbing, pulsatile nature. There is a blue or black discoloration of the involved area of the nail bed. Management depends on the area of the nail bed involved.

(1) **Subungual hematomas involving less than 25% of the nail bed.** These injuries usually require only drainage of the hematoma. The hematoma can be drained by drilling or burning a hole with the nail. A convenient way of burning a hole in the nail is to heat a paper clip in an alcohol lamp or bunsen burner until it is red hot and touch it to the nail overlying the hematoma. The paper clip will be cooled as it enters the blood in the hematoma and will not damage the nail bed. A small battery-powered electrocautery unit can also be used to burn a hole in the nail. There is almost always prompt relief of the pain when the hematoma is drained. These injuries should be followed by a hand surgeon, because there is a small risk of osteomyelitis of the distal phalanx with these injuries.

(2) **Subungual hematomas involving more than 25% of the nail bed** should be explored under digital block anesthesia with a tourniquet, because they are frequently associated with lacerations of the nail bed that need to be repaired. The nail should be gently elevated from the nail bed with either iris scissors or a freer elevator. The nail should be kept and put aside to be replaced as a splint. The nail bed should then be cleansed with saline and any lacerations repaired with 6-0 or 7-0 chromic sutures, ideally using loupe magnification. All suture knots should be left between the nail bed and the nail and not in the nail matrix. Soft tissue on the nail should be removed by scraping, and the nail replaced beneath the nail fold. The nail should then be sutured in place with 5-0 or 6-0 nylon. These injuries are best managed by a hand surgeon. Failure to properly repair these lacerations can result in a split nail deformity, irregular nail surface, or failure of the nail to adhere to the nail bed; these deformities are significant from both a cosmetic and a functional standpoint.

c. **Crushing lacerations** of the nail bed are complex and frequently result in both cosmetic and functional deformities of the nail. Proper management of these injuries is extremely important, because the results of proper early repair are always better than the results of nail reconstructive procedures. An x-ray should always be obtained since fractures of the distal phalanx are common. Crushing lacerations should be explored under digital block anesthesia using a tourniquet. If the nail is available, it should be salvaged to be used as a splint. The wound should be irrigated with saline, and careful inspection of the tissue made. If portions of the nail bed have not been avulsed, the edges should be minimally debrided and repaired (ideally under magnification) with 6-0 or 7-0 chromic sutures. Either the nail or a Silastic sheet should be used to splint the nail bed and nail fold. The patient should be placed on prophylactic antibiotics (e.g., a cephalosporin). These injuries should be managed by a hand surgeon.

d. **Fractures of the distal phalanx associated with nail bed lacerations** may be displaced or nondisplaced. If displaced, they should be properly reduced and internally fixated prior to nail bed repair. Nondisplaced fractures do not require internal fixation and can be managed by splinting with a plastic splint, such as a stack splint. Fractures associated with nail bed lacerations should be considered open fractures, and the patient should be treated with an antistaphylococcal antibiotic (e.g., cephalosporin) for 1 week.

B. **Human and animal bites.** See **Bites.**

Tendon Injuries

Tendon injuries can result from penetrating or blunt trauma.

I. **Evaluation**

A. **History.** Patients with potential tendon injuries should be evaluated by taking a good history, including the mechanism of injury (blunt or sharp trauma), extent of contamination (dirty versus tidy wounds), time of occurrence, and position of the digit at the time of injury. Since the excursion of flexor tendons is great, the position of the finger at the time of injury may markedly affect the location of the ends of the divided tendons. When there is no history of a specific injury and the patient presents with tenderness or popping consistent with de Quervain's stenosing tenosynovitis or trigger finger, an effort should be made to elicit a history of repetitive movements or repetitive trauma.

B. During the **physical examination,** the resting position of the digit and the location and nature of wounds should be noted. Fingers in which there are disrupted or divided tendons remain in an extended position, whereas uninjured digits usually remain in a semiflexed position. A thorough motor evaluation (see **Hand Examination,** sec. **III.B**) should always be performed when tendon injuries are possible. In addition, a careful sensory examination is important, since digital nerve injuries are often associated with tendon injuries.

II. Specific injuries

A. Flexor tendon injuries

1. Injuries to the flexor tendons to the **fingers** are classified into five zones.

   a. Zone I is in the distal finger at the level of the DIP joint just beyond the end of the digital sheath. Injuries here usually consist of either avulsions, as seen in football players, or lacerations. In zone I injuries the patient loses the ability to flex the distal phalanx. There is also tenderness over the digital sheath in the distal finger. In avulsion injuries there is frequently a small chip of bone seen on the lateral x-ray at the distal end of the tendon. If there is an open injury, the wound should be cleansed, debrided, and closed, proper tetanus prophylaxis administered, and the finger splinted; the patient should then be referred to a hand surgeon for immediate or early (within 2–3 days) repair. Closed injuries should be splinted and the patient referred to a hand surgeon for expeditious management. Splinting the digit in the position of function is usually best.

   b. Zone II extends from the distal interphalangeal flexion crease to the distal palmar crease. In this zone the flexor tendons are contained within the fibroosseous tunnel. Thus, repairs of tendon lacerations or disruptions in this area produce the poorest results of all zones. Digital nerve injuries are also frequently associated with these injuries. The most common cause of injury in this zone is penetrating trauma. In zone II the flexor digitorum profundus and superficialis tendons course together and either one or both may be injured. This injury can result in the inability to flex either the distal phalanx or both the distal phalanx and the PIP joint. Rarely the superficialis tendon alone will be divided, and there will be inability to flex the PIP joint with intact flexion of the DIP joint. Open injuries should be cleansed, the wound closed, and the patient referred to a hand surgeon within a few days for either immediate or delayed management. Patients with closed injuries should be promptly referred to a hand surgeon for expeditious management.

   c. Zones III, IV, and V extend from the distal palmar flexion crease to the forearm. Injuries in these zones are often associated with nerve injury. With these injuries there may be inability to flex one or more fingers at one or more joints. Disruptions of tendons in these zones are usually due to penetrating trauma. The tendons and nerves (if injured) should be repaired immediately or within several days by a person specializing in hand surgery. In zone V the results of tendon repair are usually excellent; however, the associated nerve injuries (if present) frequently produce long-term problems. Closed injuries are very rare in these zones.

2. The **thumb** is also divided into zones. Zone I extends from just proximal to the interphalangeal flexion crease to the insertion of the flexor pollicis longus tendon. Zone II extends from zone I to the MP joint, and zone III from the MP joint to the thenar muscle mass. Similar to the fingers, the flexor pollicis longus is within a fibroosseous tunnel from zone III to zone I. Since there is only one tendon within the sheath, the results of repair are usually good. Like injuries to the flexor tendons of the fingers, these injuries are usually open but may occasionally be closed avulsion injuries at the insertion of the flexor pollicis longus. They should be managed by either immediate or early repair, and care should be provided by a hand surgeon.

3. **Partial lacerations** of the flexor tendons are not uncommon, and the diagnosis is usually made by exploration of the digit. Repair is necessary only if there is a flap created by the laceration that could produce triggering or locking by catch-

ing the digital sheath. The injury should be managed by a hand surgeon, as the lacerations need to be protected for 3–6 weeks with protective splinting (in flexion), guarded physical therapy is also recommended.

B. Extensor tendon injuries

   1. Partial versus complete disruptions

   a. Partial disruptions of the extensor tendons usually result from open injuries. Whenever partial disruptions of these tendons are observed, a physician specializing in hand surgery should be contacted. The wound should then be inspected by the hand surgeon and a decision made as to whether the tendon requires repair or whether closure of the wound, splinting in extension, and closely supervised physical therapy are appropriate.

   b. Complete disruptions can result from either blunt or penetrating trauma. Closed disruptions at the level of the DIP or PIP joints are usually managed by splinting in extension for 6–8 weeks. If the injuries are open and there are no associated bony fragments, management is usually by direct repair or reinsertion of the tendons in the operating suite. If there are associated bony fragments that contain greater than one-fourth of the joint surface and are displaced, repair is by reinsertion of the bony fragments and immobilization with Kirschner wires. All of these wounds should be managed by a hand surgeon, and treatment should be either immediate or within several days.

   2. A **mallet finger deformity** (Fig. 23-2) can result from closed or open injuries. In either case there is loss of the ability to extend the distal phalanx on the middle phalanx.

   a. In **closed injuries** there may be either disruption of the extensor tendon from its insertion or avulsion of the tendon with a bony fragment. X-rays should always be obtained to determine if a bony fragment is present and, if so, how large a portion of the articular surface it contains. Essentially all of these injuries are treated by closed splinting in extension for 6–8 weeks, followed by graduated physical therapy. Injuries that involve a large portion of the articular surface or in which there is subluxation of the distal phalanx on the middle phalanx require open reduction and internal fixation by a hand surgeon.

   b. In **open injuries,** management should be immediate or early by a hand surgeon. If both tendon ends can be identified, direct repair of the tendon should be performed. This repair should be followed by internal fixation of the joint and splinting for 6–8 weeks with subsequent physical therapy.

   3. A **boutonniere deformity** (Fig. 23-3) may result from closed or open trauma to the dorsum of the PIP joint.

   a. The **mechanism** of the deformity is disruption of the central slip of the extensor tendon at the base of the middle phalanx; disruption of the central slip allows the lateral bands that normally lie dorsal to the axis of rotation of the PIP joint to drop below the axis of rotation of the joint and become paradoxical flexors of that joint. As the musculotendinous units shorten, they bring the DIP joint into hyperextension.

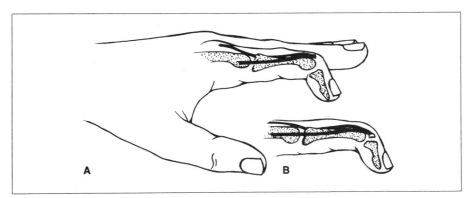

Fig. 23-2. Mallet finger deformity resulting from (A) disruption of the extensor tendon from its insertion at the distal phalanx or (B) avulsion of the tendon with a bony fragment (avulsion fracture).

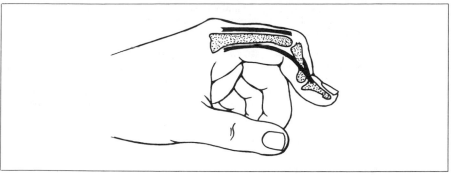

Fig. 23-3. Boutonniere deformity resulting from disruption of the central slip of the extensor tendon from its insertion at the dorsal base of the middle phalanx and subsequent volar displacement of the lateral bands yielding a flexion deformity at the proximal interphalangeal (PIP) joint.

  b. Management should be by a hand surgeon.
    (1) Acute injuries. When the injury is open, the tendon should be repaired or inserted into the base of the middle phalanx. This procedure is then followed by 6–8 weeks of immobilization and subsequent physical therapy. If the injury is closed and there is no bone chip avulsed with the tendon, treatment consists of splinting in extension for 6–8 weeks. If a large portion of the articular surface is associated with a disruption, the segment should be reattached to the base of the middle phalanx in anatomic position. If a small bone chip is avulsed and there is no subluxation of the middle phalanx on the proximal phalanx, the injury can be treated by splinting.
    (2) Patients with a **chronic boutonniere deformity** should be referred to a hand surgeon for appropriate management.
C. Nonspecific tenosynovitis
  1. De Quervain's stenosing tenosynovitis is a nonspecific inflammatory process involving the tendon sheath of the abductor pollicis longus and extensor pollicis brevis tendons.
    a. Clinical features. This tenosynovitis frequently follows minor trauma or repetitive motions. Thus, it is important to obtain an occupational history or a history of any hobby that involves repetitive motions. Patients frequently complain of pain over the area of the radial side of the dorsum of the wrist.
    b. The **diagnosis** can be established by palpable tenderness over the first dorsal compartment and by pain on extension of the thumb against resistance **(Finkelstein's test).**
    c. Management. Once the diagnosis is established, three treatment options exist: (1) injection of the tendon sheath with a steroid, (2) immobilization with a cast (3 weeks), or (3) operative release of the tendon sheath. Nonsteroidal anti-inflammatory drugs rarely work. The best initial treatment is injection of the tendon sheath with 20 mg of triamcinolone through a 27-gauge needle. If one or two injections do not relieve the symptoms within 2 weeks, the thumb and wrist should be immobilized for 3 weeks. If this treatment fails, surgical release of the tendon sheath is performed. Follow-up of these patients should be by a hand surgeon.
  2. Trigger finger or **trigger thumb** is a result of nonspecific tenosynovitis involving the flexor tendons and digital sheath. Although triggering can occur anywhere within the digital sheath, it is most common at the proximal end.
    a. Etiologies. Triggering results from blunt trauma, repetitive movements, or rheumatoid arthritis. Less commonly, it may be associated with metabolic disorders such as amyloidosis or mucopolysaccharidosis.
    b. Clinical features. Patients typically complain of two types of symptoms: (1) a popping, snapping, or locking sensation associated with the mechanical difficulty of moving the tendon through the tendon sheath and (2) pain related to the inflammation. There is usually a palpable pop or snap at the entrance to the digital sheath on physical examination. There may also be

tenderness over the proximal portion of the tendon sheath. It is not uncommon for patients to perceive the popping or locking sensation at the PIP joint; although much less common, the popping or locking sensation can also occur at the decussation of the superficialis tendons.

c. **Treatment** options consist of (1) injection of the tendon sheath with a steroid or (2) surgical release of the tendon sheath. Approximately 80% of patients will have either complete or near-complete relief of their symptoms with injection of 20 mg of triamcinolone into the tendon sheath. Although some hand surgeons recommend splinting following injection, most agree that there is no need for restriction of activity. If the injection is successful, relief usually occurs within 2 weeks. Patients who do not respond to one or two steroid injections should have surgical release of the tendon sheath.

Bone and Joint Injuries

I. **Fractures** of the bones of the hand may be closed or open (compound), single or comminuted, displaced or nondisplaced, angulated or not angulated, and with or without rotational deformity.

A. **Evaluation.** Signs suggestive of a fracture include tenderness, swelling, and deformity. The diagnosis is confirmed by appropriate radiographs that must include at least AP and lateral views. A careful physical examination is important to assess rotational alignment, which is best evaluated by observing the fingers in the flexed position, where they normally point toward the tubercle of the scaphoid and do not overlap (scissor).

B. **Specific fractures**

1. **Phalangeal fractures**

a. **Distal phalangeal fractures** are divided into those involving the tuft and the shaft.

(1) **Tuft fractures** usually result from blunt trauma, such as striking the end of the finger or thumb with a hammer. They are painful and, unless associated with an open laceration or markedly displaced, require only splinting for treatment. Healing may require as much as 3–4 months of immobilization, and these patients should be referred to a specialist for follow-up.

(2) **Fractures of the shaft of the distal phalanx** can be treated with splinting, if they are nondisplaced. If they are significantly displaced, reduction should be performed and the fragments immobilized with a splint. When they cannot be properly reduced and aligned or when the reduction cannot be maintained by closed techniques, internal fixation should be used. Open reduction is rarely necessary.

b. **Fractures of the middle phalanx,** exclusive of articular fractures, can be classified as open or closed, single or comminuted, and nondisplaced or displaced. Open fractures communicate with a wound or surface; since these fractures frequently are contaminated, the patient should be treated with an antibiotic. Due to the deforming forces exerted on the middle phalanx by the musculotendinous units that pass on the dorsal and volar surfaces, middle phalangeal fractures usually are displaced. Comminuted fractures involving multiple pieces are more prone to displacement than single fractures. Displacement of middle phalangeal fractures can be rotational or angular. In the middle phalanx there is only minimal tolerance for angulation or rotation; when either is present, the fracture should be anatomically reduced and stable immobilization established. Because of the deforming forces, it is rarely possible to maintain reduction with closed techniques, and internal fixation is usually necessary. Internal fixation offers the added advantage of allowing joint motion following reduction; motion of the joint tends to prevent joint stiffness, which is a major problem associated with closed reduction.

c. **Fractures of the proximal phalanx,** like fractures of the distal and middle phalanges, can be open or closed, single or comminuted, and nondisplaced or displaced. Also, like fractures of the middle phalanx, the musculotendinous units that pass around the bones tend to displace the fractures. Rotational deformities at the proximal phalanx produce a greater degree of overlap of the fingers on flexion (scissoring). Although this deformity can also result from middle phalangeal fractures, the more proximal the fracture occurs to the level of the metacarpal, the more scissoring is produced for any given degree of rotation. If the fractures are significantly displaced either in an angular or rotational fashion, they should be reduced and the reduction maintained by internal fixation. Fractures of the proximal phalanges require intense physical therapy following surgery. These patients should be followed by a specialist for 4–6 weeks to allow for healing, at which time the internal fixation device is removed.

2. **Metacarpal fractures** can also be open or closed, single or comminuted, and displaced or nondisplaced. Minor degrees of rotational deformity in the metacarpal produce significant overlap or scissoring on flexion. If the fractures are minimally displaced, they can be treated by closed reduction and splinting or casting. The further distal a fracture occurs, the more likely it is to be unstable and the more likely it will need reduction and internal fixation. Metacarpal fractures require 4–8 weeks to heal and should be referred to a specialist for follow-up.

   a. A **boxer's fracture** is a fracture of the neck of the little finger metacarpal. It usually results from altercations and is frequently associated with lacerations at the level of the MCP joint; these lacerations are often produced by the teeth of the other individual and are highly contaminated. These wounds should never be closed and should be treated with an antibiotic until the wound is healed, and then fracture management is initiated. Up to 40 degrees of angulation at the fracture site can be tolerated with a boxer's fracture as long as a good range of motion is maintained; these fractures can be treated with a protective splint or cast. If there is excessive angulation or rotation, a closed reduction should be performed; if the reduction is stable, the fracture can be managed by casting or splinting. If reduction is unsuccessful or cannot be maintained by closed techniques, internal fixation and occasionally open reduction are necessary. These fractures require 4–8 weeks to heal and should be referred to a specialist for treatment and long-term management.

   b. A **Bennett's fracture** is a fracture of the base of the thumb metacarpal in which the ulnar volar beak of the articular surface of the metacarpal is fractured free from the rest of the metacarpal. The abductor pollicis longus and extensor pollicis brevis pull the larger distal fragment proximally and dorsally, actively displacing it from the smaller proximal fracture fragment, which is maintained in position by the strong ligaments around the trapeziometacarpal joint. These fractures are almost always displaced because of the deforming forces and can rarely be treated without internal fixation. These fractures can usually be reduced by closed techniques and then internally fixed with Kirschner wires. Occasionally, open reduction and internal fixation are necessary. If a fracture is more than 3 or 4 weeks old, open reduction is almost always necessary.

3. **Intraarticular fractures.** The small joints in the hand have minimal tolerance for displacement of the articular surfaces. One to two millimeters of displacement of the articular surfaces can produce significant impairment of joint movement and result in early development of posttraumatic arthritis. Fractures in anatomic position should be treated by splinting and early mobilization. However, when there is displacement of the articular surfaces, open reduction and internal fixation are required, if possible. When the articular fracture is a single fracture with only two pieces, it usually can be reduced to near-anatomic position; rigid fixation can then be accomplished with internal fixation devices, such as screws or Kirschner wires. If the fracture is comminuted and there are multiple pieces that prevent anatomic reduction and internal fixation, the fracture should be treated by early mobilization and intense physical therapy. People with intraarticular fractures should be referred to a hand surgeon for treatment and follow-up.

4. **Fractures of the scaphoid.** The bone most often fractured in the wrist is the scaphoid. Typically, these patients have fallen on the wrist or have been struck on the wrist and present with tenderness in the anatomist's snuffbox. They may also have tenderness on hyperextension, flexion, and radial and ulnar deviation. Four views of the wrist including a scaphoid view should be obtained to evaluate for a fracture. Initial x-rays may fail to show a hairline fracture. If a patient has a typical history and physical findings for a scaphoid fracture, he or she should be immobilized in a short-arm thumb spica cast and referred to a special-

ist for reevaluation in 2 weeks. Usually by 2 weeks, sufficient bone resorption will occur at the fracture site to allow demonstration of the fracture radiographically. Occasionally, special studies such as magnification views, spot films, or a bone scan may be necessary to demonstrate a fracture. Since these fractures may require prolonged immobilization for as much as 4–6 months to allow healing, they should be followed by a hand surgeon. Avascular necrosis of the proximal portion of the scaphoid is a complication of these fractures.

II. **Dislocations and ligamentous injuries**
   A. **Dislocations at the DIP joint** can occur with or without a fracture and may be dorsal, volar, or lateral. The diagnosis is usually evident on physical examination and is confirmed by x-rays.
      1. **Dislocations without fractures**
         a. **Dorsal dislocations** (i.e., displacement of the distal phalanx dorsally) without a fracture are relatively common and usually can be easily reduced under digital block anesthesia by pulling the dislocated distal phalanx distally and then flexing it on the middle phalanx. Once the dislocation is reduced, the finger should be tested for flexion and extension to rule out a flexor or extensor tendon injury; the joint should also be tested for lateral stability by stressing it radially and ulnarly. An x-ray should be obtained to be certain that the reduction is complete and that there is no fracture, subluxation, or joint widening (which indicates entrapment of the volar plate in the joint). In the typical injury a portion of the volar plate will be disrupted, and the flexor and extensor tendons will be intact; in such cases, a simple reduction and splinting for 2 weeks, followed by guarded motion for an additional 2 weeks, is adequate. When there is significant subluxation, the subluxation should be corrected and the joint maintained in immobilization for 4–6 weeks with internal fixation. If entrapment of the volar plate in the joint (as evidenced by joint widening) is present, surgical exposure is necessary for repair. In injuries with lateral instability, the collateral ligament has been torn; surgical repair is necessary, followed by immobilization for 6 weeks.
         b. **Volar dislocations** of the DIP joint are usually easily reduced under digital block. After reduction, the finger should be tested for flexion and extension (to be certain that the flexor and extensor tendons are intact) and for lateral stability. If there is an associated tendon injury with this dislocation, it is usually the extensor tendon. X-rays should be obtained to confirm the reduction and to be certain there are no associated fractures. If there are no abnormalities, the finger should be splinted for 2 weeks. If it is a closed injury and the extensor tendon is disrupted (i.e., mallet finger) but there is no fracture, the finger should be immobilized with a splint (such as a stack splint) for 6 weeks (see Tendon Injuries, sec. **II.B.2**); this treatment is followed by graduated physical therapy.
      2. **Dislocations with associated fractures**
         a. **Dorsal dislocations** that are associated with fractures can be managed by splinting in flexion if the fragment is small and there is minimal displacement. When the fracture fragment is large, the fragment usually contains the insertion of the flexor digitorum profundus tendon; surgical reinsertion of the tendon and reduction of the fracture fragment are necessary, followed by 4–6 weeks of immobilization.
         b. **Volar dislocations** with associated fractures produce a **mallet finger deformity** (see **Tendon Injuries,** sec. **II.B.2**) because the extensor digitorum tendon attaches to the base of the distal phalanx. If the bony fragment is small and there is minimal displacement after reduction, the injury can be treated by splinting in extension for 6–8 weeks. If the fragment is large or significantly displaced, open reduction and internal fixation are necessary, followed by immobilization for 6 weeks.
   B. **Dislocations at the PIP joint** can be dorsal, volar, or lateral. They can also occur with or without fractures.
      1. **Dorsal dislocations** (i.e., dorsal displacement of the middle phalanx) of the PIP joint are more common than volar dislocations. In dorsal dislocation, the volar plate and a portion of the collateral ligaments are torn. These injuries usually are treated by reduction under digital block and splinting. Reduction is accomplished by applying pressure to the base of the middle phalanx and distally distracting and flexing the middle phalanx on the proximal phalanx. Following

reduction, the joint should be examined for flexion and extension and for lateral stability; it is not necessary to try to hyperextend the joint, since it will always hyperextend due to the volar plate injury. X-rays should be obtained to confirm the reduction and to rule out fractures and subluxation. If the joint surfaces are congruent, the finger should be treated by splinting in flexion for 6 weeks, gradually increasing the amount of extension. If there is an associated fracture of the volar base of the middle phalanx and it is minimally displaced, the injury can still be treated by splinting. If the fracture fragment involves more than one-fourth of the articular surface or is significantly displaced, operative reinsertion is necessary. If after reduction there is subluxation, open reduction and internal stabilization are necessary. These injuries require management by hand specialists; and although a good range of motion is usually obtained, the joints remain swollen and tender for several months.

2. **Volar dislocations** of the PIP joint frequently result in disruption of both the central slip of the extensor tendon and portions of the collateral ligaments. These dislocations usually can be reduced under digital block anesthesia. Once reduction is completed, the finger should be examined for flexion and extension and radiographs obtained. Since the central slip is usually disrupted, these injuries frequently require open reduction and reinsertion of the tendon. If open reduction and reinsertion are not accomplished, a chronic boutonniere deformity will result. The joint is kept immobilized postoperatively by internal fixation for 6 weeks, and then physical therapy is initiated. These injuries require management and follow-up by a hand specialist.

3. **Lateral dislocations** of the PIP joint involve partial or complete rupture of a collateral ligament and a portion or all of the volar plate. The collateral ligaments usually disrupt at the base of the middle phalanx. Patients have usually reduced these dislocations before they present for medical care. The diagnosis is made by noting the swollen PIP joint and observing joint tenderness on the side of the injured ligament and over the volar plate. Applying lateral stress to the joint causes the joint to open. This procedure is particularly painful, and the patient should be anesthetized with a digital block prior to performing this test. X-rays usually demonstrate soft-tissue swelling only. Disruptions of collateral ligaments are frequently partial disruptions and, if the joint is stable to lateral stress, can be treated by taping the finger to an adjacent finger for 6 weeks. If the joint is unstable to lateral stress, operative reinsertion of the ligament should be performed and followed by 6 weeks of immobilization with internal fixation and subsequent physical therapy. These injuries should be managed by hand surgeons since they require several weeks for healing, and it is several months before patients are pain-free and have normal function.

C. **MCP joint dislocations** are uncommon, with the exception of the thumb.

1. **Lateral dislocations of the thumb MCP joint.** Although dorsal, volar, and lateral dislocations can occur at the thumb MCP joint, the most common injury is that of lateral dislocation in which the collateral ligament is torn. The ligament is almost always avulsed from the base of the proximal phalanx of the thumb. The ulnar collateral ligament is torn most frequently, and this injury is called a **game-keeper's thumb.** The injury results from a radial stress applied to the thumb. The joint is swollen and more tender on the side of the torn ligament; and when the joint has a lateral stress applied to it, the joint opens. It is important to compare the two thumb MCP joints since there is significant individual variability in the laxity of the collateral ligaments. Some physicians believe that greater than 40 degrees of joint opening on lateral stress represents a complete tear of the ligament. Routine x-rays should be performed prior to stressing the joint, since occasionally there will be a bone chip avulsed with the ligament. If a bone chip is in close proximity to the base of the proximal phalanx, the injury can be treated by casting in a short-arm thumb spica cast. If the bone chip is displaced or if there is no bone chip and the joint is unstable to lateral stress, operative reinsertion of the ligament is required. This procedure requires immobilization of the joint for 6 weeks and subsequent physical therapy.

2. **Dorsal dislocations** of the MCP joint of the thumb can usually be reduced under digital block. Following relocation, the thumb should be examined for flexion, extension, and lateral stability, and x-rays obtained. It is important to demonstrate the sesamoid bones on radiographic examination, since occasionally there are fractures of these bones. These injuries can be managed by im-

mobilization with a short-arm thumb spica cast. If the joint is unstable or cannot be reduced, operative intervention is necessary. These injuries should be managed and followed by a hand surgeon.

   3. Lateral dislocations of the MCP joints of the fingers. These dislocations usually are reduced by the time patients are seen by a physician. They rarely require operative therapy and are treated by taping the finger to an adjacent finger for 6 weeks. However, when the radial collateral ligament of the index finger MCP joint is injured, lateral pinch can be unstable; in this instance, operative reinsertion of the collateral ligament should be performed.

D. Perilunate dislocation. In perilunate dislocation, the capitate and the remainder of the distal carpal row usually dislocate dorsal to the lunate. The lunate either remains in its normal position or is forced through the volar joint capsule and ligamentous structures. Because of the dorsal movement of the distal carpal bones, the median nerve is stretched over the lunate and frequently causes median nerve dysfunction (necessitating early reduction). Perilunate dislocations usually result from a severe hyperextension force acting on the hand (e.g., from violent falls). The diagnosis is confirmed by radiographs demonstrating dorsal displacement of the distal carpal row relative to the lunate and radius; the most useful x-ray for diagnosis is a lateral x-ray with the wrist in a neutral position (Fig. 23-4). When the injury is seen early, closed reduction occasionally can be performed. General anesthesia or regional block is necessary for adequate relaxation and relief of pain to allow reduction. Once reduction is completed, x-rays should be obtained to confirm the anatomic position of the carpal bones. The wrist is splinted in neutral position until swelling begins to resolve and then is casted for 6–8 weeks. If anatomic reduction cannot be accomplished by closed techniques, open reduction should be performed. This procedure usually requires internal fixation to maintain the reduction. The initial management of these injuries and follow-up should be by a hand surgeon.

E. Lunate dislocation represents a continuum along the spectrum of the perilunate dislocation; however, the lunate dislocation represents a more severe injury. These injuries are the result of disruption of the radiocarpal and intercarpal ligaments. If a hyperextension force disrupts the ligaments restraining the lunate, the lunate will dislocate volarly, impinging on the median nerve. Prompt diagnosis and reduction are necessary. Once the diagnosis is suspected, it can be confirmed with a lateral radiograph (see Fig. 23-4). Reduction should be attempted under general anesthesia or regional block, and the reduction confirmed by x-ray. If closed techniques are unsuccessful, open reduction and internal fixation are necessary. Since these wrist injuries are severe, they should be treated and followed by a hand surgeon.

III. Capsule lacerations. Lacerations of joint capsules in the hand represent open joint injuries. These injuries should be thoroughly cleansed, the overlying soft tissues closed, and the patient placed on an antibiotic. The joint capsule does not have to be closed. Closure of lacerations involving joint capsules should be performed under sterile condi-

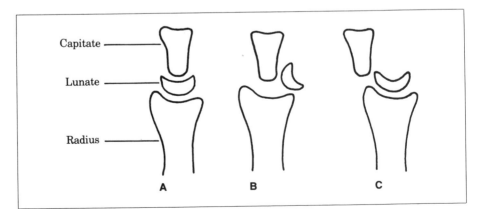

Fig. 23-4. Carpal bone dislocations. A. Normal lateral radiograph of the wrist. B. Dislocation of the lunate volarly. C. Perilunate dislocation with dorsal displacement of the capitate and the remainder of the distal carpal row.

tions with adequate anesthesia to allow proper cleansing. The patient should be referred to a hand surgeon for follow-up in 48 hours.

Arterial Injuries

Arterial injuries in the hand can be either closed or open.

I. **Closed arterial injuries** usually result from severe crushes or dislocations of either the finger joints or the wrist. These injuries produce thrombosis due to intimal damage or kinking of the blood vessels. Repeated trauma from using the hand as a hammer can also result in vascular thrombosis. The most common injury seen with this type of trauma is thrombosis of the ulnar artery at the wrist; this injury is usually very painful, and associated cold intolerance is common. Initial **treatment** of closed injuries depends on the extent of the collateral circulation and nature of the injury. If a dislocation is present, reduction and immobilization should be performed. If the injury is treated early, flow through the artery is usually restored. These patients should be admitted to the hospital for close observation for 24–48 hours. If the circulation is inadequate following reduction of the dislocation or fracture, an arteriogram should be performed to define the anatomy and localize the obstruction. If both the radial and ulnar arteries are occluded, at least one artery should be reconstituted by embolectomy (rare), direct repair, or interposition vein grafting. If one artery is occluded and if all or portions of the hand are supplied solely by that artery such that there is inadequate circulation to the hand or a part thereof, repair of the single artery is indicated. Single arterial injuries to the digits rarely require repair. However, most hand surgeons believe that when both digital arteries are occluded, one artery should be repaired or vein grafted even if the digit appears viable.

II. **Open arterial injuries.** Since the arteries in the hand are in close proximity to the nerves, it is unwise to clamp bleeding arteries. Control of bleeding can almost always be accomplished by application of pressure and a dressing. Inspection of wounds in the hand should be done in a sterile environment with proper lighting, instrumentation, and proximal control of the vessels with a tourniquet. In open injuries to the major arteries to the hand and digits, ligation or repair is recommended because false aneurysms occasionally will develop if these injuries are left unattended. If a single artery is involved and the circulation is adequate, ligation generally is performed; otherwise, repair is indicated.

III. **Ischemic hand injuries.** Major arterial injuries to the hand or crushing injuries in the hand can result in acute venous or arterial occlusion (or both) of the circulation to the intrinsic muscles or digital vessels. These injuries are analogous to Volkmann's ischemic contracture (see Chap. 26). The diagnosis is made by extending the MCP joints and passively flexing the PIP joints. If there is ischemic compromise of the intrinsic muscles, the muscles will hold the PIP joints in extension. When extension at the PIP joints occurs, the test is positive, indicating the need for decompression of the intrinsic muscles. Similarly, the carpal tunnel may need decompression. Pressure measurements have been used as guidelines for decompression; however, these measurements require special training and special equipment that may not be readily available. The presence of pulses distal to an injury does not preclude compartmental injury. Whenever there is a question of compartmental compression or acute vascular injury in the hand or wrist, a hand surgeon should be consulted.

Hand Infections

I. A **paronychia** is an infection of the soft tissue surrounding the nail bed. These infections usually begin from a hangnail or splintered nail penetrating the adjacent soft tissue. The most common infecting organism is *Staphylococcus aureus*. If the infection is not treated, it can spread further around the nail and involve the entire eponychium. Typically, there is unilateral swelling, redness, and tenderness. An early paronychia may respond to administration of an antibiotic. However, if the infection is more than 48 hours old, antibiotics alone rarely cure the infection, and surgical drainage is required. Drainage in the early stages is accomplished by dissecting the paronychial tissues away from the nail bed. If this procedure is unsuccessful, the fluctuant area is incised by advancing a scalpel away from the nail plate. If the infection extends beneath the nail, the undermined portion of the nail should be removed. Once the purulent material is evacuated, the area should be irrigated with saline, and a small wick drain inserted to facilitate drainage. An antibiotic should be prescribed, and the patient reevaluated in 2–3 days.

II. A **felon** is a deep infection in the pulp space of the finger or thumb. The most common offending organism is *S. aureus*. The most common cause of a felon is a penetrating wound, although occasionally they may follow blunt trauma. Typically, the pulp of the involved digit is swollen, red, and very tender. These infections rarely respond to an antibiotic alone. Surgical drainage should be instituted promptly; the most effective method is to make a unilateral incision that extends from one side of the finger to the opposite side. It is essential to make this type of incision because the tissue of the pulp is divided into small compartments, and all of these compartments must be entered to ensure complete drainage of the abscess cavity. The incision should be placed on the radial border of the thumb and little finger and on the ulnar border of the index, long, and ring fingers. Once the wound has been drained and irrigated, a small wick drain should be placed to facilitate drainage. An antibiotic should be instituted, and the patient reevaluated in 2–3 days.

III. **Purulent tenosynovitis** is potentially the most disabling infection involving the hand. Usually there is a history of a penetrating injury; however, the injury is often minor in nature, and the patient may be unaware of it. Although uncommon, hematogenous seeding can also occur. The infecting organisms commonly are staphylococci and streptococci. The finger typically displays four cardinal signs of tenosynovitis: (1) fusiform swelling, (2) slight flexion of the finger, (3) tenderness over the tendon sheath (particularly near the palmar surface of the MCP joint), and (4) severe pain on passive extension. These infections rarely respond to antibiotics alone; however, if symptoms and findings are compatible with a very early infection, IV antibiotics (e.g., cephalosporin) can be started and the patient reevaluated in 12–24 hours. If the infection does not respond to systemic antibiotic therapy within 24 hours, prompt surgical drainage under either axillary block or general anesthesia is necessary. Antibiotics should be continued for 7–10 days. Because of the potential for disabling and permanent impairment of hand function, management and follow-up of these patients should be by a hand surgeon.

IV. **Deep space infections.** There are four potential deep spaces in the hand: web, midpalmar, thenar, and hypothenar.

   A. The **web space, or collar button, abscess** is unique in that it has both a volar and a dorsal component. Most of the swelling and physical findings are present on the dorsal surface of the hand, but an abscess is also present on the volar surface. These abscesses can occur in any of the web spaces. The typical presentation is swelling and erythema on the dorsum of the web space, with tenderness in the dorsal and palmar aspects. Typically, there is minimal swelling on the palmar surface. The most common organism is *S. aureus*. These infections rarely respond to antibiotics alone. Incision and drainage (usually via both dorsal and volar incisions) under general or regional anesthesia by a specialist and treatment with parenteral antibiotics (e.g., cephalosporin) are essential.

   B. **Midpalmar space infections.** The midpalmar space is located beneath the flexor tendons and tendon sheaths in the midpalm. Like all space infections, it is usually the result of a penetrating injury, and *S. aureus* usually is the causative organism. Physical findings include dorsal swelling and occasionally palmar swelling. The dorsum of the hand is rarely tender or fluctuant. The palm, however, is tender and may be fluctuant. Radiographs confirm the soft-tissue swelling and rarely demonstrate gas formation. These infections rarely respond to antibiotics alone and require prompt drainage in the operating suite. Parenteral antibiotics should also be instituted. These patients should be followed by a hand surgeon.

   C. **Thenar space infections.** The thenar space is located on the radial border of the hand, along and beneath the flexor pollicis longus tendon sheath. These infections are usually the result of penetrating injuries, and the causative organisms usually are the staphylococci. Physical findings include dorsal and palmar swelling. The palmar side of the hand is exquisitely tender, but the dorsum usually is not. Thenar space infections require prompt drainage under general or regional anesthesia and institution of parenteral antibiotics.

   D. **Hypothenar space infections** are similar to thenar space infections in etiology and bacteriology. They present with palmar swelling and tenderness, as well as dorsal swelling. They rarely respond to antibiotics alone, and require prompt drainage in the operating suite and treatment with parenteral antibiotics.

V. **Subcutaneous abscesses.** The hand, like any other area of the body, can be involved with subcutaneous abscesses. There is usually a history of a penetrating injury, although hematogenous spread also occurs. Physical findings include local erythema, swelling, and fluctuance. Treatment consists of prompt drainage under local anesthesia and administration of an antibiotic. Follow-up should be in 2–3 days.

Bites

I. **Human bites** (see Chap. 22). Any time a puncture wound or laceration is seen over an MCP or PIP joint surface, the possibility of a human bite (typically from striking a tooth during an altercation) should be considered. These wounds often contain multiple organisms, in particular *S. aureus,* microaerophilic streptococci, *Eikenella corrodens,* and other anaerobes. In several large series, it has been shown that treatment with a single antibiotic is not adequate. In most cases antibiotic coverage should include penicillin plus coverage for staphylococci. In addition to institution of antibiotics, the wounds should be irrigated and debrided, and the hand placed at rest with a splint. These wounds should never be primarily sutured, but should be closed secondarily or allowed to heal by secondary intention.

Once there are clinical signs of an **infection** following a bite, cultures should be obtained and parenteral antibiotic coverage with penicillin and a cephalosporin or aminoglycoside initiated. The wound should be opened, debrided, and irrigated. Appropriate adjustments in the antibiotic coverage should be made when results of the cultures are known. Once these infections are established, significant disability can occur from joint stiffness or loss of tendon gliding or both.

II. **Animal bites**

A. **Dog bites** (see Chap. 22) usually produce lacerations or avulsions but can be simple puncture wounds. All of these wounds should be irrigated copiously and all nonviable tissue debrided. The patient's tetanus immunization status should be checked, and a booster shot given, if appropriate. Antibiotic coverage with a cephalosporin should be initiated as early as possible. If puncture wounds are present, they should not be closed. Large lacerations, when adequately debrided, can be loosely closed. A drain should be used if there is a dead space or if a flap has been elevated. A bulky dressing should be used to immobilize the hand, and the patient should be followed closely by a hand surgeon since significant disability can result if infection occurs. The Public Health Service should be notified as necessary regarding the need for rabies prophylaxis.

B. **Cat bites** (see Chap. 22) are usually small puncture wounds and rarely produce significant tissue damage. The mouths of cats are usually contaminated with *Pasteurella multocida.* This organism can cause rapid onset of a fulminant infection. Wounds should be irrigated with copious amounts of saline, and the patient started on penicillin as early as possible. The hand should be immobilized in a bulky dressing, and the patient followed in 24–48 hours by a hand surgeon.

C. **Spider bites.** See Chaps. 22 and 31.

D. **Snake bites.** See Chap. 22.

Injection Injuries

High-pressure injection injuries almost always involve either airless paint guns or grease guns. Typically, the nondominant hand and usually the index or long finger is involved. Injury usually occurs when the nozzle is being removed or the tip is being wiped, and the gun is accidentally discharged. The paint or grease is discharged from the gun under an extremely high pressure (up to 10,000 lb/sq in.). At these pressures the instrument can produce severe injuries as much as an inch or more away from the hand.

I. **Clinical features.** Initially, there is an innocuous-appearing entrance wound, with grease or paint usually oozing from the entrance site. Subsequently, the involved fingers become distended, extremely painful, and pale; the pallor is in part due to vascular compromise from the pressure of the distention of the finger and to vascular spasm secondary to chemical irritation.

II. **Treatment.** These injuries require prompt treatment by a hand surgeon. It is important to never attempt to relieve the pain by local injection of an anesthetic or by a digital block, as either can further impair circulation to the finger. The involved fingers require prompt surgical decompression under regional or general anesthesia. If prompt decompression is accomplished, the return of function, which is usually better following paint gun injuries than grease gun injuries (apparently because the paint produces less chemical irritation), may be quite good. In addition to prompt decompression, antibiotic coverage and tetanus prophylaxis, if needed, should be administered. Failure to prompt-ly decompress the involved digits uniformly results in gangrene or extensive necrosis and subsequent functional damage. Delay in treatment beyond 4–6 hours frequently results in the need for amputation.

Amputations

I. **Evaluation.** It is important to thoroughly evaluate patients following an amputation. Some of these injuries involve multiple system trauma, and patient care must not be compromised by directing attention solely to the amputation site or amputated part. This is especially true with auger injuries and other major amputations of the arms or lower extremities.

   A. The **history** should determine where and when the injury occurred, the mechanism of injury, age of the patient, and any associated or preexisting illnesses or injuries.

   B. The **physical examination** should be rapid but thorough. Particular attention should be paid to identifying any underlying or associated illnesses or injuries. The amputation site should be inspected to determine the extent and nature of the injury. A thorough inspection of the amputation site and amputated part generally will determine if replantation is feasible.

   C. **Laboratory evaluation** should include a complete blood count (CBC); serum electro-lytes, creatinine, and glucose; and a type and cross-match. X-rays of the amputated part, amputation site, and any other injured areas should be obtained.

II. **Management**

   A. **Immediate priorities.** Establishing a secure airway, maintaining adequate ventila-tion and oxygenation, and maintaining adequate circulation (through infusion of crystalloid and blood as needed) takes precedence.

   B. **Hemostasis.** Bleeding should be controlled with a pressure dressing. Clamping of blood vessels and the use of a proximal tourniquet and ligatures are to be avoided because they may cause irreversible damage to vessels, nerves, and muscle.

   C. The **amputated part** should be cleansed with saline or Ringer's lactate solution and placed in a sterile container with saline-moistened sponges. If the amputated part is small, it can be placed in a sterile plastic bag; if it is a large part such as an arm or foot, it can be placed in a Lahey bag. The bag should then be placed on crushed ice. It is important that the amputated part not be placed directly on ice or in saline to prevent freezing and maceration, respectively. It is also important not to place the part on dry ice, as this will result in irreversible damage due to freezing. If transpor-tation of the amputated part is necessary, the bag containing the part can be placed in a Styrofoam cooler (such as those used for camping) containing ice; these coolers provide adequate insulation for transportation over long distances.

   D. **Replantation.** The patient and amputated part should always be transferred to-gether and as rapidly as possible to a replantation center. Amputated digits can be replanted after as much as 36 hours of ischemia, if properly refrigerated. More proximal amputations with muscle involvement can be replanted up to 6–8 hours postamputation, if properly refrigerated; only minimal amounts of warm ischemia time are tolerated by muscle-containing tissue. Tetanus prophylaxis, if needed, and broad-spectrum antibiotic coverage should be initiated. In addition, in preparation for replantation, the patient should have an IV infusion established and an indwell-ing Foley catheter inserted, since these operations are several hours in duration.

Nerve Injuries

I. **History.** A thorough history of any prior nerve, muscle, tendon, bone, or joint injury should be obtained when evaluating a patient for a possible nerve injury. It is also important to determine the age of the patient; when, where, and how the injury oc-curred; and whether the wound is potentially contaminated.

II. **Physical examination.** Thorough inspection of the wound is necessary so that an accu-rate documentation of the extent and nature of the injury can be made. A complete sensory (including determination of two-point discrimination) and motor evaluation of all nerves in the extremity should be performed.

   A. **Median nerve injuries.** Injury to the nerve at the level of the elbow results in loss of sensation in the sensory distribution of the nerve (see Fig. 23-1) and inability to flex the IP joint of the thumb, the radialmost fingers, and the flexor carpi radialis. Isolated injury to the anterior interosseous nerve results in loss of the ability to flex the IP joint of the thumb and the radialmost fingers; in this instance sensation remains intact, as does thenar muscle function. More distal injury to the median nerve results in loss of sensation and loss of thenar muscle function. Isolated injury to the recurrent motor branch of the median nerve results in isolated loss of thenar muscle function, and injury to the sensory branches results in sensory loss.

B. Ulnar nerve injuries. Injury to the ulnar nerve in the forearm results in loss of sensation in the little finger and ulnar half of the ring finger and on the dorsum of the ulnar side of the hand. In chronic injuries, a claw-hand deformity develops in the ring and little fingers; in this deformity the MCP joints are hyperextended and the IP joints are flexed when finger extension is attempted.

C. Radial nerve injuries. Injury at or above the level of the elbow results in loss of sensation on the dorsum of the radial side of the hand and in loss of wrist and finger extension. Isolated injury to the posterior interosseous nerve results in inability to extend the wrist and fingers.

D. Digital nerves. The digital nerves are located on the volar aspect of each side of the digit and travel immediately adjacent to the digital arteries. Injury to a digital nerve results in loss of sensation on the ipsilateral radial or ulnar aspect of the finger distal to the site of injury.

III. Treatment. Nerve injuries should be treated in an operating room setting where adequately trained people and proper microsurgical instruments and microscopes are available. Ideally, nerves should be repaired as soon after the injury as is logistically convenient. Normally this means either the day of the injury or the following day. If more than a week elapses between the injury and repair, the repair should be postponed for 3 weeks. This time period allows the wound to heal and minimizes the risk of infection. It also allows easier identification of normal fascicles after resection of the neuroma and glioma. Digital nerves should be repaired as far distally as the DIP joint crease. Injuries to the nerves in the pulp of the finger are usually not repaired since sensation is usually as good without repair.

Bibliography

1. American Society for Surgery of the Hand. *The Hand. Examination and Diagnosis* (2nd ed.). New York: Churchill Livingstone, 1983.
2. Atasoy, E., et al. Reconstruction of the amputated fingertip with a triangular volar flap. *J. Bone Joint Surg.* 52A:921, 1970.
3. Edlich, R. F., Rodeheaver, G. T., and Edgerton, M. T. Airless paint gun injuries: An update. *J. Am. College Emerg. Physicians.* 7:397, 1978.
4. Farrell, R. G., et al. Conservative management of fingertip amputations. *J.A.C.E.P.* 6:243, 1977.
5. Gaul, J. S. Management of acute hand injuries. *Ann. Emerg. Med.* 9:139, 1980.
6. Gold, A. H., et al. Upper extremity replantation: Current concepts and patient selection. *J. Trauma* 21:551, 1981.
7. Haughey, R. E., Lammers, R. L., and Wagner, D. K. Use of antibiotics in the initial management of soft tissue hand wounds. *Ann. Emerg. Med.* 10:187, 1981.
8. Linscheid, R. L., and Dobyns, J. H. Common and uncommon infections of the hand. *Orthop. Clin. North Am.* 6:1063, 1975.
9. Malinowski, R. W., et al. The management of human bite injuries of the hand. *J. Trauma* 19:655, 1979.
10. Newmeyer, W. L., and Kilgore, E. S., Jr. Fingertip injuries: A simple effective method of treatment. *J. Trauma* 14:58, 1974.
11. Osterman, A. L., Hayken, G. D., and Bora, F. W., Jr. A quantitative evaluation of thumb function after ulnar collateral repair and reconstruction. *J. Trauma* 21:854, 1981.
12. Peeples, E., Boswick, J. A., and Scott, F. A. Wounds of the hand contaminated by human or animal saliva. *J. Trauma* 20:383, 1980.
13. Schoo, M. J., Scott, F. A., and Boswick, J. A. High-pressure injection injuries of the hand. *J. Trauma* 20:229, 1980.
14. Weeks, P. M. (ed.). *Acute Bone and Joint Injuries of the Hand and Wrist: A Clinical Guide to Management.* St. Louis: Mosby, 1981.
15. Westreich, M., Binns, J. H., and Posch, J. L. Emergency care of the reimplantation patient. *J.A.C.E.P.* 6:194, 1977.
16. Zook, E. G. The perionychium: Anatomy, physiology, and care of injuries. *Clin. Plast. Surg.* 8:21, 1981.
17. Zook, E. G., and Kinkead, L. R. Pressure gun injection injuries of the hand. *J.A.C.E.P.* 8:264, 1979.

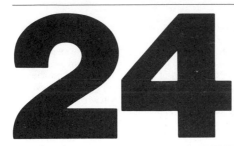

Maxillofacial and Neck Trauma

Harlan R. Muntz

Maxillofacial Trauma

The patient arriving in the emergency department with maxillofacial trauma often exhibits massive swelling and exuberant bleeding. Because of associated potential injuries to the eye, spinal cord, and brain, as well as the potential risk of airway obstruction and massive infection, immediate and rapid management with proper setting of priorities is essential.

I. **Management principles.** The management of the patient with maxillofacial trauma requires immediate evaluation and institution of therapy in a systematic manner.

　A. **Airway.** The first priority is to establish a secure airway. As the vital signs are being taken, immediate attention must be given to assess the status of ventilation. In particular, it is important to note the presence of any cyanosis, retractions, poor air movement, hoarseness, stridor, or hemoptysis. Prompt auscultation of the lungs is essential and may indicate a pneumothorax or aspiration, further comprising ventilation. If there is any evidence suggesting impending airway compromise, an airway should be established by endotracheal intubation (via the oral or nasal route with appropriate precautions in the presence of a suspected cervical spine injury), cricothyrotomy, or, if the physician is experienced, a tracheostomy in the acute setting (see Chaps. 17 and 38).

　B. **Circulation.** Blood loss is a significant consideration in that scalp and facial lacerations tend to bleed briskly. In addition, lacerations of the major arteries of the head, neck, and face can rapidly lead to a diminution in circulatory blood volume with ensuing shock. A large-bore IV catheter should be inserted in a peripheral vein and additional lines established as needed, depending on the clinical situation. Crystalloid is then infused to replete the intravascular volume. However, if there is persistent hypotension following infusion of 2 liters of crystalloid, blood should be transfused.

　C. **Control of bleeding.** Generally, application of direct pressure will terminate bleeding and can be in the form of digital pressure, packing of wounds, or application of a pressure dressing. Because of the risk of damage to vital structures, blind clamping is to be condemned. However, clamping and ligature of bleeding vessels can occasionally be performed if done cautiously under direct visualization.

　　1. **Pressure dressings.** A head or scalp laceration can be adequately dressed with a mastoid dressing. Most often in the head and neck, however, a Barton-type figure-of-eight dressing around the head and neck is needed.

　　　a. A **mastoid dressing** is essentially a "wrap-around" dressing covering one ear. This dressing covers the ipsilateral ear, traverses the forehead, and courses above the contralateral ear; it tucks posteriorly beneath and over the occiput. This pressure-type dressing can cover any unilateral scalp, ear, or anterior face laceration.

　　　b. The **Barton dressing,** on the other hand, is a figure-of-eight pressure-type dressing that is effective in controlling bleeding on the face, neck, or ear. A bolster of fluff is placed over the bleeding site; the wrap then proceeds vertically around the head and under the chin. Often it helps to cover one ear with the dressing. Further pressure can be applied with horizontal loops around the forehead and neck.

　　2. If **oral cavity bleeding** is extensive, the airway must be controlled with intubation, cricothyrotomy, or tracheostomy. The oral cavity may then be packed with gauze. Occasionally, a single bleeding point may be identified and treated with cautery, direct pressure, or ligation.

D. Cervical spine evaluation. Any time a patient has maxillofacial trauma, a cervical spine injury should be considered. The cervical spine must be immobilized (see Chap. 17) and remain so until radiologically cleared. Early in the evaluation of the patient, a cervical spine series (starting with cross-table lateral film) must be obtained to assess the integrity of the cervical spine.

E. Central nervous system (CNS) evaluation. With head and midface trauma, there is the risk of both coup and contrecoup injuries to the brain as well as an associated skull fracture. It should be noted immediately whether the patient had loss of consciousness or seizure activity. A brief neurologic examination should be carried out during the initial evaluation, with particular attention to the mental status, pupillary size and reactivity, motor activity and strength, and deep tendon reflexes. Suspected injury to the brain is an indication for neurosurgical consultation and usually computed tomography (CT).

F. Ocular evaluations. Any facial trauma must be evaluated with attention to possible ocular injury. Close examination of the lids, conjunctivae, cornea and sclera, and pupillary reactivity is essential. In addition, the extraocular motions and visual acuity should be evaluated to the extent possible. Evaluation of the anterior chamber with an ophthalmoscope and if possible a slit lamp is useful to assess for a hyphema or injury to the pupil. Unless contraindicated, the intraocular pressure should be noted. The funduscopic examination is important to determine if there is papilledema or retinal detachment. For those injuries with possible associated retrobulbar swelling, assessment of the venous pulsations is important. Any person with facial injuries involving the eye or periorbita should receive ophthalmologic consultation and frequent visual acuity checks.

G. A **complete physical examination** is essential, as is proper utilization of laboratory tests and radiologic procedures. Trauma causing significant facial injury is often accompanied by significant trauma to other body systems. In order to improve the patient's chances for survival and reduce the ensuing morbidity, the full extent of the patient's injuries must be identified. Obviously, appropriate treatment of the patient's injuries is of paramount importance.

H. Wound management. After the patient has been stabilized and potentially life-threatening injuries appropriately managed, attention should be directed to the care of the patient's wounds. Important considerations are those of function, cosmesis, and preservation of tissue. Thorough irrigation is essential to lessen the risk of infection. Careful debridement of devitalized tissue is also important. Antibiotic therapy should be instituted in cases of open fracture and gross contamination. Specific therapy will depend on the nature of the injury.

II. Facial fractures

A. Nasal fracture. Since the nose is in the center of the face and is the most projected portion of the profile, fracture of the nasal bones is the most common facial fracture. Even if the nasal bones are not fractured, the septum can be. Cartilaginous septal fractures can cause significant delayed sequelae by creating deflections of the nasal septum and hence nasal airway obstruction.

1. **Clinical features.** Initially, there often is significant swelling of the nose, with associated epistaxis or ecchymosis (or both).

2. The **evaluation** of the patient with a suspected nasal fracture includes palpation of the nose, anterior rhinoscopy, and nasal films (for objective and medicolegal documentation). Palpation of the nasal dorsum, even through significant swelling, may reveal the fracture line by a step off with depression or lateralization. Even if there is a negative nasal bone series, palpation of a step off deformity establishes the diagnosis. Dislocation of the upper lateral cartilage will not be apparent on x-ray but will give a significant deformity. Anterior rhinoscopy not only will detect fractures and deviation of the nasal septum but also will assist in the evaluation of the presence or absence of mucosal tears within the nose. Most important, rhinoscopy will establish the presence or absence of a hematoma of the nasal septum. Not infrequently in nasal trauma, bleeding beneath the perichondral lining of the nasal septum will cause a bluish-gray swelling along the septum. Since the perichondrium is a thin membrane and since the nose has significant bacterial flora, the presence of a septal hematoma places the person at great risk for formation of a septal abscess, which can lead to septal perforation, sepsis, or cavernous sinus thrombosis. The delayed sequelae includes a "saddle-nose" deformity. In addition, a septal hematoma without septal abscess may organize and have cartilage ingrowth, resulting in a significantly broadened nasal septum and nasal airway obstruction.

3. **Management**
   a. A **hematoma of the nasal septum** is either aspirated with a large-bore needle or incised and drained (or both). The nose is then packed (see Chap. 38), and dicloxacillin, 250–500 mg q6h, or erythromycin, 250 mg q6h, is administered. The patient is referred to an otolaryngologist the next day for reevaluation.
   b. **Reduction of the nasal fracture.** If there is no septal hematoma and the epistaxis is controlled, the reduction of the nasal fracture can be accomplished acutely, if swelling does not prohibit the proper palpation of the nasal fracture fragments, or the reduction can be delayed until the swelling has decreased. A child between the ages of infancy and 7 years should have the nasal fracture set within the first 4 days to prevent healing of the depressed fracture fragments prior to reduction. In the older patient, the nasal fracture can be reduced in 7–10 days.
      (1) **Closed reduction** of a nasal fracture is the most common procedure and is most often performed in the operating suite but can be done acutely in the emergency department. Anesthesia is obtained by blocking the sphenopalatine ganglion and nasociliary areas with topical cocaine. Injection of the septum and nasal dorsum with 1% lidocaine with 1:100,000 epinephrine will complete the task. The procedure involves instrumental replacement of the septum onto the maxillary crest and the elevation of fracture fragments into their proper position. Often the handle of a scalpel can be used to replace the fragments. Occasionally, these fracture fragments can be stabilized by this maneuver alone, but most often, intranasal packing (see Chap. 38) and external splinting are necessary to maintain the position of these fragments until healing occurs.
      (2) An occasional patient may need **open reduction** to properly position the fragments.
   c. Occasionally, a **nasal hematoma** is seen in the soft tissue on the nasal ala or immediately adjacent to the fracture line at the nasal dorsum. This hematoma requires urgent drainage and antibiotics as described in **a.**
   d. All patients with nasal fractures should be placed on **antibiotic prophylaxis,** including staphylococcal coverage.
   e. **Delayed complications** of nasal airway obstruction or persistent deformity may occur despite proper initial treatment. Elective rhinoplasty or septoplasty can be performed 6 weeks after injury.

B. **Mandibular fracture.** The second most common fracture of the facial skeleton is that of the mandible. The anatomy of the mandible and its relationship to the skull are such that two fracture sites usually result simultaneously. The mandibular condyle is most commonly involved.
   1. **Evaluation.** In the initial evaluation of the patient with a possible mandibular fracture, palpation of the mandible may reveal a step off, an abnormal bony prominence, or crepitance. Often soft-tissue swelling overlying the fracture site gives an indication of the location. Intraoral bleeding or a mucosal laceration is another clue to a fracture. New onset of malocclusion is another useful finding and is best assessed by having the patient close his or her mouth and examining the premolar occlusal surfaces. Often the patient complains that the teeth do not come together properly. Films of the mandible will establish the diagnosis.
   2. **Fracture types.** Two categories of fractures are established, based on their radiographic diagnosis and the angulation of the fracture. In **favorable mandibular fractures,** the pull of the muscles of mastication is in such a direction that the fracture fragments are not displaced but rather are pulled together. In contrast, **unfavorable fractures** show displacement of the fragments secondary to the pull of the pterygoids and masseter muscles. The bilateral parasymphyseal fracture is the most potentially dangerous because it may lead to life-threatening airway compromise. Swelling of the submental area and sublingual space, as well as retrusion of the symphyseal fragment secondary to the pull of the tongue musculature, may attenuate the airway.
   3. **Management**
      a. Patients with bilateral parasymphyseal fractures must be placed on **airway precautions** and, at the earliest evidence of compromise, have a secure airway established by endotracheal intubation, cricothyrotomy, or tracheostomy.

   b. Patients will be more comfortable if the mandible is stabilized by a **Barton dressing** (see sec **I.C.1.b**).

   c. The patient should be placed on a soft or liquid **diet.**

   d. Tetanus toxoid should be administered, if needed.

   e. Antiobiotic therapy. Each mandibular fracture should be treated as an open fracture. IV antibiotics covering the oral cavity flora should be started immediately; either penicillin combined with an aminoglycoside or a second-generation cephalosporin is acceptable.

   f. Since an infection at the fracture site may be caused by a periapical abscess of an involved **tooth,** such teeth should be removed at the time of surgery.

   g. Stable mandibular fractures can be treated with **intermaxillary fixation,** which assures proper occlusion. Intermaxillary fixation may be accomplished by arch bar application and banding or by the use of Ivy loops. Unstable mandibular fractures, on the other hand, must be treated not only by intermaxillary fixation but also by open reduction and internal fixation. Internal fixation can be accomplished by K-wires or figure-of-eight wire ties. A more recent advance has involved the use of compression plates for the treatment of mandibular fractures.

  4. Complications. Delayed complications occasionally stem from inattention to proper occlusion or from development of infection. The eventual outcome of an infection after a mandibular fracture may include osteomyelitis of the mandible, malunion or nonunion of the mandibular fragments, or malocclusion.

C. Blow-out fracture. The patient with an isolated orbital floor fracture generally has sustained injury to the orbit by a forceful blow directed in an anterior-to-posterior direction. This external force is transmitted through the orbit, fracturing the orbital floor.

  1. Clinical features. The patient often presents with lid edema, chemosis, subconjunctival hemorrhages, or bleeding into the sclera. Infraorbital numbness may be present, reflecting injury to the infraorbital nerve. There may be enophthalmos (i.e., retrusion of the globe into the orbit). Diplopia secondary to swelling or entrapment of extraocular muscles, if present, is most often noted on upward gaze.

  2. Evaluation of the globe is of utmost importance to detect any corneal lacerations or abrasions. A slit-lamp evaluation is useful to evaluate for a hyphema, and a funduscopic examination will reveal any vitreous bleeding or a retinal detachment. It is also wise to measure the intraocular pressure to rule out an acute glaucoma. The range of motion of the globe should also be tested by the forced duction test to assess the degree of entrapment of the extraocular muscles. This test is done by topically anesthetizing the eye and grasping the sclera inferiorly with a tissue forceps. As the globe is rotated superiorly, a crisp cessation of movement occurs if an entrapped inferior rectus muscle prevents superior rotation. Frequent visual acuity checks are essential to document vision and to enable early detection of delayed intraocular damage.

  3. Treatment. At present there is a debate as to whether early exploration is indicated or whether expectant observation is as effective. Except for severe injuries (i.e., those requiring exploration for other reasons), it is generally considered preferable to observe the patient for a period of no less than 2 weeks. This period of time allows for potential resolution of edema and hemorrhage so that any entrapment might resolve. Exploration is undertaken if entrapment persists or if enophthalmos is cosmetically unacceptable.

   a. Antiobiotic therapy. Since the blow-out fracture is open into the sinus, antibiotic therapy is required. A cephalosporin or erythromycin is adequate.

   b. Decongestants, both topical and oral, are needed if the sinus is completely opacified.

  4. Disposition. Unless there is extraocular muscle entrapment, patients with blow-out fractures may be discharged to be followed up within 2 days by an ophthalmologist or otolaryngologist.

D. Zygomatic arch fracture. The most common fracture of the zygoma is a fracture of the zygomatic arch.

  1. Evaluation. Fracture of the zygomatic arch usually can be identified by a depression in the area immediately behind the malar eminence, but this depression may be obscured by swelling in the area. A step off near the insertion of the zygomatic bone posteriorly as well as in the area immediately behind the malar eminence may be detected. Radiographic studies are diagnostic of the fracture. A submental vertex view clearly shows both arches and will demonstrate any fracture.

2. **Management.** A zygomatic arch fracture is predominantly a cosmetic problem, and effective reduction of the fracture fragments on an elective basis can restore the normal facial contour. Occasionally, with proper local anesthesia, the fracture may be reduced through the skin by grasping the arch with a sharp towel clamp and gently placing it in proper alignment. More commonly, a Gillies incision is made along the temporalis muscle in the hairline, and a urethral sound is slipped beneath the arch to elevate the fragments into proper position. Occasionally, in comminuted fractures, packing must be used to maintain the position of the bone fragments until healing begins.

E. The **tripod (trimalar) fracture** consists of a fracture through the frontozygomatic suture line, the inferior orbital rim, and the zygomatic arch. A tripod fracture results in a depressed malar eminence. If left untreated, a significant facial deformity will result.

  1. **Evaluation.** As in other periorbital injuries, associated orbital and ocular injuries must be ruled out. The inferior orbital rim fracture courses through the floor of the orbit, most often at the exit of the infraorbital nerve, and injury to the nerve with a resultant sensory deficit may occur. Although rare, there is also the potential for entrapment.

  2. **Management.** Reduction of these fractures is carried out on an elective basis. It requires an open technique, and two-point fixation is necessary. The fixation of the frontozygomatic suture line is performed through a lateral brow incision, and a rim incision can be used to reapproximate the orbital rim. Occasionally, a Gillies incision may assist in the alignment of the fracture lines and care of the arch fracture. An antibiotic (e.g., cephalosporin) should be administered because of the fracture into the maxillary sinus.

F. **Le Fort fractures.** Midface fractures are less frequent than other facial skeletal injuries. The midface essentially consists of the bones of the palate, maxillary sinuses, ethmoid sinuses, nose, and the zygoma. Le Fort divided midface fractures into three primary groups (Fig. 24-1). A Le Fort I fracture is a fracture above the level of the palate, separating the palate from the rest of the midface. A Le Fort II fracture retains the maxillary sinuses and nose with the palate; the fracture courses through the nasal bones, separating the midface from the skull at this level. A Le Fort III fracture, which is also called **craniofacial disjunction,** courses through the glabella, the orbits, and the frontozygomatic suture lines, separating the entire midface from the calvarium.

  1. **Clinical features.** On arrival in the emergency department, a patient with a midface fracture usually already has a significant amount of facial swelling. In Le Fort II and Le Fort III fractures, airway compromise may be an immediate problem. Palatal fractures, epistaxis, facial lacerations, and eye injuries are often present and may obscure the diagnosis. In addition, cerebrospinal fluid (CSF) leakage may occur.

  2. The **diagnosis** is easily made by grasping the maxillary incisors or the alveolar ridge and rocking in an anteroposterior direction. If the midface or palate moves well but the remainder of the face and skull remain still, a midface fracture is diagnosed. Palpation along the nose and frontozygomatic suture lines will establish the type of Le Fort fracture. Facial films will confirm the diagnosis. It is important to note, however, that there usually is a combination fracture (e.g., a left Le Fort II and a right Le Fort III).

  3. **Evaluation** for intracranial complications (including CSF leakage), ocular injuries, and periorbital injuries is of great importance.

  4. **Management**
     a. The **airway** is at significant risk of becoming compromised in a patient with a Le Fort II or III fracture. Endotracheal intubation is nearly impossible because the midface and palate are grossly swollen and the face will rock when pressure is placed on the maxilla by the laryngoscope. Urgent cricothyrotomy or tracheostomy is required in most of these patients.
     b. Occasionally, to **control significant bleeding** in the nasal fossa, an anteroposterior nasal pack (see Chap. 38) may be needed. If significant oral trauma has caused excessive bleeding unable to be controlled by simple pressure, the oral cavity may need to be packed after the airway is secured.

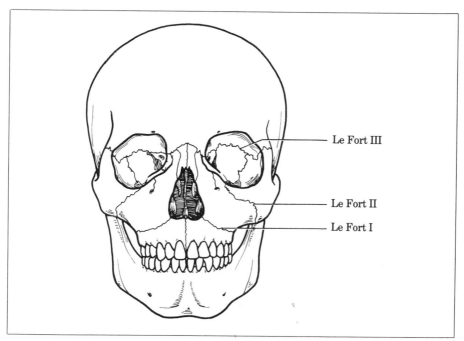

Fig. 24-1. Classification of midface fractures. Le Fort I: Fracture through the maxilla above the teeth. Le Fort II: Pyramidal fracture involving the nasal bones and maxillary sinuses, separating them from the frontal bone and zygoma. Le Fort III: Craniofacial disjunction resulting from the fracture line coursing through frontozygomatic suture lines, the orbits, and the glabella.

   c. Fracture reduction. In adults the fracture can be reduced up to 10 days after the initial injury. A major concern in the reduction of a midface fracture is to achieve appropriate occlusion, which is assisted by intermaxillary fixation. Most often, stabilization of the fracture fragments mandates open reduction and internal fixation. Palatal fractures alone (Le Fort I) may be fixed by intermaxillary fixation with circumzygomatic suspension. Le Fort II fractures require not only reduction of the nasal fracture but also wiring of the nasal bones and palate to the remainder of the stable upper midface. Le Fort III fractures are stabilized at the skull. The area of the frontal bone at the frontozygomatic suture line supports the midface by wires, and occlusion is reestablished.
   d. Prophylactic antibiotics are required.
   e. Dental abnormalities that can predispose to infection must be identified and appropriately treated.
G. Frontonasoethmoid fracture. Injuries to the nose and glabellar area may result in a complex fracture called the frontonasoethmoid fracture. Essentially there is a fracture at the glabella with retrusion of the nasal dorsum into the ethmoid bones. This fracture creates a situation called pseudotelecanthus, in which the eyes appear to be wider apart because of disruption of the bones to which the medial canthal ligaments attach. However, the interpupillary distance is within normal limits. Of primary importance in this particular fracture is potential damage to the cribriform area with resultant cerebrospinal fluid (CSF) leakage. This fracture requires open reduction and internal fixation of the entire frontonasoethmoid complex. The majority of CSF leaks in this area are stopped by adequate reduction and fixation of the fracture fragments; a dural tear, however, may occasionally need grafting. These patients are admitted for parenteral antibiotics and surgery.
H. Frontal sinus fracture. The frontal sinus is within the frontal bone, which is composed of an anterior table beneath the skin of the forehead and a posterior (internal) table adjacent to the dura. Usually a severe force is needed to fracture the frontal

sinus, and as a result, this injury is often associated with coup and contrecoup injuries to the brain. Posterior table fractures may be associated with subdural hematomas and tearing of the dura and meninges.

1. **Clinical features.** Generally these patients present to the emergency department with a depression of the forehead, often associated with lacerations, significant swelling, and ecchymosis. Because of the relation of the nose and paranasal sinuses to the anterior cranial fossa, skull and sinus radiographs may reveal free intracranial air. This radiographic finding suggests the likelihood of contamination from the nasal cavity, and such patients are at risk for developing a brain abscess or meningitis.

2. The initial **evaluation** should include assessment of the orbit and globe, including visual acuity. A detailed examination of the ears is important to determine whether there is an associated temporal bone fracture. A sinus series is the first step to ascertain the presence or absence of a fracture. Often depression of the anterior table is detected on the lateral view. Free intracranial air is a clue to more extensive damage. The presence of an air-fluid level within the sinus or fracture lines necessitates high-resolution CT of the paranasal sinuses and head to further delineate the extent of injury. CT enables an evaluation of the posterior table, ethmoid complex, and orbits, as well as the brain.

3. **Management.** High-dose antibiotics (e.g., a cephalosporin and vancomycin for CSF antistaphylococcal coverage) should be started. If the neurologic condition is stable, immediate exploration is necessary. Exploration of the frontal sinus is accomplished through a frontal sinus osteoplastic flap. The anterior table is elevated and hinged on its periosteum to allow for complete visualization of the entire frontal sinus. If a posterior table fracture is found, debridement of this area and inspection of the dura are necessary. Because of the risk of mucocele formation and nasal frontal duct obstruction following frontal sinus fractures, it is often reasonable to obliterate the frontal sinus emergently and plug the nasal frontal ducts.

III. Injury to the salivary glands and facial nerve

A. **Clinical features.** Injury to the salivary glands (i.e., parotid or submaxillary glands) or their ducts can occur secondary to deep facial lacerations and mandibular fractures. The parotid gland is at greatest risk because of its more accessible position. In addition, facial nerve injury can occur from lacerations along its course.

B. **Diagnosis.** In any facial laceration in the vicinity of a salivary gland, gentle inspection of the depth of the wound may reveal penetration of the fascia covering the gland, suggesting injury to the gland. Assessment of facial nerve function may reveal a paresis indicative of injury to the nerve.

C. **Management**

1. **Injuries to the parotid gland** must be carefully managed because Stensen's duct may also be injured. A lacrimal duct probe should be gently inserted by a specialist into an anesthetized Stensen's duct from the oral cavity as the laceration is evaluated. If there is no laceration of this duct, closure of parotid masseteric fascia and skin is accomplished. Occasionally, a small drain must be placed to allow for decompression of any salivary leakage or serous fluid accumulation.

2. If **laceration of Stensen's duct** is noted, appropriate consultation should be obtained for reanastomosis and stenting of the duct. Generally this procedure is performed in the operating suite but occasionally may be done in the emergency department.

3. Wounds near the **submaxillary gland** can be handled as described in **1.**

4. If **facial nerve injury** is noted, immediate consultation must be obtained. Care must be taken not to use electrocautery or suturing techniques for hemostasis or closure of the wound because the facial nerve stumps can be further damaged. The wound can be dressed with a Barton's dressing (see sec **I.C.1.b**), and the patient started on an antibiotic. Usually broad-spectrum coverage with a cephalosporin or erythromycin is appropriate. Tetanus toxoid should be administered as needed. The patient should then be taken to the operating suite; and, under general anesthesia without paralytic agents, the distal and proximal nerve stumps should be reanastomosed using 10-0 nylon sutures.

IV. Ear trauma. The external ear not only has a physiologic role in the amplification of sound as it enters the ear canal but is also of cosmetic importance. The pinna is a delicately sculptured piece of cartilage surrounded on both sides by thin, tightly approximated skin. The ear can be affected by blunt and penetrating trauma and physical insults.

A. **Hematoma.** Blunt trauma to the ear may cause a hematoma of the pinna, which is essentially an extravasation of blood beneath the perichondrium of the cartilage of the ear. The hematoma should be drained to prevent not only infection or perichondritis of the auricle but also organization of the clot, which leads to a "cauliflower ear" deformity. Drainage of the hematoma should be performed under sterile conditions using an antiseptic preparation. The blood can be aspirated with a large-bore needle or via a drainage incision along the antihelical fold. A mastoid dressing must then be applied to prevent the hematoma from reforming. Cotton balls soaked in mineral oil should be used to surround the ear and outline the cartilaginous framework prior to the application of the mastoid dressing. An antibiotic (e.g., dicloxacillin) must be administered prophylactically to avoid perichondritis. Reevaluation of the ear the following day has been necessary to assure that there is no reformation of the hematoma.

B. **Lacerations and soft-tissue loss**
   1. **Lacerations of the ear** should be approximated with fine, nonreactive sutures (e.g., 6-0 nylon). If the laceration penetrates the cartilage, 4-0 undyed absorbable sutures should be used to reapproximate the perichondrium (aligning the cartilage) prior to closure of the skin.
   2. If there is **loss of tissue,** reapproximation may be difficult and leave unsightly scarring. If there is full-thickness skin loss in the concha or in the area apart from the helical rim, the wound may be left to heal by secondary intention. However, if there is soft-tissue loss on the helical rim or cartilage loss, care must be taken to prevent scar contracture and notching of the pinna. If the soft-tissue loss on the helical rim is small, it can be treated in the operating suite by a wedge excision of the ear, leaving a slightly smaller helix. If the portion of the avulsed ear is intact, it should be stored in a plastic bag placed in iced saline, and the cartilage later reembedded in the posterior auricular soft tissue with the perichondrium intact. This procedure will allow for a secondary reconstruction of the auricle on an elective basis. Occasionally, elaborate flap techniques are indicated for reconstruction.
   3. If the entire **ear has been avulsed,** the cartilage should be saved for later reconstruction (see **2**). Immediate consultation by a cosmetic head and neck surgeon should be obtained.

C. **Thermal injury.** The **external ear** is prone to both heat and cold injury since it occupies a prominent position on the side of the head and is exposed on two sides. Burns and frostbite are similar in terms of their treatment. However, the depth of injury with frostbite is less easily determined at the initial presentation.
   1. **Burns** (see Chap. 21). First-degree burns are quite superficial, usually manifested by mere reddening of the skin. Second-degree burns usually show bleb formation, and deep soft-tissue injury is seen in third-degree burns. Blebs should be allowed to remain and should not be opened. Most of the time, the fluid will be resorbed spontaneously, and the skin acts as a protective coating and barrier to infection. If the bleb is open, no dressing should be applied, but application of a protective cream (e.g., silver sulfadiazine) is important. Debridement of the ear should not be done until the area of necrosis is well-defined. Care must be taken not to apply pressure to the ear with a dressing, and the patient should be instructed not to rest on that ear. Most superficial burns can be treated on an outpatient basis (unless there are associated injuries requiring admission). Deep soft-tissue injuries, however, require admission.
   2. **Frostbite** (see Chap. 31) is handled similar to burns (see **1**); however, it is difficult to establish the depth of injury in the initial setting. Usually 24–48 hours is required to delineate the depth of injury. The frostbitten ear should be warmed quickly by the use of tepid water to improve the chances of tissue survival. An antibiotic cream may be applied topically to help prevent infectious complications. Minor frostbite of the ears can be treated on an outpatient basis. Deep-tissue injury, however, requires hospitalization for close observance for infection and parenteral antibiotic therapy.

D. **Tympanic membrane perforation**
   1. **Etiology.** The tympanic membrane can be ruptured in many ways. The most common cause is insertion of a cotton-tipped swab or similar object, but a blow to the ear or closed head trauma can also cause perforation of the tympanic membrane.
   2. **Clinical features.** Perforation of the tympanic membrane usually presents as sudden hearing loss, occasionally with bleeding from the ear canal. A traumatic

perforation of this membrane most often is characterized by a mild conductive hearing loss. Almost 95% of perforations will heal within 6 months.

3. **Evaluation** of a patient who has a traumatic perforation of the tympanic membrane includes assessment for damage to the facial nerve or the vestibular system. Accurate assessment of facial nerve function by observation (e.g., movement of all facial areas, tearing, taste) is mandatory. Careful documentation of any history of vertigo at the time of the incident as well as evaluation for spontaneous or elicited nystagmus is important to assess for labyrinthine trauma. As soon as possible, formal audiometric evaluation should be undertaken to determine the extent of hearing loss. Until then, the tuning fork may be used to establish whether the hearing loss is conductive, sensorineural, or mixed. A sensorineural hearing loss indicates cochlear injury, whereas a conductive hearing loss of nearly 60 decibels is found in those with ossicular discontinuity from either a fracture or dislocation. Drainage of clear fluid from the ear canal may signify CSF, perilymph, or endolymph leakage.

4. **Management.** If there is no evidence of temporal bone fracture or sensorineural loss, the patient may be discharged with follow-up by an otolaryngologist the next day. An analgesic may be prescribed as needed, but usually no further therapy is needed. The presence of a temporal bone fracture, facial paralysis, vertigo, or sensorineural hearing loss mandates admission to the hospital.

E. **Temporal bone fractures**

1. **Types.** Temporal bone fractures are usually divided into three groups: longitudinal, transverse, and mixed.

   a. **Longitudinal fractures** are the most common and comprise nearly 75% of temporal bone fractures. They are caused by blows to the temporal area. These fractures extend along the long axis of the petrous part of the temporal bone, running lengthwise through the pyramid. Usually the fracture line does not enter the labyrinthine capsule or the cochlea but extends along the carotid canal. The major damage in longitudinal fractures is to the middle ear. Usually, a tear in the skin in the external ear canal or tympanic membrane can be seen. There may be a twisting injury to the ossicular chain with a fracture of the long process of the incus, dislocation of the incudostapedial joint, or fracture of the stapes crura with a resultant conductive hearing loss. In addition, one-fifth of patients suffering from longitudinal fractures will have a facial nerve injury.

   b. **Transverse fractures.** Twenty percent of temporal bone fractures are in the transverse orientation. The fracture line usually extends from the posterior cranial fossa into the middle cranial fossa and crosses through the otic capsule. These fractures can damage both the vestibular system and the cochlea; in addition, the facial nerve may be injured. As a result, vertigo with spontaneous nystagmus, a sensorineural hearing loss, and paralysis of the facial nerve are common. The most common cause of these fractures is a blow to the occipital area.

2. **Diagnosis.** The diagnosis can be made on clinical grounds with the finding of hemotympanum, facial nerve paralysis, vertigo, sensorineural hearing loss, or a step off in the external canal. If a patient has closed head trauma and skull films are unremarkable but hemotympanum is found, a basal skull fracture or temporal bone fracture is assumed. High-resolution CT or polytomography can be used to confirm the diagnosis. However, these sophisticated tests occasionally are unrevealing, and the diagnosis must be made on clinical grounds.

3. **Management.** Immediate otolaryngologic and neurologic consultation should be obtained. Hospitalization is indicated for observation.

   a. Occasionally, **decompression of the facial nerve** is indicated for return of function. Usually the mastoid and horizontal segment can be approached from a postauricular incision, but a middle cranial fossa approach is necessary to completely decompress the nerve. If the fracture resulted in avulsion of the nerve, a complete decompression with mobilization of the facial nerve to accomplish reanastomosis or cable grafting is required.

   b. **Fractures involving the ossicular chain** may be repaired immediately or on a delayed basis.

   c. **Transverse fractures with a damaged otic capsule** and a severe hearing loss require careful observation for perilymph, endolymph, or CSF leakage. Since meningitis in these patients is a frequent sequela, parenteral antibiotics are required. If tympanic membrane perforation exists, ear drops should be avoided until perilymph or endolymph leakage has been ruled out.

Neck Trauma

Trauma to the neck is potentially serious in that there are a vast number of vital structures within the neck. Any person with blunt or penetrating neck trauma is at risk for airway compromise from either direct injury to the airway or extrinsic compression from hemorrhage or edema. There is also the risk of esophageal injury. The jugular vein and its tributaries, as well as the carotid arteries and its major branches, are all susceptible to significant injury. The cervical spine and cranial nerves coursing through the neck may also be injured.

I. **General management principles**
  A. **Airway precautions** should be instituted in all patients with significant neck trauma. Careful observation, particularly for development of any hoarseness, stridor, retractions, or hemoptysis, is essential. Since endotracheal intubation may be difficult and dangerous if a laryngeal laceration is present, a tracheostomy may be required to establish an airway.
  B. **Cervical spine immobilization.** Since patients with neck trauma are at high risk for a cervical spine injury, the cervical spine must be immobilized (see Chaps. 17 and 25) in the proper clinical setting until cleared by appropriate radiographs.
  C. **Control of bleeding** with a Barton pressure dressing (see **Maxillofacial Trauma,** sec. **I.C.1.b**) is possible. Care must be taken, however, not to mask any enlarging hematoma.
  D. **Repletion of the intravascular volume** is necessary if significant bleeding has occurred. A large-bore IV catheter should be placed as soon as the patient arrives in the emergency department, and crystalloid and blood administered as needed.
  E. If significant injury is presumed, parenteral **antibiotics** should be started. A third-generation cephalosporin is appropriate.
  F. **Tetanus toxoid** should be administered as needed.
  G. Preparation for **endoscopic evaluation or neck exploration** (or both) may then take place.
II. **Blunt trauma.** Motor vehicle accidents have long been the chief cause of blunt trauma to the neck, usually secondary to striking the steering wheel. Other sources of injury include snowmobile, motorcycle, or sports accidents. Injuries to the underlying soft tissues predominantly include laryngeal fractures, esophageal tears, and injury to the great vessels. In addition, trauma to the neck may be associated with injuries to the cervical spine or other organ systems.
  A. **Initial assessment.** Airway precautions must be instituted while evaluation of the larynx and chest (and other body systems) is undertaken. In addition, the cervical spine must be immobilized until radiologically cleared.
    1. The **physical examination** should include a neurologic evaluation (with particular attention to the cranial nerves); palpation of the neck for pulses, hematomas, and landmarks; auscultation for bruits; and an assessment of other organ systems.
    2. **Radiographs**
      a. Anteroposterior (AP) and lateral **cervical spine films** are useful in assessing the cervical spine and in identifying both free air within the neck and soft-tissue swelling impinging on the airway.
      b. A **chest x-ray** generally will identify aspiration pneumonitis, a pneumothorax or pneumomediastinum, pulmonary contusion, and mediastinal abnormalities (suggestive of possible great-vessel injury).
    3. If there is any suspicion of laryngeal injury, indirect or direct **laryngoscopy** should be performed as soon as possible to delineate any injury and its extent. The patient with mild laryngeal trauma may undergo indirect laryngoscopy with a mirror and headlight by an experienced observer; this procedure may allow the exclusion of those with minor trauma from general anesthesia. If there is any question of the severity of injury, however, the patient should be endoscoped in the operating suite.
    4. **Esophagoscopy** should be performed if there is the possibility of an esophageal injury.
  B. **Airway management.** In patients with a neck injury and airway compromise, an emergent **tracheostomy** is indicated. A cricothyrotomy is usually less advanta-

geous, since fracture to the cricoid ring may be aggravated. Endotracheal intubation is fraught with danger, as the endotracheal tube can pass through a laceration or fracture line into the soft tissue of the neck; in addition, further damage to injured laryngeal structures can occur.

C. **Specific injuries**

1. **Laryngeal fractures**

a. The **clinical presentation** of laryngeal fractures includes one or more of the following symptoms and signs: acute airway obstruction, hemoptysis, hoarseness, dysphagia, odynophagia, hematemesis, or soft-tissue swelling. In addition, palpation of the neck may reveal free air or disruption of the normal laryngeal architecture, with either a palpable fracture line or loss of the normal laryngeal prominence. These patients must be considered at risk for sudden airway compromise.

b. **Evaluation.** Following initial stabilization, laryngoscopy should be performed to determine the nature and extent of the injury.

c. **Management** involves securing an airway (by tracheostomy) and surgical repair of the laryngeal fracture. Antibiotic therapy is also indicated.

2. **Esophageal injury.** Esophageal tears, although uncommon in blunt neck trauma, are serious because of the risk of mediastinitis. Usually these injuries are secondary to shearing of the esophageal wall with a rapid motion, since the esophagus is relatively tethered in the thorax. Most commonly, these patients present with odynophagia, dysphagia, and pooling of secretions. Radiographic evaluation often reveals cervical free air or a pneumomediastinum or pneumothorax. Endoscopy will establish the diagnosis. Treatment involves surgical repair and drainage. Administration of parenteral antibiotics is essential.

3. **Injury to the great vessels** (see Chap. 20) secondary to blunt trauma can occur and is treated similarly to great-vessel injuries resulting from penetrating neck trauma (see sec. **III.C.3**).

III. **Penetrating neck trauma** is a potentially dangerous injury. Injuries to the larynx, esophagus, great vessels, and cranial nerves are possible. It is important to note that if there is no penetration of the platysma, the risk of injury is, of course, significantly reduced. Evaluation must be prompt with an understanding that airway compromise, infection, and neurologic sequelae can develop quickly. Common inflicting instruments include ice picks, knives, and missiles. All penetrating injuries should be treated similarly. The size of the entrance wound has no relation to the extent of internal damage.

A. **Initial evaluation**

1. **Physical examination.** Since neck wounds can bleed rather profusely, even if no major vessel is injured, the extent of blood loss should be determined. In addition, any swelling must be noted and recorded to determine if there is expansion of a hematoma. Palpation of the carotid pulses and auscultation (for bruits) are important. A complete neurologic examination, with particular attention to assessment of the cranial and cervical nerves, extremity motion, motor strength, and the patient's mental status, is essential to determine whether there has been any injury to cranial or peripheral nerves, the spinal cord, or the brain secondary to direct injury or impaired blood flow.

2. An **arteriogram** or neck exploration or both should be performed if there is any question of injury to the great vessels.

3. **Esophagoscopy** is indicated if there is any suspicion of esophageal injury.

B. **Initial management** is directed at instituting cervical spine precautions as appropriate, maintaining a secure airway, controlling bleeding (usually with direct pressure), and repleting the intravascular volume. Tetanus toxoid and antibiotics should be administered as indicated.

C. **Specific injuries**

1. **Laryngeal injuries** secondary to penetrating trauma usually are manifested with signs and symptoms similar to those resulting from blunt trauma (see sec. **II.C.1.a**). In particular, hemoptysis may be present, even if other signs are not. A tracheostomy should be performed if there is airway compromise secondary to major soft-tissue injury or laceration of the mucosa of the larynx. Endoscopic evaluation of the larynx and its adjacent structures is necessary to determine the nature and extent of the injury. Open surgical procedures are often necessary to adequately close mucosal lacerations.

2. **Esophageal injuries** may go undiagnosed initially, but because of leakage of contaminated oral cavity contents into the soft tissue of the neck, an abscess usually develops rather quickly. Since the esophagus is closely related to the

prevertebral and other deep neck spaces, infection of this area is serious. During endoscopy, esophagoscopy should be performed to delineate the presence and extent of any esophageal injury. Surgical drainage and antibiotic therapy are essential.

3. **Great-vessel injuries** (see Chap. 20). Venous injuries may or may not tamponade. In the latter situation the hematoma will continue to expand. Most arterial injuries, on the other hand, will continue to bleed or be associated with an expanding hematoma. A pseudoaneurysm can also occur following blunt or penetrating trauma. An arteriogram or wound exploration is necessary if there is any suspicion of a great-vessel injury. If there is an expanding hematoma or any neurologic deficit, immediate exploration and attempted vascular repair are indicated. Prior to operative intervention, it is important to replete the intravascular volume by infusion of crystalloid and blood as needed in order to lessen the risk of neurologic sequelae. Since silent injury to the esophagus may result in a salivary fistula and subsequent infection of a vascular repair, all neck explorations must include panendoscopy.

4. **Shotgun injuries,** unlike other penetrating trauma, usually are associated with massive soft-tissue loss. A cricothyrotomy or tracheotomy for airway control and a pressure dressing for control of bleeding are the most important aspects of the initial management. A nasogastric tube should be inserted to allow for gastric decompression and subsequent feeding. Antibiotic therapy is indicated. No debridement should take place until the tissue necrosis is delineated. Tissue flaps are often needed for reconstruction.

Bibliography

1. Bailey, B. Management of maxillofacial trauma. *Resident and Staff Physician* 28(12): 57, 1982.
2. Ballantyne, J. C. Review of traumatic conductive deafness. *Proc. R. Soc. Med.* 59:535, 1963.
3. Cairns, H. Injuries of frontal and ethmoid sinus with special reference to cerebral spinal rhinorrhea and aeroceles. *J. Laryngol. Otol.* 52:589, 1937.
4. Calcatera, T., et al. Carotid artery injuries. *Laryngoscope* 82:321, 1972.
5. Dingman, R. O., and Natvig, P. *Surgery of Facial Fractures.* Philadelphia: Saunders, 1964.
6. Gros, J. C. The ear and skull trauma. *South. Med. J.* 60:705, 1967.
7. Hagan, W. E. et al. Gunshot injury to the temporal bone and analysis of 35 cases. *Laryngoscope* 89:1258, 1979.
8. Holt, J. Orbital blow-out fractures. *Ear Nose Throat J.* 62:15, 1983.
9. Hybels, R. L. Posterior table fracture of the frontal sinus. 2. Clinical aspects. *Laryngoscope* 87:1740, 1977.
10. Kettel, K. Peripheral facial palsy and fractures of temporal bone. *Arch. Otolaryngol.* 51:25, 1950.
11. Le Fort, R. Etude experimentale sur les fractures de la machoire superieure. *Rev. Chir.* 23:208, 360, 479, 1901.
12. Levine, P. A. Mandibular reconstruction: The use of open reduction with compression plates. *Otolaryngol. Head Neck Surg.* 90:585, 1982.
13. May, M. Nasal frontal ethmoid injuries. *Laryngoscope* 87:948, 1977.
14. May, M., et al. Penetrating neck wounds: Selective exploration. *Laryngoscope* 85:57, 1975.
15. May, M., et al. Shotgun wounds to the head and neck. *Arch. Otolaryngol.* 98:373, 1973.
16. Mladick, R. A. Salvage of the ear in acute trauma. *Clin. Plast. Surg.* 5:427, 1978.
17. Ogura, J. H., and Biller, H. F. Reconstruction of the larynx following blunt trauma. *Ann. Otol. Rhinol. Laryngol.* 80:492, 1971.
18. Ogura, J. H., Heeneman, H., and Spector, G. Laryngotracheal trauma: Diagnosis and treatment. *Can. J. Otolaryngol.* 2:112, 1973.
19. Stell, P. M. The fractured nose. *Clin. Otolaryngol.* 5:362, 1980.
20. Wachtel, T., et al. Management of burns of the head and neck. *Head Neck Surg.* 3:458, 1981.

25

Neurosurgical Emergencies

Arthur B. Jenny

Pain in the Neck and Back

I. General principles

A. Etiology. Pain involving the spine has multiple origins. Pain endings are found in the muscles, ligaments, periosteum, outer layer of the annulus fibrosis, and the synovium of the articular facets. Pain can arise from disease intrinsic to the spine, muscle spasm, or nerve root compression; it can also be referred from other organ systems.

B. Evaluation. The differentiation among disease of the spine, paraspinous muscles, nerve roots, and other conditions is made primarily from the history and physical examination.

  1. History. Information about what makes the pain better or worse should be sought. Pain from degenerative disk disease of the spine may radiate into the shoulder or buttock. Radicular symptoms from nerve root compression (which may be delayed after disk herniation) usually occur as pain in the arm and thigh; pain, paresthesias, or numbness in the forearm and leg; or paresthesias or numbness in the hand or foot. Changes in the gait and bladder control suggest spinal cord or cauda equina compression. Painful limitation of motion of the shoulder or hip suggests local joint disease.

  2. The **physical examination** should include observations about paraspinous muscle spasm, the extent (and pain) of voluntary range of motion, gait, distribution of weakness, distribution of sensory deficits, and reflex changes. The abdomen and the peripheral pulses should be examined in patients with low back and lower-limb pain.

  3. Lateral **x-rays** of the spine should be reviewed for alignment, narrowing of degenerated disk spaces, spondylosis, and destruction of vertebral bodies. The anteroposterior (AP) x-ray should be reviewed for erosion of the pedicles and paravertebral soft-tissue masses. More expensive diagnostic studies, such as computed tomography (CT) or magnetic resonance scanning, generally should be arranged by the patient's physician or consulting physicians.

C. The **disposition** from the emergency department depends on the diagnosis. Most patients can be discharged and followed by their physicians. Discovery or consideration of more serious disease (e.g., compression fracture from a malignancy), however, should warrant appropriate consultation, and the disposition should be according to the consultant's recommendation.

II. Specific pain syndromes

A. Neck pain

  1. Cervical disk herniation

   a. Clinical features. A common cause of acute neck, shoulder, and arm pain is lateral disk herniation in the lower cervical spine. Although there may be a history of major or minor trauma, most patients awaken in the morning with pain in the neck or rhomboid region. Pain in the neck, medial border of the scapula, or the anterior chest, however, is referred pain and is not specific for any level of disk herniation. The more distal radicular symptoms of pain in the arm or forearm and paresthesias or numbness in the forearm or hand usually develop somewhat later and usually are the result of nerve root compression. Voluntary range of motion of the cervical spine is decreased. Coughing and neck extension may make the symptoms worse, and traction and placing the forearm on top of the head may give relief of the pain. The radicular pain may be severe.

   b. The most common **levels of disk herniation** are the C5–6 (25%) and C6–7 (60%) levels.

    (1) C5 root (C4–5 disk). Pain is referred to the shoulder and lateral aspect of the upper arm. Weakness can occur in the supraspinatus, deltoid, biceps, and brachioradialis muscles. The biceps reflex is decreased or absent.

    (2) C6 root (C5–6 disk). Pain is referred to the lateral arm and dorsal forearm, and numbness involves the thumb and index fingers. The biceps muscle is weak (mild to moderate), and its reflex is decreased or absent.

    (3) C7 root (C6–7 disk). Pain is referred to the lateral arm and dorsal forearm, and numbness involves the index and middle fingers. The triceps muscle is weak (moderate to marked), and its reflex is absent or reduced.

    (4) C8 root (C7–T1 disk). Pain is referred to the medial aspect of the upper arm and ulnar forearm, and numbness involves the ring and fifth fingers. Weakness occurs in the triceps, wrist and finger extensors (except extensor carpi radialis), wrist and finger flexors (except flexor carpi radialis), and in the intrinsic muscles of the hand. The triceps reflex is absent or reduced.

    (5) T1 root (T1–2 disk). Pain is referred to the medial aspect of the arm and forearm, and numbness involves the ulnar forearm. Weakness occurs in the intrinsic muscles of the hand. There are no reflex changes, and Horner's syndrome may be present.

  c. Evaluation. The initial diagnosis of a herniated disk is made on clinical grounds. Routine x-rays should be obtained to rule out more serious disease causing neck pain and radicular symptoms (e.g., tumor, infection). Additional studies include a high-resolution CT scan of the cervical spine and cervical myelography. A CT scan is expensive and will not always show a lateral herniated cervical disk. The myelogram should be reserved as a preoperative study.

  d. Treatment

    (1) Analgesics. The radicular pain associated with disk herniation may be intense and require narcotic medication.

    (2) If muscle spasm is present, a **muscle relaxant** (e.g., diazepam, cyclobenzaprine, carisoprodol, methocarbamol) may benefit some patients.

    (3) A **cervical collar** may be helpful.

    (4) Persistent symptoms of cervical disk herniation may also respond to a trial of **cervical traction.** The response to traction, however, varies from patient to patient. It is recommended that traction be initiated with 5 lb for 5–10 minutes 3 times/day. If the pain becomes more severe, traction should be discontinued.

    (5) Surgery is beneficial in most cases when conservative treatment fails.

  e. Disposition. The presence of intractable pain, progressive neurologic deficits, or new-onset deficits with a history of trauma warrants appropriate consultation. Otherwise, conservative treatment on an outpatient basis, with arrangements for follow-up, generally is appropriate.

2. Cervical strain

  a. Clinical features. Many patients develop a stiff and painful neck that generally is unilateral and made worse with movement. Patients may awaken with symptoms, and there may or may not be a history of trauma. Paraspinous muscle spasm is present. The symptoms usually regress spontaneously over several days to 1 week and may relate to either a true muscle strain or muscle spasm associated with cervical disk herniation that does not develop radicular symptoms. X-rays generally are not needed initially; however, they should be obtained if the neurologic examination is abnormal (aside from muscle spasm), if symptoms persist, or if there are indications of more serious disease (e.g., malignancy).

  b. The **treatment** of muscular and ligamentous strains is mainly symptomatic and includes rest and avoidance of activity that worsens the pain. External moist heat and pain medication are helpful. In addition, muscle relaxants generally are useful.

3. Degenerative disk disease and stenosis

  a. Degenerative disk disease of the cervical spine is common in older patients and in some can be associated with pain and stiffness in the neck and shoulder. Bony hypertrophy may develop around the degenerated disk and facet joints and compress the nerve roots as they exit the neural foramina. The radicular symptoms are the same as those with disk herniation (see **1.b**).

  (1) **X-rays** may show narrowed disk spaces, a minor degree of misalignment or subluxation, and bony spur formation. Oblique views of the spine may appear to show encroachment of the neural foramen. A high-resolution CT scan will show bony narrowing of the neural foramen better than routine x-rays.

  (2) **Treatment** of symptomatic degenerative conditions includes administration of a nonsteroidal anti-inflammatory drug (e.g., salicylate, naproxen, sulindac, ibuprofen, indomethacin, phenylbutazone). Radicular pain may be helped with surgery if conservative measures fail.

  b. Stenosis from bony hypertrophy that bridges the posterior vertebral body on either side of a degenerated disk may become large enough to be associated with damage to the spinal cord **(myelopathy).**

  (1) **Clinical features.** Upper-limb weakness can be due to nerve root compression or degenerative changes in the spinal cord itself. Lower-limb symptoms include weakness, spasticity, increased reflexes, and gait disturbance. Neck pain and stiffness may or may not be present.

  (2) The **diagnosis** of cervical stenosis should be considered when signs and symptoms of cord compression occur with x-ray findings of severe degenerative disk disease.

  (3) **Management.** The patient should be referred for neurologic consultation. Decompressive surgery may halt the progression of symptoms, and in some patients surgery may be associated with improvement.

4. Disease in the **shoulder** (see Chap. 14) can produce pain in the neck, shoulder, and arm. Painful and decreased active range of motion of the shoulder indicates a problem with the shoulder joint, its capsule, or overlying tendons. Tendinitis and bursitis generally respond to administration of nonsteroidal anti-inflammatory agents. Inactivity related to other conditions (e.g., a cervical disk, stroke) can with time lead to a "frozen" shoulder; physical therapy is important to establish range of motion.

5. The **thoracic outlet syndrome** (superior thoracic aperture syndrome), which is mostly seen in middle-aged women, is a complex of symptoms produced by compression of the brachial plexus or subclavian artery and vein as they pass through the sites of the thoracic outlet. The syndrome is associated with cervical ribs that connect directly or by ligaments to the first rib or with anomalous positions and insertions of the anterior and medial scalene muscles.

  a. Clinical features. Neural symptoms are most frequent (95%) and include pain and paresthesias (usually in the distribution of the ulnar nerve). Weakness and wasting of the hand muscles occur in about 10%. Vascular symptoms are less common and include coldness, fatigability of the arm, a more diffuse pain, and signs of venous compression.

  b. The **diagnosis** is suggested when diagnostic maneuvers (e.g., the Adson maneuver, the exaggerated military position, and the hyperabduction maneuver) reduce the radial pulse, produce a clavicular bruit, and reproduce the neural symptoms. X-rays of the cervical spine should be examined for cervical ribs.

  c. Treatment. Most patients (60–80%) will respond to an individualized exercise program designed to improve posture and strengthen the shoulder girdle.

6. **Peripheral nerve entrapment** can sometimes simulate nerve root compression.

  a. Common syndromes

  (1) **Median nerve** compression at the carpal tunnel (see Chaps. 14 and 32) can produce pain in the shoulder, anterolateral arm, and radial forearm, in addition to pain or numbness in the thumb, index, and middle fingers. Atrophy of the thenar eminence or weakness of thumb abduction and opposition may be present. The cause is usually not determined. The possibility of hypothyroidism, amyloid deposition in the carpal ligament, rheumatoid arthritis, acromegaly, and repeated occupational trauma to the hand should be considered.

  (2) **Ulnar nerve** entrapment occurs most commonly at the elbow. There may be a history of local injury, resting the elbow on a hard surface, or frequent elbow flexion. The entrapment can be associated with pain in

the shoulder and medial arm, pain or numbness in the ulnar forearm, and numbness or paresthesias in the fourth and fifth fingers.

    b. The **diagnosis** of nerve entrapment can be confirmed in most patients by nerve conduction studies.

    c. Management. Conservative treatment includes avoidance of those activities that increase symptoms and external protection (e.g., elbow pads or pads on office desks). Surgery is generally helpful if conservative measures fail and should be considered early if significant weakness or atrophy is present to improve the chance of recovery of motor function.

  7. Causalgia is a pain syndrome that develops in about 2% of major sensory and motor nerves 1 month or longer after partial injury. The pain is a severe, diffuse, burning pain in the limb. It is made worse by light touch (e.g., by clothing or air currents) and emotional irritation, and the pain is relieved by cool water or an ice wrap. Trophic-nutritional changes (e.g., shiny, glossy skin) and vasomotor changes (e.g., vasodilatation and sweating) may occur. Initial treatment includes aggressive physical therapy and a series of stellate ganglion blocks.

  8. Reflex sympathetic dystrophy is a syndrome that can follow either a major or minor injury to a limb. It is characterized by pain, vasomotor signs (e.g., spasm, cyanosis, sweating), and trophic changes (bone demineralization, fibrosis of muscles and tendon sheaths). The pain generally is increased on cold exposure but is not made worse by emotional stimulation. Initial treatment includes stellate ganglion blocks and transcutaneous electrical nerve stimulation.

  9. Brachial neuritis (brachial plexus neuropathy) (see Chap. 32) is an unexplained illness that usually begins with severe shoulder pain and progresses to profound weakness in the shoulder and upper arm in 3–10 days. The pain often subsides as the weakness begins, and recovery usually occurs in several months. Treatment is symptomatic.

B. Thoracic pain

  1. Degenerative disk disease with disk herniation occurs rarely in the thoracic spine. Symptoms include local back pain and variable degrees of lower-limb paralysis, sensory loss, and incontinence. Thoracic spine films may show disk space narrowing at the suspected clinical level. Thoracic disk herniation may be difficult to differentiate from metastatic tumor when x-rays do not show destruction of bone. The diagnosis is made with water-soluble myelography with a CT scan.

  2. Intraspinal tumors such as neurofibroma and meningioma can present with thoracic back pain, radicular pain, and gait disturbance. Initial symptoms may be vague, and the problem can be difficult to diagnose. X-rays may show an enlarged neural foramina on the lateral view or eroded pedicles on the AP view. Appropriate consultation is indicated.

  3. Neuropathy and neuritis

    a. Notalgia paresthetica is a sensory neuropathy of the posterior rami of T2 through T6 thoracic nerves. The symptoms include paresthesias, aching or burning discomfort, and pruritis in the medial scapular region. A zone of hypesthesia occurs medial to the scapula at the level of the T2 through T6 dermatomes. The condition is benign and has no treatment.

    b. Herpes zoster is a viral infection of nerve root ganglia that occurs more frequently in the thoracic region. The presenting symptom is usually a neuralgic pain in the distribution of the affected nerve root. The vesicular eruption follows the pain in 3–4 days. Treatment is presented in Chap. 31.

    c. Diabetes mellitus can be associated with thoracic radiculopathy. The pain, which can be severe, may be described as burning, aching, or sharp and may include dysesthesias to light touch or clothing. An analgesic may offer some relief.

C. Low back pain

  1. Low back strain of the paraspinous muscles and ligaments usually follows lifting a heavy object or a sudden movement such as a fall.

    a. Clinical features. The pain is severe when the involved muscle contracts or is stretched and is relieved with rest and inactivity. Muscle spasm, tenderness, and distortion of normal posture may be present. The symptoms generally resolve over several days to 1 week. **X-rays** are not always needed initially if the history indicates a muscle strain and if there is no history of a more serious disease (e.g., malignancy).

    b. The **treatment** of muscular and ligamentous strains, which are usually self-limited, is mainly symptomatic and includes rest and avoidance of activity that worsens the pain. External heat and an analgesic are generally helpful. If muscle spasm is present, a muscle relaxant may also be helpful.

  2. **Lumbar disk herniation** is most likely to occur at the L4–5 or L5–S1 levels and is more apt to be associated with injury than is cervical disk herniation.

    a. **Radicular symptoms** from nerve root compression may be delayed. Lateral disk herniation usually compresses the nerve root below the level of the disk as the root passes laterally to exit under the pedicle of the lower vertebral body.

      (1) **L4 root.** Pain is referred down the anterolateral thigh, across the knee, and down the anteromedial leg. Weakness can occur in the quadriceps muscles; the knee reflex is usually decreased.

      (2) **L5 root.** Pain is referred to the posterolateral thigh, anterolateral leg, and medial foot. Weakness can occur in the foot dorsiflexors (i.e., foot drop on heel walking). Reflex changes, however, usually do not occur.

      (3) **S1 root.** Pain is referred to the posterior thigh, posterior leg, and posterolateral foot. Weakness occurs in the gastrocnemius and soleus muscles (toe walking). The ankle reflex is decreased or absent.

    b. **Evaluation**

      (1) There are several **tests** designed to stretch the sciatic nerve and produce radicular pain in irritated nerve roots. These tests include straight leg raising, slowly extending the flexed knee when the hip is flexed, and crossed straight leg raising. Radicular pain should be produced for the test to be positive.

      (2) **X-rays** should be reviewed for a narrowed disk space and for other underlying lesions. In thinner patients herniated lumbar disks can be demonstrated by CT scans. A myelogram, if needed, should be reserved as a preoperative study.

    c. **Treatment** includes a 7- to 10-day trial of bed rest and analgesic medication. Rapidly progressive weakness and bladder dysfunction indicate a large disk herniation and cauda equina compression; appropriate consultation should be sought immediately.

  3. **Degenerative disk disease** occurs in most persons with advancing age and is symptomatic in some patients. Stiffness and limitation of movement occur. The pain is usually increased with movement and relieved with rest. A symptomatic disk can produce pain in the back and pain laterally over a sacroiliac joint without nerve root compression. X-rays show degenerative changes. Treatment includes administration of aspirin or another anti-inflammatory medication.

  4. **Lumbar spinal stenosis.** The lumbar spinal canal can be narrowed either congenitally or secondarily by degenerative changes and hypertrophy of the ligamentum flavum and facet joints. A new-onset bulging disk may convert an asymptomatic condition to one of pain. The L3–4 and L4–5 levels are most commonly involved. Lower-limb pain may be radicular in nature or almost identical to vascular claudication. In spinal stenosis, however, the cramping, aching pain is produced by standing (or sometimes sitting), and the claudication distance is variable; the presence of peripheral pulses and toe hair go against vascular insufficiency. The clinical diagnosis can be confirmed in some patients with a CT scan. Others may require a water-soluble myelogram and CT scan to establish the diagnosis. Patients generally respond well to decompressive surgery.

  5. **Diabetic neuropathy** may occur as a painful asymmetric neuropathy involving a burning, lancinating pain in the hip, thigh, and knee. Muscle weakness is more evident in the pelvic girdle and thigh (secondary to femoral nerve involvement), and the knee reflex is decreased or absent. Recovery usually occurs with time. There is no specific therapy. An analgesic may be required for pain relief.

  6. **Abdominal disease**

    a. An **abdominal aortic aneurysm** may present with severe back pain and pain that radiates into the lower limbs. Routine examination should include palpation for an abdominal mass and lower-limb pulses and auscultation for abdominal and inguinal bruits. Surgical consultation is indicated.

    b. **Retroperitoneal and pelvic disorders.** Retroperitoneal malignancy (e.g., pancreatic carcinoma, adrenal metastasis) can be associated with low back pain. Pelvic conditions (e.g., endometriosis) and neoplastic and inflammatory conditions of the colon, kidney, bladder, and prostate also should be considered. Treatment is directed at the specific disorder.

D. **Systemic involvement of the spine**

1. **Systemic illnesses that involve the synovial membranes** and the periarticular structures and connective tissue (e.g., systemic lupus erythematosus, rheumatoid arthritis, other collagen vascular diseases) can produce neck and back pain. Treatment is directed at the underlying disease.

    Pain that radiates into the occipital area (i.e., compression of the C2 root) can be seen with atlantoaxial subluxation associated with rheumatoid arthritis; the pain may be severe and may benefit from surgery (fusion or rhizotomy).

2. **Hematogenous spread of infection** can produce osteomyelitis, disk space infection, and a spinal abscess. The patient may have symptoms and signs of spinal cord compression. X-rays may show destruction of the disk space. Appropriate consultation should be sought.

3. **Metastatic cancer** of the spine should be considered in every patient with a history of neoplastic disease. Cancer of the lung, prostate, and breast and lymphoma are the most common. Neurologic symptoms and signs of cauda equina or spinal cord compression represent an urgent situation, and immediate neurologic or neurosurgical consultation should be sought.

Head Injury

Head injuries can result from blunt or penetrating trauma. They may involve the scalp, skull, and brain, and the impact energy can be distributed in any combination. Between 2 and 10% of comatose patients secondary to blunt head trauma have a cervical spine fracture.

I. **Physiology.** The injured brain is very susceptible to further metabolic insults. Brain function is dependent on the delivery of oxygen (20% of the total oxygen consumption), which is dependent on the arterial PO_2 and cerebral blood flow.

A. The overall **cerebral blood flow** is maintained at 40–60 ml/100 gm of brain/minute (15% of the cardiac output) by autoregulatory changes in arteriole vascular resistance in response to changes in mean arterial blood pressure between 50 and 150 mm Hg. Below 50 mm Hg and above 150 mm Hg, cerebral blood flow is pressure dependent. Mean arterial pressures greater than 150 mm Hg are associated with an increased cerebral blood volume and the breakdown of the blood-brain barrier. Prolonged blood flow below 25 ml/minute is associated with ischemic damage. Vascular resistance is also responsive to the arterial PCO_2, with blood flow increasing or decreasing 1 ml/minute for each 1 mm Hg increase or decrease in PCO_2, respectively, between 20 and 80 mm Hg. Regional blood flow in the brain is controlled by metabolic autoregulation, with increased flow going to regions of increased neuronal activity.

B. The total adult **intracranial volume** is about 1200–1400 ml, divided into three basic compartments: the brain, 80–85%; cerebrospinal fluid (CSF), 8–12%; and arterial and venous blood, 3–7%. The normal intracranial pressure (ICP) is 3–13 mm Hg. The intracranial cavity accommodates mass lesions by displacing the CSF into the spinal CSF space and reducing the blood volume. With small mass lesions the ability to compensate (compliance) is adequate. However, as masses enlarge and the ICP rises above 20 mm Hg, the compliance or buffering capacity decreases. Brain shifts, including herniation of the medial temporal lobe through the tentorial notch on to the brainstem, eventually occur.

C. **Cerebral perfusion pressure** is the difference between the mean arterial pressure and the ICP. In the presence of intact autoregulation, any gradual decrease in the mean arterial pressure (and perfusion pressure) will be associated with cerebrovascular dilatation and an increased cerebral blood volume; in the head-injured patient, this cerebrovascular dilatation may lead to a high temporary ICP (plateau wave).

D. The injured brain tolerates raised **ICP** poorly. Pressures of 15–20 mm Hg are elevated, and pressure above 25 mm Hg should be treated. In severe head injuries, 50% of patients have ICPs above 20 mm Hg; one-third of these patients have uncontrollable intracranial hypertension and eventually die. The subgroup of patients with diffuse head injury has only a 30% incidence of raised ICP; in contrast, the subgroup of patients with cerebral contusion has a 70% incidence of raised pressure. Fulminant brain swelling can occur with a rapid increase in cerebral blood volume or with a loss of autoregulation of blood flow.

II. Evaluation

A. History should be sought (1) about the events leading to the head injury (e.g., syncope, seizure, chest pain) that may indicate another primary illness and (2) about the nature and severity of the head injury. In addition, information about the duration of loss of consciousness and about neurologic deficits (particularly the level of consciousness) is essential. Specific questions about neck pain and cervical radicular symptoms should be asked. The duration of retrograde and posttraumatic amnesia should be estimated by the patient's ability to remember events.

B. The **neurologic examination** (taking care to avoid moving the neck until a cervical spine fracture has been excluded) should be as thorough as possible, since it serves as a baseline for future examinations. The basic neurologic examination should include the following: (1) the level of consciousness and the patient's ability to follow commands, (2) motor strength, (3) pupillary size and response to light, and (4) eye movements. In responsive patients, orientation should be checked, and sensory testing should include smell (e.g., with hospital hand lotion or benzoin sprayed on a gauze sponge).

The level of consciousness, which is the most important indicator of the neurologic status of the patient, should be described by phrases (e.g., arousable to pain) in addition to terms such as lethargic or obtunded. **Coma** is defined as the inability to obey commands, utter recognizable words, or open the eyes. The **Glasgow coma scale** (see Table 1-2) is a 15-point grading system used by many clinicians to standardize description of head-injured patients. It combines the best response of three parameters: **eye opening** (4, spontaneous; 3, to speech; 2, to pain; 1, none); **verbal response** (5, oriented; 4, confused conversation; 3, inappropriate words; 2, incomprehensible sounds; 1, none); and **motor function** (6, obeys commands; 5, localizes pain; 4, withdraws; 3, abnormal flexion; 2, abnormal extension; 1, none). The neurologic examination should be descriptive enough to later grade the patient if desired.

C. General physical examination. The head should be examined for signs of injury (e.g., open wounds, contusion, ecchymosis, tenderness), and the ears should be checked for hemotympanum. A CSF leak can occur from the ears or nose; patients should also be asked about watery drainage down the back of their throats. The general examination should search for associated injuries.

D. Skull x-rays should be obtained in those patients who have had a concussion or who have had focal impacts. Linear fractures have well-defined margins and sharp angles where they branch. They are more radiolucent than vascular grooves since they extend through the thickness of the skull. A scalp contusion may be a clue to the side of a fracture seen on lateral x-ray. Fractures that cross the groove of the middle meningeal vessels or cross the superior sagittal sinus or transverse sinus are associated with an increased risk of intracranial hematoma. Skull x-rays on patients who did not lose consciousness or who have focal impacts have a very low yield of fracture and need not always be obtained.

E. A **CT scan** should be done as soon as possible in patients with a decreased level of consciousness or with signs or symptoms suggesting a mass lesion. It should be reviewed for hemorrhage, contusion, mass effect, size of ventricles, obliteration of cisterns around the brainstem, penetrating injuries, opacified sinuses, and depressed fractures.

Patients who are under the influence of alcohol or other drugs may have depressed levels of consciousness. Those patients who have a history or findings of head injury, have focal neurologic signs, or are unable to follow commands should have a CT scan. Judgment is required on less inebriated patients.

III. Management.

The major goals of management are to prevent additional irreversible brain injury, which can result from a secondary physiologic problem, and to evacuate mass lesions as soon as possible.

A decreasing level of consciousness is the most important indication of increasing ICP. The basic neurologic examination should be repeated at frequent intervals. Progressive coma, pupillary dilatation, paralysis, or posturing is a life-threatening situation. Emergent neurosurgical consultation should be obtained in all cases of potentially serious head injury.

A. Hypoxemia must be treated to prevent additional injury to the already impaired brain. Since patients with severe head injury may be significantly hypoxic (30% have PO_2 below 65 mm Hg), oxygen should be started at the accident site. This hypoxemia may be due to upper airway obstruction, chest injury, pulmonary shunting, atelectasis associated with the apnea of concussion, or undefined factors. Patients who are not talking or following commands should be intubated. Nasotracheal intubation is preferred in patients with suspected cervical spine injury. Positive end-expiratory pressure when needed should be limited to 10 cm H_2O, if possible, as pressures above 10 cm H_2O can elevate ICP.

B. Hypotension is not caused by head injury unless brainstem function is absent or significant blood loss from a scalp laceration has occurred. The causes of hypotension must be sought and treated appropriately. The hemoglobin should be maintained above 10–12 gm/dl to assure adequate cerebral oxygenation.

C. If there is any possibility of **injury to the cervical spine,** it must be immobilized until cleared with appropriate x-rays (see **Injury to the Spine,** sec. **IV.B** and **E**).

D. Intracranial hypertension can be due to an intracranial hematoma, focal brain swelling, or diffuse brain swelling. The mainstay of **medical treatment of intracranial hypertension** includes controlled hyperventilation and intermittent mannitol administration.

  1. Hyperventilation, which reduces cerebral blood volume by decreasing blood flow, should be initiated with regulation of the PCO_2 to around 27–30 mm Hg.

  2. Elevation of the head can be helpful in some cases of intracranial hypertension.

  3. In patients with a stable cardiovascular system, **mannitol,** 1 gm/kg IV, should be given (bladder catheterization is necessary). In the emergency department, mannitol is indicated (with neurosurgical consultation) for central nervous system (CNS) herniation or impending herniation. By increasing the serum osmolarity, mannitol draws off brain water in normal regions, thereby decreasing the ICP. Changes in the neurologic examination should be recorded; little or no improvement is a grave prognostic sign.

  4. While **steroids** have proved highly effective in the treatment of brain edema associated with tumors, their benefit in the treatment of edema associated with head injury has not been demonstrated clinically. Dexamethasone, given as 10 mg IV initially and followed by 4 mg q6h, is now considered by some to be a low-dose regimen. High-dose steroids (e.g., 100 mg q6h) also have not been shown to be beneficial. The use of steroids should be left to the discretion of the attending neurosurgeon.

  5. Although controversial, **barbiturates** are used by some physicians to try to control raised ICP that is not responsive to mannitol or hyperventilation. Barbiturates may prove to be helpful by reducing metabolic activity. Their use and dosage should be left to the attending neurosurgeon.

  6. ICP monitoring is generally used in more severe head injuries in the setting of an intensive care unit (ICU).

E. Fluid, acid-base, and electrolyte management. It is important to maintain normal serum electrolytes and to avoid overhydration and hyponatremia. Fluid replacement should begin with a crystalloid solution at three-fourths normal maintenance (i.e., 60–75 ml/hour or 1500–1800 ml/day in adults). Significant dehydration should also be avoided, and a urine output of 30 ml/hour should be maintained. Further therapy should follow basic principles of fluid and electrolyte administration.

F. Seizures (see Chap. 32) should be terminated to avoid further insults to the brain; diazepam is the drug of choice for terminating ongoing seizures. Phenytoin (or phenobarbital) generally is indicated to prevent recurrence of seizure activity, particularly in severe head injuries.

The benefit of prophylactic anticonvulsants to prevent a delayed seizure disorder in head injuries remains controversial. Patients who have evidence of cortical injury (e.g., contusion, intracranial hemorrhage), focal neurologic deficit, or early seizures (not including the first hour postinjury) have an increased risk of developing delayed seizures and should be considered for anticonvulsant therapy.

G. Hyperthermia may occur with injury to the hypothalamus and should be treated appropriately.

H. Disposition. Patients with an abnormal neurologic examination, fluctuating level of consciousness, skull fracture, or symptoms of increased ICP should be hospitalized for observation and definitive treatment. In addition, patients with a concussion generally should be admitted for observation.

I. The need for **surgery** should be based on the clinical status and radiologic findings. In general, surgery is indicated in patients with a clinically significant focal mass lesion (e.g., hematoma, anterior frontal lobe contusion). When indicated, surgery should be performed as soon as possible, as the effects of mannitol are short-lived.

IV. Specific injuries
   A. Skull fractures result from forces producing skull distortion. They can be linear or depressed and open or closed.
      1. Types of fractures
         a. Depressed fractures. High-velocity focal impacts tend to produce depressed skull fractures with possible laceration of the dura and brain beneath. Fractures that are depressed more than 3–5 mm have a greater chance of lacerating the underlying dura and brain.
         b. Linear fractures. Low-velocity impacts cause inbending of the skull at the point of impact and simultaneous outbending around the region of impact. Linear fractures (about 70% of skull fractures) begin in the region of outbending and then extend toward the point of impact and toward the base of the skull. Anterior impacts can produce linear fractures of the orbit, cribriform plate, and pituitary fossa. Occipital impacts can produce transverse parietal fractures and fractures that extend into the middle fossa and the petrous portion of the temporal bone.
         c. Basilar skull fractures generally are clinical diagnoses, since these fractures usually are not seen on x-ray. The clinical signs of basilar skull fracture include hemotympanum, ecchymosis behind the ear (Battle's sign, which may be delayed in appearance), periorbital ecchymosis not due to periorbital trauma (raccoon eyes), nystagmus, hearing loss, and decreased facial nerve function. Positional vertigo may be severe. X-rays may show clouding or air-fluid levels in the mastoid or sphenoid sinuses and intracranial air. The cleaning of blood from the ear canal may introduce infection if a basilar skull fracture with otorrhea is present.
      2. Evaluation includes pertinent physical and neurologic examinations. Skull x-rays should be obtained (see sec. **II.D**). A CT scan, in addition to identifying skull fractures, is useful in detecting parenchymal damage and intracranial hemorrhage.
      3. Management. Patients with skull fractures should be admitted for observation.
         a. The indications for exploration and elevation of **closed depressed skull fractures** remain unsettled. If the fracture involves the forehead, it may be raised for cosmetic reasons. Significantly depressed fractures should be elevated.
         b. Compound depressed fractures should undergo surgery to debride contaminated and necrotic tissue.
   B. CSF leaks usually occur through the nose (via the frontal, ethmoid, or sphenoid sinuses) in association with fractures of the frontal bone and cribriform plate or through the ear in association with petrous bone fractures and rupture of the tympanic membrane. CSF can also drain into the nose from the middle ear via the eustachian tube. The most significant complication of CSF leak is meningitis, which is due to *Streptococcus pneumoniae* in about 80% of cases.
      1. Diagnosis. The patient should be asked about watery drainage down the back of the throat. There is no reliable diagnostic test for CSF other than its characteristic spread on a gauze pad (i.e., a bloody center with a clear halo).
      2. Management of early CSF leaks is hospitalization and bed rest until the leak stops, which generally occurs between several days and 2 weeks. CSF leaks that extend beyond 2 weeks of injury or begin 2–3 weeks after injury (late CSF leaks) should be considered for surgery to repair the dural tear. The use of prophylactic antibiotics is controversial.
   C. Cerebral concussion and postconcussive syndrome
      1. Concussion is a clinical diagnosis that includes a loss of consciousness (paralytic phase) and memory loss (amnesic phase). The physiologic events that produce loss of consciousness are unknown, but the impact needs to be under 200 msec and include a rotational component. Most patients with concussion have an unremarkable neurologic examination by the time they reach the physician. The duration of unconsciousness and posttraumatic amnesia are indices of the severity of the head injury. Although the neurologic injury generally is reversible, irreversible cognitive deficits can occur. Since concussion represents a significant head injury, patients generally should be admitted for observation.
      2. The **postconcussive syndrome** is a group of nonspecific symptoms, including headache, dizziness, and nervous instability, that may follow cerebral concussion. The cause of the syndrome is unclear at present but probably represents a spectrum of organic and psychogenic factors. The headache may be generalized

or localized to the area of impact, continuous or intermittent, or aggravated by physical exertion, posture, or emotional stress. The episodes of disequilibrium are usually brief, associated with movement of the head, and, in some patients, correlated with abnormal labyrinthine function. Cognitive function and memory can be impaired, even in "minor" concussive head injury. Other symptoms are loss of self-esteem, emotional difficulty, and depression. **Treatment** is mainly supportive, including reassurance that the symptoms will usually resolve with time. Headaches should be treated with a nonnarcotic analgesic. Patients with prolonged symptoms should be referred back to their physicians.

D. Cerebral contusion and brain swelling. Cerebral contusion describes physical damage to the brain that includes small hemorrhagic areas, focal swelling, edema, and necrosis. The mechanism of brain injury after blunt head trauma remains unsettled. During head injury, the brain shifts and rotates, and sheer stresses occur on the brain where the cranial vault (particularly the anterior and middle fossae) restricts movement. This finding may explain why the frontal and temporal lobes are more frequently damaged. Contusion can occur both at and opposite the site of impact. Posttraumatic brain edema can develop during the first week of injury and extend outward from a polar injury. Contusion of the temporal and frontal lobes can be associated with significant local swelling.

1. **Clinical features.** Cerebral contusion can be asymptomatic or associated with focal neurologic signs, seizures, and a depressed level of consciousness.
2. **Management.** Patients should be admitted. Medical treatment of raised ICP is discussed in sec. **III.D.** Surgery may be required to remove necrotic brain tissue representing a life-threatening mass.

E. Intracranial hematoma. Intracranial hemorrhage can occur in the epidural space, subdural space, or within the brain. A decreasing level of consciousness is the most important sign of increasing ICP. The diagnosis is established by a CT scan. Treatment is rapid surgical evacuation unless the hematoma is clinically insignificant.

1. **Epidural hematomas** occur in approximately 1–3% of blunt head injuries and are secondary to tears in the meningeal vessels or dural sinuses. The middle meningeal artery (or vein) is most frequently involved, and the most common site is the temporal region. The patient may have had no initial loss of consciousness or a brief concussion, or may have been unconscious from the time of impact. A "lucid interval," the time between the head injury and a decreasing level of consciousness, is reported in 10–50% of patients with epidural hematomas. A lucid interval, however, can be seen with any slowly expanding mass lesion and is not diagnostic of an epidural hematoma. The mortality is about 15–25%.
2. **Acute subdural hematomas** occur with a variable amount of underlying brain injury. Subarachnoid and subdural blood from cortical lacerations or contusions generally are present with severe head injuries. The subdural hematoma, which generally arises from a torn bridging vein, can be extensive, particularly in patients with some degree of cerebral atrophy. On the other hand, the subdural hematoma may be minimal, and the major life-threatening mass may be a swollen and contused hemisphere. The mortality can be as high as 90%.
3. **Subacute subdural hematomas** refer to poorly defined entities in which the clinical signs begin between 2 days and 2 weeks of the injury.
4. **Chronic subdural hematomas** usually occur in older patients or alcoholic patients with cerebral atrophy. The hematoma develops slowly and usually follows a head injury that may be minor or forgotten. As the hematoma ages, the clot develops a membrane, turns a color and consistency of motor oil, and gradually enlarges (pathophysiology unclear). A significant brain shift can occur. The diagnosis is made on a CT scan. Hematomas 7–10 days old, however, may be of the same density as brain and appear only as a shift or obliteration of the cortical sulci. Moreover, a brain shift may not be present if the hematoma is bilateral. A CT scan with contrast may be helpful in these cases. **Treatment** is evacuation by either catheter drainage or surgery (unless the hematoma is small and asymptomatic).
5. **Intracerebral hematomas** can occur at the site of a depressed skull fracture, in association with coup or contrecoup contusions, or within the center of a lobe. The hemorrhages may be multiple and vary in size.
6. **Delayed intracranial hematomas** can occur with serious head injury. Progressive obtundation following an initial "negative" CT scan should warrant a repeat CT scan.

F. Penetrating brain injuries include open depressed skull fractures, gunshot wounds, and stab wounds. The route of entry may be hidden in the orbit, nose, or mouth. Military high-velocity gunshot wounds are associated with considerable damage and necrosis of the surrounding brain. Civilian gunshot wounds usually are low-muzzle velocity and are associated with less adjacent brain injury.

1. **X-rays and CT scans** are helpful in determining the location of indriven bone fragments and foreign bodies (wood is hypodense). Angiography may be needed to determine the relationship of a foreign body (e.g., knife blade, ice pick) to a major vessel or venous sinus.

2. **Treatment** includes removal of indriven bone fragments and foreign material, debridement of necrotic tissue, and closure of the dura and scalp. Impaled foreign bodies such as knife blades should be removed under operative exposure so that hemorrhage can be controlled. Since the incidence of posttraumatic seizures is about 40% in missile injuries and about 15% in nonmissile injuries, an anticonvulsant should be started. An antibiotic (e.g., penicillin, vancomycin, chloramphenicol, cephalosporin) generally is administered; the choice depends on the preference of the neurosurgeon.

G. Brainstem injury. The signs of midbrain injury include coma, midposition unreactive pupils, an impaired oculocephalic response, and decerebrate posturing. Hemorrhage, necrosis, and other pathologic changes can be seen in the brainstems of patients who sustain severe head injuries. It is unclear whether these changes result from the initial impact or secondarily from transtentorial herniation. The diagnosis generally is made on clinical grounds. There is no specific treatment other than that presented in sec. **III.**

H. Carotid artery occlusion can occur with head and neck injury. It begins as an intimal tear in the arterial wall and dissects to a variable degree. It most commonly occurs 1–3 cm above the bifurcation.

1. **Diagnosis.** Carotid occlusion should be suspected in patients with blunt trauma to the neck (anterior cervical region) or lower face (mandibular fracture), hyperextension and contralateral neck rotation, blunt intraoral trauma (involving the tonsillar fossa), cervical spine fracture, or basilar skull fracture (intrapetrous carotid), particularly in the presence of symptoms of transient ischemia. The hemiparesis usually develops 8–10 hours postinjury and is frequently first attributed to the head injury. Arteriography will establish the diagnosis.

2. **Treatment** (e.g., with heparin, surgery, or basic support) is individualized and depends on the duration and extent of the paralysis, the findings on arteriogram, and the severity of any associated injuries.

Injury to the Spine

Spinal cord injury is a significant social and economic problem. It occurs primarily in the young adult and is associated with motor vehicle accidents in one-third to one-half of cases. Unfortunately, once complete sensory and motor paralysis has occurred for 24 hours, recovery of motor function is unlikely; and the prognosis is dependent on symptomatic care and rehabilitation.

I. Anatomy and pathophysiology

A. Anatomy. There are three major ascending sensory systems and one major descending motor tract useful in localizing injury.

1. **Sensory systems.** Fibers carrying **pain** synapse on entry into the dorsal cord, and the bulk of the second-order fibers cross almost immediately and travel upward in the anterior cord. Fibers carrying **position** sense ascend in the posterior columns without crossing. Fibers carrying **touch** sensation are more diffusely distributed throughout the cord, and this accounts for the preservation of touch unless an extensive lesion is present.

2. The major descending **motor system** is the corticospinal tract, which crosses in the lower brainstem and continues caudally in the dorsolateral cord. Fibers involved with upper-limb movement are medial and closer to the gray matter, whereas fibers involved with lower-limb movement are more peripheral in the tract. In the adult the spinal cord usually ends at the level of L1. Injuries below L1 involve the nerve roots of the cauda equina, which are somewhat more resistant to compression.

3. Other useful points for **localization** are as follows: (1) the C4 dermatome is adjacent to the T2 dermatome about the level of the clavicle; (2) C5 and C6

innervate both the deltoid and biceps; (3) C7 lesions result in triceps weakness, and the C7 dermatome usually involves the middle finger; (4) C8 and T1 innervate the hand muscles; (5) the T1 and part of the T2 dermatomes are in the upper limb; (6) the T4 dermatome is at the nipples; (7) the T10 dermatome is at the umbilicus; and (8) the T12 and L1 dermatomes are at the inguinal ligament.

B. Pathophysiology. The spinal cord is very susceptible to injury. Experimental compressive lesions, which involve the thoracic spinal cord and produce complete sensorimotor paralysis, have to be released within minutes to obtain recovery. The cauda equina, however, is more resistant and can withstand several hours of compression and recover. The spinal cord can withstand 1 week of experimental compression and recover if some sensorimotor function remains. These experiments have outlined three groups of injury: (1) complete sensorimotor lesions, (2) incomplete sensorimotor lesions, and (3) cauda equina lesions. Patients with an immediate and complete spinal cord lesion have a bleak outlook for recovery of natural function. Patients with cauda equina lesions or incomplete cord lesions, however, may have a more favorable outcome.

II. Fractures and dislocations. The spine, which is a column of vertebral bodies linked together by disks, ligaments, and muscles, supports the body, allows complex motions, and protects the nervous system.

A. The most frequent **sites of injury** are at the C5, C6, and C7 and T12 and L1 levels, the levels of greatest mobility of the vertebral column. The disks usually can withstand high compressive loads, and in compressive injuries the vertebral bodies are the first to fail. Under bending and torsion loads, the ligaments are more likely to fail, and the disk is more apt to rupture.

    1. Fractures of the spine can be divided into three main categories: linear fractures, compression fractures, and crushing fractures. The more severe injuries may be associated with torn ligaments and dislocations as well.

        a. Linear fractures usually involve the transverse or spinous processes and generally are stable fractures.

        b. Compression fractures occur when the vertebral bodies are pinched by adjacent vertebrae and the cancellous centers give way.

        c. Crushing fractures are exaggerated compression fractures and are most apt to occur either in the lower cervical spine or at the thoracolumbar junction. Crushing fractures can be associated with posterior displacement of bone into the spinal canal and damage to the anterior portion of the cord (i.e., anterior cord syndrome).

    2. Dislocation injuries of the spine are the most serious injuries, since there is usually moderate or severe damage to the cord. Fracture-dislocations can be associated with unilateral or bilateral facet dislocations.

B. Stability of the spine is the ability to maintain vertebral alignment so that damage to the spinal canal or nerve roots does not occur, and incapacitating structural deformity is prevented. The elements that maintain stability are the anterior and posterior longitudinal ligaments and the annulus fibrosus of the disk (i.e., the anterior elements) and the facet joints, interspinous ligament, and ligamentum flavum (i.e., the posterior elements). Damage to these support elements varies with each fracture, and instability must be assessed in each case. Flexion and extension x-rays of the spine may need to be obtained to determine whether instability is present. These x-rays should be obtained only in the presence of a normal neurologic examination, only after a fracture or severe stenosis have been excluded, and generally after appropriate consultation.

    1. The **thoracic spine** has additional structural stability from the rib cage; thus, significant force is needed to produce unstable fractures. The thoracic spinal canal, however, is narrow, and fracture-dislocations usually produce total physiologic transection of the spinal cord.

    2. The **thoracolumbar junction** is a common location for fractures. Posterior displacement of bone into a spinal canal can occur. These fractures can be associated with either spinal cord or cauda equina injury or both.

III. Clinical syndromes

A. Complete functional transection can occur either with obvious destruction of cord tissue or with only minimal evidence of gross structural damage. The patient experiences an immediate flaccid paralysis, loss of reflexes, and loss of sensation below the injured level. Some reflexes (e.g., cremasteric reflex, ankle jerk, anal sphincter reflex), however, may persist for several days after the injury but do not alter the prognosis. After a period of weeks, reflexes return, and flaccidity may change to spasticity. Recovery of any function is extremely rare if complete motor and sensory paralysis has been present for a day or so after injury.

   B. **Incomplete cord injuries** can occur, and, compared with complete transection injuries, the outcome with these partial injuries is usually much better.

   1. The **anterior cord syndrome** is characterized by paralysis and loss of pain sensation below the injury but preservation of some touch and proprioception. This clinical picture can follow fractures in which a bone or disk fragment is pushed backward into the spinal canal. The anterior cord is damaged, but the dorsal columns continue to function.

   2. The **central cervical cord syndrome** is characterized by a greater motor weakness in the upper limbs than the lower limbs and variable sensory deficits. The difference in paralysis may relate to local damage to the anterior horn cells or to damage to the more medially placed fibers of the corticospinal tract that are passing off to the cervical central gray matter. This clinical picture is usually associated with extension injuries in which the cord is pinched in an anteroposterior direction. Myelograms in cadavers with cervical stenosis have shown that in hyperextension the spinal cord was compressed by the bony arthritic bar in front and by a buckled ligamentum flavum in back. Younger patients may experience only transient neurologic changes; however, damage can be much more severe in older patients with stenosis. A fracture may not be present. Surgery generally should be avoided in patients with the central cervical cord syndrome.

   3. The **Brown-Séquard syndrome** results from injury to one-half of the spinal cord and is more apt to be seen following penetrating injuries. It is characterized by ipsilateral paralysis and loss of proprioception and contralateral loss of pain and temperature.

   4. **Injuries to the lower spinal cord,** the conus medullaris, and the cauda equina can produce damage to long tracts, anterior horn cells, and nerve roots separately or in combination, so that patients may show features characteristic of both upper and lower motor neuron lesions.

   C. **Hyperextension-hyperflexion** injuries of the neck (i.e., "whiplash") most commonly are seen with motor vehicle accidents. The more severe neck pain is usually delayed 24–48 hours and can radiate into the shoulders, interscapular region, and occiput. Headache, tinnitus, and vertigo may occur. In general, few objective clinical findings are present. Prolonged symptoms may be due to a spectrum of organic, psychogenic, and other factors. **Treatment** generally is symptomatic (i.e., rest, heat, analgesics, muscle relaxants) with appropriate follow-up as needed. However, the presence of cervical radicular symptoms or signs should warrant appropriate consultation.

IV. Evaluation and management

   A. **Evaluation begins at the scene of injury.** The majority of individuals who have spinal injuries are conscious and usually have at least some symptom or sign of injury to the spine. Conscious patients must be questioned specifically about neck pain; radicular pain in the shoulders, arms, forearms, or legs; numbness or paresthesias in the forearms, hands, or legs; the ability to move; and the absence of feeling. Conscious patients with neck or back pain or neurologic complaints and all patients with a depressed level of consciousness should be assumed to have sustained a spinal injury until proved otherwise. Unless the patient is in shock from hemorrhage or in respiratory distress, he or she should not be moved until proper immobilization equipment is available.

   B. During **transfer** of patients with suspected cervical injuries, it is axiomatic to provide **head-neck-body alignment** at all times. During movement, the patient's head is held by the attendant's forearms, and the attendant's hands are placed under the patient's shoulders to maintain alignment. The neck must be immobilized during transfer and may be accomplished by applying a semirigid collar, placing sandbags adjacent to the patient's head, and taping the head to a spine board. Special straps are available on some spine boards. For patients with possible injury to the thoracic or lumbar spine, immobilization on a spine board is indicated. To avoid aspiration during vomiting, the patient may need to be log-rolled on his or her side with support under the head. Hard objects such as keys, pipes, and lighters should be removed from the patient's pockets to avoid development of pressure sores.

   C. In the emergency department, immediate attention should be given to **evaluating and stabilizing the cardiovascular and respiratory systems.** Although complete cervical lesions can present with mild hypotension (see Chap. 3) and hypothermia, the presence of shock should alert the physician to search for other causes. The surgical management of acute hemorrhage and potentially life-threatening injuries takes priority.

D. An initial thorough **neurologic examination** must be performed. It serves not only as an estimate of cord damage but also as a baseline for future examinations. An immediate and complete sensorimotor lesion should be differentiated from an incomplete or progressive lesion. Rectal tone and voluntary anal constriction should be checked.

E. **X-ray evaluation** should be performed carefully and under the supervision of both the treating physician and the radiologist. All vertebral bodies in the area of injury must be seen on x-ray.

   1. For suspected cervical spine injuries, **a lateral cervical spine film** should be performed first and checked for alignment of the posterior edges of the vertebral bodies. Since the C6 and C7 levels are frequently involved, it is imperative that all seven cervical vertebrae be visualized. Other signs of spine injury are anterior displacement of the tracheal air shadow by prevertebral swelling, increased distance between two spinous processes, and abnormal overlap of the facet joints. Unilateral facet dislocation is often difficult to see, and careful attention should be given to each facet joint. The structural continuity of the odontoid process and possibility of C1–C2 subluxation (i.e., more than a 3-mm distance between the anterior arch of C1 and the odontoid) should be checked.

      An **AP film and odontoid view** should then be obtained and inspected for lateral displacement of the lateral mass of C1 (Jefferson fracture), linear fractures at the base of the odontoid, a change in alignment of the spinous processes (indicating abnormal rotation), and fractures in the lateral masses of other cervical vertebrae. Oblique views should then be obtained to complete the spine series. Questionable findings may require further radiologic evaluation (e.g., CT scan, polytomes) in conjunction with appropriate consultation.

   2. **X-rays of the thoracic and lumbar spine** should be obtained if local pain is present or if the neurologic examination localizes injury to these areas. The films should be reviewed for alignment, compression fractures, and fractures of the spinous or transverse processes. If a compression fracture is present, spot lateral x-rays may be helpful in determining whether bone fragments have been displaced posteriorly into the spinal canal.

F. At present there is controversy regarding the use of **steroids.** There has been no clinical study demonstrating the efficacy of steroids, and some studies have shown complications of high-dose steroids. The author uses low-dose steroids (i.e., dexamethasone, 10 mg IV initially, followed by 4 mg q6h) that are started as soon as possible after injury and continued for several days.

G. **Fracture reduction and stabilization.** In addition to intrinsic injury to the spinal cord, external compression from bone, disk, or hematoma can occur. Fracture-dislocations must be reduced, and unstable fractures stabilized to prevent further injury. Appropriate consultation should be obtained with any spine fracture or neurologic deficit.

   1. **Skeletal traction** is used to reduce cervical spine dislocations and maintain alignment. Tongs are placed into the frontoparietal skull or a halo ring is applied under local anesthesia, and traction weight is applied. Traction usually begins with 3–5 lb for each cervical level above a subluxation or dislocation, and 5- to 10-lb increments are added as needed up to 40–50 lb to tire and stretch cervical muscles and establish alignment. Muscle relaxants may be helpful and are used by some physicians in lieu of increased traction weight.

   2. The incidence of a significant mass lesion (e.g., herniated disk, hematoma) following reduction of a cervial spine fracture appears to be low (8%). A cervical myelogram with iophendylate (Pantopaque) injection or cervical CT scan with water-soluble contrast (C1–C2 puncture) may be necessary to rule out such lesions, particularly if the anterior cord syndrome is present.

   3. Fractures of the **thoracic spine, thoracolumbar junction,** and **lumbar spine** warrant appropriate consultation. If neurologic deficits are present, a myelogram may need to be obtained. Treatment should be left to the consulting physician.

   4. The need for **surgery** is made on a case by case basis. Surgery is indicated when there is a progression of neurologic signs (which highlights the need for repeated neurologic examinations).

V. **Disposition.** Patients with injury to the spinal cord or with potentially significant injury to the vertebral column require hospitalization. If transfer to a specialty center (spinal cord center) is indicated to provide a higher level of care, the patient must be stabilized, the spine securely immobilized by appropriate means, and a Foley catheter (if paralyzed) inserted prior to transfer.

Peripheral Nerve Injuries

The possibility of a nerve injury should be considered with any trauma, and sensorimotor function distal to any injury should be specifically examined. As with head and spine injury, progressive deterioration can occur and may require prompt action.

I. **Pathophysiology**
   A. **Classification of injury.** Axons can react to injury in three basic ways. **Neurapraxia** is a physiologic block in conduction without anatomic interruption. It can be caused by blunt injury, stretch injury, mild compression, ischemia, and missile injuries close to the nerve. **Axonotmesis** is interruption of the axons and myelin without severe disruption of the perineurium and epineurium. Since the internal framework of connective tissue tubes is preserved, reasonably good regeneration can occur. **Neurotmesis** is the complete interruption of axons, myelin sheath, and the connective tissue framework by laceration, severe contusion, or stretch. Although the nerve may be continuous, the severe internal injury may prevent regeneration.
   B. **Nerve regeneration.** Following axon division, a neuron increases its metabolic capability in association with regeneration. Approximately 2–4 weeks are needed to begin regeneration and overcome the area of retrograde degeneration just proximal to the injury. Once the fibers have reached the distal stump, regeneration proceeds at an average rate of 1 mm/day or 1 in./month. There is also a terminal delay of several weeks or longer while axons and receptors mature sufficiently to permit function.
   Functional recovery depends on a sufficient number of proximal axons entering appropriate distal endoneurial sheaths. Reinnervation is better with mainly motor nerves (e.g., radial nerve) and proximal limb muscles than with mixed sensorimotor nerves and distal limb muscles. Functional motor recovery generally does not occur if the muscle remains denervated for more than 18 months postinjury. Sensory recovery, however, is not as severely limited by time.

II. **Evaluation of specific nerve injuries**
   A. **Median nerve** (see Chap. 23)
      1. **Median nerve injury, which most frequently occurs at the wrist,** produces inability to rotate the thumb to a position of grasp (abductor pollicis brevis, opponens pollicis); inability to flex the metacarpophalangeal (MCP) joint and extend the proximal interphalangeal (PIP) joint of the index and middle fingers (lumbricals); and loss of sensation over the palmar aspect of the thumb, index, and middle fingers and the radial half of the ring finger. The thumb should be able to be actively brought to a position almost perpendicular to the palm. The thenar muscles should be palpated during testing, as partial opposition of the thumb (trick movement) can occur using the abductor pollicis longus (radial nerve) and adductor pollicis (ulnar nerve). The autonomous sensory loss involves the tips of the index and middle fingers. Loss of finger flexion in wrist lacerations indicates a tendon laceration in addition to nerve injury.
      2. **Median nerve injury at the elbow** produces additional inability to flex the thumb and index fingers and inability to forceably flex the wrist. Forearm pronation may be present since the branches to the pronator teres originate above the elbow. The middle finger may flex normally, as it may share a proximal tendon to the ring finger (ulnar-innervated flexor profundus muscle). The anterior interosseous branch of the median nerve (motor to the long thumb flexor and the flexor digitorum profundus of the index and middle fingers) may have interconnecting branches with the ulnar nerve in the forearm (Martin-Gruber anastomosis). Thus, variable loss of additional intrinsic hand muscle function can occur.
   B. **Ulnar nerve** (see Chap. 23)
      1. **The ulnar nerve is often injured at the wrist** where it lies radial to the flexor carpi ulnaris tendon. Paralysis of the hypothenar and interosseous muscles produces inability to spread and close the fingers about the axis of the middle finger. Paralysis of the third and fourth lumbrical muscles results in inability to stabilize the flex the MCP joint independent of the long flexors to the distal digits (claw hand). Paralysis of the adductor pollicis weakens the thumb pinch.

Sensory loss involves the hypothenar eminence, volar and dorsal surfaces of the little finger, and ulnar side of the ring finger. The autonomous zone is the distal fifth finger.

2. **Ulnar nerve injury at the elbow** gives additional paralysis of flexion of the distal little finger and possible paralysis of the flexor carpi ulnaris. Flexion of the tip of the ring finger can occur, as it may share a proximal tendon with the middle finger flexor.

C. **Radial nerve** (see Chap. 23)

1. **Radial nerve injury at the elbow** produces wrist drop (some wrist function may be preserved by the brachioradialis) and loss of finger extension at the MCP joints and thumb extension at all joints. Sensation is decreased over the dorsal radial hand and forearm. There is no definite autonomous sensory zone (anatomist's snuffbox in some cases).

2. **Injury of the radial nerve at the level of the midhumerus** can occur with fractures and can cause paralysis of the brachioradialis as well. A pressure palsy at this level can also be seen after sleeping with the arm placed over the back or side of a bench, sofa, or chair (Saturday night palsy). Reinnervation of the brachioradialis by 6 weeks following injury indicates progressive regeneration.

D. **Brachial Plexus**

1. **Anatomy.** The brachial plexus originates from C5, C6, C7, C8, and T1 spinal roots. The dorsal rami innervate the paraspinous muscles, and the ventral rami combine to form an upper trunk (C5, C6), middle trunk (C7), and lower trunk (C8, T1). The trunks divide and recombine to form three cords that generally lie below the level of the clavicle. The long thoracic nerve (serratus anterior), dorsal scapular nerve (rhomboids), and suprascapular nerve (supra and infraspinatus) arise before the cords of the plexus.

2. **Injuries.** The brachial plexus can be injured by gunshot wounds, stab wounds, or severe traction on the shoulder girdle. The level of injury of the brachial plexus is determined by the path of the penetrating injury and the clinical picture. An upper trunk injury (C5, C6) involves all shoulder muscles except the pectoralis major, which is multiply innervated. The lateral cord (C5, C6, C7) gives origin to the musculocutaneous nerve (motor to the biceps and brachialis muscles) and a portion of the median nerve (mainly sensory to the thumb and index fingers); thus, injury causes paralysis of flexion and supination of the forearm. The medial cord (C8, T1) gives origin to the ulnar nerve and a portion of the median nerve (motor to forearm flexors and median-innervated hand muscles). The posterior cord (C5, C6, C7, C8, T1) gives rise to the axillary (deltoid muscle), thoracodorsal (latissimus dorsi muscle), and radial nerves. Only proximal muscles benefit from nerve suture at the plexus level.

E. **Peroneal nerve**

1. **Anatomy and function.** The superficial branch of the peroneal nerve innervates the peroneal muscles, which evert the foot, and supplies sensation to the lateral leg and dorsum of the foot (the autonomous zone). The deep branch of the peroneal nerve innervates the anterior tibial muscles, which dorsiflex the foot, and the toe extensors; and the nerve supplies sensation to the web space between the great and second toe.

2. **Injuries.** The peroneal nerve is commonly injured as it crosses the lateral popliteal space and the head of the fibula. It is susceptible to stretch, pressure, and ischemic damage; and injury to the nerve produces a disabling foot drop. Reinnervation proceeds in a sequence of foot eversion, foot extension, and toe extension. Due to the distances of regeneration, injuries to the nerve 8 in. above the head of the fibula do not respond well when sutured, and injuries capable of regeneration at mid thigh or higher fare equally poorly.

F. **Tibial nerve**

1. **Anatomy.** The tibial nerve innervates in sequence the hamstring muscles in the thigh, the gastrocnemius and soleus muscles in the calf, and the intrinsic foot muscles. The nerve provides important sensation to the sole of the foot; and since the autonomous sensory zone involves the weight-bearing surfaces, trophic ulceration of the foot will develop if sensory reinnervation does not occur.

2. **Injury** of the nerve at the popliteal fossa produces loss of plantar flexion of the foot, loss of inversion of the foot (the posterior tibial muscle tendon passes behind the medial malleolus), loss of toe flexion, and anesthesia of the sole.

G. **Sciatic nerve.** The division of the sciatic nerve into separate tibial and peroneal nerves can occur as high as the gluteal crease, and injuries in the thigh may give different degrees of injury to each nerve. Recovery of one nerve does not guarantee recovery of the other, and both must be watched for recovery.

   H. Femoral nerve. The femoral nerve innervates the sartorius muscle and the quadriceps muscles and supplies sensation to the anterolateral thigh (lateral femoral cutaneous nerve). The branches to the sartorius arise above the inguinal ligament. The branches to the quadriceps group start about 1–2 in. below the inguinal ligament, and the multiple fine branches are not amendable to suture below this level.

   I. Sacral plexus. The sacral plexus is formed from the anterior rami of L4, L5, S1, S2, and S3 that cross in front of the sacroiliac joint and converge at the greater sciatic foramen to form the sciatic nerve. Proximal branches include the superior and inferior gluteal nerves (to the hip extensors and abductors) and sensorimotor innervation to the perineum. Sciatic nerve injury does not produce sensory loss in the perianal area.

III. Management

   A. Primary repair can be considered in clean lacerations in which there is no contusion of the nerve stumps. Arguments in favor of primary suture include the ease in finding the nerve stumps, less nerve retraction, less mobilization of the nerve required during the repair, and a single operation. Relative contraindications to early surgery include gross contamination, nerve contusion in addition to laceration, and inadequate soft-tissue coverage. Arguments in favor of a delayed repair include better definition of the damage to the proximal and distal nerve stumps, presence of a thicker epineurium for suture, and neurons that are in a more optimal regenerative capacity (10–21 days). The two leading causes of failure of nerve repair are (1) insufficient debridement of scarred or contused nerve ends and (2) distraction of the suture line.

   B. Urgent surgery should be considered when a progressive nerve lesion is encountered, as with an enlarging hematoma, aneurysmal sac, Volkmann's ischemic contracture, or compression in the anterior compartment of the leg.

   C. Splints should be considered for nerve injuries with significant paralysis (e.g., wrist drop, foot drop). Patients should be referred for appropriate consultation. **Physical therapy** is extremely important for maintaining range of motion and overall recovery.

   D. Evidence of regeneration should be sought about 8–10 weeks following nerve injury. Clinical and electromyographic (EMG) signs of regeneration include return of muscle function close to the injury, conduction of evoked impulses across the injured site, polyphasic motor units, and voluntary motor units. Motor contraction in response to nerve stimulation above the injury occurs several weeks before voluntary movement. When necessary, the nerve may need to be explored and the electrical conduction across the injury tested intraoperatively.

Shunts

Hydrocephalus with increased ICP may result from tumors obstructing CSF flow (in the region of the third or fourth ventricle), impaired absorption of CSF over the convexities of the brain (secondary to meningitis, meningeal cancer, or ventricular or subarachnoid hemorrhage), or blockage of CSF flow at the aqueduct of Sylvius (due to aqueductal stenosis or unknown cause). Ventricular dilatation with normal pressure (i.e., normal pressure hydrocephalus) may be seen in older patients and may be associated with a triad of mental deterioration, gait disturbance, and incontinence.

At present, hydrocephalus generally is treated by placement of a shunt system that drains the ventricular CSF into the atrium of the heart (ventriculoatrial) or the abdominal cavity (ventriculoperitoneal). The systems are made of soft synthetic tubes and have a pressure-sensitive valve that attempts to regulate flow. Lumboperitoneal shunts are sometimes useful for treating benign intracranial hypertension. Complications of shunts are not infrequent.

   I. Shunt infections occur in about 12% of patients with shunts. Higher infection rates are associated with very old and very young patients and with multiple revisions of the shunt. Infections can occur shortly after surgery or be delayed for weeks, months, or years. The infecting organisms include *Staphylococcus epidermidis* (most common), *Staphylococcus aureus,* diphtheroids, gram-negative bacteria, alpha streptococcus, and *Candida albicans.*

   A. Clinical features. The more virulent infections usually have signs of meningeal irritation and wound infection. The less virulent and more delayed infections may be difficult to diagnose. Patients may have a low-grade fever, moderate leukocytosis, and anemia. There may or may not be clinical indication of CSF infection. Ventriculoperitoneal shunt infections may present with abdominal pain and peritonitis. Ventriculovascular shunts may be associated with nephritis; renal damage appears related to the effects of antigen-antibody complexes and the complement system.

  B. The **diagnosis** is suggested by analysis of CSF obtained by tapping the shunt and confirmed by a positive CSF culture or positive blood cultures in the presence of a ventriculoatrial shunt.

  C. **Management** includes administration of antibiotics and sometimes surgery to remove the shunt (foreign body).

II. Shunt malfunction may be related to obstruction of the system at the proximal end (ventricular catheter), the valve itself, or the distal catheter. Symptoms of malfunction are those of increasing ICP and include lethargy, irritability, headache, nausea, and vomiting. Neurosurgical consultation should be obtained. The diagnosis is made on the basis of enlarged ventricles demonstrated on a CT scan. Treatment is shunt revision.

III. Other complications. Intracranial hematomas (usually subdural hematomas) can be seen in patients with large ventricles following shunt procedures. Other complications relate to perforation by the distal catheter. Ventriculoatrial shunts can be associated with pericardial tamponade and pleural effusion, and ventriculoperitoneal shunts can produce intestinal perforation. Treatment is individualized to the problem.

Bibliography

1. Adams, R. D., and Victor, M. *Principles of Neurology* (3rd ed.). New York: McGraw-Hill, 1985.
2. Haymaker, W., and Woodhall, B. *Peripheral Nerve Injuries.* Philadelphia: Saunders, 1953.
3. Rowland, L. P. (ed.). *Merritt's Textbook of Neurology* (7th ed.). Philadelphia: Lea & Febiger, 1984.
4. Schneider, R. C., et al. (eds.). *Correlative Neurosurgery.* Springfield, Ill.: Thomas, 1982.
5. Wilkins, R. H. (ed.). *Clinical Neurosurgery (Vol. 20.).* Baltimore: Williams and Wilkins, 1973.
6. Wilkins, R. H., and Rengachary, S. S. (eds.). *Neurosurgery.* New York: McGraw-Hill, 1985.
7. Youmans, J. R. (ed.). *Neurological Surgery.* Philadelphia: Saunders, 1982.

26

Orthopedic Emergencies

William B. Strecker and
Vilray P. Blair III

General Principles

The orthopedic patient's emergency care should include (1) a careful history (with details of the accident); (2) a physical examination to determine the extent of the injuries and to identify any occult injuries (e.g., injury to the cervical spine or abdominal viscera); (3) splinting of suspected fractures to prevent further injury; and (4) dressing of any lacerations. In addition, the blood loss associated with certain fractures must be appreciated; a femoral fracture generally is associated with the loss of one to four units, and a pelvic fracture with two to ten or more units.

I. **Evaluation.** Although this chapter is limited to orthopedic considerations, careful evaluation of the entire patient is mandatory.

   A. The **history** should include the specifics of the actual traumatic event, including the time and place of the accident and the forces involved in the injury (e.g., hyperflexion, inversion). Any unusual traumatic forces, as well as potential sources of contamination (e.g., farm injuries), should be recorded.

   B. **Physical examination.** All patients require a thorough examination, with emphasis on the neurologic and circulatory status distal to sites of injury. It is also important that joints be examined for ligamentous stability. As in any assessment, the examination should include the following: (1) **observation** for deformities, swelling, ecchymoses, and skin loss or damage; (2) **palpation** for point tenderness, effusions, crepitation, and masses or palpable defects; and (3) **auscultation** for bruits, if a vascular injury is suspected.

   C. **Radiologic examination** of the injured part is indicated if there is a suspected fracture, dislocation, or foreign body. All extremities should be splinted prior to obtaining radiologic studies, which should consist of anteroposterior (AP) and lateral views and include the joints above and below the injury.

   D. **Joint aspiration** (see Chap. 38) can yield clues to the diagnosis; e.g., a hemarthrosis is present in ligamentous injuries and fractures, fat globules in fractures, and crystals in gout or pseudogout. The cell count of the fluid is important in discerning inflammatory conditions. Joint aspiration, however, generally is reserved for the evaluation of nontraumatic joint effusions (see Chap. 14).

II. **Terminology.** In the description of a fracture or dislocation, it should be kept in mind that all terms refer to the position of the distal part of the limb relative to the rest of the body. The terms most commonly used are as follows: (1) **varus**—the distal limb is angulated toward the midline of the body; (2) **valgus**—the distal limb is angulated away from the midline of the body; (3) **ventral** (anterior)—the distal limb is angulated or displaced anteriorly; and (4) **dorsal** (posterior)—the distal limb is angulated or displaced posteriorly. These terms are expressed in degrees when describing angulation.

   A. **Fractures** are described as follows (Fig. 26-1):

      1. A **buckle (torus)** fracture is one in which there is slight disruption of the cortex without any displacement.

      2. A **transverse** fracture is a complete fracture perpendicular to the shaft of the bone.

      3. An **oblique** fracture is one in which the fracture line traverses the bone at an oblique angle to the shaft.

      4. A **spiral** fracture is one in which the fracture traverses the shaft in more than one plane.

      5. A **compression** fracture is one in which a compression force produced compaction of bone trabeculae.

      6. A **segmental** fracture has at least one large fragment not attached to either the proximal or distal fragments.

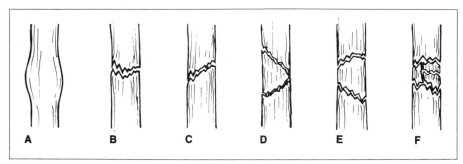

Fig. 26-1. Types of fractures. A. Buckle (torus). B. Transverse. C. Oblique. D. Spiral. E. Segmental. F. Comminuted.

7. A **comminuted** fracture has multiple fragments.
8. A **compound** (open) fracture is one that communicates either directly or indirectly with a laceration or abrasion.
B. **Ligamentous injuries** are often overlooked, since they are not apparent radiologically except for soft-tissue swelling that is asymmetric about a joint. Usually the joint is painful and difficult to examine. Sprains or ligamentous injuries can be graded into three types.
1. A **first-degree sprain** (mild), in which there is partial tearing of ligamentous fibers, is characterized by point tenderness, minimal swelling or hemorrhage, and no abnormal motion.
2. A **second-degree sprain** (moderate), in which there is further tearing of ligamentous fibers, is manifested by point tenderness, moderate swelling or hemorrhage, and slightly abnormal motion.
3. In a **third-degree sprain** (severe), there is complete disruption of the ligament; point tenderness, marked swelling and hemorrhage, loss of function, and markedly abnormal function are present.
III. **Splinting.** All areas of suspected skeletal injury or instability should be splinted prior to obtaining roentgenograms. For short periods of time (i.e., during transportation and emergency department evaluation), temporary splint immobilization may be used. These temporary splints include wood, aluminum, plastic, wire, and air devices.
A. **Extremity injuries.** The joints above and below the suspected injury should be immobilized. The splints can be held in place with well-padded wrappings of gauze or elasticized material. Frequent neurovascular checks of the affected extremity should be obtained, as temporary splinting may cause nerve compression or interfere with vascular flow. When a fracture is confirmed on roentgenograms, a more permanent plaster or synthetic molded splint should be applied to the extremity, or a final cast application should be performed. Since these splints or casts are well padded and molded to the patient's anatomy, they have a lower incidence of nerve or vascular compromise.
B. For suspected **injuries to the pelvis or spine,** backboard splints are most appropriate. Patients with possible cervical spine injuries, in particular, should have their head and neck immobilized on a backboard with a head strap and sandbags. Whenever injury to the spine is suspected, it is imperative that the spine be kept immobilized until a fracture has been completely ruled out.
C. **Hip fractures** are best immobilized by applying 5 lb of skin traction to the affected extremity. Foam boots with 5 lb of Buck's traction are usually available for application in the emergency department.
D. **Femoral fractures** are best managed by traction in Thomas splints; they can also be temporarily immobilized by being secured to the opposite uninjured extremity. Pillow splints are also effective for short periods of time. This procedure is done by securing the extremity with pillows wrapped with an ace bandage.
IV. **Anesthesia.** For the emergency physician to adequately assess or treat an injury, anesthesia of the area or limb may be required. Useful techniques (see Chap. 38 for discussion of the procedures) include (1) a joint block to anesthetize joints in order to judge ligamentous integrity; (2) a Bier (IV regional) block to anesthetize distal extremities for fracture reduction and wound debridement; (3) a hematoma block to anes-

thetize fracture sites locally for reduction; (4) peripheral nerve blocks; and (5) use of general analgesia (e.g., meperidine, which can be reversed with naloxone) for reduction of dislocations or fractures involving a proximal joint (e.g., shoulder or hip joint) where a local or regional block is not appropriate. It must be remembered that a neurologic examination should be carried out prior to the administration of any anesthetic or analgesic agent.

V. General management principles

    A. Fracture care

        1. Fracture reduction. Most fractures are reduced by reduplicating the direction of injury, with longitudinal traction being applied, and then correcting the displacement. The distal fragment is always aligned in relation to the proximal fragment. In general, residual angulation (5–10 degrees) in the plane of motion of the adjacent joint is more acceptable than residual varus or valgus deformity, which should be no greater than 5 degrees. Rotational malalignment is generally unacceptable, as is any significant shortening.

        2. Fracture immobilization can be accomplished by numerous methods including use of slings, splints, strapping, casts, or traction. The method and the duration are usually determined by the location and type of fracture. Generally, fractures of the upper extremity are immobilized 3–8 weeks, and those of the lower extremities, 6–12 weeks.

        3. An **open fracture** is one that communicates with the environment through a wound. In such instances the amount of contamination about the wound is important. Thus, wounds are classified into three types: (1) usually clean, low-energy, inside-outward wounds caused by bone, with minimal if any muscle damage; (2) wounds greater than 1 cm in length with moderate soft-tissue damage; and (3) high-energy wounds, usually greater than 10 cm in length, with extensive muscle and soft-tissue damage, and usually associated with comminuted fractures. If there is any chance that a wound communicates with a fracture, the fracture is considered open even though bone is not visible. Such wounds should be cultured in the emergency department. Open fractures with exposed bone should have sterile dressings applied, but no attempt should be made to cover the exposed bone with tissue. Large wounds with bony involvement may bleed heavily. This bleeding usually can be controlled by a local compression dressing; but if serious bleeding cannot be controlled, the use of a blood pressure tourniquet (for < 1 hour) should be considered. Open fractures require antibiotic therapy and debridement and cleansing in the operating suite.

    B. Ligamentous injuries do not require reduction (unless associated with a dislocation); however, if a second- or third-degree disruption exists, it will require either surgical repair or immobilization with the tension removed from the ligament until healing occurs. In the latter situation, immobilization with a cast for 4–6 weeks is usually required.

VI. Disposition. Patients with an open fracture or fracture of the femur, hip, pelvis, or spine usually require hospitalization, as does any patient with a fracture that will require an open reduction. Hospitalization should also be considered for patients with fractures in which there is a possibility of neurovascular compromise. Other patients can have the fracture immobilized and can be referred to an orthopedic surgeon for follow-up in 2–3 days. It is important that these patients understand the nature of their injury and potential cast complications, so that they can alert their physician or return to the emergency department should any problems develop.

Specific Injuries

I. Upper extremity

    A. Scapuloclavicular disorders

        1. Scapular fractures

            a. Mechanism of injury is usually direct trauma to the scapular region.

            b. Examination reveals tenderness about the scapula.

            c. Radiographs are diagnostic.

            d. Treatment consists of early mobilization using a sling for comfort.

            e. Complications are rare.

        2. Clavicular fractures

            a. Mechanism of injury. The clavicle is the most frequently fractured bone; it has a subcutaneous position and is usually injured by a direct blow to the clavicle or by a fall on the shoulder.

    b. Examination reveals tenderness and pain over the clavicle and pseudo-paralysis of the ipsilateral arm.

    c. Radiographs confirm the diagnosis.

    d. Treatment. Most clavicular fractures are treated with a figure-of-eight sling. Open reduction and internal fixation, however, are indicated when there is marked displacement or tenting of the skin.

    e. Complications. A brachial plexus palsy, usually of the Erb's type, may occur secondary to traction.

3. Sternoclavicular joint dislocations.

    a. Mechanism of injury is a fall on the shoulder, dislocating the medial clavicle, usually anteriorly or rarely posteriorly.

    b. Examination reveals tenderness at the sternoclavicular joint with a palpable defect.

    c. Radiographs usually require a 45-degree cephalad view or tomogram to demonstrate the dislocation.

    d. Treatment. Anterior dislocations usually are readily reduced closed by digital pressure on the proximal clavicle and then immobilized in a reverse figure-of-eight dressing, but redislocation is common. Posterior dislocations, once reduced by applying posterior pressure on the distal clavicle and pulling the medial end anteriorly, usually are maintained.

    e. Complications. In posterior dislocations, compression of the cervical vessels or trachea may occur.

4. Acromioclavicular (AC) joint dislocations

    a. Mechanism of injury. These injuries result from a direct downward blow on the shoulder.

    b. Examination reveals tenderness over the AC joint, with the distal clavicle superiorly displaced.

    c. Radiographs. AC joint separation usually is demonstrated on plain radiographs, but weighted films comparing both sides may be required.

    d. Treatment depends on the degree of displacement; minimal displacement is treated with a sling, whereas ligamentous disruption requires open reduction.

    e. Complications. Unsightly prominence and pain with active use may result.

B. Shoulder injuries

1. Dislocations. Fifty percent of all major dislocations occur at the shoulder, with 95% of these being anterior. Fifty to seventy-five percent of shoulder dislocations occur in patients under 30 years old; recurrences occur in 90–95% of patients under 30 years old but decline to 10% in patients over 40 years old.

    a. Anterior dislocations

        (1) Mechanism of injury. Anterior dislocations usually result from a combination of abduction, external rotation, and extension at the shoulder.

        (2) Examination. The patient resists any attempted motion of the shoulder. There is a loss of shoulder symmetry, with the acromion being prominent and the humeral head palpable anteriorly.

        (3) Radiographs. In all suspected dislocations, standard AP and lateral views are needed. Due to pain, it may not be possible to obtain an axillary view; in such a situation, a transscapular view is necessary.

        (4) Treatment. Reduction must be gentle, and muscle relaxation is required.

            (a) The patient is given either 50 mg of meperidine or 5 mg of morphine IV. Naloxone and resuscitation equipment should be available.

            (b) The patient is placed prone with the affected arm and shoulder hanging dependent.

            (c) Five to ten pounds of weight are secured to the arm.

            (d) Fifteen to twenty minutes are usually required to bring about reduction. If this procedure is unsuccessful, with the patient remaining in the prone position, the physician may place his or her hand in the axilla on the humeral head and apply lateral pressure while internally rotating the arm to achieve reduction.

            (e) Following reduction, the shoulder and arm are immobilized in a Velpeau dressing or sling and swathe for 3 weeks.

            (f) If it is not possible to obtain reduction in this manner, reduction should then be attempted under general anesthesia.

        (5) Complications

            (a) The most common complication is damage to nerves, either the brachial plexus or axillary nerve.

(b) Rotator cuff tears or fractures of the greater tuberosity are associated with anterior dislocations.

b. **Posterior dislocations.** Fifty percent of these injuries are missed unless a lateral radiograph is obtained. Reduction and postreduction stability are much more difficult and require an orthopedic surgeon.

2. **Acute rotator cuff tears**

a. **Mechanism of injury** usually involves a fall on the shoulder or lifting a heavy object. It is more common in older individuals because of attrition of the rotator cuff.

b. **Examination.** Shoulder abduction is either absent or weak and painful. Tenderness is usually present over the humeral tuberosities.

c. **Radiographs.** Plain radiographs usually are normal. An arthrogram is often needed to establish the diagnosis.

d. **Treatment**

(1) The young patient or a patient with a large tear usually requires surgical repair.

(2) In the older patient, treatment is symptomatic.

C. **Humeral fractures**

1. **Proximal humeral fractures.** Neer divides proximal humeral fractures into six groups, which aid in treatment. Proximal humeral epiphyseal separation is discussed in Chap. 36.

a. **Mechanism of injury** is a fall on an outstretched arm.

b. **Examination.** The patient usually presents with the complaint of pain at the shoulder and inability to use the shoulder, with varying degrees of swelling and ecchymosis.

c. **Radiographs.** As in shoulder dislocations, it is important that biplane radiographs be taken to determine the amount of displacement.

d. **Treatment** is designed to maintain glenohumeral motion and to avoid prolonged immobilization and avascular necrosis of the humeral head.

(1) Anatomic neck, surgical neck, and minimally displaced greater tuberosity fractures are usually treated by shoulder immobilization.

(2) All other proximal humeral fractures are treated by closed reduction under general anesthesia, open reduction and internal fixation, or arthroplasty.

e. **Complications**

(1) Loss of glenohumeral motion, which is secondary to the required immobilization, is common.

(2) Neurovascular damage can occur with a displaced fracture and can involve the axillary, median, ulnar, or radial nerve. Therefore, a careful neurologic examination is required.

2. **Humeral diaphyseal fractures**

a. **Examination.** The diagnosis is usually established clinically and confirmed radiographically. Most fractures occur in the middle third of the shaft. It is important that a thorough neurologic examination be carried out (with special attention to the radial nerve), with documentation of any neurologic loss and its time of onset.

b. **Treatment** consists of application of a plaster coaptation splint combined with shoulder immobilization, usually with a collar and swathe or a Velpeau dressing. Occasionally, a hanging long-arm cast is needed for severe overriding of fragments. Rarely, internal fixation is needed.

c. **Complications.** The most devastating complications, other than delayed union or nonunion, is a radial nerve injury, which can occur at the time of injury, time of reduction, or during healing of the fracture.

D. **Elbow fractures and dislocations**

1. **Supracondylar fractures** are most commonly seen in pediatric and elderly patients but can occur in any age group.

a. **Mechanism of injury.** These fractures usually result from hyperextension but can also occur with flexion.

b. **Examination.** The injury is usually self-evident clinically and is confirmed radiographically. A careful examination for neurovascular injuries must be carried out, since these injuries constitute a surgical emergency.

c. **Treatment.** In the minimally displaced fracture, closed reduction may be achieved without anesthesia. The extension injury is then casted in 100-degree flexion, while the flexion injury is placed in only 20–30 degrees of flexion. These patients should be admitted to the hospital for observation for neurovascular compromise and a compartment syndrome. In many adults, either a closed reduction under anesthesia with percutaneous pin fixation or open reduction and internal fixation is preferred in order to begin earlier motion and decrease elbow stiffness.

    d. Complications include cubitus varus or valgus deformity, a compartment syndrome, tardy ulnar nerve palsy, and loss of motion.

  2. Elbow dislocations. The most common elbow dislocation is posterior dislocation of the ulna on the humerus.

    a. Mechanism of injury is usually a fall on an outstretched hand with the elbow in slight flexion.

    b. Examination. There is marked deformity about the elbow with the olecranon usually displaced posteriorly, laterally, or both.

    c. Treatment. Usually these dislocations can be manipulated to achieve closed reduction. However, there may be associated fractures that can either block reduction or render it unstable. Reduction is performed by applying longitudinal traction manually and then correcting the lateral displacement.

    d. Complications usually follow reduction and include neurologic injury to any of the three major nerves, especially the ulnar nerve; brachial artery injury; and a compartment syndrome.

  3. Olecranon fractures

    a. Mechanism of injury is direct trauma to the olecranon or a sudden triceps contracture with the elbow being forcibly flexed.

    b. Examination reveals tenderness over the olecranon and a decrease in active elbow extension.

    c. Treatment usually involves open reduction and internal fixation to reconstitute the articular surface and allow early mobilization.

    d. Complications. The major complication is residual loss of motion.

  4. Radial head fractures and dislocations

    a. Mechanism of injury. These fractures are usually caused by a fall on an outstretched hand, forcing the radial head into the capitulum.

    b. Examination reveals tenderness over the radial head with painful pronation and supination.

    c. Treatment. If the displacement is minimal, the elbow is splinted for 7–10 days for comfort, and the patient is started on early motion. If the fracture is displaced or comminuted, the radial head is excised.

    d. Complications include some limitation of full extension and radiohumeral arthrosis.

E. Forearm injuries

  1. Radial and ulnar shaft fractures

    a. Mechanism of injury. These fractures can follow either direct or indirect forces. Since the forearm consists of two bones that function together, it is rare that an injury occurs to an isolated bone without disruption at another site; the exception to this is the nightstick fracture of the ulna from a direct blow. Thus, it is important to search for associated injuries with a careful examination and good radiographs of the adjacent joints.

    b. Types of fractures

      (1) A **Monteggia fracture** is a fracture of the ulna with dislocation of the radial head.

      (2) A **Galeazzi fracture** is a fracture of the radius with dislocation of the distal ulna.

    c. Examination reveals gross deformity of the forearm. It is important to examine for tenderness about the elbow and the distal radioulnar joint.

    d. Treatment. The dislocation can be reduced closed, but the shaft fracture requires open reduction and internal fixation.

    e. Complications include nonunion and synostosis.

  2. Distal forearm fractures

    a. Mechanism of injury

      (1) A **Colles' fracture** is a fracture of the distal radius with dorsal angulation or displacement; it is usually caused by a fall on an extended wrist.

      (2) A **Smith's fracture** is a fracture of the distal radius with volar angulation or displacement; it is caused by a fall on a flexed wrist.

      (3) A **Barton's fracture** is a dorsal rim fracture of the distal radius probably produced by dorsiflexion and pronation.

b. **Examination** discloses deformity of the distal radius, with subluxation of the wrist, and tenderness.

c. **Treatment** consists of closed reduction and application of a long-arm cast or, occasionally, external fixation or open reduction.

d. **Complications** include the carpal tunnel syndrome, malunion, and late rupture of the extensor pollicus longus.

F. **Wrist and hand injuries.** See Chap. 23.

II. **Pelvic fractures** are seen mostly in two patient populations: (1) those over the age of 60 years who sustain a fracture from a fall and (2) those of any age who are usually injured in vehicular accidents.

A. **Types.** Fractures of the pelvis can be classified into three groups based on the Key and Conwell classification, which takes into account the complexities of the injury.

1. **Type 1. Fractures of the individual bones** (including avulsion fractures) without a break in the continuity of the pelvic ring represent stable fractures.

2. **Type 2. A single break in the pelvic ring** is a stable fracture.
   a. **Ipsilateral ramus fracture.**
   b. **Fracture near or subluxation of symphysis pubis.**
   c. **Fracture near or subluxation of sacroiliac joint.**

3. **Type 3. A double break in the pelvic ring** signifies an unstable fracture.
   a. A **straddle fracture** is a fracture of all four rami.
   b. A **Malgaigne fracture** is a fracture with vertical dislocation of the hemipelvis.
   c. **Severe multiple fractures** can also occur.

B. **Examination.** In the patient with a pelvic fracture, careful assessment of the patient's hemodynamic status is essential. In addition, it is important to evaluate for rectal and perirectal lacerations, injuries to the abdominal viscera and genitourinary system, and other injuries.

C. **Radiographs** should include standard AP, 45-degree obliques, and, when indicated, 25-degree caudad and 35-degree cephalad views. A cystourethrogram or an intravenous pyelogram (IVP) or both may be required to assess the integrity of the genitourinary tract.

D. **Management.** Since pelvic fractures can cause serious hemorrhage, prompt and vigorous resuscitation may be needed, including massive volume replacement with crystalloid and blood. Application of the military antishock trousers (MAST) suit (see Chap. 38) is useful in curtailing blood loss and stabilizing unstable fractures. Occasionally, transcatheter embolization is needed to control hemorrhage. Stable fractures usually require only bed rest until the patient is comfortable, followed by protective weight-bearing. Unstable fractures require skeletal traction or open reduction with either internal or external fixation.

E. **Complications.** Early complications include hemorrhage and associated visceral injuries. Late complications include malunion and posttraumatic arthritis, usually associated with sacroiliac injuries. Delayed union and nonunion, however, are rare.

III. **Lower-extremity injuries**

A. **Hip fractures**

1. **Femoral neck fractures**

   a. **Mechanism of injury.** Femoral neck fractures are usually due to a fall in elderly patients, mostly females, who have components of osteoporosis and osteomalacia. Stress fractures, however, can occur, usually in young active patients (e.g., runners or military recruits).

   b. **Examination.** These patients usually complain of pain in the groin and medial aspect of the leg. There is also a loss of motion and pain with rotation. Patients with displaced fractures lie with the leg shortened and externally rotated. The diagnosis is confirmed by radiographs. Stress fractures, in contrast, can present with no deformity, minimal discomfort in motion, slight muscle spasm, and no radiographic changes for 10–14 days.

   c. **Treatment.** Initially, the patient is placed in 5 lb of Buck's traction in preparation for internal fixation, which most fractures of the femoral neck require. In patients under the age of 60 years, there is some degree of urgency since the incidence of avascular necrosis increases with the amount of displacement and time prior to reduction. In the young patient with a stress fracture, usually non-weight-bearing with crutches for 6 weeks is adequate, followed by partial weight-bearing for another 6-week period. In the elderly patient with comminution or marked displacement, a hemiarthroplasty is the procedure of choice.

    d. Complications. The greatest complication from a femoral neck fracture, when displaced, is avascular necrosis with late segmental collapse. The incidence of avascular necrosis has been reported to be 25% when surgery is performed within 12 hours of injury, 40% between 24 and 48 hours, and 100% after 1 week.

2. **Peritrochanteric fractures** include fractures that involve the intertrochanteric line (intertrochanteric fractures) or the proximal 3 in. of the femur (subtrochanteric) below the intertrochanteric line.

    a. Mechanism of injury

        (1) Intertrochanteric fractures are similar to femoral neck fractures in that they are usually secondary to a fall in the elderly, but the male-to-female ratio is about equal.

        (2) Subtrochanteric fractures usually result from high-velocity trauma (e.g., motor vehicle accidents) or pathologic processes.

    b. Examination. The leg usually is shortened and externally rotated, with pain on any motion.

    c. Radiographs are diagnostic.

    d. Treatment consists of open reduction and internal fixation, usually with a sliding screw-plate device. There are some indications for an intramedullary device (Zickel nail or Ender nail).

    e. Complications. Due to the advanced age of most of these patients, there usually is significant morbidity and mortality from these fractures; it is therefore important to ambulate these patients early to decrease thromboembolic complications. Nonunion may occur, but avascular necrosis is a rare complication.

3. **Hip dislocations**

    a. Mechanism of injury. Dislocations of the hip usually require a great amount of force, such as occurs in a motor vehicle accident. The dislocation can occur posteriorly, which is the most common situation, when a direct force is applied to the hip when it is flexed and adducted, such as the knee striking the dashboard. Central dislocations are associated with acetabular fractures from a force directed on the abducted hip. Anterior dislocations, which are rare, result from a force that abducts an extended hip. It is important to be cognizant of associated fractures of either the femoral head or acetabulum.

    b. Examination. As in any dislocation, the patient resists movement of the limb. In a posterior dislocation, the leg is internally rotated and adducted; and with an anterior dislocation, it is in a position of abduction and external rotation.

    c. Treatment consists of early manipulative reduction under general analgesia or anesthesia. With a posterior dislocation, the patient is placed supine with the hip flexed 90 degrees; then with traction and slight adduction, the hip is reduced. In an anterior dislocation, traction is applied and the leg is adducted, internally rotated, and flexed. If the reduction cannot be obtained, is unstable, or is associated with a significant fracture, open reduction is required. After reduction, the leg is maintained in traction for 4–6 weeks to allow for capsular healing.

    d. Complications. Injury to the sciatic nerve can occur in posterior dislocations. Avascular necrosis is associated with hip dislocations, with the incidence directly related to the length of time until reduction; this complication can appear up to 2 years following the injury. A significant incidence of late traumatic arthritis is also seen with this injury.

B. Femoral shaft fractures

1. **Mechanism of injury.** These fractures are usually caused by severe trauma, such as that sustained in a motor vehicle or motorcycle accident, and are often associated with severe soft-tissue damage and a blood loss of two to four units.

2. **Examination.** The diagnosis is usually evident on examination, but these patients must be checked for concomitant injuries, especially about the hip and knee.

3. **Radiographs,** which must always include the adjacent joints, confirm the diagnosis.

4. **Treatment** consists of application of a Thomas splint prior to any radiographs. Later the patient is usually placed in skeletal traction in preparation for intramedullary nailing. If the fracture is not applicable to intramedullary nailing or if the patient is not stable enough to undergo a surgical procedure, he or she

can be treated with balanced skeletal traction for 6–8 weeks, followed by application of a spica cast or a cast brace.

5. **Complications** include vascular and nerve damage, usually a transient peroneal nerve palsy. Also, shortening and malrotation at the fracture site can occur when the patient is treated with traction unless careful attention is paid to the alignment.

C. Supracondylar and intracondylar fractures

1. **Mechanism of injury.** In young individuals, these fractures follow a severe traumatic event and are frequently associated with neurovascular injuries. In the elderly, these fractures can result from minimal trauma, such as a fall.

2. **Examination.** Swelling and tenderness involving the distal thigh are present, along with a knee hemarthrosis. A careful neurovascular examination must be performed, and an arteriogram may be needed to evaluate the popliteal vessels.

3. **Treatment.** Nondisplaced fractures often can be treated with a long-leg cast and non-weight-bearing ambulation. Displaced fractures or intraarticular fractures, however, may require open reduction and internal fixation.

4. **Complications** are usually related to neurovascular injuries and traumatic arthrosis of the knee.

D. Knee disorders

1. **Evaluation**

a. **History.** It is important that a careful history be obtained, documenting the mechanism of injury, the location of any pain, and the time of onset of swelling.

b. **Examination.** A careful knee examination is essential.

(1) **Effusion.** It is important to document whether or not an effusion is present. An effusion can be demonstrated either by balloting the patella or, in mild effusions, by noticing the loss of the medial suprapatellar recess. It is also important to note when the effusion occurred in relation to the injury. Cruciate tears usually result in immediate effusions, whereas meniscal injuries generally are associated with delayed effusions. Complete disruptions of a collateral ligament, however, can occur without an effusion, since the effusion extravasates into the soft tissue.

(2) **Tenderness.** It is important to determine whether there is tenderness over the joint line (suggestive of a meniscal injury), over the origin or insertion of the collateral ligaments, or over the medial retinaculum and parapatellar areas (suggestive of a patellar dislocation).

(3) **Stability** is determined by applying both varus and valgus stress to the knee at full extension and 30 degrees of flexion, and noting whether there is laxity in these plains of motion suggestive of a collateral ligament injury. An anterior and posterior drawer test can be performed with the knee flexed to 90 degrees to determine whether or not the tibia subluxes anteriorly or posteriorly, suggestive of a cruciate tear.

c. **Radiographs** should be obtained in knee injuries to demonstrate the presence or absence of any fractures, but generally there are no bony abnormalities.

d. **Joint aspiration** can help lead to the diagnosis in traumatic knee disorders, since two-thirds of patients presenting with a hemarthrosis usually have an internal derangement of the knee joint. Also, the presence of fat globules within the hemarthrosis can lead to the diagnosis of an occult fracture. In those patients without a traumatic injury but with knee pain and swelling, examination of the fluid for cells and crystals can be diagnostic.

2. **Specific injuries**

a. **Patellar disorders**

(1) **Fractures**

(a) **Mechanism of injury.** The patella can be fractured from direct violence, can sustain chip fractures secondary to dislocation, or can sustain transverse fractures due to the forceful contraction of the quadriceps mechanism with the knee in flexion.

(b) **Examination** usually demonstrates a hemarthrosis with fat globules present. Direct tenderness about patella and radiographs usually confirm the diagnosis. It should be noted that, radiographically, patients may have a bipartite patella, which occurs in 3% of the population and can be confused with a fracture of the superolateral margin.

(c) **Treatment.** Extraarticular and nondisplaced fractures can be treated in a cylinder cast for 3–4 weeks with weight-bearing, followed by isometric exercises. Displaced fractures usually are treated with open reduction and internal fixation. Severely comminuted fractures require patellectomy.

(d) **Complications.** Late traumatic arthritis may occur.

(2) **Dislocations**

(a) **Mechanism of injury.** Patellar dislocations generally occur in individuals with a preexisting condition, the **patellar malalignment syndrome.** They can also be caused by direct violence to the medial side of the patella, dislocating it laterally, or, more commonly, by an indirect force, such as sudden flexion and external rotation of the knee with a contracted quadriceps.

(b) **Examination.** The knee is usually held in approximately 30–45 degrees of flexion, and the patella can be palpated laterally.

(c) **Treatment.** With simple extension of the knee, most patellar dislocations can be easily reduced. Radiographs are then needed to confirm the reduction and the presence or absence of any occult fractures. After the dislocation has been reduced, the patient should be immobilized in a cylinder cast in full extension for 4–6 weeks, allowing for healing of the medial retinacular structures.

(d) **Complications.** The two major complications that can occur from patellar dislocations are recurrent dislocations, which usually require surgical reconstruction, and chondromalacia of the patella.

b. **Meniscal injuries**

(1) **Mechanism of injury.** Meniscal injuries usually are caused by a torsion of the femur on the tibia with the foot fixed on the ground in the weight-bearing position.

(2) **Clinical features.** These patients may present with a locked knee or inability to fully extend the knee through the last 5–10 degrees of extension, complaints of buckling, or a hemarthrosis. They usually have tenderness about the meniscus along the joint line.

(3) **Plain radiographs** are not diagnostic; the diagnosis is established by an arthrogram.

(4) **Treatment** is arthroscopic meniscectomy on an elective basis.

c. **Ligamentous injuries.** There are four major ligaments about the knee joint: the anterior and posterior cruciate ligaments, and the medial and lateral collateral ligaments. These ligaments can be injured alone or in combination.

(1) **Mechanism of injury**

(a) **Anterior cruciate** tears are usually caused by a forceful rotation when the foot is planted and fixed. Many times the patient will experience a pop within the knee and a rapid onset of a hemarthrosis.

(b) The **posterior cruciate ligament** is usually injured by a hyperextension force.

(c) The **medial collateral ligament** is usually injured by having the foot fixed and a force (blow) delivered from the lateral side. This injury is commonly associated with both anterior cruciate and medial meniscal injuries.

(d) The **lateral collateral ligament** is injured by a medial blow and is less common than the medial injuries.

(2) **Examination.** If there is concern about the degree of injury, the knee can be evaluated by performing a joint block (see Chap. 38) and obtaining stress radiographs. In some patients a meaningful examination is still difficult to obtain, and these individuals require an examination under general anesthesia.

(3) **Treatment** of ligamentous injuries depends on the structures injured and the severity of the injuries. As with other ligamentous injuries (see **General Principles,** sec. **II.B**), mild tears (first-degree) can be treated with mobilization and physical therapy. Second-degree injuries require immobilization for 4–6 weeks in a cast, which relieves stress on the side of the affected joint. Complete tears, however, generally require surgical repair within 7–10 days.

    d. Baker's cysts usually occur in individuals with degenerative joint disease or rheumatoid arthritis.

        (1) Clinical features. Baker's cysts present as a swelling or mass in the popliteal fossa, usually arising from the medial posterior joint under the semimembranous tendon. Patients usually complain of an aching discomfort about the knee and a palpable mass that usually transilluminates. In patients with rheumatoid arthritis, these cysts can become quite large, extending down the posterior calf to the ankle. A ruptured cyst may mimic deep vein thrombosis.

        (2) Treatment is directed at the underlying problem, and not the cyst itself, and may involve administration of anti-inflammatory medication, meniscectomy, joint debridement, or synovectomy. On the other hand, in the pediatric patient the cyst usually is self-limiting, requires no treatment, and is not indicative of a knee derangement.

E. Leg injuries

    1. Tibial plateau fractures

        a. Mechanism of injury. These fractures usually are caused by a compressive force associated with either a varus or valgus stress.

        b. Examination should search for specific areas of point tenderness about the knee to discern any possible collateral ligament injury.

        c. Radiographs often are diagnostic, but tomograms are helpful to demonstrate minor fractures or the degree of compression of the plateau.

        d. Treatment depends on the amount of displacement of the fracture. Vertical, nondisplaced fractures through the plateau and small central depressions of the plateau of less than 3 mm can be treated with a compressive dressing for 24–48 hours, followed by a cast brace. If there is significant displacement or depression, however, open reduction and internal fixation usually are required to restore anatomic alignment to the joint surface.

        e. Complications consist of neurapraxia secondary to traction injuries of the peroneal nerve, and traumatic arthritis. Compartment syndromes of the leg can also be seen with this injury.

    2. Tibial shaft fractures

        a. Mechanism of injury. These fractures usually are the result of either direct or indirect (torsional) trauma to the leg.

        b. Treatment consists of reduction of the fracture and application of a long-leg cast. If the fracture cannot be reduced satisfactorily and there is angular or rotational malalignment or shortening exceeding 1 cm, either internal or external fixation is required.

        c. Complications. Compartment syndromes are most commonly seen with tibial shaft fractures and must always be of primary concern. These patients can also develop joint stiffness of either the knee or ankle due to the length of immobilization. Delayed union and nonunion are seen, especially in the distal third of the tibia, as is malunion due to severe angulation, malrotation, or shortening.

    3. Fibular fractures

        a. Mechanism of injury. Isolated fibular fractures are usually the result of direct blows. They can also be due to rotational forces associated with ligamentous injuries of the ankle.

        b. Examination. A thorough examination of both the ankle and knee must be performed any time a fibular fracture is confirmed on a radiograph.

        c. Treatment of isolated fibular fractures is usually symptomatic. These patients may be placed in a cylinder cast for 2–3 weeks for comfort.

        d. Complications. Rarely, a neurapraxia of the peroneal nerve occurs.

F. Ankle injuries

    1. Evaluation. As in knee injuries, the history of the mechanism of injury is important. Areas of swelling and tenderness allow the examiner to discern what structures have been injured. Radiographs, including AP, lateral, and oblique (mortise) views, are required in ankle injuries.

    2. Specific injuries

        a. Ligamentous injuries about the ankle can be divided into first-, second-, and third-degree sprains (see **General Principles,** sec. **II.B**).

        (1) Examination. It is important to document all areas of swelling and point tenderness, especially about the lateral malleolus, and to determine whether or not there is tenderness over the anterior talofibular ligament, the calcaneofibular ligament, or the posterior talofibular ligament. This examination will enable determination of the amount of instability present.

   (2) Stress radiographs are useful when a third-degree ligamentous disruption is suspected. Analgesia is usually required to enable the patient to relax so that stress views can be performed; a joint block (see Chap. 38) is usually sufficient analgesia. Radiographs are taken with forced eversion and inversion of the ankle and are compared with stress views of the opposite ankle. Tilting of the talus greater than 10 degrees compared with the contralateral side is usually indicative of a complete (third-degree) disruption.

   (3) Treatment. For treatment of first-degree sprains, strapping and early mobilization are sufficient. Second- and third-degree sprains, however, usually require immobilization in a short-leg walking cast for up to 6–8 weeks; open repair is rarely indicated with acute injury.

   (4) Complications. The most frequent complication seen is lateral talar instability, which when persistent usually requires operative measures to improve ankle function.

   b. Fractures. It should be noted that ankle fractures are interarticular injuries and therefore require anatomic reduction.

   (1) Mechanism of injury can vary, but most commonly the foot is supinated with lateral rotation of the leg. Often fractures involving the ankle are associated with ligamentous disruption, which should be sought.

   (2) Examination. Swelling and deformity are present.

   (3) Radiographs confirm the diagnosis.

   (4) Treatment is based on the location of the fracture (either medially, laterally, or both) and any associated ligamentous disruption and widening of the ankle mortise. Isolated, nondisplaced fractures without ligamentous disruption or widening of the mortise can be treated with immobilization in a short-leg cast with non-weight-bearing for 6 weeks, followed by weight-bearing for another 6 weeks. Fractures with displacement or widening of the mortise usually require open reduction and internal fixation of the ankle to assure a satisfactory result.

G. Foot injuries

 1. Fractures involving the foot result from direct blows and indirect rotational forces. These fractures usually are associated with a marked amount of swelling and ecchymosis, with maximum tenderness generally over the areas of fracture. Radiographs usually are diagnostic.

   a. Fractures of the neck or body of the talus, if displaced, require open reduction and internal fixation. If absolutely no displacement exists, these injuries can be treated with cast immobilization.

   b. Calcaneal fractures are usually secondary to a fall from a height. It is important to note that these fractures are often associated with lumbar spine injuries; therefore, careful examination of the lumbar spine should be performed. Calcaneal fractures with flattening of the articular surface of the calcaneus generally require open reduction. If there is only a compaction injury to the body of the calcaneus, a soft compressive dressing is applied to decrease the amount of swelling.

   c. Isolated fractures of the other tarsal bones are uncommon.

   d. Metatarsal fractures usually involve the base of the fifth metatarsal and are treated by either strapping or immobilization in a short-leg walking cast for 4 weeks. Metatarsal head fractures can be seen after a fall from a height and, if significantly displaced plantarward, require open reduction and internal fixation. Other metatarsal fractures, unless intraarticular, can be treated by closed manipulation and application of a short-leg cast.

   e. Phalangeal fractures are managed by taping the involved toe to an adjacent toe.

 2. Dislocations of the foot are rare.

   a. Types. Dislocations of the foot are usually divided into (1) a subtalar dislocation, in which the dislocation occurs through the subtalar and talonavicular joint, with the foot dislocated medially in relationship to the talus; and (2) a complete talar dislocation, in which the talus is dislocated from its position within the ankle mortise. Both of these dislocations are usually associated with marked disruption of the ligaments about the talus.

      b. Examination. Deformity, soft-tissue swelling, and tenting of the skin with impending skin necrosis are usually present.

      c. The **diagnosis** is confirmed by radiographs.

      d. Treatment usually consists of a closed reduction. If this method fails, open reduction is required, followed by immobilization.

      e. Complications most commonly encountered are ischemic skin loss, avascular necrosis of the body of the talus, and loss of subtalar motion.

IV. Musculotendinous injuries

  A. Ruptured biceps

    1. Mechanism of injury. The biceps brachia can be ruptured in its long head, in the muscle belly itself, or in the distal tendinous insertion. This injury can be the result of chronic tenosynovitis of the long head of the biceps in the older individual or can occur from lifting very heavy weights.

    2. Examination usually demonstrates a palpable defect and asymmetry of the muscle belly.

    3. Treatment depends on the location of the rupture. If the rupture occurs in the long head of the biceps tendon in either an elderly individual or an individual who does not require muscle power for lifting, the injury is treated nonoperatively by physical therapy and range-of-motion exercises. In the young individual or in a person who does heavy labor, however, the injury generally is repaired surgically. Complete rupture within the muscle belly or avulsion of the distal insertion are not as common but usually require surgical correction.

    4. Complications include loss of biceps strength and cosmetic deformity of the upper arm.

  B. Ruptured quadriceps

    1. Mechanism of injury. A ruptured quadriceps usually occurs in middle-aged or older individuals who experience a forceful contraction of the quadriceps muscle against a flexed knee.

    2. Examination usually demonstrates an extensor lag, with a palpable defect in the suprapatellar region.

    3. Treatment consists of surgical repair of the quadriceps mechanism.

    4. Complications include a slight extensor lag and loss of full knee flexion.

  C. Ruptured Achilles tendon

    1. Mechanism of injury. The Achilles tendon can be ruptured by a forceful contraction of the gastrocnemius-soleus complex with a dorsiflexed ankle.

    2. Examination demonstrates a palpable defect in the Achilles tendon and a positive Thomas test. The Thomas test is performed by squeezing the muscle belly of the gastrocnemius, which should cause plantar flexion of the ankle; if the ankle does not plantarflex, the tendon is ruptured. Even with an Achilles rupture, however, the patient may be able to actively plantarflex the ankle by using the plantaris tendon.

    3. Treatment requires surgical repair.

    4. Complications include some loss of ankle dorsiflexion and push-off power.

V. Compartment syndrome (Volkmann's ischemia). Most muscles within the body are contained within a closed fascial compartment. A **compartment syndrome** occurs when the pressure within the compartment is increased to a point where it compromises the circulation to the contents of that space. Typically, in the upper extremity this syndrome can involve the volar or dorsal compartments of the forearm or the interosseous compartments of the hand. In the lower extremity, the syndrome is most often seen in the anterior or deep posterior compartments of the leg.

  A. The **etiologies** of a compartment syndrome are many but basically involve a space-volume problem, i.e., either a decrease in the space of the compartment or an increase in its volume. A decrease in compartmental space can occur after applying a tight, constrictive dressing or as a result of localized external pressure, as can occur in the comatose patient. An increase in compartmental volume can occur as a result of hemorrhage; swelling due to exercise, burns, or a fracture; muscle hypertrophy; or infiltrated IV infusions.

  B. Clinical features characteristically include pain, paresthesias, paralysis, pallor, and pulselessness. Usually patients complain of pain out of proportion to the injury or of increasing pain despite analgesia, and they may have vague paresthesias of the involved nerve. Patients may also develop a pseudoparalysis of the muscles of the involved compartment. They usually have adequate capillary filling despite increased compartmental pressure and usually maintain a good peripheral pulse even in the presence of an abnormal pressure measurement.

C. **Examination.** It is important to assess the distal circulation and perform a careful neurologic examination, including testing for two-point discrimination and light touch. The passive muscle stretch test is a useful diagnostic maneuver in that it will increase the patient's pain if the involved muscle is ischemic. If there is concern about a possible compartment syndrome, the compartment pressure should be measured. This pressure can be measured either with an 18-gauge needle and a mercury manometer as described by Whitesides [7] (see Chap. 38) or with a Wick catheter. The Whitesides method, with practice, gives useful and reproducible pressure measurements without requiring any sophisticated equipment. In most instances, compartment pressures greater than 40 mm Hg are diagnostic of a compartment syndrome.

D. **Treatment.** It is imperative that compartment syndromes be recognized early and treated aggressively to avert Volkmann's ischemic contracture. Treatment includes removal of all constrictive dressings and frequent examinations. If it is apparent clinically or by a pressure measurement that a compartment syndrome exists, early surgical decompression should be performed as soon as possible.

E. **Complications.** After 12 hours from the onset of symptoms, irreversible myonecrosis is present. Due to myonecrosis, myoglobinuria and renal failure may complicate compartment syndromes.

VI. **Fat embolism syndrome**

A. **Clinical features.** The fat embolism syndrome is a form of the respiratory distress syndrome that can occur within 3 days following a fracture of a long bone. These patients have an alteration of consciousness, including confusion and delirium, and a tachycardia is common. In addition, petechial hemorrhages along the axillary folds and involving the conjunctivae of the eye usually are present. Laboratory findings usually include a PaO_2 of less than 60 mm Hg and a decreased platelet count. The serum lipase may be elevated, and fat globules can be observed in the urine. Radiographically, these patients have patchy pulmonary infiltrates.

B. **Management** consists of respiratory support with supplemental oxygen to maintain the PaO_2 between 80 and 100 mm Hg and assisted ventilation as needed. Corticosteroids (e.g., hydrocortisone, 1–2 gm in divided doses over 24 hours for 3–5 days) may be used to diminish the inflammatory process.

VII. **Cast complications.** A cast is a rigid, circumferential dressing used to immobilize fractures, dislocations, and ligamentous injuries to provide relief of pain and facilitate healing. As with any procedure, there are possible complications that should be avoided.

A. **Superficial burns.** When a plaster dressing is applied, an exothermic reaction occurs, giving off heat. Cold water should be used, since hot water increases the heat generated and can burn the patient.

B. **Skin abrasions.** The edges of the cast must be padded and trimmed so as not to abraid the patient's skin. Also, all bony prominences underneath the cast must be padded to prevent ulceration of the skin.

C. **Neurapraxia** can occur when a peripheral nerve is superficial and is compressed by the cast. The peroneal nerve at the fibular head, the ulnar nerve at the elbow, and the median nerve at the middle third of the humerus are most commonly affected. Any evidence of neurapraxia requires splitting of the cast.

D. **Compartment syndrome** (see sec. **V**). Any time the volume of a closed compartment is elevated by swelling and its space is restricted (e.g., by the application of a cast), the potential exists for a compartment syndrome. Patients must be carefully observed for this complication. Any evidence of a compartment syndrome necessitates immediate splitting of the cast and elevation of the extremity. If these procedures do not relieve symptoms within an hour, compartment pressure measurements should be obtained.

VIII. **Stress fractures** occur when the bone fatigues and cracks after repetitive loading. These fractures are frequently seen in military recruits who undergo rigorous training, but can also be seen in individuals of any age who experience excessive stress for their normal level of activity. Stress fractures most commonly involve a metatarsal bone, tibia, or the femoral neck. Patients complain of pain with activity but do not have pain at rest. Mild swelling may be present. Radiographs may be normal initially, but after 7–10 days periosteal elevation may be seen along with a fracture line. Stress fractures usually are treated with rest, decreased weight-bearing, and discontinuance of the activity that produced the fracture.

Bibliography

1. Conwell, H., and Reynolds, F. *Management of Fractures, Dislocations, and Sprains* (7th ed.). St. Louis: Mosby, 1971.
2. Lovell, W., and Winter, C. *Pediatric Orthopaedics*. Philadelphia: Lippincott, 1978.
3. Matson, F. *Compartmental Syndromes*. New York: Grune & Stratton, 1980.
4. Moore, D. C. *Regional Block: A Handbook for Use in the Clinical Practice of Medicine and Surgery* (4th ed.). Springfield, Ill.: Thomas, 1981.
5. Ogden, J. *Skeletal Injury in the Child*. Philadelphia: Lea & Febiger, 1982.
6. Rockwood, C., Jr., Wilkins, K., and King, R. *Fractures in Adults and Children*. Philadelphia: Lippincott, 1984.
7. Whitesides, T. E., et al. Tissue pressure measurements as a determinant for the need of fasciotomy. *Clin. Orthop.* 113:43, 1975.

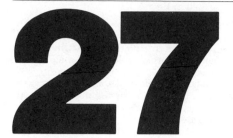

Urologic Emergencies

Russell E. Tackett and
Leonard D. Gaum

Nephrolithiasis

Nephrolithiasis is a common medical problem, with an incidence in the general population of 0.1–6.0%. It accounts for 7.4 of every 1000 hospitalizations in the United States [1]. Calcium oxalate calculi (73%) are the most common, followed by calcium phosphate and magnesium ammonium phosphate (16%), uric acid (7%) and cystine (1%) calculi. The most common sites of impaction are a renal calyx, the ureteropelvic junction, the pelvic brim, and the ureterovesical junction.

I. **Clinical features**
   A. **Symptoms.** A urinary calculus usually presents with an acute episode of renal or ureteral colic. Most patients experience flank or abdominal pain with a colicky pattern; however, location of the pain depends on the site at which the calculus obstructs the system. Impaction in the renal pelvis typically causes flank pain that may radiate into the groin. Calculi in the lower ureter may cause lower-abdominal or suprapubic pain, while calculi lodged at the ureterovesical junction often cause bladder irritability and frequency of urination.
   B. **Physical signs** accompanying urinary calculi include tachycardia, hypertension, grunting respirations, flank tenderness, and emesis. The patient frequently is writhing in pain and is unable to achieve a comfortable position. Fever and leukocytosis may be present and are particularly significant, since infection in conjunction with obstruction can quickly lead to sepsis and shock.
   C. **Laboratory data**
      1. **Urinalysis** usually reveals microscopic or gross hematuria; however, in about 5% of cases there is no hematuria. A thorough search for pyuria and bacteriuria is necessary to rule out concomitant infection. A urine culture must always be obtained. Crystalluria may indicate the type of calculus present.
      2. **Blood tests.** Serum creatinine and blood urea nitrogen (BUN) levels should be obtained to assess renal function and the state of hydration. A complete blood count (CBC) may reveal leukocytosis, often associated with calculi or infection.
      3. **Stone analysis.** For purposes of future therapy it is critical to recover any passed calculi for chemical analysis. Thus, all patients should strain their urine through gauze or a funnellike straining device and save any recovered fragments for analysis.
      4. **Metabolic workup,** if deemed necessary, is performed after the patient has recovered from the acute episode.
   D. **Radiologic procedures**
      1. **KUB** (**K**idneys, **u**reters, and **b**ladder). A plain abdominal film usually will reveal the presence of radiodensities, which may or may not be renal or ureteral calculi. Lateral and oblique projections are helpful in differentiating these densities. Approximately 90% of all renal calculi contain calcium and are radiodense; calcium oxalate calculi are easily visualized, whereas uric acid and cystine calculi generally cannot be seen.
      2. **Intravenous pyelogram (IVP)** remains the cornerstone of diagnosis. Typically, there is delayed excretion of contrast material and a dense nephrogram pattern on the film. Delayed films (up to 24 hours after the contrast material is injected) may demonstrate columning of contrast media in the ureter proximal to the point of obstruction. The delay in excretion is dependent on the grade of obstruction.
      3. **Computed tomography (CT)** is an excellent method of visualizing calculi; all stones including uric acid calculi appear radiodense on CT scanning. Thus, radiolucent stones can be distinguished from other filling defects in the renal pelvis (e.g., blood clot, tumor).

    4. Cystoscopy with retrograde pyelograms is another method for visualizing calculi in the collecting system, particularly in patients in whom an IVP is contraindicated. However, since it requires instrumentation of the genitourinary (GU) tract, cystoscopy should not be performed unless other diagnostic methods have been inconclusive or are inappropriate.

    5. Sonography is particularly helpful to evaluate patients with suspected nephrolithiasis and contrast allergies. Intrarenal stones may be visualized as sonodense areas with shadowing beyond the stone. Hydronephrosis suggestive of obstruction is readily demonstrated.

II. Differential diagnosis. Renal calculus disease often simulates biliary colic, peptic ulcer disease, appendicitis, an abdominal aneurysm, and gastrointestinal or ovarian diseases. In addition, drug abusers often give a false history of stone disease in an attempt to obtain narcotics; they frequently claim an allergy to IVP contrast material or a history of uric acid (nonvisualizing) stones. In suspected cases, narcotics should not be given until the diagnosis is established.

III. Management

    A. General supportive measures include hydration and administration of analgesics. Severe colic warrants use of narcotic analgesics, such as meperidine or morphine, prescribed on the basis of the patient's body weight and with such a frequency as to provide pain relief.

    B. Conservative versus aggressive management

        1. Conservative management of renal and ureteral calculi is warranted in most cases. The likelihood of stone passage is dependent on the size, configuration, and location of the calculus. Between 80 and 90% of calculi less than 4 mm in greatest diameter will pass spontaneously, while only 20–50% of calculi larger than 6 mm are likely to be passed. Anatomic narrowing of the urinary tract obviously will decrease the chance of spontaneous stone passage.

        2. Surgical intervention is necessary when there is evidence of renal function deterioration, bilateral high-grade urinary tract obstruction, pyelonephritis, or unremitting pain with a calculus unlikely to pass spontaneously.

        3. Urinary infection in conjunction with obstruction must be managed aggressively. Decompression of the obstruction by retrograde placement of a ureteral catheter or by percutaneous nephrostomy is required immediately. Broad-spectrum antibiotics (e.g., gentamicin and ampicillin) are administered to prevent septic shock, which can appear rapidly.

IV. Disposition. Patients who can have their pain controlled with oral analgesics and are without evidence of dehydration or infection may be managed on an outpatient basis with close urologic follow-up. However, patients with severe unrelenting colic, persistent nausea and vomiting, and fever require hospitalization for administration of IV fluids, parenteral analgesics, and, if infection is present, parenteral antibiotics.

Hematuria

Hematuria is often a sign of serious GU disease and thus requires a thorough evaluation, particularly since the degree of hematuria bears no relationship to the possible cause. Hematuria is defined as greater than 5 red blood cells (RBCs) per high-power field and can be categorized as gross or microscopic. The condition can be intermittent (in some benign disorders), or it can be either initial or terminal during voiding. Initial hematuria is seen with urethral disease, while terminal hematuria is seen with bladder neck disorders. In any case, the burden on the clinician is to rule out serious GU disease.

I. The **etiologies** of hematuria include trauma, GU tract malignancies, calculus disease, renal parenchymal disease, infections (bacterial, fungal, and viral), vascular malformations, coagulation disorders, and artifactual occurrences. **Pseudohematuria** occurs when the urine appears to contain blood, but the urinary sediment is normal. Causes of pseudohematuria include a concentrated urine or the presence in the urine of pigments from beet and berry ingestion, phenolphthalein, phenazopyridine, porphyrins, vegetable dyes, or myoglobin.

II. Evaluation. Figure 27-1 provides an algorithm for diagnosing upper versus lower urinary tract bleeding.

    A. History and physical examination. A careful history and pertinent review of systems for the GU tract are essential. The physical examination may reveal an abdominal mass, evidence of trauma, easy bruisability, or a urethral or prostate disorder.

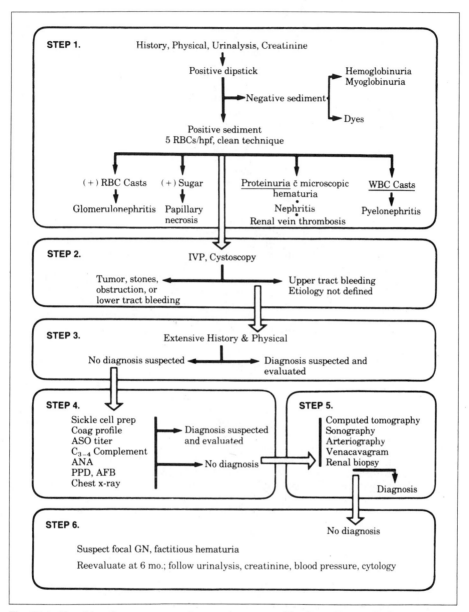

Fig. 27-1. Algorithm for upper versus lower urinary tract bleeding. (From J. E. Gottesman and M. R. Kelly, Idiopathic Renal Hematuria: Differential Diagnosis and Management of Causes. In J. J. Kaufman (ed.), *Current Urologic Therapy*. Philadelphia: Saunders, 1980. With permission.)

B. Laboratory data
1. **Urine studies.** A clean midstream voided urine or clean catheter-collected specimen is examined for the presence of white blood cells (WBCs), protein, and casts to assess for an infectious process or primary renal parenchymal disease. Urine cultures should always be obtained, including acid-fast bacillus (AFB) cultures. Urine cytologic testing is an excellent screening tool for occult malignancy.
2. **Blood studies.** Determination of coagulation parameters (prothrombin time [PT], partial thromboplastin time [PTT], platelet count), renal function (creatinine, BUN), and a CBC are essential.
C. Radiologic studies
1. When renal function is normal as determined by the serum creatinine, **IVP** with tomograms is performed to assess the function and anatomy of the urinary tract. Renal masses and collecting system defects are frequently found on urography; however, the IVP has limited sensitivity.
2. **CT scanning** and, more recently, magnetic resonance imaging (MRI) studies provide excellent resolution of renal masses. MRI is particularly helpful in detailing the pathology in the pelvis. Sonography can also detect renal and prostate masses and distinguish between cystic and solid renal masses. These modalities can also detect renal calculi not visualized on standard urograms. Arteriography and digital vascular imaging will demonstrate arteriovenous malformations.
D. Cystoscopy (appropriate only in patients without evidence of infection) will detect lower urinary tract disorders. When performed during an episode of gross hematuria, cystoscopy may also localize a source of bleeding to the upper urinary tract if hematuria is noted from one or both ureteral orifices. In patients with urinary tract obstruction or a poorly functioning kidney, retrograde pyelography during cystoscopy allows for visualization of the collecting systems. Cytologic evaluation and endoscopic biopsy of the bladder can provide tissue diagnosis.
III. Treatment consists of specific therapy directed at the underlying etiology and appropriate supportive measures.
A. IV fluid replacement and blood transfusions are given as needed.
B. Antibiotics are indicated if there is evidence of infection.
C. Anticoagulants are discontinued, if possible, in patients taking them; vitamin K, platelets, and fresh-frozen plasma may be necessary to normalize coagulation disorders.
D. Continuous bladder irrigation may be required in patients with clot retention.
IV. Disposition. Patients with gross hematuria (with the possible exception of those with hemorrhagic cystitis) require hospitalization for radiologic and cystoscopic evaluation and specific therapy. Patients with microscopic hematuria may be referred to a urologist for diagnostic workup on an outpatient basis.

Urologic Infections

I. Urinary tract infection. See Chap. 12.
II. Perirenal infection and abscess. A perirenal abscess is usually secondary to acute rupture of a renal parenchymal abscess into the perirenal space, the soft tissue of the flank, and the retroperitoneum. Renal abscesses may also arise by hematogenous spread, usually from skin infections. There is an increased incidence of renal abscesses in diabetics. Often patients have a history of recurrent urinary tract infections, renal calculus disease, or, as mentioned, skin infections. A perirenal abscess is often confused with acute pyelonephritis due to their similar presentations. It is important to make an early diagnosis, as mortality from a perirenal abscess is about 50%.
A. Clinical features
1. Typical presenting **symptoms** include abdominal and flank pain, fever and rigors, dysuria, nausea and vomiting, and weight loss. Most patients will have had symptoms for more than 2 weeks, which may be helpful in differentiating perirenal infection from acute pyelonephritis. If the abscess is associated with urinary tract obstruction, the patient may present in septic shock.
2. **Physical examination** reveals costovertebral angle tenderness or a palpable flank mass. A pointing flank abscess may be present with an advanced process. Pain with leg flexion suggests inflammation of the iliopsoas muscle.
3. **Laboratory data**
   a. A **CBC** reveals a leukocytosis with a left shift.

   b. Urinalysis usually reveals pyuria with varying degrees of bacteriuria. A urine culture should be obtained on all patients.
  4. Radiologic studies. On a KUB film there may be evidence of renal calculi, obliteration of the psoas shadow, elevation of the ipsilateral diaphragm, and scoliosis; a soft-tissue density or gas (or both) may be noted. IVP may reveal a nonfunctioning kidney, renal calculi, or a distorted collecting system.
 B. The **diagnosis** may be established by ultrasonography or CT scanning, which will demonstrate a perinephric fluid collection.
 C. Treatment
  1. The primary treatment is **surgical drainage** of the perinephric space and abscess cavity following preoperative correction of fluid and electrolyte disorders. The extent of the drainage procedure is dependent on residual renal function, the underlying cause of the renal abscess, and the condition of the patient at the time of exploration. A primary or secondary nephrectomy may be required in severe cases. In cases of localized loculated abscesses, percutaneous drainage with placement of a catheter has been successful. A perirenal abscess and pyelonephritis in the presence of urinary tract obstruction require immediate relief of obstruction and drainage of the abscess.
  2. Antibiotic regimens should be selected to cover aerobic gram-negative bacilli and *Staphylococcus aureus*. Agents of choice include an aminoglycoside and a penicillinase-resistant penicillin.
III. Prostatitis is defined as an inflammation of the prostatic acini and surrounding tissue. It may be classified as bacterial (acute and chronic types), nonbacterial, or prostatodynia.
 A. Acute bacterial prostatitis is most commonly caused by the Enterobacteriaceae.
  1. Clinical features
   a. Signs and symptoms. Patients commonly complain of low back pain and perineal pain. Fever and chills as well as symptoms of bladder irritability (i.e., urgency, frequency, dysuria) generally occur. Patients may also have varying degrees of bladder outlet obstruction and may note a urethral discharge. There is usually a concomitant cystitis. Complications include sepsis and prostatic abscess formation.
   b. Rectal examination discloses a tender, hot, often swollen prostate gland. Gentle manipulation is mandatory to prevent sepsis and ideally should be performed after an appropriate antimicrobial agent has been given.
   c. Urinalysis reveals profuse pyuria and bacteriuria, and the expressed prostatic secretion is packed with leukocytes and oval fat bodies. A urine culture should be obtained routinely and should guide the choice of an antimicrobial agent.
  2. Treatment depends on the severity of symptoms.
   a. For **severe infections** characterized by toxic systemic symptoms (e.g., fever, chills, nausea, vomiting), hospitalization and administration of IV fluids and parenteral antibiotics is required. Suggested antibiotic regimens include: (1) gentamicin, 1 mg/kg IV q8h, plus ampicillin, 0.5–1.0 gm IV q6h; (2) kanamycin, 1 gm/day IM in 4 divided doses; or (3) trimethoprim-sulfamethoxazole (TMP-SMZ), 8–10 mg/kg/day (based on the trimethoprim component) IV in 2–4 equally divided doses. Antibiotic therapy is adjusted according to susceptibility studies and continued parenterally for 1 week and then orally for 1 month.
   b. For **less severe infections,** antibiotic therapy on an outpatient basis should be adequate. Choices include: (1) trimethoprim-sulfamethoxazole, one double-strength tablet q12h; (2) tetracycline, 250–500 mg PO q6h; (3) minocycline, 100 mg PO q12h; (4) erythromycin, 250–500 mg PO q6h (in cases of penicillin allergy); (5) ampicillin, 250–500 mg PO q6h; or (6) a cephalosporin, 250–500 mg PO q6h. At present, optimum therapy appears to be a prolonged course of 1–3 months with an agent that diffuses into the prostatic fluid. Urologic referral is essential.
   c. Supportive treatment with ice packs to the perineum, analgesics, and antipyretics is indicated.
   d. For patients presenting with acute urinary retention secondary to prostatitis, urethral instrumentation should be avoided; percutaneous suprapubic cystostomy (see Chap. 38) is preferred.
 B. Chronic bacterial prostatitis is defined as recurrent episodes of documented bacterial prostatitis. Bacterial organisms implicated are the Enterobacteriaceae, *S. au-*

reus, and *Streptococcus* species. *Chlamydia* and *Ureaplasma* species also have been identified as potential pathogens.

1. **Clinical features**
   a. **Symptoms** resemble those of acute bacterial prostatitis and include back and pelvic pain, urethral discomfort, and voiding disorders. However, symptoms generally are less severe than those that occur in the acute state of the condition.
   b. **Rectal examination** reveals a boggy, tender prostate; and prostatic calculi may be noted.
   c. **Urinalysis** reveals pyuria and bacteriuria. The expressed prostatic secretion contains WBCs and oval fat bodies.
2. For accurate **diagnosis,** lower urinary tract localization cultures (i.e., a voiding bladder series [$VB_{1,2,3}$]) should be obtained [6]. The bladder urine should first be demonstrably clear of microorganisms, and patients must have discontinued all antibiotic therapy at least 7 days before the series is collected.
3. **Treatment.** Antimicrobial agents are chosen on the basis of culture and susceptibility studies. However, therapy is seldom curative due to poor drug levels achieved in the prostatic fluid. After sterilization of the bladder urine, suppressive medication is continued, with slow tapering of the dosage over 6 months to 1 year. A prostatectomy may be required in severe refractory cases and in cases associated with prostatic calculi and obstruction.

C. **Nonbacterial prostatitis (prostatosis)** is usually chronic and is the most common type of prostatitis encountered. Localizing cultures are always negative for bacteria, and true infection cannot be documented.
   1. **Clinical features.** The symptom complex and microscopic appearance of expressed prostatic secretions are similar to those associated with chronic bacterial prostatitis. Often symptoms have a variable relationship to sexual activity; testicular or groin pain is common.
   2. The **diagnosis** is based on a history of the above symptom complex and the inability to document pathologic infection.
   3. **Treatment.** Antimicrobials are not indicated, although tetracycline therapy has improved symptoms in some patients. Prostatic massage may provide symptomatic relief. Reassuring the patient regarding the benign nature of the process and its ultimate symptomatic resolution is important. In general, though, treatment of this process is extremely unsatisfactory.

D. **Prostatodynia.** The etiology of prostatodynia is unknown, but it may be related to pelvic myalgia or primary bladder neck dysfunction.
   1. **Clinical features.** Prostatodynia is a symptom complex similar to prostatosis but without evidence of an inflammatory process in the expressed prostatic secretion. Patients complain of pain in the perineum, lower back, and genitalia. Voiding disorders, particularly hesitancy and frequency, are commonly seen.
   2. **Treatment** is supportive. Physical therapy to teach habitual pelvic floor relaxation is helpful. Some conditions respond to phenoxybenzamine, 10 mg q8–12h; the duration of therapy and dosage are adjusted according to clinical response.

IV. **Urethritis** is generally categorized as specific (gonococcal), nonspecific, or idiopathic.
   A. **Specific (gonococcal) urethritis**
      1. **Clinical features.** Patients present with dysuria and a purulent urethral discharge beginning 24–48 hours after sexual exposure. Definitive diagnosis is by Gram stain of the urethral discharge with demonstration of intracellular gram-negative diplococci. Special media (Thayer-Martin or chocolate agar) are required for culture. A Venereal Disease Research Laboratory (VDRL) test should be obtained to rule out concomitant syphilis. Long-term complications of untreated cases include urethral strictures.
      2. **Treatment.** Recommended treatment is (1) amoxicillin, 3.0 gm PO, plus probenecid, 1.0 gm PO, or (2) ceftriaxone, 250 mg IM. Alternative regimens include (1) procaine penicillin G, 4.8 million units IM, plus probenecid, 1 gm PO; (2) spectinomycin, 2 gm IM; or (3) cefoxitin, 2 gm IM, plus probenecid, 1 gm PO. It is recommended that this single-dose therapy be followed by a 7-day course of tetracycline, 500 mg PO qid, or doxycycline, 100 mg PO bid, to treat possible coexisting chlamydial infection. For penicillin-resistant strains, ceftriaxone or spectinomycin is indicated. Amoxicillin, ceftriaxone, and procaine penicillin G in recommended dosages are also likely effective against incubating syphilis.
   B. **Nonspecific urethritis (NSU)**
      1. **Clinical features.** Patients suffer from dysuria, urethral itching, a watery or

white urethral discharge, and perineal, suprapubic, or testicular pain. Common bacteria isolates include staphylococcal species, *Escherichia coli, Pseudomonas,* and *Klebsiella. Trichomonas,* although rare, may be seen on a wet preparation of the urethral discharge.

   2. Treatment. The microscopic findings and cultures of the urethral discharge dictate the antimicrobial therapy. If *Trichomonas* is isolated, both the patient and sexual partner must be treated; metronidazole (Flagyl), 250 mg PO q8h for 7 days, is the drug of choice. Patients should be cautioned to avoid alcohol consumption during this therapy because of an Antabuse–alcohol-like reaction.

   C. Idiopathic urethritis, which is actually a subcategory of NSU, accounts for 75% of all urethritis cases. *Mycoplasma* species are isolated in 60% of these cases, and *Chlamydiae* in 40%. Both of these organisms are fastidious and difficult to culture. Antibiotic treatment options include (1) tetracycline, 500 mg PO q6h for 7 days; (2) doxycycline, 100 mg PO q12h for 7 days; or (3) erythromycin, 500 mg PO q6h for 7 days. Antibiotic therapy should be adjusted in refractory cases.

   D. Urethritis may be secondary to the presence of a foreign body in the urethra or self-instrumentation. This condition requires removal of any foreign body, culture of the urethral discharge, and appropriate antibiotic therapy.

V. Balanitis and posthitis. Balanitis is an inflammation of the superficial layers of the glans penis; **posthitis** is inflammation of the prepuce. The two usually occur together, and the condition is termed **balanoposthitis.** The etiology of balanoposthitis is generally poor personal hygiene, chemical irritants, or trauma. Predisposing factors include diabetes mellitus and an indwelling urethral catheter.

   A. Clinical features. Clinically, there is local itching, tenderness, and weeping from affected tissue. If the condition is untreated, severe pain can develop with a foul discharge, dysuria, edema, and phimosis of the prepuce.

   B. Treatment. Meticulous hygiene, hot baths, and use of a topical antibacterial or antifungal ointment (e.g., povidone-iodine, neomycin-polymyxin, or clotrimazole) are recommended. Powders, however, cause local irritation and should be avoided. In patients with an indwelling catheter, local care involving washing with a mild antiseptic and application of povidone-iodine or neomycin-polymyxin ointment provides prophylaxis. Surgical treatment (i.e., a dorsal foreskin split) is rarely required for urinary retention due to edema. After resolution of the acute process, circumcision will prevent recurrences. With refractory lesions, other disease entities including carcinoma of the penis should be considered and biopsied.

VI. Epididymitis and orchitis

   A. Epididymitis, which may be due to infection, trauma, or chemical irritation (sterile reflux urine), is the most common of all intrascrotal inflammations. The process may also involve the spermatic cord **(funiculitis).** Infection occurs in a retrograde fashion via the vas deferens from the posterior urethra, which is the reservoir for the organisms involved. *E. coli* is the most common organism isolated in males over 50 years of age; *Chlamydia* is the most common organism in younger patients. Traumatic epididymitis is secondary to direct trauma and generally is seen after vasectomy. Chemical epididymitis can occur with the reflux of sterile urine into the vas deferens as a result of straining to void.

   1. Clinical features. Patients generally give a history of slow onset of pain and progressive swelling and erythema of the scrotum. In addition, patients may experience pyrexia and rigors. The epididymis is exquisitely tender, and the testis lies low in the scrotum. With scrotal elevation there may be relief of pain **(Prehn's sign),** which may be helpful in distinguishing epididymitis from testicular torsion but is not diagnostic of epididymitis.

   2. Diagnosis. Since epididymitis is most commonly associated with a urinary tract infection, pyuria and bacteriuria generally are found on urinalysis. Testicular scanning, which reveals increased blood flow indicative of inflammation, will establish the diagnosis. Testicular ultrasonography reveals a paratesticular fluid collection and can rule out other disorders (e.g., testicular tumor).

   3. Management

   a. Antibiotic therapy is required. Patients with systemic toxicity require hospitalization for parenteral administration of broad-spectrum antibiotics (e.g., ampicillin plus gentamicin), IV hydration, and monitoring for sepsis. In cases unassociated with systemic toxicity, antibiotic therapy on an outpatient basis is adequate. In younger patients, amoxicillin, 3.0 gm PO, plus probenecid, 1.0 gm PO, or ceftriaxone, 250 mg IM, either followed by a 10-day course of tetracycline, 500 mg PO qid, or doxycycline, 100 mg PO bid, is recommended to treat for *Neisseria gonorrhoeae* and *Chlamydia* (see Chap. 12). In older patients, ampicillin, 500 mg PO qid for 10 days, or TMP-SMZ, two tablets PO bid for 10 days, is preferred to treat for the Enterobacteriaceae.

   b. Supportive measures include bed rest, scrotal elevation, and administration of an analgesic and anti-inflammatory agent.

   c. Refractory cases may have progressed to the formation of an abscess, which requires surgical drainage or orchiectomy. In recurrent (chronic) cases of epididymitis, epididymectomy may be indicated. Testicular tumors mimic epididymitis and may be misdiagnosed; thus, in the absence of pyuria and bacteriuria, ultrasonography of the testis is recommended to rule out carcinoma.

B. Orchitis is inflammation of the testis proper, but is rare due to the rich vascular and lymphatic drainage of the testis providing resistance to infectious processes. It usually is an extension from epididymitis and is rarely the result of hematogenous spread. Viral infections account for the majority of cases of orchitis.

   1. Clinical features. Patients have acute pain, pyrexia, and a tense, swollen, tender testis. With tissue destruction the testis may become fluctuant, resulting in an associated hydrocele. In cases secondary to spread from the epididymis, urinalysis reveals pyuria and bacteriuria. Viral orchitis may occur 4–6 days after mumps parotitis; in this setting there is testicular pain and swelling (without evidence of urinary tract infection) that generally resolve in 7–10 days, leaving an atrophic testis.

   2. Treatment. Bed rest, elevation of the scrotum, application of ice packs, and use of analgesics are recommended. Appropriate antibiotic therapy, as for epididymitis (see **A.3.a**), is indicated. A frank testicular abscess usually requires orchiectomy. Urologic follow-up is mandatory to determine resolution and assess for any underlying pathologic process.

VII. Anorectal inflammatory processes. See Chap. 30.

VIII. Soft-tissue infections of the penis, scrotum, and perineum

   A. Minor infections of the scrotum and perineum include folliculitis and infection of epidermal or sebaceous cysts. These problems are treated on an outpatient basis with antibiotics and/or incision and drainage.

   B. A periurethral abscess is the most common cause of perineoscrotal infections. Predisposing factors include those that cause obstruction to urine outflow, most commonly a urethral stricture. The route of spread of infection is through the corpus spongiosum between Buck's and Colles' fascia into the scrotum and perineum.

   1. Clinical features. Patients present with perineal swelling, soft-tissue necrosis, or fistula formation.

   2. Treatment is directed toward correcting the underlying cause, i.e., urethral stricture dilatation or incision to correct outflow obstruction. Any devitalized tissue requires debridement, and fistulas require excision. Antibiotics play a supportive role to surgical therapy.

   C. Fournier's gangrene

   1. Clinical features. Fournier's gangrene is gangrene of the male genitalia; a periurethral abscess is the most common underlying process. The syndrome results in severe toxemia and shock, with a mortality reported as high as 30–50%. Anaerobic streptococci alone or, more often, in combination with other organisms have been implicated; *E. coli*, hemolytic streptococci, *Proteus* species, and gas-forming anaerobes have also been implicated. The gangrenous process is rapid, with severe tissue destruction, and presents a true surgical emergency.

   2. Treatment

   a. Wide **surgical debridement** of necrotic tissue is mandatory; repeat debridement of devitalized tissue not apparent at first debridement may be required.

   b. Triple-antibiotic therapy with penicillin, clindamycin, and an aminoglycoside is indicated.

   c. General support with IV fluids, blood, and vasopressors is indicated.

   d. If there is urinary extravasation, diversion of the urinary stream with an **open cystostomy** is necessary.

Phimosis and Paraphimosis

I. Phimosis is stenosis of the distal foreskin (prepuce), preventing its retraction back over the glans penis. It is acquired secondary to trauma, dermatitis (e.g., diaper rash in children), or balanoposthitis. Phimosis causes hygienic problems and, in extreme cases, urinary retention. Patients often complain of painful erections and inability to engage in intercourse. Treatment is simple circumcision on an elective basis.

II. **Paraphimosis,** which is an emergent problem, is entrapment of the retracted prepuce behind the coronal sulcus, resulting in a collar ring deformity. If left untreated, it results in edema, vascular compromise, and eventually tissue necrosis distally. Paraphimosis usually can be reduced by manual decompression after adequate sedation of the patient. If manual reduction is unsuccessful, a dorsal slit of the prepuce under local anesthesia will treat the immediate problem. Circumcision should then be performed at a later date.

Hematospermia

Blood in the ejaculate may be idiopathic or secondary to bacterial infection, tuberculosis, adenomatous urethral polyps, or vascular abnormalities such as varicosities of the prostate. Patients usually are asymptomatic. Appropriate cultures of the urine and expressed prostatic secretions will assess for urinary tract infection and tuberculosis. Radiologic evaluation is not necessary. The patient should be referred to a urologist for follow-up. Since hematospermia usually is a self-limiting process, complete urologic workup (e.g., with IVP, cystoscopy) is withheld unless recurrence is a problem.

Urinary Retention

I. **Etiology.** Urinary retention may be secondary to anatomic and nonanatomic causes. In adult males, benign prostatic hypertrophy is the most common cause; in male children, posterior urethral valves and meatal stenosis may be causative; and in females, the etiology is usually psychogenic. Urethral stricture, neurologic disorders (e.g., diabetic neuropathy, multiple sclerosis, spinal injury), prostatitis, traumatic urethral disruption, and phimosis are other causes. In addition, various medications (e.g., antihistamines, anticholinergics, psychotropics) may be implicated.

II. **Clinical features**
   A. **Signs and symptoms.** Most patients present with abdominal pain and inability to void. Others may give a history of severe frequency and dribbling secondary to overflow incontinence. The physical examination reveals a distended bladder, dull to percussion and tender to palpation.
   B. **Laboratory data.** A urinalysis and urine culture should be obtained prior to catheterization, if possible, to assess for infection. A serum creatinine or BUN is necessary to assess for postobstructive renal failure. A CBC and serum chemistries are important to evaluate for secondary anemia and electrolyte disturbances, respectively.

III. **Management**
   A. **Bladder decompression** via catheter drainage is the immediate goal of therapy. However, to avoid complications (e.g., mucosal hemorrhage), only 1000 ml of urine should be removed initially, followed by drainage of 300 ml/hour until the bladder is empty.
      1. In **prostatic hypertrophy,** a standard urethral catheter can be inserted initially; however, a coudé-tip catheter may be required to pass the obstruction. Meticulous sterile technique must be used in all patients, and urethral manipulation must be gentle, with generous use of lubricant (urethral lidocaine [Xylocaine]). The use of catheter introducers and filiforms with followers should be restricted to those experienced with their use.
      2. In cases of **urethral stricture or a local inflammatory process,** urine should be diverted through a percutaneous suprapubic catheter, placed under local anesthesia (see Chap. 38).
   B. **Monitoring.** In patients with long-standing primary urinary retention, monitoring for a postobstructive diuresis following urinary tract decompression is necessary.
   C. **Definitive therapy** is dictated by the underlying disease process.
      1. **Benign prostatic hypertrophy** responds to open or transurethral resection.
      2. **Stricture disease** is handled in various ways (e.g., urethral dilatation) by a urologist.
      3. In **females who present with urinary retention,** a thorough neurologic evaluation to detect or rule out any underlying neurologic disorder is mandatory. Urodynamic evaluation is indicated if there is suspicion of neurologic disease.

Immediate treatment is intermittent self-catheterization, as the process is frequently self-limited. Psychiatric referral may be indicated.

4. **Medication-induced urinary retention.** All medications potentially responsible for urinary retention should be discontinued.

IV. **Disposition.** Hospitalization for evaluation and treatment is generally indicated for patients with urinary retention.

Priapism

Priapism, a true urologic emergency, is a condition of persistent penile erection. Often painful, it is unrelated to sexual excitation or desire. Priapism involves the corpora cavernosa only, with the glans penis and corpus spongiosum remaining flaccid. There is sludging of corporeal blood, with edema of the spongy septa and subsequent endothelial inflammation and injury. Untreated, priapism results in corporeal fibrosis and impotence.

I. **Etiology.** Priapism may be idiopathic or have specific causes. Certain drugs (e.g., phenothiazines, heparin, ethyl alcohol, antihypertensive medications, marijuana) have been linked to priapism. In addition, this condition may be secondary to sickle cell disease, leukemia, myeloma, solid tumors, pelvic or spinal trauma, neurologic disorders, and prolonged sexual activity.

II. **Management.** Urologic consultation should be sought. Either noninvasive or surgical therapy may be appropriate.

A. **Noninvasive therapy,** including sedation with narcotics (e.g., morphine) and use of ketamine anesthesia, can be tried initially. Patients with underlying sickle cell disease may respond to oxygen, blood alkalinization, and exchange transfusions. Leukemic patients may respond to chemotherapy. Caudal or spinal anesthesia may be helpful in patients with neurologic disorders.

B. **Surgical therapy** is indicated when conservative therapy fails. Immediate treatment with decompression of the corpora cavernosa best prevents fibrosis and impotence, the long-term complications of priapism. Improved venous drainage of the corpora cavernosa is the immediate treatment goal. Surgical techniques, when necessary, include large-bore needle irrigation of the corpora cavernosa with a heparinized saline solution, corpus cavernosum–corpus spongiosum shunts (open and closed), and corpus cavernosum–saphenous vein shunts.

Testicular Torsion

Testicular torsion results in vascular compromise of the testis and is a true urologic emergency, requiring prompt treatment for a successful outcome. If left untreated for more than 6–12 hours, the testis will infarct, with subsequent atrophy and total loss of spermatogenesis. Torsion can be extravaginal or intravaginal. Extravaginal torsion presents in the neonate as a painless scrotal swelling; treatment is expectant. Intravaginal torsion generally occurs during puberty, although it may occur later in life. Anatomically, there is a high insertion of the parietal layers of the tunica vaginalis testis onto the spermatic cord, creating a "bell clapper" deformity. This deformity allows increased testicular mobility, enabling the testis to twist on itself. The remaining discussion is focused on intravaginal torsion.

I. **Clinical features.** The highest incidence of intravaginal testicular torsion is among peripubertal adolescents. However, torsion can be seen in adults as well. It is characterized by the acute onset of scrotal pain and swelling. There is a variable relationship to physical activity. Physical examination reveals a high-riding testis with a thickened spermatic cord, and the epididymis is displaced from its normal posterior position in relationship to the testis proper. In addition, the cremasteric reflex is absent in torsion of the testis.

II. The **differential diagnosis** includes acute epididymitis, torsion of the appendix testis or appendix epididymis, and testicular tumor with bleeding into the tumor.

III. **Diagnosis.** The physical examination and laboratory evaluation help differentiate the disorders causing scrotal swelling. Since acute epididymitis is often accompanied by a urinary tract infection, a urinalysis generally reveals pyuria and bacteriuria. Torsion of the appendix testis or epididymis may present as a small, discolored spot on the superior pole of the testis (blue dot sign) if detected early. Testicular nuclear scans are diagnostic of epididymitis when increased perfusion is seen and may be diagnostic of torsion when there is decreased perfusion. Doppler vascular studies are usually of little help in making the diagnosis, but in some cases may show decreased blood flow to the involved testis.

IV. **Management.** Immediate urologic consultation is indicated. The urologist may recommend that manual detorsion be attempted after the administration of a local anesthetic and sedation of the patient. If this treatment is unsuccessful, immediate surgical detorsion is required, with orchiopexy of both testes due to the high incidence of contralateral torsion. As a general rule, if torsion is strongly suspected, surgery should be performed without obtaining a testicular scan. Torsion of a testicular appendage, however, does not require surgery unless testicular torsion cannot be ruled out.

Urologic Trauma

Blunt or penetrating trauma (see Chap. 17) of the GU tract is usually associated with gross or microscopic hematuria; however, significant injury can be present without it. When the history, physical examination, or urinalysis suggests injury to the GU tract, the general approach is to perform radiologic studies to define the anatomic injury. IVP and CT provide both functional and anatomic information about the upper and lower urinary tract. Retrograde urethrography and cystography provide evaluation of the lower urinary tract.

In patients with multiple trauma, associated GU tract injury should be suspected. In these cases, a single IV bolus injection of 100–150 ml of an appropriate contrast material will define baseline function and anatomy of the upper urinary tract and determine the need for exploration. In stable patients, a more thorough evaluation (including a urethrogram or cystogram or both) can be carried out as indicated.

I. **GU tract injuries**

A. **Renal injuries** most commonly result from blunt trauma, particularly deceleration-type trauma (e.g., motor vehicle accidents, falls). Penetrating injuries of the abdomen involve the GU tract in less than 10% of cases. Renal injuries can be graded according to radiographic studies as minor (i.e., no parenchymal disruption or urinary extravasation), major (i.e., parenchymal disruption or urinary extravasation), and catastrophic (i.e., avulsion of a renal pedicle, presence of devitalized tissue, or a macerated kidney).

1. **Clinical features.** Renal injuries should be suspected in cases of lower thoracic, back, or abdominal trauma. Physical findings include flank tenderness, a flank hematoma or contusion, or a retroperitoneal mass. Hematuria, gross or microscopic (i.e., > 5 RBCs/high-power field), is usually present, although significant renal trauma can occur with no hematuria. Plain radiographs may reveal a fractured lower rib or transverse spinous process, or an obscured psoas shadow.

2. **Diagnosis**

a. **IVP** is indicated in patients with suspected upper-tract urologic trauma as evidenced by gross or microscopic hematuria or signs of significant flank trauma (e.g., flank contusion or hematoma), even in the absence of hematuria. Pertinent findings on urography are delayed excretion of contrast, extravasation of contrast material (signifying disruption of the collecting system), or nonvisualization of a kidney (suggesting avulsion of the renal pedicle).

b. **Arteriography** is indicated for patients with nonvisualization of a kidney on IVP.

c. **CT** with contrast allows resolution of the renal parenchyma and thus enables assessment of tissue damage and the extent of extravasation or hematoma formation.

3. **Treatment** is determined by the patient's overall clinical condition and by the extent and severity of the renal injury. Fluid replacement and blood transfusions are given as needed.

a. **Minor renal injuries** generally are handled conservatively with bed rest and monitoring of the vital signs, hematuria, and the hematocrit.

b. **Major injuries.** Therapy is controversial, varying from conservative management to surgery; the latter generally is indicated in patients with unstable vital signs.

c. **Catastrophic injuries** require surgical intervention.

4. **Disposition.** All patients with gross hematuria or an abnormal IVP require hospitalization until the urine clears, major injury is ruled out or appropriately treated, and the clinical condition remains stable for 24–48 hours. On the other

hand, patients with a normal IVP and without gross hematuria can be treated on an outpatient basis, with urologic referral.

B. Bladder injuries. Bladder rupture is categorized as intraperitoneal or extraperitoneal. Intraperitoneal rupture occurs when a full bladder is compressed, leading to increased intraluminal pressure and rupture at the weakest point, the dome. Extraperitoneal rupture occurs with pelvic fractures and is secondary to bladder laceration by a bony spicule.

1. **Clinical features.** The hallmark of bladder injury is gross hematuria. Patients generally complain of suprapubic pain and may be unable to void. On physical examination, ecchymosis may be noted overlying the pubis. The bladder generally is nonpalpable, and signs of peritoneal irritation may be present if there is intraperitoneal rupture. X-rays of the pelvis demonstrating pubic rami fractures suggest possible bladder injury.

2. **Diagnosis.** With suspected bladder injury, an IVP is obtained first to rule out an upper tract injury. This radiograph is followed by a retrograde urethrogram (see **C.1.b**) to rule out urethral injury. Finally, a cystogram is performed with a Foley catheter in the bladder (after urethral injury has been ruled out); filling the bladder with 200–400 ml of an appropriate contrast agent by gravity is safest. If the patient is able to cooperate, his or her bladder is infused to the point of bladder discomfort. Drainage films and oblique films are always obtained to assess for a posterior injury.

3. **Treatment.** Principles of treatment include surgical repair of the bladder perforation and drainage of the bladder (with a suprapubic catheter) and perivesical space (with Penrose drains). Conservative management with indwelling urethral catheter drainage has been successful with small extraperitoneal ruptures but is not recommended.

C. Urethral injuries usually occur in males and are classified as anterior or posterior.

1. **Anterior urethral injuries** are distal to the urogenital diaphragm. They are secondary to instrumentation, straddle injuries, and, rarely, penetrating trauma. In anterior urethral rupture, extravasation of urine and associated hemorrhage generally are limited to the penis by Buck's fascia. With rupture outside of Buck's fascia, extravasation of urine is limited to the anterior abdominal wall, scrotum, and perineum by Colles' fascia and the fascia lata of the thigh. In suspected cases of urethral injury, patients should be instructed not to void until radiologic evaluation is completed.

   a. **Clinical features.** Patients complain of pain involving the penis, and swelling of the penis is noted on the physical examination. A key sign in any urethral injury is the presence of blood at the urethral meatus.

   b. **Diagnosis.** A retrograde urethrogram is diagnostic; it is performed by injecting 10–20 ml of an appropriate contrast agent via a Foley catheter inflated in the fossa navicularis (tip of the penis) or via a Brodney meatal clamp.

   c. **Treatment.** Urethral catheterization should not be attempted. Urologic consultation is indicated. Therapy consists of urinary diversion proximal to the injury by placement of a suprapubic catheter; open bladder drainage is required when there is peritoneal extravasation. In the absence of infection, lacerations can be repaired by primary anastomosis over a fenestrated catheter. Infected injuries, however, require secondary repair. Minor instrumentation (iatrogenic) injuries can be handled by Silastic urethral catheter drainage.

2. **Posterior urethral injuries.** This type of injury is usually associated with pelvic fractures and is far more severe than anterior injuries. Rupture, partial or complete, occurs between the apex of the prostate and the urogenital diaphragm.

   a. **Diagnosis.** Posterior urethral injuries should be suspected in the presence of any pelvic fracture. The diagnosis is made by a rectal examination, which reveals a displaced prostate (the so-called high-riding prostate) or a periprostatic hematoma, and is confirmed by retrograde urethrography.

   b. **Treatment.** Urologic consultation is required. Treatment consists of suprapubic urinary diversion and secondary delayed urethral reanastomosis. Urethral catheterization should not be attempted in the emergency department.

3. **Urethral foreign body.** This problem usually involves pediatric patients or patients with severe mental disorders. The patient usually presents with local inflammation, pain, and a palpable foreign body. Radiodense objects can be

localized by x-ray. Treatment consists of removal via a cystoscope or open extraction.

II. External genitalia injuries
A. Penile injuries
1. **Lacerations** of the penis without urethral involvement are treated as lacerations elsewhere.
2. **Human bites** are treated by thorough cleansing and administration of an antibiotic (e.g., a penicillinase-resistant penicillin or cephalosporin). The wound is allowed to heal secondarily.
3. **Penile amputation** requires immediate surgical repair by a urologist. Debridement of nonvital tissues is mandatory, followed by a primary urethrostomy in most cases. The goals of therapy are to preserve tissue and provide a functional urinary conduit. If the injury is too proximal, it is best to fashion a perineal urethrostomy. Reimplantation should be considered in clean injuries. The amputated segment is treated in the same manner as other amputated parts (see Chap. 23).

B. Scrotal injuries
1. Clean **lacerations** that do not penetrate dartos fascia can be repaired primarily, employing absorbable sutures. Contaminated wounds, gunshot wounds, and lacerations deep to the dartos fascia require hospitalization, surgical exploration, drainage, and antibiotic therapy. These wounds are allowed to heal secondarily.
2. **Avulsion injuries** may be partial or total; often the testes and spermatic cords are undamaged. Remnants of scrotal skin may be used for primary repair. Total scrotal avulsion injuries are best handled by placing the testes in subcutaneous thigh pouches and using skin grafts to cover bare soft-tissue areas. Secondary reconstruction is performed later.
3. **Scrotal hematoma and testicular rupture.** Blunt trauma to the scrotum may result in a scrotal hematoma or testicular rupture. A scrotal ultrasound provides excellent definition of the pathologic state. Scrotal hematomas are managed conservatively with bed rest, scrotal support, and analgesics. Testicular rupture requires surgical exploration with debridement of devitalized tissue and primary repair or orchiectomy.

Bibliography

1. Carroll, P. R., and McAnnish, J. W. Major bladder trauma. Mechanisms of injury and unified method of diagnosis and repair. *J. Urol.* 132:254, 1984.
2. Centers for Disease Control. 1985 STD treatment guidelines *M.M.W.R.* 34(Suppl.):75S, 1985.
3. Fallon, B., Noridt, J. C., and Hautrey, C. E. Urological injury and assessment in patients with fractured pelvis. J. Urol. 131:712, 1984.
4. Fraley, E. E. (ed.). Testicular tumors. *Urol. Clin. North Am.* 4:343, 1977.
5. Goldman, M. S. Repair of shattered solitary testicle. *Urology* 24:229, 1984.
6. Harrison, J. H., et al. (eds.). *Campbell's Urology*. Philadelphia: Saunders, 1978.
7. Kaufman, J. J. (ed.). *Current Urologic Therapy*. Philadelphia: Saunders, 1980.
8. Kearney, Y. P., and Coiling, P. Fournier's gangrene: An approach to its management. *J. Urol.* 130:695, 1983.
9. Krieger, J. N., Algood, C. B., and Mason, J. T. Urological trauma in the Pacific Northwest. Etiology, distribution, management and outcome. *J. Urol.* 132:70, 1984.
10. Marshall, V. F., and Fuller, N. Hemospermia. *J. Urol.* 129: 377, 1983.
11. Meares, E. M., Jr. Prostatitis syndrome: New perspectives about old woes. *J. Urol.* 123:141, 1980.
12. Medical Letter. Treatment of sexually transmitted diseases. *Med. Lett. Drugs Ther.* 28:23, 1986.
13. Peters, P. C. (ed.). Urologic emergencies. *Urol. Clin. North Am.* 9:207, 1982.
14. Resnick, I. (ed.). Surgery of stone disease. *Urol. Clin. North Am.* 10:585, 1983.
15. Stamey, T. A. (ed.). *Pathogenesis and Treatment of Urinary Tract Infections*. Baltimore: Williams and Wilkins, 1980.

28 Otolaryngologic Emergencies

Harlan R. Muntz

Upper Airway Obstruction

I. **Clinical features.** Patients with upper airway obstruction generally present in respiratory arrest or distress. Retractions on inspiration, use of accessory muscles, and/or cyanosis may be noted. Complete airway obstruction is characterized by absence of air movement. In partial obstruction, prolongation of the inspiratory phase of respiration and the presence of musical sounds on inspiration, but rarely on expiration, may be present. The presence of **stridor** (a harsh sound produced during respiration) certainly suggests upper airway obstruction, but its absence does not rule it out.

II. **Differential diagnosis.** Upper airway obstruction should be differentiated from lower airway obstruction and psychiatric disease. Lower airway disease is characterized by prolongation of expiration and expiratory wheezing. A psychogenic etiology should be considered only after organic disease has been excluded by appropriate studies (e.g., indirect laryngoscopy, soft-tissue films of the neck, endoscopy).

III. **Etiology.** The possible sites of upper airway obstruction extend from the oral cavity to the carina. The etiologies are many and primarily include infections, neoplasms, allergic phenomenon, foreign body aspiration, and trauma (Table 28-1). The obstruction may be partial or complete.

IV. **Evaluation.** Patients suspected of having a partial upper airway obstruction should immediately have soft-tissue x-rays of the neck and a chest x-ray and/or undergo indirect laryngoscopy or fiberoptic endoscopy. These studies generally will establish the diagnosis. In nonurgent situations, inspiratory flow studies can be used to define the degree of upper airway obstruction.

V. **Treatment**
   A. **Nonforeign body obstruction**
      1. **Airway.** If patient's ventilation is inadequate, immediate attention should be directed at opening the airway by properly positioning the patient (e.g., in an upright or leaning forward position unless contraindicated) and performing a standard airway maneuver, such as the head tilt–chin lift or jaw thrust with or without head tilt (see Chap. 2). In patients with suspected cervical-spine injury, the jaw thrust without head tilt technique is the safest approach to open the airway. If these attempts fail to establish an airway, immediate cannulation of the trachea is necessary. Initially, tracheal intubation via the oral or nasal route (see Chap. 38) should be attempted. The nasal route is preferred in suspected cervical spine injuries but should be avoided in the presence of a suspected cribriform plate fracture. In addition, blind nasotracheal intubation is not recommended in the presence of apnea or laryngeal edema. If an endotracheal tube cannot be placed, percutaneous transtracheal ventilation (see Chap. 38) can be used to ventilate the patient until an airway can be established by cricothyrotomy (see Chap. 38) or tracheostomy. Endotracheal intubation is a reasonable means to secure an airway in cases of oral cavity, supraglottic, glottic, or hypopharyngeal obstruction; subglottic and tracheal problems, however, generally require cricothyrotomy or tracheostomy. Cricothyrotomy is the most rapid means of securing the airway if endotracheal intubation is impossible or precluded; tracheostomy, on the other hand, although having less delayed complications, is more difficult in the relatively inexperienced.
      2. **Ancillary measures.** Low-flow oxygen with high humidity may be helpful in patients with nonforeign body obstruction. Steroids are useful in reducing edema, particularly in allergic disorders, but take several hours for this effect to be manifested. Racemic epinephrine via nebulizer may be helpful in croup or traumatic disorders. Antibiotic therapy should be initiated for infectious processes after appropriate cultures have been obtained.

Table 28-1. Etiologies of acute upper airway obstruction

I. Oropharynx
  A. Infections
    1. Ludwig's angina
    2. Peritonsillar abscess
    3. Parapharyngeal space abscess
    4. Retropharyngeal or prevertebral abscess
    5. Tonsillitis (especially due to mononucleosis)
  B. Tumor
    1. Lingual thyroid
    2. Benign and malignant neoplasia of the mouth and pharynx
    3. Tumors of the deep neck spaces
    4. Deep lobe parotid tumors
  C. Allergic reaction causing edema
  D. Foreign body
  E. Trauma
  F. Burns
II. Hypopharynx and larynx
  A. Infection
    1. Epiglottitis (supraglottitis)
    2. Croup (laryngotracheitis)
    3. Localized laryngeal infection, usually secondary to trauma
  B. Tumor
    1. Malignant and benign neoplasms of the hypopharynx and larynx (e.g., papilloma, hemangioma, soft-tissue sarcoma, epidermoid carcinoma, polyps)
    2. Vallecular cyst
    3. Laryngocele
  C. True vocal cord paralysis
  D. Foreign body aspiration
  E. Laryngospasm
  F. Allergic reaction leading to laryngeal edema
  G. Trauma
  H. Burns
III. Trachea
  A. Infection
    1. Croup (laryngotracheitis)
    2. Membranous tracheitis
  B. Tumor
    1. Duplication cyst
    2. External compression (e.g., mediastinal mass, thyroid, paratracheal adenopathy)
  C. Foreign body aspiration
  D. Trauma

    B. Foreign body obstruction. For the management of upper airway obstruction due to foreign body aspiration ("café coronary"), see Chap. 2.
  VI. Disposition. Patients with evidence of upper airway obstruction require hospitalization, usually in an intensive care unit.

Otologic Disorders

  I. Infections of the ear are common and need to be excluded in the patient with otalgia.
    A. Otitis externa ("swimmer's ear") is a common disease throughout the year, but especially in summer. It is most often related to water retention in the external canal followed by an overgrowth of bacteria. *Pseudomonas* is the usual organism, although others may be present as well.
      1. The **diagnosis** of otitis externa is suggested when pain is elicited by pulling on the pinna or by pushing on the tragus and is confirmed by visualizing a swollen, red external ear canal, often with a purulent drainage.
      2. Differential diagnosis. Consideration must be given to the possibility of malignant otitis externa, fungal otitis, and weeping tumors of the external auditory canal. Although the tympanic membrane may not be seen in the initial evalua-

tion, it must be evaluated eventually to assure that there is no perforation or cholesteatoma.

3. **Treatment**
   a. Since otitis externa is a topical infection, **topical treatment** (Table 28-2) is indicated. There are essentially two types of topical treatment, each of which is quite effective.
      (1) An **antibiotic eardrop** can be administered to eradicate the bacterial infection; gentamicin, polymyxin, colistin, or neomycin, alone or in combination, may be used. The use of a steroid in the preparation (e.g., Cortisporin Otic Suspension or Solution, 4 gtt qid) reduces swelling, thereby improving drop delivery and reducing pain. The solution is clear and translucent; in contrast, the suspension is cloudy and can obscure the view of the tympanic membrane. In a person with a tympanic membrane perforation, however, the solution may cause severe irritation and be tolerated poorly. Sometimes an ophthalmic drop may be used instead of an otic drop if sensitivity and pain are a problem.
      (2) Because the bacteria causing otitis externa are quite acid-labile, an **acidic eardrop** (e.g., VōSoL Otic Solution, 4 gtt qid) usually is an effective agent.
   b. An ear wick (commercially available or fashioned from a 2-in. segment of 0.5-in. gauze) gently inserted into the external canal will assist in the delivery of drops, especially when the canal is swollen closed.
   c. **Debridement** of the accumulated drainage by suction or with small cotton whisps on a wire applicator will reduce the bacterial load and improve the rapidity of response.

4. **Disposition.** The patient should be evaluated in 1 week to assure resolution of the process.

B. **Malignant otitis externa** is a fulminant infection (cellulitis) involving the ear canal, external ear, and surrounding tissue. It occurs in immunocompromised hosts, especially those with poorly controlled diabetes mellitus, immunodeficiency disorders, or on chemotherapy. The most common organism causing malignant otitis externa is *Pseudomonas aeruginosa.*

1. **Clinical features.** These patients usually present with deep-seated ear pain. In addition, many of the features of otitis externa (e.g., swelling and tenderness of the ear canal) are present. The diagnostic hallmark of malignant otitis externa is the presence of granulation tissue located at the bony-cartilaginous junction approximately one-third to one-half of the distance from the meatus to the eardrum. This granulation tissue houses the infection and spreads by an invasive process into the mastoid, deep neck spaces, and parotid gland and may cause an osteomyelitis of the base of the skull. Facial nerve and other cranial nerve palsies are not infrequent. Death may ensue from meningitis or a brain abscess.
   Poor prognostic signs in malignant otitis externa include (1) cranial nerve palsies (most commonly, a facial nerve palsy), (2) sensorineural hearing loss, (3) persistent pain, and (4) meningitis.

2. On immediate **evaluation** and subsequent follow-up, mastoid films should be obtained to delineate opacification or bone destruction. Later a bone scan may be done; increased activity in the mastoid or base of the skull, as well as contralateral bony involvement, may be seen and defines the need for surgical intervention.

3. **Treatment.** High-dose antibiotic therapy, with carbenicillin and an aminoglycoside (e.g., gentamicin, tobramycin, amikacin) (see Table 28-2), should be started immediately. Antibiotic ear drops to topically reduce the bacterial load are also administered. Often the use of an ear wick is helpful to facilitate drop delivery. Daily debridement of granulation tissue is necessary. If mastoid, parotid, or neck involvement is present, extensive surgical debridement is necessary.

4. **Disposition.** Hospitalization and otolaryngologic consultation are mandatory.

C. **Acute otitis media** (see Chap. 36) is a common illness in childhood but less common in adults. The most common organisms in otitis media with effusion are *Streptococcus pneumoniae* and *Haemophilus influenzae. H. Influenzae,* although less common in the adult population, must still be considered. The pathogenesis is felt to involve eustachian tube dysfunction, as suggested by the increased risk in childhood and in certain craniofacial anomalies.

1. **Clinical features.** The patient presents with ear pain that may be intense, and decreased auditory acuity is often noted. Fever may be present, particularly in children. Blood and purulent material draining from the middle ear, which represents spontaneous drainage of the otitis media, may also be noted.
2. The **diagnosis** rests with the evaluation of the drumhead. The normal drum is translucent with (1) characteristic landmarks seen on and through it, (2) a normal cone of reflected light (the light reflex), and (3) good mobility on pneumotoscopy. In early otitis media, there is a distortion of the normal landmarks, with intense hyperemia around the annulus of the eardrum coursing down the long process of the malleus. Later in the course, the eardrum becomes thick and opaque with a decrease in the mobility and a scattering of the normal cone of reflected light. Untreated, the classic description of otitis media may follow, i.e., a hot, bulging, exudative drum. The natural history leads to a perforated tympanic membrane with drainage if intervention is not prompt.
3. **Treatment**
   a. **Antibiotic therapy** should be instituted immediately. The drug of choice is ampicillin or amoxicillin (see Table 28-2). Other useful antibiotics include trimethoprim-sulfamethoxazole, erythromycin, and the cephalosporins. Amoxicillin plus potassium clavulanate (Augmentin) may be useful in cases not responding to initial antibiotic therapy.
   b. **Relief of pain** is usually accomplished with oral analgesics or eardrops or both that include a topical anesthetic (e.g., Auralgan, 3–4 gtt q3h prn).
   c. **Myringotomy** has not been shown to substantially reduce the morbidity of acute otitis media but is excellent for obtaining a culture.
4. The patient should be evaluated in 10 days to 2 weeks by an otolaryngologist or primary care physician to assure that the otitis media has resolved. If fever or severe symptoms do not resolve in 48 hours, earlier evaluation is necessary.
D. **Bullous myringitis.** The patient presents with very severe ear pain. Physical examination reveals small vesicles on the eardrum that may or may not be accompanied by an attendant acute otitis media. Although this process has been attributed to *Mycoplasma pneumoniae* or viruses, cultures have shown a distribution of organisms similar to that in acute otitis media. An elective opening of the vesicles with a myringotomy knife significantly reduces the pain. It is important to rule out herpes zoster oticus, in which complications including facial paralysis are common (Ramsay Hunt syndrome). Antibiotic treatment is as in acute otitis media (see **C.3.a**).
E. **Furuncle of the external canal.** Since the external auditory canal contains skin and normal skin appendages, including sweat glands, eccrine glands, and hair follicles, a furuncle can develop. This condition may be confused with otitis externa because of the similarity of the pain. Visualization of the ear canal reveals a single area of swelling with a pinpoint area of increased tenderness, in contrast to otitis externa, in which there is diffuse tenderness and swelling. **Treatment** consists of incision and drainage of the furuncle and placement of a small gauze wick. A culture is obtained at the time of incision and drainage, and the patient is immediately placed on an antibiotic whose spectrum includes *S. aureus* (see Table 28-2). If a cellulitis rather than an abscess is present, an antibiotic and warm compresses may resolve the problem without the need for incision and drainage. The patient should be followed up by an otolaryngologist in 2 days.
F. **Perichondritis** is an infection involving the perichondrium of the delicately sculptured cartilage of the external ear. It is a very serious complication of ear trauma, otitis externa, furuncle of the ear canal, or chronic mastoiditis. If the etiology is trauma or a furuncle, *S. aureus* must be considered; however, if otitis externa or chronic mastoiditis is the source, gram-negative organisms are commonly involved. The patient presents with severe pain and a swollen, erythematous pinna. Sepsis or necrosis of the cartilage may ensue. High-dose parenteral antibiotics should be instituted immediately. If prompt resolution of the inflammatory process does not occur during the next 24 hours, incision and drainage must be performed to preserve the cartilage of the external ear.
II. **Foreign bodies of the external ear canal** are most common in children. Foreign bodies can be inert material, vegetable matter, or insects.
   A. If the foreign body is plastic or another **inert material,** it is usually not an extreme emergency and, if desired, can be handled in a delayed setting by an otologist.
   B. **Vegetable matter,** on the other hand, can lead to otitis externa and difficulty in delayed extraction; thus, an attempt at emergent removal should be made. Removal of the foreign body is accomplished with the use of a Hartman's forceps, dull Buck's

Table 28-2. Common otolaryngologic infections and their therapy

Infection	Common organisms[a]	Treatment (adult dosage)
Otitis externa		
Acute otitis externa	Pseudomonas, other gram negative organisms	Topical antibiotic drops (e.g., Cortisporin Otic Solution or Suspension) or topical acidic drops (e.g., VōSoL HC Otic Solution)
Fungal otitis externa	Aspergillus	Acidic drops (e.g., VōSoL Otic Solution) or gentian violet
Malignant otitis externa	Pseudomonas aeruginosa	Topical drops, plus Curettage, plus Carbenicillin, 200–500 mg/kg/day IV q6h, or ticarcillin, 200–300 mg/kg/day IV q4h, plus Gentamicin, 3–5 mg/kg/day IV q8h, or tobramycin, 3–5 mg/kg/day IV q8h, or amikacin, 15 mg/kg/day IV q8h,
Acute otitis media	Streptococcus pneumoniae, Haemophilus influenzae	Amoxicillin, 250 mg PO tid[b] or trimethoprim-sulfamethoxazole, 2 tablets PO q12h, or erythromycin, 250 mg PO qid, or cephalosporin, 250 mg PO qid
Furuncle of external canal	Staphylococcus aureus	Incision and drainage, plus Dicloxacillin, 250 mg PO qid[b], or erythromycin, 250 mg PO qid, or cephalosporin, 250 mg PO qid
Acute sinusitis	S. pneumoniae, H. influenzae, S. aureus anaerobes	Amoxicillin, 250 mg PO tid[b,c] or trimethoprim-sulfamethoxazole, 2 tablets PO q12h, or tetracycline, 250 mg PO qid, or erythromycin, 250 mg PO qid, or cephalosporin, 250 mg PO qid[c], plus Topical nasal decongestant spray q4h

Nasal cellulitis	*S. aureus*	Dicloxacillin, 500 mg PO q6h[b,c], *or* erythromycin, 500 mg PO q6h, *or* cephalosporin, 500 mg PO q6h[c]
Periorbital cellulitis or abscess	*S. aureus, H. influenzae, S. Pneumoniae, Streptococcus pyogenes*	Methicillin, 50 mg/kg/day IV q6h, *plus* Chloramphenicol, 50 mg/kg/day IV q6h
Tonsillitis or pharyngitis	Viruses	Local care
	Streptococcus pyogenes	Penicillin, 250 mg PO qid[b,c], *or* erythromycin, 250 mg PO qid
	Mycoplasma pneumoniae	Erythromycin, 250 mg PO qid, *or* tetracycline, 250 mg PO qid, only if documented, protracted illness
	Neisseria gonorrhoeae	Ceftriaxone, 250 mg IM[b], *or* procaine penicillin G, 4.8 million units IM (plus probenecid, 1 gm PO), *or* trimethoprim-sulfamethoxazole, 9 tablets daily for 5 days
Deep space infections	Streptococci, anaerobes, *S. aureus*	Aqueous penicillin G, 2–4 million units IV q4h, *plus* Cephalosporin, 1–2 gm IV q4–6h, *or* clindamycin, 300–600 mg IV q6h
Laryngitis	Viral	Local care
Epiglottitis	*H. influenzae, S. pneumoniae, S. aureus*	Ampicillin, 50 mg/kg/day IV q6h, *plus* Chloramphenicol, 50 mg/kg/day IV q6h

[a] Organisms commonly producing infection. Other organisms, however, may be involved.
[b] Drug of choice
[c] More serious infection requires a larger dose of an IV preparation.

curette, or another such device. Some foreign bodies can be aspirated with a small Frazier sucker. Extreme care must be taken so that the foreign body is not pushed further into the ear canal or through the eardrum. If the foreign body is not easily removed (particularly in children), it is usually best to refer the patient to an otologist the following day for removal.

    C. A live **insect** in the external ear canal is a true emergency in that the noises from the insect are greatly exaggerated because of the proximity to the eardrum. Initial management is to kill the insect, which can be accomplished by drowning the insect with mineral oil, alcohol, eardrops, or other available fluids. It is important to note that insecticides should not be used in that they may cause a severe otitis externa. After the insect is dead, removal (see **B**) may be accomplished immediately or electively the following day.

III. Barotrauma

    A. Clinical features. Rapid changes in atmospheric pressure, most commonly seen in air flight or scuba diving, can cause severe pain in the ear. Eustachian tube dysfunction prevents equilibration of the middle ear pressure with the ambient pressure, with resultant stretching of the tympanic membrane. Often a transudate fills the middle ear cleft, and occasionally there is a hemotympanum. Hearing loss may be present.

    B. Treatment includes the use of both oral and topical decongestants. An antihistamine with or without a decongestant should be given, and phenylephrine (Neo-Synephrine) or a similar nose spray may help open the eustachian tube. In severe or persistent cases, myringotomy will reequilibrate the middle ear pressure with the ambient pressure and allow for resolution of the transudate and evacuation of any hematoma.

    C. Disposition. Since damage to the ossicular chain can occur (although rare), patients should be referred to an otologist the next day for audiometry (unless vertigo or sensorineural hearing loss is detected, for which immediate consultation is required).

IV. Sudden hearing loss.
Few events are more frightening to a patient than sudden loss of hearing. Prompt attention to the care of these patients may prevent permanent loss of hearing.

    A. Etiologies. Sudden hearing loss can occur secondary to ear canal disorders (e.g., cerumen impaction, foreign body, tympanic membrane perforation), middle ear disorders (e.g., acute otitis media, serous otitis media), inner ear disease (e.g., perilymphatic fistula), eighth nerve involvement, cerebrovascular accident, autoimmune disorders, tumor, and conversion reaction. The most common cause of acute hearing loss apart from cerumen impaction is trauma to the eardrum, usually from attempts at removing cerumen. Perilymphatic fistula should be suspected in any hearing loss occurring in relation to exercise, straining with heavy lifting, defecation, changes in ambient pressure (barotrauma), or head trauma, especially if vertigo or tinnitus is associated.

    B. Evaluation. If a patient presents to the emergency department with a sudden onset of hearing loss, the immediate concern is to establish the site of the lesion.

        1. Examination of the ear canal may reveal a wax impaction, foreign body, otitis media, or serous otitis media, all of which can be associated with a sudden onset of hearing loss.

        2. If the ear canal and eardrum are completely normal, a **sensorineural loss** must be suspected.

            a. Use of the **tuning fork tests** (with a 512-Hz tuning fork) will help establish the nature of the hearing loss.

                (1) The **Rinne test** compares air conduction (tested by holding the tuning fork just lateral to the pinna) with bone conduction (tested by placing the end of the tuning fork on the mastoid tip). The normal ear or ear with a sensorineural hearing loss will detect air conduction as being greater (i.e., louder) than bone conduction. On the other hand, in a significant conductive hearing loss, bone conduction will be greater than air conduction.

                (2) In the **Weber test,** the tuning fork is placed at the midline either on the glabella or on the central maxillary incisors, and the sound vibration is conducted through the bones of the skull. The sound normally is equal at both ears. If there is a sensorineural loss, the sound will be greater at the better ear. In contrast, a conductive loss demonstrates increased loudness at the affected ear.

b. If an acute sensorineural hearing loss is suspected, the patient should receive immediate **otologic evaluation,** including complete audiology, vestibular testing, and radiographs (most often including computed tomography [CT]).

c. A complete **neurologic evaluation** is necessary to assess for other possibly associated cranial or peripheral nerve disorders.

C. Management

1. **Cerumen impaction** should be gently removed by curettage with a Buck's curette or wire loop under direct vision. If there is no tympanic membrane perforation, irrigation with tepid water may allow effective cleaning. Alternatively, the patient may be prescribed eardrops to soften and dissolve the cerumen (e.g., carbamide peroxide [Debrox], hydrogen peroxide).

2. An **acute sensorineural hearing loss** must be treated urgently. The patient should be admitted to the hospital and placed at bed rest. Vasodilators and carbogen help dilate the cerebral vessels. Close otologic follow-up is necessary.

3. Surgical exploration to repair **perilymphatic leakage** could prevent progressive hearing loss and often allows recovery of hearing.

4. Treatment of other causes of hearing loss is specific for the underlying etiology.

Nasal Disorders

I. Epistaxis

A. Etiologies. Since the anterior septum is a highly vascularized area and prone to trauma, 95% of all nosebleeds occur in this area. Digital trauma accounts for most nosebleeds, but contributing factors include dryness of the inspired air, turbulence created by nasal septal deflections, and vestibulitis (i.e., infection of the nasal vestibule). Although epistaxis is often associated with hypertension, hypertension usually is not causal. Coagulation disorders also do not cause epistaxis but contribute to the difficulty in stopping the bleeding.

B. Evaluation. Vital signs, including orthostatic blood pressures, help evaluate the extent of blood loss. Evaluation of the nose should be done with a head light and nasal speculum. Anterior rhinoscopy is essential in locating the bleeding point. A hematocrit is useful, although equilibration does not take place for several hours. Unless there is a history of a bleeding disorder, coagulation studies are rarely beneficial.

C. Treatment

1. **Initial measures.** The most efficient way of stopping the bleeding is by application of pressure, which allows the normal clotting mechanism to effect hemostasis. The patient should blow his or her nose to remove mucus and clots. The fleshy portion of the anterior nose is then tightly pinched for 10–15 minutes; this procedure usually will terminate the bleeding. Evaluation of the nose by anterior rhinoscopy should then follow. Anterior rhinoscopy requires the use of a nasal speculum, a head light, and a suction device; the last enables the removal of blood and mucus to identify the bleeding site. Cocaine or lidocaine with epinephrine or phenylephrine may be placed on cotton pledgets and stacked in a layered fashion within the involved nasal passage from inferiorly to superiorly to effect anesthesia of the nasal mucosa and, in most cases, to diminish the bleeding.

2. **Electrocautery or chemical cautery** with trichloroacetic acid or silver nitrate may then be used to terminate the bleeding. It is important to cauterize only one side of the septum at a time because deep cautery of both sides can lead to septal perforation. Since the blood supply to the septum comes from the adjacent septum rather than perforators, cautery is carried out in a circumferential fashion ending with the bleeding point. Care must be exercised when using electrical or chemial cautery to avoid contact with the vestibular skin and lip to prevent burning and subsequent scarring.

3. **Nasal packing** (see Chap. 38) is indicated when the previously mentioned methods have failed or when a bleeding site is not seen. An anterior pack with absorbable oxycellulose, petroleum jelly gauze, or salt pork (which contains coagulation factors) is placed first. If the anterior pack fails to control the bleeding, it is removed, and a posterior pack is placed and followed by placement of another anterior pack; posterior packing always requires associated anterior packing.

4. **Artery ligation.** Unfortunately, even the combination of both anterior and pos-

terior packing occasionally fails to control the bleeding. When this treatment fails, internal maxillary artery ligation and anterior ethmoid artery ligation are indicated. These surgical procedures carry with them a certain amount of morbidity, but in the continuously bleeding patient often prove to be lifesaving.

5. **Ancillary measures**
   a. Often **hypertension,** which may be marked, accompanies epistaxis. Initial management includes sedation (e.g., with diazepam, 5–10 mg PO) and treatment of the nosebleed. Persistent hypertension following these measures may require specific antihypertensive therapy (see Chap. 6).
   b. An **antibiotic** (e.g., ampicillin or erythromycin, 250 mg q6h) should be administered to reduce the incidence of sinusitis.

D. **Disposition.** Patients requiring both anterior and posterior nasal packing should be admitted to an intensive care unit for close monitoring of the vital signs, arterial blood gases (ABGs), and electrocardiogram (ECG) because of the risk of reflex hypoxia and arrhythmias. Otherwise, those with controlled bleeding can be discharged, unless there are complicating factors (e.g., extensive blood loss), and should be followed up in a few days for removal of the packing. Recurrent epistaxis should always be evaluated by an otolaryngologist to rule out nasal, sinus, or nasopharyngeal tumors.

II. **Nasal cellulitis.** Cellulitis of the vestibule or anterior tip of the nose may be seen following trauma or a mild infection of a sebaceous gland of the skin of the nose. This infection places the patient at risk for cavernous sinus thrombosis since the veins of the midface have direct connection to the cavernous sinus. Aggressive **treatment** with an oral antibiotic with antistaphylococcal coverage (see Table 28-2) is acceptable early in the course; but if the patient appears toxic or if the cellulitis is extensive, hospital admission and administration of parenteral antibiotics are indicated.

III. **Rhinitis.** Although there are a number of varieties of rhinitis, they usually present with nasal airway obstruction and occasionally drainage.

A. **Allergic rhinitis** is heralded by a clear drainage and a high eosinophil count in the nasal smear. The nasal mucosa is boggy and often bluish. Allergic rhinitis is often well treated with an oral decongestant, antihistamine, topical nasal steroid, and/or cromolyn sodium. Allergy testing and desensitization is a reasonable alternative in the more symptomatic patient.

B. **Infectious rhinitis** is heralded by mucopus in the nose with a large number of polymorphonuclear leukocytes in the nasal smear. This condition may eventually lead to sinusitis. Infectious rhinitis may be treated with the use of salt water douches to help clear the bacteria-ladened mucus, but if this treatment is not successful within 2–3 days, an antibiotic (e.g., amoxicillin, 250 mg tid, or trimethoprim-sulfamethoxazole [TMP-SMZ], 160 mg TMP/800 mg SMZ q12h) should be used.

C. **Rhinitis medicamentosa** results from abuse of readily available over-the-counter topical nasal decongestants. This disease process has its origin in the rebound phenomenon, such that the chronic abuser gets only momentary relief of nasal congestion from the use of topical decongestants. The **treatment** of rhinitis medicamentosa is to eliminate the use of such preparations. The use of oral decongestants may afford some relief. Salt water nasal douches and occasionally the use of topical nasal steroids or cromolyn sodium may help, especially if the original problem was an allergic condition.

IV. **Nasal foreign bodies** are most often seen in children.

A. **Clinical features.** When acute, the history is usually that of a witnessed insertion of a foreign body or continual attempts at sneezing or blowing the nose. Most patients, however, present with a chronic unilateral nasal discharge. Often the foreign body will be dislodged spontaneously from the nose, but it may become firmly lodged.

B. **Treatment.** The foreign body may be observed on anterior rhinoscopy and removed with a bayonet or Hartmann's forceps. The use of topical anesthesia with either cocaine or 4% lidocaine with epinephrine is helpful in both decreasing pain and reducing nasal mucosal swelling. Rarely, general anesthesia will be required in the uncooperative patient or if the foreign body is too firmly positioned.

V. **Sinusitis.** Acute sinusitis is a very painful and potentially dangerous infection of one or more sinuses.

A. **Etiologic agents.** Bacteria frequently implicated in sinusitis include S. pneumoniae, H. influenzae, or S. aureus. An isolated sphenoid opacification is most likely due to a fungal infection, commonly aspergillosis. In the immunocompromised host or in the person with brittle, uncontrolled diabetes mellitus, mucormycosis must be considered.

B. Clinical features. The presentation is usually that of a headache or facial pain. Patients with maxillary sinusitis often present with tooth pain or midface pain, but they may have pain radiating into the frontal, temporal, or parietal areas. Patients with ethmoid sinusitis often present with pain behind the eye(s) or in the frontal area; and those with frontal sinusitis most commonly have frontal pain, but occipital pain may also be present. Patients with sphenoid sinusitis classically present with a vertex headache. The headache associated with sinusitis is exacerbated by bending over or lying down. Fever and tenderness over the involved sinus are common. It is not infrequent to see mucopus within the nasal vestibule; but with complete obstruction at the ostium, sinus drainage is prevented and the nasal passage is dry.

C. Evaluation

1. **Radiography.** Although transillumination is useful in confirming maxillary or frontal sinusitis, the diagnosis of sinusitis is established by radiography. The presence of opacification or an air-fluid level indicates sinusitis. The radiodensity of the normal frontal sinuses is similar to that of the orbit; if the density of the sinus is greater, the sinus is likely opacified. The sphenoid sinus is the most commonly misinterpreted sinus because the overlying soft tissues in each of the views can lead to the assumption that it is poorly developed but well aerated. It is important to note that the sphenoid sinus has a midline or near-midline septum; thus, an acute unilateral infectious process may not be apparent except on the submental vertex view. If there is further concern regarding the diagnosis, especially in evaluating the acute onset of a severe headache, high-resolution CT of the paranasal sinuses will completely elucidate these structures. Ultrasound is also useful in evaluating chronic infection of the maxillary sinus because of its ability to differentiate between mucoperiosteal thickening and fluid.

2. **Cultures.** Nasal cultures are of little use because the normal nasal flora consists of many microorganisms; thus, a mixed growth is not helpful. However, a relatively pure growth from a nasal culture may establish the causative organism. Nasoantral puncture or sinus washings should be reserved for the toxic patient.

D. Treatment of acute sinusitis requires antibiotic therapy and the use of a topical nasal decongestant with or without an oral decongestant-antihistamine preparation.

1. **Antibiotic therapy** (see Table 28-2). Because of the incidence of *H. influenzae*, the drug of choice in acute sinusitis in most instances is amoxicillin. The tetracyclines and sulfonamides are also quite effective because of good penetrance into the paranasal sinuses. A cephalosporin may also be used. Parenteral antibiotics are necessary only if the patient is toxic or if a complication of sinusitis is present (see **E**). Antibiotic therapy is best carried out for 3 weeks to assure resolution.

2. A **nasal decongestant** is important. Phenylephrine 1% spray or another topical decongestant is very helpful.

3. A **narcotic analgesic** may be required for pain control.

4. **Dental care.** If maxillary sinusitis results from a periapical abscess involving a maxillary tooth, treatment involves extraction of the involved tooth and antibiotic therapy. Penicillin is the drug of choice in this case.

5. **Sinus wash.** In resistant cases of sinusitis or in the more toxic patient, sinus wash is helpful, especially in maxillary sinusitis. Cultures may be obtained, and the bulk of the entrapped pus removed.

6. **Surgical drainage.** Frontal and sphenoid sinus infections are difficult to treat and not infrequently require trephination. Surgical drainage is also required if normal therapy does not control the infection or if certain complications result.

E. Complications. Infection of the paranasal sinuses, by virtue of the anatomic proximity to other vital structures, carries the risk of major complications.

1. **Periorbital and orbital cellulitis** most often results from sinusitis.

   a. **Clinical features.** Lid edema, swelling of the conjunctivae, and facial swelling are early signs. If the retroorbital area is also involved, the eye is proptotic and often restricted in its range of motion. If the origin is the frontal sinus, the eye is deviated inferiorly and laterally. Infection arising in the ethmoid sinus causes the eye to be deviated laterally, and maxillary sinus infection involving the floor of the orbit displaces the eye upward and out.

    b. Evaluation. Immediate attention should be directed to the evaluation of visual acuity and eye ground findings by funduscopic examination or retinoscopy (or both). Close checks, at least hourly, of the visual acuity are very important. High-resolution CT of the orbit and paranasal sinuses is indicated to establish the presence or absence of a retroorbital abscess.

    c. Treatment. Administration of parenteral antibiotics (e.g., chloramphenicol and methicillin) (see Table 28-2) is required.

  2. Since **retroorbital abscess** can proceed to acute blindness, immediate incision and drainage are indicated. When draining the abscess, drainage of the involved sinus is also necessary. Parenteral antibiotics (e.g., chloramphenicol and methicillin) are required.

  3. Frontal sinusitis may also present with **Pott's puffy tumor,** which is an anterior subperiosteal abscess giving a unicorn appearance. This process can proceed posteriorly through the posterior table of the frontal sinus, resulting in a subdural or epidural abscess. Treatment involves surgical drainage and antibiotic administration.

  4. Other **complications** include meningitis, brain abscesses, frontal bone osteomyelitis, and cavernous sinus thrombosis.

F. Disposition. In a routine case of sinusitis, follow-up by an otolaryngologist or primary care physician is necessary within 3 weeks. If the patient is toxic or if a complication exists, immediate hospitalization for parenteral antibiotics and an otolaryngology consultation are necessary.

Pharyngeal and Laryngeal Disorders

I. Hoarseness. Acute hoarseness is most commonly associated with vocal abuse and is of minor importance unless associated with blunt or penetrating neck trauma. Usually voice rest and humidification will alleviate this problem. If hoarseness persists over a course of two or more weeks, further evaluation by an otolaryngologist is required. Indirect laryngoscopy (using a head light and a laryngeal mirror) or fiberoptic endoscopy with visualization of the larynx will establish the diagnosis. The **differential diagnosis** includes acute onset of true vocal cord paralysis, a true vocal cord polyp, vocal nodules, acute or chronic laryngitis, laryngeal papillomas, tumors of the larynx (including epidermoid carcinoma), and other more exotic diseases of the larynx, such as sarcoidosis, pemphigus, and rheumatoid arthritis of the arytenoid. Treatment depends on the specific underlying etiology.

II. Tonsillopharyngitis is discussed in Chap. 12.

III. Epiglottitis (see Chap. 36). Adult epiglottitis is a supraglottitis caused by *H. influenzae, S. aureus,* or *S. pneumoniae.* It is a potentially life-threatening disease because of airway compromise.

  A. Presentation. There is usually a rapid onset of fever, malaise, and a sore throat with dysphagia and odynophagia. Stridor (a harsh inspiratory sound) may or may not be present. The airway may become precipitously compromised.

  B. The **diagnosis** should be suspected in patients with a sore throat out of proportion to the pharyngeal findings. It is established by a lateral soft-tissue film or laryngoscopy.

  C. Treatment involves administration of parenteral antibiotics (see Table 28-2) and airway management. Chloramphenicol should be administered along with ampicillin until blood culture reports are obtained. Airway compromise demands endotracheal intubation or a tracheostomy. Adults without airway compromise may be managed with airway precautions in an intensive care setting. All children with epiglottitis, however, require immediate endotracheal intubation or a tracheostomy.

IV. Peritonsillar abscess is a potentially life-threatening infection that follows untreated or inadequately treated tonsillitis. If left untreated, a peritonsillar abscess may dissect into adjacent deep neck spaces, including the submandibular, parapharyngeal, retropharyngeal, and prevertebral spaces.

  A. Clinical features. Usually the patient presents with a sore throat that has persisted for more than 3 days. Associated trismus, dysphagia, fever, and deep pain are often seen. Palpation of the affected tonsil may reveal fluctuance. On inspection of the oral cavity, swelling of the space behind the involved tonsil, with displacement of the tonsil and soft palate toward the midline, is noted. In addition, the uvula is often displaced toward the contralateral side. Occasionally, there is redness and swelling in the superior portion of the anterior tonsillar pillar.

B. **Evaluation.** If the diagnosis is in doubt, a large-bore needle attached to a 10-ml syringe may be advanced into the anterior tonsillar pillar near the superior pole of the tonsil using topical anesthesia (4% lidocaine). If aspiration yields pus, the diagnosis is established. If no pus is removed, a peritonsillar cellulitis is considered to be present.

C. **Management**
   1. If a **peritonsillar abscess** is either evident on clinical examination or documented by aspiration, **incision and drainage** are necessary.
      a. **Uncomplicated abscess.** If the abscess appears to be small and uncomplicated, the procedure can be carried out under local anesthesia (obtained by injecting the anterior tonsillar pillar with 1% lidocaine). With the mouth open, an incision is made vertically along the anterior tonsil pillar. A long clamp is then used to spread the tissue and enter the peritonsillar space and the abscess cavity. A culture is obtained, and the abscess cavity is thoroughly suctioned using a tonsil sucker. Since most of these infections involve mixed oral flora, penicillin (500 mg q6h) is the drug of choice. The patient should be seen the next day by an otolaryngologist.
      b. For **severe or complicated peritonsillar abscesses,** patients must be hospitalized for parenteral antibiotic therapy. Incision and drainage may then be carried out under general anesthesia.
   2. If the diagnosis is that of a **peritonsillar cellulitis** and the patient is able to swallow well, he or she may be placed on pencillin, 500 mg PO q6h, and told to gargle with warm saline. If the patient is unable to swallow, hospitalization for hydration and observation is indicated. Careful evaluation over the next few days for the presence of an abscess is important.

V. **Deep space infections of the neck** (see Chap. 29). Infections of the deep spaces of the neck in adults usually are traumatic or dental in origin, in contrast to children, in whom suppuration of lymph nodes usually is the source. A periapical abscess can dissect into the submental or submandibular space and into adjacent tissue planes. Airway compromise and mediastinitis may result, especially when the retropharyngeal or prevertebral space is involved.

A. **Clinical features.** Swelling and tenderness of the neck overlying the space is present. Occasionally, fluctuance can be detected, and the patient usually has a fever and is toxic. Stridor may be present if there is airway compromise.

B. The **diagnosis** can be made by inspection and palpation of the neck. Lateral soft-tissue x-rays, xeroradiograms, and CT also aid in establishing the diagnosis.

C. **Management.** Hospitalization is mandatory. A secure airway must be maintained, which may require endotracheal intubation or tracheostomy. Incision and drainage of the abscess under general anesthesia and parenteral antibiotic therapy (see Table 28-2) with penicillin, 2–4 million units IV q4h, and a cephalosporin (e.g., cefoxitin, 1–2 gm IV q6h) are indicated.

Foreign Substance Inhalation and Ingestion

I. **Inhaled foreign bodies** are usually those which have been placed in the mouth and, on excitement, coughing, or quick inspiration, are sucked into the airway. The upper airway often catches the foreign body, and it may become lodged at the tonsil, base of the tongue, vallecula epiglottica, or pyriform sinus; or the foreign body may course into the larynx or tracheobronchial tree. Upper airway obstruction (see **Upper Airway Obstruction**) may result.

A. **Clinical features.** The patient may complain of a foreign body sensation in the throat or neck. If hoarseness is present, it is indicative of laryngeal trauma or the presence of the foreign body in the glottic area. With foreign body aspiration there usually is marked or persistent coughing; hemoptysis or wheezing may be noted as well. Signs of upper airway obstruction may be present.

B. **Evaluation** of suspected foreign body aspiration involves a physical examination, radiologic investigation, and/or endoscopy. The approach will depend on the clinical circumstances and status of the patient.
   1. **Physical examination.** A detailed examination of the oropharynx and pharynx may reveal the foreign body lodged in the base of the tongue or tonsil. Ausculta-

tion of the chest may reveal wheezes, fluttering sounds, or absence of breath sounds, each indicating the presence of a foreign body.

2. The **chest radiograph** may show atelectasis, distal pneumonia, or distal hyperaeration. Hyperaeration is caused by the foreign body acting as a ball valve, allowing air to enter but not to escape.

3. An **indirect mirror examination** or **fiberoptic laryngoscopy** allows for visualization of the hypopharynx or larynx as possible sites of foreign body lodgment.

C. **Treatment.** Upper airway obstruction is managed as described under **Upper Airway Obstruction** (see also Chap. 2). Some pharyngeal and hypopharyngeal foreign bodies can be removed under a mirror examination using a special forceps, but often they are more safely removed at the time of laryngoscopy. Immediate rigid bronchoscopy is necessary to remove a confirmed bronchial or tracheal foreign body. If there is a history of foreign body inhalation without any accompanying signs, endoscopy is indicated to determine the presence or absence of a foreign body.

II. **Ingested foreign bodies** (see Chaps. 10 and 18)

A. **Inanimate and vegetable matter.** Such foreign bodies of the esophagus are most commonly found in small children and the geriatric population. Children not infrequently swallow a variety of inanimate objects. In contrast, foreign bodies in the geriatric population are usually poorly masticated pieces of food. Objects too large to pass through the esophagus usually will lodge at the cricopharyngeus, the entrance into the thoracic esophagus, or at the lower esophageal sphincter.

1. The **diagnosis** of esophageal obstruction is usually apparent from the presentation. The patient complains of a foreign body sensation and is unable to handle secretions, expectorating large amounts of saliva. If the foreign body is radiopaque, it usually can be visualized on a chest x-ray or on anteroposterior (AP) and lateral neck films. If the foreign body is plastic or vegetable matter, however, it may not be seen. If there is some question of a nonradiopaque foreign body, a barium swallow will establish the diagnosis.

2. **Treatment**

   a. **Removal of foreign bodies** of the esophagus may be accomplished by rigid **esophagoscopy** in an operating room setting. This procedure allows protection of the airway and the control of any sharp edges so as to prevent laceration or rupture of the esophagus. Flexible esophagoscopy has been used to remove esophageal foreign bodies but is unsatisfactory because of the inability to protect the airway and the lack of satisfactory foreign body forceps. The practice of using a Foley catheter (with the balloon inflated) to pull a foreign body from the esophagus is hazardous because esophageal rupture or loss of the foreign body into the introitus of the larynx can occur; this practice is to be condemned.

   b. **Glucagon.** By causing relaxation of the smooth muscle of the esophagus, this drug may enable passage of an obstructed foreign body. The dosage is 1 mg IV, repeated in a dose of 2 mg in 20 minutes if there is no response to the initial injection [6].

   c. Administration of proteolytic enzymes (e.g., papain) PO to dissolve the foreign body may lead to erosion of the esophageal mucosa and is to be avoided.

B. **Fish bones** commonly lodge in the upper digestive tract. A foreign body sensation in the upper aerodigestive tract is noted by the patient. Because of their very tiny and delicate nature, fish bones are often difficult to visualize on routine examination. Apart from the Buffalo fish, these bones are radiolucent and do not show up on soft-tissue films.

1. **Suspected site of lodgment proximal to the larynx.** Inspection of the tonsillar fossa, the base of the tongue, the piriform sinus, and the supraglottic larynx is necessary to assure the presence or absence of a fish bone. If found, the bone is removed. However, if detailed indirect examination does not reveal the foreign body and there is no evidence of fever, the patient may be discharged to be followed up by an otolaryngologist in 3 days. No antibiotics should be administered. Occasionally, because of a small laceration or abrasion of the mucosa, the foreign body sensation will remain for a short time. However, if the sensation remains for a period of 3 days, direct laryngoscopy must be performed to rule out the presence of a foreign body.

2. **Esophageal fish bones.** The diagnosis generally can be established with a barium swallow, including the use of barium-soaked cotton pledgets that are swallowed. Since a retained esophageal fish bone may lead to esophageal breakdown, endoscopic removal with rigid esophagoscopy is necessary.

C. Small **disk batteries** used in radios, hearing aids, or calculators can become lodged in the esophagus, usually in the upper cervical esophagus in a small child. Since these batteries contain a potent base, they can cause severe burns. Radiologically, disk batteries are easily identified on both posteroanterior (PA) and lateral views, both of which should be obtained to locate the battery. For batteries lodged in the esophagus, prompt removal with rigid esophagoscopy is essential, followed by close observation for potential ensuing mediastinitis. If these batteries pass into the stomach, they usually will pass through the gastrointestinal tract without complications. Thus, these patients can be discharged with arrangements for follow-up in a few days. Endoscopic or surgical removal, however, is indicated in symptomatic patients with peritoneal signs.

III. **Caustic ingestion.** Because of increased public awareness and child-proof packaging, the ingestion of caustic substances (see Chap. 16) has become a less frequent phenomenon in the United States today, except in suicide attempts. The most commonly ingested caustic is bleach, which can cause inflammation and reaction in the upper aerodigestive tract. Lye and strong acids, on the other hand, are stronger caustic agents and usually produce more severe injuries. Superficial burns rarely result in scarring, but burns that extend into the submucosa or muscle often cause stricture formation. If the muscularis is completely dissolved, mediastinitis and other intrathoracic complications may ensue.

A. **Clinical features.** Sore throat and drooling usually are the first symptoms of caustic ingestion. As swelling progresses, airway compromise can follow. Fever, tachycardia, and hypotension are signs of mediastinitis.

B. **Evaluation.** The caustic ingestion must be evaluated in the acute state. Endoscopy is important to confirm the presence and evaluate the depth and extent of the mucosal burn. The use of a sodium diatrizoate (hypaque) swallow may be useful in mild cases. A chest radiograph is necessary to evaluate the mediastinum.

C. **Management.** If airway compromise is present, endotracheal intubation or a tracheostomy must be performed. The use of steroids and prophylactic antibiotics is controversial; however, neutralizing solutions are to be condemned. Hospitalization is necessary in all but the most minor ingestions.

Bibliography

1. Call, W. H. Control of epistaxis. *Surg. Clin. North Am.* 49:1235, 1969.
2. Cassisi, N. J., Biller, H. F., and Ogura, J. H. Changes in arterial oxygen tension and pulmonary mechanics with the use of posterior packing in epistaxis. *Laryngoscope* 81:1266, 1971.
3. Chandler, J. Malignant external otitis. *Laryngoscope* 78:1257, 1968.
4. Chitnis, J. G. Sinusitis. *Practitioner* 227:983, 1983.
5. Fisch, U. Management of sudden deafness. *Otolaryngol. Head Neck Surg.* 91:3, 1983.
6. Glauser J., et al. Intravenous glucagon in the management of esophageal food obstruction. *J.A.C.E.P.* 8:228, 1979.
7. Goodhill, V. Sudden deafness in round window rupture. *Laryngoscope* 81:1462, 1971.
8. Henele, W., et al. Epstein-Barr virus–specific diagnostic test in infection of mononucleosis. *Hum. Pathol.* 5:551, 1974.
9. Hill, I. R. The mechanism of facial injury. *Forensic Sci. Int.* 20:109, 1982.
10. Holt, G. Peritonsillar abscesses in children. *Laryngoscope* 91:1226, 1981.
11. Knight, A., et al. Long-term efficacy and safety of beclomethasone dipropionate aerosol and perennial rhinitis. *Allergy* 50:81, 1983.
12. Laird, N., and Wilson, W. R. Predicting recovery from idiopathic sudden hearing loss. *Am. J. Otolaryngol.* 4:161, 1983.
13. McCauley, R. L., et al. Frostbite injuries: A rational approach based on the pathophysiology. *J. Trauma* 23:143, 1983.
14. Morgan, R. F., et al. Management of naso-ethmoid-orbital fracture. *Am. Surg.* 48:447, 1982.
15. Skinner, D., et al. Management of the esophageal perforation. *Am. J. Surg.* 139:760, 1980.
16. Sofferman, R. A., et al. Retrospective analysis of surgically treated Le Fort fractures. *Arch. Otolaryngol.* 109(7):446, 1983.
17. Vegealy, G., et al. Current concepts in the management of otitis media with effusion. *Am. J. Otolaryngol.* 2:138, 1981.
18. von Sydow, C., Axelsson, A., and Jensen, C. Acute maxillary sinusitis—A comparison between 27 different treatment modes. *Rhinology* 20:223, 1982.

29

Oral Surgical Disorders

Allen Sclaroff

Odontogenic Pain

Odontogenic (dental) pain results from irritation of the neural tissue within the pulp cavity of the tooth; the resultant process can be either reversible or irreversible. Since the maxilla and mandible (along with adjacent facial structures) are innervated by the second and third divisions, respectively, of the fifth cranial nerve, dental pain may localize poorly. Thus, pain originating from dental pathology can be referred to other facial structures (e.g., pain in a lower molar can be referred to the ear), and vice versa (e.g., maxillary sinusitis can cause pain and sensitivity to adjacent teeth).

I. **Etiologies.** Common causes of odontogenic pain include (1) **infection** (which may cause necrosis of neural tissue and progress to tissue abscess formation); (2) **dental caries** involving the neural tissue; and (3) **trauma** to neural tissue (e.g., fractures involving the dentin or neurovascular tissue, traumatic injuries resulting from restoration of a tooth with a high-speed dental burr). Other causes include erupting teeth (particularly in young children), poorly fitting dentures, postextraction alveolar osteitis (dry socket), and foreign bodies lodged between the teeth.

II. **Evaluation**
   A. **General principles.** The entire oral cavity and adjacent structures must be carefully examined (usually starting at an area away from the site of pain to ensure a thorough examination), including the oral mucosa, tongue, palate, tonsils, posterior pharynx, ears, nose, sinuses, salivary glands, and regional lymph nodes.
   B. The **dental examination** should include the following: (1) **inspection** for evidence of trauma, inflammation, caries, foreign bodies, and malocclusion as well as tooth displacement, eruption, or impaction (a mirror is helpful for inspecting the posterior aspect of the teeth); (2) **palpation** for evidence of tenderness, fluctuance, and loose teeth; and (3) **percussion** of the teeth with a tongue depressor or mirror handle for evidence of tenderness, which often indicates underlying dental pathology.
   C. A **panoramic radiograph** is a good screening radiograph for dental problems. It can detect periapical, periodontal, intradental (caries), sinus, and intrabony pathology [12].

III. **Treatment** usually involves the prescription of an analgesic (e.g., acetaminophen with or without codeine) and an antibiotic (e.g., phenoxymethyl penicillin, 250–500 mg PO q6h for 7–10 days) if there is evidence of infection.

IV. **Disposition.** Most cases of odontogenic pain can be referred to a dentist within 1–3 days for definitive care [9]. However, emergent consultation is recommended for (1) dental infections with deep-space involvement (see **Odontogenic Infections**, sec. **II.C**) or (2) dental trauma (see **Dentoalveolar Trauma**) with exposure of the pulp or unstable teeth necessitating emergent stabilization.

Odontogenic Infections

I. **General principles.** Most odontogenic infections are caused by penicillin-sensitive streptococci or staphylococci [5–8]. Occasionally, however, a peptostreptococcus or *Bacteroides fragilis* is the predominant offending organism.
   A. **Clinical manifestations** include a toothache, tooth mobility, and percussion tenderness (these three factors generally are present when there is a periapical abscess), gum swelling and erythema, purulent drainage, facial swelling and tenderness, and fever. Anaerobic infections are characterized by a foul-smelling purulent drainage and the presence of necrotic tissue or gas in the tissue. A **panorex** is useful in identifying abscess formation.
   B. **Treatment** includes the following: (1) incision and drainage if an abscess is present; (2) treatment of the offending tooth by endodontic therapy or extraction, if neces-

sary; (3) administration of penicillin or, in suspected anaerobic infections, clindamycin in conjunction with penicillin; and (4) hydrogen peroxide irrigation of wounds [3–6, 10, 11].

C. **Disposition.** Many odontogenic infections can be managed on an outpatient basis, with follow-up by an oral surgeon in 48 hours. Deep-space infections (see sec. **II.C**), however, generally require hospitalization for parenteral antibiotic therapy, hydration, and airway management.

II. **Specific odontogenic infections** include gingival infections, periapical abscesses, and deep-space infections.

A. **Gingival infections**

1. A **gingival abscess** is a gum boil that occurs anywhere in the gingival tissue. It is the result of periodontal disease that allows a foreign body to enter a soft-tissue pocket adjacent to an involved tooth; the impacted foreign body then becomes walled off to form an abscess. **Management** consists of administration of penicillin, 500 mg PO q6h, and follow-up by a periodontist for local debridement and curettage.

2. A **pericoronal abscess** is a gingival abscess around an erupting wisdom tooth, usually secondary to impaction of food and debris around the developing tooth. Associated factors include trauma from the erupting wisdom tooth and biting of the soft tissue overlying the wisdom tooth. **Management** of pericoronitis involves irrigation of the pericoronal tissue with saline and administration of penicillin, 500 mg PO q6h. The patient should be referred to an oral surgeon in 2 or 3 days for extraction of the offending wisdom tooth.

3. **Trench mouth** (acute necrotizing ulcerative gingivitis) is a generalized gingival infection involving mixed bacteria of normal oral flora. It usually occurs in teenagers and young adults. Affected individuals tend to have a poor nutritional status.

a. **Clinical manifestations** include painful inflamed gingivae, a grey appearance to the interdental papillae as a result of sloughing and necrosis, a foul metallic odor to the breath, and fever.

b. **Treatment** consists of the combination of antibiotic therapy and thorough cleaning of the gums and teeth. Penicillin, 500 mg PO qid, is prescribed for 10 days. Viscous lidocaine (2 tbsp), to rinse the mouth for 5–10 minutes 4–5 times daily, can be used to anesthetize the gums prior to brushing the teeth and cleaning the mouth.

c. **Disposition.** The patient should be referred to a dentist in 2 or 3 days for teeth cleaning and debridement of necrotic gingival tissue.

B. A **periapical abscess** is a localized abscess within the mandible or maxilla at the root apex of the offending tooth.

1. **Clinical features** include tooth mobility and percussion tenderness. A panoramic radiograph reveals thickening of the periodontal ligament or a large radiolucent lesion apically.

2. **Treatment** of a periapical abscess includes saline mouth rinses and the administration of penicillin and an analgesic.

3. **Disposition.** Follow-up with an endodontist should be arranged for endodontic therapy (if the tooth is salvageable) or tooth extraction (if the tooth is not salvageable).

C. **Deep-space infections** (see Chap. 28).

1. **General principles.** If untreated, a periapical abscess can perforate the buccal or labial plates of the maxilla or mandible and lead to a deep-space infection. Once an abscess has perforated the confines of the maxilla or mandible, there are a multitude of spaces and potential spaces whereby rapid spread of infection can occur, causing potentially life-threatening problems. Due to the abundant vascularity of the maxillomandibular complex, there is the potential for bacterial spread to the brain, with resultant cavernous sinus thrombosis or formation of a brain abscess. Airway compromise can also occur, depending on the site of infection.

a. **Clinical features.** These patients usually present to the emergency department with tender facial swelling, fever, dehydration, and inability to open the mouth (trismus). Occasionally, airway compromise is present.

b. **Management.** Patients with deep-space infections generally require hospitalization for hydration and parenteral antibiotic therapy (e.g., aqueous penicillin, 2–4 million units IV q4h, and cefoxitin, 1–2 gm IV q6h) (see Table 28-2). Maintaining a patent airway is essential. Definitive therapy involves incision and drainage, usually performed in the operating suite, along with extraction of the involved tooth.

2. **Specific deep-space infections**

   a. A **canine fossa (space) abscess** presents as a swelling under the upper lip from the midline to the area of the canine root tips. It results from infection of one of the six anterior maxillary teeth. There may be infraorbital or periorbital edema. Due to the vascular supply to the midface, parenteral antibiotics are necessary. Surgical drainage, accomplished through an incision in the maxillary vestibule (with care being taken not to lacerate the infraorbital nerve), is definitive therapy.

   b. A **buccal space abscess** is usually associated with the maxillary and mandibular posterior teeth, with localization beneath the buccinator muscle attachment. Clinically, there is tender swelling of the face in the maxillary or mandibular buccal vestibule. Parenteral antibiotic therapy is indicated. Incision and drainage is performed in the vestibule, with care being taken not to injure the nerves and vessels in the region.

   c. **Submandibular space abscess.** The submandibular space is located beneath the body of the mandible and is bounded laterally by the anterior and posterior bellies of the digastric muscles, roofed by the mylohyoid muscle, and based by the superficial fascia and platysma muscle [2]. A submandibular abscess usually results from a periapical abscess of a lower second or third molar. The apices of these teeth are located posterior and inferior to the mylohyoid muscle attachments, where there is direct communication with the submandibular space. There can also be involvement from a mandibular buccal space infection that dissects around the inferior border of the mandible directly into the submandibular space. Since the submandibular space communicates directly with the sublingual space at the posterior aspect of the mylohyoid muscle and posteriorly with the pharyngeal and parapharyngeal spaces, spread of infection to these spaces is possible. Clinically, the patient presents with a tender swelling beneath the lateral mandible. **Management** consists of administration of parenteral antibiotics and incision and drainage of the abscess, usually in the operating suite.

   d. **Sublingual space abscess.** The sublingual space is located in the floor of the mouth; it is bordered superiorly by the mucosa of the floor of the mouth, inferiorly by the mylohyoid muscle, and anterolaterally by the mandible [2]. Infection of this space is the result of an abscess of a lower anterior tooth or purulent dissection from the submandibular space. With sublingual space involvement, the floor of the mouth and tongue are elevated with the potential for airway obstruction. Drainage is performed intraorally with an incision parallel to the mandible, with care being taken not to lacerate the lingual nerve or submandibular duct. The incision is carried just through the oral mucosa; the remainder of the dissection is via blunt dissection. Cultures are obtained, a drain is sutured in place, and parenteral antibiotic therapy is initiated.

   e. **Pharyngeal and parapharyngeal space abscesses.** With involvement of the pharyngeal and parapharyngeal spaces, the soft palate and airway are edematous. Oral opening is difficult due to trismus secondary to medial pterygoid and masseter muscle spasm, and airway compromise may be present. The patient must be taken to the operating suite for airway management (i.e., endotracheal intubation or tracheostomy) and drainage of the abscess. Parenteral antibiotics are indicated.

   f. **Multiple deep-space abscesses.** When involvement of the submandibular, sublingual, and parapharyngeal spaces occurs simultaneously, these spaces are drained extraorally through an incision one finger's breadth below the mandible or in the most dependent area. Each space is explored by blunt dissection, drains are placed in each space, the patient's airway is artificially maintained until the swelling resolves, and high-dose parenteral antibiotics are administered.

   g. A **submental space abscess** is located beneath the chin within the area bordered by the chin, the anterior bellies of the digastric muscles, and the mylohyoid muscle superiorly [2]. The etiology is usually a lower anterior tooth abscess. The patient presents with a tender swelling under the chin. **Treatment** involves incision and drainage of the space, treatment of the offending tooth by either endodontic therapy or extraction, and antibiotic coverage.

h. Ludwig's angina is the most serious of all odontogenic infections. It is a deep-space abscess involving the submandibular and sublingual spaces bilaterally and the submental space [9].

(1) Clinical features. The patient presents with a large, hard swelling extending from the mandible into the neck, a swollen and elevated tongue, elevation of the floor of the mouth, trismus, inability to swallow, difficulty breathing, fever, and leukocytosis.

(2) Management. Ludwig's angina is a true medical emergency. A patent airway must be achieved without delay, usually by tracheostomy. Endotracheal intubation is quite difficult and generally should not be performed due to the potential for pharyngeal and parapharyngeal involvement; in addition, intubation may cause abscess perforation with aspiration of purulent material. Following airway management, incision and drainage is performed in the operating suite via three incisions, one in each submandibular space and one in the submental space, and drains are placed in all involved spaces. High-dose parenteral antibiotics (see Table 28-2) are started and later adjusted according to the culture results.

Postextraction Complications

Complications of a tooth extraction include bleeding, pain, malocclusion, loss of a tooth or root tip, and fever. Evaluation involves a careful examination of the oral cavity and a radiograph of the involved area to assess for a fracture, foreign body, or a displaced root tip or tooth.

I. **Bleeding** usually can be controlled by (1) inserting Gelfoam or Surgicel in the extraction site, (2) suturing or resuturing the soft tissue, or (3) placing gauze (or a tea bag) over the extraction site and instructing the patient to bite down to achieve pressure hemostasis; follow-up the following day by the patient's dentist is advised. A dissecting hematoma is uncommon; but when it occurs, it needs to be explored in the operating suite and the bleeding controlled by cauterization or ligation of the bleeding vessels.

II. A **dry socket** (local osteitis) presents as a severe throbbing pain approximately 3 or 4 days after a tooth extraction. Clinically, the blood clot has disappeared from the tooth socket, leaving exposed bone. **Treatment** includes irrigating the socket with saline and placing iodoform gauze saturated with oil of cloves in the socket. Oil of cloves acts as an analgesic, and pain generally disappears within 5–10 minutes. The patient should be referred to an oral surgeon the next day for changing of the pack.

III. **Malocclusion** usually is the result of swelling or a fracture. A radiograph should be obtained to assess whether there is a fracture or not. If malocclusion is due to swelling, the bite will return to normal when the swelling resolves. A fracture requires appropriate treatment.

IV. **Loss of a tooth or root tip** into the maxillary sinus or pulmonary or gastrointestinal tract may occur. Radiographs are indicated to locate the foreign body. **Therapy** depends on the site of lodgment. A tooth in the maxillary sinus can be left for a few days until the surgical wound is healed. The patient should be placed on a decongestant and antibiotic and scheduled for admission at a later date for retrieval of the tooth. A tooth in the infratemporal space or another space requires exploration in the operating suite after being isolated with radiographs. This exploration can be done electively unless there is uncontrollable bleeding, for which immediate exploration is indicated. Attempting retrieval without pinpointing the location of the tooth or root tip can cause severe soft-tissue trauma, bleeding, swelling, or infection. A tooth, root, or filling dislodged into the pulmonary tract needs to be removed via bronchoscopy. A tooth in the gastrointestinal tract should be allowed to pass spontaneously.

V. **Fever** postextraction generally signifies localized infection at the extraction site. Usually there is a prompt response to oral penicillin.

Dentoalveolar Trauma

I. **Fractures** of teeth can involve the enamel, dentin, pulp, or root. The diagnosis is made by a dental-oral examination and confirmed by radiographs.

A. An **enamel fracture** alone causes no pain, since it involves the nonvital part of the tooth. **Treatment** involves referral to a dentist on a nonurgent basis for smoothing down the fracture site or, if large enough to cause an aesthetic problem, a dental restoration [9].

   B. A fracture through the enamel into the **dentin** usually is painful, since the dentin is viable tissue that responds to hot, cold, and tactile stimulation. In the emergency department, an analgesic is prescribed. The patient should be followed up by a dentist for definitive treatment, which involves dental restoration [9].

   C. A fracture of a tooth through the enamel and dentin into the **pulp** or root canal usually is very painful, since the neurovascular bundle of the tooth is exposed to the environment. The clinical evaluation and a dental x-ray are diagnostic. There is usually blood or clot in the area of the pulp canal, and the tooth is sensitive to heat, cold, and touch. In the emergency department, an analgesic is prescribed, and the patient is referred to a dentist as soon as possible. Definitive treatment involves root canal therapy; initially, however, removal of the neurovascular supply of the root and sedative restoration will relieve the patient of pain [9].

   D. A **fracture of the root** is diagnosed by a dental x-ray. Clinically, the crown of the tooth may or may not be mobile, depending on the location of the fracture. **Treatment** of a root fracture depends on the symptoms and location of the fracture. A fracture of the root at the apical third may not require treatment and may heal on its own, require root canal therapy, or need to be stabilized against an adjacent tooth during the healing process. For a fracture at the occlusal third of the root, the crown generally is mobile, and there is not enough root above the alveolar bone for restoration; generally, these teeth require extraction. Any of the root fractures described may require root canal therapy, stabilization against adjacent teeth, or extensive restoration or extraction [9]. Clinical judgment at the time of injury is important. When in doubt, the tooth should be left in place, since the tooth can always be extracted at a later date. An analgesic and antibiotic are adjunctive therapy.

II. Subluxation and avulsion of teeth

   A. Subluxation is dislodgment of a tooth within its bony crypt. The tooth can be rotated, extruded, intruded, or displaced toward the cheek, lip, tongue, or palatal aspect of the dentoalveolus.

   1. Clinical **assessment** reveals a loose or displaced tooth. A radiograph determines whether there is any root fracture.

   2. Treatment consists of stabilizing the affected tooth against adjacent teeth with arch bars, stainless steel wires, or acrylic splints. An attempt is made to reposition the tooth in its normal anatomic position; however, proper repositioning is not always possible due to an alveolar fracture, loss of bone, hematoma formation, and the anatomic shape of the tooth. The tooth is stabilized for 4–6 weeks. The patient is informed that the prognosis is variable and may require further treatment in the future, i.e., root canal therapy or extraction [9].

   B. Avulsion of a tooth refers to traumatic removal of a tooth from its bony crypt. When applicable (primary teeth do not need to be reimplanted), the patient should be instructed to place the tooth back in the socket and proceed to the emergency department. If the tooth cannot be placed in its socket, it should be wrapped in a moist cloth and immediately brought by the patient to the emergency department. The tooth is then immediately (prior to obtaining radiographs) placed back into the socket and stabilized against adjacent teeth. It is essential that the tooth be reimplanted as soon as possible, since the success of reimplantation is inversely proportional to the length of time the tooth is out of the socket. Generally, avulsed teeth require root canal therapy, since these teeth really are compound fractures of the alveolus. Phenoxymethyl penicillin, 250 mg q6h, should be prescribed for 1 week [9].

III. Intraoral lacerations. Lacerations of the oral cavity, like lacerations elsewhere, heal better with less scarring by primary intention than by secondary intention. Deep lacerations should be debrided, if necessary, and closed in layers. Generally, for the outer layer, 3-0 or 4-0 silk is used, although resorbable suture material can also be used. Chromic or catgut sutures, however, should not be utilized as the outer layer in the tongue, since they generally work loose; Vicryl or Dexon should be used instead. Phenoxymethyl penicillin, 250 mg PO q6h, generally is indicated since the oral cavity is contaminated; and tetanus prophylaxis is provided as needed.

Oral Lesions

Patients with oral lesions usually present because of pain or fear of cancer. The most common painful lesions are herpes labialis, pharyngitis, or stomatitis; aphthous stomatitis; candidiasis; and trench mouth.

I. **Herpes simplex** (see Chap. 31) presents as small white vesicles and erosions. **Treatment** is palliative. If the mouth is painful, local anesthetic rinses are helpful. Within 10–14 days, herpetic lesions generally are healed. Occasionally, an oral herpes infection is so debilitating that the patient is dehydrated and requires hospitalization for hydration. Acyclovir (see Chap. 12) is beneficial in treating mucocutaneous infections in immunocompromised patients but not in normal hosts.

II. **Aphthous ulcers** (see Chap. 31) are small red craterous ulcers with white borders. They are extremely painful and sensitive to food. Treatment is palliative. These lesions resolve in 10–14 days.

III. **Candidal infections** present as white plaque and burning pain. These plaques are easily removed with a tongue blade. Smears are diagnostic. Mycostatin mouth rinses in a dosage of 400,000–600,000 units (4–6 ml) qid are indicated.

IV. **Trench mouth.** See **Odontogenic Infections**, sec. II.A.3.

V. **Systemic disease.** Redness, swelling, bleeding, and inflammation of the gums may be indicative of an undiagnosed systemic disease. Conditions that present as such include systemic lupus erythematosus, leukemia, diabetes mellitus, pemphigoid, pemphigus, and carcinomatous lesions. An appropriate workup, including a complete blood count (CBC) with differential count, coagulation studies, and serum chemistries, is indicated.

VI. Other lesions that are not infections should be biopsied for diagnostic purposes. Referral to an oral surgeon is appropriate.

Temporomandibular Joint Disorders

I. **Dislocation of the temporomandibular joint (TMJ)**
   A. **Clinical features.** Since TMJ dislocation results in an inability to close the mouth, the patient presents with an open mouth. Pain is also a constant feature. Clinical and radiographic evaluations reveal the mandibular condyle or condyles to be anterior to the articular eminence; the condyles can be palpated anterior to the ear and inferior to the cheek bone.
   B. **Treatment** consists of manipulating the condyles back into the fossae one side at a time. By standing in front of the patient, the attendant places his or her thumb inside the patient's mouth along the ascending ramus on the affected side, with the remaining fingers holding on to the posterior ramus and the angle of the mandible outside the mouth. The patient is instructed to close the mouth as the attendant directs the mandible inferiorly and posteriorly; usually the condyle will relocate back into the fossa [1, 9]. If the procedure is too painful, a local anesthetic (e.g., 1% lidocaine, 0.5–1.0 ml) can be injected into the capsular ligament of the mandibular condyle (by injecting directly over the condyle). In addition, the medial pterygoid and masseter muscles can be injected in the area of their attachments at the angle of the mandible. Generally, there is no difficulty manipulating the condyle back into the fossa after anesthetic injections. If needed, the procedure is then repeated for the other condyle. Postreduction radiographs are obtained to rule out a fracture, and the patient is referred to an oral surgeon for follow-up.

II. **Dislocation of the TMJ meniscus**
   A. **Clinical Features.** The patient reports a loud pop and subsequent inability to open the mouth because the mandibular condyle cannot translate across the articular eminence due to the anterior position of the meniscus and its resultant mechanical obstruction.
   B. The **diagnosis** can be established with an arthrogram.
   C. **Treatment** involves manipulating the mandible (as described in sec. I) to allow the meniscus to snap back into its normal anatomic position. A local anesthetic can be injected into the inferior joint space to aid in the manipulation. The patient is then instructed to eat soft foods and apply moist heat locally. Referral to an oral surgeon is appropriate.

III. **Hemarthrosis** of the TMJ is a bleed within the joint space secondary to a blow to the chin or TMJ directly.
   A. **Clinical features.** Patients with hemarthrosis of the TMJ usually present with a history of trauma, inability to open the mouth secondary to muscle spasm, and inability to completely close the mouth (i.e., bite the teeth together) due to blood in the joint space and TMJ capsulitis. The acute symptoms are temporary, usually lasting for 7–14 days. Radiographs are necessary to rule out a fracture.
   B. **Treatment** consists of administration of an analgesic, application of moist heat to the affected joint, a soft diet, and decreased use of the joint (for a couple of weeks)

until the acute symptoms resolve [1, 9]. The patient is referred to an oral surgeon for follow-up. Further evaluation of the TMJs may be necessary in the future.

IV. Acute TMJ pain without trauma is usually due to inflammation of the capsule secondary to bite problems and muscle spasm. Management consists of administration of an anti-inflammatory agent, a soft diet, application of moist heat to the affected joint, and follow-up with an oral surgeon [9].

Salivary Gland Disorders

The major and minor salivary glands may be affected by ductal obstruction or infection. The major glands include the submandibular, parotid, and sublingual glands.

I. Sialadenitis (salivary gland inflammation)

    A. Obstructive sialadenitis can occur in healthy adults without associated disease. It usually results from a calculus obstructing one of the salivary glands (most commonly the submandibular gland), but obstruction can also occur from strictures, inspissated secretions, or neoplasms.

        1. Characteristic manifestations include pain (or a sensation of pressure) and swelling of the affected salivary gland (especially during meals), gland tenderness, erythema and edema in the area of the duct, no salivary flow on massaging the gland, and occasionally a palpable calculus. If the obstruction is complicated by infection, pus may be expressed from the duct.

        2. Plain **radiographs** (e.g., a lateral mandible view, an occlusal view, a panoramic view) may reveal a radiopaque stone. A sialogram is useful in detecting calculi and ductal strictures but should not be performed during the acute episode due to the possibility of spreading an associated infection.

        3. Management consists of application of heat, administration of an antibiotic (e.g., phenoxymethyl penicillin, 250–500 mg q6h, since involved bacteria usually are mouth organisms), and encouraging fluid intake to maintain hydration. Follow-up with an oral surgeon within 48 hours is recommended.

    B. Purulent sialadenitis commonly occurs in patients with long-standing systemic disease (e.g., diabetes mellitus), dehydration, debilitation, or ductal obstruction.

        1. Clinical manifestations include painful swelling, erythema, and tenderness of the affected gland; fever; and often dehydration. In addition, there usually is erythema and edema of the ductal orifice, and purulent drainage may be expressed from the orifice.

        2. Treatment. A culture of any purulent drainage should be obtained, and antibiotic therapy initiated. In the case of acute suppurative parotitis, a penicillinase-resistant antibiotic is indicated because of the high incidence of involvement with *Staphylococcus aureus*; otherwise, penicillin usually is appropriate. Also, it is essential to achieve and maintain adequate hydration.

        3. Disposition. Generally, patients who are toxic (e.g., a high fever, dehydration) should be admitted to the hospital for parenteral antibiotic therapy and hydration, and patients who are nontoxic should be referred to an oral surgeon for follow-up within 48 hours.

    C. Systemic diseases associated with sialadenitis include mumps, Sjögren's syndrome, and sarcoidosis. Treatment is that of the underlying disease.

II. A mucocele is swelling of a minor salivary gland secondary to obstruction to salivary flow. It presents as a bluish-grey swelling, generally involving the lower lip but also the buccal or labial mucosa; it varies in size with eating. The patient should be referred to an oral surgeon for excision of the offending minor salivary gland.

III. A ranula is a large bluish swelling under the tongue on the floor of the mouth. By definition, it is a mucocele of the sublingual gland. **Treatment** of choice is total excision of the sublingual gland in the operating suite. Marsupialization is an alternative; however, this procedure generally results in recurrence of the ranula.

Bibliography

1. DeWeese, D. D., and Saunders, W. H. *Textbook of Otolaryngology* (6th ed.). St. Louis: Mosby, 1982.
2. DuBrul, E. L. *Sicher's Oral Anatomy* (7th ed.). St. Louis: Mosby, 1980.
3. Esenberg, M. S., Furukana, C., and Ray, G. C. *Manual of Antimicrobial Therapy and Infectious Diseases.* Philadelphia: Saunders, 1978.
4. Gabrielson, M. L., and Stroh, E. Antibiotic efficacy in odontogenic infections. *J. Oral Surg.* 33:607, 1975.

5. Gardner, A. Antibiotic therapy in the management of oral infections in dental patients. *J. Oral Med.* 36:54, 1981.
6. Greenberg, R. N., et al. Microbiologic and antibiotic aspects of infections in the oral and maxillofacial region. *J. Oral Surg.* 37:873, 1979.
7. Hunt, D. E., King, T. J., and Fuller, G. E. Antibiotic susceptibility of bacteria isolated from oral infections. *J. Oral Surg.* 36:527, 1978.
8. Hunt, D. E., and Meyer, R. A. Continued evolution of the microbiology of oral infections. *J.A.D.A.* 107:52, 1983.
9. Kruger, G. O. *Textbook of Oral and Maxillofacial Surgery* (6th ed.). St. Louis: Mosby, 1984.
10. Olson, R. E., et al. Antibiotic treatment of oral anaerobic infections. *J. Oral Surg.* 33:619, 1975.
11. Sadiston, C. B., Jr., and Gold, W. A. Anaerobic bacteria in oral infections. *J. Oral Surg.* 38:187, 1974.
12. Steiner, R. B., and Thompson, R. D. *Oral Surgery and Anesthesia.* Philadelphia: Saunders, 1977.

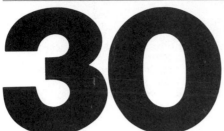

Acute Anorectal Disorders

Robert D. Fry and
Ira J. Kodner

The usual anorectal problems encountered in the emergency department include anorectal trauma, anal pain or bleeding, localized tissue protrusion or swelling, and fecal impaction. It is not unusual for the patient to be embarrassed and hesitant to discuss such symptoms. Many anorectal symptoms are frequently attributed to hemorrhoids, an impression that is often incorrect. The emergency physician should be prepared to deal with these problems in a compassionate and understanding manner, even though such problems may not represent true emergencies.

Anorectal Examination in the Emergency Department

It is mandatory that the patient with anorectal symptoms receive an adequate examination to arrive at an accurate diagnosis. The examination should be conducted as gently as possible, and usually only a few moments are required. Sedatives, anesthetics, laxatives, enemas, or suppositories are unnecessary. During the examination it is important that privacy be assured and adequate lighting be available.

The best position for anorectal examination is the knee-chest position, with the patient kneeling on the examination table, head down. The elderly or very ill patient can be placed in the left lateral decubitus (Sims') position, with the knees drawn up to the chest and the buttocks extending just beyond the table's edge.

I. **Perianal examination.** During this portion of the examination, attention is directed to the perianal region, buttocks, perineum, and sacrococcygeal region.
   A. **Inspection.** Frequently, the correct diagnosis is immediately obvious. Perianal warts, thrombosed hemorrhoids, and anal skin tags can be diagnosed on inspection. Perianal soilage, seepage, or discharge may suggest sphincteric weakness, proctitis, or an anal fistula. Skin thickening or excoriation often accompanies pruritus ani. The bulging or erythema of an abscess or the external opening of an anal fistula may be identified. Gently separating the buttocks may expose the lower edge of an anal fissure. Multiple superficial abscesses and sinuses may indicate hidradenitis suppurativa; and edematous skin tags, eccentric fissures, and multiple fistulas may suggest Crohn's disease. Exposed rectal mucosa may represent an internal hemorrhoid or procidentia. Scars from a previous operation should be noted.
   B. **Palpation.** The perianal region should be gently palpated, searching for areas of induration, fluctuance, or tenderness. Pressure may produce a drop of pus at the external opening of an anal fistula. The thickened cord of a chronic fistula is sometimes palpable.

II. **Anorectal examination.** In contrast to the usual diagnostic approach, palpation of the anorectal area precedes inspection. Since the anal sphincter reflexly contracts when touched, gentle pressure with a lubricated gloved finger should be applied at the anal orifice until relaxation occurs. The finger is then inserted in the direction of the axis of the anal canal, which is toward the patient's umbilicus.
   A. **Anal palpation.** The anal canal is quite short, with the distance from the anal verge to the anorectal junction being usually less than 3 cm. Thus, it is necessary to insert the finger only to the proximal interphalangeal joint to examine the entire anal canal. The degree of sphincter tone should be noted. Severe spasm of the sphincter suggests the presence of an anal fissure, as does tenderness in the posterior midline of the anal canal. Internal hemorrhoids usually are not palpable. Thickening and scarring of the anal canal is suggestive of Crohn's disease. The examiner should palpate the sphincter circumferentially between the index finger and the thumb, searching for areas of induration, tenderness, or fluctuance that suggest an abscess.
   B. **Rectal palpation.** After examination of the anal canal, the finger is inserted further to enter the rectum. The presence and character of stool in the rectum should be

noted, and the stool should be tested for occult blood. The prostate and seminal vesicles or cervix and uterus can be palpated anteriorly. The coccyx may be felt posteriorly, and the ischial tuberosities laterally. A rectal tumor, fecal impaction, or foreign body may be detected by digital examination.

C. **Anoscopy.** Inspection of the anal canal may be accomplished using either a tubular or slotted anoscope. The lubricated anoscope is gently inserted in the direction of the umbilicus, the obturator removed, and the anal canal inspected as the anoscope is slowly withdrawn.

1. **Internal hemorrhoids** are easily seen through the anoscope. The size of the hemorrhoids can best be appreciated by asking the patient to bear down as though to have a bowel movement. This maneuver will cause large internal hemorrhoids to prolapse into the lumen of the anoscope.

2. An **anal fissure** or an associated hypertrophied anal papilla can be seen through the anoscope. However, a fissure can usually be diagnosed without the use of an anoscope (by spreading the buttocks apart to reveal the fissure). It is then unnecessary for the patient to undergo anoscopy, which is quite painful in this condition.

3. The **Internal opening of an anal fistula** may be visible through the anoscope. Pressure applied to the perianal skin while the anoscope is inserted may cause a drop of pus to appear at the internal opening.

4. **Anal condylomata acuminata** are easily seen with the anoscope.

D. **Proctosigmoidoscopy** is usually indicated if the preceding evaluation has not defined the cause of the patient's anorectal symptoms. Enemas or suppositories are usually not required before the examination. The 20-cm rigid proctosigmoidoscope is adequate for problems requiring evaluation in the emergency department.

1. **Rectal bleeding** from a source that cannot be detected through an anoscope is an indication for immediate proctosigmoidoscopy. The rectal mucosa should be examined carefully for granularity or ulceration suggestive of inflammatory bowel disease. A rectal cancer may be detected as the bleeding source.

2. **Acute diarrhea** can be evaluated by a proctosigmoidoscopic examination. This examination allows inspection of the rectal mucosa and facilitates collection of material for culture.

3. **Anorectal trauma,** whether of a sexual nature or the result of firearms or knives, requires a careful proctosigmoidoscopic examination. The rectum should be inspected for the presence of blood as well as for mucosal lacerations.

Anorectal Trauma

Significant morbidity and mortality are associated with anorectal injuries. Gunshot wounds, knife wounds, impalement injuries, and crush injuries to the pelvis are common forms of anorectal trauma. The major effort of the emergency department staff should be aimed at diagnosing the type and severity of the injury and stabilizing the patient for definitive surgical treatment if such is required.

I. **Perineal lacerations** require careful examination to determine the extent of the injury.

A. A **history** is invaluable in determining the cause and potential severity of the perineal laceration.

B. A **sterile gloved finger** should be used to probe all perineal lacerations to determine the depth of the injury. If communication with the peritoneal cavity is found, the patient should be prepared for exploratory laparotomy.

C. **Proctosigmoidoscopy** is required if rectal injury is suspected to determine the nature and extent of injury, if any.

D. **Treatment**

1. If rectal perforation has occurred, the patient is prepared for laparotomy, colostomy, rectal washout, and presacral drainage. Broad-spectrum antibiotics should be given intravenously, and tetanus prophylaxis administered if indicated.

2. If the wound is confined to the subcutaneous tissues, it should be copiously irrigated and closed about a small Penrose drain. Sitz baths should be taken 3 times a day, and the drain removed in 24–48 hours.

II. **Laceration of the anal sphincters** can be caused by several types of trauma.

A. **Broad-spectrum antibiotics** should be given intravenously.

B. **Bleeding** is controlled by packing the wound.

C. The patient is prepared for immediate **repair** of the sphincteric injury in the operating room under general anesthesia.

III. **Rectal perforation** can occur as an isolated injury or in association with other injuries.
   A. A **careful history** is mandatory to determine the possible extent of the rectal injury and ascertain the possibility of associated injuries.
   B. A **digital rectal examination** is performed, searching for areas of tenderness. The presence of blood in the rectum should raise the suspicion of rectal perforation.
   C. An **abdominal examination** is performed. Rebound tenderness suggests intraperitoneal perforation of the rectum.
   D. **Proctosigmoidoscopy** is essential if rectal injury is suspected. A mucosal laceration, submucosal hematoma, or blood in the rectum requires further evaluation (see **E** and **F**) to rule out a perforation of the rectal wall.
   E. A **flat plate and upright film of the abdomen** should be obtained. Free air under the diaphragm suggests colonic perforation, while retroperitoneal air suggests rectal perforation.
   F. A **meglumine diatrizoate (Gastrografin) enema** should be obtained if perforation is suspected. However, a barium enema should not be obtained, because barium will aggravate the infection associated with the rectal perforation.
   G. **Management** depends on the severity of the injury. Admission and observation are appropriate if the assessment reveals that rectal perforation is possible; and this regimen applies to all but the most superficial rectal mucosal injuries. Perforation of the rectal wall requires that the patient be taken to the operating suite for definitive care. Broad-spectrum antibiotics and tetanus prophylaxis (if needed) should be administered.

Male Rape

Emergency departments are more frequently being called on to treat cases of forcible male sodomy. It must be remembered that, like female victims, male victims of sexual assault have medical, legal, and psychological needs.

I. An **accurate history** should be legibly documented. The use of force or verbal intimidation should be noted, and the patient should be specifically asked if there was penetration of any orifice. **Penetration,** not ejaculation, is the hallmark of rape or sodomy. The patient should also be specifically asked about the presence of a penile or rectal discharge, rectal bleeding, sore throat, sore mouth, or other pains that might have resulted from force. A history of any venereal disease should be noted.
II. The **physical examination** initially includes an evaluation of the airway, breathing, and circulation. The patient's condition should be stabilized before proceeding with further evaluation.
   A. The **patient's clothes** should be examined for signs of violence or traces of semen. The undergarments should be carefully examined for seminal stains. Clothes suspected of containing semen should be individually placed in paper bags, labeled, and turned over to the police.
   B. Contusions, lacerations, and any other **signs of trauma** should be carefully documented.
   C. The **oral cavity** should be examined for mucosal lacerations, a torn frenulum, broken teeth, or exudates.
   D. The **penis, perineum, and rectum** should be carefully inspected, and any signs of trauma recorded. It is most important to search for perianal contusions and anal fissures. A digital anal examination should be performed.
   E. **Proctosigmoidoscopy** should be performed in all patients suspected of having anal penetration.
III. **Laboratory examination** is determined by the type of assault that has occurred.
   A. **Pharyngeal or rectal cultures** (or both) for gonorrhea should be obtained.
   B. A **serologic test for syphilis** should also be obtained.
   C. **Rectal or oral swabs** (or both) should be inspected for motile sperm and sent for acid phosphatase, if penetration has occurred.
   D. **Samples** should be submitted to the police or pathologist as indicated. These samples include air-dried slides of swabbings from the rectum and mouth, swabs of skin areas suspected of containing semen, pubic hair combings, fingernail scrapings, and photographs.
IV. **Treatment** includes appropriate care for trauma as indicated, prophylaxis for venereal disease, and psychologic support.
   A. If oral or rectal penetration has occurred, the patient should be treated as if he were a contact of a known case of gonorrhea (see Chap. 12).

B. Psychologic support should be provided as indicated. Psychiatric treatment may be necessary, especially in younger men.

Hemorrhoids

Internal hemorrhoids are dilatations of the veins arising from the superior hemorrhoidal venous plexus and are located above the dentate line. **External hemorrhoids** drain into the inferior hemorrhoidal venous plexus and reside below the dentate line.

I. A **thrombosed external hemorrhoid** appears as a tense mass just external to the anal verge. This condition is caused by a blood clot in an external hemorrhoidal vein.

  A. Symptoms range from severe localized pain to no pain at all, as well as sensation of a perianal lump. Occasionally, spontaneous rupture occurs with extrusion of the clot, and the patient will notice bleeding.

  B. The **diagnosis** is made by inspecting the perianal region. The tense swelling is caused by a clot in the external hemorrhoidal vein, and no attempt should be made to reduce the thrombosed hemorrhoid into the anal canal.

  C. Treatment is determined by the degree of pain present.

    1. Minimal pain requires no specific therapy.

    2. Moderate pain can be treated by warm soaks. A psyllium seed preparation (Konsyl), 1 tsp dissolved in a glass of water, can be taken twice a day to keep the stool soft.

    3. Severe pain with tense swelling or a clot eroding through the skin should be treated by **excision of the thrombosed hemorrhoid.** Incision and evacuation of the clot, however, is inadequate treatment because of the high incidence of agglutination of wound edges and recurrence of the clot. Excision of the thrombosed hemorrhoid is performed as follows:

      a. A small amount of local anesthesia is injected around the site of the hemorrhoid, using a No. 25 needle.

      b. An elliptic incision is made around the base of the hemorrhoid. The incision should stop at the anal verge and not extend into the sensitive anal canal.

      c. Care must be taken to excise the entire clot.

      d. Bleeding can be controlled by several minutes of pressure. If desired, the wound edges can be electrocoagulated.

      e. It is not necessary to suture the wound closed.

      f. Aspirin or acetaminophen may be prescribed for pain.

      g. The patient should soak in a warm tub of water for 15 minutes, 3 times a day, until the pain is minimal.

      h. Stool should be kept soft by prescribing a psyllium seed preparation, 1 tsp in a glass of water twice a day.

      i. Antibiotics, topical creams, or suppositories are not necessary.

  D. Disposition. The patient should be referred to a surgeon for a follow-up examination in 3 days.

II. **Bleeding,** when caused by hemorrhoids, is almost always due to internal hemorrhoids. However, a clot in an external hemorrhoid occasionally may evacuate spontaneously, causing bleeding.

  A. The **diagnosis** is established by demonstrating the friable internal hemorrhoid with the aid of an anoscope. Rubbing the hemorrhoid with a cotton-tipped applicator will often precipitate bleeding. It is imperative that the bleeding site be visualized before making the diagnosis of bleeding from hemorrhoids. In patients over 35 years old, a proctosigmoidoscopic examination should be performed to rule out a rectal neoplasm. A hemoglobin and hematocrit should be obtained in all patients with rectal bleeding.

  B. Treatment depends on the severity of symptoms.

    1. If bleeding is minimal, satisfactory results can be obtained by keeping the stool soft with a psyllium seed preparation, 1 tsp in a glass of water twice a day.

    2. Anusol suppositories inserted in the rectum after each bowel movement are helpful.

    3. Sitz baths are of little value in the treatment of bleeding internal hemorrhoids.

    4. Pramoxine hydrochloride (Proctofoam) is helpful if suppositories are difficult for the patient to use.

  C. Disposition. The patient should be referred to a surgeon for a follow-up examination if the bleeding persists despite conservative treatment. If the hemorrhoids continue to bleed, they will require treatment by either excision or elastic ligation.

III. **Prolapsing internal hemorrhoids** are not a true emergency, although many patients seek emergency consultation due to the anxiety over the diagnosis.

   A. **Symptoms** are related to the protrusion of the internal hemorrhoids beyond the anal verge at the time of defecation. The tissue usually reduces spontaneously, although in some cases the prolapsed hemorrhoid may not reduce. Bleeding and edema may arise from the exposed, traumatized mucosa. Pruritus may result from excessive perianal moisture caused by the secretion of mucus.

   B. **Treatment** consists of prescribing a psyllium seed preparation and Anusol suppositories as described in **II.B.1 and 2**, respectively.

   C. **Disposition.** The patient should be referred to a surgeon for a follow-up examination and definitive treatment of the prolapsing hemorrhoids.

IV. **Strangulated hemorrhoids** result when the entire circumferential ring of the hemorrhoid becomes incarcerated outside the anal verge.

   A. **Symptoms** consist of severe pain associated with marked swelling of perianal tissue. The overlying tissue may become necrotic, allowing extrusion of some clots with resultant bleeding.

   B. **Treatment goals** are to reduce the edematous mass and evacuate the clots as follows.

   1. Bupivacaine 0.25% with epinephrine 1:200,000 is injected directly into the edematous, protruding mass.

   2. Firm manual pressure is applied for several minutes over the entire mass. This procedure dissipates the edema and allows reduction of the internal hemorrhoids.

   3. Clots from the external hemorrhoids are removed using elliptic incisions as described in sec. **I.C.3.**

   4. A pressure dressing consisting of several 3- × 4-in. gauze sponges are applied to the perianal skin and taped tightly to the buttocks.

   5. The following day, the patient should remove the dressing and begin taking sitz baths 4 times a day.

   6. The stool should be kept soft using a psyllium seed preparation, 1 tsp twice a day.

   C. **Disposition.** If the patient is a male with a history of urinary hesitancy, he should be admitted to the hospital because of the high incidence of urinary retention associated with this condition. Other patients should be referred to a surgeon for follow-up examination the following day.

Anorectal Abscess and Fistula

Anorectal abscesses and fistulas, in most cases, have a common etiology: infection of an anal crypt. The abscess may be considered to be the acute form of the disease, and the fistula the chronic form. However, an anorectal abscess does not invariably lead to the formation of an anal fistula.

I. **Pathophysiology and diagnosis.** There are six to eight anal glands around the circumference of the anal canal. These glands empty into the anal crypts; and since the anal crypt is the initial source of infection, the internal openings of most fistulas lie near the dentate line. Most abscesses and fistulas (see Fig. 30-1) occur posteriorly, because most anal glands reside posteriorly and drain into posterior crypts.

II. **Anorectal abscesses**

   A. **Types**

   1. **Intersphincteric abscess.** Most anorectal abscesses are initially located between the internal and external anal sphincters (intersphincteric abscesses) because the anal glands extend from the crypts through the internal sphincter to the space between the internal and external sphincters. A tender mass in the anal canal reveals the presence of an intersphincteric abscess. Pressure on the lump may produce a drop of pus from the offending crypt.

   2. A **perianal abscess** occurs when an intersphincteric abscess extends inferiorly in the space between the internal and external sphincters and expands near the anal verge. A tender, erythematous, localized swelling near the anal verge is present. Fluctuance may also be present, but is not necessary to confirm the diagnosis.

   3. An **ischiorectal abscess** occurs when an intersphincteric abscess penetrates the external sphincter and expands into the soft fat of the ischiorectal space. Tenderness and induration of the ischiorectal area indicate an underlying ab-

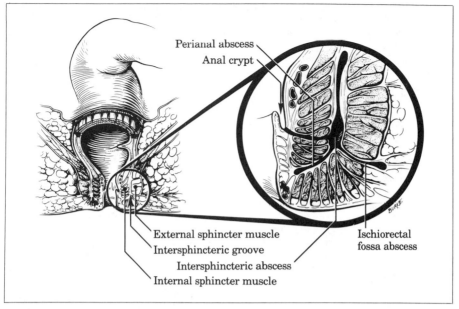

Fig. 30-1. An anorectal abscess orginates in the intersphincteric groove. An intersphincteric abscess can then extend to form a perianal abscess or an ischiorectal fossa abscess.

scess. Redness and fluctuance, however, do not develop until late in the course of this disease. An area of tender induration extending above the level of the dentate line can be detected by digital examination of the anus.

B. Management of anorectal abscesses consists of incising the overlying skin and draining the accumulated pus. To lessen the risk of complications, it is important not to wait for fluctuance to develop; incision and drainage should be performed without delay. Antibiotics are not indicated except in specific situations, such as diabetic or immunosuppressed patients.

    1. Most **perianal abscesses** can be treated in the emergency department.

        a. A local anesthetic is injected intradermally over the point of maximal swelling.

        b. To help define the anatomic limits of the abscess, a finger is inserted into the anal canal.

        c. Using a No. 15 blade, a short incision is made over the area of the abscess that is closest to the overlying skin. It is preferable to drain the abscess as close to the anus as possible, so that if a fistula should form subsequently, the tract will be short.

        d. When pus is encountered, the abscess cavity is evacuated.

        e. Adequate drainage can be assured by inserting a small (No. 10) mushroom catheter into the abscess cavity. Use of this device is less painful than packing the abscess cavity with gauze.

        f. Acetaminophen provides adequate analgesia following drainage of a perianal abscess.

        g. Follow-up. The patient should be referred to a surgeon for inspection of the wound the following day. The mushroom catheter should be removed in 2 weeks.

    2. Large **ischiorectal abscesses** should be unroofed in the operating suite under general or regional anesthesia.

III. An **anal fistula** is a chronic tract that persists about half the time following incision and drainage of an anorectal abscess. The internal opening of an anal fistula is almost always at the base of a crypt at the level of the dentate line. The external opening is usually the site at which the abscess was incised and drained.

    A. The **clinical course** of a fistula is recurring anal pain, relieved when pus drains from one of the openings.

    B. The **treatment** of an anal fistula is surgical excision of the tract, which should be performed under adequate anesthesia in the operating suite. Antibiotics and topical ointments are of no use in this condition.

Anal Fissure

I. Pathology. An anal fissure is simply a tear in the anoderm. The etiology of the fissure is unknown, but increased spasm or fibrosis of the internal anal sphincter is almost always a concomitant finding.

    A. An **anal fissure in a male** is almost always located close to the posterior midline of the anal canal.

    B. An **anal fissure in a female** is located near the posterior midline of the anal canal 80% of the time but resides near the anterior midline 20% of the time.

    C. An **anal fissure located in the lateral anal canal** is usually associated with other pathology, such as Crohn's disease, scarring from previous anorectal surgery, or trauma.

    D. A **deep, chronic anal fissure (anal ulcer)** exposes the fibers of the internal sphincter and may be accompanied by other local anatomic pathology.

        1. A **sentinel pile** is edematous skin located just below the fissure. It should not be mistaken for a hemorrhoid.

        2. A **hypertrophied anal papilla** is the result of the anal papilla above the fissure becoming edematous and enlarged. It should not be mistaken for a rectal polyp.

II. Symptoms and signs. Pain, occurring at the time of defecation and lasting for a variable time thereafter, is the most common symptom of an anal fissure; the pain is usually described as "tearing" or "burning." Bleeding frequently accompanies bowel movements. A discharge is occasionally present but usually is slight; and pruritus, which may be caused by the discharge, is sometimes present. Swelling may be noted; it simply represents the presence of an associated sentinel pile.

III. The **diagnosis** is made by gently spreading the buttocks and anal verge and visualizing the lower edge of the fissure. Anoscopy is usually not required to establish the diagnosis.

IV. Treatment is initially medical, and the great majority of fissures will heal without surgery.

    A. Warm sitz baths or warm packs help reduce sphincter spasm.

    B. A **high-fiber diet** is helpful in bowel regulation.

    C. A **stool softener,** such as a psyllium seed preparation, should be prescribed.

    D. Suppositories are of no value since they pass into the rectum, above the site of the fissure. Topical analgesic ointments provide little benefit and may cause a contact dermatitis.

V. Follow-up. The patient should be referred to a gastroenterologist or a surgeon for follow-up. **Surgical treatment** is required for a fissure that does not respond to conservative therapy and usually consists of a lateral subcutaneous internal sphincterotomy.

Pilonidal Abscess

I. Etiology. The exact cause of pilonidal disease is uncertain, but it is almost certainly an acquired condition. As the name implies (pilus, hair; nidus, nest) the disease is characterized by a cluster of ingrown hairs that is located between the buttocks in the natal cleft. Men are more commonly affected with pilonidal disease (85% of the cases) than women. Individuals between the ages of 16 and 25 years are most commonly affected, with hirsute and obese people predominating.

II. Clinical presentation. An acute abscess may be superimposed on the imbedded hairs, causing the patient to seek emergency treatment. A pilonidal abscess consists of a tender, fluctuant area located in the midline of the natal cleft. If spontaneous rupture of the abscess has occurred, the patient presents with a tender area between the buttocks, from which pus drains. Hair can usually be detected inside the abscess cavity if spontaneous rupture has occurred, or following incision and drainage. Extension of the abscess toward the anus can occur rarely, causing this disease to be mistaken for an abscess of cryptoglandular etiology.

III. Initial treatment of a pilonidal abscess is incision and drainage, which is preferred over definitive treatment in the presence of pus and adjacent cellulitis.

    A. The adjacent skin is shaved, and a local anesthetic is injected into the skin over the fluctuant abscess.

    B. The **abscess cavity is unroofed,** and the walls curetted. **All visible hairs should be removed** from the abscess cavity. Packing of the cavity is seldom necessary.

   C. Antibiotics are not a substitute for surgical drainage but should be used if cellulitis is extensive or if conditions such as diabetes mellitus or valvular heart disease are present.

   D. Warm baths, at least 3 times daily for the next few days, are recommended.

IV. Disposition. The patient should be referred to a surgeon for follow-up care, which consists of shaving the adjacent skin and debriding the wound when necessary. **Definitive surgery** to eradicate the pilonidal disease can be performed after adequate healing of the abscess has occurred.

Sexual Proctology

Changing social mores, the emergence of a homosexual population, decreasing use of the condom, and increasing use of the rectum for sexual gratification have been associated with a profound change in the prevalence and types of sexually transmitted diseases (see Chap. 12) during the past decade. The "conventional venereal diseases"—gonorrhea, syphilis, herpes simplex, and condylomata acuminata—still occur, but these conditions are now outnumbered by the common chlamydial infections (nonspecific genital infection, nongonococcal urethritis) that are more difficult to diagnose with specificity. Other conditions, formerly considered to be nonvenereal, probably occur as a result of direct or indirect oral-anal contact; such diseases include amebiasis, shigellosis, giardiasis, salmonellosis, and hepatitis (see Chap. 10). It must be emphasized that multiple simultaneous infections are common, particularly in homosexual patients. The frequent association of gonorrhea or syphilis with enteric viral or protozoal infections has led to the use of the term **gay bowel syndrome.** The acquired immunodeficiency syndrome (AIDS) (see Chap. 12) that has been recognized in homosexuals (as well as in hemophiliac transfusion recipients and a few Haitian immigrants) is caused by a virus which appears to be transmitted in a mode similar to the hepatitis B virus.

I. Anorectal gonorrhea (see Chap. 12) is transmitted almost exclusively by anal intercourse. Occasionally, it may be acquired from a vaginal or urethral discharge coming in contact with the anus.

   A. Symptoms are nonspecific and protean. Most patients are asymptomatic. Tenesmus, painful defecation, discharge, and burning, however, can occur.

   B. Signs are also nonspecfic. The proctoscopic examination may be completely normal. However, the presence of a thick, viscid, yellow pus (mucopus) is highly suggestive of gonococcal proctitis. A cryptitis may be seen, and at times the rectal mucosa may appear quite edematous and friable.

   C. Serious **complications** of untreated disease include gonococcal arthritis, meningitis, endocarditis, perihepatitis, and dissemination of disease to sexual partners.

   D. The **diagnosis** is made by culture, preferably taken through the anoscope and plated immediately on Thayer-Martin or Stuart's medium. Pharyngeal and urethral cultures also should be obtained. A Gram stain of a rectal smear will show intracellular gram-negative diplococci.

   E. A **serologic test for syphilis** should be obtained before starting treatment and repeated 3 months later.

   F. Treatment should be given if there is a high index of suspicion that the disease is present, since cultures are not positive in 100% of cases.

     1. In **women,** amoxicillin, 3 gm PO, accompanied by probenecid, 1 gm PO, or ceftriaxone, 250 mg IM, is recommended. Alternative regimens include penicillin G procaine, 4.8 million units IM, plus probenecid, 1 gm PO; spectinomycin, 2 gm IM; or cefoxitin, 2 gm IM, plus probenecid, 1 gm PO. Tetracycline, 500 mg PO qid for 7 days, or doxycycline 100 mg PO bid for 7 days, is recommended to treat possible coexisting chlamydial infection.

     2. In **men,** ceftriaxone, 250 mg IM once, is the drug of choice. Alternative therapy involves penicillin G procaine, 4.8 million units IM, plus probenecid, 1 gm PO; or spectinomycin, 2 gm IM. Since homosexual men are less likely than heterosexual individuals to have coexistent chlamydial infection, routine addition of tetracycline or doxycycline is not recommended [2].

   G. Follow-up cultures should be obtained 1 week after treatment. Treatment failure for anorectal gonorrhea has been reported to occur as often as 35% of the time. Persistent signs or symptoms with negative cultures or following treatment (see **F**) should prompt consideration of coexisting chlamydial infection or penicillin-resistant gonorrhea and institution of appropriate therapy (see Chap. 12).

II. Anorectal syphilis (see Chap. 12) is preceded by homosexual activity in 70% of primary cases.

A. Stages of disease
1. **Primary anal syphilis** presents as an indurated ulcer (chancre) in the anal canal or at the anal verge. Multiple ulcers are often present; symmetric ulcers on opposite sides of the anus are highly suggestive of primary syphilis. Severe pain usually accompanies the anal lesion, despite the classic description of a painless chancre. Inguinal adenopathy is very common. Primary healing of the chancre occurs (without treatment) in about 6 weeks.
2. **Secondary anal syphilis** appears in untreated patients 6–8 weeks following healing of the primary ulcer. **Condylomata lata** are tan or pink, flat, wartlike lesions in the perianal region; these lesions are loaded with spirochetes and are highly infectious.
3. **Tertiary syphilis** can present as anorectal disease.
    a. **Tabes dorsalis** may cause lancinating rectal pain or anal sphincter incontinence.
    b. **Gummata** may present as a mass lesion that simulates a rectal cancer; however, this finding is very rare.
B. Diagnostic tests depend on the stage of the disease.
1. The **primary chancre** contains spirochetes, but serology may be negative at this early stage.
    a. **Scrapings of the ulcer base** will reveal spirochetes on dark-field examination, if available.
    b. **Serum** from the base of an ulcer (cleansed with acetone or ether) may be dried and stained with fluorescent treponemal antibody.
2. **Condylomata lata** scrapings will always yield treponemes for dark-field microscopy or fluorescent treponemal antibody staining. The **Venereal Disease Research Laboratory (VDRL)** or **rapid plasma reagin (RPR)** test is positive in secondary syphilis, having turned positive 1–3 weeks after the appearance of the primary chancre.
C. Treatment of early syphilis (i.e., primary, secondary, or latent syphilis of less than one year's duration) consists of one of three regimens. **Penicillin G benzathine**, 2.4 million units as a single IM dose, is preferred. Alternative regimens include tetracycline, 500 mg PO qid for 15 days, or erythromycin, 500 mg PO qid for 15 days. Sexual contacts should be treated prophylactically with the same regimen. **Treatment of late syphilis** (but not neurosyphilis) involves administration of penicillin G benzathine, 2.4 million units IM weekly for 3 successive weeks. A 30-day course of tetracycline or erythromycin, 500 mg PO qid, is alternative therapy.
D. Follow-up serology is obtained 4 weeks after completing treatment, then every 3 months for 1 year, and then annually.
III. Chlamydial infections (see Chap. 12) are currently the most prevalent sexually transmitted infections in the United States.
A. "**Nonspecific genital infections**" are caused at least 50% of the time by *Chlamydia*.
1. **Lymphogranuloma venereum (LGV) serotypes** are frequently found in the more severe forms of proctitis.
2. **Non-LGV serotypes** are involved in minor forms of proctitis or asymptomatic conditions.
B. Signs and symptoms vary considerably.
1. **Non-LGV serotypes** may cause a mild proctitis or may be asymptomatic.
2. The **LGV serotypes** may cause an intense, granular proctitis associated with passage of pus and blood. In addition, a rectal stricture of variable length may be present.
C. The **diagnosis** is based on a high index of suspicion.
1. **Cultures** require a laboratory with viral and tissue culture capabilities. Rectal mucosal cells should be obtained by abrading the mucosa with a swab, and the specimen is then placed in a special transport medium.
2. **Serum** should be obtained for antibody titers.
D. Treatment should be given on suspicion alone. **Tetracycline**, 500 mg PO qid, is given for 1 week in non-LGV chlamydial infections and for 3 weeks in LGV-serotype infections. Erythromycin, 500 mg PO qid, is an alternate regimen, given for the same time periods.
IV. Anorectal herpes (see Chap. 12) is usually caused by **herpes simplex virus**, type II, although 10% of anal herpetic infections are caused by the type I virus.
A. Symptoms consist of paresthesias and pruritus in the sacral distribution, followed by severe anal pain. Fever and malaise are present half the time. Fecal impaction and urinary retention are not uncommon.

B. Examination reveals lesions at various stages of development on the perianal skin, in the anal canal, or on the rectal mucosa.

1. **Vesicles surrounded by a red areola** are the earliest visible lesions.
2. **Aphthous ulcers** are the result of ruptured vesicles.
3. A **mucosal proctitis** is usually characterized by punctate lesions and vesicles.

C. The **diagnosis** can be made by viral culture of vesicular fluid. In addition, the base of a freshly ruptured vesicle can be scraped and slides prepared as for a Pap smear or a Tzanck smear (see Chap. 38) to look for multinucleated giant cells.

D. Treatment is noncurative, and recurrent episodes are common.

1. **Acyclovir** (Zovirax), 5% topical ointment applied q4h for 1 week, is effective in promoting healing and shortening the period of viral shedding in primary disease.
2. **Acyclovir**, 200 mg PO 5 times a day for 7–10 days, reduces new vesicle formation and the healing time in primary and, to a lesser extent, recurrent disease.

E. Prevention. Sexual activity must be avoided when the lesions are present, as they are highly infectious. Oral acyclovir has prevented or reduced the frequency of recurrences of the disease.

F. Follow-up. The patient should be referred to an internist for follow-up in 1 week.

V. Perianal and anal condylomata acuminata (anal warts) are caused by a large papilloma virus. The disease is transmitted by sexual contact, is common in homosexuals, and is often associated with active gonococcal proctitis.

A. Clinical features. Anal warts vary in size from tiny, isolated polyps to large, cauliflowerlike masses. Lesions can occur in the urethra, on the penis, in the perianal region, in the anus, or on the rectal mucosa. The lesions are autoinoculable, thus requiring total destruction for a cure. Squamous cancer has been associated with condylomata on rare occasions.

B. Treatment depends on the size and location of the warts.

1. **Bichloracetic acid** may be applied to small warts located in the perianal region or low anal canal, with care taken to avoid contact of the adjacent skin with the acid. The warts turn frosty white almost immediately after bichloracetic acid is applied, allowing the physician to assess the extent of treatment.
2. **Electrocautery** under anesthesia is required to eradicate large warts or lesions located high in the anal canal.

C. Frequent **follow-up** examinations are necessary because of the high incidence of recurrence.

VI. Foreign bodies of the rectum are most common in male homosexuals. The types of items inserted anally for sexual gratification are as varied as the human imagination; but vegetables, fruits, plastic dildos, and vibrators are common.

A. Evaluation

1. **Signs of peritonitis** should be carefully sought.
2. A **digital rectal examination** will usually demonstrate the foreign body in the rectal ampulla. If not, observation of the patient for a few hours frequently will allow the foreign body to migrate back to the rectum.
3. **Abdominal x-rays** are obtained if the foreign body cannot be detected by digital examination. These radiographs will allow the location of the foreign body to be determined.

B. Management. If peritonitis is present, a colonic perforation has occurred, and the patient must be prepared for surgery. If there is no suggestion of peritonitis, the foreign body can usually be removed in the emergency department.

1. The anal canal is anesthetized locally with 1% lidocaine injected into the perianal tissue.
2. A Parks retractor is inserted into the anus to provide exposure.
3. The foreign body is grasped with a large clamp or uterine tenaculum, deflected anteriorly, and extracted.
4. The rectum should then be examined carefully with a sigmoidoscope.
5. If the foreign body cannot be successfully removed in the emergency department, the patient should be admitted to the hospital, and the foreign body extracted in the operating suite under general or regional anesthesia.

VII. Fist fornication is the insertion of a sexual partner's fist into the rectum for the purpose of sexual gratification. The practice is not uncommon in the male homosexual population.

A. Intraperitoneal transmural colonic laceration may result.

1. **Evaluation**
   a. Abdominal examination reveals signs of peritonitis, including voluntary guarding, rigidity, and rebound tenderness.

   b. An **upright chest x-ray** may reveal subdiaphragmatic intraperitoneal air.
   2. Treatment. Broad-spectrum antibiotics should be started in such cases, preparatory to emergency laparotomy. Tobramycin, 100 mg IV q8h, and metronidazole, 1 gm IV initially, followed by 500 mg q6h, provide coverage of gram-negative aerobic organisms and anaerobic organisms, respectively.
   B. Pelvic cellulitis can be caused by fist fornication.
   1. Clinical features. Fever, rectal pain, and discharge are present several hours after the incident.
   2. Evaluation. Sigmoidoscopy should be performed to rule out a transmural laceration.
   3. Management. Patients are hospitalized for close observation and parenteral broad-spectrum antibiotic therapy (see **A.2**).

Fecal Impaction

Fecal impaction is most common in elderly, debilitated patients but can occur in young active people. Predisposing conditions include recent abdominal or anorectal surgery, overuse of constipating drugs (such as codeine or other narcotics), and residual barium from a radiographic study.

I. The **clinical picture** is usually that of a patient who has had no bowel movement for several days and presents with tenesmus, urgency, and cramping abdominal pain. Paradoxical diarrhea may be present, consisting of small amounts of watery stool that pass around the hard impacted bolus, and perianal soiling may be associated with the diarrhea.

II. **Treatment** is aimed at removing the fecal bolus.
   A. Digital examination is necessary to confirm the diagnosis. An attempt should be made to mobilize the bolus at this time.
   B. Saline enemas should then be administered. Soapsud enemas, however, are irritating and should not be used.
   C. Manual removal. If enemas fail, the impaction will have to be removed manually.
   1. Local anesthesia (1% lidocaine) may be required in postoperative patients (such as posthemorrhoidectomy patients).
   2. The patient should be instructed to strain to facilitate digital removal of the impaction.
   3. After removal of the lowest portion of the impaction, a saline enema is administered to evacuate the rest.

III. **Evaluation. Sigmoidoscopy** should be performed after the impaction has been completely removed to rule out a tumor as a contributor to the impaction.

IV. **Prevention**
   A. Recurrent fecal impaction can be prevented by **eliminating factors contributing to the condition.** In particular, constipating medicines should be avoided.
   B. A **psyllium seed preparation,** 1 tsp in a full glass of water twice a day, is recommended.
   C. Enemas should be given as necessary.
   D. Lactulose, 10 ml bid, is useful in severe cases.

Bibliography

1. Brenner, B. E., and Simon, R. R. Anorectal emergencies. *Ann. Emerg. Med.* 12:367, 1983.
2. Centers for Disease Control. 1985 STD treatment guidelines. *M.M.W.R.* 34(Suppl.):75S, 1985.
3. Eisenstat, T., Salvati, E. P., and Rubin, R. J. The outpatient management of acute hemorrhoidal disease. *Dis. Colon Rectum* 22:315, 1979.
4. Goldberg, S. M., Gordon, P. H., and Nivatvongs, S. *Essentials of Anorectal Surgery.* Philadelphia: Lippincott, 1980.
5. Josephson, G. *The male rape victim: Evaluation and treatment. J.A.C.E.P.* 8:13, 1979.
6. Kodner, I. J. *Controversial Topics in Colon and Rectal Surgery.* St. Louis: Mosby, 1985.
7. MacLeod, J. H. *A Method of Proctology.* New York: Harper and Row, 1979.
8. Medical Letter. Treatment of sexually transmitted diseases. *Med. Lett. Drugs Ther.* 28:23, 1986.
9. Sohn, N., Weistein, M. A., and Robbins, R. D. Anorectal disorders. *Current Probl. Surg.* 20(1):1, 1983.

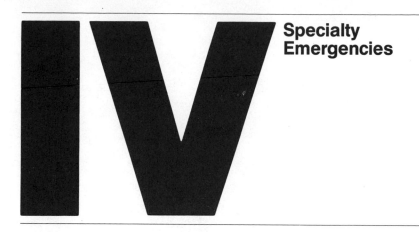

IV

Specialty Emergencies

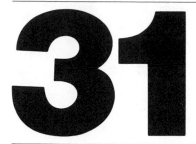

Dermatology

J. Blake Goslen and
Howard G. Welgus

General Management Principles

I. **Dermatologic diagnosis.** To properly classify cutaneous diseases, it is important to have a knowledge of the various types of **primary** and **secondary lesions.**
   A. **Primary lesions**
      1. **Macule:** a flat, cutaneous lesion with associated color change.
      2. **Papule:** an elevated, non-fluid-filled lesion that is less than 1 cm in diameter. A **plaque** is a flat-topped coalescence of papules larger than 1 cm.
      3. **Nodule:** a palpable superficial or deep skin lesion larger than 1 cm.
      4. **Vesicle:** an elevated, fluid-filled blister. A large vesicle is termed a **bulla.** Blisters can be intraepidermal or subepidermal.
      5. **Pustule:** an elevated, pus-filled lesion.
   B. **Secondary changes**
      1. **Scale:** the accumulation of stratum corneum (hyperkeratosis) on the primary lesion.
      2. **Crust:** hemorrhagic, serous, or inflammatory cell-containing material overlying an erosion or ulceration in the skin.
      3. **Excoriation:** an area where the surface of the skin has been scratched away, often leaving a superficial erosion or ulcer with overlying crust.
      4. **Lichenification:** thickened areas of skin with overlying, accentuated skin markings.

II. **Laboratory diagnosis of skin disease.** Certain simple studies are important in the diagnosis of cutaneous disease.
   A. **Potassium hydroxide preparation** (see Chap. 38). The skin is scraped, and scale is removed onto a glass slide. When searching for dermatophytes, the advancing edge of the lesion or the roof of the blister (e.g., bullous tinea pedis) supplies the best material. The specimen is treated with 10–15% potassium hydroxide and covered with a coverslip. The specimen is then lightly heated and examined microscopically. Dermatophyte infections are characterized by the presence of branching, septate hyphae. Candidal infections show nonseptate hyphae and budding yeasts. In tinea versicolor, short hyphae and spores, like "spaghetti and meatballs," are seen.
   B. **Tzanck smear.** Multinucleated giant cells are seen in herpes simplex, herpes zoster, and varicella-zoster infections. Scrapings should be obtained from the roof and base of an unroofed vesicle (see Chap. 38).
   C. **Skin punch biopsy.** A 3- to 4-mm cutaneous punch is used to remove a core of skin, which is then fixed in formalin. It is important to biopsy a primary lesion.

III. **Principles of dermatologic therapy.** Dermatologic therapy can involve topical or systemic agents or both.
   A. **Topical.** Compresses, soaks, antimicrobial drugs, and corticosteroids are the most important topical agents.
      1. **Compresses and soaks.** Soaks are generally used to cleanse and debride a wound of crusts. They are also used to dry weeping and exudative skin lesions, such as those seen in an acute contact dermatitis. Compresses may include 4- × 4-in. gauze sponges, rolled gauze bandages, or even clean linen material. They can be open-wet (continuous or wet-to-dry) or closed-wet; the latter is used less frequently because of the risk of maceration. Wet-to-dry dressings debride more thoroughly than the other types of dressings. Solutions for wet dressings are numerous and include aluminum acetate (Burow's) solution 1:10–1:40, 0.25% acetic acid compresses, or normal saline. Acetic acid is preferred by many physicians because of its anti-Pseudomonas effect and ease of preparation (½ cup of white vinegar/quart of water).

Table 31-1. Classification of topical corticosteroids by potency

High potency
    Amcinonide[a] (Cyclocort), 0.1%
    Betamethasone dipropionate[a] (Diprosone, Diprolene[b]), 0.05%
    Clobetasol propionate[a,b], 0.05%
    Desoximetasone[a] (Topicort), 0.25%
    Diflorasone diacetate[a] (Florone, Maxiflor), 0.05%
    Fluocinonide[a] (Lidex, Topsyn), 0.05%
    Halcinonide[a] (Halog), 0.1%

Intermediate potency
    Betamethasone valerate[a] (Valisone), 0.1%
    Clocortolone pivalate[a] (Cloderm), 0.1%
    Fluocinolone acetonide[a] (Synalar), 0.2%
    Flurandrenolide[a] (Cordran), 0.05%
    Hydrocortisone valerate (Westcort), 0.2%
    Hydrocortisone butyrate 0.1% (Locoid), 0.1%
    Triamcinolone acetonide[a] (Kenalog, Aristocort), 0.1%

Low potency
    Desonide (Tridesilon), 0.05%
    Hydrocortisone, 0.25–2.50%

[a] Fluorinated steroid.
[b] More potent than other class I fluorinated steroids.

2. **Topical antimicrobial agents**
    a. **Antibacterial agents.** Numerous pure antibacterial and combination antibacterial/antifungal/steroid preparations are available. Neosporin has polymyxin B sulfate, zinc bacitracin, and neomycin sulfate. It is available as an ointment, a cream, or a powder. The problem of neomycin sensitivity is obviated in Polysporin, which contains only polymyxin B and bacitracin. Ilotycin ointment contains an erythromycin base and is seldom sensitizing.
    b. **Antifungal agents.** Currently the most effective topical antifungal agents are the synthetic imidazoles (miconazole nitrate 2% [Monistat-Derm], clotrimazole 1% [Mycelex or Lotrimin], and econazole nitrate 1% [Spectazole]). All of these agents are effective against tinea versicolor, dermatophytic fungi, and *Candida albicans*. Nystatin is a polyene antimicrobial that is effective against *Candida*.
    c. **Antiviral agents.** Agents that are efficacious against cutaneous Herpes simplex infections are few. Acyclovir (Zovirax) is a purine nucleoside analogue that can be helpful in initial genital herpes infections and mucocutaneous infections present in immunocompromised hosts. It is not effective against herpes labialis or gingivostomatitis in normal hosts.
3. **Topical corticosteroids** [22, 42]. Corticosteroids are potent antiproliferative and anti-inflammatory agents.
    a. **Potency.** The potency of different corticosteroids varies widely. Changes in structure, including halogenization of key positions in the molecule, have resulted in the generation of topical steroids that are classified as to potency (Table 31-1) by means of a vasoconstrictor assay [49]. The potency is affected by the vehicle with which these drugs are compounded, how they are applied, and the type of skin on which they are applied. In general, the use of occlusive wraps (e.g., Saran Wrap, total body plastic, nylon sauna suits) or ointments (rather than the less occlusive creams, gels, lotions, or sprays) results in increased warmth and humidity of the skin, with consequent increased absorption of the drug. Application of the drugs to areas of thin skin or actively inflamed skin results in increased penetration due to a relative ineffectiveness of the epidermal barrier.
    b. **Usage.** Classically, topical steroids have been applied two or more times a day. There is evidence, however, that single daily use is just as effective [50]. A common problem with the prescription of these drugs has been an under-

Table 31-2. Dispensing of topical corticosteroids

Area to be treated	One application (gm)	bid for 1 week (gm)
Hands, head, face, or anogenital area	2	28
One arm or anterior or posterior trunk	3	42
One leg	4	56
Entire body	30–60	420–840

Table 31-3. Adverse effects of topical corticosteroids

Systemic	Local
Hypothalamic-pituitary-adrenal axis suppression	Atrophy
Iatrogenic Cushing's syndrome	Striae*
Growth retardation	Telangiectasia
	Purpura
	Impaired wound healing
	Steroid rosacea
	Perioral dermatitis
	Hypertrichosis
	Pigment abnormality (hypopigmentation)
	Glaucoma, cataracts
	Aggravation of local infections

*Irreversible even after discontinuation of the drug.
Source: Adapted from E. E. Bondi and A. M. Kligman, Adverse effects of topical corticosteroids. *Prog. Dermatol.* 14:1, 1980.

estimation of the quantity of drug needed to effectively treat a particular dermatosis. Table 31-2 provides some realistic guidelines.

  c. **Adverse effects.** The complications of prolonged topical steroid use are summarized in Table 31-3 [9]. The more lengthy the course of treatment and the more potent the drug, the greater the risk of these complications. The use of the potent, fluorinated steroids on thin-skinned areas, such as the face and genitalia, generally should be avoided.
B. **Systemic.** Systemic antihistamines, retinoids, antibiotics, corticosteroids, antimalarials, and a variety of other drugs are widely used in the treatment of skin disease.
  1. **Antihistamines** are widely used in dermatology, especially the H_1 antagonists [11]. Antihistamines function as competitive antagonists of histamine at tissue-receptor sites. A summary of the H_1 antihistamines is presented in Table 31-4. If a patient does not respond to one class of antihistamines, an agent from a different class should be selected. The tricyclic antidepressants also have antihistaminic activity and can be used instead of or in addition to the classic antihistamines [7].
  Adverse effects of antihistamines include sedation and other central nervous system (CNS) manifestations (including paradoxical hyperirritability) gastrointestinal intolerance, dry mouth, urinary retention, diplopia, and other anticholinergic effects. Since the ethylenediamine antihistamines may cross react with other drugs containing the ethylenediamine moiety (e.g., aminophylline), they are contraindicated in patients sensitive to ethylenediamine. Topical antihistamines should be avoided because of their high incidence of sensitization.
  2. **Retinoids.** Isotretinoin (Accutane) is a synthetic retinoid useful in the treatment of cystic acne. When given in a dosage of 1–2 mg/kg/day, remarkable long-term remissions of cystic acne are obtainable [38, 46]. Dose-related side effects are common and include dry skin and cheilitis in virtually all patients.

Table 31-4. Summary of H_1 antihistamines

Class	Representative examples	Usual adult oral dosage	Comments
Ethanolamine	Diphenhydramine (Benadryl)	25–50 mg q4–6h	Marked sedation; significant anticholinergic activity; less gastrointestinal intolerance compared with other antihistamines
	Clemastine fumarate (Tavist)	1.34–2.68 mg q8–12h	
Ethylenediamine	Tripelennamine hydrochloride (Pyribenzamine)	50 mg q4h	Avoid in ethylenediamine-sensitive patients; moderate gastrointestinal intolerance
Hydroxyzine	Hydroxyzine hydrochloride (Atarax)	10–25 mg q4–6h	Most effective drug in histamine-induced pruritus; cross reacts with ethylenediamine; anticholinergic effects
	Hydroxyzine pamoate (Vistaril)	10–25 mg q4–6h	
Alkylamine	Brompheniramine maleate (Dimetane)	4 mg q4h	Lower incidence of sedation, but stimulation is more frequent
	Chlorpheniramine maleate (Chlor-Trimeton)	4–8 mg q4h	
	Dexchlorpheniramine maleate (Polarimine)	2 mg q4h	
Phenothiazine	Promethazine hydrochloride (Phenergan)	1.25 mg q4–6h	Sedation; anticholinergic effects; antiemetic activity; may produce photosensitivity
Piperidine	Cyproheptadine hydrochloride (Periactin)	4 mg q4h	Cyproheptadine has antiserotonin activity; useful in cold urticaria
	Azatadine maleate (Optimine)	1–2 mg bid	
Piperazine	Chlorcyclizine hydrochloride (Fedrazil)	25 mg q6h	May cross react with ethylenediamine
	Cyclizine hydrochloride (Marezine)	50 mg q4–6h	
	Meclizine hydrochloride (Bonine, Antivert)	25 mg q6h	

Source: Adapted from O. B. Christensen and H. I. Maibach, Antihistamines in dermatology. *Semin. Dermatol.* 2:270, 1983.

Additional side effects are headache, alopecia, skin fragility, arthralgias, skeletal hyperostoses [39], and eye irritation. Laboratory abnormalities include dose-related elevations of liver function tests and hypertriglyceridemia. Most important, isotretinoin is teratogenic and should *not* be given to women in child-bearing years without the certainty of effective contraception [6].

3. **Corticosteroids.** Systemic corticosteroids (usually prednisone) are used in acute inflammatory dermatoses, such as contact dermatitis from poison ivy. In this

setting, the drug is usually given in a tapering dose over approximately 2 weeks. Long-term administration of corticosteroids for chronic dermatoses, such as psoriasis, atopic dermatitis, or alopecia areata, is difficult to rationalize and may lead to serious complications. See Chap. 14 for further discussion of corticosteroid therapy and Table 14-3 for complications of their systemic use.

4. **Antibiotics** are used to treat primary and secondary skin infections. See Chap. 12 for a discussion of systemic antibiotics.

5. **Antimalarials,** such as chloroquine, hydroxychloroquine, or quinacrine, are used in the management of certain inflammatory skin disorders [30]. Their most common use is in the treatment of lupus erythematosus and certain photodermatoses. Chloroquine in small doses (125 mg twice weekly) has been used to treat porphyria cutanea tarda. Toxicity of these agents includes skin pigmentation, leukopenia, and retinopathy. Baseline eye examinations should be done prior to therapy and every 4–6 months thereafter.

IV. **Disposition.** Most patients with dermatologic disorders can be managed on an outpatient basis. Hospitalization, however, is indicated for the therapy of widespread dermatoses such as exfoliative erythroderma or bullous disorders such as pemphigus or toxic epidermal necrolysis. Hospitalization is also warranted when the cutaneous disorder is associated with significant fever, infection, or signs of systemic toxicity or when the cutaneous disorder may compromise adequate fluid or nutritional intake.

Hypersensitivity Disorders

Hypersensitivity disorders are immunologically mediated cutaneous reaction patterns precipitated by a number of etiologic factors. These disorders include urticaria, erythema multiforme, drug reactions, toxic epidermal necrolysis, and erythema nodosum.

I. **Urticaria and angioedema**
   A. **Etiology. Urticaria** (hives) is an acute or chronic cutaneous vascular reaction pattern involving only the superficial layers of the skin. When the reaction extends into the deep dermis or subcutaneous tissue or involves the submucosa, it is called **angioedema.** In **acute urticaria,** the cause of the eruption is usually identifiable. Drugs, foods (e.g., berries, shellfish, nuts), radiocontrast media, and acute infection are often implicated. Urticaria lasting more than 6 weeks is termed **chronic urticaria.** Here a myriad of causative agents or associated disorders have been reported, including drugs, foods and food additives, focal areas of chronic infection (e.g., involving the sinuses or oral cavity), inhalants, parasitic infections, collagen vascular diseases, urticarial vasculitis, hepatitis, internal malignancies, and physical agents (e.g., heat, cold, pressure, sunlight, exercise).
   B. **Pathophysiology.** In most cases, urticaria and angioedema are immunoglobulin E (IgE)–mediated. Mast cell degranulation also can occur, however, via nonimmunologic events. Certain drugs (e.g., polymyxin B, opioids) frequently are implicated.
   C. **Clinical features.** The primary lesion is the wheal. Individual lesions are transitory and seldom persist for more than 24 hours. Tissue edema is also present and may cause respiratory compromise. Pruritis is usually a prominent feature.
   D. **Evaluation.** In most cases of urticaria, laboratory findings are normal. Nevertheless, in an effort to determine the cause of **chronic urticaria,** a complete history and physical examination should be accompanied by the following screening laboratory studies: complete blood count (CBC) and differential, stool guaiac, urinalysis, serum blood urea nitrogen (BUN) or creatinine, liver function tests, and a chest x-ray. An erythrocyte sedimentation rate, total hemolytic complement, and skin biopsy are indicated if urticarial vasculitis (i.e., individual hives lasting longer than 24 hours, areas of purpura within hives) is suspected. In this condition, a skin biopsy shows leukocytoclastic vasculitis, the total hemolytic complement is low, and the sedimentation rate is elevated [47]. In chronic urticaria, additional studies (other than perhaps dental and sinus films) are rarely useful if the above screening procedures are normal [28].
   E. **Therapy.** Acutely, patients may be given parenteral antihistamines. In addition, epinephrine, 0.3–0.5 mg of a 1:1000 solution can be given SC q20–30min for up to 3 doses (unless contraindicated), particularly if anaphylaxislike symptoms are present. For chronic therapy, antihistamines (either H_1 blockers alone or H_1 and H_2 blockers together) may be given. A short course of systemic steroids is useful in resistant cases. In addition, certain diet or other antigen elimination programs may be warranted.

Table 31-5. Drugs commonly causing cutaneous reactions

Drug	Reaction rate (reactions/1000 recipients)
Trimethoprim-sulfamethoxasole	59
Ampicillin	52
Semisynthetic penicillins	36
Erythromycin	23
Sulfisoxasole	17
Penicillin G	16
Gentamicin	16
Practolol	16
Cephalosporins	13
Quinidine	12
Mercurial diuretics	9.5
Nitrofurantoin	9.1
Heparin	7.7
Chloramphenicol	6.8
Methenamine	6.4

Source: Adapted from K. A. Arndt and H. Jick, Rates of cutaneous reactions to drugs: A report from the Boston Collaborative Drug Surveillance Program. *J.A.M.A.* 235:918, 1976.

II. Drug reactions

A. Definition and etiology. Cutaneous reactions to drugs are relatively common (Table 31-5) and can occur in 2–3% of medical inpatients [4]. The reactions may take numerous forms and can mimic other dermatoses. A partial list of the types of reactions seen and representative drugs that may cause each are presented in Table 31-6 [16].

B. Clinical features. Drug reactions have a varied presentation (see Table 31-6). The most common eruptions are urticarial and exanthematous, and they usually occur within a week of starting the drug. Some reactions (especially those involving penicillin) can begin several days after the drug has been discontinued.

C. Therapy. The offending drug should be discontinued. If there is a question as to the drug involved, all likely candidates (see Table 31-6) should be stopped or substituted for, if possible. Systemic steroids and antihistamines are often needed for resolution.

III. Erythema multiforme (EM)

A. Definition and pathophysiology. EM is a distinct hypersensitivity disorder with characteristic cutaneous features. It is immunologically mediated, most likely by an immune complex mechanism [27].

B. Etiology. The eruption may be associated with a variety of infections and drugs (see Table 31-6). Herpes simplex virus and *Mycoplasma pneumoniae* are the most commonly associated infectious agents.

C. Clinical features. EM represents a spectrum of disease from a mild syndrome having minimal mucous membrane changes **(erythema multiforme minor)** to generalized cutaneous vesiculation and necrolysis with incapacitating mucous membrane involvement **(erythema multiforme major, or Stevens-Johnson syndrome).** The more severe form of the disease may be indistinguishable from toxic epidermal necrolysis (see **IV**).

EM often presents with a prodrome of fever, malaise, and respiratory symptoms suggesting a flulike illness. Cutaneous lesions begin as symmetric, acral, erythematous papules. Vesiculation and necrosis are seen centrally (blue-gray coloration), surrounded by an erythematous border (target lesion). In more severe cases, blistering is widespread, and the mucous membranes are affected. There are erosions in the mouth and a hemorrhagic crusting of the lower lip. Ocular findings most commonly include conjunctivitis; corneal ulceration, anterior uveitis, and panophthalmitis may also occur.

Table 31-6. Common drug eruptions and important drugs that may be causative*

Acneform
  Actinomycin D
  Bromides
  Corticosteroids
  Disulfiram
  Iodides
  Isoniazid
  Lithium
  Phenytoin
  Quinine
  Thiouracil
Alopecia
  Anovulatory agents
  Anticoagulants
  Chemotherapeutic agents
  Clofibrate
  Colchicine
  Vitamin A
Erythema multiforme
  Barbiturates
  Chlorpropamide
  Furosemide
  Nonsteroidal anti-inflammatory
    agents
  Penicillin
  Phenolphthalein
  Phenytoin
  Sulfonamides
  Thiazides
Erythema nodosum
  Anovulatory agents
  Bromides
  Codeine
  Iodides
  Penicillin
  Salicylates
  Sulfonamides
Exanthematous
  Allopurinol
  Carbamazepine
  Chloramphenicol
  Erythromycin
  Gold
  Isoniazid
  Penicillin
  Phenytoin
  Sulfonamides
  Tetracycline
Exfoliative
  Actinomycin D
  Allopurinol
  Aminosalicylic acid
  Arsenicals
  Barbiturates
  Bismuth
  Chloroquine
  Chlorpromazine
  Gold
  Griseofulvin
  Iodides
  Mercury

Penicillin
Phenothiazines
Phenylbutazone
Phenytoin
Quinacrine
Quinidine
Stilbestrol
Streptomycin
Sulfonamides
Tetracycline
Thiouracil
Vitamin A
Fixed drug eruptions
  Barbiturates
  Phenolphthalein
  Phenylbutazone
  Sulfonamides
  Tetracycline
Lichenoid
  Antimalarials
  Bismuth
  Chlordiazepoxide
  Chlorpropamide
  Furosemide
  Gold
  Meprobamate
  Methyldopa
  Para-aminosalicylic acid
  Phenothiazines
  Propranolol
  Quinidine
  Thiazides
Lupuslike eruption
  Carbamazepine
  Hydralazine
  Methyldopa
  Phenytoin
  Procainamide
  Thiouracil
Photosensitive
  Amiodarone
  Griseofulvin
  Nalidixic acid
  Phenothiazines
  Psoralens
  Quinidine
  Sulfonamides
  Sulfonylureas
  Tetracycline
  Thiazides
Pityriasis rosealike eruptions
  Arsenicals
  Barbiturates
  Bismuth
  Captopril
  Clonidine
  Gold
  Metronidazole
  Tripelennamine
Porphyria cutanea tarda-like eruption
  Alcohol

Table 31-6 (continued)

Porphyria cutanea tarda-like eruption
(continued)
Estrogens
Furosemide
Nalidixic acid
Tetracycline

Psoriasiform reactions or flares of existing psoriasis
Antimalarials
Cimetidine
Clonidine
Ethanol
Gold
Lithium
Methyldopa
Nonsteroidal anti-inflammatory
agents
Propranolol

Purpura
Allopurinol
Anticoagulants
Barbiturates
Bromides
Corticosteroids
Ephedrine
Iodides
Meprobamate
Penicillin
Quinidine
Quinine
Sulfonamides
Thiazides

Toxic epidermal necrolysis
Allopurinol
Barbiturates
Hydantoins
Penicillin
Phenylbutazone
Sulfonamides

Urticaria
Allopurinol
Antimony
Antipyrines
Barbiturates
Bismuth
Chloral hydrate

Chloramphenicol
Chlorpromazine
Erythromycin
Fluorides
Gold
Griseofulvin
Iodides
Insulin
Isoniazid
Menthol
Meprobamate
Mercury
Nitrofurantoin
Nonsteroidal anti-inflammatory
agents
Opioids
Penicillin
Phenacetin
Pilocarpine
Poliomyelitis vaccine
Procaine
Promethazine
Quinine
Reserpine
Saccharin
Serums
Sulfonamides
Tetracycline
Thiamine hydrochloride
Thiouracil

Vasculitis
Allopurinol
Hydantoin
Gold
Phenothiazines
Sulfonamides
Thiazides
Thiouracil

Vesiculobullous
Barbiturates
Bromides
Furosemide
Indomethacin
Iodides
Penicillamine
Propranolol
Rifampin

*This table lists drugs more commonly associated with various drug eruptions. Other drugs, however, may produce such cutaneous reactions.
Source: Adapted from A. N. Domonkos, H. L. Arnold, Jr., and R. B. Odom, *Andrews' Diseases of the Skin: Clinical Dermatology* (7th ed.). Philadelphia: Saunders, 1982. Pp. 125–131.

D. Therapy. Supportive treatment as well as therapy for any associated infection should be instituted. Possible drug causes should be eliminated. Early ophthalmologic evaluation is important. Although controversial, systemic steroids are generally given in severely affected patients. The initial dosage is 60–80 mg of prednisone/day. Hospitalization is required for patients with severe skin and mucous membrane involvement or fever.

IV. Toxic epidermal necrolysis (TEN)

A. **Definition.** TEN is a rare but devastating cutaneous reaction in which large areas of skin become erythematous and then slough with minimal trauma.

B. **Etiology.** The eruption has been associated, in most instances, with drugs (see Table 31-6). Other etiologic factors such as viral and other infections, vaccinations, and neoplastic processes have been associated with TEN. Many cases, however, remain idiopathic.

C. **Pathology.** In TEN, there is subepidermal blister formation with epidermal cell necrosis. A similar condition seen in children, the staphylococcal scalded skin syndrome (SSSS) (see **Infectious Diseases,** sec. **II.B**), shows a subcorneal blistering process pathologically [18]. The differentiation of these two diseases is important, as the management of TEN is quite different from that of SSSS. These two conditions can be differentiated rapidly by the use of a frozen-section skin biopsy.

D. **Clinical features.** Cutaneous findings are dramatic. The skin is diffusely erythematous (scalded). Lateral finger pressure in an area of erythema produces denudation of skin **(Nikolsky's sign).** Widespread vesiculation and sloughing of the epidermis subsequently occurs. Mucous membranes of the oral cavity, eye, and gastrointestinal and respiratory tracts are affected. In addition to cutaneous disease, patients may also have fever, malaise, and symptoms suggesting a flulike illness. Pulmonary infiltrates are sometimes present. Cutaneous fluid and protein loss may lead to vascular collapse.

E. **Management.** Hospitalization is mandatory. The systemic administration of corticosteroids is helpful in a dose of 150–250 mg of prednisone/day; after new lesions cease to occur, the steroids are slowly tapered. Topical skin care includes the application of a topical antibiotic under a nonadherent dressing (e.g., Telfa) and efforts to prevent frictional injury to the skin. Intensive supportive care is necessary with careful monitoring of the fluid and electrolyte status, as well as renal and cardiopulmonary function. The high incidence of mortality from secondary infection in this disease merits aggressive administration of systemic antibiotics at the earliest signs of infection.

V. Erythema nodosum (EN)

A. **Definition.** EN is a hypersensitivity reaction in the subcutaneous fat.

B. **Etiology.** EN can be seen in association with a number of systemic infections, including deep fungal, streptococcal, mycobacterial, and *Yersinia* infections. It can also be seen with sarcoidosis, Behçet's syndrome, inflammatory bowel disease, and certain medications, especially birth control pills, sulfonamides, and halides (see Table 31-6) [8].

C. **Clinical features.** EN usually appears in the pretibial areas as red, nonulcerative subcutaneous nodules. Lesions resolve gradually, becoming bruised in appearance.

D. **Therapy.** Attempts to identify and control any underlying disease or eliminate any precipitating drug should be undertaken. Therapy may include bed rest and the use of a nonsteroidal anti-inflammatory agent or, occasionally, systemic steroids.

Papulosquamous Disorders

The papulosquamous dermatoses are typically those characterized by papular or plaquelike lesions of varying color and configuration that also show significant epidermal alteration (e.g., scaling).

I. Psoriasis

A. **Etiology and pathogenesis.** Psoriasis is a hyperproliferative reaction of the epidermis. Genetic and environmental factors are contributory [13].

B. **Clinical features.** The disorder can appear at any age. Initially, there are reddish papules and plaques with an overlying silvery scale. Occasionally, explosive development of psoriasis may present as small scaly papules that are widely distributed **(guttate psoriasis).** Common areas of distribution include the extensor surfaces of the extremities, umbilicus, scalp, and genitalia. The nails show diffuse pitting, onycholysis, or yellowish subungual spots. Occasionally, psoriasis presents with pustules that may be either localized to the palms and soles or diffusely distributed **(generalized pustular psoriasis of von Zumbusch)** [5]. There is also a erythrodermic form of psoriasis. These latter two variants are often associated with prominent systemic toxicity. Approximately 5–10% of patients with psoriasis have an associated arthritis that is most commonly an asymmetric oligoarthritis [2, 41].

C. **Differential diagnosis.** Psoriasiform lesions can be seen in certain drug reactions (e.g., secondary to B blockers, lithium, gold, methyldopa) [20]. Likewise, seborrheic dermatitis, pityriasis rosea, parapsoriasis, secondary syphilis, candidiasis (especially in intertriginous areas), subacute lupus erythematosus, and mycosis fungoides can resemble psoriasis. Pustular psoriasis can be confused with fungal infections, bacterial pyodermas, and occasionally sepsis.

D. **Therapy**
1. **Phototherapy.** Ultraviolet light therapy is widely used, alone or combined with topical tar products **(Goeckerman regimen).** Impressive clearing of plaque-type and guttate psoriasis is possible [36]. Adverse effects include the development of skin cancers in irradiated areas [48].
2. **Corticosteroids.** Systemic steroids should be avoided in psoriasis. However, topical steroids are widely used, but remissions achieved with topical steroids are short-lived. Furthermore, tachyphylaxis is common with these agents.
3. **Methotrexate** and hydroxyurea have been used in widespread, debilitating psoriasis. Dosages for methotrexate vary from 10–25 mg/week. Caution is advised because the drug has been associated with progressive cirrhosis. Liver biopsies are indicated prior to therapy and periodically thereafter [43].

E. **Disposition.** Although most cases of psoriasis can be managed on an outpatient basis, hospitalization is indicated for patients with a severe, poorly controlled flare, pustular psoriasis, or exfoliative psoriasis.

II. **Seborrheic dermatitis**
A. **Etiology and pathophysiology.** Seborrheic dermatitis is a hyperproliferative inflammatory scaling disorder of unknown cause.
B. **Clinical features.** Patients complain of excessive dandruff associated with itching. Examination reveals scaling and erythema in characteristic areas: scalp, external ear, intertriginous regions, presternal area, and face (especially the glabella, nasolabial folds, eyebrows, and beard area).
C. **Differential diagnosis.** Seborrheic dermatitis can be confused with psoriasis, tinea capitis, zinc and essential fatty acid deficiencies, lupus erythematosus, and pityriasis rubra pilaris. In children, histiocytosis X and Leiner's disease may have an appearance similar to that of seborrheic dermatitis.
D. **Therapy**
1. Treatment includes frequent **shampooing with antiseborrheic shampoos.** These shampoos may contain 2.5% selenium sulfide (Selsun), zinc pyrithione (Danex, Head and Shoulders, DHS), salicylic acid–sulfur (Sebulex, Ionil, Vanseb) or tar products (Ionil-T, T/Gel, Pentrax, Sebutone).
2. For inflammatory areas, a **corticosteroid** is useful. On the face, 1% hydrocortisone is all that is needed. For the scalp, solutions (Synalar, Fluonid) or sprays (Aeroseb) are better tolerated.

III. **Lichen planus**
A. **Etiology and pathophysiology.** The cause of lichen planus is unknown, but an epidermal autoimmune process is suspected.
B. **Clinical features.** Lichen planus is characteristically very pruritic. Lesions appear as flat-topped, violaceous, polygonal papules whose surface is laced with white striae **(Wickham's striae).** Characteristic areas for lesions are the ventral wrists, anterior thighs, and genitalia. Oral involvement is present in many patients and may be asymptomatic; usually there are reticulated white patches and, occasionally, erosions on the buccal mucosa or tongue.
C. **Differential diagnosis.** Lichen planus–like eruptions can be seen in early graftversus-host (GVH) disease and following administration of certain drugs (see Table 31-6) [16].
D. **Therapy.** Systemic or topical steroids (or both) are the most effective therapeutic agents.

IV. **Pityriasis rosea (PR)**
A. **Etiology and pathophysiology.** PR is a common, self-limited, papulosquamous process of unknown cause. It seldom occurs more than once in the same individual.
B. **Clinical features.** PR occurs in younger patients (10–35 years old). Symptoms of itching and burning are variable. Diffuse lesions are often preceded by a single, larger, scaly patch on the trunk ("herald patch"). Diffuse lesions appear reddish with a peripheral collarette of scale. They are oval and lie in the direction of skin tension lines in a Christmas tree–like pattern. Most lesions are on the trunk or proximal extremities. Spontaneous resolution occurs in 6–8 weeks.
C. **Differential diagnosis.** Other causes of a PR-like eruption include tinea versicolor,

Table 31-7. Disorders associated with exfoliative dermatitis

Preexisting dermatoses
    Eczema
    Psoriasis
    Seborrheic dermatitis
    Lichen planus
    Pityriasis rubra pilaris
    Mycosis fungoides
    Dermatophytosis
    Reiter's syndrome
Drug reactions
Internal malignancy (carcinoma, leukemia, lymphoma)
Idiopathic

    guttate psoriasis, drug reactions (see Table 31-6), and, most important, secondary syphilis.

  D. Treatment is symptomatic and includes use of topical antipruritics or steroids, systemic antihistamines, and ultraviolet B (UVB) light.

V. Exfoliative dermatitis. Exfoliative dermatitis (erythroderma) is a generalized cutaneous reaction pattern characterized by scaling and redness due to a variety of etiologies (Table 31-7) [1, 26, 34]. Problems with body temperature control and hydration can occur in severe cases. Hospitalization is warranted for all patients with exfoliative dermatitis except for those with well-tolerated, chronic exfoliative dermatitis that has been adequately evaluated. The workup generally should include a CBC with differential; urinalysis; serum BUN, creatinine, and electrolytes; a Venereal Disease Research Laboratory (VDRL) test; liver function tests; stool examination for occult blood; and a chest x-ray. Skin biopsies should be done in multiple areas; if a primary lesion is noted, it should also be biopsied. Initial therapy usually involves application of topical steroids with occlusion (with nylon or a plastic sauna suit).

Systemic Diseases and Rashes

Some systemic diseases have such characteristic cutaneous manifestations that a diagnosis can be made solely by examination of the skin. Conversely, certain dermatologic presentations can be associated with a variety of systemic illnesses.

I. Systemic diseases with specific cutaneous findings

  A. Dermatomyositis: violaceous edema of the eyelids (heliotrope), atrophic flat-topped papules over the metacarpophalangeal (MCP) joints (Gottron's papules), and periungual telangiectasias.

  B. Scleroderma: sclerodactyly, periungual and matlike telangiectasias, finger-tip ulcerations, and a confettilike hypopigmentation.

  C. Reiter's syndrome: a hyperkeratotic and pustular eruption of the palms and soles (keratoderma blennorhagicum), circinate balanitis, and mucous membrane changes involving the conjunctivae and oral cavity.

  D. Behçet's syndrome: oral and genital aphthouslike ulcerations, erythema nodosum, and pustular vasculitic lesions in areas of trauma (pathergy).

  E. Sarcoidosis: flesh- or apple jelly–colored, smooth-topped papules or plaques around the eyes, nose, and mouth.

  F. Relapsing polychondritis: red, painful, swollen ears.

  G. Nail-patella syndrome: triangular nail lunulae.

  H. Pseudoxanthoma elasticum: tan-yellow papules and plaques in flexural areas resembling plucked-chicken skin.

  I. Diabetes mellitus: atrophic, reddish-yellow plaques on the pretibial areas (necrobiosis lipoidica diabeticorum).

  J. Amyloidosis: waxy papules on the neck and around the eyes that become purpuric with mild trauma ("pinch purpura").

  K. Hyperthyroidism: moist soft skin, alopecia, onycholysis, clubbing (acropachy), and pretibial mucinous infiltration (pretibial myxedema).

  L. Hypothyroidism: macroglossia; cold, pale dry skin; and loss of dull coarse hair.

M. Hyperlipidemia: yellowish-brown papules, plaques, and nodules (plane, eruptive, striatum palmare, tendinous, or tuberous).

N. Cushing's syndrome: moonlike facies, truncal obesity with a buffalo hump, striae, acneiform eruption, and purpura.

O. Addison's syndrome: hyperpigmentation of scars, palmar creases, gingiva, and sun-exposed areas.

P. Neurofibromatosis: six or more regularly bordered hyperpigmented macules 1.5 cm in size or greater (café au lait), axillary freckling, and typical flesh-colored, pedunculated papules of various sizes (neurofibromas).

Q. Tuberous sclerosis: hypopigmented macules at birth (ash leaf macules), fleshy red-colored papules of the central face (adenoma sebaceum), and periungual fibromas.

R. Peutz-Jehgers: brownish frecklelike macules around the mouth and on the fingers.

S. Osler-Weber-Rendu syndrome: multiple telangiectatic lesions on the skin and mucous membranes.

T. Mastocytosis: brownish-red macules or papules, or macular reddish-brown areas with prominent telangiectasias (telangiectasia macularis eruptiva perstans) that urticate on scratching their surface (Darier's sign).

U. Porphyria cutanea tarda: hyperpigmentation, hypertrichosis generally; blisters and milia on the dorsal surface of the hands.

II. Cutaneous signs associated with multiple systemic illnesses

A. Pyoderma gangrenosum. This lesion is characterized by an ulceration with violaceous, tender borders that are extensively undermined. Associated systemic diseases include inflammatory bowel disease, myeloma or paraproteinemias, chronic active hepatitis, rheumatoid arthritis, leukemia, lymphoma, polycythemia vera, and myeloid metaplasia [21].

B. Pruritis without primary skin lesions: chronic renal failure, cholestatic hepatitis, polycythemia vera, lymphoma, leukemia, mastocytosis, myeloma, hyperthyroidism, carcinoid syndrome, diabetes mellitus, malignancy, old age, and a variety of drugs [23].

C. Leg ulcers: sickle cell disease and other hemoglobinopathies, rheumatoid arthritis, vasculitis, metastatic tumors, hypertension, polycythemia vera, dysproteinemia, deep fungal infections, syphilis, mycobacterial infections, diabetes mellitus, Werner's syndrome, embolic disease, and peripheral vascular disease.

D. Livedo reticularis. This cutaneous pattern consists of a brownish-red, reticulated macular eruption. Associated disorders include polyarteritis nodosa or other vasculitides, cryoglobulinemia, homocystinuria, primary oxalosis, paraproteinemias, hyperviscosity syndrome, polycythemia vera, systemic lupus erythematosus, thrombotic thrombocytopenic purpura, and thrombocytosis.

E. Leonine facies: mycosis fungoides or other lymphomas, carcinoid syndrome (later stages), and Hansen's disease.

F. Flushing reactions: pheochromocytoma, carcinoid syndrome, and mastocytosis [52].

G. Acanthosis nigricans. There is a velvety hyperpigmentation of the axillae or other intertriginous areas. The pattern may be seen with obesity, malignancies, and endocrinologic disorders such as diabetes mellitus, Cushing's syndrome, or Stein-Leventhal syndrome.

H. Generalized hyperpigmentation: Addison's syndrome, Cushing's syndrome, hemochromatosis, Whipple's disease, Cronkhite-Canada syndrome, primary biliary cirrhosis, pernicious anemia, pellagra, porphyria cutanea tarda, adrenocorticotropic hormone (ACTH)–producing tumor, and hyperthyroidism [25].

I. Hirsutism: ovarian, pituitary, or adrenal virilizing conditions; hypertrichosis lanuginosa associated with malignancy; anorexia nervosa or malnutrition; CNS disorders; and a number of porphyrias.

J. Digital gangrene: collagen vascular diseases such as scleroderma, lupus erythematosus, or vasculitis; embolic phenomenon; paraproteinemias or cryoglobulinemia; and drug-related effects from vinyl chloride, bleomycin, ergotamines, beta-blockers, alpha-adrenergic agonists, or methylsergide [12].

K. Leukocytoclastic vasculitis, urticaria, erythema nodosum, erythema multiforme, and aphthous stomatitis. These cutaneous signs are discussed elsewhere in this chapter.

III. Cutaneous disorders associated with an underlying malignancy

A. Acanthosis nigricans is a velvety thickening and hyperpigmentation of the axillae and, occasionally, other intertriginous areas. It is usually associated with an adenocarcinoma of the gastrointestinal tract.

B. Adult-onset dermatomyositis. See sec. I.A.

C. **Superficial migratory thrombophlebitis.** There is redness and tenderness over the course of superficial veins. It has been associated with carcinoma of the pancreas.

D. **Acquired ichthyosis** is an acquired drying of the skin with rhomboid-appearing scales prominent on the extremities. It has been associated with lymphoproliferative disorders.

E. **Erythema gyratum repens** refers to undulating wavy bands of slightly raised erythema involving the entire body.

F. **Hypertrichosis lanuginosa.** There is a striking increased growth of lanugo hair.

G. **Acquired pachydermoperiostosis** is a hypertrophic osteoarthropathy associated with thickened skin and acromegaloid features.

H. **Multicentric reticulohistiocytosis** is characterized by papulonodular skin lesions, commonly on the hands, associated with an arthropathy.

I. **Leser-Trélat** is characterized by the rapid onset and growth of multiple seborrheic keratoses.

J. **Acrokeratosis paraneoplastica.** There are psoriasiform-like plum-colored lesions appearing on the digits, ears, and nose. This cutaneous disorder is highly associated with tumors of the upper respiratory and gastrointestinal tracts.

K. **Necrolytic migratory erythema** is characterized by scaly, red annular lesions with peripheral bullae that appear in intertriginous areas and spread centrifugally. The pattern is seen with glucagonomas.

Infestations and Bites

A wide variety of arthropods that sting and bite can affect the integument. In addition, a host of marine life can affect the skin.

I. **Spiders, mites, and ticks**

A. **Spiders** (see Chap. 22)

1. The **black widow spider** *(Latrodectus mactans)* is the prototype of bites by the *Latrodectus* genus [14]. The female black widow is identified by a red hourglass marking on her ventral surface.

   a. **Clinical features.** The bite produces local pain with or without a prominent local reaction. Common sites are the genitalia and buttocks. Systemic symptoms begin within 15–60 minutes after the bite and consist of severe generalized muscle pains and cramping, nausea and vomiting, chills, and sweating.

   b. **Management.** Topical care includes the application of ice packs and topical corticosteroids in mild cases. In severe local reactions, application of a proximal tourniquet, incision of the bite area and suction to remove venom, and administration of horse serum antivenom (Lyovac) are indicated. Systemic reactions are treated supportively and specifically with the use of Lyovac. Muscles spasms can be managed with 10% calcium gluconate, 10 ml q4h, or methocarbamol, 10 ml IV over 5 minutes initially. Hospitalization is indicated for most severe local reactions and systemic reactions.

2. North American loxoscelism is caused by the bite of the **brown recluse spider** *(Loxosceles reclusa)*. This spider has a characteristic violin-shaped darkened area on the dorsal cephalothorax.

   a. **Clinical features.** The bite produces pain within 2–8 hours, which can be followed by an area of venom-induced ischemic necrosis that produces an angulated ulceration with an overlying dark eschar. Systemic manifestations may be negligible or may include fever, nausea and vomiting, or even shock, renal failure, or coma. There may also be evidence of hemolysis or disseminated intravascular coagulation [15].

   b. **Management.** Hospitalization is indicated for severe local and systemic reactions. Therapy with high doses of systemic steroids (e.g., 100 mg of prednisone/day) is indicated for large bites (i.e., > 2 cm in diameter) and for patients with systemic reactions. For patients with smaller lesions, intralesional steroids (e.g., triamcinolone acetonide [Kenalog-40 Injection], 20–40 mg) at the borders of the bite site may be helpful. Other reported but more controversial therapies include the use of dapsone [29] and wide surgical excision. A specific antivenom may be available in the near future [40].

B. **Mites**

1. **Scabies** (see Chap. 33) is caused by the mite *Sarcoptes scabiei.* It is transmitted by intimate personal contact with an infected individual.

   a. **Clinical features.** After an incubation period of approximately 1 month, pruritus begins. Clinical lesions (i.e., papules, papulovesicles, and pathognomonic burrows) are seen. Lesions are commonly found on the genitalia, finger webs, ventral wrists, and breasts. The head and neck are characteristically spared in adults but may be involved in young children. The organism can be seen by scraping a papule or burrow (especially the gray-black dot at one end) with a No. 15 blade and examining the material in mineral oil under low power.

    b. Treatment of adults consists of the application of gamma benzene hexachloride (Kwell) to the entire body area from the neck down; this medication is left on for 8 hours and is usually repeated in 1 week. Close contacts should also be treated. Clothing is washed in hot water or dry-cleaned. Alternative treatment consists of crotamiton (Eurax), applied for 48 hours; crotamiton is the treatment of choice in small children, because gamma benzene hexachloride has been associated with CNS toxicity in this age group.

  2. Harvest mites (chiggers). Harvest mite larvae reside in grassy areas. Bites usually appear as red papules or papulovesicles and occur in areas of restrictive clothing (belts, underwear). Lesions may be treated with topical steroids and antipruritics (e.g., pramoxine, camphor- or menthol-containing shake lotions).

  3. Other mites. Food, grain, murine, canine, or fowl mites may produce lesions similar to those of the harvest mite. A chronic course may result unless the organisms are eradicated at their source (e.g., by treating affected pets with gamma benzene hexachloride). Therapy of individual bites is as discussed under harvest mites (see **2**).

 C. Ticks. See Chap. 22.

II. Insects

 A. Lice

  1. Head louse *(Pediculosis humanus* var. *capitis)*

    a. Clinical features. Symptoms include pruritus of the scalp and neck. Examination reveals the presence of nits (i.e., whitish eggs firmly attached to the hair shaft approximately 1 cm from the scalp). Lice themselves can be seen in the hair but usually are few in number.

    b. Treatment involves the use of gamma benzene hexachloride shampoo worked into the scalp and lathered in the hair for 5 minutes. Since transmission can occur from close contact with infected individuals and from the communal use of combs and brushes, these contacts likewise should be examined and treated, and the inanimate objects soaked in gamma benzene hexachloride shampoo.

  2. Pediculosis pubis *(Phthirus pubis)* (see Chap. 33)

    a. Clinical features. In this infestation, the hairs of the pubic area and, occasionally, body and axillary hair and eyelashes are affected. Organisms and nits may be seen in infested areas. Reddish-blue macules (maculae ceruleae) may be seen on the lower abdomen and upper thighs.

    b. Effective **treatment** includes the use of gamma benzene hexachloride shampoo in the genital area in a fashion similar to the treatment of head lice (see **1.b**). Eyelash infestation can be treated by applying petrolatum to the eyelashes twice daily for 8 days.

 B. Blister beetle dermatosis is characterized by tense bullae on a noninflammatory base in areas where the beetle has been crushed against the skin. The blister is due to the vesicant cantharidin present in the beetles' genitalia. Treatment includes aspiration of the blister fluid and use of a topical antibiotic agent.

 C. Hymenoptera (see Chap. 22)

  1. Clinical features. Stings from bees, wasps, and hornets can produce a mild or severe local reaction consisting of edema, erythema, and pain at the sting site and in surrounding tissues. More serious systemic effects are seen in sensitized individuals and include anaphylaxis manifested by urticaria, angioedema, laryngeal edema, bronchospasm, abdominal cramps, and/or shock.

  2. Management

    a. Anaphylaxis (see Chap. 3).

      (1) Epinephrine is the drug of choice for treating anaphylaxis. The dosage is 0.3–0.5 mg, administered SC as a 1:1000 solution (0.3–0.5 ml) in mild cases or IV (or via an endotracheal tube) in a 1:10,000 dilution (3–5 ml) in severe cases; the dosage may be repeated as needed q20–30min (for up to 3 doses) or q5–10min, respectively.

(2) A **patent airway** must be maintained, and **IV fluids** are administered at a rate commensurate with the clinical situation.

(3) Bronchospasm is treated with IV **aminophylline;** a 6 mg/kg loading dose is administered over 20–30 minutes and is followed by an infusion of 0.5–0.9 mg/kg/hour. **Oxygen** should be administered to all patients in respiratory distress.

(4) An **antihistamine** (e.g., diphenhydramine, 50 mg PO, IM, or IV) may also be useful.

(5) **Steroids** (e.g., hydrocortisone, 500 mg IV q6h) generally are indicated for serious reactions, but their effect is delayed.

(6) A **vasopressor** (e.g., dopamine, 2–50 µg/kg/minute) is indicated to manage hypotension unresponsive to volume expansion.

(7) **Disposition.** All patients with anaphylaxis require observation for at least 4 hours. Hospitalization is indicated for patients with upper airway obstruction, hypotension, or persistent bronchospasm.

 b. **Local reactions** are managed by the use of ice packs to decrease the swelling, antihistamines, and occasionally parenteral epinephrine or systemic steroids.

 c. Patients suffering from systemic reactions, as well as those with severe local reactions, should keep an **anaphylaxis kit** readily available. In addition, desensitization should be considered for these patients.

 D. **Fleas** *(Pulex irritans, Tunga penetrans).* Flea bites often occur in groups of three and may be papular, vesicular, or pustular. **Treatment** includes the use of topical steroids, topical antipruritics (e.g., pramoxine, dyclonine hydrochloride, lidocaine), and occasionally systemic antihistamines.

III. **Coelenterates** (see Chap. 22)

 A. **Portuguese man-of-war** *(Physalia physalis)*

 1. **Clinical features.** Dermatitis results from contact with the nematocysts (venom cells) present on the trailing tentacles of the organism. The injected toxin may cause local pain and burning. Severe cases may show systemic symptoms and can progress to loss of consciousness and shock. Examination shows a series of linear papulovesicles surrounded by erythema and edema.

 2. **Treatment** includes the initial inactivation of the nematocysts by the application of alcohol, ammonia, or vinegar. Fresh water should not be applied to the sites, as it will activate the nematocysts. Subsequently, the tentacles can be scraped off with sand, flour, or talcum powder. Relief of pain can be accomplished in mild cases using a topical anesthetic (e.g., 5% lidocaine ointment); severe cases may require oral or parenteral analgesics. It may also be necessary to treat shock in severe cases (see Chap. 3).

 B. **Jellyfish dermatitis.** Linear erythematous papulovesicular lesions are seen in the areas of contact with tentacles. Local treatment is similar to that outlined for the Portuguese man-of-war dermatitis (see **A.2**).

Cutaneous Reactions to Environmental Exposure

The most common reactions to the environment occur from overexposure to the sun or excessive cold.

I. **Sunburn**

 A. **Pathophysiology.** Sunburn results from an excessive exposure to UVB light (290–320 nm). Burning is especially likely to occur in fair-skinned individuals who tan poorly. Burns can be obtained through water and wide-meshed clothing. Reflected light (e.g., that obtained from water or snow) is particularly harmful. The mediators of the sunburn reaction are multiple; however, prostaglandins are probably the most important mediators.

 Certain drugs may predispose individuals to an exaggerated sunburn reaction. These drugs include the tetracycline or sulfonamide antibiotics, thiazide diuretics, psoralens, oral hypoglycemic agents, and phenothiazines. Topical products such as the halogenated salicylanilides (soaps), musk ambrette (in certain fragrances), and the furocoumarins present in certain plants (limes, parsley, celery) may produce a localized sunburn reaction when combined with the proper wavelength of light.

 B. **Clinical features.** Diffuse erythema and edema are seen in the exposed areas, with sparing of covered areas. If the reaction is severe, bullae may be present.

 C. **Prevention.** The use of sunscreens should be encouraged [37].

D. Treatment. In mild reactions, relief can be obtained from cool compresses of water alone or milk and water in combination. Topical steroids and anesthetics (e.g., pramoxine, lidocaine, benzocaine) are also helpful. For pain relief, aspirin or indomethacin is the drug of choice; as prostaglandin inhibitors, these drugs attenuate the erythematous response. Severe reactions may be ameliorated with early therapy with systemic corticosteroids (e.g., prednisone, 40–60 mg/day).

II. Cutaneous reactions to cold

A. Pernio (chilblain) can be acute or chronic. Acute pernio presents as erythematous or cyanotic macular or bluish nodules that are bilateral and symmetric on the lower legs and feet; severe reactions may be vesicular. The areas involved may burn or itch. The reaction occurs within 12–24 hours of cold injury. Treatment includes bed rest with leg elevation. Vasodilatory drugs (e.g., nicotinic acid) may be helpful for chronic lesions.

B. Frostbite

1. **Pathophysiology.** A freezing cold injury may produce intracellular or extracellular ice crystals, which damage cells by mechanical factors as well as by producing cellular dehydration. In addition, vascular damage can occur, leading to endothelial leakage, arteriovenous shunting, and, finally, tissue necrosis.

2. **Clinical features.** Frostbite can be classified depending on the severity of injury. First-degree frostbite shows erythema and edema after thawing that resolves spontaneously within a few days. Second-degree frostbite shows vesiculation after 24–48 hours in addition to the redness and swelling. Third-degree frostbite, like a third-degree thermal burn, extends through the entire dermis and shows hemorrhagic vesicles with a longer period of erythema and edema. Fourth-degree frostbite progresses to gangrene. A deep frostbite can be predicted prethaw by the solid appearance and feel of the underlying deeper tissues.

3. **Treatment** is accomplished by rapid rewarming in a water bath (40–44°C) or by warm compresses to parts that cannot be immersed. Rewarming is continued until the area flushes pink and the tissues are pliable. Excessive heat or refreezing after the thaw will enhance the injury and must be avoided. Controversy exists as to the benefit of dextran or heparin infusions. Surgical sympathectomy or the infusion of vasodilators, such as intraarterial reserpine, has been suggested to decrease postthawing edema; however, this therapy should not be performed before 36–72 hours after injury. The use of Doppler ultrasound or digital plethysmographic studies may aid in determining a patient's potential response to intraarterial vasodilators. Surgical debridement or amputation should be delayed until demarcation of tissues occurs (usually 30–90 days).

4. **Disposition.** Hospitalization is indicated for third- or fourth-degree frostbite. A disposition should be made that takes into consideration the need to avoid refreezing the affected part. Help from social service agencies may be needed to provide suitable heat and housing to affected individuals.

Infectious Diseases

I. Viral infections

A. Hand, foot, and mouth disease is a highly contagious disease caused by different types of Coxsackie A virus. It most commonly affects young children.

1. **Clinical features.** The disease is characterized by vesicles that are 5 mm in diameter, pearly gray in color, with a narrow red areola. In the mouth the vesicles involve the palate, buccal mucosa, gums, and tongue and cause a moderately painful stomatitis. Lesions are also found on the fingers and toes, palms and soles, and along the Achilles tendon. Generally about 50 vesicles are present in total. In infants, a papular or vesicular exanthem also affects the buttocks and can be confused with diaper dermatitis. Associated mild fever and malaise are common.

2. **Diagnosis.** The presence of pearly gray vesicles with a surrounding erythematous halo in characteristic locations is sufficient to establish the diagnosis.

3. **Treatment.** The illness is mild, lasts only a few days, and does not require treatment.

B. Varicella (see Chap. 36) is a highly contagious disease caused by a Herpes virus. It is transmitted by droplet infection and most commonly affects children.

1. **Clinical features.** The prototype lesion is a clear unilocular vesicle with an umbilicated center surrounded by an erythematous halo. Such vesicles develop

from papules and progress into pustules. Typically, lesions appear first on the face, spread to the trunk, and then involve the proximal distal extremities. Vesicles occur in crops at each site, characteristically producing lesions in different stages of development, i.e., papules, vesicles, pustules, and crusts in the same area. Vesicles are commonly found in the mouth, especially on the palate. Fever and constitutional symptoms are present, and the exanthem is very pruritic. Pneumonia and encephalitis are complications of the disease.

2. **Diagnosis.** The umbilicated vesicle with surrounding erythema is characteristic, as are the centripetal distribution and polymorphism in each affected site. Unroofing a vesicle, scraping the contents of the base onto a slide, and staining with Wright's or Giemsa stain (Tzanck prep) reveals multinucleated giant cells (see Chap. 38).

3. **Treatment.** Scarring occurs only if there is secondary bacterial infection. Scarring can often be prevented by alleviating local itching by applying a drying antipruritic lotion (e.g., calamine alone or combined with 0.25% menthol and/or 1.0% phenol) or administering an oral antipruritic agent as needed. Areas of yellow crusting are best treated by application of tepid water soaks, followed by application of polymyxin-bacitracin ointment. If infected areas are widespread, systemic antibiotics should be administered.

C. **Herpes zoster** is a vesicular eruption that results from the reactivation of latent varicella virus residing in dorsal root or cranial nerve ganglion cells.

1. **Clinical features.** The appearance of the lesions is preceded by itching, tenderness, or pain in the distribution of the affected nerve. Erythematous plaques in a dermatomal distribution then appear and become studded with grouped umbilicated vesicles within 24 hours. The vesicles become purulent, crust, and fall off within 1–2 weeks. The presence of a few (10–25) vesicles outside the affected dermatome is not unusual and does not imply dissemination. Bilateral and disseminated forms are rare and may be associated with underlying malignancy. The thoracic and cervical segments are most commonly affected.

2. **Diagnosis.** Grouped umbilicated vesicles on an erythematous base in a dermatomal distribution is the clinical hallmark of herpes zoster. Scraping the base of a blister onto a slide and microscopic examination following staining with Wright's or Giemsa stain (Tzanck prep) reveals multinucleated giant cells (see Chap. 38).

3. **Management**
   a. An **analgesic** should be given as necessary. Administration of systemic steroids may also help the acute pain [51].
   b. When lesions crust, **tepid water soaks** followed by application of a topical antibiotic (e.g., Polysporin ointment) are helpful in preventing secondary bacterial infection.
   c. **Postherpetic neuralgia**
      (1) **Prophylaxis.** In patients over 50 years of age, the incidence of postherpetic neuralgia can be decreased by the use of systemic corticosteroids; in younger patients, however, the low risk of postherpetic neuralgia does not justify the use of systemic corticosteroids. The use of steroids does not affect healing, does not increase the risk of dissemination, and must be started within the first 5–7 days of the eruption. Treatment is initiated at 60 mg of prednisone/day for 1 week and then tapered over the next 2 weeks.
      (2) **Treatment of postherpetic neuralgia** is not optimal. Agents include chlorprothixene (Taractan), 50 mg PO q6h; carbamazepine (Tegretol), 600–800 mg/day, plus nortriptyline (Aventyl), 50–100 mg/day; amitriptyline (Elavil), 75–100 mg/day, plus perphenazine (Trilafon), 4 mg tid; or triamcinolone, 0.2 mg/ml SC, in the affected dermatome.
   d. **Ocular involvement** (i.e., involvement of the ophthalmologic branch of the fifth cranial nerve) demands evaluation by an ophthalmologist.

D. **Herpes simplex** (see Chaps. 12, 29, 30, and 33). Cutaneous herpes simplex infections occur in two forms: (1) the painful and disabling primary infection in previously unaffected individuals without circulating antibody and (2) the recurrent variety with periodic, less severe episodes. Recurrent herpes results from reactivation of latent virus in sensory ganglia. Triggering factors include emotional stress, physical trauma, sunburn, menses, and fever. Patients with atopic dermatitis are at risk for the development of generalized herpes simplex **(eczema herpeticum)** regardless of whether their eczema is active.

1. **Clinical features.** Primary oral and genital infections are preceded by 1 or 2 days of local tenderness or pain. Recurrent lesions are preceded by several hours of a burning or tingling sensation. Primary herpes occurs on mucosal surfaces (i.e., gingivostomatitis, vulvovaginitis, urethritis), while recurrent lesions most often affect adjacent skin. Primary disease is usually accompanied by a significant fever, regional lymphadenopathy, and constitutional symptoms; extensive numbers of vesicles rapidly form and the affected mucosa becomes eroded, macerated, and intensely painful. In recurrent infection, the lesions consist of one or a few edematous oval areas in which grouped, centrally umbilicated vesicles reside on an erythematous base.

2. **Diagnosis.** Recurrent herpes simplex is clinically identical to herpes zoster except for the lack of a dermatomal distribution. The diagnosis can be confirmed by a positive Tzanck prep (see Chap. 38) or viral culture. Recurrent oral lesions are usually confined to the hard palate; patients with recurrent painful oral erosions in other parts of the oral cavity are more likely to have aphthous stomatitis.

3. **Management.** The primary infection is extremely painful, and adequate analgesia is important. Cleansing mouthwashes soothe involved mucous membranes and decrease the incidence of secondary bacterial infection. Vulvovaginitis and genital lesions may be aided by sitz baths in tepid water. Topical anesthetics are sometimes necessary. For recurrent lesions, vesicular areas should be compressed with tepid water soaks for 10 minutes qid, and Polysporin ointment applied afterwards. Acyclovir (Zovirax) ointment 5%, applied 6 times a day for 7 days, will decrease viral shedding and the time to complete crusting of lesions in primary genital herpes only. Acyclovir, 200 mg PO 5 times daily, accelerates healing in primary genital disease and reduces the frequency of recurrences. Pregnant females with genital herpes should receive gynecologic consultation, and patients with symptoms of corneal involvement (e.g., photophobia, pain) or lesions in the periorbital area must be examined by an ophthalmologist.

E. **Childhood viral exanthems [10]**

1. **Roseola infantum (exanthem subitum)** is the most common exanthematic fever in children under 2 years of age and is presumed to be of viral origin.

   a. **Clinical features.** Fever, sometimes ranging between 39.5 and 40°C, begins abruptly, persists for 3–5 days, and is usually accompanied by few or no symptoms. As the temperature falls, an eruption of discrete rose-pink maculopapules develops on the neck and trunk and may later spread to the arms, face, and legs. After 1 or 2 days the rash fades, leaving no scaling or pigmentation.

   b. **Diagnosis.** The lack of symptoms during the febrile phase and the appearance of the eruption as the fever subsides suggest the diagnosis.

   c. **Treatment.** The course is benign, and no treatment is required.

2. **Erythema infectiosum** is a mild infectious disease, presumed to be caused by a virus, and most commonly affects children 3–10 years of age.

   a. **Clinical features.** The exanthem develops with minimal prodromal symptoms; fever is absent or slight. The face is commonly brightly erythematous, having a "slapped cheek" appearance. The trunk and extremities are affected by maculopapules, which often form in a lacelike pattern, creating arcuate rings with serpiginous borders.

   b. **Diagnosis.** The slapped-cheek appearance of the face and lacelike lesions on the trunk and extremities are characteristic.

   c. **Treatment.** The disease is entirely benign, spontaneously resolving within 2 weeks; no treatment is required.

3. **Rubella** is a exanthematous disease that has the potential for intrauterine transmission when occurring in women in the first trimester of pregnancy.

   a. **Clinical features.** After a several-day prodrome of fever, malaise, headache, and mild upper respiratory symptoms, an exanthem occurs which starts on the face as small pink macules and papules that spread quickly to the neck and trunk. Coalescence of lesions then follows. The course is usually 2 or 3 days, and clearing occurs from the head down. Suboccipital and postauricular adenopathy is usually present. Complications include an encephalitis, which may follow the rash by 2–5 days, and thrombocytopenic purpura. The neonatal rubella syndrome presents with thrombocytopenic purpura ("blueberry muffin" lesions) that is present at birth or shortly thereafter. Associ-

Table 31-8. Differentiation of rubella, rubeola (measles), and scarlet fever

	Rubella	Rubeola (measles)	Scarlet fever
Prodroma	1–2 days of mild fever and respiratory symptoms	2–4 days of fever with moderate to severe respiratory symptoms	1–2 days of fever and sore throat
Duration of rash	Average 1–2 days	Average 3–5 days	Varies with treatment
Distribution	Generalized maculopapular	Generalized maculopapular	Generalized maculopapular
Postexanthem desquamation	Occasional and branny	Common and branny	Typical and severe, often occurring on the hands and feet
Distinctive features	Striking suboccipital and postauricular lymphadenopathy	Koplik's spots (bright red spots with a central bluish-white speck on the buccal mucosa)	Circumoral pallor, "strawberry" tongue

ated systemic findings may include congenital heart disease, deafness, cataracts, mental retardation, hepatosplenomegaly, and hepatitis.

   b. Diagnosis. The clinical manifestations of the eruption are distinctive (see Table 31-8 for a comparison of rubella, rubeola, and scarlet fever). Hemagglutination inhibition and neutralizing antibody titers help confirm the presence of past or recent infection.

   c. Management

     (1) Prophylaxis may be provided by a live, attenuated rubella vaccine.

     (2) Treatment of existing disease is supportive.

  4. Rubeola (measles) (see Chap. 36) is a highly contagious myxovirus infection that presents with a characteristic exanthem.

   a. Clinical features. The incubation time is 10–11 days. Initially, fever and upper respiratory symptoms occur, followed by chills, malaise, headache, conjunctivitis, coryza, diarrhea, and cough. Small white spots (Koplik's spots) occur on the buccal mucosa during this time. The morbilliform rash starts approximately 14 days after exposure and begins on the posterior scalp and spreads first to the neck and face and then to the extremities. It fades first in the areas of initial involvement after 2 or 3 days and may produce a fine scale. Complications include encephalitis, a subacute sclerosing panencephalitis, pneumonitis, gastroenteritis, and otitis media.

   b. Diagnosis can usually be made clinically (see Table 31-8).

   c. Management

     (1) Prophylaxis can be provided using the attenuated live measles vaccine.

     (2) Treatment is usually supportive, with special attention to the therapy of secondary bacterial infections.

  5. Varicella (see **B**) is a common viral disease of childhood caused by the herpes varicella-zoster virus.

II. Bacterial infections

  A. Nonbullous impetigo is a contagious superficial bacterial infection caused by group A beta-hemolytic streptococci. It most commonly affects young children and infants.

   1. Clinical features. Small, fragile vesicopustules develop on an erythematous base, most frequently involving the face and other exposed areas. The pustules rapidly break, leaving red oozing erosions capped with a thick yellow crust that appears "stuck on."

   2. Diagnosis. The golden crusts are characteristic. Only recalcitrant or unusual cases deserve a Gram stain and culture.

   3. Treatment. Systemic antibiotic administration is indicated and may be given as follows: (1) benzathine penicillin, 600,000 units IM in children 6 years or younger or 1.2 million units IM if 7 years or older; (2) erythromycin, 30–50 mg/kg/day PO for 10 days; or (3) phenoxymethyl penicillin, 250 mg PO q6h for 10 days

[3] or, for children under 12 years of age, divided doses of 15–56 mg/kg/day. The lesions should be soaked 3 or 4 times a day in tepid tap water to remove the crusts, after which a bland antibiotic ointment can be applied.

B. **Bullous impetigo and the staphylococcal scalded skin syndrome (SSSS)** are bacterial infections most commonly affecting children; they often occur in conjunction with one another and are caused by the group II phage type 71 staphylococci. These organisms elaborate an exotoxin that induces intraepidermal separation and blister formation or epidermal denudation [18].

 1. **Clinical features.** Bullous impetigo presents as flaccid bullae that are first filled with clear and then cloudy fluid and are quickly replaced by a thin, varnishlike crust. Such bullae are usually confined to a localized area of skin. The SSSS may supervene in this setting or may arise from a staphylococcal infection elsewhere (e.g., in the nasopharynx). Widespread areas of erythematous skin enlarge rapidly and are accompanied by denudation of the overlying epidermis. Because the cleavage plane is within the granular layer of the epidermis, the process appears more superficial than the drug-induced TEN (see **Hypersensitivity Disorders,** sec. **IV**) of adults. For the same reason, pigment is retained in the areas underlying the denuded skin.

 2. **Diagnosis.** In the lesions of bullous impetigo, organisms can be identified by a Gram stain of blister fluid or by culture. The SSSS may be differentiated from drug-induced TEN by a more superficial cleavage plane on skin biopsy (i.e., subcorneal versus subepidermal, respectively).

 3. **Management**

   a. Uncomplicated **bullous impetigo** should be treated with an oral semisynthetic penicillin (e.g., dicloxacillin, 12.5–25.0 mg/kg/day) or oral erythromycin, 12.5–25 mg/kg/day. The lesions should be soaked with tepid tap water to remove crusts after the bullae have become broken [3].

   b. The **SSSS** requires hospitalization and treatment with IV oxacillin or methicillin. Because of the superficial nature of the epidermal cleavage, the prognosis is excellent and reepithelialization is often complete within 3–5 days.

C. **Cellulitis** (see Chap. 22) is an acute inflammation involving the dermis or subcutaneous tissue.

 1. **Clinical features.** An extending zone of induration is characterized by redness, warmth, and tenderness. When involving nonintertriginous skin and not associated with an ulcer, the causative organisms are largely the group A beta-hemolytic streptococci and *Staphylococcus aureus.* Erysipelas is a streptococcal cellulitis in which rapid spread and an inflammatory border sharply demarcated from normal skin are typical features. Gram-negative organisms colonize intertriginous skin and ulcerations and can cause cellulitis in these areas. *Haemophilus influenzae* can produce cellulitis in children under 3 years of age, most commonly involving the face [24]. Fever, constitutional symptoms, and lymphangitis may be present in all forms of cellulitis.

 2. **Diagnosis.** The clinical findings are characteristic. Needle aspiration of the lesions following injection of sterile saline results in a positive culture in a variable percentage of cases. Blood cultures should also be obtained.

 3. **Management.** Antibiotics appropriate for the suspected offending agent are administered orally or intravenously, depending on the toxicity of the patient and whether there are other associated medical conditions (e.g., diabetes mellitus) compromising the immune status of the patient.

D. **Scarlet fever** is a distinctive clinical syndrome caused by an erythrogenic toxin produced most commonly by group A beta-hemolytic streptococci.

 1. **Clinical features.** After a 2- to 4-day incubation period, there is the abrupt onset of headache, fever, and sore throat, followed in 1–3 days by a characteristic exanthem. Lesions are red and finely papular. They begin in intertriginous areas and then progress to the trunk and extremities. The rash fades after 3–5 days, producing a desquamating scale especially involving the palms and soles. The oropharynx may show a purulent exudate over the tonsils, and a coated tongue with prominent red papillae ("strawberry tongue") may be present.

 2. **Diagnosis.** The clinical features are distinctive (see Table 31-8). Culture of streptococci from the pharynx and a rise in serologic titers to the organism are helpful in confirming the diagnosis. The differential diagnosis includes rubella, rubeola, infectious mononucleosis, drug reactions, scarlatiniform staphylococcal infections, Kawasaki's disease, and toxic shock syndrome.

 3. **Treatment** is with penicillin (see **A.3**).

III. Sepsis (see Chap. 12) may produce skin lesions with certain common features, regardless of the specific organism involved. Generally, the lesions appear vasculitic, becoming purpuric and even necrotic in quality. Generally, hospitalization for parenteral administration of appropriate antimicrobial agents is indicated. Distinctive aspects of specific forms of sepsis are as follows.
  A. Disseminated gonorrhea. Scattered 1- to 5-mm vesicopustules, usually 20 in number, appear on the distal extremities. The lesions rapidly become purpuric and often necrotic and are sometimes accompanied by arthritis and tenosynovitis.
  B. *Pseudomonas* **(ecthyma gangrenosum).** Erythematous or purpuric macules rapidly enlarge, developing hemorrhagic bullae in their centers and often eventuating in necrosis [17].
  C. Rocky Mountain spotted fever. See **Vasculitis.**
  D. Meningococcemia. See **Vasculitis.**
  E. *Staphylococcus.* The clinical hallmark of staphylococcal sepsis is the presence of purulent purpura. Most often, such areas appear on the trunk and are several centimeters in size.
  F. *Candida.* Numerous, scattered 1- to 10-mm purpuric papules and nodules appear most commonly on the trunk. Some of the lesions may have purulent centers.
IV. Fungal infections
  A. Tinea versicolor is a common, chronic asymptomatic superficial fungal infection caused by *Pityrosporum furfur,* the pathogenic filamentous form of a fungus that normally resides on human skin.
    1. Clinical features. Hypo- or hyperpigmented, oval-to-round macular patches with overlying scale are found most commonly on the trunk. The infected areas may be darker than the surrounding skin in winter, but they do not tan and in summer become hypopigmented. Inflammation is absent.
    2. The **diagnosis** is established by potassium hydroxide examination of the fine scales, which are infected with hyphae and spores. In contrast to dermatophyte infections, a negative microscopic examination excludes the diagnosis. The causative organism, however, cannot be cultured on standard artificial media.
    3. Therapy. Topical treatment should include the entire torso from the neck to the waist, since lesions are often more widespread than is clinically apparent. A 2.5% selenium sulfide suspension (e.g., Exsel, Selsun, Iosel) is applied for 20 minutes and then removed with a harsh washcloth during bathing for 7–14 consecutive days. Clearing of the active infection (scaling) is rapid, but the pigmentary changes resolve much more slowly (over months). The frequency of relapse is very high.
  B. Dermatophytosis. The dermatophytoses are superficial infections of the skin, hair, or nails caused by three genera of fungi: *Trichophyton, Microsporum,* and *Epidermophyton.*
    1. Clinical features. Poor hygiene, warmth and moisture, and contact with infected animals, persons, or fomites all increase the likelihood of dermatophyte infections. Tinea pedis, tinea cruris, tinea barbae, and onychomycosis predominantly affect adults, whereas tinea corporis and tinea capitis usually affect children. These infections are often pruritic.
      a. Tinea corporis, or infection of the nonhairy skin, produces erythematous patches that spread outward and develop into annular or arciform lesions with a sharp, scaling, or vesicular advancing border and a healing center; hence, the eponym "ringworm."
      b. Tinea cruris, or "jock itch," affects the groin and upper inner thigh often symmetrically, producing butterfly areas of erythema and scaling with clearly defined raised margins.
      c. Tinea pedis, or "athlete's foot," most commonly produces interdigital scaling, erythema, and maceration. If involvement extends onto the sides of the feet, a well-defined polycyclic border is generally present. Some fungi can induce a vesicular or bullous eruption with large blisters on the feet.
      d. Tinea capitis, or ringworm of the scalp, produces patchy hair loss, broken hairs, and scaling. The term **kerion** describes involvement with severe inflammation and pustular folliculitis within an area of boggy swelling and purulence.
      e. Tinea barbae, or ringworm infection of the beard and moustache areas in adult men, produces inflammatory lesions akin to the kerion of tinea capitis.
      f. Onychomycosis, or tinea of the nails, is almost always accompanied by fungal infection elsewhere. The nails may become discolored (i.e., white or

yellow), thickened, brittle, crumbly, and lifted up by an accumulation of subungual keratin and debris. Fingernails are less commonly involved than toenails, and children are rarely affected.

2. The **diagnosis** is established by microscopic identification of hyphae and spores under potassium hydroxide examination of scales or hair. Infection may be confirmed or, in some instances, identified in the absence of a positive scraping by fungal culture using Mycosel or Sabouraud's artificial media; visible growth, however, requires 2–4 weeks in culture. Examination of the scalp with long-wave ultraviolet light (i.e., a Wood's lamp) is of limited value in tinea capitis, since most scalp ringworm infections are now caused by fungi that do not fluoresce.

3. **Therapy.** Infections of the skin can usually be treated by topical measures alone. Clotrimazole (Lotrimin, Mycelex), miconazole (Monistat-Derm, Micatin), or haloprogin (Halotex) solution or cream applied 3 times a day will cause involution of most superficial, scaling lesions within 1–3 weeks, but therapy should be continued for another 2–4 weeks to decrease the rate of relapse. Tinea capitis and onychomycosis require systemic therapy; ultramicrosized griseofulvin (Fulvicin), 250 mg PO bid, and ketoconazole (Nizoral), 200 mg PO qd, are equally effective. Tinea capitis is treated for a period of 6–8 weeks; onychomycosis of the fingernails and toenails, for 6–9 months and 12–24 months, respectively. Fingernails respond more readily than toenails; the latter are often unresponsive to any therapy.

C. **Superficial candidiasis.** Factors that predispose to superficial candidal infections include (1) a local environment of moisture, warmth, maceration, and occlusion; (2) obesity; (3) the systemic administration of antibiotics, corticosteroids, or birth control pills; (4) pregnancy; (5) diabetes mellitus; and (6) debilitated states.

1. **Clinical features.** Intertriginous (i.e., inframammary, groin, axillary, perianal, and interdigital) lesions are bright red, macerated, and occasionally scaly; they characteristically contain satellite erythematous papules and pustules at the periphery of their well-defined borders. *Candida* paronychiae are chronic infections that cause erythema and swelling of the posterior nail folds; the nails themselves may become ridged and discolored (green or brown). **Thrush** appears as white plaques loosely attached to an underlying bright red oral or vaginal mucosa. Perlèche produces cracked and fissured erythematous areas in the corners of the mouth.

2. **Diagnosis.** Direct examination of scrapings with potassium hydroxide reveals budding yeast forms and pseudohyphae. *C. albicans* grows readily on fungal or bacterial media, and colonies are visible within 48–72 hours.

3. **Therapy.** Topical agents effective against *Candida* include haloprogin (Halotex), miconazole (Monistat-Derm, Micatin), clotrimazole (Lotrimin, Mycelex), and nystatin (Mycostatin). The first three agents will eradicate dermatophyte fungi as well. Use of these agents 3 times a day must be accompanied by elimination of predisposing factors, especially moisture and occlusion. The drying breeze from a fan and the physical separation of skin folds are often helpful in this regard. **Thrush** can be treated with nystatin oral suspension, 4–6 ml (400,000–600,000 units) qid, held in the mouth for several minutes before swallowing; clotrimazole buccal troches, 10 mg qid; or a 1–2% solution of gentian violet.

D. **Systemic fungal infections.** In the absence of laboratory-acquired inoculation, cutaneous lesions of blastomycosis, coccidioidomycosis, histoplasmosis, and cryptococcosis imply systemic dissemination, generally from a pulmonary focus.

1. **Clinical features**
   a. Cutaneous lesions of systemic **blastomycosis** are raised, warty, vegetative, crusted plaques that often show central scarring and have a prominent nodular border.
   b. Cutaneous **coccidioidomycosis** most often presents with scattered erythematous nodules in the dermis or subcutaneous tissue.
   c. The lesions of systemic **histoplasmosis** primarily involve mucosal surfaces rather than the skin itself; large mucosal ulcerations are the usual finding.
   d. Cutaneous **cryptococcosis** is rare; lesions are variable and may include infiltrated plaques that are purpuric and of gelatinous consistency and can ulcerate.
   e. In severely immunocompromised patients with lymphoma or leukemia, *Candida septicemia* can be accompanied by disseminated skin lesions. In contrast to superficial cutaneous candidal infections, such lesions are much

deeper and typically consist of scattered erythematous nodules that are purpuric and may contain a pustular center.

2. **Diagnosis.** A skin biopsy and culture of tissue from cutaneous lesions are of great benefit in establishing the diagnosis. A deep 4 mm punch or preferably wedge biopsy of a lesion incorporating a portion of the margin is placed in formalin. The skin biopsy in deep fungal infections shows a granulomatous infiltrate in the dermis; using special stains (e.g., periodic acid-Schiff [PAS] reaction, methenamine silver), organisms can usually be identified in the tissue. An additional piece of tissue is placed in sterile saline in an aseptic container and transported immediately to the microbiology laboratory. The tissue is ground up and cultured for fungi, acid-fast organisms, and bacteria.

3. **Therapy** [31, 32] should be individualized. In general, patients with disseminated systemic deep fungal infection should be hospitalized. For blastomycosis, histoplasmosis, or coccidioidomycosis, amphotericin B in a total dose of 2–3 gm IV is usually effective. For cryptococcosis, IV (and sometimes intrathecal) administration of amphotericin B (total dose, 2–3 gm) in combination with 5-fluorocytosine, 150 mg/kg/day PO for 4 weeks, is the treatment of choice. Systemic candidiasis is usually treated with IV amphotericin B (total dose, 1.5–2.0 gm).

Alopecia

Hair loss may be caused by physical trauma (e.g., burns, chemicals, x-rays, traction), bacterial infections (e.g., syphilis, staphylococcal infections), ringworm infections, inflammatory disorders (e.g., lupus erythematosus, lichen planus, sarcoidosis), high fever (e.g., telogen effluvium), drugs (e.g., cytotoxics, anticoagulants), endocrinopathy (especially thyroid dysfunction), and factors that are less well understood (i.e., alopecia areata, male pattern baldness). For a review, the reader is referred to reference 19.

I. **Alopecia areata** is a disorder characterized by oval areas of asymptomatic, noninflammatory, nonscarring, complete hair loss most commonly involving the scalp [33]. Its association with other "autoimmune" disorders (e.g., vitiligo, thyroiditis, pernicious anemia) in approximately 5% of cases suggests a pathogenesis related to immune mechanisms. Children and young adults are most frequently affected.
   A. **Clinical features.** The lesions are well-defined, single or multiple, and round or oval areas of total hair loss. "Exclamation point hairs" may be seen at the margins; these hairs protrude about 3–10 mm above the scalp and have a dark, rough tip; a narrow, less pigmented shaft; and an atrophic root. In more severe cases, total scalp alopecia may occur, as well as loss of eyelashes, eyebrows, beard, and general body hair. Nail pitting and dystrophy occur in 10–20% of cases.
   B. **Diagnosis.** There is no evidence of scarring or inflammation, and the hair loss in involved areas is total. If the diagnosis is in question, a biopsy can be useful.
   C. **Prognosis.** Complete recovery occurs spontaneously in about one-third of patients, but in approximately another third, the hair never regrows. Onset at a young age, the presence of extensive lesions, and the presence of severe nail changes are all associated with a poor prognosis for hair regrowth.
   D. **Treatment.** There is no adequate means of treating the disorder, and additional areas of involvement can be expected to develop in approximately 50% of patients.

II. **Trichotillomania** is a disorder caused by the patient compulsively pulling out his or her own hair; children are predominantly affected.
   A. **Clinical features.** In contrast to alopecia areata, areas of hair loss are only partially thinned; and hairs can be found that are twisted, broken, and of varying lengths. Evidence of inflammation and pustular areas are often found as a consequence of physical manipulation.
   B. **Diagnosis.** Some patients will admit to pulling out their hair, but others are extremely resistant to such admission. The diagnosis can often be facilitated by a scalp biopsy.
   C. **Therapy.** Psychologic or psychiatric counseling is helpful.

Bullous Diseases

Blisters are small or large cavities, vesicles, or bullae within or just beneath the epidermis; they contain clear fluid. They are to be distinguished from blistering associated with erythema multiforme, drug eruptions, the staphylococcal scalded skin syndrome, viral and fungal infections, acute eczema, dyshidrosis, sunburn, and frostbite. Pemphigus vulgaris and bullous pemphigoid are the two most common primary bullous disorders.

I. **Pemphigus vulgaris** is a bullous disorder of middle-aged adults (fourth to fifth decades) in which blistering is produced by IgG autoantibodies to the intercellular cement substance of the keratinocytes located in the lower epidermis. Complement deposition follows, and cohesion between epidermal cells is lost, with resultant blister formation.

   A. **Clinical features.** Widespread flaccid, weeping bullous lesions produce large denuded areas of skin. Nikolsky's sign, a dislodging of the epidermis with lateral finger pressure, generally is present. The scalp, chest, umbilicus, and intertriginous areas are commonly involved. Characteristically, blisters do not become large and tense; instead, they rupture easily, leaving erosions or crusts behind. Painful erosions and ulcerations of the oral mucosa occur in more than 90% of patients and are often the presenting symptomatology. The blistered areas heal very slowly, but scarring is not a feature of the disease process.

   B. **Diagnosis.** The clinical picture must be distinguished from the other bullous diseases; and even with a typical presentation, verification by a skin biopsy is required. Immunofluorescent examination of the epidermis and serum for the presence of antibodies to the "intercellular cement substance" generally is positive.

   C. **Management.** Initial presentation and acute exacerbations of pemphigus vulgaris generally require hospitalization. In such circumstances, high-dose corticosteroids are the only effective means to control disease activity. Therapy should begin at a sufficient dose (i.e., 100–150 mg of prednisone qd) to completely suppress new blister formation. The addition of a cytotoxic agent or gold may influence disease activity but not until 6–8 weeks after their administration; these drugs ultimately may have a "steroid-sparing" effect. Topical therapy (e.g., with wet dressings, topical antibiotic ointment) is designed to prevent secondary bacterial infection.

II. **Bullous pemphigoid** is a bullous disorder of older adults (sixth to eighth decades), in which blistering is produced by IgG autoantibodies directed against the dermoepidermal basement membrane.

   A. **Clinical features.** Widespread areas of erythematous, urticarialike skin are present, on which large, tense bullae develop. The bullae may rupture, leaving denuded areas; unlike pemphigus, however, they show a good tendency to healing. Sites of predilection include the inner aspects of the thighs, the flexor surfaces of the forearms, the axillae, groin, and lower abdomen. Oral lesions occur in only one-third of patients, and despite physical maceration, intact blisters can often be observed.

   B. **Diagnosis.** The clinical presentation must be differentiated from other bullous diseases, especially bullous drug eruption; thus, a skin biopsy is required. Immunofluorescent studies of the serum and dermoepidermal junction are positive for IgG antibodies directed against the basement membrane.

   C. **Management.** Bullous pemphigoid is less of a threat to life than pemphigus vulgaris. Compared with pemphigus, the lesions of bullous pemphigoid heal more readily, in part because epidermal regeneration can begin while the blister roof is still intact. The mainstay of treatment is corticosteroids; a comparatively lower dose is required, starting with 60–80 mg qd of prednisone. A cytotoxic agent is rarely necessary but may have a "steroid-sparing" effect. Because of the age of bullous pemphigoid patients, side effects of corticosteroid treatment (see Chap. 14) are common. Hospitalization is indicated in patients with severe disease or secondarily infected lesions.

Disorders of the Mucous Membranes

I. **Aphthous stomatitis** (canker sore) is a common disorder, affecting 20% of the general population, in which recurrent, painful mucosal erosions appear on the movable mucosa of the buccal lips, gums, tongue, palate, buccal mucosa, and pharynx. The etiology has not been established but probably involves an immune mechanism [44].

   A. **Clinical features.** Tingling or burning generally antedate the onset of lesions by at least 24 hours. Aphthae appear as single or, more commonly, multiple, small (1–10 mm in diameter) shallow erosions with clearly defined borders; they are covered by a yellowish-gray membrane and surrounded by an intense erythematous halo. The lesions are extremely painful, and although healing is spontaneous, the total course usually lasts 2–3 weeks.

   B. **Diagnosis.** Recurrent, painful oral ulcerations have a high probability of being aphthae. Recurrent herpes simplex involves the vermillion border and surrounding skin; however, oral mucous membrane involvement is infrequent and is restricted to the hard palate. A biopsy is not helpful in establishing the diagnosis.

  C. **Therapy**
    1. **Controlling pain.** Topical anesthetics are effective; dyclonine hydrochloride solution (Dyclone), lidocaine (Xylocaine ointment 5% or viscous), or diphenhydramine hydrochloride (Benadryl elixir) may be used as often as needed.
    2. **Shortening the duration of lesions already present and aborting new lesions.** Topical steroids can be useful, especially if applied during the prodromal stage. Triamcinolone acetonide 0.1% in a base that adheres to mucous membranes (Kenalog in Orabase) is effective. Administration of systemic corticosteroids (e.g., prednisone, 60 mg, tapering 5 mg qd) can abort attacks if taken during the prodromal period and will usually induce healing of lesions in patients with severe erosive aphthae.

II. Several other **cutaneous disorders** can also involve the mucous membranes. These disorders include erythema multiforme, viral enanthems, herpes simplex, secondary syphilis, candidiasis, histoplasmosis, pemphigus, bullous pemphigoid, Kaposi's sarcoma, squamous cell carcinoma, lichen planus, and vasculitis. Because of constant physical trauma, lesions of the oral mucosa easily lose their original architecture and can be difficult to diagnose.

  A. **Clinical features.** Some oral presentations are characteristic. For example, lichen planus usually shows a whitish, netlike pattern on the buccal mucosa or tongue which can ulcerate. Candidiasis can present with a curdlike material overlying a red and sometimes eroded mucosa. In many other instances the physician may see only erosions or ulcerations that represent the result of a preceding infectious or blistering inflammatory process. In these cases the primary lesion is no longer visible, which may create problems in diagnosis; the clinician must then rely on other pertinent historic and physical findings to clarify the problem.

  B. **Diagnosis.** In many cases a biopsy of the oral lesion is helpful and should be obtained from an early primary lesion or, if one is not present, from the margin of an ulceration. If a blistering process is suspected, a piece of tissue should also be sent for direct immunofluorescence. Serum for indirect immunofluorescence can also be useful in this setting. If an infectious process, such as histoplasmosis, is suspected, tissue can be sent for culture as well. Potassium hydroxide preparation of any curdlike exudate is important to diagnose Candida.

  C. **Treatment** is directed toward the underlying disease. In many cases (e.g., erythema multiforme, exanthems), the process is self-limited and resolves without therapy. However, in other cases, such as pemphigus vulgaris, early diagnosis and treatment (possibly with systemic corticosteroids) is important. A topical anesthetic (see sec. **I.C.1**) can be used for relief of pain.

Eczematous Dermatoses

The morphologic and histopathologic changes in all forms of eczema (dermatitis) are similar. The factors that initiate the process, however, vary and determine the clinical type of disease (e.g., atopic dermatitis, contact dermatitis). Regardless of the inciting cause, however, the clinical morphology of the lesions is similar and can be subdivided into acute and chronic varieties. Acute eczema is characterized initially by erythema and edema; these early changes progress to vesiculation and oozing and then to crusting and scaling. Finally, if the process becomes chronic, the skin becomes thickened with prominent skin markings (lichenified), excoriated, and either hypo- or hyperpigmented. All types of eczema are very pruritic.

I. **Atopic dermatitis** is an intensely pruritic, chronic type of eczema. Its onset is early in childhood, and the condition is often associated with atopy (i.e., rhinitis, hay fever, asthma).

  A. **Clinical features.** Ninety percent of patients manifest their disease by 5 years of age. In children under the age of 3, involvement is widespread with erythematous papulovesicles and oozing. Between the ages of 4 and 10, the lesions are less acute and exudative, more scattered, and often localized in the flexor folds of the neck, elbows, wrists, and knees. Dry papules, excoriations, lichenification, and periorbital erythema and edema are common. In adolescents and adults, the lesions are primarily dry, lichenified, hyperpigmented plaques in the flexor areas and around the eyes. Patients with atopic dermatitis have, as yet, an undefined defect in cellular immunity that lowers their resistance to certain viruses, especially herpes simplex and vaccinia, predisposing them to dissemination of usually localized infections. In all phases of the disease, itching leads to scratching, and scratching further compromises the integrity of the affected skin and lowers the threshold for renewed itching. In addition, most patients have very dry skin, which also aggravates this itch-scratch cycle.

B. **Diagnosis.** The clinical history and localization of chronic eczematous lesions to the flexor areas in older children and adults are usually sufficient to establish the diagnosis.

C. **Therapy**

1. **Preventive measures** include elimination of excessive bathing (which promotes xerosis), use of a nonirritating soap (e.g., Dove, Basis, Alpha-Keri), and frequent application of bland lubricants (e.g., Lubriderm, Eucerin). Scratch and intradermal allergy tests are not useful.

2. **Treatment of active dermatitis.** The mainstay of therapy is the application of a topical steroid. Fluorinated preparations (e.g., Aristocort 0.1%, Kenalog 0.1%) should be used in adults; 1% hydrocortisone is often effective in younger children. Steroids should be applied 3 times a day, and an ointment base used for chronic, dry lesions. Since atopic dermatitis can be a lifelong disease, the long-term administration of systemic corticosteroids plays no part in its management; even short courses of prednisone are to be avoided. Oral antihistamines (e.g., hydroxyzine, diphenhydramine) are useful adjuncts to suppress pruritus.

II. **Contact dermatitis** is an eczematous eruption produced by either primary irritants or allergic sensitizers. Primary irritants (e.g., occupational chemicals) cause a nonallergic reaction, provided the concentration and duration of contact are sufficient. Allergic sensitizers (e.g., poison oak or ivy) cause a delayed hypersensitivity response, and a much lower concentration of the offending agent is sufficient.

A. **Clinical features.** Contact dermatitis appears as an acute eczematous eruption. There is erythema, edema, vesiculation, and oozing confined to the areas of contact with the offending agent, thus providing a bizarre or artificial pattern with sharp, straight margins. Areas of linear vesicles from brushing against trees and plants are the clinical hallmark of poison ivy and oak.

B. **Diagnosis.** A pruritic, acute eczematous eruption with linear, abrupt margins form the necessary criteria for diagnosis.

C. **Therapy.** Early and aggressive treatment with systemic corticosteroids is indicated in most cases of moderate to severe contact dermatitis. The initial prednisone dosage should be 60–80 mg qd, and the dose decreased only after a clinical response is observed; the total course of therapy should be 2–3 weeks. Milder variations may be treated with cool compresses, oral antihistamines, and topical fluorinated steroids. Referral to a dermatologist for patch testing is prudent once the reaction has subsided.

III. **Dyshidrotic eczema** is an acute, recurrent, or chronic vesicular eruption on the palms and soles.

A. **Clinical features.** The clinical hallmark is the presence of deeply seated clear vesicles along the sides of the fingers. Vesicles also occur on the palms and, less frequently, on the soles of the feet. In more severe cases, vesicles may become confluent and form large bullae. Erythema and scaling are minimal. Recurrent acute bouts are the expected clinical course.

B. **Diagnosis.** An acute pruritic eruption featuring deep vesicles along the sides of the fingers is sufficient to establish the diagnosis.

C. **Therapy.** Severe cases with large bullae can be treated with a tapering 2-week course of oral prednisone, starting at a dose of 60 mg. Mild to moderate episodes generally benefit from cool compresses or wet soaks and the application of a potent topical steroid 4 times a day, e.g., 0.05% fluocinonide (Lidex) cream or 0.1% halcinonide (Halog) cream.

Vasculitis (see Chap. 14)

Despite its many underlying etiologies, vasculitis manifests itself in the skin with a limited clinical spectrum of lesions [45]. The cutaneous hallmark of vasculitis is palpable purpura. Purpura represents the extravasation of erythrocytes from blood vessels and can be either inflammatory (e.g., vasculitis) or noninflammatory (e.g., thrombocytopenia) in nature. The presence of purpura is tested by applying pressure with a glass slide (i.e., diascopy), which demonstrates lesions that do not blanch or decrease in intensity. An inflammatory basis for purpura imparts the quality of palpability. Any vasculitis, regardless of the cause, can present as a palpable purpura, with the extremities (particularly the legs) as the sites of predilection; included are vasculitides due to infection (e.g., Rocky Mountain spotted fever), hypersensitivity (e.g., drug-induced allergic vasculitis), or of unknown etiology (e.g., lupus erythematosus). Necrotic lesions are another common cutaneous presentation of vasculitis, also occurring most frequently on the extremities; such areas are black in color, follow frank vessel occlusion, and may be preceded by a vesicular or purpuric component. Other cutaneous findings that commonly represent a vasculitis include hemorrhagic bullae, tender erythematous nodules, and areas of palpable erythema with circinate or arciform borders.

I. **Cutaneous manifestations of specific vasculitides**
   A. **Allergic vasculitis.** Leukocytoclastic vasculitis, typically from a drug ingestion, starts with 1-cm or smaller hemorrhagic macules on the lower extremities that rapidly become palpable [45]. The trunk and upper extremities are often involved, but the lesions characteristically are most severe on the legs. Coalescence into larger purpuric plaques and hemorrhagic bulla formation may also occur. Target lesions with a central vesicular area are common. Allergic vasculitis is the prototype condition associated with the skin lesions of palpable purpura.
   B. **Serum sickness.** A variety of cutaneous manifestations can occur, ranging from urticaria to palpable purpura. Erythematous plaques with arciform borders and erythema multiforme–like lesions are common.
   C. **Henoch-Schönlein purpura.** Crops of lesions appear, progressing from urticarial papules and plaques to frank palpable purpura. Sites of predilection are the limbs and buttocks.
   D. **Rheumatoid vasculitis.** Small reddish-brown infarcts occur near the nail folds; and larger, painful, hemorrhagic maculopapular lesions are found on the digital pads of the hands. Rheumatoid nodules and a high rheumatoid factor titer are common associated findings.
   E. **Lupus erythematosus.** The malar rash of systemic lupus erythematosus closely resembles an exaggerated sunburn. Early on, there is a blanching erythema, but in longer-standing lesions, atrophy and telangiectasias develop. A photosensitivity dermatitis involving the face and upper extremities commonly is present and is characterized by erythema, scaling, atrophy, and telangiectasias. Distal infarcts, palpable purpura, bullae, subcutaneous nodules over joints, and tender subcutaneous plaques ("lupus panniculitis") also may occur. Discoid lesions are seen in patients with discoid lupus erythematosus and also in approximately one-third of patients with systemic lupus erythematosus; these lesions are oval plaques on sun-exposed surfaces that are erythematous and atrophic and exhibit follicular plugging (scales over hair follicles) and telangiectasias. Areas of scarring alopecia are common.
   F. **Cryoglobulinemia.** Findings include purpuric plaques on exposed body parts after cooling, necrotic ulcerations involving the extremities, and Raynaud's phenomena. Lesions arise from intravascular precipitation of proteins, which often produces a concomitant vasculitis.
   G. **Polyarteritis nodosa.** Cutaneous or subcutaneous nodules, 4–15 mm in diameter, occur in groups along the course of superficial arteries, most frequently on the lower extremities. Infarcts in the skin from peripheral embolization of thrombi may produce splinter hemorrhages, Osler's nodes, tender nodules, purpuric plaques, or hemorrhagic bullae.
   H. **Wegener's granulomatosis.** Persistent crusted, hemorrhagic, granulomatous lesions involve the nostrils, nasal septum, pharynx, larynx, or trachea. Papulonecrotic, vesicular, or ulcerative lesions also may occur, particularly on the lower extremities.
   I. **Bacterial endocarditis** (see Chap. 12). Subungual splinter hemorrhages, Osler's nodes (erythematous, painful small nodules on the pads of the fingers and toes), Janeway spots (erythematous macules on the palms and soles), and scattered petechiae are frequently present. Since a variety of other factors can cause splinter hemorrhages, they are not diagnostic of bacterial endocarditis by themselves.
   J. **Rocky Mountain spotted fever** (see Chap. 12). A maculopapular eruption appears first on the wrists and ankles and spreads centrally to involve the trunk and face; the palms and soles are usually involved. The lesions rapidly become purpuric, palpable, and, in severe cases, confluent.
   K. **Meningococcemia.** Extensive areas of purpura occur on the trunk and limbs. Lesions initially may be papular and discrete but rapidly evolve into large, coalescent

hemorrhagic plaques, often assuming a livedo configuration. Differentiation from Rocky Mountain spotted fever on a cutaneous basis, however, usually is impossible.

II. Management

    A. Disposition. Hospitalization for diagnosis and therapy is generally indicated in most cases of cutaneous vasculitis, particularly for those patients who are systemically toxic, demonstrate areas of widespread necrosis (e.g., digital gangrene), have evidence of impaired vital organ function (e.g., renal failure), or are suspected of having a systemic infection, such as Rocky Mountain spotted fever or meningococcemia.

    B. Therapy is directed toward the underlying disease process. Septic vasculitis should be treated with appropriate systemic antibiotics; vasculitis associated with collagen vascular disease is often treated with prednisone in combination with an immunosuppressive agent, such as cyclophosphamide or azathioprine. The therapy of idiopathic leukocytoclastic vasculitis is variable. Useful regimens include colchicine, 0.6 mg PO bid; indomethacin, 25–50 mg PO tid; dapsone, 50 mg PO bid; oral antihistamines (see Table 31-4); topical corticosteroids (see Table 31-1); and, in severe cases with internal organ involvement, oral corticosteroids (e.g., prednisone, 1 mg/kg/day) or antimetabolites.

Bibliography

1. Abrahams, I., McCarthy, J. T., and Sanders, S. L. 101 cases of exfoliative dermatitis. *Arch. Dermatol.* 87:96, 1963.
2. Anderson, T. F., and Voorhees, J. J. Psoriasis and arthritis. *Cutis* 21:790, 1978.
3. Arndt, K. A. *Manual of Dermatologic Therapeutics: With Essentials of Diagnosis* (3rd ed.). Boston: Little, Brown, 1983. Pp. 23–27.
4. Arndt, K. A., and Jick, H. Rates of cutaneous reaction to drugs: A report from the Boston Collaborative Drug Surveillance Program. *J.A.M.A.* 235:918, 1976.
5. Baker, H., and Ryan, T. J. Generalized pustular psoriasis: A clinical and epidemiological study of 104 cases. *Br. J. Dermatol.* 80:771, 1968.
6. Benke, P. J. The isotretinoin teratogen syndrome. *J.A.M.A.* 251:3267, 1984.
7. Bernstein, J. E., Whitney, D. H., and Soltani, K. Inhibition of histamine-induced pruritus by topical tricyclic antidepressants. *J. Am. Acad. Dermatol.* 5:582, 1981.
8. Blomgren, S. E. Erythema nodosum. *Semin. Arthritis Rheum.* 4:1, 1974.
9. Bondi, E. E., and Kligman, A. M. Adverse effects of topical corticosteroids. *Prog. Dermatol.* 14:1, 1980.
10. Cherry, J. D. Viral exanthems. *D.M.* 28(8):1, 1982.
11. Christensen, O. B., and Maibach, H. I. Antihistamines in dermatology. *Semin. Dermatol.* 2:270, 1983.
12. Coffman, J. D., and Davies W. T. Vasospastic diseases: A review. *Prog. Cardiovasc. Dis.* 18:123, 1975.
13. Cram, D. L. Psoriasis: Current advances in etiology and treatment. *J. Am. Acad. Dermatol.* 4:1, 1981.
14. Crounse, R. G. Arachnidism (excluding North American loxoscelism). In D. J. Demis and J. McGuire (eds.), *Clinical Dermatology* (Vol. 4). Philadelphia: Harper and Row, 1984. Units 18-26.
15. Dillaha, C. J., Jansen, G. T., and Honeycutt, W. M. North American Loxoscelism. In D. J. Demis and J. McGuire (eds.), *Clinical Dermatology* (Vol. 4). Philadelphia: Harper and Row, 1984. Units 18-25.
16. Domonkos, A. N., Arnold, H. L., Jr., and Odom, R. B. *Andrews' Diseases of the Skin: Clinical Dermatology* (7th ed.). Philadelphia: Saunders, 1982. Pp. 97–143.
17. Dorff, G. J., et al. *Pseudomonas* septicemia. *Arch. Intern. Med.* 128:591, 1971.
18. Elias, P. M., Fritsch, P., and Epstein, E. H., Jr. Staphylococcal scalded skin syndrome: Clinical features, pathogenesis, and recent microbiological developments. *Arch. Dermatol.* 113:207, 1977.
19. Fenske, N. A., and Johnson, S. A. M. Major causes of alopecia: With suggestions for history taking, workup, and therapy. *Postgrad. Med.* 60:79, 1976.
20. Fitzpatrick, T. B., Polano, M. K., and Suurmond, D. *Color Atlas and Synopsis of Clinical Dermatology.* New York: McGraw-Hill, 1983. Pp. 46–47.
21. Fowler, J. F., and Callen, J. P. Pyoderma gangrenosum. *Dermatol. Clin.* 1:615, 1983.
22. Fritz, K. A., and Weston, W. L. Topical glucocorticoids. *Ann. Allergy* 50:68, 1983.
23. Gilchrest, B. A. Pruritus: Pathogenesis, therapy, and significance in systemic disease states. *Arch. Intern. Med.* 142:101, 1982.

24. Ginsburg, C. M. *Hemophilus influenzae* type B buccal cellulitis. *J. Am. Acad. Dermatol.* 4:611, 1981.
25. Greipp, P. R. Hyperpigmentation syndrome (diffuse hypermelanosis). *Arch. Intern. Med.* 138:356, 1978.
26. Hasan, T., and Jansen, C. T. Erythroderma. A follow-up of fifty cases. *J. Am. Acad. Dermatol.* 8:836, 1983.
27. Huff, J. C., Weston, W. L., and Tonnesen, M. G. Erythema multiforme: A critical review of characteristics, diagnostic criteria, and causes. *J. Am. Acad. Dermatol.* 8:763, 1983.
28. Jacobson, K. W., Branch, L. B., and Nelson, H. S. Laboratory tests in chronic urticaria. *J.A.M.A.* 243:1644, 1980.
29. King, L. E., and Rees, R. S. Dapsone treatment of a brown recluse bite. *J.A.M.A.* 250:648, 1983.
30. Koranda, F. C. Antimalarials. *J. Am. Acad. Dermatol.* 4:650, 1981.
31. Medoff, G., Brajtburg, J., and Kobayashi, G. S. Antifungal agents useful in therapy of systemic fungal infections. *Annu. Rev. Pharmacol. Toxicol.* 23:303, 1983.
32. Medoff, G., and Kobayashi, G. S. Strategies in the treatment of systemic fungal infections. *N. Engl. J. Med.* 302:145, 1980.
33. Mitchell, A. J., and Krull, E. A. Alopecia areata: Pathogenesis and treatment. *J. Am. Acad. Dermatol.* 5:763, 1984.
34. Nicolis, G. D., and Helwig, E. B. Exfoliative dermatitis: A clinicopathologic study of 135 cases. *Arch. Dermatol.* 108:788, 1973.
35. Orton, P. W., et al. Detection of a herpes simplex viral antigen in skin lesions of erythema multiforme. *Ann. Intern. Med.* 101:48, 1984.
36. Parrish, J. A., et al. Photochemotherapy of psoriasis with oral methoxsalen and long-wave ultraviolet light. *N. Engl. J. Med.* 291:1207, 1974.
37. Pathak, M. A. Sunscreens: Topical and systemic approaches for protection of human skin against harmful effects of solar radiation. *J. Am. Acad. Dermatol.* 7:285, 1982.
38. Peck, G. L., et al. Prolonged remissions of cystic and conglobate acne with 13-*cis*-retinoic acid. *N. Engl. J. Med.* 300:329, 1979.
39. Pittsley, R. A., and Yoder, F. W. Retinoid hyperostosis: Skeletal toxicity associated with long-term administration of 13-*cis*-retinoic acid for refractory ichthyosis. *N. Engl. J. Med.* 308:1012, 1983.
40. Rees, R., et al. Management of the brown recluse spider bite. *Plast. Reconstr. Surg.* 68:768, 1981.
41. Roberts, M. E. T., et al. Psoriatic arthritis: Follow-up study. *Ann. Rheum. Dis.* 35:206, 1976.
42. Robertson, D. B., and Maibach, H. I. Topical corticosteroids. *Semin. Dermatol.* 2:238, 1983.
43. Roenigk, H. H., Jr., et al. Methotrexate guidelines—revised. *J. Am. Acad. Dermatol.* 6:145, 1982.
44. Rogers, R. S. Recurrent aphthous stomatitis: Clinical characteristics and evidence for an immunopathogenesis. *J. Invest. Dermatol.* 69:499, 1977.
45. Sams, W. M., Jr. Necrotizing vasculitis. *J. Am. Acad. Dermatol.* 3:1, 1980.
46. Shalita, A. R., et al. Isotretinoin treatment of acne and related disorders: An update. *J. Am. Acad. Dermatol.* 9:629, 1983.
47. Soter, N. A. Chronic urticaria as a manifestation of necrotizing venulitis. *N. Engl. J. Med.* 296:1440, 1977.
48. Stern, R. S., et al. Cutaneous squamous-cell carcinoma in patients treated with PUVA. *N. Engl. J. Med.* 310:1156, 1984.
49. Stoughton, R. B. Bioassay system for formulations of topically applied glucocorticosteroids. *Arch. Dermatol.* 106:825, 1972.
50. du Viver, A. Tachyphylaxis to topically applied steroids. *Arch. Dermatol.* 112:1245, 1976.
51. Wassilew, S. W. Management of pain in herpes zoster. *Semin. Dermatol.* 3:116, 1984.
52. Wilkin, J. K. Flushing reactions. Consequences and mechanisms. *Ann. Intern. Med.* 95:468, 1981.

32

Neurologic Emergencies

Octavio de Marchena

Stupor and Coma

The terms **stupor** and **coma** are used to describe alterations in the level of consciousness. It is important to realize that coma is a sign, not a disease, and that a large number of lesions, both structural and metabolic, can affect the level of consciousness. A methodic approach to the handling of the comatose patient is essential in sorting out the many possible etiologies.

I. **Pathophysiology.** Basically, there are only two types of lesions that cause coma: (1) both cerebral hemispheres are involved or (2) the reticular activating system that is present from the tegmentum of the pons to the diencephalon is damaged. Lesions that involve only one hemisphere do not normally cause coma or even substantially impair consciousness. Metabolic anomalies usually produce coma from bilateral hemispheral dysfunction.

II. **Etiologies of coma**

A. **Supratentorial mass lesions** cause coma either by affecting both hemispheres or, more commonly, by causing injury to the upper midbrain through herniation. Specific etiologies include cerebral hemorrhage, large cerebral infarction, epidural or subdural hematoma, and brain tumor or abscess.

B. **Subtentorial lesions** cause coma through injury to the reticular formation. Specific disease processes include pontine or midbrain infarction, pontine or cerebellar hemorrhage, and tumors.

C. **Metabolic disorders or diffuse lesions** can cause coma, usually by affecting both cerebral hemispheres. Such processes include ischemia, hypoglycemia, infections (meningitis or encephalitis), electrolyte or ionic disorders, exogenous toxins or poisons, endogenous organ failure (e.g., uremia, hepatic encephalopathy), cerebral concussion, and postictal states.

III. **Assessment**

A. **History.** A careful history can be very helpful in determining the cause of the coma. Important historic features to determine are the circumstances and suddenness of onset of the decreased consciousness; whether there were any preceding symptoms such as headache, vomiting, weakness, or seizures; whether there is a history of drug or alcohol use; and whether there is any history of prior medical or psychiatric disease. Since the patient cannot assist with the history, an attempt to interview relatives, friends, or observers should be made.

B. **General physical examination.** The vital signs may provide clues about what led to the alteration of consciousness. Coma in association with an elevated blood pressure suggests (1) an increased intracranial pressure due to a mass lesion, (2) hypertensive encephalopathy, or (3) a hypertensive bleed. Cheyne-Stokes respirations (i.e., alternating tachypnea and apnea) are seen in bihemispheral dysfunction, usually of a metabolic etiology. Other respiratory abnormalities have been described with brainstem dysfunction (e.g., central neurogenic hyperventilation, apneustic breathing), but their localizing value is poor. The general physical examination can also suggest a metabolic disorder (e.g., hepatic failure) or a structural lesion (e.g., bruising about the head) associated with coma.

C. **Neurologic examination.** The initial neurologic examination should be directed toward determining if there are any findings of a brainstem lesion or whether there is damage to both hemispheres. It is also important to determine whether there is a structural or metabolic dysfunction. In most cases, the lack of a definite anatomic site for the coma or decreased consciousness suggests a metabolic etiology. The following criteria are most helpful in the initial examination:

1. **Level of consciousness** is judged by noting the patient's responses to a variety of stimuli, ranging from calling the patient's name to pain. Since terms such as stuporous or semicomatose lack precision to allow comparison of the mental status over time, it is important to describe the patient's actual responses to stimuli.
2. **Pupillary size and reactions.** The pathway for pupillary constriction is based in the midbrain and travels with the third cranial (oculomotor) nerve to the eye. Abnormalities of pupillary function suggest midbrain dysfunction or damage to the third nerve, as may occur from uncal herniation.
   a. Reactive pupils equal in size are seen normally and in comatose states in which the brainstem is not involved, as in most metabolic comas.
   b. A unilateral fixed and dilated pupil most often suggests a hemispheric mass lesion, usually ipsilateral, with herniation. It is usually accompanied by oculomotor paralysis.
   c. Small but reactive pupils are seen in metabolic lesions, but may also be seen in thalamic or pontine lesions.
   d. Bilateral dilated and fixed pupils are associated with severe anoxic damage to the brainstem or with bilateral herniation from a hemispheric mass. Occasionally, they may be seen with toxicity from anticholinergic medication or glutethimide.
3. **Eye position and movement.** The evaluation of eye position and movement is the most important part of the coma examination, since normal eye movements require functioning of a substantial portion of the brainstem.
   a. **Eye position.** Dysconjugate gaze at rest suggests the presence of a cranial nerve lesion. Abduction of one eye is seen with a third nerve lesion, whereas adduction of one eye is seen with a sixth nerve lesion. Significant vertical separation of the axes of the eyes (skew) suggests a cerebellar or pontine lesion. Eyes looking down and in are seen in lesions of the midbrain-thalamic junction, as in thalamic hemorrhage. Conjugate gaze of the eyes in one direction suggests damage to either the contralateral frontal hemispheral gaze center or the ipsilateral pontine gaze center. If the eyes look toward the hemiparesis, the lesion is pontine; if away from the hemiparesis, it is hemispheric.
   b. The circuitry for **horizontal eye movements** travels through the tegmentum of the brainstem from the eighth to the third cranial nerve. Intact functioning of this system in a comatose patient confirms bihemispheric disease as the cause of the coma. Two reflexes are used to test this system.
      (1) The **oculocephalic maneuver** (also known as the **doll's eyes maneuver**) is tested by quickly turning the head of the patient from side to side. In comatose patients with an intact brainstem, the eyes move conjugately in a direction opposite to the head turning. This test should *not* be performed in patients with a possible cervical spine injury.
      (2) If the oculocephalic test shows no horizontal eye movements, the **oculovestibular test** (also known as **ice water calorics**) should be performed. This test is carried out with the head of the patient elevated to 30 degrees above the horizontal in order to maximally stimulate the horizontal semicircular canal. After making sure that there is no tympanic membrane rupture or basilar skull fracture and that the tympanic membrane is not occluded by cerumen, approximately 30–60 ml of ice cold water is squirted into the external auditory canal. The other ear is tested after an interval of 2–3 minutes. The normal response in a comatose patient with an intact brainstem is conjugate deviation of the eyes toward the ear that is being stimulated with cold water. In a patient who is awake, nystagmus with the fast component away from the stimulated side is seen. Failure of response only on one side suggests pontine damage on that side. Bilateral failure of response suggests extensive brainstem dysfunction. A partial deficit may suggest a cranial nerve dysfunction, such as failure of abduction of one eye with a sixth nerve lesion. When there is no response, it is possible that there might be bilateral eighth nerve damage from trauma or ototoxic drugs; this possibility should be considered before definitely assuming that parenchymal brainstem damage is present.
4. **Motor responses** are of value in evaluating the depth of coma and in detecting asymmetries in the examination. Any spontaneous movements should be ob-

served to determine if they are purposeful and if one side is used more than the other. The response to pain, usually a sternal rub or pressure on the knuckles, is observed for purposefulness and symmetry. Decorticate (flexor) or decerebrate (extensor) posturing may be seen spontaneously or in response to pain. In animal preparations, decorticate posturing is said to indicate a more rostral level of dysfunction in the brainstem than decerebrate posturing; however, in humans this localization is less clear, and generally posturing suggests a rostral brainstem, diencephalic, or hemispheric dysfunction. Posturing may also be seen in metabolic dysfunctions. Deep tendon reflexes and pathologic reflexes, such as the Babinski sign, should be checked; these reflexes are most useful when asymmetric.

D. Laboratory tests

   1. Computed tomography (CT) scan. If the cause of coma is not obvious on the physical examination or early laboratory studies (e.g., serum electrolytes, glucose, creatinine, and calcium; complete blood count [CBC]; and an arterial blood gas [ABG]), the next most useful test is the CT scan. The CT scan is frequently normal in coma, since in addition to being normal in metabolic coma, it is also normal in early brain infarction and most cases of meningitis and encephalitis. In addition, the CT scan may miss isodense lesions, such as subacute subdural hematomas. However, it is very useful in excluding hemorrhagic and mass lesions and may lead to the diagnosis by default (e.g., brainstem dysfunction secondary to infarction with an initially normal CT scan versus a cerebellar hemorrhage with an initial abnormal scan). The CT scan also allows determination of whether a lumbar puncture can be safely done.

   2. Lumbar puncture. The lumbar puncture (LP) is predominantly done to diagnose meningitis, encephalitis, or subarachnoid hemorrhage and should be analyzed for protein, glucose, and cell count. A subarachnoid hemorrhage can be distinguished from a traumatic tap by early centrifugation of a specimen of cerebrospinal fluid (CSF); in a subarachnoid hemorrhage that is more than a few hours old, the supernatant will be xanthochromic. In addition, a declining red cell count from the first to the last tube obtained is helpful in identifying a traumatic tap. The procedure is presented in Chap. 38.

   3. Other tests, such as the radionuclide brain scan and angiography, can be done depending on the suspected diagnosis and availability. The radionuclide brain scan may be more sensitive in herpes encephalitis than the CT scan. Angiography may detect isodense subdural hematomas missed by the CT scan and is necessary in the management of a subarachnoid hemorrhage.

IV. Differential diagnosis

   A. The **locked-in syndrome** is caused by damage to the base of the pons without affecting the reticular activating system present in the tegmentum. It is characterized by a patient who is awake but because of bilateral corticospinal tract damage has lost the ability to move and may appear unresponsive. Usually, at least vertical eye movements are preserved, and patients may communicate by these eye movements or by blinking.

   B. Akinetic mutism, or **abulia,** can be caused by lesions in the frontal lobes, basal ganglia, or midbrain. These patients usually appear awake and have preserved voluntary eye movements, but little to no spontaneous motor movements and a poor response to painful stimuli.

   C. Catatonia is a psychiatric syndrome in which the patient may not respond to voice stimuli or surroundings. Catatonic patients usually appear awake and may appear similar to patients with akinetic mutism; however, they are not difficult to differentiate from comatose patients.

   D. Hysterical unresponsiveness is not uncommon in emergency departments. Usually it can be distinguished from coma by the patient's resistance to attempted eye opening or by an inconsistency in the motor and reflex examination. Awake patients usually do not have doll's eyes, and caloric stimulation produces nystagmus rather than conjugate deviation. Since the response to pain is variable in patients with hysterical coma, excessive reliance on the response to painful stimuli is unreliable and not needed.

   E. Delirium is an abnormal mental state characterized by disorientation, irritability, paranoia, hallucinations, delusions, and a level of alertness ranging from lethargy to hyperalertness (see Chap. 34). Frequently, there are marked variations in the level of alertness, and lucid periods may alternate with episodes of delirium.

   1. Etiologies. Delirium usually is associated with toxic or metabolic disorders but may also be seen with multifocal cerebral illness and usually implies diffuse dysfunction of brain function. Particularly in elderly patients, the cause of delirium may be multifactorial, with no one metabolic dysfunction sufficient to cause delirium; the combination of several disturbances, however, can lead to a significant mental aberration.

2. **Evaluation.** The initial evaluation includes determination of electrolytes, calcium, creatinine, and an ABG; a toxicology screen should also be obtained. The drugs that the patient has been taking should be examined and unnecessary medications discontinued. A CT scan of the head and an LP should be performed to evaluate for structural lesions or infections. Since the electroencephalogram (EEG) is usually markedly slowed in delirium, it may be helpful in distinguishing delirium from psychiatric illness.

3. The **treatment** of delirium is the identification of the underlying cause and its correction, if possible. If no cause is apparent from careful evaluation of metabolic factors, continued observation and supportive care are indicated. With few exceptions (e.g., withdrawal states such as delirium tremens), sedation should be kept to a minimum, since it frequently increases confusion. When necessary to prevent self-injury, low doses of a neuroleptic, such as haloperidol, should be used. Often reassurance, a lighted room at night, and frequent orientation will be sufficient.

V. Treatment

A. **Airway.** Except for readily reversible causes of coma (e.g., hypoglycemia, opiod overdosage), endotracheal intubation (taking care in patients with suspected cervical spine injury) is indicated to secure a protected airway. Stuporous patients with intact pharyngeal reflexes, however, may not require intubation. Supplemental **oxygen** should be administered.

B. **Circulation.** An IV line should be started. Unless it is necessary to support the circulation or blood pressure, a dextrose solution (e.g., 5% D/W) should be infused at a slow rate.

C. **Dextrose.** Since hypoglycemia can cause coma and permanent neurologic damage, either immediate determination of the blood glucose with a Dextrostix or administration of 50 ml of 50% dextrose solution IV is indicated. If dextrose is administered, it is recommended that thiamine, 50–100 mg IV, also be given to avoid precipitating a Wernicke's encephalopathy.

D. **Naloxone hydrochloride,** 0.8–2.0 mg IV, should be given if there is any suspicion of a narcotic drug overdose, and the response assessed.

E. If there is clear evidence of **increased intracranial pressure** or **impending herniation** on examination, agents to reduce the intracranial pressure, such as an osmotic agent (e.g., mannitol, 1 gm/kg IV) or steroids (e.g., dexamethasone, 10 mg IV), are indicated; otherwise, they generally should be avoided.

F. **Control of an elevated blood pressure** should be done carefully and slowly in the setting of an ischemic brain infarction or a mass lesion, such as an intracerebral hematoma. Too rapid a drop in blood pressure may exacerbate the neurologic deficit by reducing perfusion. Initially, lowering of the diastolic blood pressure to 100–110 mm Hg generally is acceptable.

G. There are increasing data regarding the use of agents to reduce neuronal damage during episodes of hypoxia or increased intracranial pressure (e.g., use of calcium channel blockers or phenobarbital coma). Their use is controversial, and the benefits are still not demonstrated; thus, they cannot be recommended for routine use.

H. **Specific and definitive therapy** depends on the suspected etiology. See other sections of this book for specific therapeutic modalities.

VI. Prognosis of nontraumatic coma.
Excellent studies are available on the prognosis of coma based on clinical criteria [19]. While the absence of pupillary light reflexes, corneal reflexes, or caloric or doll's-eye responses on admission correlate with a poor prognosis for good recovery, it is not appropriate in the emergency department setting to make decisions to stop or limit therapy on these clinical criteria alone. For example, barbiturate intoxication may present with absent brainstem reflexes and still have a good prognosis with adequate support.

VII. Brain death.
Although the diagnosis of death is frequently made in the emergency department, the diagnosis of brain death is more involved and requires several studies and the input of more than one physician. State laws and hospital guidelines vary; but most protocols require that there be a cessation of all cerebral and brainstem functions (including respiration), that the damage be irreversible, and that conditions that might interfere with the examination (such as hypothermia, drug or metabolic intoxications,

and hypovolemic shock) be excluded or corrected. Radionuclide studies showing no cerebral blood flow or an EEG that shows no electrocerebral activity usually are required, in addition to the neurologic examination.

Seizures

Seizures are one of the major signs of central nervous system (CNS) dysfunction and can be caused by a variety of neurologic and systemic disorders. Seizures represent an abnormal, paroxysmal electrical discharge of neurons. The manifestations of a seizure depend on the location and spread of this abnormal activity. Therefore, seizures may present with (1) an altered consciousness, (2) motor activity, and/or (3) sensory, autonomic, or psychic symptoms. **Epilepsy** is defined as recurrent seizures. When seizures are due to an underlying process or lesion (e.g., hypoglycemia, drug withdrawal, tumor), they are called **secondary seizures.**

I. **Classification.** Since the pathophysiology of seizures is still largely unknown, the most useful classification uses the clinical symptomatology of the seizures. Seizures can be classified into two types: partial and generalized. Those that have clinical or EEG evidence of a focal onset are called **partial seizures,** and those that show synchronous involvement of both hemispheres are called **generalized seizures.**

II. **Clinical appearance**

   A. **Generalized seizures.** Since both hemispheres are involved, consciousness is impaired.

      1. **Absence seizures** are manifested as brief episodes of loss of consciousness associated with 3 cps (Hz) spike-and-wave discharges on the EEG. They usually begin in childhood and most frequently resolve or change to another seizure type in adult life. The attacks last for 5–30 seconds in duration and appear as blank staring with rhythmic blinking, chewing, or lip smacking. There is no aura, and recovery of consciousness is abrupt with no postictal confusion.

      2. **Generalized tonic-clonic seizures** begin with a sudden loss of consciousness with major motor activity. Initially, the whole body becomes rigid, sometimes associated with a cry (the tonic phase), and is followed by clonic jerking of the face, body, and extremities that slows and eventually stops. There may be associated tongue biting, cyanosis or brief apnea, and bowel or urinary incontinence. Consciousness returns slowly with a postictal period of confusion, headache, or lethargy. While premonitory symptoms of malaise or irritability may be present, there is no true aura.

   B. **Partial or focal seizures** arise from a particular area of the brain. These seizures may remain partial or spread to involve other areas of the brain and become generalized. When generalization occurs, the symptoms preceding the generalization are known as the **aura**; an aura occurs only in partial epilepsy. A **postictal (Todd) paralysis** also suggests a focal onset.

      1. **Simple partial seizures** present with simple symptoms, such as simple movements, primary sensations, or autonomic symptoms without a disturbance of consciousness.

      2. **Complex partial seizures** may have purposeful activity and amnesic or psychic phenomena. These seizures have also been called **psychomotor,** or **temporal lobe,** seizures, since they frequently arise from abnormalities in the temporal lobe. They may appear as absences with staring and automatisms, which are purposeless repetitive movements such as smacking of the lips or fingering of buttons in clothing; in addition, hallucinations and affective disturbances may be present.

      3. **Partial seizures with secondary generalization.** Many generalized tonic-clonic seizures may actually be partial seizures with secondary spread. This distinction is important since partial seizures are associated with focal brain disease, while true generalized seizures usually are not.

III. **Etiologies.** Seizures are usually divided into two categories: idiopathic and acquired (or secondary).

   A. **Idiopathic.** When no etiology is found for a seizure, the seizure is said to be idiopathic, although a variety of causes (some even genetic) are likely to be present, but are not discernible with present diagnostic techniques.

   B. **Secondary.** Structural abnormalities, diseases of the nervous system, and toxic or metabolic disorders may produce seizures.

      1. **Head injuries** can be a cause of secondary epilepsy or seizures. Seizures may

occur just after the head injury or as a late complication. The latter are more likely to become part of a seizure disorder.

2. **Brain tumors** are an important cause of seizures, particularly in the adult population. A focal seizure may be the first manifestation of a brain tumor, particularly if the tumor is in the hemispheres. Both primary brain tumors (e.g., astrocytomas, meningiomas) and metastatic tumors can be associated with seizures.

3. **Cerebrovascular disease** is a common cause of new-onset seizures in older people. While seizures can occur acutely during an ischemic infarct, they most frequently follow the development of a chronic scar. Both intracerebral and subarachnoid hemorrhages are associated with acute and delayed seizures.

4. **Degenerative and demyelinative diseases** (e.g., Alzheimer's disease, various storage diseases) can be associated with seizures.

5. **Toxic and metabolic disorders** are a very common cause for new and, less commonly, for recurrent seizures.

   a. **Hypoglycemia,** particularly in patients with a history of diabetes mellitus, should be suspected in any patient with a seizure.

   b. **Hyponatremia,** particularly in association with inappropriate antidiuretic hormone secretion, use of diuretics, hemodilution from hypotonic IV fluids, or water intoxication, is associated with seizures.

   c. **Hypocalcemia,** with or without hypoparathyroidism, may produce seizures. Hypomagnesemia is an uncommon cause of seizures but is seen occasionally in alcoholics or patients with poor nutrition.

   d. **Hypoxia** may produce seizures acutely during the hypoxic event (e.g., secondary to cardiac arrhythmias producing hypotension) or as a delayed effect in hypoxic encephalopathy.

   e. **Drug intoxication or withdrawal** may produce seizures. Some drugs are associated with seizures (e.g., amphetamines), while other drugs, such as the barbiturates and alcohol, produce seizures during withdrawal from chronic use.

   f. **Chronic renal or hepatic dysfunction** is associated with seizures, frequently myoclonic in type.

6. **Encephalitis, meningitis, and brain abscess** can all be associated with seizures, acutely and during healing. An infectious process should always be considered in new-onset seizures.

7. **Congenital abnormalities and perinatal trauma and asphyxia** are causes of seizures in childhood and, less commonly, of later epilepsy.

8. **Febrile seizures** are a type of seizure seen in childhood, associated with a high fever, but not with direct infection of the nervous system. The differentiation between meningitis and a febrile seizure may require performing an LP.

IV. **Evaluation.** It is essential to determine if the episode truly was a seizure, the type of seizure, and whether there is an underlying cause.

   A. **History.** Since patients with seizures frequently cannot remember the event, a reliable observer is helpful. Any factors suggesting focal onset, such as an aura prior to the onset of the seizure, onset of the seizure focally with later spread, eye deviation, or automatisms, should be sought. Postictal changes also are important, particularly the presence of a postictal deficit such as a Todd paralysis, which suggests a focal onset. Other important historic information includes a history of drug abuse, alcoholism, or previous head injuries. A history of diseases that can be associated with seizures (e.g., diabetes mellitus with hypoglycemia, previous meningitis, or encephalitis) or a family history of seizures should be sought.

   B. **Physical examination.** The general physical examination is frequently normal in patients with seizures. The emphasis should be directed toward evidence of diseases that can cause seizures, such as evidence of cardiovascular, renal, hepatic, or neoplastic disease. Examination of the skin is useful in detecting evidence of trauma, neurofibromatosis, and other neurocutaneous syndromes. The neurologic examination is valuable in demonstrating any neurologic diseases that can be associated with seizures and, particularly, in detecting any possible asymmetry of function that can suggest a focal onset.

   C. **Laboratory tests**
   1. **First seizure.** Patients who experience a seizure for the first time require evaluation of the underlying cause. In addition to the examination, important tests include the following:

Table 32-1. Anticonvulsant drugs according to type of seizure

Generalized seizures		Partial (focal seizures)		
Tonic-clonic	Absence	Simple	Complex	Secondary generalization
Phenytoin	Ethosuximide	Phenytoin	Carbamazepine	Phenytoin
Phenobarbital	Valproate	Phenobarbital	Phenytoin	Carbamazepine
Carbamazepine		Carbamazepine	Phenobarbital	Phenobarbital
Valproate		Valproate	Valproate	Valproate
			Primidone	

> **a. Biochemical tests** include serum electrolytes, creatinine, calcium, and glucose; liver function tests; CBC; and a sedimentation rate. Occasionally, serologic tests, such as a Venereal Disease Research Laboratory (VDRL) test or antinuclear antibody (ANA) determination, may be necessary.
>
> **b. CT scan.** Most patients with generalized or partial seizures should have a CT scan as part of their initial evaluation to search for a structural lesion that may have produced the seizure.
>
> **c.** An **LP** is essential if infection is a possibility. Fluid should be sent for cell counts, glucose, protein, serologies, and culture.
>
> **d.** A **toxicology screen** should be obtained if there is any possibility of drug ingestion or withdrawal.
>
> **e.** An **EEG** is useful in determining the seizure type. However, since the EEG usually is obtained interictally, it may be normal in up to one-third of patients with seizure disorders.
>
> **2. Recurrent seizures.** Patients with a known seizure disorder who present with recurrent seizures do not require extensive evaluation, unless there has been a change in the seizure type or in the examination. The reason for the recurrence (e.g., noncompliance, intercurrent illness) should be determined, if possible. Metabolic screening and drug levels are helpful in management, but other testing usually is not necessary.

V. Management

A. General principles. Treatment depends on the cause (e.g., hypoglycemia) and type of seizure. If a cause can be found for the seizure, correction of that cause is the correct treatment. If the seizure is idiopathic or if the cause is not directly treatable, anticonvulsant therapy (Table 32-1) is indicated. Once an anticonvulsant has been started, the dose is increased until the seizures are controlled, a therapeutic level is achieved, or symptoms of toxicity appear. If there has been no decrease in the seizure frequency with the anticonvulsant, the drug should be replaced by another drug. If a partial response is noted, however, a second drug should be added to the first. Although multiple anticonvulsants may be necessary to control seizures in a given patient, the complications of this type of therapy are substantial; thus, it is desirable to use as few drugs as possible to maintain good control.

B. Specific situations

> **1. Status epilepticus** consists of either continuous tonic-clonic seizures or recurrent seizures so frequent that normal consciousness does not return interictally. It is a neurologic emergency requiring immediate treatment and hospitalization, usually in an intensive care unit.
>
> **a. General measures**
>
> > **(1)** A secure **airway** must be maintained and aspiration prevented. Supplemental oxygen is administered.
> >
> > **(2) Vital signs** and the electrocardiogram (ECG) are monitored.
> >
> > **(3)** Baseline **blood tests** are drawn, preferably before therapy is initiated. These tests include serum electrolytes, CBC, glucose, calcium, and an ABG.
> >
> > **(4) Dextrose,** 50 ml of a 50% solution, is given IV. Since the nutritional status of the patient is not always known, it is recommended that thiamine, 50–100 mg IV, be administered at the same time to prevent precipitating Wernicke's encephalopathy.

Table 32-2. Treatment of adult status epilepticus*

Agent	Dosage	Rate
Step 1: Diazepam (Valium)	5–15 mg IV	5-mg boluses
Step 2: Phenytoin	18 mg/kg IV	< 50 mg/min
Step 3: Phenytoin	7 mg/kg IV	< 50 mg/min
Step 4: Phenobarbital	15 mg/kg IV	5 mg/kg IV q20–30min
Step 5: Lidocaine	1 mg/kg IV push, then 1–4 mg/min	Over 1–2 min, then drip infusion
Step 6: General anesthesia		

*Appropriate airway management is essential.

- **b. Drug treatment (Table 32-2)**
  - **(1) Diazepam,** initially 5-10 mg IV, is administered. Diazepam produces high initial brain levels and thus frequently will terminate seizures. However, because cerebral levels rapidly decline, seizures can recur. In addition, diazepam is a respiratory depressant and, by causing lethargy, makes postictal evaluation difficult. Because of these disadvantages, a total dosage exceeding 15 mg generally should be avoided.
  - **(2) Phenytoin.** The initial dosage is 18 mg/kg IV. The rate of administration should be no greater than 50 mg/minute; and ECG monitoring and frequent blood pressure checks during administration are necessary, since both arrhythmias and hypotension can occur with IV infusion. Since phenytoin precipitates in glucose solutions, only a normal saline drip should be used during phenytoin infusion. The CNS penetration is rapid. If seizures persist after the initial loading dose, an additional 7 mg/kg can be given, for a total dose of 25 mg/kg. This last step should be taken with caution in patients who are already taking phenytoin. However, the initial loading is justified in patients already on phenytoin, since the most common cause of status epilepticus in known epileptics is noncompliance.
  - **(3) Phenobarbital.** The dosage is 15 mg/kg, and the rate should be no faster than 100 mg/minute. Generally, doses of 5 mg/kg IV can be given 20 minutes apart until the loading dose is reached or the seizures stop. Since phenobarbital is a respiratory depressant, especially in combination with diazepam, endotracheal intubation and possibly respiratory assistance should be considered during phenobarbital loading.
  - **(4) Paraldehyde** IV or per rectum can be administered if seizure activity persists after phenytoin and phenobarbital loading.
  - **(5) Lidocaine,** 1 mg/kg IV as a loading dose, followed by an infusion of 20–60 μg/kg/minute (1–4 mg/minute), may be helpful.
  - **(6) General anesthesia** with a short-acting barbiturate, such as sodium amytal, may be required to terminate the seizure. Rarely, paralyzing agents may be needed to stop the muscle activity when it interferes with ventilation or when acidosis is severe; EEG monitoring is necessary in these cases to determine whether electrical seizures are still present.
- **2. Partial status and non-tonic-clonic status.** Patients may present with focal continuous seizure activity involving one side, a single extremity, or even a portion of a limb. Since these seizures do not always generalize to both sides of the brain, consciousness may be retained during the seizure. These seizures may be very persistent when not treated **(epilepsia partialis continua).** Patients may also present with **partial complex status;** during these seizures, consciousness is not normal, and the individual may have continuous automatisms, staring spells, or unusual behavior. While both of these seizures represent continuous seizure activity, they are not life-threatening and do not require as rapid an intervention as in status epilepticus. Initial treatment is similar to that of status epilepticus (see **1**), with small doses of diazepam and phenytoin loading, although the rate of loading can be slower. If additional drugs are needed, oral loading is safer and usually satisfactory.
- **3. Febrile seizures** (see Chap. 36) are brief, generalized seizures in a child, usu-

ally below 5 years of age, who is febrile prior to the seizure and has no evidence of CNS infection. The seizures should be short and nonfocal; the neurologic examination after the seizure should be normal; and laboratory studies, including serum glucose, electrolytes, creatinine, calcium, phosphate, and magnesium, should also be normal. An LP is required in most cases to rule out meningitis. The initial treatment is lowering the temperature with acetaminophen or cool baths. Generally, febrile seizures do not require anticonvulsant therapy; however, frequent recurrent febrile seizures may require prophylactic treatment with oral phenobarbital.

4. **Alcohol withdrawal seizures** (rum fits) typically occur when prolonged alcohol intake (usually for weeks) is decreased or stopped. The seizures usually occur 12–48 hours after the decrease or cessation of drinking. Although some patients may have several seizures, most patients have one or two seizures that are short in duration and require no treatment. Since patients who are alcoholics are prone to having seizures from electrolyte imbalances, hypoglycemia, trauma, or meningitis, a thorough neurologic examination, metabolic screening, and a period of observation (for at least 6 hours) in the emergency department are warranted. If the seizure is a first seizure, an evaluation (usually as an inpatient) is necessary, even if there is a clear history of alcohol withdrawal. If no cause is found other than alcohol withdrawal, no treatment with chronic anticonvulsants is indicated.

VI. Disposition. Patients who present with a first seizure usually require hospitalization for evaluation of the underlying etiology. On the other hand, patients with a known seizure disorder who present with recurrent seizures may be discharged with appropriate arrangements for follow-up, unless there are complicating factors (e.g., persistent seizures, change in seizure pattern, fever).

Cerebrovascular Disease

Cerebrovascular disease ranks as a leading cause of death and disability in developed countries. Vascular disease of the brain takes two major forms: ischemic disease and hemorrhage.

I. Anatomy of the cerebral circulation. The brain is perfused by two pairs of arteries: the carotid and vertebral arteries. The anterior circulation is fed by the two carotid arteries. The left carotid artery originates from the aortic arch and divides in the anterior neck into an internal and external branch; the internal branch enters the skull and then divides into the anterior and middle cerebral arteries. The right carotid usually originates from the innominate artery, but otherwise has the same course as the left carotid artery. The posterior circulation starts with two vertebral arteries that originate from the left and right subclavian arteries; they enter the skull through the foramen magnum and then join at the pontomedullary junction to form the basilar artery. The basilar artery, in turn, divides into the two posterior cerebral arteries. Collateral circulation is present through the circle of Willis, which connects the right and left circulations and the anterior and posterior circulations. Unfortunately, the ability of this collateral circulation to compensate for occlusion of major branches frequently is inadequate.

II. Features of anterior and posterior circulation disease. Since the carotid and vertebral arteries feed different areas of the brain, it is frequently possible to differentiate between anterior and posterior circulation disease on the basis of the symptoms and neurologic findings. This differentiation is of more than academic interest, since the handling of disease in these two areas is different.

A. **Manifestations of anterior circulation disease** are secondary to involvement of the portion of the cerebral hemisphere fed by the carotid artery. These manifestations include (1) a contralateral hemiparesis and hemisensory loss and (2) ipsilateral amaurosis fugax. Aphasia suggests involvement of the dominant hemisphere and is not seen with posterior circulation disease. Nondominant hemisphere involvement may present as neglect or denial of the contralateral side.

B. **Posterior circulation signs and symptoms** are secondary to ischemia of the brainstem, the occipital cortex, or portions of the temporal lobe. They include visual field loss, cortical blindness (from bilateral involvement of the occipital cortices), diplopia, ataxia, vertigo, sensory changes, and cranial nerve findings. Hemiparetic and hemisensory defects from involvement of descending and ascending tracts may also be seen, usually "crossed" to the cranial nerve findings (e.g., a left peripheral facial paresis with a right hemiparesis).

III. Ischemic cerebrovascular disease. In ischemic damage to the brain, there is interruption of the circulation to the brain tissue, either from generalized or focal decreases in blood flow. There are many causes of ischemia (e.g., atherosclerosis with occlusive disease of the intracranial or extracranial cerebrovascular circulation with artery-to-artery embolization, embolization from the heart). Other etiologies include small intracerebral vessel disease (lacunar infarctions), vasculitis, polycythemia, thrombocytosis, and hypotension.

A. Types of disease

1. **Transient ischemic attack (TIA).** A TIA is a transient neurologic deficit of vascular origin. By definition, the deficit resolves in 24 hours, although most TIAs are considerably shorter. The importance of TIAs is that approximately one-third of patients developing a TIA will go on to have a stroke, many of them within the first month after the first TIA. Transient ischemic neurologic deficits lasting longer than 24 hours are termed **reversible ischemic neurologic deficits (RINDs)** or **prolonged reversible ischemic neurologic deficits (PRINDs).** There is no prognostic or pathophysiologic difference between these neurologic deficits and other TIAs, with the exception that some of the former may actually represent small completed strokes. It is important to be sure that the transient episode represents a vascular phenomenon, since cardiac arrhythmias, orthostatic hypotension, hypoglycemia, seizures, and mass lesions (e.g., tumors, subdural hematomas) can also present with transient symptoms.

2. **Stroke in evolution (progressive stroke)** refers to the progression of a neurologic deficit, either from the history or physical examination during a period of observation. Anterior circulation strokes tend to reach maximum deficit faster, usually over a 24-hour period. In contrast, posterior circulation strokes may progress over 72 hours.

3. A **completed stroke** refers to a stroke in which the neurologic deficit has stabilized. While no intervention is likely to help the infarcted brain, if the deficit is small or there is still significant brain tissue at risk for further damage, intervention (see **D**) may prevent further strokes.

4. **Lacunar strokes** are small infarcts produced by the occlusion of small arteries within the brain. They are seen most commonly in the basal ganglia, thalamus, pons, cerebellum, or subcortical white matter. Hypertension seems to be the predominant risk factor, although these strokes may be seen with other diseases causing small-vessel disease. Some specific vascular syndromes are associated with lacunar infarcts, including a pure motor hemiparesis, pure hemisensory deficit, clumsy hand dysarthria, and ataxic hemiparesis. Multiple lacunar infarcts may produce a pseudobulbar state from bilateral damage to corticobulbar fibers.

5. **Cardiac embolization.** Emboli from the heart are a significant cause of ischemic stroke. Common sources of emboli are mural thrombi forming after a myocardial infarction or in akinetic segments of the ventricle. Atrial fibrillation, with or without valvular heart disease, is a significant risk factor for stroke from cardiac emboli. In addition, mitral valve prolapse may occasionally increase the risk of emboli.

B. Evaluation of cerebral ischemia

1. **History.** When a patient presents with a transient or still present neurologic deficit, the history should be directed toward the following:

   a. **Prior episodes.** Frequent, similar neurologic dysfunction tends to point toward a problem in one vascular distribution or in one area of the brain. Dissimilar episodes involving different areas of the brain suggest either multifocal disease or other etiologies (e.g., cardiac emboli).

   b. **Systemic illnesses.** Some illnesses may suggest possible etiologies. Diabetes mellitus is associated with both early atherosclerosis and small-vessel disease; both can cause ischemic strokes. However, diabetes can also be associated with hypoglycemia that can mimic TIAs. Cardiac disease (particularly a recent myocardial infarction, arrhythmias, or valvular disease) is associated with cardiac embolization. Hypertension can increase the risk of both intracerebral hemorrhage and lacunar infarction.

   c. **Mode of onset of symptoms.** Most strokes present with sudden or rapid onset of symptoms and focal neurologic signs. However, the initial symptoms may be mild, and the deficit may progress over a period of hours. A history of paresis, aphasia, diplopia, vertigo, or other symptoms may be useful in localizing the area of deficit, particularly if the symptoms and signs have resolved by the time the patient is examined. A history of headache, fever, malaise, or other illness preceding the onset of the neurologic deficit may suggest other diagnoses (e.g., meningitis or encephalitis).

2. **Physical examination.** The general physical examination can help in distinguishing between cerebrovascular lesions and other causes of stroke or neurologic dysfunction. Fever or a stiff neck suggests infection or subarachnoid hemorrhage. The presence of a murmur or atrial fibrillation suggests cardiac emboli as a possible cause. Evidence of neoplastic disease suggests metastatic disease to the brain. The neurologic examination is useful in determining the level of consciousness. A depressed mental status is not seen in stroke unless there is extensive involvement of the brainstem or bilateral hemispheric disease. Depression of the mental status occurs more frequently with seizures, mass lesions affecting both hemispheres (e.g., intracerebral hematoma), or metabolic derangements (e.g., hypoglycemia). The neurologic examination should also attempt to determine the extent and location of the dysfunction.

3. **Laboratory tests**

   a. Initial laboratory tests should include a serum glucose, electrolytes, and creatinine; CBC; platelet count; and coagulation studies. An ECG also should be obtained.

   b. The **CT scan** of the brain is a very useful initial test. Acute ischemic strokes do not show on the CT scan; they require a few hours to days to appear as a hypodense area. However, many other potentially confusing lesions do appear on the CT scan, particularly intracerebral hemorrhages, brain tumors, and most cases of subarachnoid hemorrhage. The CT scan also shows any significant mass effect that might be a contraindication to an LP.

   c. **LP.** The need for an LP in the evaluation of stroke is controversial. It is diagnostic in encephalitis and meningitis presenting as a stroke. It may also detect small subarachnoid hemorrhages missed by the CT scan. However, an LP followed by heparin anticoagulation increases the risk of spinal epidural hematomas. In general, an LP should be done when there is anything atypical or unusual about the presentation (see Chap. 38).

C. **Differential diagnosis.** A variety of conditions can present with transient neurologic dysfunction and appear as a TIA; these conditions need to be considered.

   1. A **mass lesion** (e.g., tumor, brain abscess, subdural hematoma) can present as transient neurologic dysfunction. CT can exclude most of these lesions.

   2. **Seizures** can produce focal neurologic dysfunction. A Todd paralysis (transient dysfunction of the area of the brain involved in a focal seizure, usually clearing within 24 hours) can be confused with a TIA, particularly if the seizure activity was not observed.

   3. A **migraine** can produce focal neurologic dysfunction as part of the aura of the migraine or during the headache phase in hemiplegic migraine. In **classic migraine,** the visual aura is characteristic enough to allow distinction from ischemia of the brain. In **hemiplegic migraine** and other complicated migraine (e.g., vertebrobasilar, ophthalmoplegic), this distinction can be more difficult, particularly if there is no history of prior episodes.

   4. **Hypoglycemia** can occasionally produce focal neurologic deficits that are reversed rapidly with correction of the hypoglycemia.

D. **Management.** In the emergency situation, it is frequently not possible to determine whether a given deficit represents a TIA, a stroke in evolution, or a completed stroke. When this determination cannot be made, all three conditions are managed the same way initially.

   1. **General measures**

      a. The **airway** should be secured as needed, and supplemental **oxygen** administered.

      b. **Blood pressure control.** It is important to correct hypotension, if present. On the other hand, hypertension, while a risk factor for stroke, should be treated very cautiously in the setting of an ischemic deficit. Since cerebral autoregulation is impaired during ischemia, rapid correction of hypertension may worsen the deficit and should be avoided. Unless there is evidence of hypertensive encephalopathy, the blood pressure should be lowered over a period of several hours to days.

      c. **Metabolic derangements,** such as hyper- or hypoglycemia or hyponatremia, should be corrected.

      d. If the CT scan and LP do not show evidence of bleeding and there are no other strong contraindications, most neurologists would start **heparin** with the aim to keep the partial thromboplastin time (PTT) at 2–2½ times control.

2. Specific measures

a. TIAs

(1) Anterior circulation TIAs. If the symptoms of a TIA are those of the anterior circulation, the next decision is whether to evaluate the carotid circulation with angiography. The importance of angiography is that as many as 50% of anterior circulation TIAs are secondary to a surgically correctable lesion; however, there is a 1–3% risk of stroke from angiography and carotid endarterectomy each. Usually there is time to evaluate for other causes of TIAs, such as cardiac emboli, before angiography is done. Angiography is performed as an emergency procedure only when there is progression of neurologic deficit despite aggressive medical therapy and only if there is a surgical team available to act on the results of the angiogram. Angiography also should be reserved for patients who might be surgical candidates. Most neurologists would recommend carotid endarterectomy if an appropriate lesion is found. If the patient is not a surgical candidate, the choice is between antiplatelet agents and warfarin.

(a) Antiplatelet agents. Aspirin, in dosages ranging from 900–1300 mg/day has been shown to reduce the risk of stroke after a TIA or small stroke by as much as 50%. Laboratory evidence suggests that for the antiplatelet effect much lower doses are necessary, perhaps as little as 1 mg/kg/day; however, the lower doses, although widely used, have not yet been examined for the same clinical effect. Other antiplatelet agents, such as sulfinpyrazone or dipyridamole, have not been shown to have any added advantage to aspirin alone.

(b) Warfarin. There is little controlled evidence to suggest that warfarin anticoagulation helps in cerebrovascular disease, in contrast to its benefit in cardiac embolization. However, many physicians feel that it is of benefit. Because of the risk of chronic anticoagulation with coumadin, it is worthwhile to try antiplatelet agents first. If warfarin is started, attempts to convert the patient over to aspirin should be made after a few months of therapy.

(2) Posterior circulation TIAs. The management of TIAs in the posterior circulation is the same as that of TIAs in the anterior circulation except that angiography is rarely indicated, since there is no current surgical approach to vertebrobasilar disease. Since vertebrobasilar TIAs involving the basilar artery seem to have a worse prognosis than those involving its end branches, many physicians will anticoagulate with warfarin rather than with antiplatelet agents when basilar artery disease is apparent.

b. Stroke in evolution.
When there is actual progression of neurologic symptoms during the period of initial observation, heparin anticoagulation should be instituted as soon as an intracranial bleed is ruled out. Progression of anterior circulation symptoms after heparin treatment is an indication for angiography.

c. Completed stroke.
When a patient has a completed stroke, the management is dependent on the amount of brain tissue still at risk in that vascular distribution. If the deficit is small, the management is the same as for a TIA (see **a (1)**), although there is little evidence that chronic anticoagulation helps completed strokes. For larger strokes, the emphasis should be on good nursing care to prevent aspiration pneumonia, contractures, urinary tract infection, and thrombophlebitis; early physical therapy and evaluation and correction of risk factors, such as hypertension, also are important.

Complications of completed strokes can occur, particularly in large strokes. Infarcted brain tissue becomes edematous and can produce a mass effect. When a hemisphere is infarcted, the swelling can be severe enough to cause herniation. Unfortunately, swelling from fluid entering dead brain tissue is not responsive to treatment with steroids. Hyperosmolar agents such as mannitol have only a transient effect. Generally, preventing fluid overload is the only available management. However, it is a different matter with cerebellar infarctions. Because of the limited space in the posterior fossa, infarction of a cerebellar hemisphere can lead to delayed deterioration of mental status from pressure on the brainstem. In such a situation, surgical evacuation of the infarcted cerebellum can be lifesaving.

    d. Lacunar strokes. The treatment of lacunar strokes is to control hypertension. Anticoagulation is rarely required unless there is doubt as to the true etiology. Small embolic strokes may resemble lacunes and should be handled as TIAs or cardiac embolic disease.

    e. Cardiac embolic disease should be considered in most TIAs or strokes as a possible etiology. The presence of atrial fibrillation, valvular heart disease, a recent myocardial infarction, or any cardiomyopathy should increase the suspicion of the heart as the source of emboli to the brain. Although echocardiography rarely demonstrates the thrombus, it frequently reveals the underlying cardiac disorder. Holter monitoring to demonstrate otherwise inapparent arrhythmias is also of value. Heparin anticoagulation, followed by administration of warfarin, is the treatment of choice for most cardiac emboli and should be maintained while the cardiac problem is present. Cardiac emboli can produce what is known as a "red," or hemorrhagic, infarct; this condition represents blood seepage into infarcted brain tissue. In most cases this infarct can be distinguished from an intracerebral hematoma, since the density of the blood is less in a hemorrhagic infarct. If the CT suggests a hemorrhagic infarct and the clinical picture is consistent with cardiac emboli, anticoagulation should be instituted even when some blood is present on the CT scan, since the rate of reembolization is high and can be reduced by early anticoagulation. The risk of increasing bleeding and producing a mass effect is small.

IV. Hemorrhagic cerebrovascular disease is usually divided into subarachnoid and intracerebral hemorrhages. In a subarachnoid hemorrhage, bleeding is into the subarachnoid space, producing a bloody spinal fluid. In intracerebral hemorrhage, bleeding is into the brain parenchyma, producing a hematoma within the brain. Occasionally, the two conditions are present together (e.g., when an intracerebral hematoma ruptures into a ventricle).

    A. Intracerebral hemorrhage

        1. Etiologies. The most common underlying cause of intracerebral hemorrhage is hypertension. The most common sites are the same as those of lacunar infarcts, namely, the basal ganglia, brainstem, cerebellum, and subcortical white matter. Other causes include arteriovenous malformations, aneurysms, mycotic aneurysms, blood dyscrasias (including anticoagulation), and tumors.

        2. Clinical features. In an intracerebral hemorrhage, blood at arterial pressure is introduced into the brain parenchyma. The result is the rapid development of a space-occupying lesion in the brain. This lesion is associated with headache, vomiting, and frequently a change in mental status. The type of deficit depends on the location of the hemorrhage. For basal ganglia or thalamic hemorrhages, there is usually a dense contralateral hemiparesis and hemisensory defect. The eyes frequently have a gaze preference toward the side of the lesion. Because of the mass effect affecting the deeper structures of the other hemisphere, patients are lethargic, whereas patients who have an ischemic stroke affecting only one hemisphere are not. For cerebellar or pontine hemorrhages, changes in mental status are even more prominent from damage to the reticular activating system, either directly or from a mass effect. In small cerebellar hemorrhages, ataxia with difficulty walking may be prominent.

        3. The **diagnosis** of an intracerebral bleed is suggested by the acute onset of a focal neurologic deficit with a change in mental status. The CT scan is the test of choice for diagnosis of an intracerebral hemorrhage. Angiography is indicated if there is suspicion of an arteriovenous malformation or if the bleed is atypical in some way (e.g., an intracerebral bleed in a normotensive patient).

        4. Treatment

            a. If signs of **herniation** are present, therapy is aimed at reducing the intracranial pressure with steroids (e.g., dexamethasone, 10 mg IV initially, followed by 4 mg q6h) and osmotic agents.

            b. Hypertension usually is present and should be treated if excessive; the blood pressure is not necessarily restored to normal, however, since the perfusion pressure may be reduced if there is too radical a reduction in the blood pressure. Diastolic pressures in the range of 110 mm Hg are satisfactory in the initial management. Nitroprusside has the advantage of rapid titration of blood pressure and is the drug of choice for initial treatment.

   c. **Cerebellar hemorrhages** and superficial temporal hemorrhages in the nondominant hemisphere can be surgically evacuated; and in the case of cerebellar hemorrhages, evacuation of the clot may be necessary to prevent herniation with irreversible damage to the brainstem. However, deep hemorrhages are not usually surgically accessible without unacceptable neurologic damage.

B. Subarachnoid hemorrhage

   1. Etiologies. Subarachnoid blood can be caused by a variety of lesions, including aneurysms, arteriovenous malformations, head trauma, and tumor. Large subarachnoid hemorrhages most commonly are caused by a "berry" aneurysm, which is a congenital defect in the media and internal elastic membrane of arteries, predominantly at the base of the brain. Aneurysms may produce symptoms as mass lesions. Posterior communicating artery aneurysms may compress the third nerve and produce a third nerve palsy with a dilated and fixed pupil. However, most aneurysms are asymptomatic until they rupture.

   2. Clinical features. With leakage of blood into the CSF there usually is a sudden onset of a very severe headache, vomiting, focal neurologic deficits, and changes in mental status. Nuchal rigidity follows in a few hours. Intracerebral blood may also be present and produce a mass effect of its own with focal findings.

   3. Diagnosis. The CT scan will demonstrate subarachnoid blood and any intracerebral hematoma in moderate to large subarachnoid hemorrhages. If there is CT evidence of blood in the CSF, an LP is not necessary. However, when a subarachnoid hemorrhage is suspected and the CT scan is normal, an LP is necessary to check for blood in the CSF. In subarachnoid hemorrhage, the CSF will have red cells, and the freshly spun fluid will be xanthochromic. Xanthochromia and a persistently elevated red cell count in the several tubes obtained are important features to distinguish a subarachnoid hemorrhage from a traumatic tap. Angiography should be performed early to allow localization of the aneurysm and should include both carotid arteries and the posterior circulation, since there may be more than one aneurysm present.

   4. Management. Initial management is aimed at controlling the elevated intracranial pressure, reducing the risk of rebleeding, and supporting the patient until surgery can be done.

      a. General care of the patient includes bed rest with sedation, treatment of cerebral edema with dexamethasone, and control of hypertension.

      b. Antifibrinolytic agents such as aminocaproic acid (Amicar) are used in the hope of delaying rebleeding. Doses range from 24–36 gm/day IV. Their use is complicated by pulmonary emboli and rarely a myopathy.

      c. The **timing of surgery** for aneurysms varies with the clinical state of the patient. Generally, the operative results are better with patients who are neurologically normal. However, waiting too long increases the risk of rebleed during the waiting period.

      d. Treatment of complications. In addition to a rebleed, vasospasm of cerebral vessels can cause additional neurologic damage. There is no good treatment for vasospasm currently available, although the calcium channel blocker, nimodipine, has been reported to be helpful.

      e. Arteriovenous malformations can be treated by surgical removal or by angiographic embolization.

Headache

I. Pain-sensitive structures. The brain parenchyma is insensitive to pain, as are most of the intracranial contents except for the large proximal blood vessels, the venous sinuses, and portions of the basal dura and the tentorium. This relative insensitivity of the intracranial structures explains why large parenchymal lesions usually produce no pain until they displace the pain-sensitive structures. In contrast, the pericranial tissues, including the fascia, muscles, scalp, and extracranial blood vessels, are all pain-sensitive, as are the nearby structures that may refer pain to the head (in particular, the eyes, teeth, nasal sinuses, and cervical spine).

II. Evaluation of the patient with headache

   A. History. A careful history will frequently identify the headache type. It is important to inquire about the quality of the headache; its duration, frequency, and location;

and premonitory or associated symptoms. From the point of view of separating dangerous from benign headaches, chronic or recurrent headaches are much more likely to be benign than acute or recent-onset headaches.

B. Physical examination. The general physical examination should be directed toward a possible systemic cause for the headache and should include an examination of the surrounding structures. In particular, fever and meningismus suggest meningitis, and tender temporal arteries in an elderly patient suggest temporal arteritis; a red painful eye may be sign of angle closure glaucoma. The neurologic examination, with few exceptions, should be normal in patients with uncomplicated headache, and any abnormalities should dictate further evaluation. If the neurologic examination is normal, further neurologic evaluation is not necessary unless the history suggests a particular diagnosis (e.g., positional headaches suggesting a mass lesion), the headaches have changed in character, or some features of the headaches are atypical (e.g., new onset of vascular headaches in a 70-year-old person).

C. Laboratory tests are reserved for patients with an abnormal examination or when the history suggests a particular diagnosis that may need further confirmation.

1. The **CT scan** is an excellent test for determining whether any mass lesions are present. It should be performed in patients with an abnormal neurologic examination or when the history suggests the presence of a mass lesion (e.g., positional headaches). In most cases, a CT scan should be done before performing an LP.

2. The **LP** in evaluating headache has two purposes: (1) to measure the CSF pressure and (2) to evaluate for blood and inflammatory or carcinomatous changes in the CSF. While in some situations an LP may be done as the first test (e.g., a suspected bacterial meningitis when a rapid diagnosis is essential), usually a CT scan is done first to make sure no mass lesion is present that might increase the risk of herniation.

3. **Other tests** depend on the suspected cause of the headache. Sinus, dental, or cervical spine films may be helpful in the evaluation of referred pain. A sedimentation rate is essential in the elderly patient with a new headache.

III. Headache syndromes

A. Vascular headaches

1. **Migraine headaches** are usually defined as severe intermittent headaches that are usually throbbing in character. Although usually thought to be unilateral, they may be bilateral or change sides. Most patients with migraine headaches are women. Onset of the headache is usually in adolescence or young adulthood, although onset in childhood and later life is possible.

   a. Types of migraine

   (1) **Classic migraine.** This variant is characterized by the presence of a visual aura before the onset of the headache. Usually this aura takes the form of a **scintillating scotoma,** which is an area of decreased or absent vision surrounded by bright zig-zag lines that may wander through the visual field. In other cases, patients may just describe blurriness or waviness of the vision. After the aura, which lasts from 10–30 minutes, the headache begins. The headache is usually unilateral, throbbing in character, and frequently associated with nausea, vomiting, and photophobia. The duration varies from 4–24 hours but may occasionally be longer.

   (2) **Common migraine.** As the name suggests, this variant is the most common form of migraine. Unlike classic migraine, no aura is present. The first warning of the onset of the headache is the beginning of pain. The headache can be unilateral or bilateral. The quality of the pain and associated symptoms are the same as for classic migraine. Patients with classic migraine may also have common migraine.

   (3) **Complicated migraine.** Several less common migraine variants are characterized by associated neurologic deficits other than the visual symptoms seen in classic migraine. These neurologic deficits may precede the headache or appear with and persist with the headache. These complicated migraines include **hemiplegic migraine** (with a hemiparesis or hemisensory defect), **ophthalmoplegic migraine** (with variable loss of extraocular muscle and pupillary function), and **basilar artery migraine** (with vertigo, diplopia, and ataxia). Rarely, the neurologic deficit may appear without the headache **(acephalgic migraine).**

b. The **mechanism of migraine** is not known. In classic migraine, the blood flow to the brain appears to be decreased during the aura and then increased in both the intracranial and extracranial vessels during the headache, presumably from vasoconstriction and dilation, respectively. What triggers this cycle and how this produces pain is not yet apparent. Patients with migraine, however, seem to be more sensitive to a variety of stimuli. These people may respond with headache to stimuli that would not produce a headache in a patient without migraine. For example, a history of ice cream headache, a brief throbbing bifrontal headache produced by the application of cold to the palate, can be elicited in almost 90% of patients with migraine but in less than 30% of patients who do not have migraine.

c. Treatment

(1) Symptomatic therapy. Unfortunately there is little that can be done for the acute migraine attack once the headache begins. For mild cases, aspirin, acetaminophen, or one of the nonsteroidal anti-inflammatory agents may be helpful. Combinations of aspirin, caffeine, and small amounts of barbiturate (e.g., Fiorinal) may also provide some relief. For severe migraines, narcotics may be necessary along with antiemetics, such as promethazine or prochlorperazine. Some physicians have suggested the use of a nonsteroidal anti-inflammatory agent in combination with metoclopramide to speed absorption and reduce nausea. Sedation may also be helpful.

(2) Abortive therapy involves administration of medication at the onset of a migraine to prevent the headache phase. These medications work best when taken immediately before the onset of the headache. When taken during the headache phase, they are essentially ineffective. They are the treatment of choice for patients who have an aura or infrequent migraines. Because the treatment is episodic, they are worth a trial in most patients who have migraine headaches. Ergotamine is the most widely used agent for aborting migraines and comes in a variety of preparations containing caffeine and sedatives. When the oral route cannot be used because of nausea or delayed absorption, rectal, sublingual, and inhaled forms are available. Ergotamine is contraindicated in the presence of peripheral arterial disease or coronary artery disease, as well as in pregnancy. To prevent ergotism, the dose/migraine attack should not exceed 6 mg, and no more than 12 mg should be used each week.

(3) Prophylactic therapy is usually very effective, but it requires taking medicine daily and therefore should be used only in those patients who have very frequent migraines or severe migraines not responsive to ergotamine.

(a) Propranolol, 40–320 mg/day in divided doses, is a very effective method for preventing the onset of migraine attacks, including the aura. The mechanism of action is uncertain. While the effectiveness may vary, other beta-blockers have also been shown to be effective, including nadolol (40–160 mg/day), atenolol (50 mg/day), and metoprolol (100–300 mg/day).

(b) Amitriptyline, 25–75 mg at bedtime, is another effective regimen. The antimigraine effect appears to be independent of the antidepressant action and frequently occurs at doses that are not thought to be sufficient to be antidepressant. Because amitriptyline is also effective in tension headaches, it is useful in patients with mixed tension-vascular headaches, a not uncommon occurrence. Other tricyclic antidepressants also may be helpful, although experience with them is more limited.

(c) Methysergide, 4–8 mg/day in divided doses, is another effective prophylactic agent. Unfortunately, its use is restricted by a rare complication: retroperitoneal, cardiac, or pulmonary fibrosis. This complication appears to be dependent on the length of time the patient is on the drug and rarely occurs before 6 months of use. Since migraine is a chronic illness, methysergide is rarely used in migraine. In severe cases responsive only to methysergide, discontinuing the drug every 4–6 months seems to lower the risk of fibrotic complications.

(d) **Ergotamine.** Some patients may respond to daily ergotamine in doses of 1 mg bid as a prophylactic agent. With daily dosing, care should be taken to avoid ergotism.

(e) **Other agents.** Phenytoin at therapeutic levels may serve as an effective prophylactic agent in some patients; it seems to be more effective in childhood migraine. New drugs that may prove helpful are the calcium blocking agents, although experience with them is still limited; diltiazem, verapamil, and nifedipine have been reported as effective in migraine prophylaxis.

2. **Cluster headaches** are relatively rare vascular headaches that, in contrast to migraine, are more common in men than in women.

a. **Clinical features.** Typically the headaches are unilateral and are usually localized in the periorbital area. The pain is very severe and is usually described as jabbing or boring. Each episode of pain is relatively brief, lasting from 15 minutes to 1–2 hours and then resolving. No aura is present. More than one episode of pain can occur daily, with up to three to eight episodes possible. The name cluster comes from the temporal clustering. Patients have daily headaches that last from 3 weeks to 3 months. Then the headaches resolve, and the patient may remain headache-free for months to years. A fortunately rare variant is **chronic cluster,** which has the same characteristics as regular cluster headaches, but the episodes of pain occur chronically.

b. **Treatment.** The short duration of cluster headaches makes symptomatic treatment difficult because the headache may resolve before oral analgesics become effective.

(1) **Abortive therapy.** Ergotamine, particularly if taken sublingually (Ergostat) or inhaled (Medihaler Ergotamine Aerosol) occasionally may abort an attack of pain. Inhaled oxygen also has been reported to be useful in aborting an attack, presumably by inducing vasoconstriction.

(2) **Prophylactic therapy.** More useful are medications that tend to prevent cluster headaches rather than those that abort the individual episodes of pain; preventive medications include the following:

(a) **Prednisone** in doses of 40–60 mg/day, given for a week to 10 days and then tapered over 3 weeks, is effective in stopping clusters, although the headaches may return as the prednisone is lowered.

(b) **Methysergide** in doses of 4–8 mg/day is effective in up to 75% of patients with cluster headaches. The long-term complications of methysergide need to be kept in mind, but usually the duration of clusters is brief enough so that the drug can be given safely.

(c) **Lithium carbonate** in doses of 300 mg tid or qid can be used in refractory cases of cluster headaches. It actually seems to be most useful in chronic clusters. Since the toxicity of lithium can be substantial, frequent monitoring of serum levels is indicated.

(d) **Calcium blocking agents** have also been reported to be useful in cluster headaches, although the optimal agents and dosages have not yet been determined.

(e) **Indomethacin,** 25–50 mg tid, has been reported to be useful in a clusterlike syndrome called **chronic paroxysmal hemicrania.** This syndrome differs from cluster headaches predominantly in the number of daily attacks, which may reach up to 18/day.

B. **Tension headaches**

1. **Clinical features.** In their mild form, tension headaches are intermittent, frequently related to stressful events, and easily relieved by mild analgesics, such as aspirin or acetaminophen. When they become chronic, however, they can be severe and produce significant distress. Patients with severe tension headache describe the pain as a tight sensation (like a "band" around the head) or a pressure sensation (like a "balloon blowing up") within the head. In addition, patients frequently complain of a stiff neck. When a patient reports that a headache has been present for months or years and is present continuously throughout the day from arising until going to sleep at night but rarely, if ever, interferes with sleep, the diagnosis is almost certainly a tension headache. Patients with severe tension headaches frequently are depressed and anxious, although the etiology of the depression may not always be obvious. Tension headaches can coexist with other headaches. A not unusual headache pattern is

tension headaches with intermittent migraines; some investigators have pointed out that there is no sharp dividing line between patients with tension headaches and those with migraine headaches and that the two populations frequently blend.

2. **Treatment.** It is important to establish rapport with the patient and provide reassurance that no life-threatening process, such as a brain tumor, is present.

   a. Initially, **mild analgesic** (e.g., aspirin, acetaminophen) should be tried. Often this treatment is effective. Narcotic analgesics should be avoided.

   b. **Mild tranquilizers,** such as the benzodiazepines, may be useful for short-term treatment of tension headaches. However, they are rarely useful for the chronic variety and may exacerbate depression. Diazepam, 10–30 mg/day, may be given in conjunction with a mild analgesic, such as aspirin or acetaminophen. The duration of treatment should be well defined.

   c. The **tricyclic antidepressants** probably are the most effective agents in severe chronic tension headaches. Amitriptyline is the most frequently used agent, although other antidepressants likely are equally effective. As in migraine, the doses required are lower than those thought necessary to treat depression. For amitriptyline, this usually means doses in the range of 25–75 mg/day, usually given at bedtime to reduce the sedating effect of the medication.

   d. **Relaxation techniques** such as biofeedback, muscle relaxation exercises, meditation, and hypnosis may prove helpful in some patients and should be tried in patients with refractory headaches or in those who cannot tolerate other medications.

   e. In patients with clinical depression, psychiatric referral is of benefit.

C. **Headache of mass lesions.** Mass lesions displacing the dura or vascular structures can cause headache. Unfortunately, there is little specific about these headaches. Approximately 60% of patients with a brain tumor complain of headache; however, in only 30% is it the major complaint. Tumors in the posterior fossa, because of the limited space and because they obstruct CSF pathways early, produce headache more frequently. When present, the headache of a mass lesion is described as a deep, steady, dull ache that rarely is throbbing. Occasionally, the pain is severe, but most of the time it is only moderate in intensity. Frequently, it is aggravated by coughing, straining at stool, or exertion. If there is any variation in severity, the headache is worse in the morning. In particular, features of a headache that suggest a mass lesion include (1) an abnormal neurologic examination, (2) positional or exertional exacerbation of the headache, and (3) a paroxysmal onset. The last refers to a headache that has a very sudden onset, reaching a maximum intensity within seconds to a few minutes, and is typical for a headache that is caused by obstruction of CSF pathways; the pain is bifrontal or generalized and may be associated with nausea, vomiting, or loss of consciousness, and moving the head may relieve or bring on the headache. An emergent CT scan is indicated. CT scanning is also indicated in the presence of an abnormal neurologic examination. Otherwise, referral to a neurologist is appropriate.

D. **Headache due to CNS bleed**

   1. **Clinical features.** The sudden onset of a violent headache, with or without a change in mental status or focal findings, suggests a subarachnoid hemorrhage. While a stiff neck is frequently present with this hemorrhage, it may take a few hours to develop and thus may not be present initially. Patients describe the headache as the worst headache of their life or as "something exploded" in their head. Malaise, photophobia, or an abnormal neurologic examination may be present.

   2. **Evaluation.** Patients with a suggestive history and an abnormal neurologic examination should have a CT scan of the head performed to evaluate for the presence of a parenchymal hematoma or subarachnoid blood; a normal CT scan generally should be followed by an LP. Patients with a normal examination, except possibly for a stiff neck, should have an LP to evaluate for the presence of red blood cells or xanthochromia.

E. **Headache due to CNS infection.** The presence of headache, fever, and a stiff neck suggests the presence of meningitis or encephalitis. An immediate LP is indicated for diagnostic purposes.

F. **Temporal arteritis** (also called **giant-cell arteritis**) is an inflammatory disease of predominantly the extracranial portions of the cerebrovascular circulation.

   1. **Clinical features.** The disease affects older patients and is very rare before age

50. Typically, it presents with malaise, a low-grade fever, weight loss, and headache. Since it is frequently seen in association with polymyalgia rheumatica, patients may also complain of proximal joint or muscle pains. The laboratory hallmark is a markedly elevated sedimentation rate, usually greater than 60 but frequently as high as 100. Temporal arteritis is rarely fatal, but a feared complication is visual loss, which may be bilateral, due to ischemia to the optic nerves from involvement of the ciliary arteries by the inflammation. The headache in temporal arteritis is nonspecific. There may be tenderness over the temporal arteries, but this feature is not reliable.

   2. **Evaluation.** Essentially, any new headache in an elderly patient warrants obtaining a sedimentation rate. If the sedimentation rate is elevated, the diagnostic test of choice is a temporal artery biopsy to look for granulomatous arteritis.

   3. **Treatment.** In suspicious cases, particularly when there is any suggestion of visual involvement, treatment with high-dose steroids should be started even before the biopsy is obtained. Prednisone, in dosages of 60–100 mg/day in divided doses, usually is recommended for initial treatment. Since temporal arteritis is a self-limited illness, the steroids can be tapered after a few months to a year.

G. **Postconcussion syndrome.** Following head injury, patients frequently complain of dizziness, headache, malaise, poor concentration, and depression. Usually this syndrome is associated with head injuries severe enough to produce loss of consciousness but may be seen with less severe injuries. The neurologic examination is normal; and laboratory tests, including the CT scan, are frequently normal, although occasionally subtle abnormalities of vestibular function can be demonstrated. The duration of the syndrome is variable and is poorly correlated with the severity of the head injury. Generally, reassurance and administration of a mild analgesic is sufficient. Rarely, treatment with antidepressants or psychotherapy may be necessary.

H. **Post-LP headache.** A headache that occurs after an LP typically is mild to absent when the patient is lying flat but becomes severe and may be associated with dizziness or nausea when the patient stands. It is thought that the headache is secondary to a persistently low CSF pressure from leakage of the CSF into the epidural tissues through the spinal needle puncture site. The headache usually can be managed by bed rest and administration of a mild analgesic but, if prolonged, may require an epidural patch with autologous blood.

I. **Trigeminal neuralgia**
   1. **Clinical features.** Also known as **tic douloureux,** trigeminal neuralgia is a syndrome characterized by sudden, severe jabbing pains in the distribution of one of the branches of the trigeminal nerve. The pain occurs as brief, very severe stabs of pain that may be precipitated by touching a specific area in the mouth, lips, or cheek. Talking or eating may also trigger the pain. Each episode of pain lasts only for a few seconds, but multiple episodes may occur, producing pain for hours. Generally, the neurologic examination is normal. Evidence of significant sensory loss in the trigeminal distribution should prompt a search for structural disease of the nervous system.

   2. **Treatment.** Carbamazepine is the drug of choice for trigeminal neuralgia. The patient is started at doses of 200 mg bid, and the dosage is increased slowly until either relief of symptoms is obtained or side effects intervene. Because of the rare incidence of aplastic anemia and a dose-dependent reversible leukopenia, frequent CBCs are recommended. For patients who derive inadequate relief from carbamazepine, baclofen, as an additional drug, may be helpful. In patients in whom drug therapy is no longer helpful, surgical therapy can be tried and usually consists of either selective injuries to the gasserian ganglion or decompression of the gasserian ganglion through a posterior fossa craniotomy.

J. **Benign intracranial hypertension,** also known as **pseudotumor cerebri,** is a condition in which the CSF pressure is elevated without any mass lesion or obstruction to CSF pathways being present. Although usually idiopathic, the condition has also been described with excessive vitamin A ingestion, as a side effect of tetracycline use, or, occasionally, in association with steroid treatment. The cause is uncertain but is thought to be due to defective CSF absorption at the level of the arachnoid villi.
   1. **Clinical features.** Patients present with a generalized headache and papil-

ledema. Most patients are young obese women without any obvious cause. The neurologic examination is usually normal, with the exception of papilledema, although unilateral or bilateral sixth nerve palsies may be present.

2. The **diagnosis** requires demonstration of a normal CT scan (or one showing small ventricles) and an elevated CSF pressure measured by LP.

3. **Initial treatment** is repeated LPs to reduce the CSF pressure. If the elevated pressure does not resolve, treatment with a diuretic, such as acetazolamide, may be necessary. On rare occasions, lumboperitoneal CSF shunting may be needed to prevent blindness.

Dizziness

Dizziness is a common complaint in the emergency department and, like many other symptoms, may be benign or portend more severe illness. A problem with the evaluation of the dizzy patient is the vagueness of the term *dizzy*; several different conditions can be implied when a patient complains of dizziness. Important distinctions are between central and peripheral causes of vertigo, lightheadedness, syncope, and imbalance. In many cases, careful history taking enables the clinician to distinguish between these different forms.

I. **Types of dizziness**

A. **Vertigo** is a sensation of either the patient or the environment moving. The sensation usually is rotational, although in some cases the patient may describe a sensation of being hurled to the ground. Severe vertigo usually is accompanied by nausea, vomiting, and an unstable gait. Milder forms may be difficult to distinguish from lightheadedness. Rotational vertigo usually signifies disease of the vestibular system, either the peripheral apparatus or its central connections.

B. **Faintness** or impending loss of consciousness is another form of dizziness. Pallor, diaphoresis, a roaring sensation in the ears, and dimming of vision frequently are described. This dizziness usually implies a diffuse decrease in cerebral blood flow, as seen in orthostatic hypotension, vasovagal episodes, or cardiac arrhythmias with hypotension. Less commonly, it suggests a widespread metabolic dysfunction, such as hypoglycemia.

C. **Imbalance, or disequilibrium,** is another type of dizziness. This sensation is of a loss of balance without an abnormal sensation of movement. Patients with imbalance have disorders of motor control, on the basis of motor system disease, cerebellar dysfunction, and/or sensory deficits.

D. **Lightheadedness** other than vertigo is another form of dizziness. Patients usually complain of vague symptoms that cannot be clearly identified as the other types of dizziness. This sensation may represent milder forms of vertigo or imbalance. However, it may also be seen in depression, anxiety, hyperventilation, or multiple sensory deficits, particularly in the elderly.

II. **Evaluation of the dizzy patient**

A. **History.** The history should be aimed at distinguishing between the different types of dizziness. In particular, the abruptness or duration of symptoms and precipitating factors, such as head motion or changes in position, should be elicited. In addition, a history of any acute or underlying illnesses and use of drugs should be sought.

B. **Physical examination.** The general physical examination may reveal evidence of an acute or underlying disease process (e.g., dehydration, cardiac arrhythmia, otitis media). The neurologic examination may enable distinction between central and peripheral vestibular involvement. It may also reveal features suggestive of brainstem involvement or sensory impairment. In addition, a variety of bedside tests are useful in the evaluation of dizziness. Reproduction of the patient's symptoms with one of these maneuvers may be very helpful in determining the cause of the dizziness, especially when the history is vague or inconclusive.

1. **Orthostatic hypotension** (see **Syncope,** sec. **II.C.2**). The blood pressure and pulse are measured with the patient lying down and then after standing for 1 minute. Additional measurements may need to be taken after the patient has been standing for a few minutes. A drop in systolic pressure of more than 20 mm Hg or an increase in the pulse rate of at least 20 beats/minute, particularly if associated with the appearance of symptoms, suggests orthostatic hypotension as the cause of the dizziness.

2. **Neck twist.** The patient twists the head in each direction. Dizziness in this test can be seen with labyrinthine disease, carotid sinus hypersensitivity, central positional vertigo, or even with cervical spine disease.

Table 32-3. Positional nystagmus with Nylen-Bárány maneuver

Sign	Peripheral	Central
Latency before onset of nystagmus	2–30 sec	None
Duration	1 min or less	Persists
Fatigues on repetition	Yes	No
Direction of nystagmus	One direction/head position	May change

3. **Carotid sinus stimulation** requires ECG monitoring and an IV line in place. This maneuver should be used with care in elderly patients and in those with cardiovascular disease. The appearance of dizziness or syncope suggests carotid sinus hypersensitivity (see **Syncope**, sec. **II.C.4**).
4. **Walking and turning.** The patient walks in one direction and then quickly turns. Patients with cerebellar disease, multiple sensory abnormalities, or labyrinthine disease will have difficulty with this maneuver.
5. **Nylen-Bárány, or head-hanging, maneuver.** The patient is taken from a seated position to a lying down position with the head extended over the edge of the bed 45 degrees below the horizontal and turned 45 degrees to the right or left. The onset of vertigo with nystagmus suggests positional vertigo of either a peripheral or central etiology (Table 32-3).
6. **Hyperventilation** for 3 minutes. Dizziness in this setting suggests anxiety as the etiology.
   C. **Laboratory tests.** In the emergency department, an ECG, CBC, and serum electrolytes, glucose, and creatinine should be obtained. More sophisticated tests include electronystagmography with caloric stimulation of the vestibular canals, audiometry, and brainstem-evoked responses; these tests are useful in determining the site of the lesion. A CT scan may show the presence of a vascular or mass lesion of the posterior fossa.
III. **Specific states of dizziness**
   A. **Vertigo.** In patients with vertigo, the most important distinction is between central or peripheral disorders. Particularly important in this distinction is neurologic evidence of involvement of surrounding brainstem structures indicative of central lesions.
      1. **Peripheral vertigo**
         a. **Types of peripheral vertigo**
            (1) **Acute peripheral vestibulopathy** (also known as **acute labyrinthitis** or **vestibular neuronitis**) presents as a single episode of spontaneous vertigo, sometimes with a sudden onset, that lasts for hours or a few days. Although attacks may follow minor respiratory or viral infections, the relationship to infections is not always present. With the vertigo, there are symptoms of nausea, vomiting, and instability of gait. Patients usually appear ill, are often diaphoretic, and have prominent nystagmus. Generally, symptoms improve after a couple of days, but a sensation of instability may persist for weeks. There is no impairment of hearing, but caloric testing shows impairment of function of the vestibular system on one side.
            (2) **Acute and recurrent peripheral vestibulopathy.** This entity is clinically similar to the acute form but consists of multiple bouts of vertigo that may occur over a period of years. Generally, patients with this condition are older than those with the single episodes. Again, there is no auditory impairment.
            (3) **Benign positional vertigo** is a common cause of vertigo. Typically, the patient experiences vertigo when making sudden head movements, such as turning over in bed. The vertigo is worse when the affected ear is underneath, may be accompanied by nausea or vomiting, and generally lasts only seconds to minutes. When there is no precipitating head movement, the patient is free of vertigo. The presence of benign positional vertigo can be determined by the Nylen-Bárány maneuver (see **II.B.5**) and usually can be differentiated by this test from positional vertigo caused by central lesions (see Table 32-3).

(4) **Ménière's disorder.** Although Ménière's disorder is considered a common cause of dizziness, it is actually infrequently seen. It usually occurs in adults and consists of bouts of vertigo associated with hearing loss and tinnitus. The hearing loss may precede the first episode of vertigo and is initially unilateral in most patients. Each episode of vertigo lasts from hours to days and recurs at variable intervals. The diagnosis is made from the history and characteristic findings on audiometry.

(5) **Toxic damage to the labyrinths.** A variety of drugs can cause temporary or permanent vestibular dysfunction. These drugs primarily include antibiotics of the aminoglycoside group; the toxicity usually is dose-related and may be reversible if detected early. Although vertigo may be present, the more disturbing symptom is imbalance due to the loss of vestibular function. Salicylates can also cause tinnitus and vertigo as a sign of toxicity. Alcohol intoxication produces vertigo and imbalance, in addition to its other CNS effects. Several anticonvulsants in toxic doses can produce vertigo and ataxia, which usually are reversible when the level drops.

(6) **Posttraumatic syndrome.** Head trauma frequently is followed by positional or persistent vertigo. Although usually of the benign positional variety, it may consist of vague unsteadiness or lightheadedness. Like other features of the posttraumatic syndrome, there is frequently an overlay of neurosis that may complicate the diagnosis.

b. **Treatment of peripheral vertigo.** Management of the above disorders is similar. If the vertigo is very severe or disabling, bed rest is necessary. When nausea and vomiting are severe, hospitalization may be required. Meclizine, 25 mg PO tid or qid, helps to reduce vertigo and nausea, and sedation with diazepam, 5–10 mg PO, controls the anxiety associated with severe vertigo. Occasionally, scopolamine hydrobromide, 0.6 mg PO q6h or in the transdermal administration form, may be helpful instead of meclizine. Severe nausea sometimes requires the addition of a phenothiazine, such as promethazine (25 mg PO q6h) or prochlorperazine (10 mg PO q6h). The treatment of acute attacks of Ménière's disorder is the same as that of the other acute peripheral disorders; a variety of surgical and medical treatments to prevent recurrence have been tried with controversial results.

2. **Central vertigo**

a. **Cerebrovascular disease.** Ischemia in the distribution of the vertebrobasilar system may produce vertigo by damage to the vestibular nuclei or their connections. If a stroke has occurred, it is rare for surrounding structures not to be affected; as a result, persistent vertigo in the absence of other neurologic abnormalities is not usually seen. TIAs may produce vertigo. If the patient is not examined during the symptomatic period, the etiology of the vertigo may be difficult to determine. A history of associated neurologic abnormalities (e.g., diplopia, dysarthria, or a visual field defect), however, suggests brainstem dysfunction as the etiology of the vertigo. See **Cerebrovascular Disease, sec. III.D** for management.

b. **Cerebellopontine angle tumors** are a rare cause of vertigo. Most of these tumors are benign acoustic neuromas that predominantly arise from the vestibular portion of the eighth cranial nerve in the internal acoustic meatus. They usually present with vague unsteadiness, tinnitus, and decreased hearing rather than with vertigo. When they enlarge enough to involve the nearby brainstem, facial numbness, weakness, or central vertigo may develop. Caloric testing reveals markedly decreased vestibular function on the side of the tumor. A CT scan of the posterior fossa may reveal the tumor, or tomograms of the internal auditory canals may reveal bony erosion. Other mass lesions of the posterior fossa may also cause vertigo, again with associated neurologic findings. Treatment is surgical excision.

c. **Other causes of central vertigo**

(1) **Migraine** (see **Headache, sec. III.A.1**) can occasionally produce vertigo either prior to the onset of the headache (as a manifestation of the aura) or even during the headache phase. **Treatment** during the period of vertigo is symptomatic for the nausea, vertigo, and headache. Prophylactic treatment of the migraines should also control the vertigo.

(2) **Partial complex seizures** (see **Seizures, sec. II.B.2**) may rarely present as brief episodes of vertigo.

B. **Faintness and syncope** (see **Syncope**). Dizziness can precede loss of consciousness from hypotension, either from cardiovascular etiologies (i.e., decreased cardiac output from arrhythmias, valvular disease, or myocardial dysfunction) or from other etiologies (e.g., vasovagal reactions, orthostatic hypotension, carotid sinus hypersensitivity, cough and micturition syncope). Treatment is directed at the underlying etiology.

C. **Disequilibrium or imbalance.** Although patients with imbalance may complain of dizziness, they often describe a feeling of imbalance when questioned about the sensation. Several conditions can produce this sensation. Cerebellar lesions can produce an unsteady, wide-based gait; if the cerebellar lesion is midline, the gait may be disproportionately impaired. Parkinson's disease, by impairing postural reflexes, bradykinesia, and retropulsion, frequently produces a sensation of imbalance. Apraxia of gait is seen in the elderly, particularly in association with lacunar states, normal pressure hydrocephalus, or other bilateral hemispheric lesions. In this disorder, the patient's gait is slow, with small steps and a great deal of difficulty in initiating walking movements. On neurologic examination, the strength, sensation, and coordination are normal; and the patient can perform complicated maneuvers with the legs in bed (e.g., bicycling), but the gait is still abnormal. Patients with sensory ataxia from peripheral neuropathy also frequently complain of unsteadiness. Treatment is aimed at the underlying disorder.

D. **Lightheadedness.** Complaints of lightheadedness, frequently vague, may comprise the most common form of dizziness in the general population. Mild forms of vertigo or other types of dizziness are often described as lightheadedness, particularly by poor observers.

1. **Hyperventilation** is the most common cause of dizziness in younger patients. Patients present with episodes of shortness of breath, lightheadedness, paresthesias involving the mouth and distal extremities, palpitations, and panic. Having the patient hyperventilate in the emergency department will reproduce the symptoms and establish the diagnosis. **Treatment** involves having the patient rebreathe carbon dioxide (by breathing into a paper bag) and reassurance. Frequent or recurrent episodes may be part of the syndrome of "panic attacks" and may require psychiatric consultation.

2. **Multisensory deficit.** As a common cause of dizziness in the elderly, multisensory dizziness occurs when several sensory modalities are impaired. Since the patient cannot properly orient to the environment, attempting to walk produces a sensation of dizziness and instability. Sitting or lying down corrects the instability. A common combination of sensory impairment includes a peripheral neuropathy (with impaired touch and proprioception), decreased vision, and some vestibular dysfunction. Patients may improve if one of the sensory deficits, particularly vision, can be corrected. A cane to provide additional proprioceptive input can also be helpful.

E. **Physiologic dizziness.** Dizziness can be present even in normal individuals in conditions where there is inadequate sensory information, stimulation that exceeds the capacity of the sensory systems, or a discrepancy in the information obtained from different sensory modalities. Motion sickness is an example of physiologic dizziness. This condition typically occurs when a person is subjected to vestibular stimulation in a setting where visual and tactile stimuli report that there is no motion (e.g., in the back seat of a car or in a closed cabin in a ship). Patients report nausea, increased salivation, fatigue, and, when severe, vomiting. The sensation can be reduced by fixating on the surroundings to give a visual input to the movement. Prevention is useful; and meclizine, 25 mg PO, or scopolamine, 0.4–0.8 mg, taken before travel can prevent the onset of motion sickness.

Syncope

Syncope is a transient (i.e., < 30 minutes) loss of consciousness. Generally, causes of syncope can be divided into (1) a critical reduction of oxygen or glucose delivered to the brain (e.g., cerebral hypoperfusion, hypoxia, hypoglycemia), and (2) primary CNS dysfunction (e.g., seizures, concussive head injuries, subarachnoid hemorrhage).

I. **General principles.** There are many diverse causes of syncope. In one series [6], the etiology of syncopal attacks was identified as benign causes (e.g., vasovagal, hysterical, postural hypotension, hyperventilation, micturition) in 40% of the cases, seizures in 29%, an undetermined etiology in 13%, cardiac syncope in 8%, drug or metabolic causes in 7%, and other CNS disorders (e.g., cerebrovascular accident, migraine headache) in 3%.

A. Assessment. The history and physical examination can identify the etiology in about 85% of diagnosable syncopal attacks; furthermore, the history and physical examination suggest the etiology in most of the other 15% of cases that require diagnostic tests to establish the cause of the syncopal episode [6]. Thus, diagnostic tests generally should not be performed routinely but only as indicated by the initial assessment of the patient.

1. **History.** It is important to obtain historic information from the patient and from witnesses to the occurrence. The following are important historic features:

   a. **Age.** Patients over 50 years of age are at an increased risk of syncope from malignant causes (e.g., cardiac arrhythmia, cerebrovascular occlusive disease, abdominal aortic aneurysm, aortic dissection).

   b. **Warning period.** Vasovagal and hypoglycemic syncope are usually preceded by weakness, dizziness, yawning, nausea, vomiting, epigastric discomfort, diaphoresis, dimming of vision, or changes in hearing. Hyperventilation syncope is usually preceded by paresthesias of the hands or face, and, occasionally, by carpopedal spasm. A brief or absent warning period is characteristic of cardiac syncope, pulmonary embolus, seizures, subarachnoid hemorrhage, postural hypotension, carotid sinus syncope, and micturition syncope.

   c. **Position at onset of attack.** Most syncopal episodes occur in the standing or sitting position. Recumbent syncope suggests cardiac arrhythmia, seizures, hypoglycemia, or hyperventilation.

   d. **Description of syncopal attack.** Generally, syncopal episodes related to seizures are characterized by tonic-clonic motor activity, tongue biting, urinary or fecal incontinence, and facial cyanosis. In contrast, syncope not due to seizures is characterized by flaccidity (however, tonic-clonic motor activity may occur due to cerebral anoxia or hypoglycemia but is usually of briefer duration than that due to seizures), no tongue biting, no incontinence (however, urinary incontinence can occur in nonseizure syncopal episodes), and pallor.

   e. **Duration of loss of consciousness.** Generally, syncopal patients recover consciousness shortly after assuming a supine position. More prolonged episodes of loss of consciousness can occur with hypoglycemia (loss of consciousness may not resolve until glucose is administered), hyperventilation syncope, and seizures.

   f. **Recovery period.** Unless the patient has suffered a prolonged anoxic or hypoglycemic episode, recovery of mental status after a syncopal attack is usually rapid. Seizures, however, are characteristically followed by a postictal alteration in mental status of varying duration.

   g. **Predisposing factors.** Factors that often predispose patients to a syncopal attack include conditions that reduce a patient's tolerance to hypoxia (e.g., anemia, organic heart disease, cerebrovascular disease, fatigue, recent physical illness, age over 60 years) or predispose the patient to postural hypotension (e.g., an upright posture, a warm environment, poor physical condition, alcohol ingestion, reduced oral intake, or certain drugs such as propranolol or diuretics).

   h. **Situational syncope.** Situations that are associated with syncopal episodes include exertion (in persons with aortic stenosis, hypertrophic cardiomyopathy, congenital heart disease, mitral stenosis, pulmonic stenosis, or pulmonary hypertension); emotional stress (vasovagal syncope); standing (postural hypotension); anxiety (hysterical syncope or hyperventilation syncope); head turning, neck extension, or wearing a tight collar (carotid sinus syncope); and coughing (cough syncope). Syncope that occurs in the bathroom may be due to postural hypotension secondary to standing after a period of recumbency, arising from a warm bath, or standing in a warm shower; decreased venous return to the heart as a result of straining at the stool (Valsalva maneuver); or micturition syncope. Syncope that occurs at church may be due to postural hypotension as a result of standing after a period of sitting or kneeling (particularly in elderly persons), a Valsalva maneuver associated with singing, or a vasovagal episode secondary to an emotional experience.

   i. **Associated symptoms** may include chest pain (e.g., myocardial infarction, pulmonary embolus, aortic dissection), dyspnea (pulmonary embolus), abdominal pain (abdominal aortic aneurysm), headache (subarachnoid hemorrhage), or palpitations (e.g., arrhythmia, hyperventilation, hypoglycemia). Severe pain in itself may lead to vasovagal syncope.

j. Associated trauma. Syncope either can be caused by a traumatic injury (e.g., head injury, acute blood loss, vasovagal reaction) or can cause a traumatic injury (e.g., from a fall, a motor vehicle accident, or near-drowning). It is important to establish a cause for traumatic injuries with a loss of consciousness, particularly in patients over 50 years old. Generally, a preceding syncopal attack should be suspected in patients with traumatic injuries when there is either a loss of consciousness of undetermined cause or no attempt by the patient to avoid the accident or to protect himself or herself from injury.

k. A **past history** of cardiac disease (e.g., ischemic heart disease, congestive heart failure, valvular heart disease, arrhythmia, pacemaker), seizure disorder, or diabetes mellitus and a **drug history** are often helpful in establishing a diagnosis of syncope.

2. A complete **physical examination** is essential in evaluating patients with syncope. The following specific aspects of the physical examination are particularly useful in establishing a diagnosis of syncope:

a. A **blood pressure** and **pulse** taken while the patient is first lying and then standing (for at least one minute) will detect postural hypotension.

b. Cardiac examination. A heart murmur may suggest hypertrophic cardiomyopathy, aortic stenosis, pulmonary stenosis, mitral stenosis, congenital heart disease, or aortic insufficiency (from aortic dissection). A midsystolic click with associated syncope should suggest the diagnosis of mitral valve prolapse. An arrhythmia may be detected on cardiac auscultation.

c. Neurologic examination. Focal neurologic deficits may be found in patients with occlusive cerebrovascular disease, intracranial bleeds, hypoglycemic episodes, or postictal states. Nuchal rigidity suggests a subarachnoid hemorrhage.

d. Abdominal examination. A tender pulsatile mass may be found in patients with an abdominal aortic aneurysm. Blood in the stool or vomitus (gastric aspirate) suggests a gastrointestinal bleed.

e. Physical maneuvers. Induced hyperventilation and neck turning or gentle carotid massage (with ECG monitoring and an IV line in place) are useful in assessing for hyperventilation syncope and carotid sinus syncope, respectively.

3. Diagnostic tests may be useful in establishing a cause for syncope in selected cases.

a. Cardiac tests. An initial ECG and cardiac monitoring have the highest yield of diagnostic tests in establishing a cause for syncope [6, 12]. However, an initial ECG and inhospital monitoring may be unrevealing, since rhythm disturbances are often transient and may subside with rest and reduction in catecholamines. Studies have found major arrhythmias on Holter monitoring in 10–62% of patients with the complaint of syncope or dizziness and an unremarkable standard ECG [6]. Holter monitoring is recommended for patients with syncope of unknown etiology in the following circumstances: a history or physical findings suggestive of cardiac syncope, an age over 50 years, recurrent syncopal episodes, or a rhythm disturbance discovered on an initial ECG or by inhospital monitoring. Other useful cardiac tests, depending on the clinical circumstances, include electrophysiologic studies, echocardiography, stress testing, and cardiac catheterization.

b. CNS tests include electroencephalography, a CT scan, an LP, and cerebral angiography. Use of these tests will depend on the clinical situation.

c. Ventilation-perfusion lung scanning or **pulmonary angiography** should be performed if a pulmonary embolus is suspected.

d. Blood tests. A CBC may reveal a low hematocrit secondary to blood loss. Dehydration can cause an elevated hematocrit, an elevated BUN, and electrolyte abnormalities. Hypoglycemia is diagnosed by a blood sugar less than 40 mg/dl. Seizures may be caused by an electrolyte disturbance (e.g., hypocalcemia, hyponatremia); also, seizures usually produce a lactic acidosis that persists for about 1 hour postseizure [20].

B. Treatment
   1. **General principles.** Patients with syncope should be placed in a supine position, and measures to protect the airway (e.g., airway maneuvers, suctioning of secretions, insertion of an oro- or nasopharyngeal airway) and maintain an adequate blood pressure (e.g., application of the military antishock trousers [MAST] suit, volume infusion) instituted as appropriate. Administration of supplemental oxygen, IV catheter placement, and cardiac monitoring are generally recommended.
   2. **Definitive therapy** should be directed at the etiology of the syncopal episode (e.g., glucose administration for hypoglycemia; anticonvulsants for seizures; atropine, isoproterenol, or pacemaker insertion for bradycardia; antiarrhythmic agents or electrical cardioversion for tachycardia; volume infusion for hypovolemia).
C. Disposition
   1. The disposition of patients with **known or suspected causes of syncope** is based on the etiology. In general, patients with vasovagal syncope, hyperventilation syncope, hysterical syncope, micturition syncope, or cough syncope can be discharged home. Patients with cardiac syncope, pulmonary embolus, or vascular causes of syncope (e.g., abdominal aortic aneurysm, aortic dissection, subarachnoid hemorrhage, or cerebrovascular occlusive disease) require admission to the hospital. Depending on the clinical circumstances, patients with hypoglycemia or seizures may require hospitalization.
   2. Patients with **syncope of undetermined etiology** have a low incidence of recurrence of syncopal episodes [25] and constitute a low-risk subgroup for major morbidity or mortality [6]. However, due to an increased incidence of malignant causes of syncope, hospitalization is recommended for patients with syncope of undetermined etiology with the following: (1) an age exceeding 70 years [6], (2) a brief or absent warning period prior to loss of consciousness [20], (3) recumbent syncope, (4) recurrent episodes of syncope, or (5) underlying cardiac disease [20].
II. Specific etiologies of syncope
A. Cardiac syncope
   1. **Arrhythmias** (see Chap. 4). Syncope associated with a decreased cardiac output as a result of alteration in the cardiac rate or rhythm is referred to as a **Stokes-Adams attack.** Common causes include ventricular tachycardia, complete heart block with an inadequate ventricular response, and prolonged (i.e., > 3 seconds) asystole. These attacks are characterized by the sudden loss of consciousness, usually without warning. These patients warrant admission to a monitored bed for observation and further evaluation.
   2. **Pacemaker malfunction** (see Chap. 4) may be manifested by cessation of pacing, alteration of the pacing rate, improper sensing (which may result in the pacemaker firing on the T wave and precipitating ventricular tachycardia or ventricular fibrillation), extracardiac stimulation (e.g., diaphragmatic stimulation), or alteration in spike or timing characteristics. However, pacemaker malfunction may be intermittent and may not be seen on an ECG taken in the emergency department. Thus, patients with a pacemaker implant who present with unexplained syncope should be admitted to the hospital and evaluated for pacemaker malfunction [18].
   3. **Myocardial infarction** (see Chap. 5) can cause syncope as a result of arrhythmias, pump failure, or a vasovagal episode induced by pain and anxiety.
   4. **Obstruction to blood flow** (see Chap. 5) can cause syncope as a result of diminished cardiac output.
     a. **Hypertrophic cardiomyopathy** may be associated with exertional syncope as a result of outflow obstruction or arrhythmias.
     b. **Aortic stenosis** may be associated with exertional syncope as a result of an inability to increase the cardiac output to meet the demands of skeletal muscle vasodilation or arrhythmias. Syncope in a patient with aortic stenosis often indicates significant stenosis and the need for surgical intervention.
     c. Other causes of syncope from blood flow obstruction include pulmonic stenosis (usually exertional syncope) and severe mitral stenosis (syncope secondary to exertion or atrial fibrillation with a rapid ventricular response). Sudden onset of syncope may also occur with prosthetic valve malfunction, a left atrial ball-valve thrombus, or a left atrial myxoma.

5. **Congenital heart disease** with a right-to-left shunt may be associated with exertional syncope as a result of increased blood flow through the shunt with exercise, leading to systemic hypoxia.

B. **Pulmonary causes of syncope**

1. **Pulmonary hypertension** is associated with exertional syncope as a result of either a relatively fixed cardiac output or possibly a vasovagal reflex from dilation of the pulmonary artery.

2. A massive **pulmonary embolus** (see Chap. 7) causes syncope in more than 10% of cases [26]. The mechanism is believed to be (1) transient occlusion of the pulmonary artery with interruption of blood flow to the left side of the heart and systemic circulation or (2) a vasovagal reflex.

C. **Autonomic dysfunction**

1. **Vasovagal (vasodepressor) syncope** is a common type of syncope that occurs from a vagal reflex (leading to cardiac slowing) or a depressor reflex (resulting in hypotension from a sudden decrease in peripheral resistance due to skeletal muscle and splanchnic vasodilation) or both.

a. **Clinical manifestations.** Vasovagal syncope occurs in response to an emotional stress that is threatened, real, or imagined (e.g., venipuncture, the sight of blood, painful stimuli, excitement, anxiety). A pure vagal response may be associated with distension of an intestinal viscera (e.g., from an endoscopic procedure), irritation of the pleura or peritoneum, or lesions of the mediastinum or larynx. Factors predisposing to vasovagal syncope include a long period of standing upright, a hot environment, a crowded room, fatigue, hunger, fasting, a recent illness, poor physical conditioning, alcohol ingestion, prolonged bed rest, mild blood loss, anemia, and underlying organic heart disease.

b. **Treatment** consists of placing the patient in a recumbent position and elevating the legs to increase venous return to the heart. Atropine is useful in preventing or treating vagal-mediated responses but is not useful in treating depressor-mediated responses.

c. **Disposition.** Although morbidity or mortality can occur in patients with underlying heart disease, vasovagal syncope is generally a benign condition, and patients can generally be discharged home from the emergency department.

2. **Orthostatic (postural) hypotension** is a fall in blood pressure associated with dizziness or syncope occurring upon standing or when standing motionless in a fixed position.

a. **Etiologies**

(1) **Poor postural adjustment.** This condition is associated with a tall asthenic habitus, age over 60 years, pregnancy, poor physical state, physical exhaustion, exposure to hot weather, prolonged standing, and prolonged recumbency.

(2) **Hypovolemia** is a common cause of orthostatic hypotension and may be secondary to dehydration or blood loss.

(3) **Drugs,** particularly psychotropic agents (e.g., phenothiazines), antihypertensive agents (e.g., guanethidine, alpha methyldopa, prazosin, diuretics), and nitroglycerin, may cause orthostatic hypotension.

(4) **Idiopathic orthostatic hypotension** includes orthostatic hypotension in a pure form or in combination with neurologic manifestations (Shy-Drager syndrome).

(5) Orthostatic hypotension may result from **endocrine disorders** (e.g., diabetes mellitus, amyloidosis, adrenal insufficiency, pheochromocytoma, primary aldosteronism) or **neurologic disorders** (e.g., tabes dorsalis, syringomyelia, Wernicke's encephalopathy, multiple cerebral infarcts, peripheral neuropathy, Landry-Guillain-Barré syndrome).

(6) Miscellaneous disorders (e.g., chronic hemodialysis, electrolyte disturbances, surgical sympathectomy) may be associated with orthostatic hypotension.

b. **Diagnosis.** Various criteria exist for diagnosing orthostatic hypotension. These criteria include the following changes in going from a recumbent to a standing position: (1) a decrease in systolic blood pressure of more than 30 mm Hg or in diastolic blood pressure of more than 10 mm Hg [25]; (2) a decrease in systolic blood pressure of more than 25 mm Hg associated with dizziness or syncope or a decrease in systolic blood pressure of 10 mm Hg or more when associated with a decline in systolic pressure to less than 90 mm Hg [13]; (3) a pulse increase of 30 beats or more/minute or the appearance of severe symptoms [15]; or (4) a decrease in systolic blood pressure of more than 20 mm Hg [20] or a rise in pulse of more than 20 beats/minute in the presence of clinical symptoms (e.g., presyncope, syncope). Orthostatic measurements should be taken first with the patient in the supine position for at least 2–3 minutes and then in the standing position for at least 1 minute (if tolerated by the patient). If the patient is unable to stand, the blood pressure and pulse can be taken with the patient in a sitting position with the legs dangling; however, this technique is less reliable [15]. Unless patients are taking a beta-adrenergic blocking agent or are elderly, a pulse increase is usually seen with postural hypotension due to hypovolemia [15]. Other forms of postural hypotension, however, may not manifest an orthostatic pulse increase.

   c. **Treatment** depends on the particular form of postural hypotension present. Hypovolemia is treated with volume repletion. Implicated drugs may need to be discontinued. Chronic forms of postural hypotension may be treated by educating these patients about arising from a recumbent position gradually, using support stockings, maintaining a high sodium intake, and the use of alpha fluorohydrocortisone, as appropriate.

   d. **Disposition.** Generally, patients with poor postural adjustment, chronic forms of postural hypotension, or mild to moderate dehydration in whom fluid replacement can be achieved in the emergency department can be discharged home. Admission is recommended for patients with orthostatic hypotension on the basis of blood loss, patients with associated conditions requiring admission to the hospital, and severely symptomatic patients.

3. **Micturition syncope** is syncope that occurs during or immediately after urination, usually in persons rising from bed in the evening or early morning hours following consumption of alcohol. Micturition syncope is a benign disorder requiring no specific therapy. Thus, these patients can generally be discharged from the emergency department.

4. **Carotid sinus syncope** (see Chap. 4) usually occurs in patients over the age of 60 years and is due to a hypersensitive carotid sinus that may cause a vagal response or a depressor response. Syncope may be precipitated by phenomena that produce stimulation of the carotid sinus (e.g., head turning, neck extension, a tight collar, coughing, sneezing, straining at stool); in addition, digitalis increases carotid sinus sensitivity.

   a. The **diagnosis** can be confirmed by producing asystole for 3 seconds or by a drop in systolic blood pressure of more than 50 mm Hg with carotid sinus massage, which **in this setting should be performed only with an IV catheter in place and ECG monitoring.**

   b. **Treatment** includes the use of (1) an alpha-adrenergic agent for treating the depressor-mediated response and (2) an anticholinergic agent or a transvenous pacemaker or both for treating the vagal-mediated response.

   c. **Disposition.** Patients with suspected carotid sinus syncope are usually admitted to the hospital to substantiate the diagnosis and plan an appropriate treatment regimen.

5. **Glossopharyngeal neuralgia** is characterized by severe pain in the oropharynx, tonsillar fossa, base of the tongue, or ear precipitated by coughing, chewing, or swallowing. This pain may be followed by syncope due to a vagal reflex mechanism. **Treatment** consists of pharmacologic management with carbamazepine or, in refractory cases, nerve root section. Bradyarrhythmias may require administration of atropine or, occasionally, transvenous pacemaker insertion [11]. Patients with severe discomfort or arrhythmias require hospital admission.

D. **CNS causes** (see appropriate sections of this chapter and Chap. 25) of syncope include seizures, subarachnoid hemorrhage, and traumatic head injuries (e.g., concussion, intracranial bleeds). Other less common causes include cerebrovascular occlusive disease and migraine headaches.

E. **Vascular causes of syncope**
1. **Aortic arch syndromes.** Diseases affecting the aortic arch can cause syncope as a result of coronary or carotid artery occlusion.
   a. **Aortic dissection** (see Chap. 5) may cause syncope as a result of occlusion of a coronary or carotid artery, rupture into the pericardium with resultant

pericardial tamponade, rupture through the adventitia with resultant profound hypovolemia, or as a result of a vasovagal reaction.

   b. Takayasu's disease (pulseless disease) is a rare cause of syncope due to arteritis of the aorta and great vessels. The disease characteristically affects young Oriental females. Clinical manifestations include a prodrome of fever, malaise, myalgias, arthralgias, and anorexia, followed by manifestations of arterial insufficiency (e.g., coronary artery ischemia, cerebrovascular insufficiency, absent peripheral pulses). The diagnosis is confirmed by angiographic study of the aorta. Although steroids may be of benefit, the disease usually is progressive and fatal.

   2. An **abdominal aorta aneurysm** (see Chap. 20) may cause syncope as a result of (1) profound hypovolemia from rupture into the peritoneum or (2) a vasovagal reaction from a leaking aneurysm.

   3. The **subclavian steal syndrome** occurs when there is occlusion of the subclavian artery proximal to the origin of the vertebral artery, leading to retrograde blood flow from the opposite vertebral artery. This syndrome is characterized by vetebral-basilar artery insufficiency (see **Cerebrovascular Disease** sec. **II.B**) induced by exercise of the arm supplied by the retrograde blood flow from the vertebral artery. Other clinical manifestations include a blood pressure difference of greater than 10 mm Hg between the arms, a supraclavicular fossa bruit, and ischemia of the affected arm. Management consists of localization of the occlusion by arteriography, followed by endarterectomy.

F. Hyperventilation can cause syncope due to hypocapnia and respiratory alkalosis, leading to cerebral arteriolar vasoconstriction and peripheral vasodilation. Hyperventilation syncope usually occurs in response to an emotional stress in an anxious patient. The diagnosis usually can be established by reproducing the syndrome by having the patient hyperventilate in the emergency department. This condition is benign, and reassurance is usually all that is necessary.

G. Hysterical syncope characteristically occurs under dramatic circumstances in the company of the patient's friends or family and with no traumatic injury occurring as a result of the syncopal episode. The diagnosis is suggested by a normal physical examination and the bizarre nature of the syncopal attack. If necessary, feigned unconsciousness can be proved by the response to a noxious stimulus (e.g., aromatic spirits of ammonia placed next to the patient's nose), an intact lash reflex (i.e., stroking the eyelash and causing a reflex blink), or cold water caloric testing revealing horizontal nystagmus with a fast component away from the lavaged ear. This condition is benign, and these patients can generally be discharged home with a referral to a psychiatrist as needed.

H. Cough syncope is syncope that occurs during paroxysms of coughing, usually affecting older patients with underlying chronic obstructive pulmonary disease (COPD). It is probably caused by an increased intrathoracic pressure during coughing, resulting in a decreased venous return to the heart. There is no specific treatment other than cough suppression, if appropriate.

I. Hypoglycemia (see Chap. 7) can cause an altered mental status with seizures, syncope, or coma. The diagnosis is confirmed by a blood glucose less than 40 mg/dl. Treatment consists of administration of glucose.

J. Drug-induced syncope may occur due to arrhythmias (e.g., digitalis, quinidine, sympathomimetics, anticholinergics), postural hypotension (e.g., phenothiazines, antihypertensives), CNS depression (e.g., opioids, sedatives, hypnotics), hypoglycemia (e.g., insulin, oral hypoglycemics, alcohol, salicylates), anaphylactic reactions, or seizures (e.g., tricyclic antidepressants, antihistamines, stimulants). Management consists of supportive and specific measures as needed. Overdosage management principles (see Chap. 16) should be applied as appropriate.

K. Hypoxia-induced syncope may occur from anemia, high-altitude exposure, barotrauma, or transient inhalation of toxic gases (e.g., carbon monoxide, carbon dioxide, hydrogen sulfide, arsenic, cyanide, methane). Management consists of administration of oxygen, maintenance of ventilation, and specific measures directed at the etiology as needed.

Neuropathies

Peripheral neuropathies include diseases that primarily affect peripheral nerve function. Symptoms include weakness, sensory changes, and autonomic dysfunction, depending on the relative involvement of these components. Diabetes mellitus and leprosy are the most common causes of neuropathies worldwide; however, many other etiologies have been described. Indeed, in many neuropathies, no underlying cause is found.

I. **Mononeuropathy**

A. **Cranial nerves.** A variety of diseases can affect the function of the cranial nerves.

1. **Olfactory nerve.** Involvement of the olfactory nerve causes anosmia. Because of the importance of smell in taste, patients frequently complain of also losing taste, although formal testing of primary taste sensations will show that they are still intact. Most patients who complain of anosmia actually have disease of the olfactory mucosa rather than the nerve. However, head trauma (by distracting the olfactory bulbs from their attachments through the lamina cribrosa) or tumors at the base of the anterior fossa along the olfactory groove can produce true anosmia.

2. **Optic nerve.** The optic nerve can be injured along its course by mass lesions, vascular disease, trauma, inflammatory disease, or toxins. Lesions distal to the chiasm produce unilateral visual loss; midline chiasmatic lesions produce bitemporal hemianopsia; and lesions proximal to the chiasm produce homonymous defects involving a visual field. Common distal lesions include the following:

   a. **Mass lesions** affecting the optic nerve (e.g., meningiomas, optic nerve gliomas, metastatic tumors in the orbit) can cause blindness in the affected eye. Chiasmatic lesions include pituitary adenomas, craniopharyngiomas, and other perisellar lesions.

   b. **Inflammatory diseases** of the nerve, such as optic neuritis, usually are caused by demyelinating disease. When the inflammation is close to the retina, swelling of the optic nerve head can be seen on funduscopic examination. More proximal intrinsic lesions (e.g., retrobulbar neuritis) do not initially affect the appearance of the optic disk. Temporal arteritis can also affect the optic nerve, producing an ischemic optic neuritis, presumably from vasculitis involving the ciliary arteries that feed the nerve.

3. **Oculomotor, trochlear, and abducens nerves.** A variety of diseases can affect the motor nerves to the eyes, causing diplopia. These diseases include vascular disease, mass lesions compressing the nerves, neoplasms, inflammatory disease, and diabetes mellitus.

4. **Trigeminal nerve.** Decreased sensation to the face is more likely to be due to disease within the brainstem than to trigeminal nerve lesions. However, loss of sensation limited to one of the three branches suggests more distal involvement caused by tumor, trauma, infection, or collagen vascular disease. **Trigeminal neuralgia** is discussed under **Headache**, sec. **III.I.**

5. **Facial nerve** disorders above the level of the facial nerve nucleus tend to spare movement of the upper part of the face because of bilateral innervation. Lesions of the nucleus or distal to the nucleus produce equal paralysis of the upper and lower face. Parenchymal lesions within the brainstem also usually lead to involvement of the abducens nerve.

   Bell's palsy is a peripheral facial nerve palsy of unknown etiology. Frequently, the onset of the palsy is preceded by an upper respiratory infection and by a day or two of retroauricular pain. The onset is rapid, with the development of weakness within a day or two. Because of the facial weakness, the lower face appears "drawn" toward the uninvolved side. Weakness of the upper face leads to impairment of eye closure. Since the localization of the damage appears most frequently to be at the site of entry of the nerve at the internal auditory canal, taste is often decreased on the side of the palsy. The prognosis for recovery is good. Approximately 75–85% of these patients have complete recovery; about 5% have no recovery; and the remainder have some recovery, although incomplete. Poor results are seen more commonly in the elderly and in patients with diabetes mellitus. While steroids have not been shown to change the prognosis, they appear to shorten the course of the recovery and should be used in patients who have no contraindication. Usually prednisone, 40–60 mg/day, is given for 4 or 5 days and then tapered over an additional 7–10 days. Because of the inability to completely close the eye (even during a blink) on the side of the palsy, the cornea is at risk from damage; thus, the eye should be patched in patients who cannot close the eye completely. Even in patients with nearly complete eye closure, the eye may remain open during sleep, requiring patching at night.

Patients who have a good recovery do not need further evaluation. However, failure of recovery within 4–6 weeks requires investigation for compressive lesions of the nerve.

B. Compression and entrapment syndromes. The peripheral nerves in the limbs are particularly susceptible to damage by compression against bony prominences or by fascial planes. Diabetes mellitus, malnutrition, and a variety of other neuropathies increase the likelihood of an entrapment becoming symptomatic.

   1. Carpal tunnel syndrome. Median nerve compression as the nerve passes through the canal formed by the carpal bones and ligaments is the most common entrapment syndrome.

      a. Clinical features. The disorder is seen most commonly in middle-aged women. Tingling, numbness, and pain most commonly with the thumb, palm, and first three fingers are the initial symptoms. Initially, these symptoms may be intermittent and typically are present when the patient wakes up from sleep. The discomfort can be relieved initially by changing position. Occasionally, patients complain of discomfort extending proximally up the arm. The neurologic examination may reveal sensory loss in the distribution of the median nerve in the hand. In severe cases, thenar atrophy or weakness of the hand muscles innervated by the median nerve may be seen. Patients with carpal tunnel entrapment may feel tingling or pain when the wrist over the median nerve is percussed **(Tinel's sign)** or have an increase in numbness with forced flexion of the wrist **(Phalen's sign).** Nerve conduction measurements reveal slowing of conduction across the wrist.

      b. Treatment. Mild cases should be treated conservatively with reduction of aggravating activities (such as frequent flexion of the wrist) and the use of a nighttime wrist splint. Occasionally, patients respond to steroid injections into the wrist. If these measures do not provide relief of symptoms, surgical release should be done.

   2. Tardy ulnar palsy. The ulnar nerve is vulnerable to damage as it passes the elbow in the ulnar groove. Repeated traumatic injury leads to tingling and numbness in the ulnar portion of the palm and the fourth and fifth fingers. Since the ulnar nerve innervates most of the intrinsic muscles of the hand, weakness and atrophy of these small muscles can occur. The **treatment** of choice is avoiding further injury (e.g., avoiding excessive leaning on the elbows). In severe cases, mobilizing and transplanting the ulnar nerve anterior to the medial epicondyle can prevent further damage.

   3. Radial nerve palsy. The radial nerve is vulnerable to compression in the upper arm at the level of the spiral groove. The most common cause of compression is external pressure on the lateral aspect of the arm, as in the "Saturday night" palsy where a sleeping patient, often intoxicated with alcohol, has compressed the nerve between the humerus and a chair. The patient presents with a wrist and finger drop. Sensory abnormalities may be seen over the dorsum of the thumb at the base. Recovery usually occurs over 6–8 weeks. A cockup splint for the wrist may help with hand function until recovery occurs.

   4. Peroneal nerve palsy. The peroneal nerve can be injured where it crosses the head of the fibula, particularly with fractures of the fibula. Crossing the legs frequently puts pressure at this point, and the nerve can also be injured by multiple flexions of the knee. Weight loss seems to predispose to peroneal palsy. Typically, there is weakness of the motor distribution of the peroneal nerve, which presents as a foot drop and lack of toe extension and ankle eversion. Ankle inversion, however, is spared. Although the peroneal nerve does have a sensory distribution, this branching is not as severely affected.

   5. Meralgia paresthetica. Patients with a pendulous abdomen, pregnant women, and patients wearing tight belts can develop compression of the lateral femoral cutaneous nerve at the level of the inguinal ligament. Symptoms include tingling, burning, and sometimes pain in the lateral thigh above the knee. Weight loss or relief of the precipitating circumstance relieves the discomfort. When no obvious precipitating cause is present, treatment may be more difficult, since surgical release is not frequently performed.

C. Mononeuritis multiplex refers to involvement of several different individual peripheral nerves at the same time. The presumed etiology is involvement of small arteries in the epineurium of nerve trunks. It is a pattern that can be seen in vasculitis, such as periarteritis nodosa. It may occasionally be seen in diabetes mellitus. Typically, patients develop pain, paresthesias, or weakness in the distribution of a peripheral nerve that rapidly progresses. Other nerves may follow within a short period of time. Recovery is variable and dependent on the underlying disease, against which treatment is directed.

D. **Plexal neuropathies**

1. The **brachial plexus** can be injured by trauma, by compression, or by neoplasm with variable degrees of arm weakness, sensory loss, pain, and atrophy. **Brachial plexitis** is an illness of unknown etiology. Cases have been related to vaccination and intercurrent infections, but many cases have either no apparent predisposing circumstance or only a minor nonspecific illness. The illness begins with aching pain in the shoulder or forearm, and progresses rapidly with the onset of weakness, sometimes with atrophy. Sensory loss is much less impressive than the motor weakness. Any part of the brachial plexus can be affected, although the upper portion is affected more than the lower. The prognosis for recovery is good, although it may take weeks to months. The differential diagnosis is mainly between brachial plexitis and cervical radiculopathy. Generally, the more extensive involvement of brachial plexitis (extending beyond a single root) will establish the diagnosis, although in unclear cases a myelogram may be necessary. Occasionally, diffuse infiltration of the brachial plexus by tumor may mimic brachial plexitis, although the course is slower and the lower plexus is involved more often in neoplastic infiltration. There is no specific treatment for brachial plexitis, although an analgesic for relief of pain and physical therapy may be needed.

2. The **lumbar plexus** may be involved by mechanisms similar to those affecting the brachial plexus. The most common lumbar plexus involvement is seen in patients with diabetes mellitus and is known as **femoral neuropathy.** It is actually an upper lumbar plexus involvement affecting predominantly the distribution of the femoral nerve. The patient presents with pain in the anterior thigh extending into the medial part of the leg and with weakness of the iliopsoas and quadriceps muscles. The etiology is unknown but is possibly vascular in origin. Recovery is slow and may be incomplete. There is no specific treatment.

II. **Polyneuropathy.** The term *polyneuropathy* refers to diffuse involvement of the peripheral nervous system. Typically, polyneuropathies produce symmetric weakness, atrophy, sensory impairment, diminished deep-tendon reflexes, and autonomic dysfunction. Functionally, they are classified as motor, sensory, or autonomic; and pathologically they can be divided into axonal or demyelinative. Frequently, the polyneuropathies are also divided into acute, subacute, or chronic depending on the time course of development of symptoms. Muscle weakness and atrophy are commonly seen in neuropathies but are also encountered in upper motor neuron lesions, neuromuscular diseases, and myopathies. Generally, an association of weakness with sensory symptoms, decreased deep-tendon reflexes, and a distal distribution of symptoms suggest a neuropathy. Sensory symptoms are typical of a neuropathy and may consist of positive symptoms such as complaints of tingling, tightness, burning, or tenderness; these abnormal sensations may actually be worse at night or during inactivity. Negative symptoms are secondary to decreased sensory information available because of damage to the nerves; these symptoms consist of numbness, clumsiness, unsteadiness when walking, and painless injuries. Autonomic symptoms, such as postural hypotension, anhidrosis, and loss of bladder and bowel control, are seen in some neuropathies.

A. **Acute inflammatory polyradiculoneuropathy** (Landry-Guillain-Barré syndrome) is the most common acute polyneuropathy.

1. **Clinical features.** Approximately one-half of patients give a history of a mild infection a week or two prior to the onset of the neuropathy. Although no specific virus or other infective agent has been consistently identified, the syndrome has followed infectious mononucleosis, measles, influenza, herpes zoster, hepatitis virus infection, and enterovirus infection. In the classic description, the illness presents with an ascending paralysis that develops over the course of several days, reaches a plateau, and after a few weeks begins to improve. However, patients can present with both distal and proximal weakness. In severe cases, the cranial nerves can also be involved, although the first, second, and eighth nerves are spared and the cranial nerves controlling eye movements are rarely affected. The deep-tendon reflexes usually are absent at an early stage. Although motor symptoms predominate, most patients complain of sensory involvement with numbness, tingling, or pain; these symptoms usually involve the feet or hands but may extend upward. Involvement of the autonomic

nervous system may appear as autonomic instability, cardiac arrhythmias, or orthostatic hypotension. Forms in which either the sensory symptoms or autonomic symptoms predominate have been described. With deterioration, the axial muscles are involved, with resultant respiratory distress.

2. **Pathogenesis.** The cause of this syndrome is unknown but is suspected to be autoimmune, with the involvement of viruses being indirect. Pathology reveals perivascular inflammatory infiltrates in capillaries of nerves, edema, and segmental demyelination, which can be spottily distributed.

3. **Laboratory studies.** The diagnosis of Landry-Guillain-Barré syndrome can be confirmed by the CSF findings and nerve conduction studies. The CSF is usually relatively acellular with less than 5 mononuclear cells; the protein, however, is usually markedly elevated, although this finding may not occur in the first week of the illness. In over 60% of cases there is slowing of the conduction velocities of nerves in the limbs. Occasionally, distal nerve conduction velocities are normal, but proximal velocities are prolonged or show a proximal block.

4. **Differential diagnosis.** The Guillain-Barré syndrome must be differentiated from the acute neuropathies caused by diphtheria, porphyria, and collagen vascular diseases. In the early stages it may be necessary to consider myelopathies from cord compression or intrinsic disease. Some toxic exposures (e.g., with triorthocresyl phosphate) may also present with an acute neuropathy. Polioencephalitis is associated with inflammatory cells in the spinal fluid.

5. **Management.** Hospitalization is indicated in all cases of suspected or diagnosed Landry-Guillain-Barré syndrome, since the progression to respiratory insufficiency can be rapid.

   a. **Respiratory assistance.** Frequent determinations of the vital capacity should be performed until the disease has stabilized. If respiratory function is insufficient, endotracheal intubation and respiratory assistance should be provided.

   b. Since cardiovascular complications from autonomic abnormalities can occur, **cardiac monitoring** and appropriate treatment as needed are indicated.

   c. The role of **steroid therapy** has not been established. Controlled studies have failed to demonstrate any benefit in the acute form of the illness, although steroids appear to be of benefit in the chronic relapsing form. Nevertheless, many neurologists use steroids during the early phase of the illness.

   d. **Plasmapheresis** may shorten the duration of weakness, particularly if started early in the illness.

6. The overall **prognosis** for recovery is good, with most patients making a complete or near complete recovery. However, convalescence may take weeks to months and in severe cases may require prolonged hospitalization and physical therapy.

B. **Diabetic neuropathy.** Diabetes mellitus may be associated with various types of neuropathy. Approximately 15% of patients with diabetes complain of symptoms of neuropathy, and as many as 50–60% may have some evidence of neuropathy on examination. The incidence of neuropathy rises with increasing age of the patient and duration of the disease.

   1. **Classification**

      a. **Distal neuropathy.** A common pattern of diabetic neuropathy is the development of a diffuse, symmetric distal neuropathy affecting particularly the lower extremities. This condition is frequently seen in older diabetics, even with mild disease. In mild cases, only a nonpainful numbness of the toes and feet is present. However, patients with a distal neuropathy may also have a burning discomfort of the skin of the toes, feet, and legs; this discomfort may be particularly severe at night. The ankle and, less commonly, knee jerks are either absent or decreased. Touch, pain, and position sense are variably decreased in the distal lower extremities. When severe, gait instability from impaired sensation may be present (sensory ataxia). Autonomic involvement is frequently seen along with painful diabetic neuropathy and, in addition to orthostatic hypotension, may produce impotence and bowel and bladder dysfunction.

      b. **Proximal neuropathy.** This form of diabetic neuropathy affects predominantly the **lumbar plexus** and has been variously known as femoral neuropathy, diabetic amyotrophy, and diabetic lumbosacral plexus neuropathy (see sec. **I.D.2**). The etiology is not known but has been presumed to be secondary to ischemia of the plexus or roots.

    c. Rarely, **cranial mononeuropathies** can occur in diabetes. The oculomotor nerve is most frequently involved with the development of an ophthalmoplegia without involvement of pupillary function. In contrast, compression of the oculomotor nerve by a mass lesion or during herniation is associated with a pupillary abnormality. Again, the cause is not known but is presumed to be vascular.

  2. Treatment. Currently, there is little preventive treatment available for the diabetic neuropathies. While the general clinical impression is that good control of the blood glucose is useful in preventing diabetic complications, there has been relatively little evidence that neuropathy is prevented or ameliorated by good control. Since there is some evidence that the distal neuropathies may be caused in part by sorbitol deposition in the peripheral nerves during periods of hyperglycemia, clinical trials are in progress to ascertain whether inhibitors of sorbitol production are of help. Currently, only symptomatic treatment is available.

    a. The **painful component** of the neuropathy may be helped by amitriptyline in low doses, 25–75 mg PO qhs, although at the risk of worsening any orthostatic hypotension that may be present. Occasionally, phenytoin or carbamazepine may also help.

    b. The treatment of **autonomic symptoms** is usually unsatisfactory and requires salt loading and the use of leg stockings (e.g., Jobst stockings) to reduce venous pooling in an attempt to maintain standing blood pressures.

C. Neuropathy with systemic illness. Neuropathies may be seen in association with other systemic illnesses, including uremia, amyloidosis, and carcinoma. Treatment should be directed at the underlying illness.

D. Neuropathy in association with drugs and toxins. A variety of drugs can produce neuropathies. The vinca alkaloids, especially vincristine and vinblastine used in cancer chemotherapy, can produce a primarily sensory neuropathy that may be painful. Nitrofurantoin can produce a neuropathy, particularly in patients with poor renal function. Metronidazole, when used in large doses, can also produce a sensory neuropathy, ataxia, and dysarthria. Isoniazid produces a neuropathy at high doses, which can be prevented with pyridoxine supplementation. Industrial and chemical agents regularly associated with a neuropathy include acrylamide monomer, hexacarbons (such as *n*-hexane and *n*-butyl ketone), triorthocresyl phosphate, methyl bromide, arsenic, lead, and thallium. In cases of subacute polyneuropathy, the possibility of a toxic exposure should be considered. Excessive alcohol intake is frequently associated with a distal neuropathy, although the role of the alcohol versus nutritional deficiency in the cause of the neuropathy is still not known. Treatment consists of discontinuing or avoiding the offending agent.

Neuromuscular Diseases

The **motor unit** consists of the motor neuron, the axon of the neuron, the neuromuscular end plate, and the muscle fibrils that are innervated by the neuron. Commonly, neuromuscular disease is classified by the portion of the motor unit that is predominantly involved. The predominant symptom in diseases of the motor unit is weakness, although patients frequently complain more of what they are unable to do because of their weakness rather than of weakness itself. Other common symptoms in neuromuscular disease include myalgias, myotonia (persistent contraction of a muscle from delayed relaxation after a contraction), and muscle cramps. The diagnosis of neuromuscular disease requires evaluation of the symptoms, the findings of the physical examination, the results of selected laboratory tests, and historic features, such as the age of onset, rate of progression, and genetics.

I. Motor neuron diseases. In amyotrophic lateral sclerosis (ALS), there is degeneration of motor neurons throughout the nervous system. Both upper and lower motor neurons are affected; thus, in addition to the signs of lower motor neuron dysfunction characterized by atrophy, fasciculations, and weakness, there is spasticity and hyperreflexia, indicating involvement of upper motor neurons. However, significant sensory involvement is lacking; and there is no involvement of eye movements, bladder and bowel control, or intellectual functioning. The disease is fatal, varying from 2–3 years in most patients to 7–10 years in some. Treatment is supportive care.

II. Diseases of the neuromuscular junction

A. Myasthenia gravis is a disease that appears to be caused by antibodies to the acetylcholine receptors at the muscle end plate. The prevalence is about 33/million individuals.

1. **Clinical features.** The illness can be seen at all ages but occurs most frequently in the third and fourth decades. Younger cases have a female predominance; however, in cases with later onset, men and women are affected equally. The presenting symptoms particularly involve weakness of the eye muscles, with development of ptosis or diplopia. The pharyngeal muscles also are involved early, with resultant difficulty chewing, dysarthria, and dysphagia. Limb weakness is usually proximal, but the distal musculature can also be involved. The weakness may fluctuate widely and can even change during an examination. Involved muscles fatigue easily, and prolonged activity can precipitate or exacerbate the weakness. Reflexes are reduced but present, and sensory abnormalities are absent. In about 20% of patients, the physical findings remain limited to the ocular muscles. In the rest, the disease follows a variable course with remissions and relapses, the latter frequently precipitated by systemic infections. The weakness may be severe enough to cause respiratory insufficiency and require ventilatory support.

2. **Diagnostic studies.** The diagnosis may be suspected from the observation of fatigable weakness. The patient is asked to maintain an upward gaze. As fatigue develops, ptosis increases. This test is frequently done in conjunction with edrophonium (Tensilon) injection.

   a. **Tensilon test.** Edrophonium chloride (Tensilon) is a short-acting anticholinesterase medication that, when given IV, acts within a minute and wears off in 5–10 minutes. Usually a test dose of 1 mg is given, and the patient is observed for any untoward reaction. Then 9 mg is injected, and the patient's fatigability is retested. A marked improvement in strength is a positive response.

   b. **Electromyography (EMG).** In myasthenia gravis, there is a decrease in the muscle action potential with repetitive stimulation because of the failure of neuromuscular transmission. This decrease is referred to as a **decremental response.**

   c. **Acetylcholine receptor antibodies.** A substantial number (85%) of patients with myasthenia gravis have measurable serum antibodies to the acetylcholine receptor. Although disease activity is poorly correlated with the level of antibodies, the presence of these antibodies is useful in confirming the diagnosis.

   d. **Chest CT scan.** Approximately 10% of patients with myasthenia gravis have an associated thymoma. Chest x-rays with oblique views will show most of these tumors, but the CT scan has a lower percentage of false-negatives.

3. The **treatment** of myasthenia gravis is either symptomatic (i.e., improving strength without changing the course of the illness) or directed toward producing a remission.

   a. **Anticholinesterases.** By preventing the breakdown of acetylcholine in the region of the neuromuscular junction, these medications can provide a transient increase in strength. Their use is accompanied by cholinergic side effects, including excessive salivation, abdominal cramps, and diarrhea. In addition, prolonged use tends to make myasthenics "brittle" and susceptible to life-threatening episodes of weakness with infections. Too much cholinergic effect can also produce a **cholinergic crisis,** with additional medication increasing weakness rather than helping it. Most neurologists currently use anticholinesterases either for mild myasthenia or as an adjunct to other therapy.

      (1) **Pyridostigmine** is available in 60-mg tablets, as a parenteral preparation, and also in a slow-release capsule of 180 mg. There is no standard dose, since the dosage is titrated to the patient's response. Some patients may require as little as 30 mg tid. Since it is rare to be able to reverse all symptoms with anticholinesterase medications, excessive doses should be avoided.

      (2) **Neostigmine** is available in a 15-mg tablet, which is equivalent to 60 mg of pyridostigmine. Most patients prefer pyridostigmine, because it

has a longer duration of action and has less cholinergic side effects. Neostigmine is also available in a parenteral form.

b. Steroids and immunosuppressants. Steroids are now commonly used in the treatment of myasthenia. A substantial number of myasthenics treated with steroids will have a remission of their symptoms. Most neurologists use prednisone in doses of 80–100 mg every other day. Once a remission is obtained, the dose is lowered slowly over a period of 1–2 years. Other immunosuppressants have been used in steroid–resistant patients; however, data on their effectiveness are still limited.

c. Thymectomy. Approximately two-thirds of patients with myasthenia gravis improve after a thymectomy, whether a thymoma is present or not. However, the improvement can be delayed significantly.

d. Plasmapheresis. Removal of circulating antibodies by plasmapheresis appears to transiently improve patients with myasthenia gravis, although the degree of improvement bears a poor relationship to the reduction in titer. The technique is expensive and is used predominantly to transiently improve the patient's condition in preparation for other procedures, such as thymectomy, or to shorten a myasthenic crisis.

e. Management of myasthenic crisis. Patients with myasthenia gravis may rapidly develop weakness with respiratory failure and require mechanical ventilation. Most commonly, this complication is triggered by infection. If there is any doubt about the ability of the patient to maintain adequate respirations, a cuffed endotracheal tube should be inserted, and assisted ventilation implemented. Anticholinesterase medication is stopped, and the cause of the crisis is sought and treated, if identified. After a few days, medications can be restarted, and the patient weaned off the ventilator.

B. Eaton-Lambert sydnrome (also known as **myasthenic syndrome**) is seen as a perineoplastic syndrome, usually in association with oat cell carcinoma of the lung. In contrast to myasthenia gravis, there is a defect in the release of acetylcholine. On the EMG, repetitive stimulation may produce an incremental response. Symptoms consist of weakness, usually mild with more proximal involvement. The ocular muscles, however, are spared. Guanidine hydrochloride may help the weakness.

C. Botulism is a rare form of neuromuscular blockade caused by the effect of botulin, a neurotoxin produced by *Clostridium botulinum*. The toxin binds to the presynaptic terminal of cholinergic neurons, blocking acetylcholine release. The two most common types are foodborne botulism and infant botulism. In foodborne botulism, the toxin is ingested; usually poorly preserved canned foods in which bacteria have grown are involved. In infant botulism, the bacteria produce the toxin within the child's intestine. Several hours after ingestion of the toxin, the patient develops nausea and vomiting. Over the next few hours, neurologic symptoms develop, including dilated and fixed pupils, paralysis of eye movements, pharyngeal dysfunction, and paralysis of limbs and respiratory function. Patients frequently also complain of a dry mouth and severe constipation. Mentation remains normal. Infant botulism is of slower onset since the toxin is slowly absorbed, and progression for several days is not unusual. The diagnosis of botulism is established by detection of the toxin in the stool and serum. In addition, EMG can show an incremental response at rapid stimulation (50 Hz). Recovery is slow, and treatment is predominantly supportive. Antitoxin to the toxin is available and should be given once the diagnosis is established.

III. Myopathies. A variety of illnesses affect skeletal muscle, including the genetic dystrophies, inflammatory myopathies, metabolic myopathies, and endocrine and toxic myopathies.

A. Dystrophies. A variety of muscular dystrophies have been identified, although the cause for the muscle dysfunction is unknown. Treatment is supportive.

B. Endocrine myopathies. Muscle is sensitive to a variety of systemic disturbances. Both hypo- and hyperthyroidism can lead to a disturbance of muscle function. Hypothyroidism is likely to present with muscle aches and pain and very mild weakness; the creatine phosphokinase (CPK) level is frequently elevated. In hyperthyroidism, CPK levels are usually normal, but significant proximal weakness may be present. Hypo- and hyperadrenalism can also produce weakness, although not usually severe. Hyperparathyroidism can produce muscle weakness, pain, and fasciculations and can be confused with motor neuron disease. Treatment is correction of the underlying metabolic disturbance.

C. **Toxic myopathies.** A variety of substances can cause muscle damage. Most common of these substances is alcohol, which can produce acute muscle damage in the form of alcoholic rhabdomyolysis. Muscle tenderness, swelling, and weakness are associated with markedly elevated CPK levels and myoglobinuria that may cause renal failure. Because myoglobin reacts with reagents used to test for blood in the urine, an indication of myoglobinuria is a positive test for blood in the urine, in the absence of red cells seen on microscopic examination. In addition to the acute form, alcohol can also cause a chronic proximal muscle weakness. **Treatment** of the acute episode involves administration of IV fluids and correction of any electrolyte imbalances.

D. **Periodic paralyses** are diseases characterized by recurrent attacks of flaccid paralysis associated with high or low potassium concentrations. Cases are frequently familial. In the hypokalemic form, attacks frequently are triggered by a large carbohydrate meal. Both types frequently occur during rest after exercise. An attack begins with weakness of the legs, is followed by weakness of the arms, and lasts from hours to a day. Some persistent proximal weakness between attacks is also present. Acute attacks can be treated by correcting the potassium abnormality by either giving potassium or treating with glucose and insulin for the hyperkalemic form. Acetazolamide in small doses, 250 mg PO bid or tid, serves as a prophylactic agent for both forms.

E. **Malignant hyperthermia.** A fortunately rare but serious complication of general anesthesia is the syndrome of malignant hyperthermia, for which there is a familial tendency. It can be triggered by several of the inhaled anesthetics and the muscle relaxant, succinylcholine. In susceptible individuals, exposure to one of these substances leads to a tachycardia, muscle rigidity, autonomic abnormalities, and a rapid increase in body temperature. In untreated cases, acidosis, hyperkalemia, and rhabdomyolysis develop; and death from cardiac arrhythmias may follow. Immediate **therapy** is necessary and includes discontinuation of the anesthetic agent, rapid cooling of the body, and administration of dantrolene sodium in a dose of 1–2 mg/kg q5–10min to a total dose of 10 mg/kg.

Bibliography

1. Aminoff, M., and Simon, R. Status epilepticus: Causes, clinical features and consequences in 98 patients. *Am. J. Med.* 69:657, 1980.
2. Barnett, H. J. M. The pathophysiology of transient ischemic attacks. *Med. Clin. North Am.* 63:649, 1979.
3. Brandt, T., and Daroff, R. The multisensory physiological and pathological vertigo syndromes. *Ann. Neurol.* 7:195, 1980.
4. Brooke, M. *A Clinician's View of Neuromuscular Disease.* Baltimore: Williams and Wilkins, 1977.
5. Byer, J., and Easton, J. D. Therapy of ischemic cerebrovascular disease. *Ann. Intern. Med.* 93:742, 1980.
6. Day, S. C., et al. Evaluation and outcome of emergency room patients with transient loss of consciousness. *Am. J. Med.* 73:15, 1982.
7. Delgado-Escueta, A., Treiman, D., and Walsh, G. The treatable epilepsies. I. and II. *N. Engl. J. Med.* 308:1508, 1576, 1983.
8. Drachman, D., and Hart, C. An approach to the dizzy patient. *Neurology* 22:323, 1972.
9. Earnest, M. P. *Neurologic Emergencies.* New York: Churchill Livingstone, 1983.
10. Easton, J. D., and Sherman, D. G. Management of cerebral embolism of cardiac origin. *Stroke* 11:433, 1980.
11. Greeson, S. D., and Linden, C. H. Glossopharyngeal neuralgia. *Ann. Emerg. Med.* 10:656, 1981.
12. Kapoor, W. N., et al. Syncope of unknown etiology. The need for a more cost-effective approach to its diagnostic evaluation. *J.A.M.A.* 247:2687, 1982.
13. Kapoor, W. N., et al. A prospective evaluation and follow-up of patients with syncope. *N. Engl. J. Med.* 309:197, 1983.
14. Kapoor, W. N., et al. Micturition syncope. A reappraisal. *J.A.M.A.* 253:796, 1981.
15. Knopp, R., et al. Use of the tilt test in measuring acute blood loss. *Ann. Emerg. Med.* 9:72, 1980.
16. Lance, J. Headache. *Ann. Neurol.* 10:1, 1981.
17. Lance, J. *The Mechanisms and Management of Headache* (4th ed.). London: Butterworth, 1982.

18. Leung, F. W., and Oill, P. A. Ticket for admission: Unexplained syncopal attacks in patients with cardiac pacemakers. *Ann. Emerg. Med.* 9:527, 1980.
19. Levy, D., et al. Prognosis in non-traumatic coma. *Ann. Intern. Med.* 94:293, 1981.
20. Martin, G. J., et al. Patient's evaluation of syncope. *Ann. Emerg. Med.* 13:499, 1984.
21. Penry, J. K., and Newmark, M. E. The use of antiepileptic drugs. *Ann. Intern. Med.* 90:207, 1979.
22. Plum, F., and Posner, J. B. *The Diagnosis of Stupor and Coma* (3rd ed.). Philadelphia: Davis, 1980.
23. Ross-Russell, R. W. Pathogenesis of transient ischemic attacks. *Neurol. Clin.* 1:279, 1983.
24. Shaumburg, H., Spencer, P. S., and Thomas, P. K. *Disorders of the Peripheral Nerves.* Philadelphia: Davis, 1983.
25. Silverstein, M. D., et al. Patients with syncope admitted to medical intensive care units. *J.A.M.A.* 248:1185, 1982.
26. Simpson, R. J., et al. Vagal syncope during recurrent pulmonary embolism. *J.A.M.A.* 249:390, 1983.
27. Thomas, J. E., et al. Orthostatic hypotension. *Mayo Clin. Proc.* 56:117, 1981.
28. Toole, J. *Cerebrovascular Disorders* (3rd ed.). New York: Raven, 1984.

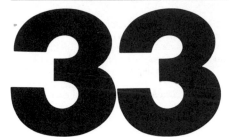

Obstetric and Gynecologic Emergencies

Diane F. Merritt

General Principles in the Evaluation of Obstetric and Gynecologic Emergencies

The underlying principle of management in obstetrics and gynecology, as in all of medicine, is to make a presumptive clinical diagnosis based on the history and physical examination and to commence therapy. However, objective laboratory verification (e.g., with hematologic, bacteriologic, and ultrasonic tests) of the clinical diagnosis is mandatory. Therapy based on symptoms alone without a diagnosis is not considered acceptable.

I. **Evaluation of pain**
   A. **History.** The accurate evaluation of abdominal pain demands detailed information concerning the onset, location, quality, duration, aggravating and relieving factors, and associated symptoms (e.g., anorexia, nausea, vomiting, diarrhea, dysuria, fever, chills, syncope) [18]. Any woman of reproductive age who presents with abdominal pain must be evaluated for pregnancy or a complication thereof, pelvic infection, and ovarian disorders, in addition to intraabdominal disease processes (e.g., appendicitis). Whenever pelvic pain is associated with missed or atypical menstrual periods or vaginal bleeding, the diagnosis of ectopic pregnancy must be considered. Pelvic inflammatory disease (PID) as a cause of pain may be chronic in nature or may appear a few days following sexual contact with an infected partner; in addition, asymptomatic cervical infections often progress to PID in the week following the last menstrual period.
   B. **Pelvic examination.** Whenever a patient complains of pelvic pain, a pelvic examination (see sec. **IV**) is a mandatory and essential part of that patient's evaluation.
   C. **Laboratory evaluation.** A pregnancy test (see sec. **III.C**), complete blood count (CBC), and urinalysis are important studies in the evaluation of patients with pelvic pain.

II. **Evaluation of vaginal bleeding.** Cyclic vaginal bleeding (menstruation) is normal in women of reproductive age. However vaginal bleeding may be irregular or abnormal in amount relative to the usual menses. In addition, vaginal bleeding in premenarchial and postmenopausal women is abnormal and may signify serious underlying disease.
   A. **Definitions**
      1. **Menorrhagia, or hypermenorrhea,** is excessive or prolonged menstrual bleeding.
      2. **Metrorrhagia** refers to uterine bleeding independent of the menstrual cycle.
      3. **Menometrorrhagia** refers to irregular or excessive bleeding during and between menstrual periods.
      4. **Polymenorrhea** is increased frequency of menstrual bleeding; **oligomenorrhea** is decreased frequency of menstrual bleeding.
   B. In taking **a menstrual history,** the following factors must be considered: (1) the patient's age at the onset of menstrual periods, the interval between periods (from the first day of flow to the first day of flow in the next cycle), and the duration of flow; and (2) the dates of the patient's last menstrual period (LMP) and previous menstrual period (PMP). It is also important to determine whether these factors were normal for her and to determine the character of the flow. Pregnancy should be suspected when there is a missed period (amenorrhea) or an abnormal last period and associated symptoms of nonspecific abdominal pain, morning sickness, fatigue, breast tenderness, and urinary frequency.
   C. A **pelvic examination** (see sec. **IV**) is an essential part of the evaluation of vaginal bleeding. The only exception is in the third trimester of pregnancy when vaginal bleeding may be a sign of placenta previa; in such a situation, a speculum examina-

tion is contraindicated because it can inadvertently cause fatal maternal hemorrhage.

D. Laboratory tests. A pregnancy test (see sec. **III.C**) is essential. A hematocrit and type and cross match, including Rh determination (see **Obstetric Emergencies,** sec. **III.C.1**), may also be indicated.

III. Diagnosis of pregnancy

A. Subjective symptoms of pregnancy include amenorrhea, nausea (with or without vomiting), urinary frequency, breast fullness or tenderness, fatigue, abdominal enlargement, and fetal movements.

B. Objective signs

1. **Breast enlargement,** an increase in breast nodularity, and enlargement of the nipples and areolae with hyperpigmentation and elevation of the sebaceous glands (Montgomery glands) are noted.

2. The **uterus** is palpable above the symphysis pubis at 12 weeks, at one-half the distance to the umbilicus at 16 weeks, and at the umbilicus at 20 weeks. The fundic height is measured with a centimeter tape from the symphysis pubis to the top of the fundus.

3. **Fetal movement** (quickening) may be appreciated in the fourth or fifth month of pregnancy. **Fetal heart tones** can be heard with a Doppler stethoscope as early as 12–14 weeks and with an obstetric stethoscope after 20 weeks.

4. **Uterine changes.** Six to eight weeks after the onset of the last period, the uterine isthmus (i.e., the junction between the cervix and corpus) softens (Hegar's sign), and the vagina and cervix may have a blue discoloration (Chadwick's sign).

C. Diagnostic tests for pregnancy

1. **Human chorionic gonadotropin (HCG)** is a glycoprotein normally produced by the syncytiotrophoblast cells shortly after implantation of the fertilized ovum into the uterine wall. Detectable concentrations of HCG appear in the serum within 7 days of conception (i.e., prior to the missed menstrual period). An **intrauterine pregnancy (IUP)** is the most common source of HCG in the serum; but other conditions, including an ectopic pregnancy, trophoblastic tumors, and other malignancies (e.g., embryonal cell cancer, seminoma, adenocarcinoma of the ovary or pancreas, hepatoma, lung cancer, melanoma, leukemia, lymphomas), may also produce HCG and therefore lead to an erroneous diagnosis of IUP [9].

   Urinary pregnancy tests are less sensitive than serum HCG assays but, depending on the sensitivity of the assay, may be positive as early as 1–2 weeks after the missed period; false-positive results, however, may be obtained if there is protein or blood in the urine.

2. **Ultrasonography** may demonstrate an intrauterine gestational sac at 5–6 weeks from the LMP and the fetal pole with fetal heart movements at 7 weeks. Measurements of gestational sac diameter, crown-rump length, biparietal diameter, and femur length have been used to estimate gestational age.

IV. Pelvic examination. Patients are best examined with an empty bladder.

A. Examination of the prepubertal child. Infants are best examined in their mothers' laps, and young children are best examined in the supine position with the hip and knees flexed and the heels together. The child is draped, if appropriate, and asked to drop her knees to the side. Perineal structures may be easily visualized in this way and examined for the stage of development (Tanner classification) and for evidence of trauma or infection. Any vaginal discharge should be cultured and examined by microscope; a urethral swab or plastic eye dropper is very useful in obtaining samples of vaginal discharge. Any foul discharge should be cultured for *Neisseria gonorrhoeae* and mandates inquiry as to possible sexual abuse. Nasal specula and special instruments (Cameron Miller prepubertal vaginoscope) allow visualization of the vagina and may be done without anesthesia or under general anesthesia by persons with experience in pediatric gynecology. The bimanual examination in young children is best performed by the rectoabdominal route.

B. Examination of the woman of reproductive age. An examination table with stirrups is necessary.

1. **Inspection.** The external genitalia are inspected for escutcheon (pattern of pubic hair distribution), evidence of inflammation, lesions, and signs of trauma. The labia are separated, and the clitoris, hymen, and urethra are examined.

2. **Speculum examination.** The vaginal speculum comes in many sizes and makes (e.g., Huffman, Pederson, Graves). Most young women are easily examined with

a medium Pederson speculum. If the vaginal walls are redundant or if the patient is obese, the Graves speculum can be used. Prior to insertion, the blades of the speculum are moistened with warm water, the blades are closed, and the speculum is directed downward toward the rectum to avoid unnecessary pressure and trauma to the urethra. The walls of the vagina are inspected for estrogen status (i.e., pink color, mucosal rugae) and evidence of inflammation. Any purulent discharge from the cervix should be cultured for *N. gonorrhoeae; Chlamydia trachomatis* is now another prominent organism associated with pelvic infections but requires special culture techniques. Specimens of any vaginal discharge (i.e., wet and potassium hydroxide preparations) should be collected for microscopic evaluation in patients complaining of vaginitis. Any fetal or placental tissue in the cervical os is presumptive evidence of a spontaneous abortion and should be saved for pathologic examination.

3. **Vaginal examination.** The gloved, lubricated index and middle fingers are gently inserted into the vagina, and any masses present in the introitus or vaginal walls are noted. Purulent material may be expressed from the paraurethral (Skene's) glands if they are infected. The cervix can be outlined; cervical softening suggests pregnancy. While performing the vaginal examination, the hand that is on the patient's abdomen, with the fingers slightly flexed, may be used to outline the uterine contours and adnexa (bimanual examination). Normal ovaries are usually 2.5–3.0 cm in size and usually are not palpable; direct bimanual pressure on a normal ovary may elicit pain, but excessive pain on light palpation suggests an inflammatory condition. A vaginal examination is contraindicated if there is vaginal bleeding in late pregnancy (see **Obstetric Emergencies, sec. VII**).

4. The **rectovaginal examination** allows for palpation of the rectovaginal septum, uterosacral ligaments, and cul-de-sac; anal masses may also be noted. The bimanual rectovaginal examination may better detail cul-de-sac masses.

C. **Postmenopausal women** are examined as in **B**. Occasionally, women with back problems are more comfortable if the head of the examination table is elevated.

Pelvic Pain of Gynecologic Origin

I. **Mittelschmertz** refers to ovulatory pain. This pain is secondary to distention of the ovarian capsule by a developing follicle or by follicle rupture or bleeding.

A. **Clinical features.** Mittelschmertz typically occurs in ovulatory patients 2 weeks before their expected menstrual period. The patient experiences a sudden or gradual onset of pain that is usually mild and lasts a few hours to 2 or 3 days. Clear fluid or sanguineous fluid may be present in the cul-de-sac.

B. **Diagnosis.** The midcycle timing and recurrent nature of the pain tend to confirm the diagnosis. Since these patients may have unilateral adnexal tenderness, an ovarian cyst or ectopic pregnancy should be considered in the differential diagnosis.

C. **Management.** The patient may be released on a mild analgesic once the diagnosis is confirmed; she should be reassured that this pain is part of a normal menstrual cycle.

II. **Dysmenorrhea,** or pain during the menstrual period, is a common cause of recurrent pelvic pain.

A. **Primary dysmenorrhea** is believed to be caused by local prostaglandin production and is associated with regular ovulatory cycles, fertility, and a normal pelvic examination.

1. **Clinical features.** Primary dysmenorrhea is characterized by a delayed onset (of a few months to years) after the initial menstrual period and by recurrence with each period. The pain may precede or follow the onset of bleeding and is usually worst when the flow is heaviest (i.e., on the first or second day); the pain may be crampy and localized to the suprapubic area, lower back, or thighs. Nausea, vomiting, increased frequency of bowel movements or diarrhea, palpitations, headache, and dizziness may be associated with the pain and are felt to be secondary to the systemic effects of the prostaglandins. The abdomen is soft, bowel sounds are present, and the pelvic examination is normal.

2. **Treatment.** Prostaglandin synthetase inhibitors, e.g., ibuprofen (Motrin), 200–600 mg PO q6h prn; naproxen sodium (Anaprox), 550 mg PO initially, followed by 275 mg PO q6h prn; or mefenamic acid (Ponstel), 500 mg PO, then 250 mg PO q6h prn, may be effective. The patient should be reassured that the pelvic examination is normal and should be given a gynecologic referral.

B. Secondary dysmenorrhea, characterized by pain before or during menses, is associated with some form of pelvic pathology, such as anomalies of müllerian development, adhesions, endometriosis, myomas, adenomyosis, or PID. The pelvic examination may be abnormal, reflecting such pathology. If prostaglandin synthetase inhibitors and ovulation suppression do not afford relief, diagnostic laparoscopy is useful to diagnose underlying pelvic pathology.

III. PID. See **Gynecologic Infections, sec. III.**

IV. Ovarian tumors

A. Ovarian enlargement. Inflammatory and dysfunctional enlargements of the ovary commonly produce pain or menstrual irregularities, whereas neoplastic lesions rarely are associated with clinical manifestations until late in their course [13].

1. **Follicular cysts** are follicles that have degenerated. They are usually tiny and numerous but can reach 8–10 cm in size. Large follicular cysts usually present with pain, and risk of torsion may complicate the picture. They may be associated with irregular or late menstrual periods or prolonged bleeding. The natural course is that of spontaneous regression. Ultrasound evaluation can confirm the finding of a single, simple, fluid-filled cyst. Simple follicular cysts may be suppressed with a trial of birth control pills or medroxyprogesterone acetate, 10 mg PO daily for 3–4 weeks. These patients must be referred to a qualified gynecologist in case resolution does not occur in 3–4 weeks.

2. **Lutein cysts and corpus luteum cysts.** Following ovulation, the granulosa and theca cells undergo luteinization, and a central cavity may form and become filled with blood (hemorrhagic corpus luteum); gradual resorption of blood over weeks may leave a cavity filled with fluid (lutein cyst). If ovulation is abnormal, there may be persistent function of the corpus luteum, which may result in delayed menstruation followed by persistent bleeding. This clinical picture is often associated with palpation of an enlarged and tender adnexal mass, which raises the possibility of the diagnosis of ectopic pregnancy (see **Obstetric Emergencies, sec. IV**). However, if the pregnancy test (serum HCG) is negative, the mass is unlikely to be an ectopic pregnancy; the patient should be referred for gynecologic follow-up. If the pregnancy test is positive, either an intrauterine or ectopic pregnancy exists. Often a pelvic ultrasound is useful to determine the location of the pregnancy. Gynecologic consultation is required if an ectopic pregnancy is suspected.

3. **Theca lutein cysts.** These ovarian cysts are found in response to elevated HCG and may coexist with a normal pregnancy (rarely), hydatidiform mole, or choriocarcinoma. They can reach massive sizes (up to 20 cm in diameter) and usually regress when the pregnancy is terminated or when HCG levels fall. Gynecologic consultation is indicated.

4. **Polycystic ovaries** can be enlarged up to 2 times normal size and be associated with oligomenorrhea, anovulation, infertility, and obesity and, occasionally, with mild virilism, hirsutism, and clitoromegaly. Polycystic ovaries are rarely a source of abdominal pain, as they are incidental findings in the above clinical picture. However, these patients may present to the emergency department with menorrhagia following a prolonged period of amenorrhea (see **Vaginal Bleeding of Gynecologic Origin, sec. I**). Referral to a gynecologist for evaluation is appropriate.

5. **Endometriomas** (see sec. **V**).

6. **Ovarian malignancies.** Discussion of these malignancies is beyond the scope of this chapter. Any time ovarian enlargement is found, malignancy must be excluded by mandatory gynecologic follow-up.

B. Accidents due to ovarian tumors [5]

1. **Ovarian torsion** can occur any time there is ovarian enlargement, whether the cause of the enlargement is benign or malignant. The long pedicle of a nonadherent cystic or solid growth may undergo torsion as a result of uneven growth or exercise. The pedicle of a fixed tumor, however, usually does not become twisted.

   a. In **chronic torsion,** twisting of the ovarian pedicle may occur slowly, causing few symptoms. There may be moderate discomfort resulting from a low-grade peritoneal inflammatory reaction and formation of adhesions. The physical examination generally reveals a low-grade fever, mild leukocytosis, and a tender abdominal or pelvic mass.

   b. **Acute torsion** often presents a dramatic clinical picture with the abrupt onset of pain, which is usually unilateral in the lower abdomen. The tumor, if palpated, is exquisitely tender. Once torsion occurs, the blood supply to the ovary is obstructed, leading to edema, hemorrhage, and gangrene. Peritonitis develops with rebound tenderness, guarding, abdominal distention, and signs of an ileus. The patient may have nausea and vomiting, tachycardia, leukocytosis, and fever.

    c. The **differential diagnosis** includes intestinal obstruction, volvulus, intussusception, and acute appendicitis.

    d. Treatment. The diagnosis of torsion of an ovarian cyst or tumor is an indication for prompt surgical intervention.

  2. Hemorrhage into a follicle cyst or corpus luteum is common and may result in moderate to acute distress. The involved ovary is large and tender on palpation. Symptoms may resemble torsion, ectopic pregnancy, or appendicitis; but as a rule, there is no leukocytosis, fever, or gastrointestinal symptoms. A positive pregnancy test suggests an ectopic pregnancy or an IUP associated with a hemorrhagic corpus luteum. If hemoperitoneum is present (caused by hemorrhage into the cyst or corpus luteum and subsequent rupture), culdocentesis is positive. Diagnostic laparoscopy may be necessary to properly diagnosis the condition. Brisk bleeding requires prompt surgical intervention.

  3. Rupture. Large ovarian cysts may rupture spontaneously or as a sequel to torsion. Follicular cysts, corpus luteal cysts, thin-walled adenomas, endometriomas, and benign cystic teratomas are prone to rupture. The patient presents with the sudden onset of severe abdominal pain, peritoneal irritation, and signs of shock. Culdocentesis may be diagnostic. Prompt laparoscopy or laparotomy is mandatory in such cases.

V. Endometriosis is characteristically a disease of reproductive age women, with the greatest incidence in the third and fourth decades. Endometriosis may occur in any menstruating patient and be a cause of abdominal and pelvic pain, dysmenorrhea, dyspareunia, premenstrual spotting, hypermenorrhea, infertility, or pain with defecation [13]. The disease is due to the presence of aberrantly occurring tissue resembling uterine endometrium in various sites, including the ovaries, uterine ligaments, rectovaginal septum, pelvic peritoneum covering the uterus, fallopian tubes, rectum, sigmoid colon, bladder, umbilicus, laparotomy scars, hernial sacs, appendix, vagina, vulva, cervix, and lymph nodes. The etiology is unknown but is postulated to be caused by retrograde menstruation, hematologic or lymphatic spread, or vestigial (congenital) ectopic location.

  A. Ovarian endometriosis. Ovarian involvement may range from superficial implants of endometrial tissue to endometrial cysts several centimeters in diameter (chocolate cysts). Even small punctate lesions may be associated with severe symptoms. The cysts can perforate and cause the ovary to adhere to any contiguous structure, usually the uterus or broad ligaments. Rupture of an ovarian endometrioma may result in sudden severe pain and present as an acute surgical abdomen requiring laparoscopy or laparotomy and copious pelvic lavage to prevent severe adhesion formation.

  B. Pelvic endometriosis

    1. Clinical features. The patient frequently complains of severe rectal and sacral pain, especially before and during menses. Involvement of the bowel may cause obstruction or rectal bleeding. Adhesions may form, fixing the uterus in a retroflexed position in the cul-de-sac. On pelvic examination, tender, firm blue nodules may be visible on the cervix or in the vaginal mucosa. Implants of endometrial tissue on the uterosacral ligaments may be palpable on rectovaginal examination as firm tender nodules. Infertility may result from very mild, as well as severe, cases of pelvic endometriosis.

    2. Definitive **diagnosis** requires laparoscopy to exclude other causes of pelvic pathology.

    3. The **differential diagnosis** of pelvic endometriosis includes primary dysmenorrhea, PID, pelvic adhesions, ovarian cysts and neoplasms, and gastrointestinal disorders.

    4. Management. If the presumptive diagnosis of pelvic endometriosis is made on clinical examination, gynecologic referral for long-term management and follow-up is indicated.

      a. Medical management. Ovulation suppression with birth control pills or progestins may be tried. If laparoscopy documents the presence of endometriosis, women who wish to maintain their fertility may receive significant relief of pain and resolution of adhesions caused by endometriosis by ovulation suppression with danazol (Danocrine) in a dosage of up to 800 mg PO daily for 6–8 months; however, with these high doses of danazol, menses are suppressed and the patient may suffer from androgenic side effects (i.e., acne, hirsutism, vaginal dryness).

b. Endometriosis is often managed by **conservative surgery** in which adhesions are lysed and endometriomas are removed using microsurgical techniques or laser surgery to minimize adhesion formation. Severe disease in symptomatic women who are not interested in childbearing can be treated by total abdominal hysterectomy and bilateral salpingo-oophorectomy.

Vaginal Bleeding of Gynecologic Origin

I. Dysfunctional uterine bleeding is abnormal bleeding that has no clear organic cause, such as a neoplasm, coagulation disorder, or pregnancy. The bleeding results from a disturbance in the usually finely synchronized hormonal activities that result in normal menstrual periods. Dysfunctional bleeding may occur in anovulatory as well as ovulatory cycles. Differentiation of ovulatory versus anovulatory bleeding often requires an outpatient evaluation with basal body temperature charting, progesterone levels, and endometrial biopsies. Most patients presenting in the emergency department with dysfunctional bleeding can be managed as outpatients, but it is the duty of the emergency department physician to rule out organic causes (e.g., pregnancy, neoplasm, trauma, coagulation disorder) by a careful history, physical examination, and, if indicated, pregnancy test or clotting profile.

A. Anovulatory dysfunctional bleeding. Patients should be referred to a gynecologist for outpatient management. Therapy depends on the patient's goals. If pregnancy is not desired, birth control pills will result in cyclic periods. If oligomenorrhea is the problem, medroxyprogesterone acetate, 10 mg PO daily for 10 days, should cause withdrawal bleeding within 10 days of the last tablet. If pregnancy is desired, therapy should be directed toward ovulation induction with agents such as clomiphene citrate or exogenous gonadotropins.

B. Control of severe dysfunctional bleeding can be gained rapidly by IV administration of a conjugated estrogen (Premarin), 25 mg q4h. At the same time, an oral conjugated estrogen, 2.5–7.5 mg/day, is begun and continued for 3 weeks; an oral progestin is added for the last 10 days. Withdrawal bleeding will follow after therapy is discontinued.

II. Perimenopausal and menopausal bleeding. The likelihood of an organic etiology increases as the patient progresses beyond the perimenopausal state. It is important to remember that vaginal bleeding in a postmenopausal woman is due to malignancy until proved otherwise (conversely, any gynecologic malignancy can present as abnormal vaginal bleeding).

A. Etiologies. The most frequently diagnosed causes of postmenopausal bleeding include endometrial and cervical polyps, atrophic vaginitis, atrophic endometrium, and endometrial cancer.

B. Evaluation. A careful history and pelvic examination is required of the emergency physician, who may find an obvious cause of the vaginal bleeding. Referral to a gynecologist or hospitalization is indicated to assess for a malignancy. A dilatation and curettage (D and C) or office curettage is mandatory prior to initiation of therapy.

III. Trauma to the genital organs is best diagnosed by a careful history. In young children and adolescents, vulvar trauma can occur from falling onto a protruding object, bicycle bar, or gymnastic equipment. For the sake of the child with anal or genital trauma, the possibility of sexual abuse must be assessed by appropriate careful questioning of both the child and guardian and by a thorough examination (see **Victim of Alleged Rape**). Generally, an examination under anesthesia is necessary to determine the full extent of genital injuries in children. Genital trauma resulting from injuries of childbirth is discussed in **Obstetric Emergencies, sec. IX.**

IV. Foreign bodies

A. Children. Foreign bodies are sometimes introduced into the vagina by children. Common items include wads of paper, chalk, crayons, and small pieces of plastic, metal, or wood. Such children present with a serosanguineous drainage or foul discharge. The rectal examination may be helpful in outlining a foreign body. An abdominal x-ray will reveal metal objects, such as paper clips and safety pins. Examination with a nasal speculum or vaginoscopy may be attempted but often requires general anesthesia.

B. Adults may also introduce foreign bodies into the vagina. The most common object is a forgotten tampon that causes a foul-smelling dark brown discharge and can be visualized high in the vagina on speculum examinations. Other objects may be introduced vaginally and then become lodged. Removal of the foreign object generally can be accomplished with a uterine forceps.

Gynecologic Infections

I. **Vulvar infections**
   A. **Pediculosis pubis** (see Chap. 31) is a contagious infestation caused by the "crab" louse, *Phthirus pubis*. This louse is found principally on pubic hairs after contact with an infected individual. The adult louse is 1–2 mm in length and appears as a rusty spot on the skin. The tiny nits, which are oval, whitish, transparent ova about 0.5 mm in length, generally can be found attached to the bases of hair shafts.
      1. **Diagnosis.** The patient presents complaining of severe itching. Confirmation of the diagnosis is made by observing a nit or adult form.
      2. Effective topical **treatment** less toxic than lindane is with pyrethrins with piperonyl butoxide (RID) [11]. This liquid is applied to the infected area for 10 minutes and then removed with warm water and soap. Dead lice and nits can then be removed with a fine-toothed comb. The lotion should be reapplied in 7–10 days to kill any newly hatched lice. Alternative medications include malathion lotion 0.5% and lindane (Scabene, Kwell). Clothing and bed linens should be washed in boiling water or dry-cleaned.
   B. **Pubic scabies** (see Chap. 31) is a highly contagious infestation caused by *Sarcoptes scabiei*, which varies from 0.2–0.4 mm in length. The mite is transmitted by intimate contact with an infected individual or by infested clothing. The impregnated female mite burrows into the skin to deposit eggs, which hatch into larvae in 3–4 days.
      1. The clinical **diagnosis** is suspected by complaints of severe pruritus and the presence of burrows (rarely larger than 1 cm in length and visible to the naked eye as elevated threadlike lines with a whitish vesicle at the end), papules, vesicles, urticarial wheels, or nodules. Confirmation of the diagnosis is made by a skin biopsy of a burrow; finding the adult, larva, or nymph under low-power microscopic examination is diagnostic.
      2. **Treatment** of scabies involves topical application of 10% crotamiton (EURAX) [11]. Alternative therapy includes application of lindane (Scabene, Kwell), benzyl benzoate, or sulfur in petrolatum. Clothing and bed linens should be washed in hot water or dry-cleaned.
   C. **Genital herpes simplex** (see Chaps. 12, 30, and 31)
      1. **Clinical features.** About 7 days after inoculation, usually by sexual contact, an initial infection of genital herpes may occur characterized by a prodrome of itching and tingling and followed by development of painful blisters or pustules that progress to ulcerative lesions. The entire time course until healing occurs may be 20 days, and viral shedding can occur during the entire time course of the infection.
      2. The **diagnosis** is presumptive from the clinical findings in the case of initial or recurrent infection but must be documented by a positive tissue culture, since the medical, psychological, social, and obstetric implications are serious.
      3. **Management.** In the first clinical episode, the patient may apply 5% acyclovir ointment to the lesions q3h for 7 days, begun as early as possible after the onset of the symptoms. This treatment reduces viral shedding and the duration of disease in patients with primary initial infection but does not prevent recurrences. The recommended dosage of oral acyclovir for treatment of genital herpes simplex infections is one 200-mg capsule PO five times daily for 7–10 days for treatment of initial disease or for 5 days for treatment of recurrent disease. The dosage recommended for suppression is one 200-mg capsule PO 2 to 5 times daily for up to a maximum of 6 months. The long-term safety of acyclovir is not known. The drug is not recommended for pregnant or lactating women.
II. **Vaginal and cervical infections**
   A. *Trichomonas vaginalis* is characterized by a vaginal discharge and itching and by minute punctate red lesions on the cervical and vaginal mucosa.
      1. The **diagnosis** is established by finding motile protozoa on a wet mount preparation.
      2. Recommended **treatment** is administration of metronidazole, 2.0 gm PO at one

time, with the same dose given to the sexual partner(s). Recurrences can be treated with metronidazole, 250 mg PO tid or 500 mg PO bid for 7–10 days. In pregnancy, clotrimazole vaginal suppositories, 100 mg daily for 7 days, may provide some relief to symptomatic patients; metronidazole is not a safe drug for use in the first two trimesters of pregnancy.

B. *Candida albicans* produces a vulvovaginitis that is characterized by a white cheesy discharge and vulvovaginal itching. Dysuria may also be a prominent feature. Predisposing factors include pregnancy, use of oral contraceptives, antibiotic therapy, use of corticosteroids, menstrual cycle changes, and diabetes mellitus.

   1. The **diagnosis** is established by finding spores and hyphae on a potassium hydroxide smear.

   2. Recommended **treatment** is administration of miconazole nitrate 2% vaginal cream or suppositories for 7 days or clotrimazole 1% cream for 7–14 days.

C. Nonspecific vaginitis can be recognized by signs of vaginal discharge and odor. *Gardnerella vaginalis* and anaerobic bacteria are associated with this infection, which is best treated with metronidazole, 500 mg PO bid for 7 days. Ampicillin, 500 mg PO qid for 7 days, is an acceptable alternative therapy when metronidazole cannot be used [10]; however, patients should be warned that the use of ampicillin can predispose them to candidal vaginitis.

D. Mucopurulent cervicitis may be caused by *N. gonorrhoeae* or *Chlamydia* (see Chap. 12). There is a mucopurulent discharge from an often friable cervix. **Treatment** is based on the culture reports. In the absence of culture results, however, uncomplicated infections are best treated with (1) a single dose of amoxicillin, 3 gm PO, plus probenecid, 1 gm PO, to slow renal excretion of the semisynthetic penicillin, or (2) ceftriaxone, 250 mg IM, either followed by tetracycline, 500 mg PO qid for 7 days, or doxycycline, 100 mg PO bid for 7 days. This regimen has the advantage of single-dose effectiveness against gonorrhea, combined with effectiveness against *Chlamydia*. In pregnant or lactating women, erythromycin, 500 mg PO qid for 7 days, should be substituted for tetracycline or doxycycline [10]. Tetracyclines are not recommended in pregnancy because of possible adverse effects on the teeth and bones of the fetus.

E. Toxic shock syndrome (TSS) (see Chap. 12)

   1. Clinical features. TSS is an uncommon condition characterized by rash, fever, hypotension, desquamation of skin, and multisystem involvement. The syndrome most commonly occurs in menstruating women. Use of tampons has been implicated as a predisposing factor. The etiology of TSS appears to be a toxin produced by *Staphylococcus aureus*.

   2. Evaluation. The definitive diagnosis of TSS is one of exclusion, but the index of suspicion should remain high in the menstruating population. A complete history, physical and pelvic examinations, and a standard laboratory workup (including a CBC with differential, blood cultures, and vaginal and cervical cultures) should be part of the emergency department evaluation of any woman of reproductive age who presents with a fever, rash, and hypotension.

   3. Management. If a tampon is found, it should be removed and cultured. After the vagina and cervix are cultured, the vagina should be irrigated profusely with saline. Hospitalization and IV administration of a penicillinase-resistant penicillin are indicated. Patients should be advised not to use tampons in the future if TSS is documented.

III. PID is an often made clinical diagnosis that is seldom substantiated by objective laboratory data. In Jacobson and Weström's study of 814 cases clinically diagnosed as having PID, only 65% were found to have PID by laparoscopic criterion; the others were found to have either a normal pelvis (23%) or other pathologic conditions (12%) that included acute appendicitis, pelvic endometriosis, ectopic pregnancy, ovarian cysts and tumors, pelvic adhesions, and mesenteric lymphadenitis [6].

PID may begin as an asymptomatic cervical infection. The infection, however, is often noted to spread into the upper genital tract following menstruation (probably because the menstrual endometrium serves as an excellent bacterial medium) and cause endometritis, salpingitis, and peritonitis. An episode of PID may follow a vaginal delivery, cesarean section, or abortion. In addition, any gynecologic manipulation, such as a hysterosalpingogram, can cause a flare of existing PID. The incidence of PID is 3–7 times greater in women using an intrauterine device (IUD) as their primary form of contraception [8, 20]. A variety of organisms are responsible for pelvic infections, and it is up to the clinician to prove by culture whether the infection is gonococcal or nongonococcal in nature.

A. Salpingitis is an inflammation of the fallopian tube and can be acute or chronic.

   1. The etiologic agent may be *N. gonorrhoeae, C. trachomatis,* or polymicrobial in nature. Gonococcal salpingitis is more likely in the initial episode when the symptoms appear during or shortly after a menstrual period. In addition, fever is more common and response to antibiotics more rapid in gonococcal salpingitis compared with polymicrobial salpingitis. Salpingitis caused by *Chlamydia* is often very mild in clinical presentation.

   2. Clinical features

      a. History. The presenting complaint is lower abdominal pain, which is often bilateral; the pain gradually increases in severity and is worse with movement. There may be an increase in menstrual flow or intermenstrual bleeding and associated fever, chills, and anorexia.

      b. On **physical examination,** there is often fever and a tachycardia. The patient may walk shuffling and bent over and lie with her knees flexed if peritonitis is present. The abdomen may be tender in the lower quadrants, with rebound tenderness, guarding, and decreased bowel sounds. The pelvic examination may reveal a purulent cervical discharge and presence of cervical and adnexal tenderness. An adnexal mass or cul-de-sac fullness may suggest a pyosalpinx, hydrosalpinx, or tuboovarian abscess.

      c. Laboratory evaluation. The white blood cell (WBC) count generally is elevated with a left shift. The hemoglobin and hematocrit are normal (unless the patient is dehydrated), as is the urinalysis. The cervix should be cultured for *N. gonorrhoeae* and *C. trachomatis.* If there is a poor clinical response to antibiotics or if the diagnosis is in question, diagnostic laparoscopy may be useful.

   3. The **differential diagnosis** includes ectopic pregnancy, which is usually associated with a missed menstrual period, positive pregnancy test, and a normal WBC count; in addition, culdocentesis is often positive in the presence of an ectopic pregnancy. Appendicitis must also be differentiated from PID; the former, however, is usually characterized by an initial periumbilical pain that subsequently localizes to the right lower quadrant and is associated with anorexia, nausea, and vomiting. Other diagnoses include endometriosis, diverticulitis, torsion of the bowel or ovary, an ileus, urinary tract infection, acute intermittent porphyria, and tuberculous peritonitis, which may be present with clinical signs similar to those of PID.

   4. Management. Aggressive management of properly diagnosed PID is necessary to prevent subsequent infertility caused by adhesions, tubal damage, or formation of tuboovarian abscesses.

      a. Mild, uncomplicated salpingitis. Compliant patients with mild, uncomplicated salpingitis may be managed as outpatients. Recommended antibiotic schedules include (1) cefoxitin, 2.0 gm IM, plus probenecid, 1.0 gm PO, or (2) ceftriaxone, 250 mg IM. Alternative regimens include (1) amoxicillin, 3.0 gm PO, plus probenecid, 1.0 gm PO; (2) ampicillin, 3.5 gm PO, plus probenecid, 1.0 gm PO; or (3) aqueous procaine penicillin G, 4.8 million units IM, plus probenecid, 1.0 gm PO. Cefoxitin and ceftriaxone have the advantage of being effective against penicillin-resistant strains of *N. gonorrhoeae.* This initial dose should be followed by doxycycline, 100 mg PO bid for 10–14 days, or tetracycline hydrochloride, 500 mg PO qid for 10 days. If there is no clinical response in 48–72 hours, the patient should be hospitalized to reassess the diagnosis. If an IUD is present, it should be removed.

      b. Severe or complicated salpingitis. Patients with a fever of 101°F or more, persistent nausea and vomiting, signs of peritonitis, an adnexal mass, or the possibility of a surgical emergency (e.g., appendicitis, ectopic pregnancy) should be hospitalized for parenteral therapy and observation. Patients who are unreliable, fail outpatient therapy, have an underlying medical disease (e.g., valvular heart disease, diabetes mellitus), are immunocompromised, or are pregnant must also be hospitalized. Recommended antibiotic regimens include the following: (1) cefoxitin, 2.0 gm IV qid, in combination with doxycycline, 100 mg IV bid, until improvement is noted and then followed by doxycycline, 100 mg PO bid for 10 days; or (2) clindamycin, 600 mg IV qid, combined with gentamicin, 2.0 mg/kg IV followed by 1.5 mg/kg IV tid, until improvement occurs and then followed by clindamycin, 450 mg PO qid, to complete a 10–14-day course of therapy [10, 15]. Pregnant patients may be treated with the second regimen; tetracyclines are not recommended in pregnancy because of possible adverse effects on the teeth and bones of the fetus. If an IUD is in place, it should be removed. Ovulation suppression with birth control pills may prevent tuboovarian abscesses.

If during the hospitalization the patient fails to improve, diagnostic laparoscopy may be done to confirm the diagnosis and assess for other disease processes.

B. Tuboovarian abscess

1. **Pathophysiology.** A tuboovarian abscess (TOA) evolves as a sequela of acute or chronic salpingitis. It is thought that ovulation allows access of bacteria into the disrupted ovarian capsule. Hematogenous spread may also carry bacteria into the ovary. The tubal damage may be subtle, with disruption of the ciliated endothelium, or extensive, resulting in a pyosalpinx (i.e., a distended tube filled with purulent discharge) or hydrosalpinx (i.e., a distended tube filled with sterile fluid) with clubbing of the tubes and loss of patency. Infertility and chronic pelvic pain may result.

2. **Clinical features**

   a. **Presentation.** The patient presents with pelvic pain. Sudden, severe, and diffuse pain suggests rupture of a TOA. There may be associated vaginal bleeding, fever, nausea, vomiting, pain with defecation, tenesmus, or diarrhea; and the patient may appear toxic. A ruptured TOA may lead to bacteremia and septic shock.

   b. On **physical examination,** the patient may have a subnormal body temperature or be hyperthermic with temperature spikes as high as 40°C (104°F). A tachycardia and hypotension may be present. The abdominal examination may reveal abdominal distention; hypoactive or absent bowel sounds may be noted secondary to an ileus, and guarding and rebound tenderness may be present secondary to peritoneal irritation. Purulent discharge may be present in the cervical os, and the cervix may be deviated by the abscess; cervical motion is very painful. Since TOAs, which can be unilateral or bilateral, are very tender, they may be best palpated in the cul-de-sac on rectal examination. Adhesions of bowel and omentum may add to the apparent size of the mass.

   c. **Laboratory assessment.** The WBC count is elevated with a marked left shift. Blood cultures should be obtained along with aerobic and anaerobic cervical cultures and possibly cul-de-sac cultures. Abdominal radiographs may demonstrate the presence of a mass, a foreign body (e.g., IUD), and signs of an ileus. Ultrasonography can be very useful in documenting the size and location of the abscess.

3. **Management.** These patients should be hospitalized, aggressively cultured, rehydrated, and started on parenteral antibiotics.

   a. **Antibiotic therapy.** Since the cause is often polymicrobial, antibiotic therapy may be the same as that of severe salpingitis (see **A.4.b**) or involve triple antibiotic coverage: penicillin G, 3–5 million units IV q4h; gentamicin, 60–80 mg IV q8h; and clindamycin, 450–600 mg IV q6–8h. Once specific bacterial culture results are available, antibiotic coverage should be adjusted accordingly.

   b. **Nasogastric suction** is indicated if an ileus is present.

   c. **Laparoscopy or laparotomy.** Patients must be followed closely, particularly with regard to their general condition, temperature, serial WBC counts with differentials, and serial assessment of the size and tenderness of the mass. If the patient does not improve, if the mass fails to reduce in size or ruptures, or if the diagnosis is in question, exploratory laparoscopy or laparotomy is indicated. Depending on the pelvic findings, the patient's condition, and the desire for future childbearing, a total hysterectomy and bilateral salpingo-oophorectomy or, occasionally, a unilateral salpingo-oophorectomy may need to be performed.

C. Perihepatitis. Curtis was the first to describe "violin-string" adhesions between the anterior surface of the liver and the anterior abdominal wall in patients with PID [2]. Fitz-Hugh later described the clinical syndrome, which is now known as the Fitz-Hugh–Curtis syndrome, or perihepatitis [4].

1. **Clinical manifestations.** There is often a prodrome of low abdominal pain, abdominal distention, fever, and perhaps abnormal menses. This prodrome may be followed by right upper quadrant rigidity and tenderness. The pain is worse with coughing and movement of the trunk. A friction rub (crunching to-and-fro

sound) is sometimes noted over the anterior abdominal wall. There may be a leukocytosis and mild elevation of liver function tests. The acute time course may run 3–6 weeks, or the patient may be totally asymptomatic.

2. **Diagnosis.** Perihepatitis can occur following genital infection with *C. trachomatis* as well as *N. gonorrhoeae* [12]; therefore, isolation of either of these organisms on cervical cultures in the proper clinical setting supports a presumptive diagnosis of the syndrome. A normal chest x-ray, negative gallbladder studies, and a normal ventilation-perfusion scan aid in eliminating the alternatives. The diagnosis, however, can be established by laparoscopy.

3. The **differential diagnosis** includes acute cholecystitis, pneumonia, pleurisy, a subdiaphragmatic abscess, and pulmonary embolism or infarction.

4. **Management** of perihepatitis in its acute phase includes administration of appropriate antibiotics (see **A.4.a**) and pain medication.

Obstetric Emergencies

I. **General principles of pregnancy**
A. Pregnancy is associated with a multitude of **anatomic, physiologic, and endocrine adjustments** [14] in response to the developmental needs of the fetus and placenta and directed toward creating the optimum environment for the growing fetus.

1. **Uterine and fetal changes.** The uterus enlarges from a strictly pelvic organ at 12 weeks of gestation to become an abdominal organ, displacing the intestines laterally and superiorly and coming into direct contact with the abdominal wall; the uterus ultimately rises to reach the liver at term, achieving a capacity that is 500–1000 times greater than in the nonpregnant state. Movement of the fetus is perceived by most women at 16–20 weeks gestation, while fetal heart tones are audible at a rate of 120–160 beats/minute by Doppler as early as 12 weeks from the last menstrual period.

2. **Cardiovascular effect.** During normal pregnancy, the mother's resting heart rate increases about 10–15 beats/minute, while the vascular resistance and arterial blood pressure decrease; the blood pressure reaches its nadir during the second trimester or early third trimester and then rises toward the prepregnancy level. The maternal blood volume increases nearly 45% during pregnancy to meet the demands of the enlarged uterus as well as to protect against supine hypotension (from the enlarged uterus impeding venous return to the heart) and the blood loss associated with delivery. The increase in blood volume results from an increase in both plasma and erythrocytes, with the increase in the former usually predominating. Each of these factors, along with the increase in basal metabolic rate that occurs during pregnancy, affects the cardiac output, with the net effect being that the cardiac output at rest (when measured in the lateral recumbent position) increases significantly during the first trimester and remains elevated during the second and third trimesters. Typically, cardiac output in late pregnancy is less when the woman is in the supine position, since in that position the uterus often impedes venous return to the heart. Other cardiovascular changes noted during pregnancy include (1) displacement of the heart upward and to the left, giving rise to an enlarged cardiac silhouette on chest radiograph and slight deviation of the electrical axis to the left on the electrocardiogram (ECG), and (2) an increased femoral venous pressure and decreased blood flow in the legs (except in the lateral recumbent position) predisposing the woman to dependent edema and to the development of varicose veins and hemorrhoids. In addition, a systolic murmur is present in 90% of pregnant women.

3. **Respiratory effects.** Although the respiratory rate and vital capacity change little during pregnancy, the tidal volume and minute ventilatory volume increase considerably as pregnancy advances. These increases, in turn, give rise to a mild respiratory alkalosis, which is partially compensated for by a decline in the plasma bicarbonate concentration.

4. **Genitourinary effects.** Glomerular filtration rate (GFR) and renal plasma flow (RPF) increase during pregnancy, the former by as much as 50% at the beginning of the second trimester and the latter to a lesser extent. The increased GFR results in decreased plasma concentrations of urea and creatinine. Glucosuria may occur during pregnancy in the absence of diabetes mellitus from increased glomerular filtration and impaired tubular resorptive capacity. However, proteinuria is an abnormal finding during pregnancy (except during or soon after

vigorous labor) and may be a sign of preeclampsia. Ureteral dilatation above the pelvic brim occurs during pregnancy from compression by the uterus and is usually more marked on the right side; this hydronephrosis and hydroureter predispose the pregnant woman to development of pyelonephritis.

5. **Gastrointestinal effects.** During normal pregnancy, the tone and motility of the gastrointestinal tract are usually decreased, which prolongs gastric emptying and intestinal transit time; thus, esophageal reflux is a frequent occurrence, causing heartburn.

6. **Hematologic changes.** Although the erythrocyte volume increases during normal pregnancy by an average of about 33% from accelerated production (reflected by an increased reticulocyte count) if exogenous iron is made available to the mother, the hematocrit and hemoglobin concentration decline, the latter to about 12.1–12.5 gm/dl on the average at term, from expansion of the plasma volume. Because of the needed increase in maternal circulating erythrocytes and demands by the developing fetus, the iron requirements of normal pregnancy total about 1 gm. Unless exogenous iron is made available to the mother, the desired expansion in maternal erythrocyte volume will not occur, and the hematocrit and hemoglobin concentration will decline appreciably as the maternal plasma volume increases; a hemoglobin concentration of less than 11.0 gm/dl is likely due to iron deficiency. The blood leukocyte count usually varies from 5000–12,000/mm^3 during normal pregnancy, increasing during labor and the early puerperium to 14,000–16,000/mm^3 on the average and, occasionally, up to 25,000/mm^3 or more. Plasma fibrinogen and several other coagulation factors are increased during pregnancy. The increase in fibrinogen concentration contributes to the increase in sedimentation rate (ESR) found in normal pregnancy.

7. Other effects of pregnancy. The average total weight gain in pregnancy is 25–30 pounds. Although increased water retention is a normal physiologic alteration of pregnancy, marked water retention with the development of edema may be a sign of preeclampsia (see sec. **XII**). In healthy pregnant women, the fasting plasma glucose concentration is typically lower than in non-pregnant women. However, pregnancy is potentially diabetogenic; diabetes mellitus may be aggravated by pregnancy, and clinical diabetes may occur in some women only during their gestation. The enlarging breasts and uterus during pregnancy shift the woman's center of gravity and exaggerate lordosis, often leading to complaints of back pain during pregnancy. Headaches can also be quite common during pregnancy and, if persistent and severe, mandate a good evaluation as well as exclusion of preeclampsia.

B. **Approach to the pregnant patient.** In evaluating and treating a pregnant woman with an illness, injury, or possible complication of pregnancy, it is important to consider the anatomic and physiologic changes of pregnancy. It is also essential for the physician to keep in mind that there are two patients, the mother and the fetus, and that the well-being of the latter depends, to a large extent, on the well-being of the former. Thus, whenever a pregnant woman is ill or injured, every effort should be made to maximize her care and, during this time, to monitor the status of the fetus (e.g., by monitoring the fetal heart tones, as appropriate). In addition, the potential benefits to the mother and fetus of diagnostic procedures and therapeutic modalities must be carefully weighed against the possible risks, and potentially injurious interventions must be avoided, if possible. Although unnecessary radiographs should be avoided during pregnancy, radiographs needed to properly manage a pregnant woman should be obtained, since in this situation the potential benefits to the mother (and indirectly to the fetus) outweigh the potential risks to the fetus. Since drug use during pregnancy can interfere with embryogenesis, resulting in congenital anomalies, it is accepted practice in pregnant women to avoid drugs, particularly during the first trimester when the risk of teratogenesis is greatest, unless absolutely necessary to maintain the pregnancy or the health of the mother. Table 33-1 classifies some relatively common drugs with regard to their safety for use during pregnancy. In caring for a pregnant woman in the latter stages of pregnancy, it is wise to place the patient in the left lateral decubitus position, unless contraindicated, to avert the supine hypotension syndrome (resulting from compression of the inferior vena cava by the uterus).

II. **Nausea and vomiting of pregnancy and hyperemesis gravidarum**

A. **"Morning sickness"** has been accepted as one of the natural discomforts of early pregnancy. The typical course of nausea, vomiting, and food aversion is usually mild, self-limiting, and present only for a few weeks in the first trimester.

Table 33-1. Safety of drug use in pregnancy[a]

Type of medication	"Safe"[b]	Relatively safe	Some risk	Contraindicated[c]
Analgesics	Acetaminophen Meperidine[d,e] Morphine[d,e] Codeine[d,e]	Hydrocodone[d,e]	Salicylates	Indomethacin
Antacids	Aluminum hydrochloride Calcium carbonate Magnesium compounds			Sodium bicarbonate
Antibiotics	Ampicillin Cephalosporins Erythromycin Penicillin Semisynthetic penicillins	Clindamycin Gentamicin	Amphotericin B Chloramphenicol[f] Isoniazid Kanamycin[g] Nitrofurantoin[h] Streptomycin[g] Sulfonamides[i] Tobramycin Vancomycin[g]	Metronidazole[j] Tetracycline
Anticoagulants	Heparin[k]		Warfarin[l]	
Anticonvulsants	Magnesium sulfate	Phenobarbital	Diazepam[d] Ethosuximide Phenytoin Primidone	
Antiemetics		Metoclopramide hydrochloride Trimethobenzamide		
Antifungal agents	Clotrimazole Miconazole Nystatin			Griseofulvin
Antihypertensives	Hydralazine Methyldopa	Propranolol		Clonidine Diazoxide Guanethidine Reserpine Sodium nitroprusside
Bronchodilators	Aminophylline Theophylline	Beclomethasone Cromolyn sodium Terbutaline[m]	Epinephrine Metaproterenol	

Cardiac drugs	Digoxin Lidocaine	Atropine Quinidine Verapamil	Procainamide	Disopyramide[n]
Cold, cough, and allergy medications	Guaifenesin (Robitussin)	Dextromethorphan Pseudoephedrine	Chlorpheniramine Diphenhydramine[o]	
Corticosteroids		Dexamethasone[p] Hydrocortisone[p] Methylprednisolone[p] Prednisone[p]		
Diuretics			Furosemide[q] Ethacrynic acid[q] Spironolactone[q] Thiazide diuretics[q]	Mercurial diuretics
Gastrointestinal preparations	Anusol suppositories Bran Carboxymethylcellulose Cascara Dioctyl sulfosuccinate Kaopectate Methylcellulose Milk of Magnesia Senna	Cimetidine Docusate sodium Psyllium preparations		Mineral oil[r]
Hypoglycemics	Insulin			Oral hypoglycemic agents
Obstetric and gynecologic preparations	Ritodrine hydrochloride[s]		Progestins	Bromocriptine mesylate Clomiphene citrate Diethylstilbestrol Estrogens Oral contraceptives
Psychiatric medications			Phenothiazines Tricyclic antidepressants	Lithium
Sedatives		Phenobarbital Secobarbital	Diazepam[d]	
Thyroid preparations	Thyroxine		Methimazole[t]	
Vaccines	Polio[u] Rabies Tetanus	Hepatitis B Influenza[v] Yellow fever[w]		Mumps Rubeola Rubella

Table 33-1. (Continued)

Type of medication	"Safe"[a,b]	Relatively safe	Some risk	Contraindicated[c]
Other	Ferrous sulfate Naloxone hydrochloride	Probenecid	Allopurinol Methadone[d,e]	Aminocaproic acid Amphetamines Antineoplastic drugs Ergotamine tartrate Ethanol Marijuana Potassium iodide Tobacco

[a]This table is only a guide. The decision to use a particular drug must be based on careful consideration of the potential therapeutic benefit to be derived versus the risk of possible adverse effects on the fetus or uterus. Generally, drugs should be avoided during the first trimester (unless absolutely necessary) and used sparingly (only if indicated) thereafter.

[b]Although these drugs are generally considered to be safe, no drug can be used with assurance that there will be no adverse effects associated with its use.

[c]These drugs have been associated with adverse fetal effects and should not be used in pregnancy.

[d]Possible neonatal depression when used intrapartum.

[e]Possible neonatal addiction and withdrawal with long-term use.

[f]Avoid during third trimester unless absolutely necessary because of risk of the "gray syndrome" in neonates.

[g]Can cause ototoxicity in utero.

[h]Avoid use at term because of risk of hemolytic disease in the newborn with glucose-6-phosphate dehydrogenase deficiency.

[i]Avoid during third trimester because of risk of kernicterus in neonates.

[j]Contraindicated during first and second trimesters.

[k]Drug of choice for anticoagulation during pregnancy because it does not cross the placenta.

[l]Avoid during first trimester because of risk of congenital anomalies and avoid after 36 weeks of gestation or whenever delivery is imminent to avoid hemorrhagic complications during delivery.

[m]Inhibits uterine activity in second and third trimesters; can be used to manage premature labor.

[n]Associated with initiation of uterine contractions.

[o]Associated with cleft palates.

[p]Can cause neonatal adrenal suppression with long-term use.

[q]Not indicated for pregnancy-induced hypertension because of risk of depletion of maternal intravascular volume and, rarely, neonatal thrombocytopenia.

[r]Interferes with vitamin absorption.

[s]Contraindicated before the twentieth week of pregnancy.

[t]May induce goiter or cretinism.

[u]Not recommended for routine prophylaxis during pregnancy.

[v]Recommended only for the pregnant woman with serious underlying disease.

[w]Recommended only for the pregnant woman at high risk for the disease.

Source: Adapted from D. A. Skor, Patient Care in Internal Medicine. In M. J. Orland and R. J. Saltman (eds.), *Manual of Medical Therapeutics* (25th ed.). Boston: Little, Brown, 1986.

1. **Differential diagnosis.** Not all nausea and vomiting in pregnancy is related to the pregnancy. Physicians must remain alert to the possibility of other etiologies, e.g., acute gastroenteritis, cholecystitis, hepatitis, pancreatitis, diabetic ketoacidosis, and gestational trophoblastic disease.

2. **Laboratory findings.** Simple nausea and vomiting of pregnancy are not associated with any laboratory abnormalities other than those associated with pregnancy itself.

3. **Treatment.** The patient should be instructed to eat small carbohydrate meals frequently and to avoid greasy foods and any food that the patient finds disturbing. Since the safety of antiemetics in pregnancy has not been established, they should not be used for mild nausea and vomiting. The patient should be monitored closely for signs of weight loss or evolution into hyperemesis gravidarum.

B. **Hyperemesis gravidarum** refers to a condition of persistent and severe vomiting in pregnancy, resulting in nutritional deficiencies or fluid and electrolyte disturbances.

   1. **Laboratory findings.** Loss of fluid and electrolytes is reflected by elevation of the hematocrit, blood urea nitrogen (BUN), serum and urinary osmolalities, and urine specific gravity. In addition, acetonuria (ketonuria) and decreases in the urinary volume and creatinine clearance are encountered. Because of the persistent vomiting, the patient has hyponatremia, hypokalemia, hypochloremia, and a metabolic alkalosis. If the illness is not treated, jaundice and hypoalbuminemia will ensue.

   2. **Management.** All patients with persistent vomiting, weight loss, or dehydration must be hospitalized. IV fluids are administered. When oral intake is tolerated, the patient is given 1 oz of water/hour; the amount of water is gradually increased, and juices and tea are added as tolerated. The diet is then advanced from liquids to a full diet as the patient tolerates. These patients may benefit from sedation (e.g., with phenobarbital, 30 mg PO q6h while awake). If necessary, an antiemetic (e.g., trimethobenzamide hydrochloride [Tigan]) may be added if the nausea and vomiting are so serious and intractable that, in the judgment of the physician, drug intervention is required and the potential benefits outweigh possible hazards. Administration of all drugs, however, must be reassessed frequently and not used more often than needed. The patient's daily weight should be recorded; once the weight loss has ceased and the patient is tolerating her diet, she may be discharged from the hospital.

   3. **Complications** of vomiting include aspiration pneumonia, gastrointestinal hemorrhage due to mucosal tears at the gastroesophageal junction, esophageal rupture, electrolyte depletion, acid-base disturbances, and dental erosions.

III. **Abortion.** Abortions can be spontaneous or induced. The majority of pregnancies spontaneously aborted in the first trimester have morphologic or chromosomal abnormalities.

A. **Types**

   1. **Threatened abortion.** The patient presents with an IUP, uterine bleeding, and possibly abdominal cramping pain and is found to have an enlarged uterus consistent with the date of her last menstrual period, a closed cervix (not permitting passage of a ring forceps), and bleeding from the external os. The patient should be reassured that 60% of such pregnancies go on to deliver a viable infant. Bed rest, avoidance of intercourse, and avoidance of vigorous physical activity is encouraged. The patient should be instructed to return if the bleeding and cramping increase or if tissue is passed. Any tissue should be saved by the patient and brought in for examination. An ultrasound examination to document fetal viability is a reasonable option, if available; if fetal heart motion is documented by ultrasonography in a threatened abortion at 7–10 weeks, 90% of these fetuses will survive [7].

   2. **Inevitable abortion.** The patient presents with excessive or prolonged vaginal bleeding and continuous and progressive dilatation of the cervix without expulsion of the products of conception. Treatment in the first trimester is uterine evacuation by suction curettage.

   3. **Incomplete abortion.** The products of conception are in the vagina or have been expelled, but trophoblastic tissue remains in the uterus. To prevent further bleeding and the possibility of infection, uterine evacuation by suction curettage is indicated.

   4. **Complete abortion.** All trophoblastic elements have been completely expelled spontaneously. An intact sac with no further uterine bleeding suggests curettage is unnecessary.

5. Septic abortion is an infected abortion in which there is dissemination of microorganisms and their products into the maternal circulation.

a. Clinical features

(1) A septic abortion can follow either a spontaneous or induced abortion. There may be evidence of an illegally induced abortion (e.g., lacerations of the cervix or vagina).

(2) The patient presents with local and systemic complaints, including fever, tachycardia, and pelvic or abdominal tenderness. A leukocytosis with a left shift is common.

(3) In its most severe form, a septic abortion is characterized by profound hypotension, renal failure, disseminated intravascular coagulation (DIC), a paradoxically low body (core) temperature, and leukopenia.

b. Evaluation. Cervical and blood cultures (aerobic and anaerobic) should be obtained in all cases. The causative organisms cultured from the blood and cervix may include gram-negative enteric aerobic and anaerobic pathogens, including clostridial species. A Gram stain of the tissue or endocervical smear is useful in directing initial antibiotic choice, pending culture and sensitivity results.

c. Treatment

(1) Treatment of septic shock may require rapid and large **volume infusion** of normal saline. Thus, a central venous pressure line or Swan-Ganz catheter may be needed. A Foley catheter must be placed to evaluate the urinary output.

(2) Blood replacement may be required for blood loss caused by the abortion or hemolysis.

(3) A **vasopressor** (e.g., dopamine, norepinephrine) may be required to manage fluid-resistant hypotension.

(4) Corticosteroids may be beneficial if given in the first 24 hours; methylprednisolone, 30 mg/kg, or dexamethasone, 3 mg/kg, may be given IV [16].

(5) Antibiotic therapy is administered immediately pending the results of the cultures. A common drug regimen includes penicillin, 20 million units/day IV; gentamicin, 5 mg/kg/day IV; and clindamycin, 25 mg/kg/day IV. If *Clostridium* is identified, chloramphenicol, 50–75 mg/kg/day IV, is substituted for clindamycin.

(6) Surgical therapy. Infected tissue must be removed as soon as the patient is stable. Dilation and curettage (D and C) may suffice for removal of tissue; but if there is extensive necrosis, a hysterectomy and adnexectomy may be required.

B. Complications of induced abortion. Suction curettage is legally performed to induce abortion in the first trimester. Cervical lacerations from forceful dilation can occur. The uterus is occasionally perforated, resulting in vaginal or concealed (intraperitoneal or retroperitoneal) hemorrhage or injury to the bowel. If the procedure is incomplete, a second procedure is needed to evacuate the uterus. The patient may not have had an IUP but instead an ectopic pregnancy; in such a situation, very little tissue will be obtained from the uterus, and the pregnancy test will remain positive. These complications demand gynecologic consultation.

C. General management measures of first-trimester abortion

1. Blood type and Rh determination. All patients seen in the emergency department for a first-trimester abortion should have a blood type and Rh determination. $Rh_o(D)$ immune globulin (RHIG) (RhoGAM) is given to all Rh-negative patients who are unsensitized following a spontaneous or induced abortion or termination of an ectopic pregnancy. The blood type and RHIG administration must be documented in the hospital record. The recommended dose of RHIG following spontaneous abortion, induced abortion, ectopic pregnancy, or amniocentesis is 50 mg IM; preterm or term deliveries require 300 mg IM; more than 300 mg IM is required for large transplacental hemorrhage or a mismatched blood transfusion.

2. Control of bleeding. In cases of spontaneous abortion, bleeding can be controlled with oxytocin (synthetic), 20–40 IU/liter at 10 ml/minute, and the patient may be discharged on methylergonovine maleate (Methergine), 0.2 mg PO tid for 3 days. To minimize the increased risk of endometritis after abortion, tetracycline, 250 mg PO qid for 5 days, is also administered.

3. **Suction curettage** to complete uterine evacuation is done in either the operating suite or the emergency department, depending on the hospital policy and individual physician preference. All tissue obtained by curettage or spontaneously passed by the patient should be sent for histologic evaluation. An immediate impression can be obtained by immersing the tissue in saline; it should float and have a frondlike appearance that is characteristic of placental tissue.

D. **Management measures for abortion beyond the first trimester.** Spontaneous abortion in the second trimester requires evaluation of fetal viability and gestational age. If the fetus is no longer viable, IV infusion of oxytocin (see **C.2**) facilitates uterine contractions and decreases blood loss. Care must be taken, when evacuating the uterus, not to allow fetal parts (e.g., fragments of skull or long bones) to lacerate the uterus; fetal tissue should be allowed to pass spontaneously with uterine contractions, rather than be forcibly removed (see sec. **VI**).

IV. **Ectopic pregnancy.** An extrauterine or ectopic pregnancy (EP) refers to implantation of the blastocyst in a site other than the endometrial cavity. Ninety-five percent of all EPs are in the fallopian tube. Other sites include a primary ovarian pregnancy and, rarely, an abdominal pregnancy. The most widely accepted mechanism for EP is failure of the ovum to pass through the fallopian tube in the properly timed sequence that allows for proper uterine implantation. A major risk factor includes partial tubal obstruction following previous tubal infection, intraabdominal or tubal surgery, or tubal ligation. Use of an IUD or a low-dose progesterone agent is also associated with EP [3]. A woman who has had one EP has a 12–15% chance of having another.

A. **Clinical features.** The diagnosis of EP may be difficult to establish before rupture occurs. Vaginal bleeding, present in about 95% of EPs, is usually less than that seen in first-trimester abortions and characteristically involves "irregular spotting." Lower abdominal pain is present in 95% of cases. On examination, more than 50% of patients have a tender, usually unilateral adnexal mass. Early signs of pregnancy (e.g., breast changes, nausea, fatigue) may or may not be present. With tubal rupture, the patient may present with syncope; severe, sharp lower abdominal and pelvic pain; and hypotension.

B. **Diagnosis**
1. A **positive pregnancy test** will help distinguish a tubal pregnancy from other adnexal pathologic conditions.
2. **Culdocentesis.** Aspiration of the pouch of Douglas (see Chap. 38) is very helpful if positive for nonclotting blood, which signifies a tubal rupture, tubal abortion, or rupture of a corpus luteum cyst or other viscus. Return of clotting blood may indicate a traumatic tap or very active concurrent bleeding. When no blood is found on aspiration, there is the possibility that a tubal pregnancy, as yet unruptured or unaborted, is present.
3. **Ultrasonography** may visualize an intrauterine gestational sac at or after 5 weeks of gestation. Documentation of a normal IUP generally rules out an EP, although there is a 1 in 30,000 chance of a dual intrauterine and ectopic pregnancy.
4. **Diagnostic laparoscopy** may be required to document a suspected EP.

C. **Differential diagnosis.** A ruptured corpus luteum cyst with intraperitoneal hemorrhage and associated with an early IUP is easily confused with an EP. Appendicitis and salpingitis, both inflammatory conditions, generally are characterized by fever, leukocytosis, and a negative pregnancy test. Rupture of an abdominal viscus or torsion of an ovary might produce the same or similar symptoms.

D. **Treatment** is surgical once the diagnosis is made. Conservative surgery (salpingostomy) versus salpingectomy is the correct management. Blood transfusion may be required. All Rh-negative patients should receive RHIG.

V. **Gestational trophoblastic disease.** The diagnosis of trophoblastic disease should be considered when a patient with a positive pregnancy test presents with vaginal bleeding and uterine enlargement abnormally large for the date of conception. Trophoblastic disease is also a diagnosis of exclusion when there is irregular and persistent bleeding following any pregnancy.

A. **Molar pregnancy.** Hydatidiform mole (molar pregnancy) is a complication of 1 in 5000 pregnancies; there is neoplastic proliferation of the trophoblast, edema of the villous stroma, and usually absence of a fetus.
1. **Clinical features.** Uterine bleeding is usually the first sign of this complication. On examination, the uterus is larger than expected; ovarian enlargement may also be noted due to the presence of theca lutein cysts. Fetal heart tones and

fetal movement are usually absent. Nausea and vomiting may be severe, and signs of preeclampsia (i.e., hypertension and proteinuria) and hyperthyroidism may occur. Grapelike vesicles may pass spontaneously.

2. **Diagnosis.** Ultrasonography and documentation of markedly elevated HCG levels are useful in establishing the diagnosis.

3. The **differential diagnosis** includes a spontaneous abortion, an error in dating, and a uterus enlarged by myomas, hydramnios, or multiple fetuses.

4. **Management.** Patients must be admitted for management. Treatment includes stabilization of any concurrent preeclampsia and thyroid dysfunction and termination of the molar pregnancy by curettage. Long-term follow-up is mandatory for surveillance for the development of choriocarcinoma.

B. **Choriocarcinoma** can develop following a molar pregnancy, abortion, ectopic pregnancy, or normal pregnancy.

1. **Clinical features.** The most common sign is irregular bleeding and subinvolution of the uterus; the bleeding may be continuous or intermittent, with sudden and sometimes massive hemorrhage. Pelvic structures invaded by a choriocarcinoma may be fixed and tender, suggesting PID.

2. **Diagnosis.** Persistent or rising titers of HCG in the absence of pregnancy are indicative of a trophoblastic neoplasm.

3. **Management.** All cases of unusual bleeding following a pregnancy or abortion should be investigated by a physical examination, curettage, and quantitative measurement of chorionic gonadotropin. Suspected cases must be referred to a gynecologic oncologist for workup and, if documented, long-term management and chemotherapy.

VI. **Preterm labor**

A. Known **predisposing conditions** of preterm labor include spontaneous rupture of membranes, local infection, cervical incompetency, uterine anomalies, an overdistended uterus, anomalies of the fetus, faulty presentation, a retained IUD, fetal death, and serious maternal disease (e.g., pyelonephritis, peritonitis). In the majority of cases, however, the cause of preterm labor is unknown [14].

B. **Diagnosis of preterm labor.** It may be difficult to differentiate true preterm labor from false labor. Uterine contractions that occur prematurely at least every 10 minutes and last for 30 seconds or more identify preterm labor [14]. Dilatation of the cervix is diagnostic of labor.

C. **Treatment.** Before attempting to arrest preterm labor, the physician must determine if the fetus is better off in the uterus or delivered. This decision is best made by an obstetrician who is most familiar with (1) survival statistics for gestational age and (2) the benefits and risks to the mother and fetus of an early delivery compared with attempts to arrest preterm labor.

1. Accepted methods of **treatment of preterm labor** include bed rest and administration of a progestational agent, magnesium sulfate, beta-adrenergic agonist, narcotic, and/or sedative.

2. Documented urinary tract infection should be treated with an appropriate antibiotic.

3. Continuous electronic **fetal monitoring** must be utilized.

4. **Treatment of the apparently incompetent cervix** is surgical. A reinforcing suture (cerclage procedure) is placed in the cervix after the first trimester. Bleeding and uterine contractions are contraindications to surgery.

D. **Disposition.** Hospitalization is mandatory. If the hospital is not equipped to handle preterm infants in the nursery, maternal transfer to a medical center with a high-risk nursery is required.

VII. **Placenta previa** is the condition in which the placenta implants in the lower uterine segment, encroaching on or covering the internal cervical os. Frequency at term is 1 in 167 to 1 in 260 pregnancies.

A. **Predisposing conditions** include increased parity, increased maternal age, multiple births, a previous cesarean section, previous D and Cs, prior abortions, and a previous placenta previa.

B. **Signs and symptoms.** The most characteristic event is painless hemorrhage in the latter half of pregnancy. The initial bleeding, however, is rarely profuse enough to be fatal [14].

C. The **diagnosis** of placenta previa as a cause of uterine bleeding in the latter half of pregnancy can be established by ultrasonography.

D. The **differential diagnosis** includes placental abruption and bloody show in active labor.

E. **Management.** These patients should be evaluated by an obstetrician. Examination of the cervix is never performed unless the woman is in the operating suite and prepared for immediate cesarean section. Management of placenta previa depends on the stage of maturity of the fetus, whether labor is in progress, and the degree of hemorrhage. Fetal monitoring and replacement of blood loss is appropriate.

VIII. **Placental abruption** is separation of the placenta from its site of implantation in the uterus prior to delivery of the fetus. Various degrees of placental abruption can occur, ranging from an area of a few millimeters in diameter to the entire placental surface. The incidence ranges from 1 in 78 to 1 in 206 deliveries. The incidence of severe abruption resulting in fetal death is 1 in 500 deliveries.

A. **Predisposing factors** include trauma, shortness of the umbilical cord, sudden decompression of the uterus, pregnancy-induced or chronic hypertension, and a previous history of placental abruption.

B. **Clinical features.** The hemorrhage may be concealed behind the adherent membranes, or vaginal bleeding may be present. Patients in the latter half of pregnancy usually complain of severe uterine tenderness and rigidity.

C. **Evaluation.** Ultrasonography is often helpful in verifying the diagnosis and determining the gestational age of the fetus. Since placental abruption is the most common cause of a consumptive coagulopathy in pregnancy, clotting parameters (i.e., prothrombin time [PT], partial thromboplastin time [PTT], platelet count, DIC screen) must be obtained.

D. The **differential diagnosis** includes placenta previa.

E. **Management.** These patients need to be typed and cross-matched and transferred immediately to the care of an obstetrician.

1. **Blood transfusion.** The hemorrhage from the abruption may require massive blood replacement.

2. The **gestational age** of the fetus must be determined to assess extrauterine viability.

3. **Delivery.** If the fetus is alive, rapid delivery of the fetus by cesarean section is mandated, preferably when the mother is stabilized. If the fetus is dead, vaginal delivery is preferred unless the hemorrhage is so brisk that it cannot be managed by vigorous blood replacement or there are other obstetric complications that contraindicate vaginal delivery.

IX. **Postpartum hemorrhage**

A. **Immediate causes**

1. **Uterine atony.** Predisposing causes of uterine atony include an overdistended uterus, prolonged or precipitous labor, high parity, and use of general anesthesia. Immediate treatment is infusion of oxytocin (20 IU/liter at 10 ml/minute until the uterus is firm), fundal massage, and volume replacement. The obstetric service should be notified immediately.

2. **Abnormally adherent placenta.** If the placenta does not spontaneously separate from its implantation site, it should not be removed in the emergency department. The placental villi may be abnormally invading the uterine wall (placenta accreta), and improper attempts to manually remove such a placenta may lead to uterine inversion or massive bleeding. Thus, the patient should be transferred to the labor and delivery area where manual removal of the placenta can be accomplished under controlled conditions.

3. **Lacerations of the birth canal.** If the uterus is well contracted, injuries to the birth canal (i.e., cervix, lower uterine segment, and vagina) may be a source of persistent postpartum bleeding. Vaginal and vulvar hematomas may cause increasing pain and require surgical intervention. Birth canal injuries are best repaired in the operating suite where good lighting, assistance, and anesthesia backup are available.

4. **Coagulation defects.** Preexisting defects in coagulation (e.g., von Willebrand's disease, idiopathic thrombocytopenic purpura) and acquired defects (e.g., secondary to preeclampsia, sepsis, fetal death syndrome, placenta accreta, uterine rupture, massive blood volume replacement, placental abruption, amniotic fluid embolism) will intensify all of the previously mentioned causes of immediate postpartum hemorrhage. Documentation of coagulation status is an appropriate initial step in the management of massive or unexplained postpartum hemorrhage.

B. **Delayed causes of postpartum hemorrhage**

1. **Return of menses.** The first menstrual period after childbirth is often abnormal. It may be profuse, with clots, and stop and restart.

a. For **nonnursing mothers,** the earliest menstruation is usually at 4 weeks postpartum, and 90% of women are menstruating by 3 months postpartum.

b. **Nursing mothers** may describe a persistent light vaginal spotting, which is not menstrual flow but rather bleeding from an undifferentiated or hypoproliferative endometrium, for 1 or 2 months following delivery. Reassurance is indicated. The majority of women who nurse report return of their menses at 5–6 months postpartum; however, menstruation may be absent as long as lactation continues.

2. **Subinvolution of the uterus** is an arrest of the process by which the postpartum uterus is restored to its normal proportions. The causes of subinvolution are retention of placental fragments and infection. As retained placental tissue necroses, hemorrhage occurs as the tissue detaches from the endometrium.

a. **Clinical features.** Lochia may be prolonged, and profuse hemorrhage can occur. On examination, the uterus will be enlarged and softer than normally expected.

b. **Evaluation.** The index of suspicion for the diagnosis of retained placental tissue is raised when there is a history of manual removal of the placenta. If the patient is febrile, cultures of blood and endometrium are indicated. In all cases of delayed postpartum hemorrhage, documentation of a negative HCG excludes gestational trophoblastic disease.

c. **Treatment.** Oxytocin infusion, curettage, and antibiotic administration are appropriate in the management of this condition.

X. **Uterine inversion.** Although uterine inversion can occur spontaneously, complete inversion of the uterus is most often caused by strong traction on the umbilical cord prior to placental separation. Profuse hemorrhage makes inversion a serious and rapidly fatal complication.

A. The **diagnosis** should be suspected by the presence of a vaginal or perineal mass, severe abdominal pain, hypotension, and tachycardia.

B. **Treatment** of uterine inversion consists of immediate reduction of the malpositioned uterus while restoring lost blood volume. Continued firm pressure against the uterus from inside the uterus is necessary for reduction. If the uterus has begun to contract, reduction without adequate anesthesia is difficult. If the uterus cannot be reinverted by vaginal manipulation, immediate laparotomy is indicated.

XI. **Uterine rupture** can occur spontaneously but usually occurs in the setting of oxytocin overstimulation or prolonged labor with a large fetus, or in patients who have had a previous cesarean section or operative scarring. The patient complains of severe abdominal pain. Vaginal bleeding may or may not be present. Intraabdominal hemorrhage and fetal distress may occur and demand prompt diagnosis and immediate abdominal exploration. If fetal demise is documented by the absence of fetal heart tones or by the lack of fetal cardiac motion on ultrasonography, exploratory laparotomy is still required to repair the uterine defect and control hemorrhage.

XII. **Preeclampsia and eclampsia** (see Chap. 6)

A. **Definitions**

1. **Preeclampsia** is the development of hypertension with proteinuria and edema (or both) due to pregnancy or the influence of a recent pregnancy. It commonly occurs after the twentieth week of gestation but may develop before this time in the presence of trophoblastic disease. Preeclampsia is predominantly a disorder of primigravidas but can occur in multiparous patients.

2. **Eclampsia** is the occurrence of one or more convulsions, not attributable to other cerebral conditions, such as epilepsy or cerebral hemorrhage, in a patient with preeclampsia [14].

B. **Clinical features.** Although the causes of preeclampsia are still unknown, the clinical course is well described. The most dependable warning sign of preeclampsia is elevation of the diastolic blood pressure. Other signs include weight gain, edema, proteinuria, headache, visual disturbances, and epigastric pain. An ominous sign includes elevation of the systolic blood pressure (SBP) by 30 mm Hg or of the diastolic blood pressure (DBP) by 15 mm Hg; the degree of elevation is more significant than any absolute value. Other criteria for the diagnosis of severe preeclampsia include an SBP greater than 160 mm Hg or a DBP greater than 110 mm Hg on two readings 6 hours apart, proteinuria of 5 gm or more/24 hours, oliguria with a urinary output of less than 40 ml/hour, cerebral or visual disturbances, pulmonary edema or cyanosis, and the **HELLP syndrome** (i.e., **h**emolysis, **e**levated **l**iver function tests, and a **l**ow **p**latelet count) [19].

C. **Differential diagnosis of eclampsia.** To establish the diagnosis of eclampsia, all other causes of seizures must be ruled out, including epilepsy, subarachnoid hemorrhage, meningitis, toxicity of local anesthetics, electrolyte disturbances, cerebral brain thrombosis, thrombotic thrombocytopenic purpura, amniotic fluid embolism, pheochromocytoma, hypoglycemia, hyperventilation, and hypoxia.

D. Management

1. **Preeclampsia.** Management of preeclampsia depends on the severity of the disease, the gestational age of the fetus, and the condition of the cervix (can labor be induced?). A patient with severe preeclampsia should be admitted to the obstetric service for evaluation and therapy. The currently accepted therapy of severe preeclampsia and the prevention of eclampsia is magnesium sulfate. The commonly used dosage of magnesium sulfate is a loading dose of 4 gm IV or 10 gm IM, followed by a maintenance dose of 1–3 gm/hour IV or 5 gm IM q4h. To prevent magnesium toxicity, the patellar reflexes, urinary output, and respirations are monitored along with maternal blood pressure and fetal heart rate. Serum magnesium levels should also be followed; therapeutic levels are 4–7 mEq/dl.

2. **Eclampsia**

   a. **Seizures.** It is generally accepted in obstetric circles that eclamptic seizures are treated with magnesium sulfate as in **1**, rather than with diazepam, phenobarbital, or phenytoin. These agents, while excellent anticonvulsants, are known to cause respiratory depression and hypotonia in the neonate and generally should be avoided if delivery is imminent.

   b. **Hypertension.** When hypertension is severe and the DBP reaches 110 mm Hg, hydralazine can be administered IV in 5- to 10-mg doses at 15- to 20-minute intervals until the DBP approaches 90 mm Hg. Placental perfusion will be compromised, however, if the DBP declines below 90 mm Hg.

XIII. Emergency delivery. Despite original plans for a hospital delivery, the first stage of labor may progress so rapidly that a woman may present in the emergency department about to deliver. If it is clear that there is time to transfer the patient to the labor and delivery area, it should be done efficiently with a suitably skilled person (i.e., one who can deliver the baby, if necessary) accompanying the patient. However, if the woman is straining, as if to have a bowel movement, or if the fetal head is visibly bulging at the vaginal opening, delivery is imminent.

A. Procedure. The woman should be reassured and instructed to lie supine. If possible, pillows or a roll of blankets can be placed under the buttocks to facilitate delivery of the baby's head and shoulders. The birth attendant must continue to reassure the woman and place a hand over the advancing fetal head to prevent the head from popping through the vagina. To prevent the mother from bearing down too hard, she should be asked to take deep breaths through her mouth. If necessary, an episiotomy can be performed, preferably with the use of local anesthesia. Once the head is delivered (see Fig. 33-1), mucus should be removed from the mouth and nose with a bulb syringe, if available. At this point, the physician should check for the presence of the umbilical cord around the neck and gently lift the cord over the head, if present. Delivery of the shoulders is facilitated by gentle downward traction on the baby's head (see Fig. 33-2). Once the baby is delivered, he or she should be kept at the same level as the uterus until the cord is clamped; the baby is placed on dry blankets or towels on the bed (or floor) between the mother's legs. The baby should be dried (as heat loss by evaporation cannot be well compensated for by the baby) and wrapped in a clean dry towel or blanket. The umbilical cord is then doubly clamped or tied and severed between the two clamps or ties. The birth time should be recorded, and the infant can be given Apgar scores at 1 and 5 minutes of life.

B. Complications of vaginal delivery

1. **Nuchal cord.** The umbilical cord may be so tightly wound around the baby's neck that it will have to be clamped and divided to allow for the delivery.

2. **Shoulder dystocia.** The incidence of shoulder dystocia is 0.15%–0.60% of all deliveries. Risk factors include maternal obesity, maternal diabetes, and large babies (i.e., with weights exceeding 4000 gm). After the head is delivered, the shoulders may become lodged behind the pubic symphysis. Quick action on the part of the birth attendant can prevent significant damage to the baby. The attendant should (1) call for help, (2) cut a generous episiotomy, and (3) rotate the posterior shoulder by applying pressure with the index and middle fingers over the anterior aspect of the baby's lower shoulder. Usually this shoulder can then be delivered after a 90- or 180-degree rotation. If this procedure fails, an attempt can be made to deliver the posterior shoulder and arm. The use of

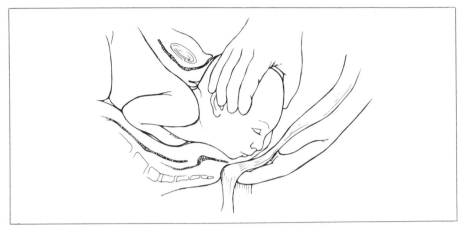

Fig. 33-1. Delivery of the fetal head by the modified Ritgen maneuver. Moderate upward pressure is applied to the fetal chin by the posterior hand while the suboccipital area of the fetal head is held against the symphysis pubis. (From J. A. Pritchard, P. C. MacDonald, and N. F. Gant, *Williams Obstetrics* (17th ed.). Norwalk, Conn.: Appleton-Century-Crofts, 1985. With permission.)

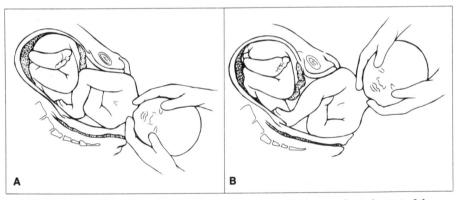

Fig. 33-2. Delivery of the shoulders. Gentle downward traction brings about descent of the anterior shoulder (A), followed by gentle upward traction to deliver the posterior shoulder (B). (From J. A. Pritchard, P. C. MacDonald, and N. F. Gant, *Williams Obstetrics* (17th ed.). Norwalk, Conn.: Appleton-Century-Crofts, 1985. With permission.)

fundal and suprapubic pressure by an assistant is controversial but may be helpful.

3. **Breech presentation.** The incidence of all breech presentations is 3–4%. Under ideal circumstances, this delivery should not be allowed to become an emergency.

   a. **Management.** Every attempt should be made to rapidly transport the mother to the labor and delivery area for proper assessment and delivery. For a favorable outcome with any breech delivery, the birth canal must be sufficiently large to allow passage of the fetus without trauma, and the cervix must be completely effaced and dilated. If these conditions are lacking, a cesarean section is always the more appropriate method of delivery. If it is a medical emergency and necessary for the emergency physician to perform the delivery without the assistance of an obstetrician, the patient should be positioned in stirrups, and a generous episiotomy should be performed. Delivery is easier and perinatal morbidity and mortality are reduced if the fetus is allowed to deliver spontaneously. No attempt should be

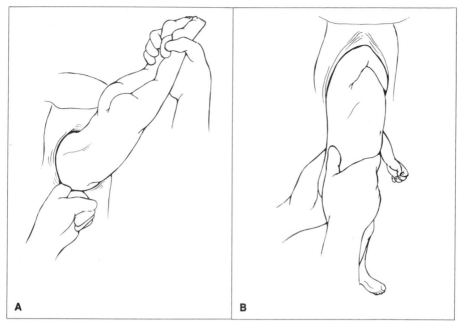

Fig. 33-3. Breech presentation. A. Delivery of the posterior shoulder by upward traction on the fetus, followed by digital freeing of the arm. B. Delivery of the anterior shoulder by downward traction. (From J. A. Pritchard, P. C. MacDonald, and N. F. Gant, *Williams Obstetrics* (17th ed.). Norwalk, Conn.: Appleton-Century-Crofts, 1985. With permission.)

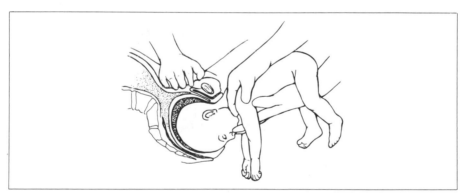

Fig. 33-4. Breech presentation. Delivery of the aftercoming head by the Mauriceau maneuver. During delivery of the fetal head, flexion of the head is maintained by suprapubic pressure provided by an assistant and simultaneously by pressure on the maxilla by the operator as traction is applied. (From J. A. Pritchard, P. C. MacDonald, and N. F. Gant, *Williams Obstetrics* (17th ed.). Norwalk, Conn.: Appleton-Century-Crofts, 1985. With permission.)

made to deliver the shoulders or arms until an axilla becomes visible. Either shoulder may then be delivered first, and the body of the fetus is rotated to deliver the other shoulder and arm (see Fig. 33-3). Once the shoulders are delivered, the Mauriceau maneuver is used to assist in the delivery of the head (Fig. 33-4). While the fetal body rests on the operator's hand and forearm, the index and middle finger rest on the fetal maxilla. With two fingers of the other hand hooked over the fetal neck and grasping the shoulders, downward traction is applied until the suboccipital region appears under the symphysis. The body of the fetus is then elevated toward the mother's abdomen, and the rest of the head is delivered with gentle traction exerted by the fingers over the shoulders. An assistant may apply gentle suprapubic pressure to help deliver the head [14].

   b. **Complications.** Occasionally, especially with small preterm fetuses, an incompletely dilated cervix may result in entrapment of the aftercoming head. When entrapment occurs, an attempt should be made to slip the cervix over the occiput. If this maneuver is not readily successful, incisions can be made in the cervix corresponding to the hours of 2, 6, and 10 on the face of a clock. This is one of the few indications for this procedure in modern obstetrics [14].

4. **Cord prolapse**
   a. **Clinical features.** The incidence of cord prolapse is about 1 in 300 deliveries and is associated with any cause of poor application of the presenting part onto the cervix, such as prematurity, twins, polyhydramnios, a transverse lie, or breech or shoulder presentation. Fetal hypoxia results from compression of the umbilical cord between the presenting part and the pelvic tissue.
   b. **Management.** As soon as a patient is seen with the umbilical cord in the vagina, the physician should summon help. An immediate vaginal examination is performed to check for the presence of cord pulsations, which indicate that the baby is alive. The cervix is then checked for the degree of dilation. If there are no cord pulsations, the physician checks for fetal heart tones and assesses cardiac activity with ultrasonography, if immediately available. If the baby is alive, the best chance for survival depends on the fastest route of delivery (vaginal or cesarean). In order to elevate the presenting part and thereby remove pressure from the cord, the mother should be placed in the knee-chest or steep Trendelenburg position. Vaginal delivery, however, should not be attempted through an incompletely dilated cervix; in this situation, cesarean section is usually the fastest route. Oxygen should be administered to the mother. If no underlying complications are present and the baby is dead, intervention is not required and the baby is allowed to be delivered spontaneously.

XIV. **Medical and surgical problems in pregnancy**
   A. **Exacerbation of asthma** (see Chap. 7)
      1. **Assessment.** Initial steps require documentation of the respiratory rate, blood pressure, heart rate, pulsus paradoxus, and chest examination. An arterial blood gas and pulmonary function tests are important in assessing the severity of the attack. A chest x-ray (with the uterus shielded) is recommended only in patients with clinical signs of pneumonia or pneumothorax; at term, the chest x-ray of a normal pregnant patient usually demonstrates an elevated diaphragm, increased anteroposterior diameter, and increased lung markings [1].
      2. **Treatment**
         a. **Oxygen** should be administered to keep the maternal arterial oxygen tension greater than 70 mm Hg [1]. Patients with an elevated $PaCO_2$ and decreasing PaO_2 may require endotracheal intubation and assisted ventilation.
         b. **Aerosol bronchodilator** therapy (e.g., with metaproterenol) is administered on a periodic basis as needed.
         c. **Hydration** with 0.5 normal saline at 100–125 ml/hour is instituted. IV fluid rates must be carefully monitored, however, to avoid fluid overload.
         d. **Aminophylline** therapy is initiated with an appropriate loading dose (see Chap. 7), given IV over 20 minutes, and followed by a maintenance dose of 0.2–0.5 mg/kg/hour. Theophylline can also be given PO as appropriate.
         e. **Corticosteroid** therapy may be administered with methylprednisolone, 0.5 mg/kg IV q6h, if needed (especially in cases of prior steroid dependence).
         f. **Beta stimulants.** Terbutaline or epinephrine can be given subcutaneously, if needed. Terbutaline or metaproterenol can be administered orally to treat asthma in pregnancy if the potential benefit to be derived justifies the potential risk to the fetus.
   B. **Thrombophlebitis** (see Chap. 20)
      1. **Evaluation.** Tenderness and pain in the leg are nonspecific signs common in normal pregnancies. The physician should take a meticulous history and weigh all available evidence before requesting radiologic assessment of possible thrombophlebitis.
      2. Precise **diagnosis** requires phlebography (venography) with shielding of the

uterus. Noninvasive methods such as Doppler ultrasonography or impedance plethysmography are alternative diagnostic studies.

3. Treatment

a. Symptomatic treatment with moist heat, elevation of the extremity, and bed rest is appropriate.

b. Heparin is the anticoagulant of choice in pregnancy. Coumadin, aspirin, and most anti-inflammatory agents are contraindicated in pregnant and lactating women.

C. Pulmonary embolism (see Chap. 7)

1. Diagnosis. If warranted by the history, physical examination, and arterial blood gas, a suspected pulmonary embolism may be diagnosed by ventilation-perfusion lung scanning; appropriate uterine shielding is mandatory. If the scan cannot be reliably interpreted or is indeterminant, pulmonary angiography is required, if clinically warranted.

2. Treatment

a. Appropriately diagnosed pulmonary embolism in pregnancy is treated by systemic anticoagulation with IV **heparin** and bed rest for the first 5–7 days. The patient must then be maintained on heparin (usually minidose) for the duration of her pregnancy.

b. If heparin anticoagulation is contraindicated or fails to control recurrence of pulmonary embolism, surgical interruption of the vena cava should be considered.

D. Diabetes mellitus (see Chap. 9)

1. Diagnosis

a. The normal fasting plasma glucose in a pregnant patient is less than 100 mg/dl. Diabetes is likely in a pregnant woman if the fasting plasma glucose exceeds 100 mg/dl or if a 2-hour postprandial glucose is more than 150 mg/dl.

b. Glycosuria frequently occurs in healthy women during pregnancy because of increased glomerular filtration and less effective renal tubular resorption than in the nonpregnant state. Thus, in pregnancy the diagnosis of diabetes cannot be made by glycosuria. Serum glucose levels must be obtained to evaluate glycosuria.

2. Clinical significance

a. All pregnant diabetic patients should be enrolled in prenatal care and must be followed closely.

b. Preeclampsia and urinary tract infection (especially pyelonephritis) are bad prognostic signs in pregnant diabetic patients and require obstetric consultation and probable admission. Any infection in diabetic patients should be appropriately cultured and then aggressively treated.

c. Diabetic ketoacidosis (DKA) is associated with great risk to the mother and fetus. Fetal death associated with maternal DKA ranges from 50–90%. The diagnosis is established if the urine is strongly positive for glucose and ketones, if the arterial pH is below 7.30 with the $PaCO_2$ not above 35 mm Hg, and if undiluted serum is strongly positive for ketones. Once the diagnosis of DKA is established, the patient must be admitted to the obstetric service for management.

E. Trauma (see Chap. 17). Pregnant women may sustain blunt or penetrating traumatic injuries that can jeopardize their well-being and that of their fetus.

1. Evaluation

a. The presence or absence of fetal heart tones, fetal movement, contractions, and vaginal bleeding should be assessed and documented in the emergency department record. Vaginal bleeding may be a sign of placental abruption.

b. If any **x-ray studies** are indicated by the history and physical examination, uterine shielding is recommended.

2. Management. When a pregnant woman presents to the emergency department having sustained a traumatic injury, it is essential to remember that the life of the fetus depends on the maintenance of hemodynamic stability of the mother and her survival. Advanced trauma life support guidelines should be followed.

a. Stabilization. In order to maximize the chance for fetal survival, it is essential to establish and maintain acceptable hemodynamic parameters in the mother through control of hemorrhage and administration of crystalloid and blood as needed. Maintenance of adequate oxygenation is also vital.

    b. Surgical procedures. Minor lacerations can be repaired under local anesthesia. Any procedure that requires general anesthesia, however, requires consultation from the obstetric service.

F. Abdominal pain (see Chap. 19). Common symptoms of early pregnancy (e.g., anorexia, nausea, vomiting, vague abdominal pain) may also be early signs of an acute surgical emergency. Surgery that is delayed until unequivocal signs of an acute abdominal emergency have developed poses a greater hazard to the mother and fetus than does early operative intervention.

    1. Pathogenesis. The pregnant uterus grossly interferes with the normal defense mechanisms of the abdomen. Since the omentum is displaced cephalad and is no longer free to wall off inflammation, progression from localized disease to frank peritonitis may be extremely rapid.

    2. Causes of abdominal pain that may require surgical intervention during pregnancy include appendicitis; torsion, hemorrhage, or rupture of an ovarian tumor; EP; intestinal obstruction; renal stones; and cholecystitis.

    3. Complications. Shock and frank peritonitis increase the chance of premature labor and perinatal and maternal mortality.

    4. Evaluation involves a careful history and physical examination (including a pelvic examination) and appropriate use of laboratory studies. Radiographic studies deemed necessary to properly evaluate the patient should be obtained, with shielding of the abdomen to the extent possible. Since the pregnant uterus displaces intraabdominal structures from their normal location and since pregnancy may be associated with a leukocytosis, a careful evaluation and a high index of suspicion are required to correctly diagnose the cause of abdominal pain in pregnancy.

    5. Management is directed at the etiology of the abdominal pain. Potentially serious disorders require obstetric consultation as well as surgical consultation.

XV. Fetal death

A. Diagnosis

    1. In early pregnancy, the diagnosis of fetal death is suspected when the uterus fails to grow on repeated examinations.

    2. A positive pregnancy test that becomes negative is suggestive of fetal death. On the other hand, since the placenta may produce HCG for several weeks after the death of a fetus, a positive pregnancy test is not diagnostic of a viable pregnancy.

    3. In the latter half of pregnancy, absence of fetal movements alerts the mother to the possibility of fetal death in utero.

    4. Absence of fetal heart tones on auscultation by stethoscope or Doppler stethoscope suggests fetal death.

    5. Ultrasound examination failing to demonstrate fetal heart motion is definitive evidence of fetal death.

    6. Radiologic signs of fetal death include overlap of the skull bones, exaggeration of the curvature of the fetal spine, and demonstration of gas in the fetus.

B. Management

    1. These patients should be referred to the obstetric service for counseling and management of pregnancy termination.

    2. Since coagulation disorders thought to be mediated by thromboplastin from the dead products of conception are sometimes seen, coagulation studies should be obtained on all of these patients as part of their initial evaluation.

    3. Induction of labor with oxytocin is most successful near term. Prostaglandin E_2 (PGE_2) vaginal suppositories are useful in inducing labor after the first trimester. Suction curettage is used to evacuate the uterus in the first trimester.

XVI. Postmortem cesarean sections are rare; there are less than 200 case reports in the English literature. In the tragic situation where emergency department personnel are confronted with a fatally injured pregnant patient, an immediate decision must be made regarding cesarean section. The survival of the infant depends on the duration and nature of the mother's fatal injuries, how soon the fetus is extracted, the maturity of the infant, the performance of postmortem cardiopulmonary resuscitative measures on the mother, and the availability of neonatal intensive care.

A. Indications. The decision to perform a postmortem cesarean section should be made by the senior obstetrician or physician in attendance based on (1) the family's wishes, (2) the gestational age of the fetus, and (3) the maternal status. If maternal viability cannot be maintained, the survival of a fetus 26–28 weeks or older is likely great enough to justify postmortem cesarean section. The duration of gestation, however, may not be available if the patient is moribund. Estimation of fetal age by palpation of the abdomen requires considerable experience. However, after the twentieth week of gestation, the uterine fundal height in centimeters corresponds roughly to the gestational age in weeks for singleton pregnancies. Thus, a 28-cm fundus corresponds approximately to a 28-week gestation. Similarly, at 28 weeks the fundus is midway between the umbilicus and the costal margin. These simple measurements may provide guidelines in the emergency situation.

B. Procedure. While a senior obstetrician is being immediately summoned, the emergency department staff should continue all possible resuscitative measures for the pregnant woman, including cardiopulmonary resuscitation, if indicated. To avoid the supine hypotensive syndrome, a wedge or roll of sheets may be placed under the right hip to displace the gravid uterus from the inferior vena cava and improve venous return, cardiac output, and placental perfusion. The presence of fetal heart tones should be documented; a portable fetal monitoring unit or bedside ultrasound unit can provide continuous evaluation of the fetal status. If the fetus is alive, an attempt should be made to document the gestational age of the fetus by contacting any family members for such information or by ultrasound evaluation. If the decision by the senior obstetrician in attendance is to proceed with cesarean delivery, it is of the utmost importance that full resuscitative measures, including cardiopulmonary resuscitation, be continued for the mother during the delivery. In addition, minimizing the elapsed time is crucial. The abdomen need not be prepped. A vertical midline incision from the epigastrium to the symphysis pubis is carried through all layers of the abdominal wall to the peritoneal cavity. A vertical incision is then made into the anterior wall of the uterus from the fundus to the bladder reflection. This long incision allows rapid removal of the fetus with minimal trauma. After delivery, the umbilical cord should be doubly clamped and divided. The pediatric staff should be in attendance to resuscitate the infant.

Victim of Alleged Rape

I. Definition. Rape is unlawful sexual intercourse through force or deception and without consent. This definition includes any orifice: oral, anal, or vaginal. Whether rape has occurred is a **legal matter** for court decision and not a medical diagnosis. Medical evidence, however, may be necessary to verify penetration, ejaculation, and any injuries sustained.

II. Patient rights. When a woman who is allegedly the victim of rape is seen in an emergency department, she has special medical, psychologic, and legal needs. The patient has a right to request or refuse medical treatment and examination for collection of legal evidence. The patient should give written, witnessed informed consent for physical examination, collection of laboratory specimens, photographs, release of information to the proper authorities, and medical treatment.

III. Evaluation

A. History. Questioning and examination of the patient should always be done in the presence of a witness. The patient's history should be kept to a minimum to avoid conflicts in later detailed testimony. The time, place, and degree of penetration should be noted. The patient should be asked if she has bathed, douched, changed clothing, or taken any medication since the alleged assault. The date of her last menstrual period and details of contraceptive usage aid in evaluation of pregnancy risk.

B. Physical examination

1. **General examination.** The patient's general appearance, emotional state, and behavior and appearance of clothing are noted. The skin is inspected for signs of trauma, i.e., abrasions, contusions, lacerations, and scratches. If dried seminal stains are found on the skin, they should be removed with saline-moistened swabs, which are then preserved in envelopes or stoppered test tubes. The oral cavity is examined; if fellatio occurred, a gonorrhea culture is taken from the pharynx. Polaroid photographs are taken to document any injuries.

2. **Pelvic examination.** The external genitalia are inspected for evidence of trauma. The pubic hair is combed for foreign material; hairs containing seminal stains are trimmed out and preserved as evidence. The examiner may be directed to seminal fluid stains by use of a Wood's light examination, since the seminal fluid stains will fluoresce. The condition of the introitus is described. In prepubertal children, the normal vaginal introitus measures 2–10 mm; penetration is suggested by trauma or a markedly dilated introitus. Adult women

may have no lacerations present; however, a nonlubricated, water-moistened speculum is placed in the vagina and any injuries are noted. The following specimens are obtained: (1) secretions in the vaginal fornix for evidence of semen, (2) a cervical culture for gonorrhea, (3) a cytologic smear of the cervix for sperm, and (4) saline vaginal washings (with 4 ml of normal saline) for evidence of semen. A bimanual examination is done to check for preexisting pregnancy, infection, and trauma. If the patient has reported anal penetration, an anal culture for gonorrhea is taken.

   C. Laboratory documentation. Laboratory tests include (1) cervical, rectal, and oral cultures for gonorrhea as indicated, (2) vaginal washings for semen, (3) analysis of pubic hairs, (4) a pregnancy test, and (5) a serologic test for syphilis. All specimens obtained by the physician in the presence of an attendant, who acts as a witness, must be identified and dated and personally placed in the hands of a pathologist, laboratory technician, or police officer to maintain the chain of evidence. The hospital record should show the names of the witness and the person to whom the laboratory specimens, clothing, and photographs were delivered.

IV. Diagnosis. The physician should not express any conclusions or opinions in the medical record; only phrases such as "suspected rape" or "alleged assault" should be used. However, any specific diagnosis of traumatic injury or preexisting pregnancy and treatment given must be recorded. A statement as to whether the examination is consistent with the victim's story is useful.

V. Management

   A. Psychologic support from a nonthreatening medical staff is important. Details of the examination and procedures should be explained clearly. Medication for anxiety may be indicated.

   B. Lacerations and physical injuries should be appropriately treated. Some child victims will require examination under general anesthesia to fully assess and repair injuries.

   C. Since the assailant may have gonorrhea or a chlamydial infection, the patient should be offered **prophylactic antibiotic therapy,** i.e., (1) amoxicillin, 3.0 gm PO, plus probenecid, 1 gm PO; (2) ceftriaxone, 250 mg IM; or (3) procaine penicillin G, 4.8 million units IM, plus probenecid, 1 gm PO; each followed by a 7-day course of tetracycline, 500 mg PO qid, or doxycycline, 100 mg PO bid. Although any of these regimens likely will abort incubating syphilis, a follow-up serology test for syphilis is recommended at 4 weeks. If positive, benzathine penicillin G, 2.4 million units IM, is given.

   D. If the patient is not pregnant and not using contraceptive methods, the possibility of pregnancy resulting from the sexual assault, as well as the benefits and risks of antipregnancy measures, should be discussed with the patient. Adequate postcoital contraception may be achieved by administration of estrogen in large doses (e.g., diethylstilbestrol, 25 mg PO bid for 5 days, starting within 72 hours of exposure or preferably within 24 hours; conjugated estrogen, 30 mg PO daily for 5 days; ethinyl estradiol, 5 mg PO daily for 5 days; or norgestrel and ethinyl estradiol [Ovral], 2 tablets q12h for 2 doses [17]) along with an antiemetic for control of gastrointestinal symptoms.

Bibliography

1. Berkowitz, R. (ed.). *Critical Care of the Obstetric Patient.* New York: Churchill Livingstone, 1983.
2. Curtis, A. A cause of adhesions in the right upper quadrant. *J.A.M.A.* 94:1221, 1930.
3. Eschenbach, D. A., and Daling, J. R. Ectopic pregnancy. *J.A.M.A.* 249:1759, 1983.
4. Fitz-Hugh, T. Acute gonococcic peritonitis in the right upper quadrant in women. *J.A.M.A.* 102:2094, 1934.
5. Huffman, J., Dewhurst, C. J., and Capraro, V. *The Gynecology of Childhood and Adolescence* (2nd ed.). Philadelphia: Saunders, 1981.
6. Jacobson, L., and Weström, L. Objectivized diagnosis of acute pelvic inflammatory disease. *Am. J. Obstet. Gynecol.* 105:1088, 1969.
7. Jouppila, P., Huhtamiemi, I., and Tapanginem, J. Early pregnancy failure: Study by ultrasound and hormonal methods. *Obstet. Gynecol.* 55:42, 1980.
8. Kaufman, D., et al. The effect of different types of intrauterine devices on the risk of pelvic inflammatory disease. *J.A.M.A.* 250:759, 1983.
9. Main, D., and Main, E. *Obstetrics and Gynecology: A Pocket Reference.* Chicago: Yearbook, 1984.

10. Medical Letter. Treatment of sexually transmitted diseases. *Med. Lett. Drugs Ther.* 28:23, 1986.
11. Medical Letter. Drugs for parasitic infections. *Med. Lett. Drugs Ther.* 28:9, 1986.
12. Müller-Schoop, J. W., et al. *Chlamydia trachomatis* as possible cause of peritonitis and perihepatitis in young women. *Br. Med. J.* 1:1022, 1978.
13. Novak, E., and Woodruff, J. D. *Gynecologic and Obstetric Pathology with Clinical and Endocrine Relations* (8th ed.). Philadelphia: Saunders, 1979.
14. Pritchard, J. A., MacDonald, P. C., and Gant, N. F. *Williams Obstetrics* (17th ed.). Norwalk, Conn.: Appleton-Century-Crofts, 1985.
15. Sanford, J. P. *Guide to Antimicrobial Therapy 1986.* San Antonio: Antimicrobial Therapy: 1986.
16. Schumer, W. Steroids in the treatment of clinical septic shock. *Ann. Surg.* 184:333, 1976.
17. Speroff, L., Glass, R., and Kase, N. *Clinical Gynecologic Endocrinology and Infertility* (3rd ed.). Baltimore: Williams and Wilkins, 1982.
18. Taber, B. Z. *Manual of Gynecologic and Obstetric Emergencies* (2nd ed.). Philadelphia: Saunders, 1984.
19. Weinstein, L. Syndrome of hemolysis, elevated liver enzymes, and low platelet count: A severe consequence of hypertension in pregnancy. *Am. J. Obstet. Gynecol.* 142:159, 1982.
20. Weström, L., Bengtsson, L. P., and Mårdh, P. A. The risk of pelvic inflammatory disease in women using intrauterine contraceptive devices as compared to non-users. *Lancet* 2:221, 1976.

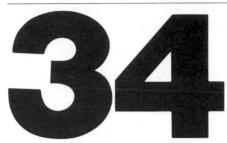

Psychiatric Emergencies

Mark S. Zoccolillo

Patients with an altered mental state or behavioral disturbance frequently present to emergency departments. The emergency physician must identify those patients who have an altered mental state due to a serious medical disorder and those patients with psychiatric disorders who present a serious danger to themselves or others. The emergency physician must also be familiar with community resources to make the necessary referrals for those patients who do not require hospitalization but need continuing care.

Approach to the Psychiatric Patient

As in other specialties of medicine, the treatment and disposition of psychiatric patients depend on reaching an **accurate diagnosis.** Psychiatric disorders can be diagnosed as reliably as common medical disorders [10]. The psychiatric diagnosis is useful in predicting the course of the illness and in choosing an appropriate treatment plan.

I. **General considerations.** Most psychiatric patients are cooperative and present no danger to themselves or others. However, some patients can be dangerous, particularly those who exhibited violent or threatening behavior prior to arriving at the emergency department. It is the responsibility of the emergency department staff to take appropriate precautions.

A. **All patients, no matter how threatening or bizarre, should be approached in a nonthreatening manner** and as patients who are ill and whom the physician is trying to help. The physician should never use threats or become angry.

B. A **secure, locked room,** with only a mattress on the floor, should be readily available for dangerous patients. This room should contain no other furnishings or equipment and should have inaccessible electrical outlets.

C. Patients who are brought to the emergency department in restraints should remain in restraints until fully evaluated.

B. **Potentially violent patients should never be approached alone.** Patients who must be subdued should be handled by several staff members. **A show of force** is often effective in preventing violence.

E. A **designated team** should be available at all times to cope with violent patients.

F. **Restraints should be used for violent patients.** Patients should be restrained face down to prevent aspiration from vomiting. Restraints, wide enough to allow circulation and padded to avoid self-injury, should be placed on the wrists and ankles and released as soon as possible. **An attendant should be present at all times with any patient in restraints,** and vital signs recorded frequently.

G. **Until evaluated, no sedating drugs should be given.**

H. **Any potentially violent patient should be searched for weapons and drugs.** The least threatening way to do this is to put the patient in a hospital gown.

I. **Patients with an altered mental state are prone to escaping** from the emergency department, even when cooperative. A family member, friend, or staff member should be responsible for watching the patient at all times; if this is not possible, the patient should be locked in a secure room until the final disposition is made.

II. The **psychiatric evaluation.** The psychiatric evaluation should focus on three questions: (1) Does the patient have an acute brain syndrome requiring medical treatment? (2) Does the patient have a psychiatric disorder? and (3) What are the patient's current social circumstances?

A. **Chief complaint.** The chief complaint of the patient and accompanying personnel should be recorded; it is often the latter complaint that is the most important.

B. **History of the present illness.** Since the physical examination and laboratory tests seldom are diagnostic, the history is the most important tool. Because psychiatric patients are often unreliable, other informants must be used, including the family and any available records.

1. **Onset of symptoms.** Psychiatric disorders usually present over weeks to months, while acute brain syndromes develop over hours to days. Psychiatric disorders are often chronic; in these patients any recent change in the patient's usual condition should be noted.

2. **Symptoms.** The following should be asked about: change in mood, sleep, appetite, energy, or sex drive; change in social function (e.g., more withdrawn, unable to work or keep house); bizarre behavior; delusions; hallucinations; suicide attempts or threats; violent acts or threats toward others; disorientation, memory impairment, or speech difficulties; and alcohol and drug use.

3. **Past psychiatric history.** Since most psychiatric disorders either are chronic or have recurrent episodes, patients often have a history of psychiatric admissions or psychiatric treatment. If the patient is currently under care, compliance with medications should be ascertained.

4. **Past medical history and review of systems.** Patients with medical illnesses are prone to develop acute brain syndromes, and patients with psychiatric disorders often have intercurrent medical illnesses. It is particularly important to ask about current medications and medical illnesses. The review of systems should be as thorough as possible.

C. **Mental status examination.** The purpose of the mental status examination is to elicit symptoms necessary to establish the diagnosis, assess suicidal or violent thoughts, and assess the severity of the illness. Psychiatric symptoms are best elicited by allowing the patient to relate his or her story, followed by direct questioning. It is best to interview the patient after the history has been obtained from other informants, so that specific questions can be asked of the patient.

1. **General appearance and behavior.** The patient's hygiene, dress, motor activity (increased or decreased), and any bizarre mannerisms should be noted. Poor hygiene and a disheveled appearance are common in schizophrenia but can be seen in other disorders and generally indicate severe illness. Bizarre mannerisms (such as posturing or repetitive motor movements) can be seen in mania and schizophrenia but also in neurologic disorders (such as partial complex seizures) and acute brain syndromes. Decreased motor movement must be distinguished from the stupor of an acute brain syndrome.

2. **Orientation and recent memory.** Decreased or fluctuating levels of consciousness, disorientation, and memory impairment are indicative of an acute brain syndrome. The patient should be asked the date and the place and to remember three objects (words) for 3 minutes. Other useful tests include asking the patient to draw a clock (patients with an organic brain syndrome are often unable to do this correctly, whereas patients with a psychiatric disorder often draw bizarre and elaborate clocks) and perform simple arithmetic computations (adjusting for the patient's education). An impaired sensorium is rare in psychiatric disorders but diagnostic of an acute brain syndrome.

3. **Speech.** It is important to distinguish between aphasic speech and psychotic speech. Aphasic patients often cannot comprehend, and their speech may be unintelligible. Patients with a psychiatric disorder can always comprehend; and their speech, while bizarre, is intelligible. Push of speech (i.e., inability to stop talking) is common in mania, whereas slow speech is common in depression. Tangential speech (i.e., no obvious connection from subject to subject) is common in schizophrenia and mania.

4. **Hallucinations.** Auditory hallucinations are common in psychiatric disorders but may also occur in acute brain syndromes. Visual hallucinations can be present in psychiatric disorders but are more suggestive of acute brain syndromes, particularly those due to drugs. Hallucinations common to psychiatric disorders include those from the radio or television.

5. **Affect** is the patient's emotional state as it appears to the examiner. A euphoric affect is most common in mania, a sad effect in depression, and a flat affect in schizophrenia; but there is considerable overlap. A labile affect is suggestive of an acute brain syndrome but is also common in psychiatric disorders.

6. **Delusions.** Common delusions are persecutory (e.g., being followed or spied on), grandiose, of excess guilt, religious, of being controlled or influenced by outside forces, and of reference (e.g., certain objects or actions having special meanings). Delusions occur in acute brain syndromes, drug psychoses, schizophrenia, mania, and major depression.

   7. Suicidal and violent thoughts. Plans, methods, and intent should be asked about in detail.
   8. Insight and judgment. It is useful to assess the patient's understanding of his or her condition and whether he or she would act on irrational beliefs.
   D. Physical examination. A thorough physical examination, including vital signs, should be performed on all patients. Positive physical findings suggest an organic etiology.
   E. Social circumstances. Emergency department visits by patients with a chronic psychiatric disorder are often precipitated by social circumstances. The usual pattern, particularly in schizophrenia, is for the family to tolerate considerable bizarre behavior before seeking hospitalization for the patient. It is important to assess the family's and the community's ability to tolerate the patient when deciding on hospitalization. Requests for hospitalization can also be precipitated by the patient not having a place to stay. It is often useful to assess the patient's social circumstances (since patients familiar with hospitals may exaggerate symptoms to seek hospitalization when they have no place to stay or are unhappy with their current living situation). Patients should be asked were they live, with whom they live, how they are supported, and if there have been any recent changes in their living situation.
III. Psychiatric medications. The most commonly used psychiatric medications in the emergency department are the antipsychotic and benzodiazepine classes of drugs. Because of the delayed onset of action and the need for careful monitoring, the antidepressants and lithium carbonate are not appropriate for emergency department use. Any prescribed medication should be only a 2- to 3-day supply to avoid a possible lethal overdosage. Emergency department physicians should be familiar with these drugs and their side effects.
   A. Antipsychotic medications are divided into two broad classes: (1) high-dose, low-potency agents (e.g., chlorpromazine, thioridazine), and (2) low-dose, high-potency agents (e.g., haloperidol, thiothixene, fluphenazine). These drugs specifically treat psychosis. Because of the lower incidence of cardiovascular and anticholinergic side effects, low-dose, high-potency antipsychotic medications should be used in the emergency department. Haloperidol has been studied extensively and has been shown to be safe for emergency use because of its minimal effects on the blood pressure [6].
      1. Indications. These drugs control the psychotic symptoms and violent behavior of schizophrenia, mania, psychotic depression, drug psychosis, and acute brain syndrome.
      2. Dosage. Antipsychotic medications are much more sedating and rapidly acting when given IM, compared with PO, with an onset of action of around 20 minutes. The usual dose of haloperidol or thiothixene is 5–10 mg PO (for patients not requiring much sedation or rapid action) or IM, repeated every 30–60 minutes until the patient is controlled or sedated. Patients with an acute brain syndrome or underlying dementia require lower doses of 1–2 mg PO or IM, repeated every 30–60 minutes. Usually only one or two doses are required in the emergency department, but there is no absolute ceiling; sedation and hypotension are the usual limiting factors acutely, while anticholinergic and parkinsonlike symptoms are limiting effects chronically. Fluphenazine decanoate is a long-acting (up to several weeks) injectable antipsychotic medication that is commonly used to prevent relapse of symptoms in patients with schizophrenia.
      3. Side effects. The only significant side effects of acute use of haloperidol and thiothixene are dystonic reactions (common), sedation, and hypotension (uncommon). A more comprehensive summary of side effects of these and other antipsychotic medications is as follows:
         a. Anticholinergic side effects are a dry mouth, constipation, urinary retention, an ileus, and, rarely, delirium (usually in the elderly).
         b. Cardiovascular side effects include hypotension and tachycardia. All patients receiving an antipsychotic medication intramuscularly should have their blood pressure checked every 15 minutes. Electrocardiographic (ECG) changes consisting of an increased QT interval and flattened T waves occur with the phenothiazines and, most commonly, with thioridazine. These changes are usually not clinically significant.
         c. Dystonic movements (uncoordinated spasmodic body movements involving the tongue, mouth, neck, back, limbs, and eyes), **akathisia** (restlessness), **parkinsonlike symptoms,** and **sedation** are relatively common side effects. Dystonic movements, akathisia, and parkinsonlike signs are uncomfortable

to the patient; they are easily treated with benztropine (Cogentin), 1–2 mg IM, followed by an oral maintenance dose of 2 mg PO daily; or diphenhydramine (Benadryl), 50 mg IM, followed by a maintenance dose of 50 mg PO daily. The patient's antipsychotic medication should not be stopped.

  d. Antipsychotic medications may lower the seizure threshold.

  e. The **neuroleptic malignant syndrome,** consisting of fever, rigidity, hypertension, and coma, is a rare but potentially fatal complication. Bromocriptine, amantadine, and dantrolene may be effective therapeutic agents [3] along with vigorous intensive care.

  f. Phototoxicity and heat stroke are occasional complications of antipsychotic medication.

  g. Tardive dyskinesia is a complication of long-term antipsychotic therapy.

B. Antidepressants. There are several classes of antidepressants. Because these drugs take several days to weeks to relieve symptoms, they are not useful in the emergency setting.

  1. Indications. Antidepressants are specific for major depression and panic disorder. Emergency use is not indicated (unless discussed with the patient's physician).

  2. Side effects include **anticholinergic** manifestations (see **A.3.a**), **cardiovascular** effects (e.g., tachycardia, hypotension, arrhythmias, intracardiac conduction defects), seizures, and skin rashes.

C. Lithium is an effective medication for manic-depressive illness. There are no emergency indications for this drug. Since the margin of safety with this medication is low, serum levels of lithium must be monitored to achieve the right dose and assess side effects. The usual dose range is 900–1500 mg/day in divided doses. The therapeutic blood level is 0.6–1.2 mEq/liter. Dehydration, thiazide diuretics, or nonsteroidal analgesics increase serum lithium levels. Toxic effects of lithium (see Chap. 16) usually occur at levels exceeding 1.5 mEq/liter but can occur at therapeutic levels. Lithium may be teratogenic and should not be used in pregnant women.

D. Monoamine oxidase inhibitors (MAOIs), such as tranylcypromine, phenelzine, and pargyline, are useful second-choice drugs for major depression and phobic disorders.

  1. There are no emergency indications for MAOIs.

  2. Side effects. Orthostatic hypotension and dizziness are the most common significant side effects of MAOIs. Other autonomic side effects include epigastric distress, urinary difficulties, constipation, dry mouth, and sexual dysfunction. The most worrisome side effects are **hypertensive crises and the adverse interaction of MAOIs with numerous medications.** MAOIs and tyramine, found in many foods, can cause a hypertensive crisis. The MAOIs also potentiate or interact adversely with numerous drugs, including analgesics (especially meperidine), methyldopa, ganglionic blocking drugs, procaine and other anesthetics, chloral hydrate, aspirin, tricyclic antidepressants, and sympathomimetics (including those in over-the-counter cold preparations and appetite suppressants). Treatment of the hypertensive crisis includes immediate administration of an alpha-adrenergic–blocking drug, such as phentolamine.

E. Antianxiety drugs (benzodiazepines)

  1. Indications. These drugs are useful for controlling the symptoms of alcohol withdrawal, anxiety and panic disorder, and insomnia. Only a 2- to 3-day supply should be prescribed from the emergency department. Diazepam, 5–15 mg PO qd, and flurazepam, 30 mg PO qhs for insomnia, are commonly used agents.

  2. Side effects. Sedation occurs commonly and may be severe in patients with liver or preexisting brain disease and in patients who are taking another sedating medication or drug (including alcohol). Respiratory depression may occur in patients receiving IV administration of a benzodiazepine or having underlying lung disease. Hypotension occurs occasionally.

  3. Withdrawal. Seizures have been reported on withdrawal of therapeutic doses of short-acting benzodiazepines (e.g., lorazepam, oxazepam, alprazolam) [8, 12]. Minor withdrawal symptoms have been reported on withdrawal of therapeutic doses of long-acting benzodiazepines (e.g., diazepam, chlordiazepoxide); however, withdrawal from high doses is similar to barbiturate withdrawal. The benzodiazepines should never be discontinued abruptly.

IV. Disposition. The disposition of the psychiatric patient depends on the diagnosis and the patient's social circumstances.

A. Patients with an acute brain syndrome should have the underlying cause treated. Medical or neurologic intensive care is often needed.

B. Psychiatric hospitalization (or an emergency psychiatric consultation) is indicated for patients who are a **danger to others** (particularly psychotic patients), are a **danger to themselves** (particularly suicidal patients who are psychotic or severely depressed or who have made a serious suicide attempt or retain suicidal ideas), or have psychiatric disease and **cannot be adequately cared for as outpatients** (e.g., psychotic patients who have become acutely ill and have few social supports or are not compliant with medication). **Social circumstances** (e.g., the family can no longer tolerate the patient's disruptive behavior) will often dictate admission; a brief hospitalization will often restore family harmony and prevent the family from permanently abandoning the patient.

C. Outpatient psychiatric referral is indicated for patients who are not a danger to themselves or others and are able to be adequately cared for as outpatients. Such patients include psychotic patients who are compliant and have adequate social supports, depressed or anxious patients who are not suicidal, and patients who are substance abusers (but not at risk for life-threatening drug overdosage or withdrawal).

D. Violent patients who are not psychotic and have either a personality disorder or no personality disorder are often difficult disposition problems, and a psychiatric consultation should be obtained. If no consultation is available, the physician should attempt to secure a temporary solution, such as hospitalization, to allow social agencies to ameliorate the situation. If these patients are under arrest, incarceration may be the appropriate solution.

E. Civil commitment may be indicated, depending on state law. The physician should first decide if hospitalization is indicated and then determine if criteria for commitment apply. Generally, patients who are psychotic or have an affective disorder and are a danger to themselves or others and refuse voluntary hospitalization are candidates for commitment. Psychiatric consultation should be obtained if possible; however, if psychiatric consultation is not available, the physician should initiate commitment proceedings. The emergency physician must be familiar with the state's commitment law, as improper commitment not only exposes the physician to liability but may also jeopardize continued treatment and hospitalization for the patient. The emergency physician should comply with the law but in questionable cases should err on overcommitment.

Specific Behavioral Disturbances

I. Acutely psychotic patient. Psychosis is defined as the presence of hallucinations, delusions, or bizarre (but not aphasic) speech and is seen in a number of medical, neurologic, and psychiatric disorders. The emergency physician must make a careful diagnostic evaluation of the patient to determine the appropriate diagnosis and treatment and at the same time prevent the patient from harming himself or herself or others.

A. Evaluation. The initial evaluation should ascertain if the patient has an **acute brain syndrome,** a **drug-induced psychosis,** or a **psychiatric disorder (i.e., schizophrenia, mania, or psychotic depression)** (Table 34-1). A careful history and thorough physical examination, including the recording of vital signs, is essential in differentiating these disorders.

1. An **acute brain syndrome** can be caused by many illnesses and toxins (Table 34-2). There are no particular laboratory tests or physical findings that can be relied on as screening tools to distinguish an acute brain syndrome from other disorders. However, **the acute onset of symptoms (over hours to days)** and

Table 34-1. Differential diagnosis of acute psychosis

Characteristic	Acute brain syndrome	Drug-induced psychosis	Psychiatric disorder
Vital signs	Often abnormal	May be abnormal	Normal
Onset	Abrupt	Abrupt	Gradual
Disoriented or impaired memory	Yes	Maybe	Rarely
Age > 40 years	More likely	Less likely	Less likely

Table 34-2. Some causes of acute brain syndrome

Drug and alcohol withdrawal	Medications and drugs
Hypo- and hyperglycemia	Hypoxia
Inadequate brain perfusion	Electrolyte abnormalities
CNS infections	Anemia
Remote infections	Brain tumor
(especially in the elderly or demented)	Endocrine disorders
Seizures	Hepatic encephalopathy
Uremia	Vitamin deficiencies
Wernicke-Korsakoff syndrome	

disorientation and impairment of memory indicate an acute brain syndrome. Whereas tachycardia and mild hypertension are common in psychotic patients, fever often indicates an acute brain syndrome. The **elderly** and **patients with a preexisting brain disease** (such as dementia) are particularly prone to develop an acute brain syndrome, even from relatively minor illnesses such as a urinary tract infection.

2. **Drug-induced psychosis** (see Table 34-11) should be suspected in young patients with a psychosis of acute onset (over several hours) and a history of drug ingestion. Disorientation and memory impairment may be present. The route of ingestion, type of drug, and time of ingestion should be obtained. Often other informants are needed, as these patients are often unreliable historians. Since the treatment, evaluation, and prognosis of drug psychosis differ from those of the other acute brain syndromes, drug psychosis is useful as a distinct category.

3. **Psychiatric disorders usually have an onset over weeks to months, and orientation and memory are not impaired.** Although it is often difficult to distinguish among psychiatric disorders in the emergency department and the emergency treatment is the same, physicians should be familiar with the diagnostic criteria for these disorders (see **Specific Disorders** secs. **II, III,** and **IV**).

B. **Management.** Accurate evaluation must precede management. Sedating medication should be avoided until the initial evaluation is completed, to avoid masking a deteriorating mental status. The safety of the patient and staff and prevention of patient elopement must be assured (see **Approach to the Psychiatric Patient,** sec. **I**).

1. The **acute brain syndrome** is managed by correcting the underlying cause.
    a. **Combative behavior** can be controlled with haloperidol or thiothixene, 1–2 mg IM, repeated q30–60min until the patient is calm; the dose can be increased up to 10 mg if no effect is seen. There is no upper limit to the total dose that can be given, but oversedation should be avoided. Vital signs should be monitored frequently.
    b. **Delirium tremens and sedative-hypnotic withdrawal** should be treated with a benzodiazepine or barbiturate (see Chap. 16).

2. **Drug psychosis.** Acutely intoxicated patients are managed according to the type of drug ingested, route of ingestion, and level of intoxication. Overdosage management principles should be followed (see Chap. 16). Management is then symptomatic. Haloperidol or thiothixene, 5–10 mg IM q30–60min, can be used to control psychotic symptoms or combative behavior. Patients intoxicated with alcohol should also be given thiamine, 100 mg IM. The patient's vital signs and mental status must be evaluated frequently.

3. Patients with **schizophrenia, mania, or agitated psychotic depression** should be treated with haloperidol or thiothixene, 5–10 mg IM q30–60min until the patient is calm or sedated. The blood pressure should be checked every 15 minutes.

C. **Disposition**
1. Patients with an **acute brain syndrome** should be admitted to a medical or neurologic service; they often require intensive care.
2. Patients with a **drug psychosis** should be observed in the emergency department (if possible) or on a medical service until they are no longer intoxicated. If the psychotic symptoms persist, psychiatric consultation should be obtained, and psychiatric hospitalization or outpatient follow-up with a psychiatrist within a few days should be arranged.

Table 34-3. Criteria for antisocial personality disorder

I. Current age at least 18
II. Three or more of the following before age 15:
   A. Truancy
   B. Expulsion or suspension from school for misbehavior
   C. Delinquency
   D. Running away from home overnight at least twice
   E. Persistent lying
   F. Repeated sexual intercourse in a casual relationship
   G. Repeated drunkenness or substance abuse
   H. Thefts
   I. Vandalism
   J. School grades markedly below expectations
   K. Chronic violations of rules at home or at school
   L. Initiation of fights
III. At least four of the following since age 18:
   A. Inconsistent work behavior (e.g., too frequent job changes, significant unemployment, serious absenteeism from work)
   B. Poor parenting (i.e., inadequate care and supervision of children)
   C. Any of the following: repeated thefts, illegal occupation, multiple arrests, or a felony conviction
   D. Two or more divorces or separations, desertion of spouse, or promiscuity
   E. Repeated physical fights or assaults, including spouse or child beating
   F. Failure to honor financial obligations
   G. Wandering from place to place or lack of a fixed address
   H. Repeated lying, use of aliases, or "conning" others for personal profit
   I. Driving while intoxicated or recurrent speeding
IV. A pattern of continuous antisocial behavior in which the rights of others are violated, with no intervening period of at least 5 years without antisocial behavior between age 15 and the present time
V. Antisocial behavior not due to either severe mental retardation, schizophrenia, or mania

Source: Adapted from the American Psychiatric Association, *Diagnostic and Statistical Manual of Mental Disorders* (3rd ed.). Washington, D.C.: American Psychiatric Association, 1980. Pp. 320–321. With permission.

   3. Patients with **schizophrenia, mania, or psychotic depression** should be managed as described under **Specific Disorders**, secs. **II, III,** and **IV.**
II. **Violent/assaultive patient.** The physician must first gain control of the patient and then perform a diagnostic assessment to effectively manage the violent patient.
   A. **Evaluation.** Violent behavior is not specific to any particular diagnosis. It can be a manifestation of an acute brain syndrome, drug intoxication, schizophrenia, mania, depression, or antisocial personality disorder; in addition, violent behavior can occur in the absence of any psychiatric disorder.
      1. **Psychotic patients** should be evaluated as in sec. **I.A.**
      2. **Drugs and alcohol** are frequent causes of violent behavior.
      3. **Antisocial personality disorder** (Table 34-3) is frequently associated with violence. Often intoxication and repetitive antisocial behavior coincide.
      4. The **social circumstances** of the violent patient are important. Pertinent questions are the seriousness of the violent act, the intent of the patient, the intended victim, whether this is a chronic pattern, and if criminal charges are pending.
   B. **Management.** Both the diagnosis and the social circumstances determine the management of the violent patient.
      1. The **patient must be secured** to prevent harm to himself or herself and the staff and to allow for adequate evaluation (see **Approach to the Psychiatric Patient,** sec. **I.**).
      2. **Psychotic and intoxicated patients** are managed as described in sec. **I.B.**
      3. **Violent patients who are neither intoxicated nor psychotic** and have either repetitive antisocial or criminal behavior or no psychiatric disorder should not be medicated. Often these patients will respond to firmness and a show of force. If the patient remains a threat, **restraints** or **physical confinement** should be used.

C. **Disposition**
   1. **Psychotic patients** who are violent usually should be hospitalized on a psychiatric service or receive emergency psychiatric consultation.
   2. **Intoxicated patients** should be observed until they are no longer intoxicated (see sec. I.C.2). Patients under arrest should not be sent to a jail facility until free of intoxication.
   3. **Patients without a psychiatric disorder or with an antisocial personality disorder** are difficult disposition problems. If criminal charges are pending, the patient should be released to jail. If the violence is intrafamilial, efforts should be made to place the affected family members in a protective shelter. As a last resort, the patient can be hospitalized, even if it is not medically or psychiatrically indicated, as this allows time for family and social agencies to ameliorate the situation. If a specific victim is being threatened, efforts should be made to protect the victim, such as warning the victim and contacting law enforcement agencies.
   4. **Civil commitment** should be used for psychotic or acutely intoxicated patients who refuse hospitalization, depending on state law. In many jurisdications, however, civil commitment cannot be used for violent patients without a psychotic disorder or for those with antisocial personality disorder.

III. **Suicidal patient.** Most patients who attempt suicide and almost all successful suicides have a diagnosable and often treatable psychiatric disorder [19, 23]. Many have been under the care of a physician close to the time of the suicide attempt. All patients who make a suicide attempt or present with suicidal thoughts must receive a thorough psychiatric evaluation. The patient's psychiatric diagnosis is the most important factor in the patient's disposition from the emergency department.
   A. **Evaluation.** Because suicide is a rare event, even in psychiatrically ill patients, suicide cannot be predicted without a high rate of false-positive or false-negative errors [22]. However, certain diagnoses are much more commonly associated with completed suicides, while other diagnoses are rare in successful suicides but are common in those who attempt suicide.
      1. **Psychiatric diagnoses**
         a. **Major depression and alcoholism** occur commonly in successful suicides [23]; the emergency physician must inquire specifically about these disorders.
         b. **Schizophrenia** occurs less commonly but is a high risk factor; hallucinations and delusions, particularly any that may be involved in the patient's suicide attempt, must be asked about and the presence of a concurrent depression assessed.
         c. **Somatization disorder and antisocial personality disorder** are common diagnoses among patients who attempt suicide but occur rarely in patients who successfully complete suicide; the presence of a coexisting major depression or substance abuse increases the risk of suicide.
      2. **Patients who threaten or have attempted suicide** should be questioned about the **intent, method,** and **access to method.** The conditions surrounding the suicide attempt should be assessed. Specifically, the intent of the patient, the possibility of rescue, the lethality of the attempt, and obvious precipitating factors are important. However, these factors are additional to the diagnosis.
   B. **Management.** While in the emergency department, patients who have suicidal ideations or have made a recent suicide attempt are at risk for suicide. Thus, these patients should be placed in hospital garb, have someone in constant attendance in a secure area away from lethal objects, and be prevented from elopement.
   C. **Disposition.** All attempted suicides and patients with serious suicidal thoughts should have an emergency psychiatric consultation, if possible. If psychiatric consultation is not available, the guidelines listed in Table 34-4 should be followed. As a small proportion of suicides occur in patients released from emergency departments en route to other hospitals, the emergency department physician must ensure secure transportation for patients being transferred and impress on accompanying personnel the seriousness of the situation.

Specific Disorders

I. **Acute brain syndrome.** The presence of disorientation, impaired memory, and other disorders of cognition occurring acutely is diagnostic of the acute brain syndrome. In at least 90% of the cases there is a recognizable neurologic or medical cause.

Table 34-4. Disposition of suicidal patients

Must be admitted	Can be released (with psychiatric follow-up)
Medically serious attempt	Patients with antisocial personality or somatization disorder but without major depression
Psychiatrically serious attempt (e.g., patient clearly intended to die, no possibility of rescue)	
Patients with major depression	Patients who do not have a psychiatric disorder, and the attempt was not serious
Patients with alcoholism	
Psychotic, demented, or intoxicated patients	
Patients who are still suicidal	
Patients over the age of 40	

    A. Clinical characteristics. While disorientation and memory impairment are diagnostic, a variety of other symptoms can be present, including hallucinations, delusions, bizarre behavior, depression, impaired judgment, and suicidal and homicidal behavior. Patients may be quietly confused or highly agitated. The level of consciousness may fluctuate over minutes to hours, as may any of the other symptoms.

    B. Differential diagnosis. Rarely, severely depressed or manic patients may appear to have an acute brain syndrome. Misdiagnosing an acute brain syndrome as a psychiatric disorder can have severe consequences; therefore, the emergency physician should beware of diagnosing patients with the characteristics mentioned in **A** as having a psychiatric illness.

    C. Predisposing characteristics. The elderly and patients with preexisting brain disease (such as dementia) are particularly prone to develop an acute brain syndrome, even from relatively minor illnesses such as a urinary tract infection.

    D. Etiology. There are many causes of the acute brain syndrome (see Table 34-2). The emergency physician must use the history and physical examination to search for the cause. The physician should concentrate on immediately life-threatening conditions, such as hypoxemia, hypoglycemia, and electrolyte abnormalities. Often the cause is not neurologic; in the elderly and in patients with preexisting brain disease, remote infection, medications, and dehydration are common causes of the acute brain syndrome.

    E. Management of this syndrome is determined by the underlying cause. Combative patients can be managed by rapid tranquilization (see **Specific Behavioral Disturbances, sec. I.B.1**). If the cause of the acute brain syndrome is not determined in the emergency department, the patient should be admitted to an intensive care unit because the syndrome carries a high mortality.

  II. Schizophrenia is a chronic illness that begins in young adulthood. It is characterized by hallucinations, delusions, tangential speech, and social deterioration.

    A. Clinical features. The criteria for this diagnosis are given in Table 34-5. Usually these patients are unable to work and often live with family members, in boarding homes, or on the streets. Major depression frequently complicates this disorder, and 10% of all deaths among schizophrenics are by suicide.

    B. Differential diagnosis. Mania and psychotic depression can be indistinguishable from this disorder acutely. It is the course of the illness that distinguishes among these disorders. Because schizophrenia almost always begins before the age of 45, patients presenting for the first time with psychotic symptoms after the age of 45 are likely to have some other diagnosis.

    C. Emergency department presentation. Patients with schizophrenia usually visit emergency facilities because of a violent act or threat or a social crisis. Discontinuation of medication is often a precipitating factor. Often families have tolerated considerable distress before bringing the patient to the emergency department.

    D. Treatment. Long-term management of schizophrenia involves administration of antipsychotic medication and adequate social support. Acute worsening of psychotic symptoms should be treated with antipsychotic medication (see **Specific Behavioral Disturbances, sec. I.B.3**). Patients who are not violent and not in acute distress can be treated with the oral concentrate of haloperidol or thiothixene, 10 mg q2–4h,

Table 34-5. Diagnostic criteria for schizophrenia

I. At least one of the following during a phase of illness:
  A. Bizarre delusions, such as being controlled, thought broadcasting, thought insertion, or thought withdrawal
  B. Somatic, grandiose, religious, nihilistic, or other delusions without persecutory or jealous content
  C. Delusions with persecutory or jealous content, if accompanied by hallucinations of any type
  D. Auditory hallucinations in which either a voice keeps up a running commentary on the individual's behavior or thoughts, or two or more voices converse with each other
  E. Auditory hallucinations on several occasions, with content of more than one or two words, having no apparent relation to depression or elation
  F. Incoherence, marked loosening of associations, markedly illogical thinking, or marked poverty of content of speech if associated with at least one of the following: blunted, flat, or inappropriate affect; delusions or hallucinations; or catatonic or other grossly disorganized behavior
II. Deterioration from a previous level of functioning in such areas as work, social relations, and self-care
III. Continuous signs of the illness for at least 6 months at some time during the person's life, with some signs of the illness at present
IV. A full depressive or manic episode, if present, developed after any psychotic symptoms, or was brief in duration relative to the duration of the psychotic symptoms
V. Onset of illness before the age of 45
VI. Not due to any organic mental disorder or mental retardation

Source: Adapted from the American Psychiatric Association, *Diagnostic and Statistical Manual of Mental Disorders* (3rd ed.). Washington, D.C.: American Psychiatric Association, 1980. Pp. 188–189. With permission.

until the hallucinations and delusions are improved or the patient becomes sedated. Patients who are not admitted to the hospital should be continued on antipsychotic medication (haloperidol or thiothixene, 10–30 mg/day in 1 or 2 doses) and referred to a psychiatrist.
  E. **Disposition.** The decision to hospitalize these patients depends on the patient's clinical condition and social circumstances. The family should be consulted to help determine the disposition. Violent or suicidal schizophrenics should be hospitalized. Patients who have exhausted the family's or community's tolerance, are very delusional, or have marked hallucinations and are not compliant should also be hospitalized. Civil commitment should be used if necessary.
III. **Bipolar disorder (manic-depressive illness)** is defined as one or more episodes of mania. Usually these patients will also have episodes of major depression. Bipolar disorder, however, is a separate disorder from major depression alone. It has a later age of onset than schizophrenia, but the first episode of illness can occur at any age. The disorder is usually episodic with normal behavior between episodes. Patients with bipolar disorder usually do not show social deterioration.
  A. **Clinical characteristics.** Mania is characterized by a euphoric or irritable mood and characteristic symptoms (Table 34-6). Hallucinations, delusions, and bizarre speech may be present. Severely manic patients can be violent and difficult to control because of irritability, excess physical energy, hallucinations, or delusions. Major depression is discussed in sec. **IV.**
  B. The reasons for emergency department presentation are similar to those of schizophrenic patients (see sec. **II.C.**).
  C. **Differential diagnosis.** An acute brain syndrome, drug intoxication, and schizophrenia can also present with manic symptoms. The patient's history helps distinguish these conditions. For purposes of emergency care, distinguishing an acute brain syndrome and drug intoxication from a manic episode is important, whereas distinguishing between schizophrenia and mania is not. Patients presenting with psychotic symptoms for the first time after the age of 45 and who do not have an acute brain syndrome most likely will have mania or psychotic depression.
  D. **Treatment.** Emergency treatment of manic patients is with antipsychotic medication (see **Specific Behavioral Disturbances,** sec. **I.B.3**). Long-term treatment of this

Table 34-6. Diagnostic criteria for mania

I. One or more distinct periods with a predominantly elevated, expansive, or irritable mood; the elevated or irritable mood must be prominent and relatively persistent, although it may alternate or intermingle with a depressive mood
II. Duration of at least 1 week, with at least three of the following symptoms:
   A. Increase in activity (socially, at work, or sexually) or physical restlessness
   B. More talkative than usual or pressure to keep talking
   C. Flight of ideas or subjective experience that thoughts are racing
   D. Inflated self-esteem or grandiosity that may be delusional
   E. Decreased need for sleep
   F. Distractibility
   G. An unrecognized excessive involvement in activities that have a high potential for painful consequences, such as buying sprees, sexual indiscretions, foolish business investments, reckless driving
III. Hallucinations and delusions may be present
IV. Not superimposed on schizophrenia
V. Not due to any organic mental disorder or substance intoxication

Source: Adapted from the American Psychiatric Association, *Diagnostic and Statistical Manual of Mental Disorders* (3rd ed.). Washington, D.C.: American Psychiatric Association, 1980. Pp. 208–209. With permission.

Table 34-7. Diagnostic criteria for major depressive episode

I. Persistent dysphoric mood (depressed, sad, hopeless, irritable) or loss of interest or pleasure in almost all usual activities or pastimes
II. At least four of the following symptoms present nearly every day for a period of 2 weeks:
   A. Increased or decreased appetite or significant weight loss or weight gain
   B. Insomnia or hypersomnia
   C. Psychomotor agitation or retardation
   D. Loss of pleasure in usual activities or decrease in sex drive
   E. Loss of energy or fatigue
   F. Feelings of worthlessness, self-reproach, or excessive or inappropriate guilt
   G. Complaint or evidence of diminished ability to think or concentrate
   H. Recurrent thoughts of death, suicidal ideation, wish to be dead, or suicide attempts
III. Not due to any organic mental disorder or uncomplicated bereavement
IV. Hallucinations and delusions may be present

Source: Adapted from the American Psychiatric Association, *Diagnostic and Statistical Manual of Mental Disorders* (3rd ed.). Washington, D.C.: American Psychiatric Association, 1980. P. 213. With permission.

disorder is with lithium carbonate. Because lithium takes several days to be effective in controlling mania and has a low margin of safety, it is not a drug to be used in the emergency department.
   E. Disposition. Because of the episodic nature of the illness, the potential severity of symptoms, and the need for lithium carbonate, patients who are manic should be hospitalized on a psychiatric service or receive emergency psychiatric consultation.
IV. **Major depression.** Patients often present to the emergency department with complaints of depression and anxiety. While a depressed mood is common, a persistently depressed mood with certain symptoms (Table 34-7) is not. Major depression can be severely debilitating and life-threatening, with a lifetime suicide rate of about 15%. However, it is usually treatable. Symptoms of depression can be caused by a number of medical disorders, and major depression can be a complication of medical disorders. Major depression frequently complicates other psychiatric disorders.
   A. Clinical characteristics. A persistently depressed mood and characteristic symptoms for at least 2 weeks are necessary for the diagnosis of major depression (see Table 34-7). Vague somatic symptoms may be the chief complaint, and only specific questioning will elicit symptoms of depression. Hallucinations and delusions may be present.

B. Differential diagnosis. Major depression with hallucinations and delusions can be indistinguishable in the emergency department from schizophrenia; however, if the patient is more than 45 years of age with a first episode, schizophrenia can essentially be excluded. An acute brain syndrome may also present initially with major depression. Medical disorders, including cancer, hypothyroidism, other endocrine disorders, and a number of medications, can produce depressive symptoms. Usually a careful history will distinguish between major depression and depressive symptoms secondary to a medical illness. Patients may report depression, but careful questioning will reveal that they are complaining of malaise or fatigue. If the physical symptoms of depression, such as weight loss or fatigue, are the predominant symptoms, a medical cause should be suspected.

C. Emergency department presentation. Suicide attempts or suicidal thoughts are common presentations. Anxiety, nervousness, insomnia, or vague somatic symptoms may also be the initial complaint.

D. Treatment. Antidepressant medication is an effective treatment, as are certain types of psychotherapy. Severely depressed patients may require electroconvulsive therapy. Patients with hallucinations or delusions are also treated with antipsychotic medication. Because antidepressant medication and psychotherapy take 1–3 weeks to be effective, they are not emergency department treatments. The emergency department physician should initiate treatment only after consulting with the physician who will continue the patient's care. Even if the patient's major depression appears understandable in light of the patient's social circumstances, the patient should be referred for treatment because major depression, regardless of the presumed etiology, is debilitating.

E. Disposition. Depressed patients who do not have hallucinations or delusions, who are not suicidal, and who are able to care for themselves can be treated as outpatients. Treatment of these patients can be initiated by the emergency department physician after consulting with the physician who will be following the patient. If no immediate consultation is available, the emergency department physician can prescribe a 2- or 3-day supply of flurazepam, 30 mg qhs, if insomnia is a problem, and refer the patient to a psychiatrist or to the primary care physician. Patients who are suicidal, have hallucinations or delusions, or are so profoundly depressed that they cannot provide for their basic needs should be hospitalized on a psychiatric service or receive emergency psychiatric consultation.

V. Grief (bereavement). The symptoms of grief (following the death of a loved one) can be indistinguishable from those of major depression. Most grief reactions, however, do not require treatment. Patients with prolonged grief (lasting more than several months), marked functional impairment, morbid preoccupation with worthlessness, suicidal thoughts (other than thoughts of wishing to have died with the person who died), marked psychomotor retardation, or a history of major depression should be referred to a psychiatrist. Uncomplicated grief can be treated with reassurance and, if insomnia is a major problem, flurazepam, 30 mg qhs for 2 or 3 nights. Help from the bereaved individual's family and friends should be obtained.

VI. Anxiety disorders. Complaints of anxiety, tension, and nervousness are common. A specific syndrome, **panic disorder,** has been well described. Panic disorder is commonly seen in the emergency department and resembles a number of medical disorders. This disorder usually begins before age 35 and often coexists with phobias and generalized anxiety.

A. Clinical characteristics. A panic attack is an acute episode of anxiety with an abrupt onset and termination and characteristic somatic symptoms (Table 34-8). During the attack the patient may believe he or she is having a heart attack and often presents to the emergency department complaining of chest pain. The patient's symptoms may not be apparent on physical examination.

B. Differential diagnosis. Many physical disorders can present with a similar picture (Table 34-9). Since this disorder usually begins before age 35, patients who are middle-aged or older and present with these symptoms for the first time should be considered to have a medical illness and worked up accordingly. Panic attacks can complicate other psychiatric illnesses, particularly major depression.

C. Emergency department presentation. The patient often presents convinced of a serious medical disorder.

D. Treatment. Hyperventilation and tetany can be treated by rebreathing into a bag. An oral benzodiazepine (e.g., diazepam, 5 mg PO) can help abort the attack. Reassurance that the patient is not suffering from a medical disease is very important. Since the panic attack is not medically serious, the emergency physician should

Table 34-8. Diagnostic criteria for panic disorder

I. At least three panic attacks within a 3-week period under circumstances other than marked physical exertion or a life-threatening situation, with the attacks not precipitated only by exposure to a circumscribed phobic stimulus
II. Attacks manifested by discrete periods of apprehension or fear, with at least four of the following symptoms during each attack:
   A. Dyspnea
   B. Palpitations
   C. Chest pain or discomfort
   D. Choking or smothering sensations
   E. Dizziness, vertigo, or unsteady feelings
   F. Feelings of unreality
   G. Paresthesias (tingling in hands or feet)
   H. Hot and cold flashes
   I. Sweating
   J. Faintness
   K. Trembling or shaking
   L. Fear of dying, going crazy, or doing something uncontrolled during an attack
III. Not due to a physical disorder or another mental disorder, such as major depression, somatization disorder, or schizophrenia

Source: Adapted from the American Psychiatric Association, *Diagnostic and Statistical Manual of Mental Disorders* (3rd ed.). Washington, D.C.: American Psychiatric Association, 1980. Pp. 231–232. With permission.

Table 34-9. Medical conditions mimicking panic disorder

Pulmonary embolism	Cardiac arrhythmias
Alcohol and sedative-hypnotic withdrawal	Hyperthyroidism
Hypoglycemia	Parathyroid disease
Angina pectoris	Drug intoxication
Pheochromocytoma	

refrain from overmedication. Imipramine is an effective medication on a long-term basis but should not be prescribed from the emergency department unless discussed with the patient's primary physician.
   E. Disposition. Unless complicated by another psychiatric illness, these patients do not require hospitalization. They should be referred to their primary care physician or a psychiatrist and given a 2- or 3-day supply of a benzodiazepine (e.g., diazepam, 5 mg PO bid or tid).
VII. Unexplained physical symptoms. Physical symptoms for which there is no obvious medical cause can be placed in two general categories. The first category includes symptoms occurring in a patient who does not have a psychiatric diagnosis. The second category includes physical symptoms in a patient with a psychiatric diagnosis.
   A. Unexplained physical symptoms in a patient without a psychiatric diagnosis
      1. From 13–33% of patients thought to have false neurologic symptoms were found on follow-up to have an organic disorder that explained the false neurologic symptom [16]. When a symptom appears to be without a medical basis, the physician frequently can expect to be found wrong on follow-up.
      2. Patients with known medical disorders may complain of symptoms in the absence of clinical indicators of disease (e.g., patients with a known seizure disorder frequently have pseudoseizures).
      3. When confronted with unexplained physical symptoms in a patient without a psychiatric diagnosis, the physician should explain to the patient that no cause can be found for the patient's symptoms; the patient should be followed up because of the possibility of occult disease.
      4. Invoking psychologic explanations as a cause of these symptoms is not helpful and may obscure the clinical picture, even if the patient appears dramatic or to have an "obvious" psychologic explanation for his or her symptoms.

Table 34-10. Diagnostic criteria for somatization disorder

I. A history of physical symptoms of several years' duration beginning before the age of 30

II. Complaints of at least 14 symptoms for women and 12 for men from the 37 symptoms listed below. To count a symptom as present, the symptom must have caused the individual to take medicine (other than aspirin), alter his or her life pattern, or see a physician; and the symptom must not be adequately explained by physical illness or injury and not be a side effect of medication, drugs, or alcohol. The symptom need not actually be present; report of the symptom is adequate. Records and other informants can be used to obtain these symptoms:

   A. Sickly: believes that he or she has been sickly for a good part of his or her life
   B. Pseudoneurologic symptoms: difficulty swallowing, loss of voice, deafness, double vision, blurred vision, blindness, fainting or loss of consciousness, memory loss, seizures, paralysis or muscle weakness, urinary retention or difficulty urinating
   C. Gastrointestinal symptoms: abdominal pain, nausea, vomiting (other than pregnancy-related), bloating, intolerance of a variety of foods, diarrhea
   D. Female reproductive symptoms: painful menstruation, menstrual irregularity, excessive bleeding, severe vomiting throughout pregnancy or causing hospitalization during pregnancy
   E. Psychosexual symptoms (for the major part of the individual's life after opportunities for sexual activity): sexual indifference, lack of pleasure during intercourse, pain during intercourse
   F. Pain: back, joints, genital area (other than during intercourse), on urination, other pain
   G. Cardiopulmonary symptoms: shortness of breath, palpitations, chest pain, dizziness

Source: Adapted from the American Psychiatric Association, *Diagnostic and Statistical Manual of Mental Disorders* (3rd ed.). Washington, D.C.: American Psychiatric Association, 1980. Pp. 243–244. With permission.

B. **Unexplained physical symptoms in patients with a psychiatric diagnosis.** Specific psychiatric disorders can be associated with unexplained physical symptoms. The strength and usefulness of this association is determined by the specific diagnosis.

   1. **Somatization disorder** is a chronic polysymptomatic disorder that begins early in life (usually in the teens), chiefly affects women, and is characterized by recurrent, multiple, and medically unexplainable somatic complaints (Table 34-10). These patients have 2 or 3 times as many operations and hospitalizations as medically ill patients or patients with anxiety or depressive disorders. Follow-up studies of these patients have not found an increase in mortality or medical or neurologic illness that explain their symptoms.

      a. The **diagnosis** of this disorder depends on the presence over a period of time of medically unexplainable physical complaints involving several organ systems, with the onset in the teens or twenties. These complaints must have led to doctor visits, been disabling, or required pain medication other than nonprescription analgesics. Headache, backache, abdominal complaints, gynecologic complaints, and neurologic symptoms are common complaints. A variety of psychiatric symptoms, including suicide attempts, also commonly occur. In addition, these patients often have chaotic social situations. Since patients with somatization disorder may deny previous complaints, old records, other physicians, and family members should be consulted. Women with unexplained complaints who do not give a history of polysymptomatic complaints or whose complaints begin after the age of 30 years should not be diagnosed as having somatization disorder.

      b. The optimal **management** of these patients is to limit their medical workups and prevent unnecessary surgery. The emergency department physician should (1) explain to these patients that they are ill but that their symptoms will not lead to medical deterioration and (2) refer them to a primary care physician or a psychiatrist. Insistent or disruptive patients should receive psychiatric consultation. An important part of the management of these patients is to restrict their care to one physician to prevent multiple evaluations.

   2. **Malingering and factitious disorder.** These patients present to the emergency

department with false physical symptoms for gain. Drug abuse, evasion of the police, and worker's compensation are some common reasons. To diagnose malingering, the physician must have clear evidence (1) that a false physical sign or symptom with obvious gain to the patient is present and (2) that the patient knows the symptom is being faked. A good history (including the use of previous records and other informants) and physical examination are the means to establish the diagnosis. Antisocial personality disorder and drug abuse are commonly associated. The **management** of this disorder is to confront the patient with the evidence. Depending on the circumstances, it may be important to alert other emergency departments in the area.

3. **Münchausen syndrome (chronic factitious disorder).** A small group of patients make a career of seeking hospitalization and undergoing surgery and medical procedures. These patients are clearly in control of their symptoms and have a great deal of medical knowledge. Unlike malingering, there is no obvious gain to the patient's symptoms. Dramatic presentations, multiple surgical scars, and the absence of family or friends (as these patients often travel around the country) are diagnostic clues. Obtaining a history from other informants or hospitals is essential to establish the diagnosis. Psychiatric consultation may be helpful in clarifying the diagnosis. There is no treatment for this disorder. Confronting the patient with the disorder usually results in the patient moving elsewhere.

4. **Major depression** can present with somatic symptoms, particularly in the elderly. Conversion symptoms, however, are not usually associated with uncomplicated major depression; their presence requires a careful evaluation and consideration of somatization disorder or an organic illness. Since major depression can be caused by physical disorders, the emergency physician should be careful in ascribing physical symptoms to major depression.

5. **Psychotic patients** may complain of delusional somatic symptoms. Asking the patient the belief as to the cause of the symptom is diagnostic. However, psychotic patients may give delusional reasons for real symptoms, and psychotic patients as a group are more prone to physical disorders.

6. **Alcoholism** can cause certain symptoms, particularly gastrointestinal symptoms.

7. **Panic disorder** is discussed in sec. **VI.**

VIII. **Substance abuse.** A variety of drugs and substances are commonly abused, with resultant effects peculiar to each agent (Table 34-11). Physicians should suspect drug abuse in patients who present to the emergency department and request narcotics or sedative-hypnotic medications, especially if they ask for these drugs by name. Even in seemingly legitimate circumstances, emergency physicians should prescribe only a 2- or 3-day supply of these drugs at any one time, preferably with the concurrence of the

Table 34-11. Most clinically significant drug problems by class

Class of drug	Panic	Flash-backs	Toxicity[a]	Psychosis[b]	Acute brain syndrome[c]	Withdrawal
Depressants			+ +	+ +	+ +	+ +
Stimulants	+		+	+ +	+	+
Opioids			+ +		+	+ +
Cannabinols	+	+	+		+	
Hallucinogens	+ +	+ +	+	+	+	
Solvents	+		+		+ +	
Phencyclidine	+	?	+ +	+ +	+ +	?
Over-the-counter			+		+ +	

Key: + = Drug is capable of producing the adverse effect listed; + + = Drug may produce a more serious adverse effect; ? = Unclear whether the drug can produce the effect listed
[a] Seriously compromised vital signs.
[b] Hallucinations or delusions without a clouded sensorium or unstable vital signs.
[c] Clouded sensorium with stable vital signs; hallucinations or delusions may be present.
Source: Adapted from M. A. Schuckit, *Drug and Alcohol Abuse* (2nd ed.). New York: Plenum, 1984. P. 10.

Table 34-12. Diagnostic criteria for alcohol abuse and dependence

I. Abuse
  A. Pattern of pathologic use: need for daily use of alcohol for adequate functioning; inability to cut down or stop drinking; repeated effort to control or reduce excess drinking by "going on the wagon" or restricting drinking to certain times of day; binges (remaining intoxicated for at least 2 days); occasional consumption of a fifth of spirits or its equivalent in wine or beer; amnesic periods for events occurring while intoxicated; continuation of drinking despite a serious physical disorder aggravated by drinking; drinking of nonbeverage alchohol
  B. Impairment in social or occupational functioning due to alcohol use, e.g., violence while intoxicated, absence from work, loss of job, legal difficulties (such as traffic accidents while intoxicated), arguments or difficulties with family or friends
  C. Duration of disturbance of at least 1 month
II. Dependence
  In addition to the criteria listed in I, diagnostic criteria for alcohol dependence require either tolerance (need for markedly increased amounts of alcohol to achieve the desired effect or markedly diminished effect with regular use of the same amount) or withdrawal symptoms

Source: Adapted from the American Psychiatric Association, *Diagnostic and Statistical Manual of Mental Disorders* (3rd ed.). Washington, D.C.: American Psychiatric Association, 1980. Pp. 169–170. With permission.

patient's primary physician. Emergency department management of substance abusers depends on the class of the substance abused.
  A. Opioid abusers often present to emergency departments requesting opioids for pain relief or demanding treatment for withdrawal. In the former instance, it is important to recognize that the patient is feigning a pain syndrome (e.g., migraine headache, ureteral colic) and not to administer or prescribe an opioid. The patient should be confronted with the evidence of abuse, and other emergency departments in the area should be alerted. Since withdrawal from opioids is self-limiting and not life-threatening, patients undergoing withdrawal can be referred to a drug treatment center; emergency treatment is not necessary. Furthermore, such patients are often not interested in terminating their abuse but only in obtaining more opioids. These patients may be dramatic in their pleas, but it is in their best interest to refer them to a treatment center and not to prescribe any opioids. The use of methadone is restricted to specially licensed facilities and should not be prescribed from the emergency department. While most opioids do not produce hallucinations or delusions, pentazocine can produce psychotic symptoms, which should be treated with antipsychotic medication (see **Specific Behavioral Disturbances,** sec. **I.B.2**).
  B. Ethanol is the most common drug of abuse. Intoxicated, belligerent, and violent patients can be treated as described under **Specific Behavioral Disturbances,** sec. **I.B.2.** Alcohol withdrawal is treated as presented in Chap. 16. Alcoholism frequently presents with medical complications; the presence of such disorders as gastritis, bleeding from the upper gastrointestinal tract, unexplained diarrhea, aspiration pneumonia, unexplained trauma, or neuropathies should alert the physician to ask about alcoholism. Alcohol abuse also complicates other psychiatric disorders, and major depression is common in alcoholics. Patients with a suspected diagnosis of alcoholism (Table 34-12) should be referred to a psychiatrist or an alcohol treatment program.
  C. Sedative-hypnotic abuse. This class of drugs includes the benzodiazepines, barbiturates, and a number of sleeping medications. Addiction to a long-acting benzodiazepine (e.g., diazepam, flurazepam) occurs at the equivalent dose of 40 mg of diazepam a day. The short-acting benzodiazepines (e.g., lorazepam, oxazepam, alprazolam) may have serious withdrawal symptoms at high but therapeutic doses. Barbiturates are addictive at the equivalent dose of 400 mg of pentobarbital or more/day.
    1. Patients presenting with early signs and symptoms of withdrawal (e.g., tremulousness, tachycardia, hypertension, hyperreflexia, anxiety, malaise) are at risk of progressing to life-threatening delirium. Management is presented in Chap. 16.
    2. Patients addicted to a sedative-hypnotic drug but not showing signs of with-

drawal should be referred to a drug treatment program. The emergency physician can prescribe a 2- or 3-day supply of a drug in a dosage equivalent to the dose of the drug the patient is abusing, but there is always the risk that the patient will abuse this drug. Patients who refuse referral for drug treatment should not be prescribed any medication. The risk of a serious withdrawal should be explained to the patient.

3. **Sedative-hypnotic drugs (including benzodiazepines), even at therapeutic doses, should always be tapered slowly** to prevent withdrawal symptoms.

D. **Amphetamines** can cause an acute and chronic psychotic illness.
1. **Acute psychosis** can be treated with antipsychotic medication (see **Specific Behavioral Disturbances**, sec. **I.B.2**).
2. **Chronic psychosis** is treated by stopping the amphetamine and administering antipsychotic medication. These patients require psychiatric consultation.
3. **Amphetamine withdrawal** can be followed by a severe suicidal depression; such patients should be hospitalized or receive an emergency psychiatric consultation.

E. **Cocaine** can present with problems similar to those of amphetamines (see **D**), but most symptoms are self-limiting due to the short half-life of cocaine.

F. **Phencyclidine (PCP) or hallucinogen** abuse usually presents to the emergency department as an acute psychosis, which should be treated with antipsychotic medication (see **Specific Behavioral Disturbances**, sec. **I.B.2**). PCP can produce a psychosis that lasts several weeks. These patients should be hospitalized or receive emergency psychiatric consultation.

G. **Inhalants.** A wide variety of inhalants are abused, including gasoline, toluene, glue, aerosols, and other organic solvents. They can produce an acute psychosis or acute brain syndrome, which should be treated with antipsychotic medication (see **Specific Behavioral Disturbances**, sec. **I.B.2**). In addition, these patients should be evaluated for respiratory and cardiac complications. Gasoline can produce lead poisoning, which may require chelation therapy.

H. **Marijuana** rarely leads to a psychiatric emergency. However, it can cause an acute self-limiting panic state that may last several hours. This panic state can be treated with reassurance, solitude, and diazepam, 5 mg PO. Marijuana smokers who develop a psychosis most likely have smoked marijuana adulterated with PCP or have an underlying psychotic illness, usually schizophrenia.

Bibliography

1. Adams, R. A., and Victor, M. *Principles of Neurology* (2nd ed.). New York: McGraw-Hill, 1981.
2. American Psychiatric Association. *Diagnostic and Statistical Manual of Mental Disorders* (3rd ed.). Washington, D.C.: American Psychiatric Association, 1980.
3. Ayd, F. J. Neuroleptic malignant syndrome: New therapies. *Int. Drug Ther. Newsletter* 18:3, 1981.
4. Bernstein, J. G. *Handbook of Drug Therapy in Psychiatry.* Boston: John Wright-PSG, 1983.
5. Bornstein, P. E., et al. The depression of widowhood after thirteen months. *Br. J. Psychiatry* 122:561, 1972.
6. Donlon, P. T., Hopkin, J., and Tupin, J. P. Overview: Efficacy and safety of the rapid neuroleptization method with injectable haloperidol. *Am. J. Psychiatry* 136:273, 1979.
7. Dubin, W. R., Weiss, K. J., and Zaccardi, J. A. Organic brain syndrome: The psychiatric imposter. *J.A.M.A.* 249:60, 1983.
8. Gelenberg, A. J. (ed.). Benzodiazepine withdrawal. *Biol. Ther. Psychiatry* 7:14, 1984.
9. Goodwin, D. W., and Guze, S. B. *Psychiatric Diagnosis* (3rd ed.). New York: Oxford University Press, 1984.
10. Helzer, J. E., et al. Reliability of psychiatric diagnosis. II. The test/retest reliability of diagnostic classification. *Arch. Gen. Psychiatry* 34:136, 1977.
11. Hollister, L. E. *Clinical Pharmacology of Psychotherapeutic Drugs.* New York: Churchill Livingstone, 1978.
12. Howe, J. G. Lorazepam withdrawal seizures. *Br. Med. J.* 280:1163, 1980.
13. Khantzian, E. J., and McKenna, G. J. Acute toxic and withdrawal reactions associated with drug use and abuse. *Ann. Intern. Med.* 90:361, 1979.
14. Klein, D. R., et al. *Diagnosis and Drug Treatment of Psychiatric Disorders: Adults and Children* (2nd ed.). Baltimore: Williams and Wilkins, 1980.
15. Lader, M. Dependence on benzodiazepines. *J. Clin. Psychiatry* 44:121, 1983.

16. Lazare, A. Current concepts in psychiatry. Conversion symptoms. *N. Engl. J. Med.* 305:745, 1981.
17. A. J. Lishman. *Organic Psychiatry.* Boston: Blackwell, 1978.
18. Lipowski, Z. J. Transient cognitive disorders (delirium, acute confusional states) in the elderly. *Am. J. Psychiatry* 140:1426, 1983.
19. Murphy, G. E. Problems in studying suicide. *Psychiatr. Dev.* 4:339, 1983.
20. Murphy, G. E., and Robins, E. Social factors in suicide. *J.A.M.A.* 199:303, 1967.
21. Pearlson, G. D. Psychiatric and medical symptoms associated with phencyclidine (PCP) abuse. *Johns Hopkins Med. J.* 148:25, 1981.
22. Pokorny, A. D. Prediction of suicide in psychiatric patients. *Arch. Gen. Psychiatry* 40:249, 1983.
23. Robins, E., et al. Some clinical considerations in the prevention of suicide based on 134 successful suicides. *Am. J. Public Health* 49:888, 1959.
24. Schmidt, E., O'Neal, P., and Robins, E. Evaluation of suicide attempts as a guide to therapy: Clinical and follow-up study of 109 patients. *J.A.M.A.* 155:549, 1954.
25. Schuckit, M. A. *Drug and Alcohol Abuse* (2nd ed.). New York: Plenum, 1984.
26. Smith, K., Pumphrey, M. W., and Hall, J. C. The "last straw": The decisive incident resulting in the request for hospitalization for 100 schizophrenic patients. *Am. J. Psychiatry* 121:228, 1963.
27. Wesson, D. R., and Smith, D. E. *Barbiturates: Their Use, Misuse, and Abuse.* New York: Human Sciences Press, 1977.

35

Ocular Emergencies

Lawrence A. Gans

Evaluation of Ocular Emergencies

The emergency physician is frequently called on to diagnose and initiate treatment on a wide range of ocular emergencies, most often ocular trauma and infection. Less often, patients will present with primary ocular disease or with ocular symptoms of a systemic or remote disorder. The ability of the physician to recognize a true emergency promptly and initiate appropriate therapy may directly affect the patient's ultimate visual function. Table 35-1 lists the chief complaints associated with those ocular emergencies that require immediate diagnosis and ophthalmologic consultation; suggestions for appropriate initial action are also included.

I. **History.** A detailed history is fundamental to the selection of appropriate diagnostic procedures and the planning of effective therapy in ocular emergencies. The eye findings may represent only a part of a more generalized illness or a complex of injuries. Ocular symptomatology is frequently helpful in narrowing the differential diagnosis for many common, nontraumatic eye emergencies (Table 35-2).

II. **Visual function** is the major ocular "vital sign." Visual function should almost always be tested prior to examination or initiation of therapy, so that the patient cannot attribute visual loss to treatment or neglect. The only exception is the treatment of an acute chemical injury where rapid irrigation of the eye is extremely important.

A. **Acuity** should be measured in each eye separately. A hand card or wall acuity chart provides standardized lines of characters for this purpose. The distance from the patient to the chart, as well as the smallest line of characters easily read, should be noted in the medical record. If the patient sees better with glasses, they should be worn during testing, and the acuity noted "with correction." A tiny pinhole in an opaque card will focus distant rays of light; if the patient's glasses are not available or if his or her decreased vision is related to a refractive problem, the acuity will be improved by holding the pinhole in front of the eye while testing. If the patient cannot see letters or symbols on an acuity chart, the distance at which the examiner's fingers can be counted should be noted (e.g., counts fingers [CF] at 2 ft). Hand motion (HM) or light perception (LP) describes lesser degrees of function. If the brightest light available is not seen, the vision is recorded as "no light perception" (NLP). Even when the patient cannot or will not open the eyelids, vision can be assessed by the perception of light through the closed eyelid or by observing pupil constriction in the opposite eye by consensual reflex.

B. **Visual field** assessment is particularly important in the evaluation of alterations in visual function, ocular motility, headache, and other neurologic disorders. Confrontation fields can be performed rapidly. The visual field above, below, and to either side of the point of fixation should be tested separately in each eye. More precise information can be obtained by having the patient compare the color of two red-top (dilating) eyedrop bottles held to either side of the examiner's head. The patient is instructed to stare at the examiner's nose. Alteration in color or brightness perception across the horizontal or vertical midline of the visual field is a significant finding that requires prompt consultation from an ophthalmologist or neurologist.

III. **Pupillary activity** is another of the ocular "vital signs." The pupil is affected by trauma (ocular, head, or neck), ocular inflammation, medications (therapeutic, drug abuse, poisons), tumor, vascular disease, glaucoma, and systemic diseases (e.g., syphilis, diabetes mellitus).

A. The **afferent arc of the pupillary reflex controls both pupils symmetrically** and is tested by the "swinging flashlight" test. Light directed at one eye should cause both pupils to constrict equally. If the afferent visual system in one eye is significantly disturbed (e.g., optic neuritis, retinal detachment, central retinal vascular occlu-

Table 35-1. Ocular emergencies

Chief complaint	Rule out	Findings	Immediate action
Sudden profound loss of vision	Central retinal artery occlusion	Retinal edema (milky and translucent)* Afferent pupillary defect* Cherry-red spot Optic disk pallor	Intermittent digital pressure on the globe Immediate ophthalmologic consultation for administration of retrobulbar anesthetic and paracentesis of the anterior chamber
Profound loss of vision with pain	Endophthalmitis	Hypopyon (layered anterior chamber pus)* Cloudy vitreous*	Immediate ophthalmologic consultation
Pain and halos around lights	Acute angle-closure glaucoma	Intraocular pressure > 30 mm Hg* Closed anterior chamber angle* Middilated, poorly reactive pupil Moderately red eye	Acetazolamide (Diamox), 250 mg IV Mannitol, 1–2 gm/kg IV
Pain and diplopia	Intracranial aneurysm	Fixed pupil Third cranial nerve palsy	Immediate neurosurgical consultation
Pain and swelling	Orbital cellulitis	Orbital edema and erythema* Proptosis* Decreased vision Ophthalmoplegia	Immediate ophthalmologic and otolaryngologic consultation CT scan for orbital abscess and sinusitis Open and culture any previous skin laceration IV antibiotics
Chemical splashed into eye	Significant toxic injury	Cloudy cornea* Epithelial staining (with fluorescein)* Conjunctival ischemia (white, avascular)	Irrigate eye with saline (several liters) Remove foreign matter with a cotton swab
Purulent ocular discharge	Hyperacute bacterial conjunctivitis	Copious discharge* Venereal disease *Neisseria* on smear	Scrape the conjunctiva for culture and smear Parenteral and topical antibiotics
	Neonatal conjunctivitis	Purulent discharge*	Scrape the conjunctiva for culture and smear Sepsis workup Topical and IV antibiotics
Ocular injury	Penetrating trauma	Intraocular pressure < 5 mm Hg Shallow anterior chamber Laceration, irregular pupil Blood in anterior chamber and/or vitreous	Protect the eye with a metal or plastic shield Evaluate for possible retained foreign body
	Ruptured globe	Intraocular pressure < 5 mm Hg*	Protect the eye with a metal or plastic shield

Table 35-1 (continued)

Chief complaint	Rule out	Findings	Immediate action
		Vitreous blood* Subconjunctival hemorrhage	
	Hyphema	Anterior chamber blood*	Measure intraocular pressure and treat for acute glaucoma if over 35 mm Hg Protect the eye with a metal or plastic shield

*Invariably present finding.

Table 35-2. Ocular symptomatology

Symptom	Likely diagnosis
Itch	Allergy
Photophobia	Keratitis Iritis
Scratch	Foreign body Blepharitis Conjunctivitis Keratitis
Crusting	Blepharitis
Eye pain	Significant inflammation Endophthalmitis Scleritis Optic neuritis Keratitis Acute glaucoma
Floaters	Retinal hemorrhage or tear Posterior vitreous separation
Smokey vision	Uveitis Vitreous hemorrhage
Flashes	Retinal traction Migraine

Lines
  Wavy
  Zigzag
	
	Macular disease
	Migraine

sion), both pupils should remain equal. Light directed at the normal eye will cause both pupils to constrict. If the light is then directed at the diseased eye, both pupils will dilate. The test is performed by swinging a light from one eye to the other while observing the pupil size of either eye. This test can even be used through swollen eyelids by observing the reflex in the opposite pupil when a very bright light is employed.

B. The **efferent arc of the pupillary reflex controls each pupil separately,** producing unequal pupils (anisocoria) when an abnormality exists. Lesions affecting the third cranial nerve can produce mydriasis, ptosis, and weakness in elevation and adduction of the eye. Involvement of the sympathetic fibers can produce Horner's syndrome (ipsilateral ptosis, miosis, anhidrosis). The difference in pupil size is enhanced in dim room lighting.

C. **Ocular conditions causing pupillary abnormalities** include iris injury (trauma can produce spastic miosis or paralytic mydriasis, atrophy, incarceration in a wound, inflammatory synechia to the lens capsule, or sphincter rupture), medications (myd-

Table 35-3. Abnormal ocular alignment

Cranial nerve palsy	Position of the affected eye	Diplopia*	Other features
Oculomotor (third nerve)	Down and out	Crossed and vertical	Ptosis, dilated and nonreactive pupil
Trochlear (fourth nerve)	Higher	Vertical	Head tilted away from the affected side, chin down
Abducens (sixth nerve)	Inward	Uncrossed	Head turned toward the affected side

*If a red filter is placed in front of the right eye and the patient describes the red image to the left of the normal image, the diplopia is said to be crossed. If the red image is to the same side as the red filter (right side), the diplopia is uncrossed. If the red image is above or below the normal image, the diplopia is vertical.

riatics, cycloplegics, miotics), glaucoma (acute angle closure, miotic therapy), intraocular foreign body, post–laser photocoagulation, and congenital iris abnormalities.

    D. Pharmacologic testing in diagnosing pupillary abnormalities

        1. Small pupil. Cocaine 4% dilates the pupil poorly in Horner's syndrome when the lesion involves the second- or third-order neuron. Hydroxyamphetamine 1% dilates the pupil poorly in third-order neuron Horner's syndrome. Both drugs will dilate a normal pupil. Most third-order neuron lesions are benign, whereas 84% of adults with first- or second-order neuron lesions will be found to have a malignancy.

        2. Middilated or poorly reactive pupil. Pilocarpine 1% will not constrict a pupil under cycloplegic block (e.g., atropine). Pilocarpine 0.125% or methacholine 2.5% will constrict Adie's tonic pupil but not a normal pupil. **Adie's tonic pupil** is a benign condition that usually occurs in young women and is often associated with the loss of deep tendon reflexes.

IV. Motility. Ductions, i.e., movements made by one eye alone, are tested by having the patient cover one eye and look up, down, and to each side. **Alignment** is the ability to direct the visual axes of both eyes to the same point in space. Alignment is tested in several ways. With significant deviations, the misaligned eye can be noted on inspection. If the patient is instructed to look at an object and each eye is individually covered and uncovered, the deviating eye will move to point toward the fixation target when the nondeviating eye is covered. For complete testing, alignment is measured in up, down, right, and left gaze as well as in the primary position at distance and near. In congenital strabismus, there is little difference in measurements for each field of horizontal gaze (comitant deviation). In acute palsies, the deviation is greater in the field of action of the affected muscle (e.g., the eyes will be more crossed in right gaze when a right abducens palsy is present) (Table 35-3).

V. Slit-lamp examination. The slit lamp is a biomicroscope designed for the examination of the eye. By altering the illumination, different structures can be highlighted or seen in optical cross section.

    A. The **conjunctiva** is a highly reactive vascular tissue with excellent lymph drainage to the preauricular and submandibular nodes. The conjunctiva reacts to irritation in several characteristic ways; the most common reaction is hyperemia, the typical "red eye."

    B. The **cornea** has three structural layers: the epithelium, which rests on its basement membrane and Bowman's layer; the stroma; and the endothelium, which rests on Descemet's membrane. The surface cells of the epithelium form a lipid barrier. When trauma or disease alters the corneal epithelium, this barrier is disrupted. A sterile paper strip of fluorescein dye touched to the tear film allows the dye to dissolve in the tears and bathe the corneal surface; if the epithelial surface is disrupted, the dye will penetrate and stain the deeper layers. When blue light hits fluorescein, a green glow highlights the affected area. If the cornea has been perforated, the dye will rapidly stain the stroma and enter the aqueous humor. In contact lens abrasions, flash burns, keratoconjunctivitis, hairspray keratitis, and other conditions, the green staining may require the slit-lamp microscope for detection.

C. The **Seidel test** is used to test for leakage of aqueous humor through a wound. If a corneal perforation is suspected, fluorescein is placed directly over the anesthetized wound site with a sterile paper fluorescein strip. Under blue light, the aqueous streaming from a perforation will dilute the fluorescein and be readily visible.

D. **Anterior chamber reaction** can be judged by examination of the slit beam as it crosses the chamber. A bright, tiny beam of light is directed obliquely across the chamber in front of the dark pupillary space. Cells are seen under high-power magnification as they pass through the beam. Protein content in the aqueous produces "flare," a glow in the normally transparent fluid. The presence of cells and flare in the anterior chamber is an abnormal finding and is a measure of ocular inflammation. In severe inflammatory reactions, white cells settle to the bottom of the anterior chamber, forming a layer known as a **hypopyon.** Bleeding into the anterior chamber, a **hyphema,** also produces cells and flare and may form a layer of red cells at the bottom of the chamber, by which the severity of the hyphema is graded (e.g., 2 mm or 20% layered hyphema). The presence of a hypopyon or hyphema can usually be established by penlight inspection of the anterior chamber.

E. The **iris** should be inspected for signs of injury in blunt or penetrating trauma. In corneal perforations, the iris is frequently drawn up to the wound and may internally seal it. Adhesions (synechiae) may also form between the iris and lens capsule in the presence of iritis. The pupil may become fixed and irregular. Iris vessels are normally radial, and the blood column is rarely seen. With iris neovascularization (rubeosis iridis), a membrane of nonradial vessels covers the iris and often leads to glaucoma and hyphema.

F. The **lens** is best examined through a dilated pupil. Lens opacity can be generalized or discrete. In penetrating trauma the opacity begins in the area of penetration and may spread to produce an opaque cataract within several hours. Any form of trauma can lead to the development of a cataract at some later time.

VI. **Tonometry** is described in Chap. 38.

VII. **Examination of the fundus** is critical to the complete examination of the eye. It is especially important in the diagnosis of alterations of visual function and in the location and identification of retained intraocular foreign bodies.

A. **Direct ophthalmoscopy** provides a magnified view of the posterior pole. The disk should be examined for pallor, edema, cupping, hemorrhage, and loss of the nerve fiber layer (notching). The macula should be inspected for foveal reflex, pigment changes, edema, hemorrhage, exudate, and subretinal fluid. The vessels should be examined as they emerge from the disk and form the arcades that sweep around the macula. Vascular proliferation, crossing changes, emboli, aneurysms, and any other abnormalities should be noted on a drawing of the fundus.

B. **Indirect ophthalmoscopy** provides a low-power, wide-field view of the fundus, including the far anterior periphery, especially when assisted by scleral depression. This technique is most useful in locating and diagnosing retinal tears, intraocular foreign bodies, and peripheral retinal pathology.

Ophthalmic Medications

I. **Topical anesthetics** afford rapid relief from pain in patients with superficial trauma (e.g., corneal abrasion, superficial keratitis, flash burns) and are helpful in providing sufficient comfort to allow a complete eye examination. However, their repeated use delays epithelial healing and may allow additional trauma to the anesthetized cornea. Prolonged use has led to corneal ring abscesses and is absolutely contraindicated. Proparacaine 0.5% has a duration of about 15 minutes, while tetracaine 0.5% lasts about 30 minutes. Both have an onset in less than 20 seconds.

II. **Topical antibiotics** (Table 35-4) provide a high concentration of drug to the ocular surface and anterior segment of the eye. At these levels, a drug may be very effective against organisms that are resistant by standard disk sensitivity testing. Thus, for superficial infections (e.g., conjunctivitis, sty), most topical antibiotics will be effective against the vast majority of causative organisms. Ointments prolong the contact of the drug with the ocular surface but also blur the vision. They are best used (1) at bedtime, (2) in eyes with already poor vision, or (3) when an eye pad will be used to apply pressure and keep the eyelids closed. When serious infections (e.g., bacterial corneal ulcer) are treated with topical antibiotics, solutions of higher drug concentration than

Table 35-4. Topical ophthalmic antibiotics

Agent	Standard preparation	Fortified eyedrops*
Bacitracin	500 units/gm ointment	10,000 units/ml
Cefazolin		50 mg/ml
Chloramphenicol	5 mg/ml eyedrops	
Erythromycin	5 mg/gm ointment	
Gentamicin	3 mg/ml eyedrops	9–15 mg/ml
	3 mg/gm ointment	
Methicillin		50 mg/ml
Penicillin G		100,000 units/ml
Sulfacetamide	100 mg/ml eyedrops	
	100 mg/gm ointment	
Sulfisoxazole	40 mg/ml eyedrops	
	40 mg/gm ointment	
Tetracycline	10 mg/ml eyedrops	
	10 mg/gm ointment	
Tobramycin	3 mg/ml eyedrops	9–15 mg/ml
	3 mg/gm ointment	
Vancomycin		50 mg/ml

*See Table 35-5.

commercially available should be prepared by the physician or hospital pharmacist (Table 35-5).

III. **Antiviral agents** (Table 35-6) are indicated for the treatment of epithelial herpetic keratitis. Their therapeutic activity is related to blocking viral replication, but they also delay epithelial healing and thus prolong morbidity in lesions of the corneal epithelium not related to the herpes simplex virus.

IV. **Mydriatic-cycloplegic eyedrops** (Table 35-7) are used to dilate the pupil and paralyze accommodation. Anticholinergics also have a role in reducing inflammation by inhibiting the formation of cyclic guanosine monophosphate (GMP), thereby reducing the release of histamine from mast cells. Pupil dilation and accommodative paralysis significantly blur the vision, and it is important to advise patients of the duration of this effect. Specific agents are available with durations ranging from hours to weeks. By convention, cycloplegic eyedrops come in bottles with red tops.

V. **Glaucoma medications** (Table 35-8) can be divided into four classes: miotic agents, osmotic agents, carbonic anhydrase inhibitors (CAIs), and other agents.

A. **Miotic agents** come in a bottle with a green top by convention and are either cholinergic agonists (e.g., pilocarpine, carbachol) or anticholinesterases (e.g., physostigmine, demecarium, echothiophate, isoflurophate). These topical agents constrict the pupil, limiting the ability both to test pupillary function and to visualize the fundus. Since miotic agents increase inflammation in the eye, they should not be used to lower intraocular pressure (IOP) when significant iritis is present. These agents may also have systemic side effects, including headache and signs of cholinergic stimulation of the smooth muscle of the gastrointestinal tract, lungs, and cardiovascular system.

B. **Osmotic agents** are employed to withdraw fluid from the eye by creating an osmotic gradient between the eye and the vascular system. They include mannitol 20%, glycerin 50–100%, and isosorbide solution 45%. These agents produce a significant volume load and should be used with caution in patients with cardiac or renal disease.

C. **Systemic CAIs** block the formation of aqueous humor by the ciliary body. Renal effects of the CAIs include diuresis and bicarbonate loss. Common side effects include fatigue, anorexia, and paresthesias.

D. **Other agents** include epinephrine, dipivefrin, and timolol. These topical medications may have systemic effects on the blood pressure, heart rate, heart rhythm, and pulmonary tract.

Table 35-5. Preparation of fortified topical antibiotics

To make:	Use:	Commercial drug for parenteral use available as:	Plus:	Commercial drug for topical use available as:	Further dilute:
Gentamicin, 9 mg/ml	1 ml	40 mg/ml solution	5 ml	3 mg/ml	None
Tobramycin, 9 mg/ml	1 ml	40 mg/ml solution	5 ml	3 mg/ml	None
Cefazolin, 50 mg/ml	1 ml	1 gm in 5 ml sterile water	None	None	3 ml sterile water
Methicillin, 50 mg/ml	1 ml	1 gm in 5 ml sterile water	None	None	3 ml sterile water
Vancomycin, 50 mg/ml	10 ml	500 mg in 10 ml sterile water	None	None	None

Table 35-6. Ophthalmic medications for herpetic keratitis

Agent	Dosage	Schedule
Idoxuridine	1.0% eyedrops	q1–2h
	0.5% ointment	q4–5h
Vidarabine	0.3% ointment	q4–5h
Trifluridine	1.0% eyedrops	q2–4h

Table 35-7. Medications for pupillary dilation

Agent	Usual concentration	Cycloplegia	Average duration
Phenylephrine hydrochloride	2.5%		3 hours
Tropicamide	1.0%	+	6–8 hours
Cyclopentolate hydrochloride	1.0%	+ + +	24 hours
Homatropine hydrobromide	5.0%	+ +	1–3 days
Scopolamine	0.25%	+ +	3–7 days
Atropine sulfate	1.0%	+ + + +	1–2 weeks

Key: + = slight; + + = mild; + + + = moderate; + + + + = marked.

Table 35-8. Glaucoma medications

Agent	Dosage	Usual schedule
Topical miotic agents		
Pilocarpine	0.5–6.0%	qid
Carbachol	0.75–3.00%	tid
Echothiophate iodide	0.06–0.25%	bid
Demecarium bromide	0.125–0.250%	bid
Other topical agents		
Epinephrine	0.25–2.00%	bid
Dipivefrin	0.1%	bid
Timolol	0.25–0.50%	bid
Systemic carbonic anhydrase inhibitors		
Acetazolamide	125–250 mg PO or IV	qid
	or 500-mg Sequels PO	bid
Methazolamide	50–100 mg PO	tid
Dichlorphenamide	50–100 mg PO	tid
Systemic osmotic agents		
Mannitol	1–2 gm/kg IV	q6h prn
Glycerol	1.0–1.5 gm/kg PO	q4h prn
Isosorbide	1–2 gm/kg PO	q6h prn

VI. **Topical corticosteroids** should be used with great caution by the emergency physician. If used inappropriately, corticosteroids can lead to blindness from glaucoma, produce cataracts, worsen infections due to viral and fungal organisms, or increase the chance that a corneal ulcer will perforate. The use of topical steroids should be limited to specific conditions where the diagnosis is established with certainty. Follow-up by an ophthalmologist is essential.

VII. **Ocular lubricants** are available in the form of eyedrops, ointments, and sustained-release inserts. Eyedrops (e.g., artificial tears) may be used as needed for tear deficiency states. Ointments (e.g., Duolube, Duratears, Lacri-Lube S.O.P.) are used at bedtime or, more frequently, for corneal exposure when there is incomplete lid closure (e.g., Bell's palsy). Sustained-release inserts of hydroxypropyl cellulose are small pellets that are placed under the eyelid to effect a slow release of lubricant.

VIII. **Topical decongestants** are effective in reducing symptoms and redness from minor eye irritation and allergy. They are safer than steroids and may relieve symptoms until an ophthalmologic consultation can be obtained for definitive diagnosis. The major component of the majority of these agents is either naphazoline hydrochloride or tetrahydrozoline hydrochloride.

Red Eye

A red eye can result from many diverse causes, including trauma, infection, allergy, glaucoma, hemorrhage, and vascular abnormalities. The specific characteristics of the redness, along with the associated symptoms and findings, help the physician to make a provisional diagnosis and begin appropriate emergency therapy. Redness can be diffuse (conjunctivitis), discrete (nodular scleritis, episcleritis), vascular (arteriovenous [AV] fistula), zonal (ciliary flush with iritis), or hemorrhagic (subconjunctival hemorrhage) (Table 35-9).

I. **Conjunctivitis.** The conjunctiva is a highly reactive mucous membrane that is sensitive to almost any form of ocular insult. Conjunctivitis is typically a benign self-limited condition. Conjunctival erythema, however, can be the overt manifestation of a more serious intraocular process (e.g., acute glaucoma, penetrating foreign body) for which prompt management may be vital. A complete ocular examination is essential to assure the accurate diagnosis of conjunctivitis.

A. **Viral conjunctivitis**
1. **Clinical features.** Viral conjunctivitis presents acutely with erythema, edema, a watery discharge, and a foreign body sensation. Viral conjunctivitis is commonly bilateral, although asymmetric. A follicular conjunctival reaction with many fine 0.5- to 2.0-mm lymphoid aggregates in the loose conjunctiva of the inferior fornix is typical and can be noted by penlight examination. Other findings include preauricular or submandibular adenopathy and, occasionally, subconjunctival hemorrhage, lid edema, or ecchymosis. With corneal involvement, fluorescein staining will demonstrate superficial punctate erosions, epithelial abrasion, or multiple discrete subepithelial opacities. With severe infections, a membrane of fibrin and leukocytes may form on the inner surface of the eyelids. When there are no systemic symptoms of a viral syndrome, these findings are characteristic of **epidemic keratoconjunctivitis (EKC),** an infection produced by adenovirus types 8 and 19. **Pharyngoconjunctival fever (PCF)** has eye findings similar to those of EKC along with viral pharyngitis, more generalized adenopathy, and fever. PCF can be caused by almost any of the adenoviral types. Both of these forms of conjunctivitis are highly contagious. Respiratory transmission may spread the virus to the eye, but more commonly it is passed by contact with contaminated materials (e.g., face cloth, tissue, hands). Since the virus can be isolated from the conjunctiva for up to 14 days after the onset of symptoms, patients should be advised to avoid situations or activities likely to expose others to infection over this period. Viral conjunctivitis is generally a self-limited disease with a 2-week course.
2. **Treatment** is directed toward symptomatic relief and prevention of complications. Cold moist compresses and decongestant eyedrops (e.g., naphazoline 0.1% q4h) are beneficial. Topical steroid therapy is reserved for patients with severe visual disability or membrane formation.

B. **Bacterial conjunctivitis** begins with nonspecific irritation and redness and progresses to include a mucopurulent discharge. Concomitant blepharitis is frequently found. Staphylococci account for the vast majority of cases. Hypersensitivity to staphylococcal antigens may result in marginal corneal ulcers, typically noted as small whitish infiltrates within 1–2 mm of the limbus. *Haemophilus aegyptius* is a common cause of infection in young children. Cultures of the conjunctival discharge may be misleading because the resident conjunctival flora can include both pathogenic and nonpathogenic organisms. A more accurate yield results from culturing the material obtained by scraping the surface of the conjunctiva lightly with a sterile spatula. However, cultures rarely are needed for mild cases, since they are self-limited, lasting 1–2 weeks. Prompt clinical improvement results from topical antibiotic therapy q4–6h (see Table 35-4).

Table 35-9. Differential diagnosis of the red eye

	Conjunctivitis	Iritis	Acute glaucoma	Keratitis	Scleritis/episcleritis
Erythema	Diffuse	Circumcorneal	Diffuse	Diffuse	Discrete area
Discharge	Watery-mucopurulent	None	None	Watery	None
Blurring of vision	None	None to mild	Moderate to marked	Mild to moderate	None
Symptoms	Irritation	Photophobia	Pain	Photophobia	Tenderness
Pupil size/reactivity	Normal/normal	Small/poor	Middilated/poor	Normal/normal	Normal/normal
Cornea	Clear	Clear	Slight haze	Hazy-cloudy	Clear
Intraocular pressure	Normal	Variable	> 30 mm Hg	Normal	Normal

C. **Hyperacute bacterial conjunctivitis** usually is caused by *Neisseria gonorrhoeae* or, rarely, *Neisseria meningitidis*.

1. **Clinical features.** A unilateral or bilateral copious purulent discharge, chemosis, and lid swelling develop rapidly. Preauricular adenopathy may be prominent. Marginal corneal infiltration and ulceration may develop because of the ability of the organism to penetrate intact corneal epithelium. Serious corneal scarring can result from inadequate treatment.

2. **Evaluation. Laboratory evaluation of hyperacute bacterial conjunctivitis is mandatory.** Conjunctival scrapings should be examined and cultured on appropriate media (e.g., blood agar and chocolate agar in 4–10% carbon dioxide at 37°C). Precise identification of these infections is vital, since sepsis and meningitis may develop; and public health considerations require prompt attention.

3. **Management** combines systemic antibiotics directed at gonorrhea (e.g., in adults, aqueous penicillin G, 10 million units IV daily for 5 days; cefoxitin, 1.0 gm IV qid for 5 days) with topical antibiotic therapy (e.g., penicillin G, 100,000 units/ml, or bacitracin eyedrops, 10,000 units/ml, every hour). Purulent debris should be irrigated from the eye with saline prior to eyedrop instillation. Hospitalization is required.

D. **Chlamydial (adult inclusion) conjunctivitis** is a mucopurulent follicular conjunctivitis. There is often concomitant chlamydial urethritis or cervicitis, which is transmitted through sexual contact. The symptoms are similar to mild viral conjunctivitis except that the discharge is more mucoid than watery. The onset is gradual, and adenopathy is not present. If untreated, a chronic remittent course ensues, although scarring and visual loss do not occur. Topical antibiotic therapy is not completely effective. Systemic tetracycline, erythromycin, or a sulfonamide is combined with topical antibiotic therapy for simultaneous treatment of eye and urogenital disease.

E. **Neonatal conjunctivitis** presents within the first few weeks of life with erythema, edema, and a copious purulent discharge.

1. **Bacterial infections** from *N. gonorrhoeae* and, less commonly, *Staphylococcus aureus, Streptococcus pneumoniae, Haemophilus influenzae,* and coliforms have their onset from 3–10 days after birth. The patient should be hospitalized, and the possibility of systemic involvement should always be investigated. Examination and culture of conjunctival scrapings are mandatory. Both systemic and topical antibiotics (e.g., penicillin G eyedrops, 100,000 units/ml qh for *Neisseria*) should be used.

2. **Neonatal chlamydial conjunctivitis** is another form of acute purulent conjunctivitis and occurs 5–12 days after birth. Examination of conjunctival scrapings shows basophilic intracytoplasmic inclusions in Giemsa-stained epithelial cells. Fluorescent antibody staining using monoclonal antibodies to detect chlamydial antigens is more sensitive and can rapidly confirm the diagnosis. Topical therapy with tetracycline or sulfacetamide ointment 4 times a day for 4 weeks is often effective for the ocular surface infection, but systemic therapy with oral erythromycin is recommended because of the possibility of associated chlamydial respiratory tract infection. Hospitalization is recommended.

F. **Allergic conjunctivitis** is typically related to pollens, grasses, molds, animals, cosmetics, shellfish, and some topical eyedrops. Patients complain of burning and tearing, but the most prominent symptom is itching. The conjunctiva is pale and boggy. Papillae, i.e., elevated cobblestone-shaped areas of perivasculitis in the conjunctiva adherent to the tarsus, can often be seen with eversion of the upper eyelid. Use of a topical decongestant (e.g., naphazoline 0.1% q4h) and cool, moist compresses provides adequate emergency treatment. Topical steroid therapy should be employed only under the strict observation of an ophthalmologist because of the frequent complications related to overuse by patients.

G. **Episcleritis or scleritis** typically presents as a unilateral tender or painful area on the eye. There is a discrete patch of injected vessels in the conjunctiva overlying larger dilated vessels in the episclera or sclera. There is no discharge, and follicles and papillae are absent. With scleral involvement, the area takes on a more violet hue, and the conjunctiva may be elevated by the inflamed nodule of sclera. The etiology is unknown, but association with systemic collagen vascular diseases is frequent. Oral nonsteroidal anti-inflammatory agents frequently relieve the pain. Complete evaluation by an ophthalmologist should be scheduled within several days.

II. **Eyelid infections** are frequently associated with concomitant conjunctivitis and keratitis, producing a red eye with symptoms relating to all three tissues.

A. Staphylococcal blepharitis produces crusting and scaling of the eyelid margins. It may be unilateral or bilateral and is often recurrent in patients with tear film deficiencies. Dried secretions may cause the lids to stick together on awakening. Fibrin is typically seen encircling the bases of the lashes. The staphylococcal organisms produce an exotoxin that becomes concentrated in the tears when the eyelids are closed and produces a toxic, superficial keratoconjunctivitis with burning and irritation on awakening. **Treatment** combines the administration of a topical antibiotic with frequent cleansing of the eyelids to remove crusts and debris. Warm, moist compresses are applied to soften dried secretions, and the lid margins are then gently scrubbed with cotton swabs soaked in diluted baby shampoo. When the eyelids are clean, topical antibiotic eyedrops or ointment is applied.

B. Hordeolum or sty. Focal infection of an eyelid gland at the lid margin produces the sty or external hordeolum. An internal hordeolum results from infection of the Meibomian glands deep within the eyelid tarsus. While usually benign and self-limited, these infections cause both discomfort and cosmetic difficulties. If 2 weeks of frequent warm, moist compresses and topical antibiotic therapy has not produced spontaneous drainage and resolution, surgical drainage may be required.

C. Chalazion. Retained secretions in an obstructed Meibomian gland may produce a chalazion, which is a nodule of chronic granulomatous inflammation. Chalazia may be single or multiple and may involve several lids. Initial therapy of chalazia is similar to that of sties (see **B**); however, many chalazia require incision and curettage.

D. Parasitic infestations of the eyelids may occur with generalized scabies or pediculosis (commonly *Phthirus pubis*). Nits are found on the eyelashes more often than the parasites themselves. Impetiginous skin lesions and blepharoconjunctivitis may also be present. **Treatment** involves mechanical debridement to remove parasites and nits. Pediculocides for general skin therapy should not be used on the eyes. Anticholinesterase eyedrops or ointment (e.g., echothiophate iodide [Phospholine Iodide]) can be used to poison the parasites in extensive infestations.

III. Keratitis may be a primary corneal process; or it may be related to diseases of the skin, eyelids, or conjunctiva. Since the cornea is the major refracting surface of the eye, anything that alters its surface contour or clarity will adversely affect vision.

A. Superficial keratitis may result from a wide variety of conditions, the most common being blepharitis, conjunctivitis, tear deficiency, aberrant eyelashes, drug toxicity, radiation exposure, and exposure to environmental pollutants. Photophobia, blurred vision, and tearing are prominent symptoms. If the etiology can be determined, specific therapy can be planned. Symptomatic relief may be obtained with an ocular decongestant (e.g., naphazoline 0.1% q4h) until an ophthalmologist is consulted.

B. Contact lens complications. The most common contact lens problem is the **contact lens overwear syndrome.** With prolonged wearing of hard (and some soft) contact lenses, the central corneal epithelium becomes hypoxic and is damaged. While the lens is in place, the patient is often asymptomatic. Several hours after removal of the lens, the injured epithelium sloughs, and increasingly severe pain develops. Fluorescein will stain the epithelial defect and confirm the diagnosis. **Therapy** with a short-acting cycloplegic (e.g., cyclopentolate) and a topical antibiotic, followed by covering the eye with a firm double patch, will usually allow healing within 24 hours. Contact lens wear may be restarted after 3 days, but for short periods, gradually working up to a full wear schedule. If the integrity or fit of the contact lens is in doubt, it should be examined by the prescribing eye care specialist prior to reinsertion.

C. A **bacterial corneal ulcer** may occur after trauma but is more frequently related to other ocular diseases (e.g., dry eyes, blepharitis, corneal exposure from incomplete eyelid closure) or contact lens wear.

    1. Clinical features. Common symptoms include blurred vision, a mucopurulent discharge, photophobia, a variable amount of eyelid swelling with erythema, and a foreign body sensation to frank pain. Examination with fluorescein will demonstrate the extent of the ulceration. An infiltrate of white blood cells in the corneal stroma usually rings the ulcer, and a plaque of leukocytes may also be seen on the inner surface of the cornea at the ulcer base. **Hypopyon,** a layering of white cells in the anterior chamber, is also frequently present; the hypopyon is a sterile reaction to the infection. The ulceration may progress until Descemet's membrane balloons forward **(descemetocele)** and ultimately ruptures.

    2. Evaluation. Material for culture and smear should be obtained by scraping the ulcer base and edges with a sterile spatula prior to beginning any therapy.

Debridement of necrotic stroma is accomplished, simultaneously promoting better penetration of topical antibiotics and providing a smoother, cleaner surface for reepithelialization. Bacterial and fungal media should be inoculated, and smears examined for the presence of organisms.

3. **Management.** Patients with bacterial corneal ulcers are hospitalized to provide nursing care for frequent antibiotic administration and general assistance while vision is poor. As soon as diagnostic samples have been obtained, intensive broad-spectrum local antibiotic therapy is started. Commercially prepared ophthalmic antibiotics should be fortified, or solutions of specific concentrations should be prepared (see Tables 35-4 and 35-5). Fortified topical antibiotics (e.g., gentamicin, 9 mg/ml, and cefazolin, 50 mg/ml) are administered q30–60min. Subconjunctival antibiotic injections (e.g., gentamicin, 20 mg, with either cefazolin, 100 mg, or vancomycin, 25 mg) may be given q12–24h when nursing considerations make frequent topical instillations difficult or uncertain. Systemic therapy is unnecessary when the infection is confined to the cornea because of the high tissue levels obtained with local antibiotic administration. Nonspecific supportive therapy includes administration of an analgesic for pain, frequent cleansing of the eyelids and eyelashes to remove crusts and discharge, and instillation of a cycloplegic for iritis and ciliary spasm.

D. **Herpes simplex** can cause a variety of ocular diseases.

1. **Clinical features.** Primary infection usually occurs during childhood and produces a unilateral follicular conjunctivitis and characteristic vesicular blepharitis. This infection is frequently associated with a viral syndrome of fever, adenopathy, and malaise. Half of the cases with ocular involvement have an epithelial keratitis with punctate staining, microdendrites, or a frank dendritic ulcer. Dendrites can occur anywhere on the cornea and may be single or multiple. Recurrent disease may take the form of vesicular lesions of the eyelids, conjunctivitis, or uveitis, but the most common form is the dendritic corneal ulcer. Recurrences can occur at any age and are most common in fall and winter months. Patients complain of a foreign body sensation, watery discharge, photophobia, and blurred vision when the visual axis is involved.

2. **Evaluation.** In most cases, herpetic infection is diagnosed from its clinical appearance. Primary herpetic blepharoconjunctivitis has a characteristic vesicular dermatitis and a follicular conjunctival reaction. The corneal infection of primary or recurrent disease is diagnosed by the pathognomonic epithelial dendrite. Fluorescein staining will highlight the typical branching pattern of this epithelial defect. With multiple recurrences, corneal nerve involvement leads to partial or complete anesthesia. Decreased corneal sensation, however, is not a pathognomonic finding for herpetic keratitis because it is common in many acute corneal inflammatory conditions and in contact lens wearers.

3. **Management.** Topical antiviral therapy with vidarabine, trifluorothymidine, or idoxuridine is effective treatment for dendritic keratitis. The recurrence rate is not altered by therapy, but prompt epithelial healing is common in uncomplicated cases. Patients treated with an antiviral agent should have a follow-up examination by an ophthalmologist within several days. Corticosteroids are contraindicated in epithelial herpes keratitis because they promote viral replication, prolong morbidity, double the recurrence rate, and can lead to serious complications.

IV. **Uveitis** is a nonspecific inflammation of the uveal tract. If the inflammation is confined to the anterior segment, it is called **iritis** or **anterior uveitis**. When it involves the posterior segment, it is termed **posterior uveitis**. A wide variety of ocular and systemic diseases are associated with uveitis.

A. **Iritis**

1. **Clinical features.** Iritis typically produces progressive photophobia, pain, and blurred vision. "Ciliary flush," i.e., hyperemia of the conjunctival and episcleral vessels surrounding the cornea for 2–3 mm (overlying the ciliary body), is frequently present. Although glaucoma may be associated with iritis, the IOP is typically low when the eye is inflamed. **Keratic precipitates (KPs)**, i.e., white cell deposits on the endothelial surface of the cornea, and aqueous cells and flare are present. The iris may become adherent to the lens capsule (posterior synechia), resulting in an irregular, poorly reactive pupil.

2. **Management.** Since nontraumatic iritis is commonly recurrent and requires skilled evaluation and follow-up, it is best treated by an ophthalmologist. Appropriate emergency department care for iritis with a low IOP is topical cyclo-

plegia (e.g., with cyclopentolate 1% qid) with follow-up by an ophthalmologist within 24 hours. If the IOP is elevated, angle-closure glaucoma may be present, either as a primary process with secondary iritis or as a secondary process from synechiae associated with the iritis. In either case, the glaucoma should be treated with topical timolol, systemic acetazolamide, or an osmotic agent (see Table 35-8), and ophthalmologic consultation should be obtained immediately.

B. Herpes zoster may cause vesicular lesions of the eyelids, dendritic corneal ulcers, and uveitis. Involvement of the nasociliary nerve leads to the frequent association of lesions on the tip of the nose and uveitis **(Hutchinson's sign). Treatment** of herpes zoster of the eyelids involves application of an antibiotic ointment to the eyelid skin for the prevention of superinfection. Antiviral therapy is of no benefit for keratitis or uveitis; cycloplegic therapy (e.g., with cyclopentolate 1% qid) constitutes adequate emergency care. Outpatient management is appropriate, with prompt ophthalmologic consultation for keratitis or uveitis.

C. Posterior uveitis typically presents with progressively blurred or smoky vision in one or both eyes. Slit-lamp examination may demonstrate cells in the anterior vitreous. Examination of the fundus is difficult because of the hazy media, but focal choroidal lesions may appear as yellowish-white patches with retinal hemorrhages and exudate present. Prompt ophthalmologic evaluation to determine appropriate therapy for specific uveitis syndromes is indicated. The urgency for referral is determined by how severely vision has been affected and by the proximity of any focal lesions to the macula or optic nerve.

D. Endophthalmitis is typically a bacterial infection inside the eye occurring after trauma, surgery, or perforation of a corneal ulcer. A profound loss of vision occurs early in the course of the infection with increasingly severe pain. A hypopyon is present; and the eyelids, conjunctiva, and orbit are inflamed and swollen. Patients are hospitalized, and prompt ophthalmologic consultation is vital. Material for culture must be obtained from the vitreous, and antibiotics must be injected into the vitreous cavity in order to control the infection. Systemic antibiotics alone are not sufficient. The prognosis is related to the virulence of the organism involved and the immediacy of treatment.

V. Glaucoma is visual loss from optic nerve damage associated with an elevated IOP. Glaucoma is classified by the specific mechanism producing the pressure elevation; it may be primary, secondary, or congenital. Secondary glaucomas result from trauma, inflammation, medications, or tumor.

A. Pathophysiology. Aqueous humor is produced by the ciliary body. It flows between the iris and lens, through the pupil, across the anterior chamber, and through the trabecular meshwork located at the apex of the "angle" made by the iris insertion into the corneal-scleral junction (limbus) and exits the eye through a canal that drains into the episcleral venous system. Blockage of fluid flow at any of these points may cause an elevated IOP.

B. Classification

1. Open-angle glaucoma. If the access of aqueous humor to the trabecular meshwork is unrestricted and the "angle" is wide, the glaucoma is termed open angle. **Chronic open-angle glaucoma** is commonly associated with moderate elevations in the IOP, leading to progressive, asymptomatic loss of the visual field over a period of several years. This condition requires emergency treatment only when the IOP reaches a level that threatens to occlude a major retinal vessel. This level is detected by observing pulsations in the central retinal artery coming out of the optic disk. These pulsations usually will not occur unless the IOP is in excess of 40 mm Hg, although systemic hypotension, atherosclerosis, or heart failure can produce this finding at a lower level. Prompt lowering of the IOP with systemic acetazolamide or an osmotic agent is indicated (see Table 35-8).

2. Angle-closure glaucoma. If the angle is narrow, as in small or farsighted eyes, the iris may occlude the trabecular meshwork resulting in angle closure.

a. Clinical features. Angle-closure glaucoma may be asymptomatic; but, more commonly, the dramatic rise in IOP produces corneal edema with red and blue halos around lights, photophobia, a red eye, nausea, and headache or eye pain. Extreme elevations of the IOP can cause acute damage to optic nerve fibers and may be associated with retinal vascular occlusions. In angle-closure glaucoma, the anterior chamber is shallow peripherally; and the pupil is typically middilated (3–4 mm), slightly irregular, and not reactive.

b. Management. Initial therapy for acute glaucoma includes an osmotic agent (e.g., mannitol, 1.0–1.5 gm/kg IV), a CAI (e.g., acetazolamide, 250 mg IV), and a topical miotic (e.g., carbachol 3% gtts q15min until the pupil constricts and the attack is broken). Definitive therapy for angle-closure glaucoma is the creation of a peripheral iridotomy, either by laser or surgical excision, to provide an alternate access route for the aqueous to reach the trabecular meshwork. This procedure can be electively performed on an outpatient basis if medical management promptly breaks the acute attack. In any case, immediate ophthalmologic consultation is necessary.

VI. Acute bacterial dacryocystitis occurs when the lacrimal outflow system is obstructed by a congenital anomaly, stenosis, tumor, or lithiasis. Painful swelling and erythema develop in the area of the lacrimal sac just nasal and inferior to the eye. Conjunctivitis and tearing may be associated findings. Oral and topical antibiotics, combined with warm, moist compresses, are usually effective treatment. Hospitalization is not generally required. When the acute infection has resolved, further studies and therapy to relieve the obstruction should be undertaken by an ophthalmologist.

VII. Preseptal cellulitis is a bacterial infection in the potential space between the eyelid skin and orbital septum, bounded by the superior and inferior orbital rims.

A. Etiology. The most common organism in posttraumatic cases is *S. aureus,* although streptococci and anaerobes are frequent after human or animal bites. In the absence of trauma, children develop preseptal cellulitis from localized infections (e.g., a sty) or in association with a respiratory tract infection. *H. influenzae* type B is a frequent cause of preseptal cellulitis in young children. Detection of its capsular polysaccharide by latex agglutination in the blood or urine rapidly identifies this possible etiologic organism.

B. Clinical features. Preseptal cellulitis causes a rapidly progressive swelling of the soft tissues surrounding the eye, with erythema and a mucopurulent conjunctival discharge. Mild fever and leukocytosis may also be present. The vision is normal, although lid swelling may make testing difficult. There is no proptosis or motility disorder.

C. Differential diagnosis. The distinction between preseptal and orbital cellulitis is critical, because the latter can rapidly cause blindness and may lead to septic thrombosis of the cavernous sinus and intracranial complications. Computed tomography (CT) is very helpful in ruling out orbital involvement.

D. Management. Mild infections can be treated with an oral antibiotic (e.g., ampicillin, cephalexin, or erythromycin) and warm compresses. All other cases should be hospitalized for parenteral and possibly surgical therapy. With massive edema, a fluctuant area of abscess formation may require drainage. Traumatic wounds should be explored, cultured, and drained. When constitutional symptoms are present, sepsis is frequently associated and hospitalization is required. Cultures of the blood, nasopharynx, and conjunctiva should be obtained. Most young children with *H. influenzae* type B cellulitis should undergo a lumbar puncture to rule out meningitis. IV antibiotics (e.g., penicillin G, methicillin, and gentamicin in adults; methicillin and chloramphenicol in children) are required for serious infections, especially in the presence of tissue necrosis or orbital fracture.

VIII. Orbital cellulitis is a bacterial or fungal infection of the soft tissues surrounding the globe behind the orbital septum.

A. Bacterial cellulitis is either posttraumatic or secondary to paranasal (especially ethmoidal) sinusitis. Staphylococci and streptococci are the most frequent pathogens in adults; *H. influenzae* is common in young children.

1. Clinical features. Physical examination demonstrates proptosis along with periorbital swelling, restricted motility, and pain on attempted eye movement. Fever and leukocytosis are often present. As the orbital swelling increases, pressure on the globe produces stria in the choroid and retina. Optic nerve function may rapidly deteriorate with resulting blindness. Cavernous sinus thrombosis produces increased headache, nausea, vomiting, toxemia, and altered consciousness.

2. Evaluation. Cultures of the nasopharynx, conjunctiva, and any orbital wound should be obtained for aerobic and anaerobic bacteria and for fungi. Roentgenographic studies are always indicated to diagnose sinus disease in cases without a history of trauma and to investigate the possibility of a retained orbital foreign body in posttraumatic cases. CT is useful in detecting abscess formation and in assessing the status of the globe after trauma.

3. Management. Hospitalization and immediate consultation with an ophthalmologist and otolaryngologist are required. Treatment for bacterial orbital cellulitis involves administration of IV antibiotics and prompt surgical drainage of paranasal sinusitis or any orbital abscess. Corneal exposure from proptosis may require protective care with an antibiotic ointment and a moisture chamber.

B. Orbital mycosis is the most feared form of orbital cellulitis. *Mucor* or *Rhizopus* infections may develop in patients with diabetes mellitus (particularly with ketoacidosis) and in patients debilitated by extensive burns, malignancy, or other disease. These organisms produce a thrombosing vasculitis and ischemic necrosis of the orbital and sinus tissues. Rapid visual loss due to central retinal vascular occlusion and cranial nerve involvement **(orbital apex syndrome)** in a debilitated, dehydrated, or acidotic individual is a typical presentation. Lesions of the nasal mucosa covered by eschars of blackened blood may demonstrate the branching hyphae on smear or biopsy. **Management** involves prompt surgical debridement of all necrotic tissues, parenteral antifungal therapy (e.g., with amphotericin), and correction of any metabolic abnormalities. Hospitalization is mandatory.

Disturbances in Vision

Visual loss can result from both reversible and irreversible processes, the latter requiring prompt, appropriate treatment if vision is to be preserved. Even more subtle visual symptoms can be the initial sign of life-threatening disease.

I. Retinal artery occlusion can involve the central retinal artery or any of its branches. Common etiologies include emboli, thrombi, and arteritis.

A. Clinical features

1. Retinal artery occlusion. Sudden, painless loss of vision occurs over a few minutes in one eye and is associated with optic disk pallor and retinal edema. The swollen retina becomes translucent ("milky") and obscures the normal orange hue of the choroid, except in the fovea where a "cherry-red spot" may be seen. With **central retinal artery occlusion**, retinal edema is seen throughout the fundus, although it may be patchy in the initial stage. In **branch retinal artery occlusion**, the retinal edema is limited to the distribution of the affected vessel. Occasionally, a glistening embolus can be seen at the bifurcation of a proximal arteriole.

2. Amaurosis fugax. Embolic disease occurs most frequently in patients with valvular heart disease or carotid artery disease. These patients have episodes where vision is transiently lost due to retinal ischemia. Emboli briefly become lodged at a vessel bifurcation (where they may be visible on funduscopic examination) and then travel distally, allowing restored circulation and visual recovery. The patient experiences a period where the vision becomes gray in the distribution of the affected vessel. The disturbance may last as long as several hours.

B. Evaluation of the heart and major vessels of the chest and neck should be undertaken. In patients over age 45, an erythrocyte sedimentation rate should be obtained immediately to assess for the possibility of giant-cell arteritis.

C. Management. The diagnosis of retinal artery occlusion must be made rapidly, since only prompt treatment to restore the retinal circulation will be effective. Intermittent pressure on the globe will lower the IOP and may dislodge an embolus. If a physician capable of performing a paracentesis of the anterior chamber is readily available, this procedure should be undertaken to lower the IOP and enhance perfusion. Immediate ophthalmologic consultation and hospitalization are indicated.

II. Retinal vein occlusion can involve the central retinal vein or any of its branches. Profound visual loss follows **central retinal vein occlusion**, while visual acuity and only a portion of the visual field will be lost from a **branch retinal vein occlusion**. Occlusion occurs in the nerve head or at AV crossings where the vessels share a common adventitia. Systemic hypertension, glaucoma, and hyperviscosity states are commonly associated with vein occlusions. Extensive intraretinal hemorrhage in the distribution of the occluded vessel is present ("blood and thunder fundus"). There is no effective therapy for venous occlusions, but patients should have an evaluation for associated systemic diseases that may require treatment. Referral to an ophthalmologist for possible photocoagulation to prevent the later onset of neovascular glaucoma is appropriate.

III. Ischemic optic neuropathy (ION) presents in adults between the ages of 45 and 80 years with the sudden onset of painless, irreversible, nonprogressive visual loss. Usually the upper or lower half of the visual field in one eye is affected, although the entire visual field may become involved. The optic nerve appears pale, milky, and edematous with occasional nerve fiber layer hemorrhage. Ophthalmologic consultation is required, although treatment rarely restores lost vision.

Giant-cell arteritis, a treatable disease that may cause ION and often involves the second eye and other parts of the body, should be considered in all patients in this age group having unexplained visual loss. Associated symptoms include jaw claudication, headache, proximal muscle aches, and scalp tenderness. An erythrocyte sedimentation rate should be obtained immediately; and if elevated, the patient should be hospitalized and started at once on high-dose corticosteroid therapy (e.g., prednisone, 100 mg/day to prevent progression). A temporal artery biopsy should be obtained within several days to confirm the diagnosis.

IV. **Optic neuritis** presents with progressive loss of vision in patients between 20 and 50 years of age. It is often associated with pain behind the eye or on eye movement. Vision may vary over a wide range, but patients note desaturation of color and decreased intensity of light in the affected eye compared with the unaffected eye. A relative afferent pupillary defect is present. Acutely, the optic nerve head may be swollen, although in retrobulbar neuritis it may appear either normal or atrophic from previous attacks. Optic neuritis is usually unilateral, although bilateral cases can occur. A detailed history and neurologic examination may disclose other defects compatible with a diagnosis of multiple sclerosis, secondary syphilis, viral illness, or collagen vascular disease. Optic neuritis is generally self-limited and requires no therapy. Corticosteroids may hasten recovery and are reserved for the treatment of cases with bilateral involvement or poor vision in the opposite eye. Ophthalmologic referral is indicated.

V. **Retinal or vitreous hemorrhages** occur in a wide variety of conditions. Small, isolated intraretinal hemorrhages are usually asymptomatic when associated with diabetes mellitus or hypertension. Nerve fiber layer hemorrhage at the optic disk may be associated with glaucoma, optic nerve drusen, papilledema, or optic neuropathy. When intraretinal hemorrhage is localized to the distribution of a retinal vessel, a branch retinal vein occlusion should be suspected. Inflammatory conditions of the retina and uvea can produce hemorrhage associated with exudate and changes in the uniform appearance of the retinal pigment epithelium. Patients with vitreous hemorrhage often complain of smoky vision or seeing cobwebs, the result of blood casting a shadow on the retina. Funduscopic examination may be impossible with diffuse vitreous hemorrhage. The red blood cells can be seen by focusing on the anterior vitreous through the dilated pupil with the slit lamp or ophthalmoscope. The absence of an afferent pupillary defect is good evidence for an intact anterior visual system despite the inability to view the fundus. Patients with diffuse vitreous hemorrhage are promptly evaluated with ultrasonography by an ophthalmologist and are treated with bed rest (usually in the hospital) with the head elevated. With clearing of the hemorrhage, specific indicated treatment should be undertaken.

VI. **Retinal detachment** occurs when the neurosensory retina becomes separated from the underlying retinal pigment epithelium (RPE). This detachment is termed **rhegmatogenous** when liquid vitreous seeps through a retinal break causing the detachment, and **tractional** when the retina is pulled from the RPE by contracting membranes, as in diabetes mellitus. When the retina is detached, the receptors no longer function, and a visual field defect is present. With large detachments, a relative afferent pupillary defect will be found. On funduscopic examination, the retina appears translucent gray with a wrinkled surface. The retinal vessels are elevated, and the normal choroidal pattern cannot be seen. If the macula is still attached, immediate referral to an ophthalmologist for surgery may preserve good visual function. Treatment for a retinal detachment involves the surgical closure of retinal breaks and often drainage of subretinal fluid. Bed rest (usually in the hospital) is indicated until repair can be performed.

VII. **Macular degeneration** typically produces a gradual deterioration in visual acuity with increasing age. Occasionally, patients will notice the onset of metamorphopsia, where straight lines become wavy and distorted. This finding may indicate the development of subretinal neovascularization. Examination of the fundus may disclose a "dirty gray" patch with subretinal hemorrhage. Prompt ophthalmologic evaluation for possible photocoagulation is important.

VIII. **Double vision** is usually caused by a misalignment of the two eyes. If double vision remains when one eye is covered, it may be due to macular disease, refractive changes, or malingering, and the patient should be referred promptly for evaluation. Acute nontraumatic misalignment of the eyes in adults may be due to a cranial nerve palsy, thyroid ophthalmopathy, or myasthenia gravis. Acute onset of pain with a partial or complete third cranial nerve palsy may result from an aneurysm of the internal carotid or posterior communicating artery and should have immediate neurosurgical evaluation. Vasculopathic third nerve palsies in diabetics do not involve the pupil and resolve after several weeks.

IX. Blindness from hysteria or malingering presents a formidable problem to the emergency physician. Evaluation to rule out organic causes of visual loss requiring emergent attention must be undertaken. Several objective tests are helpful. The finding of normal pupillary responses without an afferent defect rules out most lesions of the anterior visual system requiring emergent care. Careful examination of the anterior segment, fundus, and visual fields is essential. If these examinations prove normal, the emergency physician may elicit **optokinetic nystagmus (OKN)** by moving the stock pages of a newspaper in front of both of the patient's eyes. This large target is difficult for the malingerer to avoid, and a normal OKN response is good evidence against profound visual loss. Blind patients have no trouble touching the tips of their fingers, looking at their hands, or signing their names. Persons feigning blindness often demonstrate difficulty with these tasks.

Trauma

I. Lacerations of the eyelids produce both a functional and a cosmetic injury. Careful examination of the lacrimal drainage system should be undertaken for all medial lacerations. Complicated lacerations of the lid margin and lacerations involving the canalicular system require a detailed closure which can be performed electively within 24–72 hours if the wound is kept moist and clean. End-to-end anastomoses of the canaliculus and lid margin are performed, with intubation of the lacrimal system to maintain patency during healing. Lacerations of the upper lid may require exploration of the levator aponeurosis if ptosis is present. Horizontal lacerations of the eyelid skin can be closed with 6-0 silk or nylon suture.

II. Corneal abrasions produce severe pain, photophobia, foreign body sensation, and tearing. Fluorescein staining of the abraded epithelium aids in defining the area of trauma. An abrasion does not penetrate Bowman's layer and typically will heal within 24–48 hours without scarring. A short-acting cycloplegic (e.g., cyclopentolate) will decrease painful ciliary spasm, and an antibiotic ointment will lubricate the epithelial surface and reduce bacterial flora during healing. A firm double patch over the closed eyelid for 24–48 hours will promote reepithelialization.

  A. Recurrent erosions of the corneal epithelium occur in some patients several weeks after minor trauma. The patient typically is awakened by eye pain and a foreign body sensation, which gradually improve after several hours. Examination shortly after the onset of symptoms discloses fluorescein staining in the area previously abraded. If sufficient healing has taken place prior to the examination, only very subtle intraepithelial lines or inclusions will be found. **Treatment** of the recurrent lesions is the same as that of traumatic abrasions; occasionally, troublesome lesions require a bandage contact lens to cover the epithelium for up to 3 months. The use of hypertonic saline 5% ointment at bedtime may prevent recurrence.

  B. Corneal abrasions associated with contact lens wear fall into two categories: those associated with anoxia and those associated with lens manipulation or lens debris. Treatment of either condition includes discontinuation of contact lens wear for several days, instillation of a topical antibiotic, and application of a firm eyepatch over the closed eyelid to promote healing. The lenses should be cleaned and sterilized. Any discomfort on reinsertion indicates the need for the lenses to be examined by the dispensing specialist.

III. Ocular lacerations can occur alone or in combination with other facial and head injuries. Careful examination is necessary to ensure that all injuries are identified. When injury is work-related, it is important to document whether safety glasses were worn at the time of injury. The prognosis is always uncertain with penetrating ocular injuries, because late complications may profoundly affect the outcome of even minor lacerations. Tetanus prophylaxis should not be neglected in any penetrating ocular injury.

  A. Conjunctival lacerations indicate the possible presence of a retained foreign body or injury to the globe. Fluorescein will highlight a conjunctival laceration, but frequently these injuries can be seen without difficulty with the slit lamp. When the examination has been completed, the eye should be covered with a protective metal or plastic shield. If the possibility of a retained foreign body cannot be ruled out by a detailed history and examination, x-ray (i.e., scout film and CT scan) or ultrasound studies should be obtained. Small (i.e., < 1 cm) conjunctival lacerations will heal without repair. If the laceration is large or if a laceration of the globe cannot be excluded, an ophthalmologist should explore the globe and close the laceration.

  B. Corneal lacerations can be penetrating or perforating.

   1. A **penetrating corneal laceration** is confined to the epithelial and stromal layers. The laceration is clearly defined by fluorescein staining. The anterior chamber is deep and the iris and pupil are normal. The Seidel test (see **Evaluation of Ocular Emergencies, sec. V.C**) demonstrates no leakage of aqueous through the wound. These injuries can be treated with antibiotic drops (not ointment, which may be incarcerated in the wound and delay healing) and a firm double eye patch.

2. With a **perforating corneal laceration,** the anterior chamber may be collapsed or shallow. The iris is frequently incarcerated in the wound or may plug the wound internally, allowing spontaneous reformation of the anterior chamber. The pupil typically is pulled toward the laceration by the incarcerated iris. The Seidel test will show streaming of aqueous through the wound. After examination for other injuries and retained foreign body is completed, a protective shield should be placed over the eye, and microsurgical repair by an ophthalmologist should be planned. Topical antibiotic eyedrops should be used only if a significant delay in surgical repair is anticipated; ointments should be avoided.

C. A **scleral laceration** or **ruptured globe** should be suspected in all cases of trauma with subconjunctival hemorrhage. The sclera is weakest at the limbus, under the rectus muscle insertions, and around the optic nerve, so occult scleral rupture can occur easily. Vitreous hemorrhage and a low IOP are frequently found. With scleral laceration, it is likely that retinal injury may be present or may develop as a late complication. The eye should be covered with a protective shield, and prompt ophthalmologic repair under general anesthesia planned.

IV. **Hyphema,** or bleeding into the anterior chamber, can occur with blunt or penetrating trauma.

A. **Clinical features.** Vision may be decreased by the blood in the visual axis or by an associated injury. Examination typically finds a layer of blood settled in the anterior chamber; and with a slit lamp, red cells can be seen circulating throughout the entire chamber. Acute bleeding may clear within hours, whereas continued or recurrent bleeding often remains for days. Occasionally, recurrent hemorrhage occurs as late as 7 days following the original injury and is often more severe.

B. **Management.** All acute traumatic hyphemas should be treated with bed rest and daily ophthalmologic follow-up during the week following injury. A protective shield should cover the eye to prevent further injury. Hospitalization and treatment with an antifibrinolytic agent (e.g., aminocaproic acid, 100 mg/kg/day in divided doses q4h up to a maximum of 5 gm/day) should be considered for children with severe contusion injury where recurrent hyphema is likely.

C. **Complications**

1. **Glaucoma.** With a severe hyphema or recurrent bleeding, the IOP may rise dramatically, resulting in acute glaucoma. Initial management includes administration of acetazolamide, 250 mg IV (5 mg/kg in children), and mannitol, 1.5 gm/kg IV. However, acute glaucoma from a hyphema responds poorly to medical management and may require surgical evacuation of the hyphema. A significant percentage of patients will develop glaucoma many years after injury.

2. **Optic atrophy.** Patients with sickle hemoglobin may be at increased risk for optic atrophy following hyphema with an increased IOP.

V. **Foreign bodies**

A. **Foreign bodies loosely embedded in the corneal epithelium** can be removed at the slit lamp with a cotton swab following instillation of a topical anesthetic. For removal of recalcitrant foreign bodies, a needle (held tangentially to the cornea) can be used. Careful examination of the conjunctival fornix and eversion of the upper eyelid should confirm the removal of all surface foreign bodies. Application of a topical antibiotic ointment, followed by a firm patch for 24 hours, typically results in prompt healing. A rust ring requires ophthalmologic referral within 1 week for removal.

B. **Penetrating foreign bodies** may occur, particularly in patients who were hammering metal on metal or working with power tools. There may be little initial discomfort and minimal signs of inflammation with a significant penetrating injury.

1. **Evaluation.** Direct visualization of a retained intraocular foreign body provides the most accurate localization and assessment of the degree of injury involved. An early dilated funduscopic examination may enable direct visualization of the foreign body before lens clouding or hemorrhage obscures the fundic details. Radiographic studies with both plain films and CT are essential to assure identification of all foreign bodies and to localize them when the ocular media is opaque.

2. **Management.** A culture of the conjunctiva should be gently obtained with a swab; and broad-spectrum IV antibiotic therapy (e.g., with a penicillinase-resis-

tant penicillin and an aminoglycoside) and tetanus prophylaxis (if indicated) should be administered. The eye should be covered with a protective shield, and the patient kept NPO while being referred to an ophthalmologist for surgery.

VI. Chemical injury. The prognosis for vision and the survival of the eye after chemical injury is directly related to the nature of the chemical involved and the immediacy of treatment. Acids precipitate proteins on the ocular surface and tend to be less toxic than alkalis, which penetrate the eye immediately and cause more severe injury. Immediate, copious irrigation with water or saline is mandatory, superseding the need to measure vision. Then, following instillation of a topical anesthetic, any toxic matter should be swabbed from beneath the eyelids, and the pH of the conjunctiva tested for any persistent abnormality (normal tear pH = 7.3–7.7). A white, ischemic conjunctiva or marbleized, hazy cornea indicates a poor prognosis. Cycloplegic eyedrops may be instilled and systemic analgesics administered, while ophthalmologic consultation for more specific therapy is obtained.

VII. Radiation injury from the ultraviolet light of a sunlamp or welder's arc produces a painful superficial keratitis, which develops several hours after exposure. Diffuse corneal punctate staining with fluorescein can be seen on slit-lamp examination. Therapy includes instillation of a short-acting cycloplegic (e.g., cyclopentolate) and a topical antibiotic and application of a firm double patch. A systemic analgesic is appropriate for control of pain. Healing typically is complete after 12–24 hours. Care should be taken to avoid repeated administration of a topical anesthetic, as this will delay epithelial recovery.

VIII. Contusion injury to the globe produces a wide range of injury.

    A. Mild contusions can produce a **traumatic iritis** with a few cells and flare in the anterior chamber. Instillation of a short-acting cycloplegic (e.g., cyclopentolate) is adequate therapy; steroid therapy is rarely necessary.

    B. Blunt trauma may damage or dislocate the lens with resulting refractive change or the formation of a cataract. Examination by an ophthalmologist within 24–48 hours is necessary to assess the need for surgery, if the lens capsule has been ruptured. When the natural lens is dislocated, surgery is rarely indicated; however, dislocation of an intraocular lens implant requires urgent ophthalmologic consultation and prompt surgical correction.

    C. Retinal edema is usually seen as a gray translucent area. No specific therapy is required. Follow-up by an ophthalmologist should be planned within a few days.

    D. Transmitted energy can result in a **retinal tear or dialysis** requiring surgical repair. Detection of these posterior injuries requires a dilated fundus examination with scleral depression. **Retinal detachment** may follow a retinal tear or dialysis, but detachment rarely occurs immediately with blunt trauma; it can be prevented from developing as a late complication by timely ophthalmologic referral for evaluation and possible treatment. This detailed examination is usually performed within several days of the injury when swelling and tenderness have lessened; for young children, it is performed under general anesthesia.

Bibliography

1. Bohigian, G. M. *Handbook of External Diseases of the Eye* (2nd ed.). St. Louis: DAC Medical Publishing, 1982.
2. Burde, R. M., Savino, P. J., and Trobe, J. D. *Clinical Decisions in Neuro-Ophthalmology.* St. Louis: Mosby, 1985.
3. Dawson, C. R., and Togni, B. Herpes simplex eye infections: Clinical manifestations, pathogenesis, and management. *Surv. Ophthalmol.* 21:121, 1976.
4. Forster, R. K., Abbott, R. L., and Gelender, H. Management of infectious endophthalmitis. *Ophthalmology* 87:313, 1980.
5. Freeman, H. M. *Ocular Trauma.* New York: Appleton-Century-Crofts, 1979.
6. Glaser, J. S. *Neuro-Ophthalmology.* Hagerstown, Md.: Harper and Row, 1978.
7. Grant, W. M. *Toxicology of the Eye* (2nd ed.). Springfield, Ill.: Thomas, 1974.
8. Kolker, A. E., and Hetherington, J., Jr. *Becker-Shaffer's Diagnosis and Therapy of the Glaucomas* (5th ed.). St. Louis: Mosby, 1983.
9. Paton, D., and Goldberg, M. F. *Management of Ocular Injuries.* Philadelphia: Saunders, 1985.
10. Pavan-Langston, D. (ed.). *Manual of Ocular Diagnosis and Therapy.* Boston: Little, Brown, 1980.
11. Peyman, G. A., Carroll, C. P., and Raichand, M. Prevention and management of traumatic endophthalmitis. *Ophthalmology* 87:320, 1980.

36

Pediatric Emergencies

Joseph G. Gibbons and
Robert M. Kennedy

Neonatal Care

In possibly the most crucial moments of life (i.e., the few minutes following delivery), a complex transition is made from fetal, placenta-based circulation to postnatal, lung-based circulation. Relaxation of the pulmonary vasculature and closure of the ductus arteriosus is induced by an increase in the arterial PO_2 and pH; thus, this transition is intimately tied to the establishment of adequate ventilation and circulation.

I. **Assessment** of the newborn in the delivery room is best carried out by observation of the parameters outlined in the Apgar scoring system (Table 36-1). This system provides a rapid, dependable, and familiar measurement of the infant's physiologic status. The 1-minute score correlates well with the pH of the umbilical cord arterial blood, whereas the 5-minute score correlates better with subsequent neurologic outcome.

II. **Initial management**
   A. **Infants with Apgar scores of 8, 9, or 10** exhibit no evidence of asphyxia and merely need to be dried, warmed, and gently suctioned using a bulb syringe in the nares and mouth. A suction catheter should not be used (except when there is thick meconium), as it may induce apnea or arrhythmias due to the extremely active vagal reflexes present at delivery.

   B. **Infants mildly asphyxiated** (i.e., Apgar scores of 5, 6, or 7). In addition to the above measures, these infants may benefit from free-flow oxygen held by the infant's face; however, unwarmed oxygen blown in the infant's face at a high flow rate may diminish the respiratory and heart-rate reflexes.

   C. If the infant does not respond to free-flow oxygen after a couple of minutes or initially exhibits **cyanosis, a weak tone, or a heart rate of less than 100/minute,** the infant is ventilated at a rate of 40/minute with a bag and mask using 100% oxygen and enough pressure to move the chest. Ventilation is continued until the infant is pink and the heart rate exceeds 100.

   D. **Neonatal cardiac arrest** (see **Cardiac Arrest**). If the infant is **deeply cyanotic and flaccid with a heart rate less than 60–80/minute,** endotracheal intubation is performed (after initially ventilating the infant with a bag-valve-mask device) using a 2.5-mm endotracheal tube (ETT) in an infant less than 1000 gm, or a 3.0-mm ETT in an infant greater than 1000 gm. Ventilation is then carried out using 100% oxygen at 40–60 breaths/minute and enough pressure to move the chest wall. Proper ETT placement should be verified by listening for good breath sounds bilaterally and later checking a chest radiograph. Simultaneously, external cardiac massage is begun at 120/minute with the fingers encircling the infant's chest and the thumbs compressing the sternum at a point just below a line drawn between the nipples. Often, adequate ventilation will be enough to revive the infant. However, if the heart rate continues to be low (i.e., < 80/minute) or absent, an assistant should place an umbilical venous catheter (UVC). This procedure is performed by cutting the umbilical cord 1–2 cm from the abdominal wall; identifying the large umbilical vein (the two arteries are smaller and in spasm); and after the prepping the umbilical stump with povidone-iodine, inserting a 3.5 or 5.0F UVC only 2–3 cm, so as not to inject hypertonic solutions directly into the small hepatic veins or the liver itself. After the catheter is secured, epinephrine, 0.01–0.03 mg/kg (0.1–0.3 ml/kg of a 1:10,000 solution), and sodium bicarbonate, 1 mEq/kg as a half-strength solution (0.5 mEq/ml), are administered as needed (Table 36-2). Dextrose, 0.5 gm/kg (2 ml/kg of 25% D/W), is given, since the neonatal glycogen reserves are small. Naloxone hydrochloride, 0.01 mg/kg IV, ETT, or IM, is administered if the mother received a narcotic analgesic prior to delivery. In the presence of suspected hypovolemia, volume expansion is indicated and may be accomplished by delivering 10 ml/kg of

Table 36-1. Apgar scoring system

Sign	0 points	1 point	2 points
Heart rate	0	< 100/min	> 100/min
Respiratory effort	Absent	Slow, irregular	Good, crying
Color	Blue, pale	Pink body, blue extremities	Pink
Muscle tone	Limp	Some flexion	Active movement
Reflex irritability (to catheter in naris)	None	Grimace, avoidance	Cry, cough, sneeze

normal saline of Ringer's lactate solution and blood (if needed) through the UVC over 5–10 minutes.

III. Specific problems

A. Persistent fetal circulation (PFC). If hypoxemia and acidosis develop after delivery, the fetal circulatory pattern may persist, bypassing the lungs via the foramen ovale and patent ductus arteriosus (PDA). PFC is a very serious situation with a high morbidity and mortality, and is most often seen in the term or postterm infant with meconium aspiration–induced hypoxia. At delivery, the infant appears ill with cyanosis, tachypnea, grunting, and acidosis. Tentative confirmation of PFC can be made by demonstrating a right-to-left shunt at the level of the ductus arteriosus. This shunt is demonstrated by finding a marked difference in PO_2 from arterial blood proximal and distal to the ductus arteriosus (e.g., arterial blood gases [ABGs] from the right radial artery and umbilical artery). The PO_2 will be significantly lower distal to the PDA due to the admixture of blood bypassing the lungs. Hyperventilation with 100% oxygen will often relax the pulmonary vasculature and result in an increased PO_2, demonstrating that the cyanosis is not due to a fixed shunt from a congenitally malformed heart. Once the diagnosis of PFC is seriously considered, mechanical hyperventilation should continue, keeping the PO_2 at or above 150 mm Hg and the pH above 7.45. A neonatologist should be consulted, and arrangements made for transfer to a neonatal intensive care unit (ICU).

B. Meconium aspiration by the newborn can be reduced by obstetric suctioning of the infant's hypopharynx after delivery of the head but prior to delivery of the thorax. If the meconium is thick (of pea-soup consistency), the infant should be intubated and suctioned below the vocal cords as rapidly as possible. Ten percent of infants with meconium below the vocal cords develop pulmonary air leaks with a pneumomediastinum or pneumothorax. If there is any evidence of respiratory distress, the infant should be observed and treated in a neonatal ICU.

C. Blood loss. Rarely, the newborn is hypovolemic from intrapartum blood loss from placental separation, avulsion of the umbilical cord from the placenta, placenta previa, an anterior placenta at cesarean section, twin-twin transfusion, or rupture of the liver or spleen due to a difficult delivery. The baby is tachycardiac (with a heart rate at or above 180/minute), tachypneic, and hypotensive with poor capillary refill and weak pulses. Initially, the hematocrit may be normal. Transfusion with O-negative packed red blood cells (RBCs) may be given emergently in a volume of 5–20 ml/kg over several minutes via a UVC. If blood is not immediately available, autologous cord blood from the placenta may be obtained emergently.

D. Infection. The neonate poorly localizes infection and is especially prone to sepsis. Common pathogens are group B streptococcus, *Escherichia coli, Klebsiella,* and *Staphylococcus aureus.* Indications for blood, cerebrospinal fluid (CSF), and urine cultures and for administration of IV antibiotics are fever or hypothermia, persistent respiratory distress, rupture of the amniotic membranes for more than 24 hours prior to delivery, unexplained lethargy or irritability, or almost any other abnormal sign. Recommended initial antibiotics are usually ampicillin and kanamycin or gentamicin. Herpes simplex infection can also be devastating to the neonate. Suspected infection or exposure requires immediate consultation with a neonatologist.

E. Respiratory distress (i.e., a respiratory rate > 60/minute) is a common symptom in the newborn. Infection, aspiration, malformation, obstruction, and pneumothorax are a few of the problems that can cause tachypnea and grunting respirations. Fortunately, many of these babies have transient tachypnea that resolves over 4–12

Table 36-2. Cardiac drugs in children

Drug	Route	Dose	Indication	Untoward effects	Comments
1. Atropine sulfate	IV, EIT	0.02 mg/kg (minimum of 0.1 mg/dose and maximum of 1.0 mg/dose) q5min prn to a maximum total dose of 1.0 mg in a child or 2.0 mg in an adolescent	Bradycardia accompanied by poor perfusion or hypotension, symptomatic bradycardia with AV block, ventricular asystole, vagally mediated bradycardia during intubation	Paradoxical bradycardia, tachyarrhythmias	It is important to give a vagolytic dose, since smaller doses may produce a paradoxical bradycardia
2. Bretylium tosylate	IV	5-mg/kg bolus, followed by 10 mg/kg q15min prn to a maximum of 30 mg/kg	Refractory ventricular fibrillation, refractory ventricular tacycardia	Nausea, vomiting, hypotension, bradycardia, arrhythmias	Bretylium should be considered a secondline drug behind lidocaine in the treatment of ventricular fibrillation or tachycardia
3. Calcium Calcium chloride 10%	IV	20 mg/kg (0.2 ml/kg) (maximum of 200 mg/dose) q10min prn (preferably according to calcium measurements)	Hypocalcemia, hyperkalemia, hypermagnesemia, calcium-channel blocker overdose	Asystole, potentiation of digitalis-related arrhythmias, bradycardia	Efficacy in electromechanical dissociation and asystole is lacking; calcium must be infused slowly
Calcium gluconate 10%	IV	100 mg/kg (1 ml/kg) (maximum of 1 gm/dose) q10min prn (preferably according to calcium measurements)			
4. Dextrose	IV	0.5–1.0 gm/kg (2–4 ml/kg of 25% D/W), followed by infusion of 5–10% D/W	Hypoglycemia	Hyperglycemia, hyperosmolality	
5. Dobutamine hydrochloride	IV	Usually 5–15 μg/kg/min, titrated to desired effect*	Poor myocardial function with decreased cardiac output	Ventricular ectopy, tachyarrhythmias	Dobutamine increases myocardial contractility with little change in peripheral vascular resistance

Drug	Route	Dose	Indication	Adverse effects	Comments
6. Dopamine hydrochloride	IV	Usually 2–20 µg/kg/min, titrated to desired effect*	Hypotension or poor perfusion with good electrical activity	Ventricular ectopy, tachyarrhythmias, nausea, vomiting, vasoconstriction	Alpha-adrenergic action predominates at 15–20 µg/kg/minute
7. Epinephrine	IV, ETT	0.01 mg/kg (0.1 ml/kg of 1:10,000 solution) (maximum of 5 ml/dose) q5min prn; also, infusion of 0.1–1.0 µg/kg/min, titrated to desired effect*	Asystole, hemodynamically significant bradycardia, hypotension, ventricular fibrillation (to enhance defibrillation)	Ventricular ectopy, tachyarrhythmias, ventricular fibrillation, vasoconstriction compromising tissue perfusion	Epinephrine infusion is useful in the treatment of (1) hypotension or poor perfusion (following restoration of spontaneous circulation) or (2) hemodynamically significant bradycardia resistant to atropine; epinephrine may be preferable to dopamine in the child (particularly an infant) with marked circulatory instability
8. Isoproterenol hydrochloride	IV	0.1 µg/kg/min initially, followed by increasing the infusion by 0.1 µg/kg/min q10min prn to a maximum of 1.0 µg/kg/min*	Hemodynamically significant bradycardia resistant to atropine, severe bronchospasm	Hypotension, tachyarrhythmias, myocardial ischemia	As a pure beta-adrenergic agonist, isoproterenol decreases coronary perfusion pressure and increases myocardial oxygen demand; it has no role in the treatment of asystole
9. Lidocaine	IV, ETT	1.0 mg/kg as an initial bolus, repeated q5–10 min prn to a maximum of 5 mg/kg or 225 mg and followed by an infusion of 20–50 µg/kg/min*	Ventricular tachycardia, ventricular fibrillation, premature ventricular complexes	Nausea, vomiting, altered mental status, seizures, myocardial depression, heart block	The infusion rate should be reduced in the presence of shock, congestive heart failure, liver disease, or cardiac arrest because of impaired drug clearance in these conditions
10. Naloxone hydrochloride	IV, ETT, IM	0.01 mg/kg prn	CNS depression, respiratory depression, or hypotension secondary to opioids	None	Since the duration of action of opioids may exceed that of naloxone, continued surveillance of the child is required

Table 36-2. (continued)

Drug	Route	Dose	Indication	Untoward effects	Comments
11. Norepineph-rine bitar-trate	IV	0.1 µg/kg/min initially, titrated to desired effect (0.1–1.0 µg/kg/min)*	Poor perfusion with good electrical activity	Ventricular ectopy, tachyarrhythmias	
12. Oxygen	Mask, ETT	100%	All arrests	None	Adequate ventilation is essential and of primary importance
13. Sodium bicarbonate	IV	1 mEq/kg q10 min prn (preferably according to ABGs)	Metabolic acidosis (with adequate ventilation), hyperkalemia	Metabolic alkalosis, hypernatremia, hyperosmolality	
14. Verapamil	IV	0.1 mg/kg over 2 min, repeated in 10–30 min prn	Supraventricular tachycardia	Hypotension, bradycardia, tachycardia	Contraindicated in the presence of severe hypotension, congestive heart failure (unless secondary to a tachycardia amenable to verapamil therapy), atrial fibrillation or flutter in association with an accessory bypass tract, or recent IV administration of a beta-adrenergic blocking agent

*Infusion rates/body weight are presented in Appendix C.
Source: Adapted from American Heart Association, Standards and guidelines for cardiopulmonary resuscitation (CPR) and emergency cardiac care (ECC). *J.A.M.A.* 255:2905, 1986.

hours, and the infants show no other untoward signs of illness. The etiology may be slow alveolar clearing of aspirated fluid or lack of mechanical expulsion of fetal pulmonary fluid following cesarean delivery.

F. **Hyaline membrane disease** occurs in 0.5–1.0% of all deliveries and is seen in at least 10% of premature infants, especially those weighing 1000–1500 gm. Insufficient pulmonary surfactant results in atelectasis and decreased lung compliance. Many of the infants have trouble initiating normal respiration or begin grunting in an attempt to open collapsed alveoli. Cyanosis on room air, nasal flaring, and intercostal retractions are all commonly seen. A chest radiograph reveals a reticulogranular ground-glass appearance with air bronchograms; because this appearance cannot be distinguished from pneumonia, antibiotics usually are employed. If hood oxygen is inadequate in correcting hypoxemia, hypercapnia, and acidosis, intubation and assisted ventilation are required. Since the respiratory distress usually worsens over the next 3 or 4 days before improving, the infant should be transferred to a neonatal ICU for further care.

G. Neonatal **seizures** can be quite subtle due in part to the lack of anatomic cortical organization needed to propagate and sustain a generalized seizure and in part to the possibility that inhibitory synapses develop earlier than excitatory ones. Seizures in the neonate generally are not associated with serious respiratory or circulatory compromise, but prolonged electrical activity can seriously impair the brain's metabolism and the development of its deoxyribonucleic acid (DNA) and ribonucleic acid (RNA) content.

1. **Etiologies. Hypoxia** is the largest identifiable cause of seizures in the newborn. Other common etiologies of seizures during the first day of life include hypo- or hyperglycemia, effects from drugs used during labor and delivery, intra- or extrauterine infection, and subarachnoid hemorrhage from birth trauma. Subsequently, drug withdrawal from maternal addiction, developmental malformations, intracranial hemorrhage, and metabolic disorders (e.g., hyponatremia, hypocalcemia, urea cycle defects) are likely causes.

2. **Evaluation** usually includes determination of a complete blood count; serum electrolytes, calcium, phosphorus, magnesium, glucose (including a Dextrostix determination), and ammonia; and an ABG. In addition, cultures of blood, CSF, and urine are obtained. Further evaluation using an electroencephalogram (EEG) and ultrasound or computed tomography (CT) scan of the head is usually indicated after the seizures are controlled.

3. **Treatment**

   a. Seizures are controlled with administration of appropriate **substrates** as indicated. For hypoglycemia (with a serum glucose < 30 mg/dl), dextrose, 200 mg/kg, is given IV as a bolus and followed by 250–500 mg/kg/hour as indicated. Because hypoglycemic seizures can be stopped with anticonvulsants, measurement of the serum glucose with Dextrostix is crucial as the initial evaluation. Hypocalcemic seizures are treated with calcium gluconate, 200 mg/kg IV over 15 minutes. If routine laboratory tests are normal, a trial dose of pyridoxine (vitamin B_6), 100 mg IV, may be used, although pyridoxine deficiency is rare.

   b. **Anticonvulsants.** If seizures persist, phenobarbital, 20–30 mg/kg IV, or phenytoin, 20 mg/kg IV, is administered; this loading dose is followed by a maintenance dose of 3–5 mg/kg/day IV, given q12h. Because of differing hepatic and renal function in the neonate, serum anticonvulsants levels are essential.

   c. Because of the risk of infection, **antibiotic coverage** is initiated, pending culture results.

IV. **Referral to a neonatal specialty center.** When the decision is made that the infant is in need of more specialized care, a neonatologist at a specialty center is contacted. In preparation for transport, particular care is taken to correct hypoxia, hypovolemia, and acidosis; and a neutral thermal environment is provided. Copies of the mother's and infant's charts, 5 ml of the mother's clotted blood, and copies of x-rays are sent with the infant. Whenever possible, the best means of transport is in utero.

Cardiac Arrest (See Chap. 2)

Cardiac arrest in children is often secondary to a primary respiratory arrest. In contrast to adults, primary arrhythmias as a cause of arrest in children are rare. Common causes of respiratory arrest include pneumonia, aspiration, bronchiolitis, asthma, epiglottitis, and foreign body obstruction. Central nervous system (CNS) disorders (e.g., trauma, meningitis, seizures) and cardiovascular disorders (e.g., septic shock, congenital heart disease, severe dehydration) account for the majority of the other causes of childhood cardiorespiratory arrest. Over half of these patients are less than 1 year of age. If the arrest occurs while under close medical supervision (i.e., in the hospital), the survival rate may be greater than 50%. Outpatient victims do much worse, with a 3–30% survival rate without sequelae.

I. **Primary priorities** in children, as in adults, include establishment of an airway, breathing, and circulation. Determination of a cardiorespiratory arrest in the child is made by noting cyanosis or pallor, lack of respiratory effort, and lack of a palpable pulse in the brachial or femoral areas.

A. **Airway management.** Because airway obstruction is frequently the precipitating cause of the arrest, particular attention should be paid to securing the airway.

1. **Initial maneuvers.** The child is placed in the supine position (with care if a cervical spine injury is suspected), and the airway is opened by performing a standard airway maneuver (i.e., head tilt–chin lift or jaw thrust); the jaw thrust without head tilt is the safest technique when neck injury is possible. In opening the airway, hyperextension of the neck should be avoided, as it is unnecessary and may cause tracheal collapse in young children. Rescue breathing is then initiated in the nonbreathing child by the mouth- or mask-to-mouth technique. In the very young child, both the mouth and nose are covered by the rescuer's mouth or mask. Two slow breaths (1.0–1.5 seconds/breath) are given, using chest wall movement to judge patency of the airway and efficacy of ventilation. If the child makes no spontaneous respiratory attempts after these initial rescue breaths, preparation is made for endotracheal intubation while rescue breathing continues at the rates described in **B.**

2. **Endotracheal intubation** (see Chap. 38). In the infant, the larynx is located more anteriorly and cephalad, and the epiglottis is relatively shorter than in the adult. For intubation, the child is placed in the supine "sniffing" position. A laryngoscope with a No. 1 straight Miller blade is generally adequate for a term newborn up to 2 years of age; a No. 2 straight Miller blade is used thereafter until adolescence. Care is taken to protect the fragile gums or teeth as the laryngoscope is introduced with the left hand. The tip of the blade may be positioned either in the vallecula or directly under the epiglottis, keeping the tongue well to the left. The laryngoscope is then lifted, without tilting, revealing the glottic opening. Gentle downward pressure exerted externally on the larynx may help bring the vocal cords into view. Because of the natural subglottic narrowing in infants and children, an uncuffed ETT is used until the age of 8–10 years. The proper ETT size in millimeters can be estimated by taking the patient's age in years, adding 16, and then dividing that sum by 4 (e.g., a 4-year-old child would take a 5.0-mm inside-diameter [ID] ETT). A term newborn requires a 3.0-mm ID ETT, and a 6-month old infant requires a 3.5-mm ID ETT. The ETT size can also be estimated by the size of the child's little finger. Endotracheal tubes larger and smaller by 0.5-mm increments should also be immediately available when attempting intubation. Care is taken when inserting the ETT that undue pressure is not used to force it through the vocal cords. The ETT is inserted only a short distance (usually 3–4 cm) beyond the vocal cords in order not to pass the carina and enter a mainstem bronchus (a common error). Correct positioning of the tube should then be checked by auscultating the chest for equal breath sounds, visualizing chest wall movement versus stomach distention, and, as soon as is practical, obtaining a chest radiograph. With an uncuffed tube, a small air leak through the vocal cords is desirable at ventilatory pressures greater than 20–30 cm H_2O. A nasogastric tube is inserted after intubation to relieve gastric distention and remove gastric contents.

B. **Ventilation.** A ventilatory bag with 100% oxygen is used initially, generating enough pressure to move the patient's chest wall. The rescue ventilatory rate is approximately 20/minute in the infant and 16–20/minute in the child. Often hyperventilation is useful initially to counter the combined respiratory and metabolic acidosis.

C. **Circulation.** If ineffective cardiac output is determined by pallor and lack of a palpable pulse (at the brachial, carotid, or femoral artery), **external cardiac massage** is begun. A precordial chest thump is not used in children because of the higher risk of internal organ damage. Cardiac compressions in infants are performed on the sternum at a site centered about 2 fingerbreadths below a line connecting the nipples; compression to a depth of about 1.3–2.5 cm can be accomplished either by applying 2 or 3 fingers to the sternum with the patient on a backboard or by encircling the chest with both hands and compressing the sternum with both thumbs. In young children, compressions to a depth of about 2.5–3.8 cm are performed with the heel of one hand placed on the sternum, with the lower edge of the hand about 1 fingerbreadth above the lower costosternal notch. In children older than about 8 years, cardiac compressions should be performed as described for adults (see Chap. 2). Care must be taken to stay on the sternum and not be overly vigorous with compressions, as separation of the ribs from their cartilage can occur with perforation of a lung or the liver. Compression rates are generally 100–120/minute for infants and 80–100/minute for children. Ventilation (1.0–1.5 seconds/breath) is interposed after every fifth compression.

II. Secondary priorities

A. IV access is essential for support of the cardiovascular system with stimulant drugs and isotonic solutions. However, venous access in infants and children can be difficult; and in a cardiopulmonary arrest, time should not be wasted by persistence in trying to gain percutaneous access if this is not readily accomplished. In this situation, the saphenous or femoral vein should be cannulated via a cutdown. Temporary access for administration of fluids and drugs can be achieved via the **intraosseous route** by placing a large-bore metal needle directly into the medullary cavity of the proximal tibia. Since subclavian and internal jugular lines are difficult to place and fraught with complications in younger children, they should be avoided.

B. Fluid and drug therapy (see Chap. 2). After IV access is established, the cardiovascular system is supported using (1) the drugs listed in Table 36-2 as needed and (2) isotonic solutions, such as lactated Ringer's (LR) or normal saline (NS), each with 5% dextrose added. Initially, a bolus of 5% D/WLR or 5% D/WNS at 20–30 ml/kg of the patient's body weight is given intravenously to treat hypotension. This bolus is repeated as indicated by serial blood pressures. When the blood pressure returns to the normal range, the rate of infusion of fluid is decreased to the maintenance rate (i.e., 1500 ml/M^2/day), and the electrolyte content is altered as indicated by the measured serum electrolytes. Supplemental potassium is withheld from the IV fluids until urine production is confirmed and serum potassium levels are determined to be normal or low. Of note is that epinephrine, lidocaine, and atropine are well absorbed when delivered via the ETT and may even have a more sustained effect than when given intravenously. Thus, these drugs can be given initially via the ETT while IV access is being established.

C. Defibrillation (see Chap. 2) is rarely needed in pediatric cardiac resuscitation due to the rarity of ventricular fibrillation. However, if required, 4.5-cm diameter paddles are used for infants, and 8-cm diameter paddles for older children. An initial dose of 2 joules/kg is used. If this dose is ineffective, it can be doubled, and defibrillation attempted again. If still ineffective, drug therapy (e.g., administration of epinephrine, sodium bicarbonate, and/or lidocaine is also required.

Foreign Body Obstruction (see Chap. 2)

In infants and children, aspiration of a foreign body is a common occurrence and may lead to cardiac arrest. In fact, cardiac arrest from airway obstruction is much more common than from primary cardiac causes. It is important to differentiate upper airway obstruction due to a foreign body from other causes (e.g., epiglottitis, croup) in order to initiate proper therapy. This differentiation can usually be made on clinical grounds, with foreign body obstruction being suspected in the previously healthy child who choked while eating or playing with small toys.

I. Upper airway obstruction with adequate ventilation. In this situation, the child usually is capable of breathing, making sounds, and coughing. Attempts at removing the foreign body under these circumstances may convert a partial airway obstruction into a complete obstruction and are not recommended. Appropriate diagnostic tests (e.g., soft-tissue neck x-rays) and specialty consultation are indicated.

II. Upper airway obstruction with inadequate ventilation

A. Conscious victim

1. In the **conscious child** older than 1 year of age, abdominal thrusts (see Chap. 2) are delivered in rapid sequence until the foreign body is dislodged or the child becomes unconscious. In small children, abdominal thrusts must be performed gently.

2. In the **conscious infant** less than 1 year of age, four back blows are delivered by straddling the infant over the rescuer's arm with the head positioned below the

trunk and applying the back blows with the heel of the rescuer's hand between the infant's shoulder blades. If this series of back blows is unsuccessful, the infant is turned over and four chest thrusts are delivered in the same manner as external chest compressions but at a slower rate. This sequence of back blows and chest thrusts is repeated until the victim becomes unconscious or the airway obstruction is relieved.

B. In the **unconscious victim,** an attempt should be made to open the airway by performing a standard airway maneuver (see Chap. 2) and to ventilate the patient. If this procedure is unsuccessful, in children older than 1 year of age, 6–10 abdominal thrusts are delivered. In infants less than 1 year of age, four back blows followed by four chest thrusts are delivered. If there is no response and proper equipment is readily available, removal of the obstructing foreign body with a clamp or forceps under direct visualization with a laryngoscope should be attempted. In the absence of proper equipment, manual removal should be attempted only if the foreign body can be visualized after performing a tongue-jaw lift maneuver (see Chap. 2); blind manual removal of a foreign body (by finger sweeps) is not recommended in infants and children. If these attempts fail, an airway must be established without delay distal to the site of obstruction by percutaneous transtracheal catheter ventilation (see Chap. 38), cricothyrotomy (see Chap. 38), or tracheostomy.

Asthma

Asthma is a syndrome of complex reversible airway obstruction due to diffuse hyperreactivity of the lower airways in response to various stimuli (e.g., extrinsic allergens, viral respiratory infections, cigarette smoke, exercise).

I. Pathophysiology

A. Pathophysiologic changes. Asthma is characterized by bronchial smooth muscle spasm; edematous mucosa; and excessive, tenacious secretions, all hindering airflow through the bronchi and bronchioles. Since the conductance of the airway is proportional to the radius raised to the fourth power, a small decrease in the already narrow airways in children causes a large increase in resistance. Moreover, the young child has only a small reserve for gas exchange and often presents to the emergency department in a more serious condition than older children. Children under 2 years of age tend to be more resistant to initial bronchodilator therapy, because edema of the bronchial mucosa and mucous secretions tend to predominate over bronchospasm.

B. Ventilatory and acid-base effects. Early in the acute asthma attack, diffuse but unevenly distributed airway narrowing tends to result in areas of alveolar hyper- and hypoventilation, creating ventilation-perfusion mismatching and subsequent hypoxemia. The concurrent hyperventilation initially results in hypocapnia and respiratory alkalosis; thus, early in the attack the child likely will have a low arterial PO_2, low arterial PCO_2, and a normal or elevated arterial pH. The respiratory alkalosis may be tempered by a metabolic acidosis resulting from decreased oral intake and increased lactic acid production resulting from the increased work of breathing. As airway obstruction progresses and the child begins to tire, alveolar hypoventilation worsens, leading to increased carbon dioxide retention; thus, an elevated or even normal arterial PCO_2 in asthma is an ominous sign indicating impending respiratory failure.

II. Differential diagnosis. In young children who present with their initial (or even subsequent) episode of sudden onset of wheezing or respiratory distress, other diagnoses must be entertained, e.g., bronchiolitis, aspiration of a foreign body, cystic fibrosis, and extrinsic airway compression from vascular rings or tumor. As in adults, a prior history of wheezing, a family history of asthma, absence of fever, and a chest radiograph revealing only hyperinflation help confirm a diagnosis of asthma.

III. Assessment

A. History. Important historic parameters include the duration of the attack, precipitating factors, current therapy, and a history of prior asthma and the course of those episodes.

B. Physical examination. Attention should be directed to the child's general appearance, activity, and mental status. Subjective dyspnea, wheezing, and the duration of expiration need to be assessed; however, they are not necessarily accurate indices of the severity of disease (e.g., an increase in wheezing may actually indicate improvement with increased air exchange). Sternocleidomastoid contraction and supraclavicular retraction appear to correlate with the degree of airway obstruction. When

Table 36-3. Respiratory scoring system

Parameter	0 points	1 point	2 points
PaO$_2$ (mm Hg)	70–100	≤ 70 in room air	≤ 70 in 40% O$_2$
Cyanosis	None	In room air	In 40% O$_2$
PaCO$_2$ (mm Hg)	< 40	40–65	> 65
Use of accessory muscles of respiration	None	Moderate	Marked
Air exchange	Good	Fair	Poor
Mental status	Normal	Depressed or agitated	Coma

Score
0–4: No immediate danger
5–6: Impending respiratory failure
7 or greater: Respiratory failure

Source: Adapted from D. W. Wood, J. J. Downes, and H. I. Lecks, A clinical scoring system for the diagnosis of respiratory failure. *Am. J. Dis. Child.* 123:227, 1972.

auscultating the chest, the degree of air movement and quality of breath sounds should be noted; distant or absent breath sounds in a patient with marked respiratory distress is an ominous sign. Pulsus paradoxus may be a useful indicator of airway obstruction but is often difficult to obtain in a frightened child. A moderate tachycardia prior to epinephrine administration is to be expected, but rates exceeding 150 beats/minute may indicate severe hypoxia or prior abuse of adrenergic drugs. Table 36-3 summarizes a scheme for evaluating respiratory distress.

C. **Laboratory studies**
   1. **ABGs** should be obtained from the child with moderate to severe obstruction, particularly if there is no improvement after initial therapy. As noted, a PCO$_2$ greater than 35 mm Hg and a pH less than 7.40 may be evidence of impending respiratory failure and the need for a more vigorous approach.
   2. A **serum theophylline level** should be obtained if the patient is taking a theophylline preparation. The therapeutic range is 10–20 μg/ml.
   3. A **complete blood count (CBC)** may reveal evidence of infection. However, an elevated white blood cell (WBC) count with neutrophilic predominance may be a response to epinephrine or steroids.
   4. A **chest x-ray** is usually needed only in the child with a severe attack, unless there is evidence of a pulmonary abnormality, such as unequal breath sounds or rales. In such situations, a chest radiograph may detect a pneumothorax, pneumomediastinum, evidence of foreign body aspiration, or pneumonia. Atelectasis is often present, making pneumonia difficult to diagnose.
   5. **Spirometry** is usually very difficult to perform in a frightened child and consequently is of little use.
   6. **Cultures** are obtained as indicated.
   7. **Serum electrolytes and BUN** may be helpful in severe attacks to evaluate the state of hydration. Although rare, the syndrome of inappropriate antidiuretic hormone (SIADH) has been noted in acute asthma attacks.

IV. **Emergency department management.** All therapy should be administered with close observation of the patient.
   A. **Oxygen.** Since all patients have some degree of hypoxia with the acute attack, all but the least ill, most playful children with acute wheezing will benefit from oxygen delivered by a face mask or nasal cannula. In the small child, parental help and reassurance are often required to keep the mask in place.
   B. **Fluids.** Since most children with acute asthma have had a decreased intake of fluids, the child is usually somewhat dehydrated. Encouraging fluids (e.g., juices) by mouth may be adequate in the mild or moderate attack. If it is determined from the history and physical examination that the child is dehydrated and unable to be rehydrated by increased oral intake, 20–30 ml/kg of 5% D/WLR or 5% D/WNS should be given intravenously over 30–60 minutes and followed by 5% D/W0.2% NaCl with 30–40 mEq/liter of potassium added, at a maintenance rate of 2.4 liters/M^2/day until the urine output is reestablished at 1–2 ml/kg/hour. There is no good evidence, however, that excessive hydration enhances removal of thickened bronchial secretions.

Table 36-4. Aerosolized beta agonists

Drug	Dose	Treatment interval
Isoetharine 1%	0.03 ml/kg (maximum, 0.5 ml)	q2–4h
Isoproterenol 1:200	0.02 ml/kg (maximum, 0.5 ml)	q4–6h
Metaproterenol 5%	0.01 ml/kg (maximum, 0.3 ml)	q4–6h

C. **Bronchodilators**
1. **Epinephrine.** A dose of 0.01 ml/kg to a maximum of 0.3–0.5 ml of a 1:1000 solution is given subcutaneously and repeated q20min as needed for a maximum of 3 doses. Children often react with restlessness, vomiting, and anxiety. If the child clears of wheezing, a sustained-release epinephrine (Susphrine), 0.005 ml/kg SC, can be given. Epinephrine should not be repeated earlier than 4–6 hours after the Susphrine dose.
2. **Aerosolized adrenergic agents.** Isoetharine (Bronkosol), isoproterenol (Isuprel), and metaproterenol (Alupent, Metaprel) are all commonly used bronchodilator aerosols. Although there are no clear, controlled standard treatment regimens for these agents, the commonly accepted dosages and intervals listed in Table 36-4 have been used successfully. Each agent is diluted in 1–2 ml of normal saline and delivered by aerosol with oxygen. Treatment is discontinued if the pulse exceeds 200/minute. Positive-pressure delivery should be avoided, since it can induce greater bronchospasm, a pneumothorax, or pneumomediastinum. Far more important than the agent or dosage is close monitoring of the pulse, chest examination, and subjective response to treatment.
3. **Theophylline.** Xanthine derivatives, especially theophylline, have long been used in the treatment of asthma and are thought to work by inhibiting phosphodiesterase degradation of cyclic adenosine monophosphate (cAMP), leading to relaxation of bronchial smooth muscle.
   a. The **therapeutic range** of theophylline has been found to be 10–20 μg/ml. Since individual pharmacokinetics vary widely with this drug and toxic reactions can be serious (e.g., seizures, arrhythmias), serum drug levels are essential for optimal usage of theophylline. Nausea and restlessness are often seen when the level approaches 20 μg/ml, but these symptoms are unreliable indicators of impending serious toxicity.
   b. **Dosages.** For persistent wheezing following initial therapy with beta agonists, administration of IV aminophylline is indicated. A general guideline is that 1 mg of aminophylline/kg body weight will raise the serum concentration by 2 μg/ml. Thus, if the patient is not taking theophylline, a loading dose of 5.0–7.5 mg/kg of aminophylline given IV over 20 minutes will result in a serum level of 10–15 μg/ml. A constant infusion of 0.65 mg/kg/hour in a child under 1 year of age, 0.85–1.00 mg/kg/hour in a child 1–10 years of age, or 0.85 mg/kg/hour after 10 years of age should maintain a constant serum theophylline level. If the patient is already on a theophylline preparation, a constant infusion can be started while awaiting the serum theophylline level. A repeat serum level 4–6 hours after the constant infusion is begun can be used to decide if the infusion rate needs to be changed or another bolus given. If a theophylline level cannot be obtained and the patient is on a low outpatient theophylline dosage (i.e., less than 6 mg/kg q6h), a loading dose of 2–3 mg/kg of aminophylline usually can be safely given IV over 20 minutes, and a constant infusion then begun.
4. **Steroids.** The mechanism by which steroids aid in combating asthma is still not clear, but several possibilities exist, e.g., an anti-inflammatory effect with reduction in airway edema, increased beta-adrenergic receptor activity, or prevention of reaccumulation of histamine in mast cells. The effects tend to take 12–24 hours to become clinically apparent. A short course of steroids is indicated in children receiving chronic theophylline therapy who have an acute exacerbation of asthma or in children in whom the attack is severe enough to require hospitalization. Dosages are listed in Table 36-5. Since a short course (i.e., < 1 week) of steroids does not cause significant adrenal suppression, they can be discontinued abruptly.
5. **Isoproterenol IV.** This drug has been found to be very effective in severe status

Table 36-5. Steroid therapy of asthma

Drug	Dose
Prednisone	1–2 mg/kg/day PO
Hydrocortisone hemisuccinate	10 mg/kg IV loading, followed by 10 mg/kg/day IV divided q6h
Methylprednisolone	1–2 mg/kg IV loading, followed by 1–2 mg/kg/day IV divided q6h

asthmaticus in children who fail to respond to conventional therapy. However, it should be used only by those experienced in its use because of the potential for producing serious arrhythmias and possibly myocardial necrosis. The electrocardiogram (ECG) and ABGs must be carefully monitored, and preparations made for immediate intubation and assisted ventilation, if required. The initial isoproterenol dose is 0.1 µg/kg/minute as a constant infusion. The infusion is increased in increments of 0.1 µg/kg/minute until (1) the arterial PCO_2 (monitored q20min) becomes less than 55 mm Hg or decreases by at least 10% from preinfusion levels, (2) the heart rate exceeds 200 beats/minute, or (3) arrhythmias develop.

6. **Mechanical ventilation.** The child with an arterial PCO_2 rising above 55 mm Hg and failing to respond to the above medical therapy may require ventilatory assistance. The dangers of a pneumothorax, pneumomediastinum, and extubation are great. Paralyzation and sedation of the child are usually required. Consultation with an anesthesiologist is recommended.

7. Sedatives are contraindicated, except in the intubated patient, because they impair the patient's mental status and respiratory drive.

V. **Disposition.** Most children with persistent wheezing after administration of subcutaneous epinephrine, one or two trials of an aerosolized beta agonist, and attaining an adequate serum theophylline level will require hospitalization. Other children generally can be discharged with arrangements for close follow-up.

VI. **Outpatient management.** Spirometry has demonstrated that even after wheezing has cleared, significant airway obstruction persists for up to 1 week after the acute attack. Therefore, the patient who clears of wheezing while in the emergency department should be maintained on a bronchodilator for at least 1 week. The usual bronchodilator of choice is theophylline. If the patient is already receiving adequate theophylline therapy as demonstrated by a serum level, metaproterenol, albuterol, or prednisone may be added. Cromolyn may be used prophylactically in the child old enough to inhale medications. In all cases, close follow-up is necessary for continued control.

A. **Theophylline.** Short-acting theophylline preparations (i.e., elixirs, chewables, non-sustained-release preparations) are well absorbed orally, with peak serum levels occurring in 1–2 hours.

1. **Dosages and preparations.** Patients 8–12 months old need 4 mg/kg q6h, children 1–9 years old need 5–6 mg/kg q6h, and those over 10 years of age need 4 mg/kg q6h. Since theophylline clearance is significantly prolonged in neonates, in children taking erythromycin, and in children with hepatic or cardiac disease, the maintenance dose should be reduced in such cases. Serum theophylline levels aid in adjusting dosages, especially in infants and adolescents. Elixirs and chewable preparations generally are bitter to taste and are often rejected by children. For those too young to swallow pills intact, an alternative in the form of sustained-release granules is now available. These granules can be mixed with a small amount of food, thus increasing patient compliance. However, 48 hours or more is required when using these preparations to reach a steady-state therapeutic level (five half-lives = 2.5 days). To overcome this problem, a short-acting preparation of 6 mg/kg and a sustained-release preparation (e.g., Somophyllin CRT, Theo-Dur Sprinkle, Slo-Phyllin Gyrocaps) in a dose of 8 mg/kg can be given concurrently as the initial dose in the patient not previously on a theophylline preparation or in one who has a serum theophylline level of less than 5 µg/ml. The patient can then be maintained on the sustained-release preparation at 8 mg/kg q12h, with a maximum dose of 300 mg q12h. Patients started on a sustained-release preparation should have the serum level checked in 1–2 weeks and periodically thereafter.

   2. Toxicity includes restlessness, vomiting, seizures, and arrhythmias.
B. **Metaproterenol,** a beta-adrenergic bronchodilator, is an alternative for children who tolerate theophylline poorly. It can also be used in conjunction with theophylline for better control of an acute attack; a sustained-release theophylline preparation can be used for chronic control, and metaproterenol added for exacerbations. The elixir is generally palatable to children. The dosage is 10 mg PO q6–8h in the child weighing less than 30 kg and 20 mg PO q6–8h in the child heavier than 30 kg. Toxicity is rare and consists of restlessness and a mild tachycardia.
C. **Albuterol,** a relatively selective beta$_2$-adrenergic bronchodilator, is rapidly gaining favor as a primary or secondary bronchodilator of choice because of its efficacy, palatability in liquid form, and low incidence of side effects. The dosage is 0.1 mg/kg PO q6-8h.
D. **Steroids.** A course of prednisone in a dose of 1–2 mg/kg/day for less than 1 week can be quite effective. Alternate-day therapy must be considered if chronic use is required; however, even this regimen may cause growth disturbances and is to be avoided if possible. Regular outpatient follow-up is essential if chronic steroid usage is prescribed.

Seizures

I. **Febrile seizures** are brief (i.e., < 15 minutes in duration), generalized, tonic-clonic seizures with loss of consciousness. The seizures often occur with the initial rise in the child's temperature and may be the first sign of illness. The correlation between the degree of fever and the likelihood of seizures is uncertain. Two to five percent of children will have at least one febrile seizure. The age range for these seizures is 4 months to 5 years, with a peak occurrence at 24 months. To qualify as a simple febrile seizure, there must be (1) no CNS infection, (2) no systemic metabolic disorder, and (3) no prior afebrile seizure disorder. Simple febrile seizures increase the risk of subsequent development of afebrile seizures (i.e., epilepsy) by two- to three-fold. The risk of later epilepsy is increased by up to 20-fold in those patients with a preexisting neurologic abnormality, a family history of afebrile seizures, or a febrile seizure that was prolonged (i.e., > 20 minutes in duration) or focal. The risk of a recurrent febrile seizure is 30–50%, with 90% of recurrences occurring within 18 months of the first seizure. Recurrences of simple febrile seizures only slightly increase the risk of later epilepsy.
A. The **differential diagnosis** includes meningitis, hypoglycemia, electrolyte abnormalities (especially hyponatremia and hypocalcemia), head trauma, poisonings, and idiopathic epilepsy.
B. **Assessment**
   1. **History.** The convulsion is often the first sign of illness in the child. Information concerning other etiologies of seizures (e.g., exposures, diarrhea, water intoxication, drugs in the household) should be sought.
   2. **Physical examination.** Usually by the time the child is seen in the emergency department, the short postictal period is past, and the child appears alert and active, although febrile. The cause of the fever is often otitis media or a nonspecific viral syndrome. A bulging fontanel and resistance to neck flexion should especially be sought.
C. **Laboratory studies.** A CSF examination; serum electrolytes, glucose, and calcium; and a CBC are usually performed. Electroencephalography (EEG) is not usually done, as it generally is not helpful in predicting recurrent seizures or subsequent epilepsy. A frankly epileptiform EEG obtained several days after the seizure, however, suggests a diagnosis of epilepsy.
D. **Treatment**
   1. If the history, physical examination, and appropriate laboratory studies confirm that the convulsion was indeed a simple febrile seizure, **treatment of the source of fever and proper use of antipyretic agents** are usually all that is needed. The parents should be reassured and given first-aid instructions for possible subsequent seizures.
   2. **Anticonvulsants prophylaxis.** If the child is at significantly increased risk for later epilepsy (because of a neurologic abnormality, family history of epilepsy, or a prolonged or focal seizure), anticonvulsant prophylaxis with phenobarbital, 3–5 mg/kg/day, is advocated. The physician may also occasionally elect to begin anticonvulsant treatment when a child has had multiple febrile seizures or when the seizures occur in an infant under the age of 12–18 months. Prophylaxis is usually continued for at least 2 years or for 1 year after the last seizure,

whichever is longer. Intermittent phenobarbital therapy, which is started during febrile episodes, is ineffective, as several days are required to reach a therapeutic blood level.

E. **Disposition.** Hospitalization is usually required only for the child who has had a prolonged, complex seizure requiring IV anticonvulsants for control. These patients should be handled as described in the section on status epilepticus.

II. **Status epilepticus** (see Chap. 32) is defined as seizures that are so frequently repeated or prolonged as to create a fixed and lasting epileptic condition, usually of at least 30 minutes duration without recovery of consciousness between the episodes. Status epilepticus can involve any seizure type, but it is usually only the generalized seizures that represent a true medical emergency because of compromise of respiration, the CNS, and other vital functions.

A. **Etiologies.** Status epilepticus occurs in 5–10% of children with epilepsy. The peak incidence is within the first 3 years of life. In one large series of children with status epilepticus, 26% had an acute insult to the CNS in the form of infection, trauma, anoxia, or a metabolic or toxic derangement [1]. In 21% of the children, status epilepticus occurred in conjunction with a chronic encephalopathy or rapid discontinuation of anticonvulsants; in the remaining 53% of cases, no obvious etiology was uncovered, but approximately half of the children had fever secondary to a non-CNS-related infection [1]. Tumor or vascular insult as a cause of status epilepticus in children is rare.

B. **Prognosis.** The mortality in children with status epilepticus ranges from 5–25%, with death being secondary to the underlying disease, respiratory or cardiac insufficiency, or excessive use of medication. Neurologic sequelae in previously normal children can be as high as 50% and include mental retardation, focal motor deficits, behavioral disorders, and chronic epilepsy. In general, the younger the child, the more likely severe disability will result.

C. **Evaluation**

1. **History.** Information (preferably obtained by an assistant during the resuscitation) should be sought from the child's parents concerning possible etiologies. Particularly important are a history of prior seizures and anticonvulsants taken.

2. **Physical examination.** Evidence of trauma, cyanosis, or cardiac insufficiency is initially sought.

3. **Laboratory studies.** Immediate determination of the blood glucose with a Dextrostix or Chemstrip is indicated. Other tests generally include a serum glucose, electrolytes, calcium, magnesium, and creatinine. An ABG, CBC, and toxicology screen are also sent, if indicated. If the patient is already taking an anticonvulsant medication, rapid determination of the serum level of that medication will be helpful in management of the patient. Further laboratory studies as indicated by the history and physical examination (e.g., CSF examination, head CT scan) may be obtained after the seizures are controlled and the patient is stable.

D. **Management**

1. An adequate **airway** must be established. The child is placed on the side, an oral airway is inserted, secretions are cleared, and oxygen is administered by mask. Endotracheal intubation and assisted ventilation may be required.

2. **Monitoring.** The vital signs and cardiac rhythm are monitored closely.

3. An **IV line** is established, and an infusion of 5% D/WNS is begun.

4. If the Dextrostix reading suggests the presence of hypoglycemia, **dextrose,** 0.5–1.0 gm/kg (2–4 ml/kg of 25% D/W), is administered.

5. **Precautions** (e.g., padding the bed railings) are taken to prevent the child from injury from seizure activity.

6. **Anticonvulsant therapy.** Many pharmacologic agents exist for seizure control with varying combinations advocated. For generalized or focal motor status epilepticus compromising vital functions, the following approach generally enables control of the seizures without significant respiratory or cardiovascular depression. Since the goal is to control the seizures as rapidly as possible without further detriment to the patient, the drugs should be administered intravenously, allowing enough time between doses for an effect to take place.

a. **Diazepam (Valium).** Maximum brain concentration of diazepam is reached 1 minute after IV injection. However, redistribution out of the brain results in lower concentrations 45–60 minutes later. Diazepam, therefore, is short acting and must be followed by a longer-acting anticonvulsant, such as phenytoin or phenobarbital in a full loading dose. The dosage of diazepam is 0.2–0.5 mg/kg IV, given over a 2-minute period, with a maximum dose of 10 mg/injection. Side effects include sedation, hypotension, respiratory depression, laryngospasm, and cardiac arrest. Respiratory depression may be accentuated in a patient who has also received phenobarbital. The dose can be repeated in 15 minutes if the seizures are not terminated.

   b. **Phenobarbital.** Whether phenobarbital or phenytoin is used next depends on personal preference. The maximum brain concentration of phenobarbital occurs 3 minutes after IV injection, and clearance from the brain is slow. The dosage is 10 mg/kg IV, given at a rate not greater than 30 mg/minute; the dose can be repeated in 20 minutes. If seizures are still occurring after another 20 minutes, a third dose can be given for a total of 30 mg/kg. This amount inevitably causes significant sedation, and the patient should be monitored closely for respiratory depression. Initial maintenance therapy should be started later at 3–5 mg/kg/day. The therapeutic range for serum levels is 10–30 µg/ml.

   c. **Phenytoin (Dilantin)** is not highly sedative and thus enables a more accurate mental status evaluation. However, it may not be effective in controlling status epilepticus resulting from trauma, anoxic or metabolic encephalopathy, stroke or vascular disease, or a CNS tumor. The maximum brain uptake is 6 minutes after IV infusion. The dosage is 20 mg/kg IV infused slowly at a rate not greater than 30 mg/kg/minute. Side effects include hypotension and cardiac arrest from artrioventricular (AV) nodal block; however, cardiac arrhythmias are rare in children without preexisting heart disease. The initial maintenance dose is 5–7 mg/kg/day.

   d. If the combination of diazepam, phenobarbital, and phenytoin does not interrupt the status epilepticus, **lorazepam,** 0.05 mg IV (to a maximum of 2.0 mg/injection), may be used; the dose can be repeated in 15 minutes, if needed. Because of its rapid brain uptake and longer lasting brain levels, this benzodiazepine is also useful as a first-line drug (instead of diazepam) to control status epilepticus. The complications of its use are similar to those of diazepam (see **a**).

   e. **Paraldehyde** may be of benefit in terminating refractory seizures. The dosage is 0.3 ml (300 mg)/kg/dose dissolved in vegetable oil and given per rectum q4–6h. A glass syringe and red rubber rectal tube must be used. A discolored solution should not be used. Paraldehyde may cause cardiorespiratory depression. It is contraindicated in patients with hepatic or pulmonary disease.

   7. **General anesthesia.** Rarely, if the patient has severe lactic acidosis or hyperkalemia or if the motor activity impairs therapy, paralyzation with a curare agent may be required to stop the motor activity. Persistent brain electrical activity is then terminated with barbiturates. EEG monitoring is essential.

   E. **Disposition.** Admission and further evaluation and treatment are imperative.

Infectious Diseases

I. **Approach to the febrile child**
   A. **Fever** is defined as a rectal temperature greater than 38°C (100.4°F), an oral temperature greater than 37.8°C (100°F), or an axillary temperature greater than 37.2°C (99°F).

   1. **Temperature measurement.** The rectal thermometer is the most reliable and accurate means of measuring the body temperature. However, use of a rectal thermometer in uncooperative or active infants carries a risk of thermometer breakage and rectal perforation by the retained portion. In general, the axillary temperature is a reliable way to detect fever in all age groups. Forehead temperature strips, however, are not reliable.

   2. **Treatment of fever.** The main reason to treat a fever is to make the child more comfortable. Fever, by itself, is seldom harmful to the child. Untreated fevers do not continue to rise, and they do not cause brain damage. First-time febrile seizures (see **Seizures,** sec. I) are probably not preventable.

      a. An **antipyretic** should be used in the uncomfortable child with a fever. **Acetaminophen** and aspirin are available; both act by lowering the hypothalamic set point for body temperature, and both have equal antipyretic activity. However, acetaminophen is preferred by most pediatricians, be-

Table 36-6. Dosages of acetaminophen*

Age	Acetaminophen drops (80 mg/0.8 ml)	Acetaminophen elixir (160 mg/5 ml [tsp])	Chewable tablet (80 mg)	Adult tablet (325 mg)
0–3 mo	0.4 ml			
4–11 mo	0.8 ml	½ tsp		
12–23 mo	1.2 ml	¾ tsp	1½ tab	
2–3 yr	1.6 ml	1 tsp	2 tab	
4–5 yr	2.4 ml	1½ tsp	3 tab	
6–8 yr		2 tsp	4 tab	1 tab
9–10 yr		2½ tsp	5 tab	1¼ tab
11–12 yr		3 tsp	6 tab	1½ tab

*Doses can be repeated 4 or 5 times daily.

cause it is available in a liquid preparation for infants and young children and does not have the toxicity of aspirin in excessive doses. In addition, the American Academy of Pediatrics and the Centers for Disease Control do not recommend the use of aspirin in children with influenzalike illness or varicella because of a possible role in the etiology of Reye syndrome. There is no indication to use both acetaminophen and aspirin together or to alternate their use. Dosages of acetaminophen preparations are listed in Table 36-6.

    b. Sponging is also a useful way to reduce fever in infants. Thirty minutes after an antipyretic is given, the child should be placed in a shallow pool of lukewarm water (at 29.4°–32°C) and sponged with a wet washcloth. The child should not be immersed in the water. Rubbing alcohol should not be used for sponging because it is absorbed through the skin.

B. Febrile child less than 2 months of age

    1. General principles. The febrile child in this age group requires careful evaluation for serious and potentially life-threatening infections, including meningitis, pneumonia, urinary tract infection, and sepsis. Less commonly, cellulitis, septic arthritis, otitis media, omphalitis, congenital disseminated viral infections, and gastroenteritis cause fever in children this age. The following considerations apply to these infants:

        a. Since the **immune system** is immature in the newborn, the newborn is more likely to acquire infection and to have infection disseminate throughout the body. In particular, bacterial infection is seldom limited to one focus; multiple foci, including the blood, CSF, urinary tract, middle ear, and joints, are more common.

        b. Most **organisms** associated with serious infection are unique to this age group. These organisms include the following:

            (1) Group B streptococcus *(Streptococcus agalactiae)* is a gram-positive, chain-forming coccus found frequently in the healthy female gastrointestinal tract and vagina. Transmission to the infant most commonly occurs during passage through a colonized birth canal; chorioamnionitis also occurs with subsequent colonization and infection of the fetus. Group B streptococcus is the most common bacterial cause of sepsis, pneumonia, and meningitis in this age group.

                (a) Clinical features. Disease occurs in both an early-onset and a late-onset fashion. **Early-onset disease** occurs within the first week of life; and infants with a low birth weight, prematurity, or prolonged rupture of the amniotic membranes are at an increased risk for infection. The infant presents with respiratory distress, lethargy, shock, or other nonspecific signs of serious illness (Table 36-7). The chest x-ray usually reveals pneumonia, although the findings may be indistinguishable from the "ground glass" appearance of hyaline membrane disease. Meningitis and sepsis are also frequently present at diagnosis. **Late-onset disease** usually occurs in the first month of life and is uncommon beyond 2 months of age; it usually

Table 36-7. Signs and symptoms of infection in newborns*

Apnea	Hypothermia	Respiratory distress
Decreased activity	Hypotonia	Seizures
Decreased appetite	Inconsolability	Tachypnea
Fever	Irritability	Tachycardia
Full or bulging fontanel	Lethargy	
(with the infant held upright)		

*Less than 8 weeks of age.

presents with meningitis as its predominant feature, although sepsis and pneumonia are frequently also present.

    (b) Treatment. The organism is sensitive to penicillin and ampicillin. Some studies have shown synergistic activity with ampicillin and gentamicin.

   (2) *Escherichia coli* and other gram-negative enteric bacilli, including *Klebsiella pneumoniae,* cause neonatal sepsis and meningitis; *E. coli* is the second most common cause of meningitis in newborns. Transmission occurs by passage through a colonized birth canal; prolonged rupture of the membranes and a low birth weight are risk factors for infection. Disease is most common in the first 2 weeks of life and is rare in the normal host after 2 months of age. The antibiotic of choice depends on the sensitivities of the organism. The combination of ampicillin and an aminoglycoside or ampicillin and cefotaxime may be used as initial therapy. Many experts prefer the use of cefotaxime over an aminoglycoside because the former achieves higher concentrations in the CSF.

   (3) *Listeria monocytogenes* is a small gram-positive rod that causes sepsis and meningitis in neonates. Transmission is most commonly from a mother with *Listeria* chorioamnionitis or vaginitis. Ampicillin and an aminoglycoside should be used as initial therapy.

   (4) Herpes simplex virus, type I and type II, causes severe disseminated infection involving multiple organs, including the liver, eyes, skin, and brain. Transmission can occur transplacentally, during passage through an infected vagina, or postnatally by contact with a person with active oral lesions. Signs resemble those of bacterial sepsis. Infants with vesicular skin lesions, conjunctivitis, or a history of exposure should be evaluated for this disease. Present treatment consists of adenosine arabinoside; acyclovir is currently being evaluated in clinical trials. Since the morbidity and mortality in these infections are high, infants suspected of having this infection require referral to a tertiary care center for diagnostic evaluation and treatment.

   (5) Enteroviruses also cause disseminated infection in newborns. Infection can be acquired either congenitally or nosocomially, with a presentation similar to that of bacterial sepsis. Therapy involves supportive care; antiviral agents are usually not successful in reducing the morbidity and mortality.

  c. The **signs of infection** in newborns (see Table 36-7) are limited and frequently subtle. Any of these signs alone may represent severe illness.

2. Evaluation

  a. The **history** should include information about maternal vaginal infections, duration of rupture of amniotic membranes, and exposure to illnesses in the nursery or at home. Recent changes in activity, appetite, and sleep patterns should also be noted.

  b. Physical examination. The most important aspect of the evaluation is prolonged observation of the general behavior, feeding, and activity of the child while being comfortably held in the parent's arms. The vital signs are recorded, and the fontanel, eyes, ears, neck, lungs, heart, abdomen, joints, and skin are examined for signs of focal infection.

  c. Laboratory evaluation. All children less than 8 weeks of age with fever or other signs of illness require a urinalysis, chest radiograph, and blood cultures. A lumbar puncture (LP) must be performed on all of these patients; it is the only way to assess for meningitis in this age group. The WBC count and differential are not sensitive enough to be used as a screening test in these infants; however, leukopenia, leukocytosis, or thrombocytopenia may be an early sign of infection.

3. **Management.** Most pediatricians believe that the infant with fever or any other sign of illness should be hospitalized, given parenteral antibiotics, and observed for other symptoms, even if all the laboratory tests are normal. In general, ampicillin and an aminoglycoside are administered and continued for 2 or 3 days, pending a change in the infant's status and the results of the urine, CSF, and blood cultures. Specific treatment of various illnesses is discussed in other parts of this chapter.

C. **Febrile child older than 2 months of age**

1. **General principles.** Evaluation of these children is directed at identifying severe and life-threatening infections (especially meningitis, sepsis, and epiglottitis), other bacterial infections, and characteristic viral infections. Several considerations apply to children in this age group.

   a. **Organisms** responsible for severe infection in the infant and child include the following:

      (1) *Haemophilus influenzae* **type B** is a small gram-negative coccobacillus. It is the most common cause of bacterial meningitis in childhood. This organism is also one of the more frequent causes of pneumonia, septic arthritis, periorbital cellulitis, facial cellulitis, and epiglottitis in children from 1 month to 5 years of age. Infection begins when the child acquires the organism from another human by respiratory transmission and the nasopharyngeal mucosa is colonized. The organism then invades the bloodstream and may enter the CSF, lungs, or synovial fluid. Since as many as 30% of *H. influenzae* type B organisms are resistant to ampicillin, patients with suspected *H. influenzae* type B disease are usually placed on ampicillin and chloramphenicol, pending results of cultures and a beta-lactamase determination. Recently, cefuroxime, cefotaxime, and ceftriaxone have been used to treat *H. influenzae* type B infections, but experience with these newer agents is limited.

      (2) *S. pneumoniae* is a gram-positive diplococcus that can cause otitis media, pneumonia, sepsis, arthritis, and meningitis in children. It is sensitive to penicillin, erythromycin, and chloramphenicol; penicillin is the drug of choice in the nonallergic patient.

      (3) *Neisseria meningitidis* is a gram-negative diplococcus that causes sepsis and meningitis, frequently progressing rapidly to shock and death. Fever, petechiae, and purpura may be the only presenting signs. The organism is sensitive to penicillin or ampicillin; chloramphenicol is the drug of choice in the penicillin-allergic patient. All patients suspected of having *N. meningitidis* sepsis must be hospitalized and placed on an antibiotic, pending culture results.

   b. A syndrome of **bacteremia** exists in children 6–24 months of age. The pathogen, usually *S. pneumoniae* or, less commonly, *H. influenzae* type B, circulates in the bloodstream, causing fever and malaise in the child. In most cases, the organism is removed from the bloodstream by the body's immune system without antibiotic treatment. Occasionally, however, especially with *H. influenzae* type B, the organism continues to multiply, causing sepsis, or spreads to other areas of the body, causing meningitis, pneumonia, or septic arthritis. Approximately 5% of all febrile children between 6 months and 24 months of age who have a WBC count greater than 15,000/mm^3, an erythrocyte sedimentation rate (ESR) greater than 30 mm/hour, a fever greater than 40°C (104°F), or a combination of these factors have bacteremia. The indications for laboratory tests on febrile children are not well defined, and the disposition of the potentially bacteremic child is even more controversial. Use of oral antibiotic prophylaxis in children at high risk for bacteremia has had equivocal results.

   c. **Signs of serious illness** in children greater than 2 months of age are usually less subtle and more specific than in younger children. Nevertheless, it is often difficult to detect the degree of illness in fussy, febrile children. The following variables, when moderately or severely impaired, should be considered an indication of potentially severe illness: looking at the observer, looking around the room, sitting, moving arms and legs on a table or lap, movement in the mother's arms, vocalizing spontaneously, playing with an object, sucking a bottle, reaching for objects, stops crying when held by a parent, crying with noxious stimuli, smiling, crying with mild stimuli, and color [19].

2. Evaluation

    a. The **history** should include details of symptoms (e.g., respiratory distress, cough, otalgia, abdominal pain, dysuria) and the course of the illness. Exposure to illness and use of medications should also be recorded.

    b. Physical examination. The most important aspect of the physical examination is the overall assessment of the child's behavior while being comfortably held by a caretaker. This assessment should be performed over a sufficiently long period of time to ensure an accurate evaluation; a repeat examination after administering an antipyretic agent and/or after sponging the child is often extremely useful. After the overall assessment is completed, the fontanel, ears, throat, skin, neck, lungs, heart, abdomen, and other parts of the body are examined for signs of infection.

    c. Laboratory evaluation. The most common laboratory test ordered by pediatricians in evaluating a febrile child is a WBC count with differential. It must be emphasized that this test is an adjunct to the physical examination; a normal WBC count and differential does not rule out severe illness. A sedimentation rate (ESR) can be obtained when the WBC counts exceeds 15,000/mm^3 or when sepsis is a possibility. An LP should be performed in all children with a stiff neck, bulging fontanel, Brudzinski's or Kernig's sign, lethargy, or other signs of serious illness (see **1.c**). Other tests useful in localizing the source of a fever include a chest x-ray, throat culture, and urinalysis. Blood cultures generally are recommended for children with a temperature greater than 40°C (104°F), a WBC count greater than 15,000/mm^3, or an ESR greater than 30 mm/hour because of potential occult bacteremia.

3. Management

    a. Management of the **child with fever without a source** is controversial. The following recommendations are offered:

        (1) Children at risk for bacteremia (see **1.b**) but without signs of serious illness (see **1.c**) generally can be discharged but require close follow-up; parents should be given specific instructions regarding serious signs and instructed to return with the child at once if these develop. Infants with noncompliant parents should be hospitalized and observed.

        (2) Febrile children with signs of serious illness (see sec. **1.c**) should be considered as possibly septic; admitted to the hospital; evaluated with blood cultures, a chest x-ray, urinalysis, and an LP; and placed on antibiotics. Ampicillin and chloramphenicol or cefuroxime alone is most often used to assure coverage of *S. pneumoniae, H. influenzae* type B, and meningococcus. Antibiotics are usually continued until the blood cultures have had no growth for at least 2 or 3 days and the clinical course has improved.

        (3) Infants with a positive blood culture for *H. influenzae* type B or at high risk for infection with this organism (i.e., a positive latex agglutination test, positive outpatient blood culture, or recent significant exposure to *H. influenzae* type B) should be hospitalized; evaluated with blood cultures, a chest x-ray, urinalysis, and an LP; and given IV antibiotics effective against the organism.

    b. For the **child with fever and an identifiable source** of infection, treatment is directed at the source (see other sections of this chapter for specific therapeutic recommendations).

D. Antibiotic dosages for neonates and children are given in Tables 36-8 and 36-9, respectively.

II. Specific infections

    A. Pharyngitis (see Chap. 12)

        1. Etiology. Group A beta-hemolytic streptococcus *(Streptococcus pyogenes)* is the only common bacterial cause of pharyngitis. Viruses commonly associated with pharyngitis include the adenovirus, parainfluenza viruses, and Epstein-Barr (EB) virus (infectious mononucleosis). Infection with *Corynebacterium diphtheriae, N. gonorrhoeae,* or *Mycobacterium tuberculosis* is uncommon.

        2. Specific infections

            a. Streptococcal pharyngitis occurs most commonly in school children and

Table 36-8. Antibiotic dosages for neonates

	0–7 days of age		7–28 days of age	
Drug	Dosage[a,b] (mg/kg/day)	Dosing schedule (divided doses)	Dosage[a,b] (mg/kg/day)	Dosing schedule (divided doses)
Ampicillin				
Meningitis	150	3	200	4
Other diseases	75	3	100	4
Cefotaxime	100	2	150	3
Gentamicin	5	2	7.5	3
Kanamycin	20	2	30	3
Methicillin				
Meningitis	150	3	200	4
Other diseases	75	3	100	4
Moxalactam	100	3	150	3
Oxacillin	75	3	150	4
Nafcillin	50	3	75	4
Penicillin G				
Meningitis	150,000 units/kg/day	3	200,000 units/kg/day	4
Other diseases	50,000 units/kg/day	3	100,000 units/kg/day	4
Tobramycin	4	2	6	3

[a] All dosages listed are for IV use.
[b] Dosages apply only to infants greater than 2000 gm.
Source: Adapted from G. H. McCracken, Jr., and J. D. Nelson, *Antimicrobial Therapy for Newborns* (2nd ed.). New York: Grune & Stratton, 1983.

    rarely in children less than 2 years of age. It is most frequent in the winter and spring, especially in temperate and cold climates. The patient complains of a sore throat, mild malaise, and fever. On examination, the tonsils are enlarged, inflamed, and covered with a whitish-yellow exudate. The soft palate may have petechiae, and the anterior cervical lymph nodes are often enlarged and tender. An erythematous, blanching, sandpaperlike exanthem occurring on the trunk 24–48 hours after the onset of symptoms; the absence of laryngitis and rhinorrhea; the presence of tender, enlarged anterior cervical lymph nodes; or close contact with a person with proved streptococcal pharyngitis suggests a streptococcal etiology. Complications of streptococcal pharyngitis include a peritonsillar abscess, acute glomerulonephritis, and acute rheumatic fever. A throat culture generally should be obtained on all patients suspected of having streptococcal pharyngitis.

  b. Infectious mononucleosis, which is due to the EB virus, is associated with a mild headache, malaise, fever, and a sore throat. The tonsils are markedly enlarged and covered with exudate. Extensive lymphadenopathy occurs frequently in the anterior and posterior cervical chains, and splenomegaly may also be present. The presence of atypical lymphocytes in the peripheral blood or a positive serologic study (i.e., heterophile agglutinin or Monospot) confirms the diagnosis.

3. Treatment

  a. All patients with a throat culture positive for **group A beta-hemolytic streptococcus** should be treated with penicillin to prevent rheumatic fever. A single IM injection of benzathine penicillin (50,000 units/kg) or a full 10-day course of oral penicillin (25–50 mg/kg/day in 3 or 4 divided doses) is used. Oral erythromycin, 40 mg/kg/day in 4 divided doses to a maximum of 1–2 gm/day, is used in the penicillin-allergic patient. It is controversial whether treatment with penicillin changes the early course of the disease and whether treatment should be initiated prior to the culture results. Initiation of treatment should be on an individual basis, as determined by the likelihood of the diagnosis and the availability of the patient for follow-up.

Table 36-9. Antibiotic dosages for children

Drug	Route	Dosage (mg/kg/day)	Dosing schedule (divided doses)	Daily maximum dose (grams)
Amoxicillin	PO	30–40	3	2–3
Ampicillin				
Meningitis	IV	200–400	4–6	8–10
Other diseases	IV	100–200	4–6	8–10
	PO	50–100	4	2–3
Cefaclor	PO	40	3	1–2
Cefotaxime	IM, IV	100–200	3–4	8–10
Cefoxitin	IM, IV	80–160	4–6	8–12
Cefuroxime				
Meningitis	IV	200–250	4	4–6
Other Diseases	IM, IV	75–150	3	4–6
Cephalexin	PO	25–50	4	2–3
Cephalothin	IV	75–125	4–6	8–10
Chloramphenicol				
Succinate	IV	50–100	4	2–4
Palmitate	PO	50–100	4	2–3
Dicloxacillin	PO	12–25	4	1–2
Erythromycin	PO	40	4	1–2
Gentamicin	IM, IV	3.0–7.5	3	0.3
Kanamycin	IM, IV	15–30	3	0.75–1.00
Methicillin	IV	150–200	4	8–10
Moxalactam	IV	150–200	3–4	8–10
Nafcillin	IV	150	4	8–10
Oxacillin	IV	150–200	4	8–10
Penicillin G				
Benzathine	IM	50,000 units/kg	1 dose	2.4 million units
K^+ or Na^+	IV	100,000–250,000 units/kg/day	6	20 million units
Procaine	IM	25,000–50,000 units/kg/day	1–2	4.8 million units
Penicillin V	PO	25–50	3–4	2–3
Sulfisoxazole	PO	120–150	4–6	4–6
Tobramycin	IM, IV	3–6	3	0.3
Trimethoprim-sulfamethoxazole	PO	6–12/30–60	2	0.32/1.60

Source: Adapted from J. D. Nelson, *1985 Pocketbook of Pediatric Antimicrobial Therapy* (6th ed.). Baltimore: Williams and Wilkins, 1985.

    b. Patients with **infectious mononucleosis** are treated with bed rest and an analgesic, if needed. Ampicillin is avoided, because it may produce a maculopapular rash in these patients. If splenomegaly is present, abdominal trauma should be avoided. Rarely, steroids are given if the enlarged tonsils cause airway obstruction.

B. Acute suppurative otitis media (ASOM) (see Chap. 28)
    1. Etiology
      a. Children under 2 months of age
        (1) A sterile middle ear effusion is present in all children at birth, usually resolving within the first 10 days of life.
        (2) Bacteria. *S. pneumoniae*, *H. influenzae* (both nontypeable strains and type B), and group A beta-hemolytic streptococcus cause most infections. Less commonly, especially in premature infants and infants who have been on a ventilator in an intensive care unit, *E. coli*, *K. pneumoniae*, other gram-negative bacilli, or *Staphylococcus aureus* can cause infection.
      b. Children older than 2 months of age

(1) **Bacteria.** The most common agents are *S. pneumoniae* and *H. influenzae* (nontypeable strains and type B). Other organisms, including *S. pyogenes,* occur much less frequently.

(2) **Viruses** and **mycoplasmas** are rare causes of ASOM.

(3) **Sterile.** No organism can be recovered in as many as 50% of purulent effusions.

2. **Clinical features**

   a. **Signs and symptoms**

      (1) **Infants** most commonly present with mild irritability or fever. Asymptomatic infection is also common.

      (2) **Older children** most frequently complain of symptoms localized to the ear, especially otalgia.

   b. **Physical findings.** Visualization of the tympanic membrane is frequently difficult in the small child but can be enhanced by applying downward and inward traction on the ear lobe in infants and upward and outward movement on the auricle in older children. The tympanic membrane in ASOM is dull and bulging, with erythema of its borders and peripheral vessels. The light reflex is not present, and light is scattered diffusely across the membrane. There is little or no movement of the tympanic membrane with insufflation. Lack of mobility of the tympanic membrane may be the only sign of infection in neonates.

3. **Treatment**

   a. **Antibiotics.** A 10-day course of any of the following drugs can be used:

      (1) **Amoxicillin,** 30–40 mg/kg/day in 3 divided doses to a maximum of 2–3 gm/day, is the most commonly prescribed drug for ASOM. Ampicillin, 50–100 mg/kg/day in 4 divided doses to a maximum of 2–3 gm/day, may also be used.

      (2) **Trimethoprim-sulfamethoxazole (TMP-SMX).** TMP, 6–12 mg/kg/day, and SMX, 30–60 mg/kg/day, in 2 divided doses to a maximum of 320 mg of TMP/day and 1.6 gm of SMX/day offers coverage for ampicillin-resistant *H. influenzae* but does not eradicate *S. pyogenes* from the throat.

      (3) **Erythromycin-sulfisoxazole.** Erythromycin (40 mg/kg/day in 4 divided doses to a maximum of 1–2 gm/day) plus sulfisoxazole (120–150 mg/kg/day in 4 divided doses to a maximum of 4–6 gm/day) is available in a single suspension of 200 mg of erythromycin equivalent and 600 mg of sulfisoxazole equivalent/5 ml (Pediazole).

      (4) **Cefaclor,** 40 mg/kg/day in 3 divided doses to a maximum of 1–2 gm/day, covers ampicillin-resistant *H. influenzae* as well as *S. pneumoniae.*

   b. Since the signs of otitis media in neonates are indistinguishable from the signs of severe infection and since infection can spread rapidly in the newborn, these children should have (1) diagnostic tympanocentesis to assess for gram-negative enteric infection and (2) an LP and blood cultures to assess for spread to the spinal fluid and blood. IV antibiotics, initially ampicillin and an aminoglycoside, should be initiated, pending culture results, and continued for at least 10 days.

4. **Complications** of treated ASOM are uncommon. Either *S. pneumoniae* or *H. influenzae* type B in middle ear effusions can seed the bloodstream and produce bacteremia, sepsis, or meningitis. Children with continuing fever and children who develop other signs of serious illness (see sec. I) should be reexamined for these illnesses. Other complications of ASOM include tympanic membrane perforation, hearing loss, and mastoiditis.

5. **Disposition.** Neonates with ASOM require hospitalization. All others require follow-up in 2 weeks to demonstrate resolution of the effusion. They should be reevaluated sooner if their symptoms persist.

C. **Croup (laryngotracheobronchitis)** is a common disease of childhood characterized by inspiratory stridor and respiratory distress. It occurs in the first to fourth years of life, primarily in the autumn and winter. Pathologically, there is a variable degree of subglottic inflammation and fibrinous exudate in the larynx and trachea.

   1. **Etiology.** Parainfluenza (types I, II, and III) is the major cause of the infection. Influenza A and B, respiratory syncytial virus (RSV), and adenovirus occur less commonly.

   2. **Clinical features.** The disease begins with several days of a mild upper respiratory tract infection that progresses to tachypnea and inspiratory stridor. The most prominent symptom is a "croupy" cough, which resembles the bark of a

seal. Severe retractions, restlessness, anorexia, pallor, and cyanosis may develop and are signs of worsening distress. Decreased retractions and stridor with listlessness also suggest worsening disease.

3. The **differential diagnosis** includes a tracheal foreign body, esophageal foreign body, epiglottitis, bacterial tracheitis, and congenital anomalies of the airway. In particular, croup is distinguished from epiglottitis by a lack of the following (all of which are characteristic of the latter): drooling, an erect and forward head position, and rapid progression of symptoms. **Spasmodic croup** is a poorly understood entity that is probably not associated with direct viral infection of the subglottic area. The infant usually awakens suddenly at night with dyspnea, a cough, and stridor and is usually afebrile. The symptoms tend to recur on successive nights, with few symptoms present during the daytime. Gentle comfort and mist therapy relieve the distress in most cases.

4. **Radiographs,** although not necessary in most cases, should be obtained in children with moderate to severe distress and in children with unusual historic or physical features. In such situations, posteroanterior (PA) and lateral radiographs of the neck can be used to confirm the diagnosis and exclude other causes of actue stridor. In croup, the normal "squared" configuration of the subglottic area on the PA x-ray is replaced by a "steeplelike" narrowing directly distal to the vocal cords; all other structures, particularly the distal trachea and epiglottis, are normal in appearance.

5. **Treatment.** Most cases resolve with little special care.
   a. **Comforting the infant** in the arms of a caretaker often dramatically reduces respiratory distress.
   b. **Mist therapy** is very effective. At home, this treatment can be accomplished with a cold-water vaporizer or by placing the child near a steamy shower.
   c. **Humidified oxygen** is administered by tent or mask, if necessary. Endotracheal intubation and mechanical ventilation may be necessary in the most severe cases.
   d. **Racemic epinephrine** 2.25%, 0.3–0.5 ml in 2.5 ml of normal saline, administered by nebulized aerosol via a face mask q2–4h prn is considered efficacious by some physicians. Since its use is limited by a brief duration of action and a potential for rebound obstruction, it should be used only in hospitalized patients. The child's heart rate must be closely monitored during administration.
   e. Antibiotics are given only if a concurrent bacterial infection is present.
   f. Steroids are not of proved therapeutic value.
   g. Hospitalized patients are placed either in the arms of a caretaker or in a mist tent.

6. **Disposition.** Moderately to severely dyspneic children should be admitted to the hospital. Others require close follow-up.

D. **Epiglottitis (supraglottitis)** (see Chap. 28) is a disease characterized by acute inflammation of the epiglottis, the aryepiglottic folds, and the arytenoids. The disease progresses rapidly to total airway obstruction if untreated. It occurs most frequently between 3 and 7 years of age but has been described in all age groups; however, it is rare in the first year of life. Epiglottitis is always a medical emergency.

1. **Etiology.** Almost all cases in the pediatric age group are caused by *H. influenzae* type B. Rare causes include *S. pneumoniae* and *S. aureus*.

2. **Clinical manifestations.** The time from onset of symptoms to severe distress is usually less than 24 hours. The child first develops a severe sore throat; dysphagia, drooling, and respiratory distress soon follow. The patient is febrile, appears toxic and anxious, and sits forward with the neck extended and the jaw and chin protruded; the mouth is open, and drooling and stridor are usually prominent.

3. The **diagnosis** is established by the clinical features. However, if the diagnosis is in doubt and the patient is not in severe distress, a lateral x-ray of the neck may be performed with a physician in attendance. Three features are noted: (1) the epiglottis, which is usually thin and leaflike, is enlarged and convex on both sides (the thumb sign); (2) the aryepiglottic folds are thickened; and (3) the vallecula is obliterated. Subglottic edema similar to that seen in croup may also be seen in epiglottitis.

4. **Treatment** is guided by the fact that any manipulation of the patient, particularly placing the patient in a supine position and examining the oropharynx, may produce sudden and total airway obstruction. Unnecessary procedures,

including obtaining an ABG, venipuncture, and attempts to view the pharynx, must be avoided. The treatment of epiglottitis consists of two equally important aspects: placement of an artificial airway and antibiotic therapy.

   a. Securing the airway. Since the airway in these patients is vulnerable to rapid and unpredictable total obstruction from the epiglottic edema, aspirated secretions, and laryngospasm, an artificial airway is always placed, even in patients with mild disease. This procedure is usually performed in a prearranged fashion by a team composed of an anesthesiologist, an otolaryngologist or general surgeon, and a pediatrician. Under mask anesthesia, direct laryngoscopy is performed to confirm the diagnosis. A nasotracheal tube is then placed by an experienced endoscopist. A surgeon is present to perform a tracheostomy if intubation is not possible or if total airway obstruction develops. The nasotracheal tube remains in place until the epiglottis has decreased in size, usually after 3–5 days of antibiotic therapy.

   b. Antibiotic therapy. After establishing the airway and obtaining a surface culture of the epiglottis and blood cultures, ampicillin (150 mg/kg/day in 4–6 divided doses to a maximum of 8–10 gm/day) and chloramphenicol (50–75 mg/kg/day in 4 divided doses to a maximum of 2–4 gm/day) or cefuroxime alone (75 mg/kg/day in 3 divided doses to a maximum of 4–6 gm/day) is promptly initiated intravenously. Antibiotic therapy is later adjusted according to sensitivity reports and is continued for a total of 10 days.

   5. Disposition. Admission to an intensive care unit is mandatory.

   6. Prophylaxis against *H. influenzae* type B disease is indicated for close contacts (see **H.7.a**).

E. **Bronchiolitis** is a disease of lower airway obstruction, manifested by wheezing and respiratory distress. It is most common in the winter and spring and is virtually absent during other times of the year. The disease usually occurs in infants from 2–8 months of age and is almost limited to the first year of life. Bronchiolitis may be life-threatening, but most cases are mild and require little special therapy.

   1. Etiology. RSV is responsible for almost all cases and is essentially the only virus isolated during the epidemic season. Other viruses implicated in bronchiolitis include parainfluenza viruses and adenovirus. There is no evidence of a bacterial etiology.

   2. Clinical manifestations

   a. Symptoms and signs. Usually, the illness begins with a mild upper respiratory tract infection, which lasts several days and changes acutely to respiratory distress and wheezing. The infant is afebrile or has a low-grade fever; is tachypneic; and may have coryza, a cough, grunting respirations, and retractions. The degree of respiratory distress is variable. Auscultation of the lungs reveals fine, high-pitched wheezes predominantly during expiration. Evaluation of the degree of respiratory distress may be difficult in the small infant. A rapidly increasing respiratory rate, retractions, lethargy, or inability to feed should suggest worsening distress.

   b. Laboratory data. The chest x-ray shows hyperinflated lungs and, occasionally, streaky infiltrates. Lobar consolidation is uncommon and may represent bacterial pneumonia. Viral cultures and immunofluorescent antibody techniques, if available, can confirm the etiology.

   3. Differential diagnosis includes an aspirated foreign body, asthma, airway anomalies, gastroesophageal reflux, and pneumonia.

   4. Treatment

   a. Humidified oxygen is the only agent that is consistently therapeutic in bronchiolitis. However, mist tents are not useful and may interfere with observation of the infant. Assisted ventilation may be necessary for the most severely affected infants.

   b. Adequate **hydration** is an important aspect of therapy. IV fluids should be given to infants unable to hydrate themselves orally because of a rapid respiratory rate or moderate to severe respiratory distress.

   c. Bronchodilators, such as epinephrine, isoetharine, and aminophylline, have not been demonstrated to be of therapeutic value in bronchiolitis and are infrequently used. However, a careful trial in the hospitalized patient with moderate to severe distress has been advocated by some physicians. Aminophylline, in particular, must be used with caution in infants due to its erratic metabolism and high potential for morbidity in the very young (see **Asthma**).

  d. Corticosteroids have not been shown to be efficacious in treating bronchiolitis.

  e. Antibiotics are used only if a concurrent bacterial infection, such as otitis media or bacterial pneumonia, is suspected.

  f. Ribavirin is presently being investigated for use by nebulization in the treatment of bronchiolitis.

 5. Disposition. At least three groups of children should be considered at high risk for the development of severe respiratory distress from bronchiolitis and should be hospitalized: (1) infants with a chronic illness, especially congenital heart disease; (2) infants with a past history of prematurity or chronic lung disease; and (3) infants less than 2 months of age. Other children with mild respiratory distress may be treated as outpatients, with instructions for a prompt return to the hospital if worsening distress develops. Since bronchiolitis is very contagious, hospitalized patients should be isolated from infants with other diseases.

F. Pneumonia (see Chap. 12)

 1. Clinical manifestations vary with the age of the patient.

  a. Newborns may present with fever, tachypnea, poor feeding, or other nonspecific generalized signs of illness. Pulmonary symptoms may be minimal or even absent, and auscultation frequently is not revealing. Lethargy, cyanosis, or inactivity suggests severe disease.

  b. Infants generally have a cough and tachypnea as the most prominent signs; retractions and dyspnea are also frequently present. Auscultation may reveal only minimal findings, including decreased breath sounds, rales, and rhonchi. Grunting respirations, poor feeding, lethargy, or cyanosis suggests severe involvement.

  c. Older children have clinical findings similar to adults, including fever, a cough, tachypnea, and retractions. Percussion may reveal dullness, and auscultation may reveal decreased breath sounds, rales, or rhonchi. Signs of severe disease resemble those seen in adults.

 2. Etiologies and related features

  a. Bacteria. In the newborn period, group B streptococcus and gram-negative enterics, particularly *E. coli* and *Klebsiella,* predominate. In the child from 2 months to 5 years of age, *S. pneumoniae* and *H. influenzae* (type B) are the most common. In the child over 5 years of age, *S. pneumoniae* is the most frequent bacterium. *H. influenzae* pneumonia is uncommon beyond 8 years of age. *S. aureus* pneumonia is rare, occurring most commonly in the newborn or immunocompromised patient; its features include severe respiratory distress and rapid progression with formation of pneumatoceles, abscesses, or empyema. The other bacteria tend to produce similar clinical features, including an abrupt onset, high fever, toxic appearance, productive cough, and pleuritic chest pain. Rapid progression generally occurs in the untreated. In most cases, the chest x-ray reveals lobar consolidation and hyperaeration. The leukocyte count is usually elevated with a left shift.

  b. Viruses are responsible for most pediatric pneumonias. RSV is the most common agent, especially in the very young, and also causes bronchiolitis in the first year of life. Parainfluenza (types I, II, and III), influenza A and B, adenovirus, and rhinovirus also occur. Viruses usually produce milder disease than bacteria (except in the newborn period) and generally present as a gradually worsening upper respiratory tract infection with a low-grade fever, cough, and tachypnea. Progression to severe disease is uncommon in older children. Auscultation reveals diffuse, frequently nonlocalized findings and/or wheezing. The chest x-ray shows either diffuse perihilar or interstitial infiltrates. The WBC count usually is only mildly elevated.

  c. *Chlamydia trachomatis* causes an afebrile pneumonia in infants 4–12 weeks of age. The infant has a gradually evolving illness with tachypnea, mild respiratory distress, a staccato cough, and few systemic signs. A history of eye drainage in the child or venereal disease in a parent may be present. The chest x-ray reveals hyperinflation with diffuse, patchy interstitial and alveolar infiltrates. It rarely causes severe disease.

  d. *Mycoplasma pneumoniae* is the most frequent cause of pneumonia in adolescents and occurs in children as young as 2 years old. In general, it presents with a gradual onset of fever, cough, malaise, and headache, with a sore throat and abdominal pain occasionally reported. The physical examination reveals dry rales and, occasionally, a mild pharyngitis. There are no typical radiographic findings; either lobar consolidation or diffuse perihilar infiltrates may be seen. Elevated cold agglutinins in the serum support the diagnosis. Progression to severe disease occasionally occurs.

  e. *M. tuberculosis* should be considered in any child with pneumonia.

3. Laboratory evaluation

  a. Sputum may be Gram-stained in search of a predominant organism. Sputum cultures in children, however, are not reliable because of the difficulty in obtaining appropriate specimens (many organisms that cause bacterial pneumonia are present in normal mouth flora).

  b. Tracheal aspirates and **percutaneous lung punctures or biopsies** are reserved for severely ill patients who fail to respond to routine management.

  c. Blood cultures are obtained on all hospitalized patients prior to treatment; they can be obtained on outpatients as well.

  d. An **LP** is performed on all newborns and young infants and on any children in whom the severity of illness makes the absence of meningeal signs unreliable.

  e. ABGs should be obtained in patients with moderate or severe respiratory distress.

  f. A **tuberculin skin test** should be placed on all patients with pneumonia.

  g. Immunofluorescent techniques and cultures are availble in some laboratories for *C. trachomatis*.

4. Treatment

  a. Antibiotic therapy. Moderately to severely ill patients and those with symptoms of bacterial pneumonia should be treated with antibiotics. When either penicillin or ampicillin is used in outpatients, the initial dose may be given intramuscularly to produce a high serum level and assure initiation of treatment. Antibiotic treatment is usually continued for a minimum of 7–10 days in uncomplicated cases.

   (1) Newborns. Ampicillin and an aminoglycoside are indicated.

   (2) Age 2 months to 6 years. Amoxicillin (30–40 mg/kg/day in 3 divided doses to a maximum of 2–3 gm/day) is the most commonly used drug for outpatient therapy despite the fact that up to 30% of *H. influenzae* type B organisms are resistant to it. Because of this incidence of drug resistance, many physicians now use cefaclor (40 mg/kg/day in 3 divided doses to a maximum of 1–2 gm/day) to improve coverage against this organism, but the drug has not been studied in a conclusive fashion for the treatment of bacterial pneumonias. Parenteral treatment consists of ampicillin (150 mg/kg/day in 4 divided doses to a maximum of 8–10 gm/day) and chloramphenicol (50–75 mg/kg/day in 4 divided doses to a maximum of 2–4 gm/day). Alternatively, cefuroxime (75 mg/kg/day in 3 divided doses to a maximum of 4–6 gm/day) may be used. A penicillinase-resistant semisynthetic pencillin (i.e., nafcillin, oxacillin, or methicillin), 150 mg/kg/day in 4 divided doses to a maximum of 8–10 gm/day, is used if *S. aureus* is suspected.

   (3) Age greater than 6 years. Penicillin V (25–50 mg/kg/day PO in 4 divided doses to a maximum of 2–3 gm/day) or penicillin G (100,000–250,000 units/kg/day IV in 6 divided doses to a maximum of 20 million units/day) is the drug of choice for presumed pneumococcal pneumonia.

   (4) Patients with suspected *M. pneumoniae* are treated with erythromycin, 40 mg/kg/day in 4 divided doses to a maximum of 1–2 gm/day.

   (5) Patients suspected of having pneumonia caused by *C. trachomatis* are treated with erythromycin, 40 mg/kg/day in 4 divided doses to a maximum of 1–2 gm/day.

  b. Adequate **hydration** must be maintained, using IV fluids if necessary.

  c. Humidified **oxygen** is given when indicated.

5. Disposition. Patients requiring hospitalization include newborns and young infants, moderately to severely ill patients, and patients not responding to outpatient therapy. Also, infants less than 6 months of age with pneumonia are highly susceptible to apneic episodes and need close observation. Children with suspected bacterial pneumonia treated as outpatients should be reevaluated in 24 hours by a physician. Failure to respond promptly to an oral antibiotic suggests worsening disease, and parenteral therapy should be considered. In particular, patients not responding to ampicillin or amoxicillin should be considered as possibly having infection due to *H. influenzae* type B resistant to ampicillin;

these patients should be hospitalized, and chloramphenicol or cefuroxime added for expanded coverage.

G. Urinary tract infection (UTI) (see Chap. 12) is a common but frequently unrecognized problem in infancy and childhood.

    1. Etiology. The most common organism in all age groups is *E. coli*, accounting for 80% of all infections. Other pathogens include *Klebsiella, Proteus* species, enterococci, and *Pseudomonas.*

    2. Clinical features

        a. Newborns. Males predominate in this age group, and infection is acquired hematogenously in most cases. Signs of infection are frequently subtle and are often not recognized early. Irritability, weight loss, jaundice, or vomiting may be the initial symptoms of a UTI. Any newborn with unexplained fever or signs of systemic illness (see sec. **I.B**) requires an evaluation for a UTI.

        b. Infants. Females predominate in this group, and infection is acquired in an ascending fashion. Again, signs and symptoms are frequently subtle and often are not generally attributed to the urinary tract. Frequent damp diapers, difficulty initiating a stream, a weak stream, dribbling, and prolonged voiding are early signs of infection. Other manifestations include abdominal pain, irritability, unexplained fever, hematuria, and urinary frequency. The physical examination occasionally reveals an abdominal mass or abdominal tenderness.

        c. Older children. Again, females predominate and infection is acquired in an ascending fashion. Signs and symptoms in this age group include enuresis, nocturesis, dribbling, frequency, urgency, dysuria, hematuria, flank pain, and a high fever. The physical examination may demonstrate suprapubic tenderness, flank tenderness, or an abdominal mass.

    3. Laboratory. A high index of suspicion and prudent use of the laboratory are required.

        a. Urinalysis

            (1) Bacteriuria. Any bacteria seen under the microscope in fresh, uncentrifuged urine at high magnification in a wet prep or on oil immersion in a Gram-stained specimen correlates well with the presence of a UTI.

            (2) Pyuria. Ten or more WBCs/high-power field in the sediment of centrifuged urine also correlates with a UTI. The significance of fewer WBCs must be evaluated in light of the clinical situation.

            (3) Hematuria without pyuria may be due to a UTI, especially in females.

        b. Urine culture. A urine culture must be performed on any child suspected of having a UTI.

            (1) Collection methods include the following:

                (a) Suprapubic puncture (SPP) is the most reliable method of collection in the young infant.

                (b) Urethral catheterization. The complication of urethral laceration in males and the difficulty in performing urethral catheterization in infant females limits it use to experienced personnel.

                (c) Midstream, clean-catch urine collection. This method is useful (but slightly less accurate than the above methods) in older children and adults. Serial cultures increase the specificity.

                (d) Adhesive bags. Although adhesive bags are probably the most common method used to obtain urine from newborns and infants, the urine is frequently contaminated.

            (2) Any **growth of pathogens** in a urine culture obtained by SPP or urethral catheterization indicates a UTI. In clean-catch or adhesive-bag urines, a growth of greater than 100,000 organisms/ml of urine is significant.

    4. Localization of infection. No laboratory tests reliably distinguish infection limited to the bladder from infection that also involves the renal parenchyma, pelvis, and calices. In the newborn, the infection is frequently acquired by hematogenous spread, and all infections should be considered to involve both the upper and lower urinary tracts. In older children, fever, flank pain, signs of systemic infection, and an elevated WBC count suggest renal involvement. Due to the limited number of signs and symptoms of a UTI in the infant and the frequent inability to distinguish the extent of infection, symptomatic infants are frequently presumed to have an upper tract infection.

5. Management
  a. Newborns are hospitalized and treated with parenteral antibiotics. In general, parenteral ampicillin and an aminoglycoside are started; parenteral antibiotics are continued for at least 2 weeks. Blood and CSF cultures should be obtained prior to treatment.
  b. Infants under 1 year of age with symptomatic infection are usually hospitalized and treated with ampicillin (150 mg/kg/day IV in 4–6 divided doses) and an aminoglycoside (gentamicin, 3.0–7.5 mg/kg/day in 3 divided doses, or tobramycin, 3–6 mg/kg/day in 3 divided doses), pending organism identification and sensitivity results.
  c. Children
    (1) Lower tract disease. Children over 1 year of age without signs of upper tract or systemic disease can be treated as outpatients. The following drugs may be used: ampicillin (50–100 mg/kg/day in 4 divided doses to a maximum of 2–3 gm/day), amoxicillin (40 mg/kg/day in 3 divided doses to a maximum of 2–3 gm/day), trimethoprim-sulfamethoxazole (TMP, 6–12 mg/kg/day, and SMX, 30–60 mg/kg/day, in 2 divided doses to a maximum of 320 mg/day of TMP and 1.6 gm/day of SMX), or sulfisoxazole (120–150 mg/kg/day in 4 divided doses to a maximum of 4–6 gm/day). The duration of treatment is controversial. In the pediatric population, most physicians recommend 10–14 days of treatment for the first UTI.
    (2) Patients with signs of **upper tract disease** should be treated with parenteral ampicillin (150 mg/kg/day in 4–6 divided doses to a maximum of 8–10 gm/day) and an aminoglycoside (gentamicin, 3.0–7.5 mg/kg/day in 3 divided doses to a maximum of 300 mg/day, or tobramycin, 3–6 mg/kg/day in 3 divided doses to a maximum of 300 mg/day), pending culture and sensitivity results. A total duration of 2 weeks is recommended for uncomplicated cases.
  6. Follow-up. All children with a UTI require close follow-up, as they are at high risk for recurrence of both symptomatic and asymptomatic infections. They should have frequent cultures taken at regular intervals for at least 1 year after their first infection. Radiologic studies should be performed on all newborns with a UTI, any male after the first UTI, all females under 3 years of age after their first or second infection, and all females less than 10 years of age after the second infection.
H. Acute bacterial meningitis (see Chap. 12) is an inflammation of the meninges, in particular the pia mater and arachnoid, secondary to bacterial invasion of the CSF. It is usually caused by hematogenous seeding of the CSF during bacteremia. Other causes, including direct invasion from a contiguous site (such as ear or sinus infection) or a dural tear from a skull fracture, are much less common in children. Bacterial meningitis occurs most frequently between the ages of 6 months and 3 years of age, with most cases occurring in the first year of life.
  1. Etiology
    a. Infants less than 2 months of age. Group B streptococcus and *E. coli* account for the majority of infections, with *L. monocytogenes, Klebsiella, Enterobacter* species, *S. aureus,* group D streptococcus, and *Pseudomonas aeruginosa* occurring much less commonly.
    b. In children from 2 months to 5 years of age, *H. influenzae* type B is the most common agent, with *S. pneumoniae* and *N. meningitidis* occurring less frequently.
    c. In children over 5 years of age, *S. pneumoniae* and *N. meningitidis* are more common, with *H. influenzae* type B occurring less frequently.
  2. Clinical manifestations are age dependent and extremely variable.
    a. Newborns and young children with bacterial meningitis seldom have signs or symptoms localized to the CNS. Instead, these patients are usually first noted to have decreased activity, poor feeding, fever, or other nonspecific signs of illness (see sec. **I.B.**). These signs may seem mild in nature at first and may not even suggest severe illness. If untreated, the infant will rapidly develop a bulging fontanel, hypothermia, apnea, lethargy, and shock. Meningeal signs are not usually present in newborns with bacterial meningitis.
    b. Older children with this infection may have a fever, irritability, inconsolability, lethargy, a high-pitched cry, or headache. Meningeal signs, includ-

ing a stiff neck, Kernig's sign (i.e., with the patient in the supine position with the hips flexed, passive extension of the knees is painful and difficult), or Brudzinski's sign (i.e., with the patient in the supine position, flexion of the neck causes flexion of the legs), may be present; their absence, however, does not necessarily exclude meningitis, especially in the very young.

3. **Diagnosis.** All patients suspected of having meningitis must have an LP, unless contraindicated by apneic episodes, focal neurologic signs, or the potential to interfere with respiration. Laboratory evaluation of the CSF includes a cell count with differential, determination of glucose (and a simultaneous serum glucose) and protein, a Gram stain, and bacterial cultures. Simultaneous blood cultures should be obtained. The diagnosis of bacterial meningitis is suggested by the following findings: a CSF glucose less than 50% of the serum glucose, an elevated CSF protein, and a pleocytosis with a predominance of polymorphonuclear cells. The diagnosis is confirmed by the identification of organisms on a Gram stain or by growth of organisms on culture.

4. **Complications** that may occur during the course of the disease include apnea, hypotension and shock, seizures, SIADH, subdural effusions, and hypoglycemia. Concurrent infections including pneumonia, otitis media, septic arthritis, and pericarditis may also be present.

5. **Treatment**
   a. **IV Antibiotics** must be given promptly and should not be withheld if the physician is unable to perform an LP. Ampicillin (200–300 mg/kg/day in 4–6 divided doses to a maximum of 8–10 gm/day) and chloramphenicol (75–100 mg/kg/day in 4 divided doses to a maximum of 2–4 gm/day) is the currently recommended drug regimen for children over 2 months of age. Alternatively, cefotaxime (200 mg/kg/day in 4 divided doses) can be given. Antibiotic therapy for infants less than 2 months of age is controversial; a combination of either ampicillin and gentamicin or ampicillin and cefotaxime is used. Immediate consultation with a referral center for assistance in antibiotic choice and management is necessary for these infants.
   b. The patient's **airway** and respirations must be carefully evaluated. ABGs should be obtained if respiratory distress is present. Endotracheal intubation and mechanical ventilation may be required.
   c. **Fluid therapy** is administered in two phases. First, isotonic solutions are given if the child is poorly perfused, usually in 10-ml/kg increments until adequate perfusion is achieved. Second, fluid infusion is limited to 800–1200 ml/M²/24 hours to minimize the effects of SIADH, which frequently develops. Serial weights, urinary output, and the serum sodium are monitored closely.
   d. Critically ill infants are especially vulnerable to develop **hypoglycemia.** The serum glucose is monitored closely, and glucose is infused in quantities sufficient to prevent hypoglycemia.
   e. Generalized **seizures** are not uncommon in early meningitis. Seizures are treated with either phenytoin or phenobarbital (see **Seizures**). Both hyponatremia secondary to SIADH and hypoglycemia must be considered in these children.

6. **Disposition.** Hospitalization, often in an ICU, is mandatory. These children should be isolated from other children for 24 hours.

7. **Prophylaxis**
   a. *H. influenzae* **type B.** Prophylaxis of contacts remains controversial. The most recent recommendations of the American Academy of Pediatrics are as follows [5]:
      (1) Rifampin (20 mg/kg/day to a maximum of 600 mg/day as a single dose for 4 days) should be given to all household contacts (defined as individuals, including adults, either living in the residence of the index case or having spent more than 4 hours a day with the index case for 5 of the 7 days preceding hospitalization of the index case) if there is any contact less than 49 months of age in the household who either has not been immunized with the Haemophilus B polysaccharide vaccine or received the vaccine at less than 24 months of age or within the preceding 3 weeks. Prophylaxis is not recommended in pregnant women, and a dose has not been established for very young infants, although some experts use a dose of 10 mg/kg/day during the first month of life.
      (2) The risk of secondary cases in a daycare center with a single index case is unknown, and specific recommendations are not available. However,

most experts recommend rifampin prophylaxis for all children and supervisory personnel in daycare centers when two cases of *H. influenzae* type B disease occur within a 60-day period.

 b. *N. meningitidis.* All household contacts and daycare center contacts are given rifampin (20 mg/kg/day in 2 divided doses to a maximum of 1200 mg/day) for 2 days. Infants less than 1 month old are given 5 mg/kg/dose bid for 4 doses.

 c. The **index cases** of both *H. influenzae* disease and meningococcal disease should receive rifampin prophylaxis at the end of their antibiotic therapy.

I. Cervical lymphadenitis is characterized by infection of one or more lymph nodes in the neck.

 1. Clinical presentation. The involved lymph node is enlarged, with erythema and edema of the overlying skin surface. The node is markedly tender and may be fluctuant. Fever may be present. Other systemic symptoms, however, are usually absent. The submandibular and anterior and posterior cervical lymph nodes are most commonly involved.

 2. Etiology

  a. Bacteria. *S. aureus* and *S. pyogenes* are the two most common organisms isolated. Anaerobic bacteria (usually related to dental disease) and *Francisella tularensis* occur less frequently.

  b. Mycobacteria. Atypical mycobacteria occasionally cause cervical lymphadenitis; infection with *M. tuberculosis* is much less common.

 3. Differential diagnosis

  a. Cervical adenitis must be differentiated from **cervical lymphadenopathy,** a nonsuppurative condition caused by viral disease or adjacent bacterial infection. In general, erythema, edema, and fluctuance are not present in cervical lymphadenopathy. Common agents include EBV and adenovirus. Cytomegalovirus may produce a syndrome clinically similar to that due to the EBV but is Monospot-negative.

  b. Infected neck masses that are frequently mistaken for cervical lymphadenitis include thyroglossal duct cysts (located in the anterior midline), branchial cleft cysts (located most frequently at the anterior border of the sternocleidomastoid muscle and presenting as a skin dimple), and cystic hygromas.

  c. Cervical lymph node enlargement may be due to Hodgkin's disease, leukemia, or other lymphomas. Cat scratch disease produces tender cervical lymph node enlargement.

 4. Evaluation

  a. The **history** should emphasize the presence of previous skin lesions and masses, dental disease, exposure to animals, and exposure to tuberculosis.

  b. Needle aspiration. Fluctuant lymph nodes should be aspirated with a large-bore needle, and the contents cultured for aerobic and anaerobic bacteria and mycobacteria. Gram and acid-fast stains should also be performed on the aspirate.

  c. A **tuberculin skin test** should be placed. In general, induration and erythema greater than 10 mm in diameter is associated with disease caused by *M. tuberculosis,* and a reaction between 5 and 10 mm is associated with atypical mycobacteria. Specific skin tests for atypical mycobacteria are not performed at the initial evaluation.

 5. Management

  a. Antibiotics. Children with systemic symptoms and young infants should be hospitalized and treated with IV oxacillin or methicillin (150–200 mg/kg/day in 4 divided doses to a maximum of 8–10 gm/day). Other children are treated on an outpatient basis with cephalexin (50 mg/kg/day in 4 divided doses to a maximum of 2–3 gm/day) or dicloxacillin (12–25 mg/kg/day in 4 divided doses to a maximum of 1–2 gm/day) for a 10- to 14-day course. Antibiotic therapy is later adjusted based on culture and skin test results.

  b. Drainage. Fluctuant lymph nodes should be incised and drained if tuberculosis is ruled out. Patients should be followed daily at the onset of treatment for development of fluctuance.

  c. Total **excision** of atypical mycobacterial lymph nodes is the treatment of choice.

J. Measles (rubeola) (see Chap. 31)

 1. Etiology. A single RNA virus strain is responsible for measles.

 2. Clinical features. Infection usually occurs in winter and spring. The disease previously was most common in children from 5–9 years of age; but with the use of vaccine, it now occurs in young adults and others who have been inadequately immunized. The clinical course has three phases:

    a. The **incubation period** is approximately 10 days long.

    b. The **prodromal period** lasts 3 days. Malaise; a cough, coryza, and conjunctivitis (the three "Cs"); and a high fever predominate. The cough is harsh and brassy and may have a croupy quality; it worsens over the next 3 days and persists for the next week. The fever worsens over the prodromal period and is highest at the time the rash develops. Koplik spots, a characteristic feature of rubeola, appear at the onset of the prodromal period. They are small whitish papules usually no more than 1 mm wide, with an intensely erythematous base. The spots begin on the buccal mucosa adjacent to the mandibular molars and may spread to involve the entire buccal and labial mucosa. They resolve within a day of the onset of the rash.

    c. The **exanthem period** begins at the peak of the prodromal symptoms. The rash is described as small, irregular, erythematous macules, often with a fine papular component. It appears first in the postauricular area and on the forehead at the hairline. Within the next 3 days, the rash spreads sequentially to involve the face, chest, back, arms, buttocks, and legs. The rash then becomes more confluent, being most prominent on the face. After 3–4 days, it fades in the same sequence that it developed, leaving a coppery color to the skin. The total duration of the rash is about 1 week. The fever does not continue beyond the third day after appearance of the rash unless complications develop.

  3. **Complications** include pneumonia, which is most frequently due to the measles virus but also may be due to bacterial superinfection with *S. pneumoniae*, *H. influenzae* type B, group A streptococcus, or *S. aureus*. Otitis media, laryngotracheobronchitis, and laryngitis may also occur. Most serious is the development of encephalitis, which occurs in approximately 1 in 1000 cases; symptoms and signs begin during the exanthem period and include seizures, irritability, and coma. Sequellae occur in 20–40% of patients.

K. Chickenpox (varicella) (see Chap. 31)

  1. **Etiology.** The varicella-zoster virus, a herpesvirus, is the etiologic agent.

  2. **Clinical features.** The disease occurs most commonly in children between 5 and 10 years old during late winter and early spring. The typical skin lesion begins as a small erythematous macule a few millimeters wide. Over the next 24 hours, it rapidly changes to a small papule and then becomes a vesicle with an erythematous base. The contents of the vesicle are clear at first but soon develop a cloudy appearance. Within a few days, the lesion becomes crusted and heals without scarring. The lesions first appear in clusters on the trunk and over the next 3–4 days spread to the face, scalp, and extremities. The rash is very pruritic. At the height of the disease, all the different stages of development of the lesions usually are present on a single patient. Systemic symptoms are mild and include malaise and a low-grade fever. However, immunocompromised children and newborns are vulnerable to rapid dissemination of the virus to the skin, lungs, brain, and liver; the mortality is high if untreated.

  3. The **diagnosis** is usually not difficult. It is based on a history of exposure and on the characteristic lesions and progression of the rash.

  4. **Treatment** involves only supportive care in the normal host.

    a. **Pruritus** may be relieved with oral diphenhydramine hydrochloride, 5 mg/kg/day in 4 divided doses.

    b. **Fever.** Acetaminophen can be used in its usual dosages. However, aspirin should *not* be given to children with varicella, as its use during the course of this disease has been implicated as a possible factor in the etiology of Reye syndrome.

    c. **Immunocompromised children** exposed to varicella need prompt referral for consideration of immunoglobulin, vaccine, or antiviral therapy.

  5. **Complications.** The most common complication is bacterial superinfection of the vesicles, usually by *S. aureus;* superinfection is manifested by purulence in the vesicle and by increased erythema at the base of the lesion. Treatment is with an antibiotic effective against *S. aureus,* either dicloxacillin (12–25 mg/kg/day in 4 divided doses to a maximum of 1–2 gm/day) or cephalexin (25–50 mg/kg/day in 4 divided doses to a maximum of 2–3 gm/day). Other complications include pneumonia and postinfectious encephalitis or cerebellitis. Also, approximately 10% of all cases of Reye syndrome are preceded by varicella.

L. Mumps
1. The **etiology** is a single paramyxovirus strain.
2. **Clinical features.** The incubation period is usually 16–18 days, but ranges from 12–25 days. As many as 30% of cases may be subclinical. Parotid swelling is the most common sign of the disease; it can be unilateral or bilateral, and swelling on one side may precede swelling on the other side by several days. The swelling continues for 7–10 days, and the patient may be contagious for up to 7 days after the onset of swelling. Anorexia, headache, abdominal pain, and a low-grade fever may also be present.
3. The **diagnosis** is usually suggested by parotid swelling; other viruses associated with parotitis include influenza, parainfluenza, and cytomegalovirus. Mumps should be distinguished from purulent parotitis, which is associated with marked erythema, tenderness, and the presence of pus draining from Wharton's duct.
4. **Complications.** The most serious complication is orchitis, which occurs more frequently in postpubescent males and is heralded by fever and testicular tenderness at the end of the first week of the illness. It is most commonly unilateral but infrequently may be bilateral. Sterility can occur in bilateral disease. Other complications include aseptic meningitis and, less commonly, encephalitis.
5. **Treatment** involves supportive care.
6. **Vaccine.** The American Academy of Pediatrics recommends that all children be immunized against mumps at 15 months of age; this immunization is usually part of a measles-mumps-rubella (MMR) combination vaccine. The vaccine is a live attenuated virus, and approximately 90% of persons develop antibody with 1 dose. The antibody persists for at least 12 years, and immunity may last for life.

Diarrhea and Dehydration

I. **Diarrhea** (see Chap. 10) and **dehydration** are common problems in pediatrics.
   A. **Etiologies and related features**
   1. **Viruses.** The most commonly implicated virus is rotavirus, with the enterovirus, adenovirus, and Norwalk-like agent occurring less commonly. In general, rotavirus infection presents during the winter with loose, watery stools and vomiting in children 6–36 months old. Dehydration is very common, especially in children less than 12 months of age.
   2. **Bacteria.** The most common causes of bacterial gastroenteritis include nontyphoid *Salmonella, Shigella, Campylobacter fetus ss. jejuni,* and *Yersinia enterocolitica.*
      a. Nontyphoidal *Salmonella* causes a syndrome of cramping abdominal pain with profuse, watery, foul-smelling stools, occasionally containing blood or mucus. A low-grade fever and chills occur frequently. Infection is most common during summer and autumn. Although human-to-human transmission occurs, contaminated foods, particularly meat and poultry, are the most common sources of infection. *Salmonella* gastroenteritis may be associated with a bacteremia that is transient in the normal host. Children with sickle cell disease and neonates are at an increased risk for metastatic infection (especially involving bones) and sepsis.
      b. *Shigella* presents as the acute onset of small-volume, watery stools with blood or mucus, associated with a high fever and, occasionally, vomiting. Human-to-human transmission is the most common means of infection.
      c. *Y. enterocolitica* produces a watery, nonbloody diarrhea with cramping abdominal pain, frequently prominent in the right lower quadrant. Both human-to-human transmission and infection by contact with contaminated animals occur.
      d. *C. fetus ss. jejuni* causes diarrhea with abdominal pain, with or without fever. The stools are frequently contaminated with blood and mucus. Sources include contaminated foods and milk and infected humans and animals.
   3. **Protozoa.** *Giardia lamblia* is the most common intestinal parasite in children, producing loose, foul-smelling, watery stools with associated nausea and cramp-

ing abdominal pain. In young children, it may cause chronic diarrhea, malabsorption, and profound weight loss, mimicking celiac disease.

4. **Noninfectious causes** of diarrhea occur less commonly and include lactase deficiency, cystic fibrosis, and inflammatory bowel disease.

B. **Evaluation of hydration status.** Infants are very vulnerable to dehydration due to more frequent vomiting (limiting the amount of oral fluids the child is able to tolerate), a greater percentage of both total body water and extracellular fluid than in the adult, and a decreased renal concentrating ability.

1. The **history** should include information about the child's activity, the child's appetite, the type of fluids the child is currently taking, the amount of vomiting, and the frequency of urination.

2. **Physical examination.** The most sensitive sign of dehydration in the child is weight loss on comparison of recent weights. Signs of dehydration on physical examination are frequently subtle and nonspecific. They include the following:

   a. **Mild dehydration** (i.e., < 5% weight loss) is characterized by a slight decrease in skin turgor, mild dryness of the mucous membranes, no change in blood pressure, and a slight increase in the heart rate.

   b. **Moderate dehydration** (i.e., 5–10% weight loss). These patients present with very dry mucous membranes, a further decrease in skin turgor, sunken eyes, no change in blood pressure, an increase in heart rate, and oliguria.

   c. **Severe dehydration** (i.e., 10–15% weight loss) is manifested by weak, thready peripheral pulses, tachypnea, lethargy, tenting of the skin, mottled skin, decreased blood pressure, and a marked tachycardia.

C. **Laboratory evaluation**

1. **Stool cultures** should be obtained in children with moderate to severe dehydration, bloody stools, or cramping abdominal pain and in neonates with diarrhea.

2. **Enzyme-linked immunosorbent assay (ELISA)** techniques are available in many laboratories to identify rotavirus in stools.

3. **Microscopic examination of stool** stained with methylene blue for leukocytes suggests the diagnosis of bacterial infection if sheets of white cells are seen.

4. Both **wet prep and concentration techniques** should be performed on stools if *Giardia* is suspected. Because the protozoan is intermittently shed, stool specimens from at least three different days should be examined.

5. Laboratory tests available to evaluate the presence and extent of dehydration include the hematocrit, serum electrolytes, and BUN.

D. **Treatment**

1. **Rehydration**

   a. **Oral rehydration** may be used in infants with mild to moderate dehydration. Solutions available include the World Health Organization Oral Rehydration Solution (with 90 mEq of sodium/liter), Pedialyte RS (with 75 mEq of sodium/liter), and Pedialyte (with 45 mEq of sodium/liter). The use of sodas, juices, and other similar liquids is not recommended as primary rehydration solutions, as they do not contain sufficient sodium and potassium to replace losses. Home-mixed salt solutions, especially boiled milk, are frequently hypertonic and may cause hypernatremic dehydration; they should be avoided.

   b. **IV hydration** is indicated in children with moderate to severe dehydration and in children with frequent vomiting and inability to tolerate oral feedings. The fluids are given in two phases:

      (1) **Reestablishing perfusion to vital organs** is the goal of the first phase (0–1 hour). A glucose-containing extracellularlike solution (e.g., 5% D/WLR, 5% D/WNS) is generally used, and 10–20 ml/kg is infused. Alternatively, some authors recommend a solution containing 10% glucose, 75 mEq/liter of sodium, 55 mEq/liter of chloride, and 20 mEq/liter of bicarbonate. Clinical response is judged by the return of peripheral pulses, a decrease in tachycardia, and an increase in activity. Repeated boluses may be necessary to accomplish the goal.

      (2) **Correction of water and electrolyte deficits while replacing ongoing losses** is the goal of the second phase.

         (a) In **isotonic and hypotonic dehydration,** sodium is given as 0.20–0.45% sodium chloride with 5% dextrose. A fluid rate of 2500–3500 ml/M^2/day (which is twice the usual maintenance rate) is recommended. The acute deficit is replaced within the first 24 hours of treatment, with half of the deficit corrected in the first 8 hours.

(b) **Hypertonic dehydration.** Caution must be exercised in treating hypertonic dehydration (with a serum sodium > 150 mEq/liter). Rapid infusion of hypotonic solutions may be associated with cerebral edema and seizures. Many authorities recommend a solution of 5% dextrose with a sodium concentration of 40 mEq/liter at a slower ($2000-2500$ ml/M^2/day) infusion rate in the patient with mild hypertonic dehydration.

c. Neonates and young infants are particularly vulnerable to dehydration and require close attention with frequent serial weights and examinations. Regular formula feedings should not be withheld for a prolonged time, as the infant will be deprived of necessary nutrition.

d. Lactose should not be given to patients who have gastroenteritis, as the diarrhea produces a transient lactase deficiency. In older children, cow's milk should be withheld; in infants fed exclusively with formula, a non-lactose-containing formula, such as Isomil or Prosoybee, should be substituted for a lactose-containing formula, such as Enfamil, SMA, or Similac, until the diarrhea abates.

2. **Antibiotics**
   a. *Shigella* gastroenteritis generally resolves without antibiotic treatment. In the patient with prolonged symptoms TMP-SMX (10 mg/kg/day of TMP and 50 mg/kg/day of SMX in 2 divided doses to a maximum of 320 mg/day of TMP and 1.6 gm/day of SMX) can be used.
   b. *Campylobacter* gastroenteritis is treated with oral erythromycin (40 mg/kg/day in 4 divided doses to a maximum of 250–500 mg q6h).
   c. No recommendations are available concerning the antibiotic treatment of *Yersinia* gastroenteritis.
   d. Nontyphoidal *Salmonella* gastroenteritis is usually self-limited and is not treated with antibiotics in the normal host, because such treatment (e.g., with ampicillin) may prolong the carrier state.
   e. There is no ideal drug for the treatment of *G. lamblia*. Currently, three drugs are available:
      (1) Quinacrine (6 mg/kg/day in 3 divided doses to a maximum of 100 mg q8h for 7 days) is inexpensive and efficacious but unavailable in an oral suspension.
      (2) Furazolidone (5–8 mg/kg/day in 4 divided doses to a maximum of 100 mg q6h for 7–10 days) is available in both liquid and tablet forms but is not as efficacious as quinacrine or metronidazole.
      (3) Metronidazole (15 mg/kg/day in 3 divided doses to a maximum of 250 mg tid for 5–7 days) is available in tablets only. However, because it is mutagenic in bacteria and oncogenic in experimental animals, it is not approved by the Food and Drug Administration for the treatment of *Giardia*-related diseases.

3. Antiemetics and antimotility agents are generally not used in the treatment of uncomplicated pediatric gastroenteritis.

Reye Syndrome

Reye syndrome is a noninflammatory encephalopathy with elevated serum transaminases and a characteristic clinical course in the untreated patient. Early recognition of the syndrome is essential, because treatment may halt the progression of the disease.

I. The **etiology** is not known. Due to the controversial role of salicylates in the pathogenesis of Reye syndrome, the Centers for Disease Control and the American Academy of Pediatrics recommend that aspirin *not* be given to children with varicella or influenzalike illness.

II. **Clinical features.** The patient is usually between 5 and 14 years of age, although the disease has been described in all pediatric age groups. The patient develops a mild prodromal viral illness, most commonly due to influenza A, influenza B, or varicella. During the recovery phase of this illness, frequent pernicious vomiting begins and lasts for 12–24 hours. The child then develops neurologic changes and, if he or she is untreated, may progress through the following stages [17]:

A. **Stage I:** lethargy, vomiting, sleepiness, and laboratory evidence of liver dysfunction.

B. **Stage II:** disorientation, delirium, combativeness, hyperventilation, hyperactive reflexes, and appropriate responses to noxious stimuli.

   C. Stage III: coma, decorticate rigidity, and preservation of the pupillary light reaction and oculovestibular reflexes.

   D. Stage IV: deepening coma, decerebrate rigidity, loss of oculocephalic reflexes, and fixed and dilated pupils.

   E. Stage V: seizures, loss of deep tendon reflexes, flaccidity, and respiratory arrest.

 III. The **diagnosis** is based on the characteristic clinical course of a prodromal viral illness and recurrent vomiting and on the laboratory finding of a serum glutamic oxaloacetic transaminase (SGOT, or aspartate aminotransferase [AST]), serum glutamic pyruvic transaminase (SGPT, or alanine aminotransferase [ALT]), or serum ammonia (NH$_3$) greater than 3 times normal without another more reasonable explanation [6]. A liver biopsy will reveal characteristic changes and may be used in establishing the diagnosis. Patients with a prodromal illness and vomiting should have serum transaminases checked, even when there is no change in mental status.

 IV. Other **laboratory findings** include a normal serum bilirubin, a prolonged prothrombin time, and the absence of abnormalities in the CSF. An LP should be performed only on patients in stage I or II of the disease and only when there are no signs of increased intracranial pressure. Hypoglycemia is occasionally seen in children under 5 years of age.

 V. The **treatment** of Reye syndrome must be delivered by an experienced multispecialty team in a referral center. The role of the emergency physician is to make a preliminary diagnosis, stabilize the patient, and arrange for referral to an appropriate center. Intensive supportive care and treatment of increased intracranial pressure appear to reduce the morbidity and mortality.

Poisoning and Overdose

In children, poisoning usually results either from accidental ingestion of a variety of medications or household products or from unintentional misuse of medicine. Adolescents, however, may intentionally overdose on drugs for recreational purposes or in a suicide attempt. **Management principles** are the same as for adults (see Chap. 16). However, because of the smaller body mass of children, certain modifications are made in their management. The dose of syrup of ipecac is 15 ml in children over 1 year of age and 5–10 ml in children younger than 1 year old. If gastric lavage is performed (because of CNS depression, seizures, or failure of ipecac to induce emesis), the largest possible gastric tube should be used (e.g., 12–16 F in young children, up to 36 F in older children); lavage is carried out with saline at 100–300 ml/pass (depending on the size of the child) until the return is clear. The dose of activated charcoal is approximately 10 times the amount ingested or 15–50 gm, depending on the size of the child. Catharsis is usually induced with magnesium or sodium sulfate, 250 mg/kg PO. Antidotes are administered as indicated, with the dosages adjusted according to the child's body weight. Supportive and invasive measures are instituted as needed. The possibility of child abuse (see **Child Abuse**) should be considered. Parents should be given instructions regarding poison prevention as appropriate.

Child Abuse

  I. Child abuse includes any maltreatment of children, including nonaccidental physical trauma, sexual abuse, neglect of basic needs, and emotional torment. It occurs in all socioeconomic groups and is more prevalent than previously recognized. It is the responsibility of all physicians to diagnose child abuse and initiate aid to its victims.

   A. Diagnosis. Child abuse should be suspected in children with unexplained or inadequately explained injuries, children with poor growth without organic disease, children with frequent visits to physicians for seemingly trivial problems, and children with inappropriately violent or passive behavior.

   B. Evaluation and reporting. It is important of record all objective findings in detail in the patient's medical chart. Photographs should be included, when appropriate. Coagulation studies and radiographs are obtained as indicated. The physician is obligated to report any concerns regarding child abuse to the appropriate authorities for further investigation.

   C. Treatment. Appropriate therapeutic intervention is provided as needed.

   D. Disposition. The greatest responsibility of the physician who discovers an abused child is referral of the entire family to a child abuse team. This group, consisting of specially trained physicians, nurses, social workers, and psychologists, can then

begin the process of treatment. Children felt to be at risk for further injury should be hospitalized until safety can be assured; a judicial holding order may be needed.
II. **Sexual abuse** should be considered in the child with frequent or vague complaints involving the genitals or in the adolescent with venereal disease or pregnancy. The dynamics are complex. The adult is almost always known to the child, and the abuse is frequently not discovered early.
   A. **Evaluation and reporting** (see Chap. 33). A sensitively performed history and physical examination are essential. The body is examined for other stigmata of abuse, and the genitals are examined for lacerations, discharge, and bruises. Laboratory tests performed should include a wet prep for sperm; a rapid plasma reagin (RPR) or Venereal Disease Research Laboratory (VDRL) test; pregnancy test; and oral, vaginal, and rectal cultures for gonorrhea. Pulled pubic and scalp hair are sent for police analysis when appropriate. Prophylaxis for pregnancy and gonorrhea is given if indicated. Precise documentation and reporting to the proper authorities is mandatory.
   B. **Management.** A well-organized multidisciplinary treatment program should be offered to the victim and the family.

Surgical Abdomen

Acute **abdominal obstruction** in the pediatric patient may be difficult to diagnose in the child unable to communicate his or her symptoms. Of particular interest in the infant or young child are malrotation and midgut volvulus, pyloric stenosis, and intussesception.
I. **Malrotation.** Rotational anomalies occur when the fetal midgut fails to complete the necessary 270-degree counterclockwise rotation in its return to the abdominal cavity at 10–12 weeks of gestation. Clinically significant malrotation occurs when the duodenojejunal loop remains to the right of the spine, while the colonic loop rotates 180 degrees but fails to descend to the right lower quadrant. This anomaly leaves the two points of fixation of the small-bowel mesentery almost superimposed on one another, resulting in a narrow base of attachment and the likelihood of **volvulus.** Peritoneal bands also course over the malpositioned duodenum, often causing obstruction. Because of the resultant bowel ischemia, volvulus of the midgut is considered a critical surgical emergency.
   A. **Clinical features.** Most infants with malrotation or volvulus present early in life, with 60–80% of cases being diagnosed prior to 1 month of age. Virtually all of these patients present with bilious vomiting and bloody stools, but often with little or no abdominal distention. The vomiting may be spontaneous or associated with feeding.
   B. **Diagnosis.** Abdominal radiographs may reveal the site of obstruction, especially if it is at the duodenum; however, a normal plain film may be present when (1) the duodenum is emptied by vomiting or suction, (2) the infant is too ill to swallow air, or (3) the volvulus is intermittent. A more definitive diagnosis can be made by a barium enema or upper GI series, which reveals displacement of the cecum or duodenum, respectively.
   C. **Treatment.** Once the diagnosis is made, **rapid surgical correction** is usually critical to the infant's survival.
II. **Pyloric stenosis.** Congenital hypertrophic pyloric stenosis occurs as often as 1 in 150 male infants of Scandinavian descent but rarely occurs in children of African heritage. Male infants are 4 times more frequently affected, especially those that are firstborn.
   A. **Clinical features** usually present between the third and sixth week of life, with gradual or, occasionally, sudden onset of vomiting in a previously well infant. Vomiting usually is nonbilious, soon becomes projectile, and occurs directly after feeding; the infant feeds eagerly again after vomiting. With persistent vomiting, the infant fails to gain weight and becomes dehydrated, developing a hyponatremic, hypokalemic, hypochloremic alkalosis. In addition, constipation generally is seen. On examination, characteristic gastric peristaltic waves are seen, especially after feeding. With the stomach empty, the olive-sized pyloric mass usually can be palpated 3–5 cm below the right costal margin and just lateral to the right rectus muscle. If necessary, an upper GI series with barium can be used to show elongation and narrowing of the pyloric channel.
   B. **Management.** Prior to surgery, gastric decompression, IV rehydration, and correction of electrolyte imbalances are crucial. After initial isotonic correction of hypovolemia with normal saline (usually 20–40 ml/kg), a solution of 5% dextrose and 0.45% saline with 30 mEq/liter of potassium chloride added, administered at a

maintenance rate for 12–24 hours, will usually normalize the serum pH and electrolytes. Pyloromyotomy is then performed, and oral feedings of clear liquids can be started as early as 8–12 hours postoperatively.

III. **Intussusception** is the most common cause of bowel obstruction in children less than 2 years old. It usually occurs between 4 and 12 months of age, has a slightly male predominance, and rarely (in < 10% of cases) has a demonstrable mechanical cause or "lead point." The older the patient, the greater the likelihood of discovering a lead point, such as a polyp, Meckel's diverticulum, duplications, or a lymphosarcoma. Ileocolic intussusception (i.e., beginning at or near the ileocecal valve) is the most common form.

A. **Clinical features.** The child usually presents with a history of sudden onset of severe, intermittent, abdominal cramping pain and nonbilious vomiting progressing to bilious vomiting. In between the episodes of colic, the child is usually comfortable, although often somewhat lethargic. Bloody ("currant jelly") stools are sometimes seen in younger children as the telescoping intussusception causes venous stasis, then ischemia, and finally gangrene of the bowel wall. By then the child has become pale, is lethargic, and is in a shocklike state. A palpable abdominal mass may be noted, along with an emptiness in the right colonic gutter.

B. **Management.** Once the diagnosis is suspected, isotonic IV hydration is begun, and surgical and radiologic consultations are obtained. Plain abdominal radiographs may appear completely normal. A barium enema not only confirms the diagnosis, but in about 75% of cases, the enema will reduce the intussusception, averting the need for surgery. The patient is usually then observed for 24 hours in the hospital for possible recurrence (about a 5% incidence). Barium enema reduction is less successful if (1) the intussusception is present for more than 48 hours, (2) necrotic bowel is present, or (3) there is a mechanical lead point. The enema is contraindicated in the patient with suspected peritonitis.

Trauma

I. **Multiple trauma.** Trauma is the leading cause of death in children over 1 year of age. Blunt trauma predominates, being associated with 80% of serious injuries. Child abuse (see **Child Abuse**) is a relatively frequent source of injuries in children.

A. **Unique features** pertaining to the traumatized child include the following:
1. **Vital signs** in children vary with age, as do various tube sizes (Table 36-10).
2. The **blood volume** in children is small, being 8–9% of the body weight (i.e., 80–90 ml/kg). Thus, loss of a small amount of blood can lead to significant hemodynamic compromise.
3. Adequate **urinary output** is 1–2 ml/kg/hour in infants and 0.5–1.0 ml/kg/hour in older children (and adults).
4. **Heat loss** can readily occur in children as a result of the large body surface relative to the body mass.
5. A **paralytic ileus and acute gastric dilatation** (from aerophagia) commonly occur in injured children and can lead to respiratory compromise from elevation of the diaphragm.
6. **Congenital anomalies** (e.g., cardiac defects) may be present and affect management of the child.
7. **Psychologic development** in children is limited.

B. **Management principles** for traumatized children are the same as for adults (see Chap. 17). However, because of the size and developmental differences, there are special considerations in the management of these children.
1. **Airway.** If endotracheal intubation is required, a tube of appropriate size (see Table 36-10) without a cuff (for children < 8 years old) is used. Surgical cricothyrotomy should be avoided in children less than 12 years of age, if possible.
2. **Circulation**
   a. **Venous access.** At least one peripheral IV line should be established by percutaneous venipuncture, using the largest catheter possible. If it is not possible to establish a percutaneous line, a venous cutdown (see Chap. 38) should be performed on the greater saphenous vein at the ankle, the basilic vein at the elbow, or the external jugular vein. Percutaneous placement of a central venous line generally should be avoided because of the associated increased risk of complications; however, if necessary (for monitoring purposes), these lines can be placed in children over 2 years of age using a standard technique (see Chap. 38) and appropriately sized catheters.
   b. **MAST suit.** An appropriately sized pediatric MAST suit (see Chap. 38) may

Table 36-10. Vital signs and tube sizes

Age	Weight (kg)	Heart rate	Respiratory rate	Blood pressure Systolic	Blood pressure Diastolic	Endotracheal tube ID (mm)	Endotracheal tube Length (cm)	Suction catheter (F)	Chest tube (F)
Premature	<1	145		42 ± 10	21 ± 8	2.5	10	6	8–10
Newborn	1–2			50 ± 10	28 ± 8	3.0	11	6–8	10–12
Newborn	2–3	130	30–60	60 ± 10	37 ± 8	3.0	12	6–8	
1 mo	4	120		80 ± 16	46 ± 16	3.5	13	8	
6 mo	7			89 ± 29	60 ± 10	3.5	14	8	
1 yr	10	115	22–38	96 ± 30	66 ± 25	4.0	15	8–10	16–20
2–3 yr	12–14	110	20–30	99 ± 25	64 ± 25	4.5	16	10	
4–5 yr	16–18	100		99 ± 20	65 ± 20	6.0	17	10	20–28
6–8 yr	20–26	90	18–24	100 ± 20	65 ± 15	6.5	18	10	
10–12 yr	32–42	85	18–22	115 ± 20	75 ± 15	7.0	20	12	28–32
>14 yr	>50	75	12–20	125 ± 20	75 ± 15	7.5–8.5	24	12–14	32–42

Source: Adapted from R. M. Barkin and P. Rosen (eds.), *Emergency Pediatrics.* St. Louis: Mosby, 1984. P. 696.

be used (1) to raise the blood pressure in hypovolemic patients, (2) to splint pelvic and femoral fractures, and (3) to tamponade bleeding.

   c. **Fluid resuscitation.** In the hypovolemic child, 20 ml/kg of LR is administered by rapid IV infusion. If there is no improvement, a second 20-ml/kg bolus is given. If the child is still hypotensive, 20 ml/kg of blood (i.e., cross-matched blood, type-specific blood, or type O–Rh-negative packed cells, in that order depending on availability) is administered. Additional blood is given as needed. Once the blood volume is repleted, LR is infused at a maintenance rate of 1500 ml/M^2/day (unless fluid restriction is indicated).
3. The child's **body temperature** must be maintained at 36–37°C (96.8–98.6°F) during the resuscitation by the use of blankets, an overhead heat lamp, or a thermal blanket, as needed.
4. A **nasogastric tube** is necessary in potentially seriously injured children to decompress the stomach, thereby lessening the risk of aspiration and allowing for improved ventilation and a more reliable abdominal examination.
5. **Peritoneal lavage.** Because of the increasing use of nonoperative management of children with blunt trauma, peritoneal lavage (see Chap. 38) is used less often in children than in adults. If used (for the same reasons as in adults), the lavage fluid is normal saline in the amount of 15 ml/kg (up to a maximum of 1000 ml).
6. **Child abuse** must always be considered in the traumatized child and, if suspected, be appropriately managed (see **Child Abuse**).
7. Appropriate **psychologic support** is essential for the frightened traumatized child. The child should be comforted and, if appropriate, should be told what has happened and what is about to happen.

II. **Fractures.** In children a unique condition exists with the presence of the epiphyseal plate (physis), which allows for longitudinal growth.
   A. **Special considerations**
      1. **Epiphyseal plate**
         a. The weakest site of bones in a child is the area of the epiphyseal plate called the zone of provisional calcification on the metaphyseal side of the physis. This area is where most fractures occur, at least in part.
         b. Growth can remodel residual angulation as long as it is in the plane of motion of the adjacent joint. Malrotation or residual varus or valgus deformity cannot be accommodated by growth.
         c. It is much more common to have an epiphyseal injury than a ligamentous injury, especially at the knee. A child with a suspected ligamentous injury may require stress radiographs to determine whether or not such an injury or a physeal fracture is present. Stress radiographs may demonstrate an occult fracture.
         d. Any fracture that traverses the physis can cause a longitudinal growth disturbance. This disturbance can be either a total cessation of longitudinal growth or a partial one, which will lead to the development of an angular deformity with time.
      2. **Radiographs.** If there is doubt regarding the presence of a fracture in a child because of the varying development of the ossification center of the epiphysis, radiographs of the other extremity should be obtained for comparison.
      3. **Description of fractures.** The Salter-Harris classification is as follows (Fig. 36-1):
         a. **Type I.** This fracture passes through the zone of provisional calcification, usually without displacement. Radiographs are usually normal. Growth disturbances are rarely seen.
         b. **Type II.** This is a metaphyseal fracture passing through the physeal plate. Growth abnormalities are rarely seen.
         c. **Type III.** This is a physeal fracture with extension into the epiphysis. This type of fracture crosses the germinal layers of the epiphyseal plate; thus, growth abnormalities are unpredictable. It must also be appreciated that these fractures are intraarticular and therefore must have anatomic reduction.
         d. **Type IV.** This fracture extends from the metaphysis through the physis and epiphysis. These fractures have a much higher incidence of growth disturbance and require anatomic reduction. Many of these fractures require open reduction and internal fixation
         e. **Type V.** This is a crush injury to the physis and usually results in growth arrest.

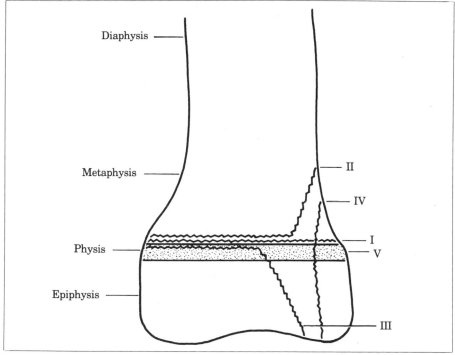

Fig. 36-1. Salter-Harris classification of fractures involving the physis. Type I: separation of the physeal-metaphyseal junction. Type II: separation of the physeal-metaphyseal junction along with a triangular metaphyseal fragment. Type III: fracture extending transversely through a portion of the physis and then longitudinally across the epiphysis into the joint space. Type IV: fracture traversing the epiphysis (with joint involvement), physis, and a portion of the metaphysis. Type V: crush injury to the physis or a portion thereof.

4. **Reduction of fractures.** It must be remembered that reduction of fractures in this group of patients cannot be too vigorous, since damage to the physis can occur. If reduction cannot be achieved in the emergency department with gentle manipulation, it is best performed in the operating room under general anesthesia.
B. **Special fractures and dislocations**
   1. **Supracondylar elbow fractures** usually are produced by a hyperextension force and rarely by hyperflexion.
      a. **Examination** reveals minimal to marked swelling about the elbow with tenderness. Radiographs may not be diagnostic in nondisplaced fractures but can be suggestive if a posterior fat pad is present. Attention must be paid to the neurovascular status.
      b. **Treatment** consists of closed reduction or open reduction with or without internal fixation. Occasionally, these fractures are treated in traction. Since reduction can often be difficult, it should be left to someone with experience. If there is uncertainty as to whether or not a fracture exists, it is best to immobilize the child's arm in a posterior splint with the elbow flexed to 90 degrees and reexamine the arm in 7–10 days for an occult fracture. The parents must be instructed about the warning signs of a compartment syndrome.
      c. **Complications.** A compartment syndrome (see Chap. 26) may evolve. Late complications include (1) an angular deformity due to malunion or epiphyseal injury and (2) a tardy ulnar nerve palsy.
   2. **Proximal humeral fractures** usually occur from a fall on an outstretched hand, resulting in a Salter-Harris type I epiphyseal separation. Care must be taken in reducing these fractures to avoid further damage to the physis. Most often the

humeral head is in varus angulation and external rotation and can be reduced by abducting and externally rotating the arm and then slowly bringing the arm down to the side and internally rotating it. The shoulder should then be immobilized for 3 weeks in a Velpeau dressing. If reduction is lost when adducting the arm, the shoulder must be maintained in the "Statue of Liberty" position for several weeks with a cast.

3. **Slipped capital femoral epiphysis** is seen in the adolescent population, usually in obese children but also in tall, thin children. It can be seen after a minor traumatic event. The child complains of knee or medial thigh pain. The diagnosis of a mild slip may be difficult to make radiographically unless both anteroposterior (AP) and true lateral radiographs are taken. An acute slip, when diagnosed, constitutes a surgical emergency and needs to be reduced under anesthesia and internally fixed.

4. **Radial head dislocation,** or nursemaid's elbow, is usually seen in the 1- to 5-year-old age group. It usually occurs after pulling on a child's extended pronated arm. The child refuses to use the arm and has a pseudoparalysis. The radial head is reduced by supinating the forearm and then flexing it at least 90 degrees. Often the dislocation is reduced by the radiology technician in attempting to obtain radiographs. Once relocation has been achieved, the child will begin to purposefully use the arm. Usually no immobilization is required unless there have been previous dislocations.

III. **Burns.** The same fluid resuscitation and monitoring guidelines used in adults (see Chap. 21) are followed in children. However, because of the larger surface-area-to-body-weight ratio in infants and small (i.e., < 20 kg) children, fluid resuscitation requirements may be somewhat greater for them than adults; these adjustments are best made after the initial response to fluid therapy (calculated on the basis of body weight) is evaluated. Other burn management principles are the same as for adults. Indications for hospitalization are presented in Table 21-1; in addition, minor superficial burns of the face, perineum, or genitalia in infants and small children are often best managed in the hospital for a few days.

Bibliography

1. Aicardi, J., and Chevrie, J. Convulsive status epilepticus in infants and children: A study of 239 cases. *Epilepsia* 11:187, 1970.
2. American Heart Association. Standards and guidelines for cardiopulmonary resuscitation (CPR) and emergency cardiac care (ECC). *J.A.M.A.* 255:2905, 1986.
3. Barkin, R. M., and Rosen, P. (eds.). *Emergency Pediatrics* (2nd ed.). St. Louis: Mosby, 1986.
4. Behrman, R., and Vaughan, V. (eds.). *Nelson's Textbook of Pediatrics* (12th ed.). Philadelphia: Saunders, 1983.
5. Brunell, P. A., et al. (Committee on Infectious Diseases). Revision of recommendation for use of rifampin prophylaxis of contacts of patients with *Haemophilus influenzae* infection. *Pediatrics* 74:301, 1984.
6. Centers for Disease Control. Follow-up on Reye syndrome—United States. *M.M.W.R.* 29:321, 1980.
7. Cole. C. (ed.). *The Harriet Lane Handbook* (10th ed.). Chicago: Yearbook Medical Publishers, 1984.
8. Committee on Accident and Poison Prevention, American Academy of Pediatrics. First aid for the choking child. *Pediatrics* 67:744, 1981.
9. Dickerman, J., and Lucey, J. (eds.). *Smith's The Critically Ill Child, Diagnosis and Medical Management* (3rd ed.). Philadelphia: Saunders, 1985.
10. Feigin, R., and Cherry, J. (eds.). *Textbook of Pediatric Infectious Diseases*. Philadelphia: Saunders, 1981.
11. Fleisher, G., and Ludwig, S. (eds.). *Textbook of Pediatric Emergency Medicine*. Baltimore: Williams and Wilkins, 1983.
12. Hughes, W. T., and Buescher, S. (eds.). *Pediatric Procedures* (2nd ed.). Philadelphia: Saunders, 1980.
13. Hurwitz, S. *Clinical Pediatric Dermatology*. Philadelphia: Saunders, 1981.
14. Klaus, M., and Fanaroff, A. (eds.). *Care of the High-Risk Neonate* (3rd ed.). Philadelphia: Saunders, 1986.
15. Klein, J. O. (ed.). *Report of the Committee of Infectious Diseases. The Red Book* (20th ed.). Evanston, Ill.: American Academy of Pediatrics, 1986.

16. Lewis, A. J., et al. *A Manual for Instructors of Basic Cardiac Life Support*. Dallas: American Heart Association, 1981.
17. Lovejoy, F. H., Jr., et al. Clinical staging in Reye syndrome. *Am. J. Dis. Child.* 128:36, 1974.
18. Lovell, W., and Winter, C. *Pediatric Orthopaedics*. Philadelphia: Lippincott, 1978.
19. McCarthy, P. L., et al. Further definition of history and observation variables in assessing febrile children. *Pediatrics* 67:607, 1981.
20. McCracken, G. H., and Nelson, J. D. *Antimicrobial Therapy for Newborns* (2nd ed.). New York: Grune & Stratton, 1983.
21. Nelson, J. D. *1985 Pocketbook of Pediatric Antimicrobial Therapy* (6th ed.). Baltimore: Williams and Wilkins, 1985.
22. Ogden, J. *Skeletal Injury in the Child*. Philadelphia: Lea & Febiger, 1982.
23. Randolph, J., et al. (eds.). *The Injured Child: Surgical Management*. Chicago: Yearbook Medical Publishers, 1979.
24. Winters, R. *Principles of Pediatric Fluid Therapy* (2nd ed.). Boston: Little, Brown, 1982.
25. Wood, D. W., Downes, J. J., and Lecks, H. I. A clinical scoring system for the diagnosis of respiratory failure. *Am. J. Dis. Child.* 123:227, 1972.

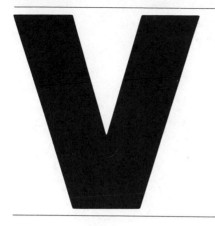

Issues and Procedures

37

Medicolegal Issues

Kathryn Kottemann Wire

General Medicolegal Principles

I. **Medical malpractice** is a form of negligence in which a patient may recover from a physician if the four factors discussed in **A–D** occur simultaneously.

   A. Duty is an obligation imposed by law on one person to behave in a certain way toward another. In any negligence case, the defendant must owe a duty to the plaintiff. In medical malpractice, the physician's duty to the plaintiff can arise from one of several sources.

      1. Physician-patient relationship. In most malpractice cases, the duty arises because the plaintiff is a patient. The "patient" must have presented for treatment, and the physician must have directly or indirectly agreed to treat the patient. However, there generally is not an obligation to treat a nonpatient.

      2. Many states have **Good Samaritan statutes** that protect medical personnel from liability for malpractice if they choose to treat a nonpatient with an emergency illness or injury. Generally, these statutes do not require medical personnel to deliver treatment but are intended to encourage it in an emergency. A physician continuing treatment beyond the emergency would establish a physician-patient relationship that could create an ongoing duty. Good Samaritan laws, however, do not apply to an emergency department, because it has a separate obligation to treat, as discussed below (see **Medicolegal Issues,** sec. I).

      3. Where a duty exists, it requires a certain level of skill, often referred to as the "standard of care."

   B. Breach of the standard of care. The plaintiff must prove a breach of the standard of care, i.e., that the defendant physician failed to use the appropriate level of skill. The level of skill required varies but usually is the same level of skill that a reasonably skillful physician would exercise under the same or similar circumstances.

      1. Some courts apply a standard based on the prevailing skill level in the physician's locality. Now, though, most courts apply a national standard of skillfulness that varies with the specialty and training of the physician. A specialist is expected to treat the patient with a higher standard of care due to his or her additional level of training and skill in the chosen field. Increasingly, both specialists and nonspecialists are expected to be aware of medical developments on a national scale. In addition, the nature of the facility involved has some impact on the expected level of care.

      2. The standard of care in a particular case is usually established with the testimony of experts for both sides. These witnesses tell the jury what "reasonable care" was required. In a small number of cases where the alleged negligence is really not medical in nature but rather involves common knowledge and experience, the courts will allow the patient to prove negligence without expert testimony establishing the standard and its breach. For example, if a patient having abdominal surgery comes out of surgery with a broken arm or a pair of scissors in the abdomen, the court will relieve the plaintiff of bringing in medical experts to prove a breach of duty [14, 17].

      3. When hospital policies are used to establish the standard of care, hospital staff must follow them. A patient may be able to make a malpractice case without expert testimony by using hospital policies to set the standards [11].

   C. Injury. A plaintiff cannot recover unless there is an injury. Even the worst care cannot result in liability for malpractice if the patient suffered no harm. The law previously required physical injury but has increasingly allowed recovery for infliction of emotional distress to patients and family members without any actual physical injury.

741

    D. Proximate cause of the injury. The breach of duty to the patient must be the proximate cause of the injury. The negligence need not be the only cause but must contribute significantly to the injury. For example, improper use of equipment by a physician combined with malfunction of the equipment may create liability, whereas neither alone would have caused the eventual injury.

II. Informed consent. Patients have a **right to physical integrity.** Physicians must honor this right and will be liable to the patient if it is violated. The basic rule is that competent adult patients have a right to control their treatment. The special problems of incompetent patients are discussed below (see **Medicolegal Issues,** secs. **III.C** and **D** and **IV.E).** A violation of the patient's right to give informed consent to treatment can result in two types of liability.

    A. Battery is offensive and unpermitted touching. The most skillful treatment can be a battery, if performed without actual or implied consent of the patient for the actual physical contact.

    B. Medical malpractice liability may occur if the patient consents to treatment without being adequately informed of the risks of the procedure. Standards for the required level of information vary significantly; physicians must know the standard for their area. Some courts judge this standard by what a "reasonable medical practitioner" would disclose; others look to what a typical patient would want to know. The latter standard does not depend on medical expert testimony and reflects the majority of recent rulings on the issue.

Medicolegal Issues

I. Duty to treat. Emergency department personnel have a special duty to treat those who present for treatment. Personnel in attendance should assume that they will be liable for any unexcused failure to treat that results in an injury. For example, one hospital had a policy prohibiting emergency department treatment of patients of private doctors without contacting the private physician first. The rule was designed to avoid conflicts regarding patient management. When a patient did not receive necessary treatment because the hospital could not reach the private physician, the hospital was held liable [19]. Hospitals also have been held liable for failure to treat patients in immediate need because they had no means to pay for the treatment [8].

    A. Acute care hospitals must offer some level of emergency care to be accredited by the Joint Commission on Accreditation of Hospitals (JCAH) [6]. Once a hospital offers emergency care, it assumes a duty to treat those who request its services.

    B. Even in the absence of outside standards, such as the JCAH requirements, some courts have held that hospitals "hold themselves out" as places in which the sick and injured can obtain care. Those courts hold that the institution must fulfill the public expectation of available emergency treatment. Thus, the facility and its staff will have a duty to strangers beyond that applicable to physicians generally.

    C. Other duties may arise from requirements of government-funding agreements (e.g., the Hill-Burton Act) and other relationships between a facility and the entities around it, such as health maintenance organizations [5]. Some states have financing or licensing requirements that limit a hospital's freedom to refuse to treat a patient. Hospital policies should specify any of these special requirements. The hospital or its staff may be liable for failure to treat a patient when the hospital has specifically agreed to do so.

II. Patient transfer. If hospital policy or a lack of facilities or medical expertise requires transfer of a patient, emergency department personnel have a duty to use reasonable skill in effecting the transfer safely.

    A. Stabilization. It is mandatory to do whatever is necessary immediately to preserve the life and health of the patient.

    B. Documentation. If the transfer is for medical reasons, they must be documented in detail. If the transfer is for other reasons, it is essential to document in detail why the transfer is an acceptable alternative.

    C. JCAH standards prohibit transfer from a hospital that has reasonable resources for the patient unless the transfer will not endanger the patient and the receiving hospital has consented to the transfer [6]. A reasonable record of the patient's immediate care must accompany the patient in transfer [6].

III. Consent to treatment. A physician must have consent to treat any patient. Consent can be oral or written, although written documentation is crucial in case of a later dispute.

    A. Implied consent. In some cases consent may be implied, but it is still necessary.

Implied consent occurs when (1) a delay in treatment poses a serious threat to the patient and (2) the patient is not able to give valid consent and there is no family member available. In such a situation, the law assumes the patient would consent to treatment and thus implies consent; however, the need for "patient" consent is not waived. Accordingly, even if the conditions listed above exist, if the physician knows the patient would not have consented, then implied consent is not available.

B. Minors. In all states, parents may give consent for treatment of their children, based on the theory of "substituted" judgment, which presumes that a parent will choose in the best interests of the child. If a parent is not available, the implied consent analysis outlined in **A** applies. If the parents do not agree to needed treatment or with each other, the physician should consider obtaining a court order. If the parents are divorced, it is important to know who has custody and the legal right to determine major treatment decisions, if the state distinguishes those powers in custodial and noncustodial parents.

C. Unconscious or incompetent adults. Most states recognize a "substituted judgment" consent from a close family member. The order in which to consult family members, as well as the validity of such consents, varies among states; thus, it is important to know the local law. However, this substituted judgement will not overcome patient refusal expressed while the patient was competent.

D. Determining competence. The standard for "competence" is not the same as the standard required for guardianship proceedings or psychiatric commitment. Instead, it focuses on the patient's ability to comprehend his or her immediate condition and the options for treatment. Competence can be affected by disease, medication, emotional status, extreme fatigue, and many other factors. Consent from an incompetent patient (with an impaired ability to comprehend) may be invalid. A safe approach if competence is in question is to obtain the informed consent of both the patient and the next of kin.

E. Brain-dead patients do not require consent for treatment. The institution's procedures for declaration of brain death should be followed carefully. The only consent issues for such patients relate to autopsy and organ donation. Of course, nonlegal considerations indicate a need for close communication with the families of such patients. Because it takes some time to properly obtain a declaration of brain death, brain death generally will not be an emergency department issue; the patient should be admitted to the hospital for evaluation of brain death.

IV. Refusal of treatment

A. Right to refuse treatment. All competent patients have the right to refuse treatment. Interference with that decision may lead to liability.

B. Release of patients. Even though patients generally may not be treated without consent, emergency department staff may be liable if they release a patient with an illness or injury (such as drug intoxication or a head injury) that could render the patient's judgment about leaving the department suspect and could later endanger the patient. In such a situation, the staff must choose between two potential liabilities: abandonment and battery (treating without consent); generally, the courts will look more favorably on the latter, if it is in the best interest of the patient. Any patient who leaves against medical advice should sign a form to that effect, and the physician should outline in detail the information made available prior to discharge to the patient and the family about the patient's condition and potential risks to the patient.

C. Some courts will appoint a guardian to consent to treatment of an adult if the death of the patient will affect small children or some other "interest" recognized by the state. However, this doctrine is very limited, not universally recognized, and not expanding; even when this doctrine applies, it requires a court order of guardianship [1, 4, 9, 12, 18]. Physicians should be aware of issues relating to maternal/fetal life in late pregnancies, as the courts have recognized a right of the unborn child in late pregnancy that may outweigh the mother's right to refuse necessary treatment [3, 15].

D. Court order. If parents refuse necessary treatment for their children, courts frequently are willing to intervene on behalf of the child, appointing a guardian with the power to consent. If possible, court approval should always be obtained in advance of treatment.

E. Incompetent patients

1. Living wills. The physician should look first to any expressed intention of the patient made when he or she was competent, i.e., living wills. Some states have statutes that require health care providers to follow a living will. A court's analysis of these situations, even in the absence of living-will legislation, almost always tries to determine what the patient would have wanted.

2. Without actual knowledge of the patient's wishes, the decision is more difficult; but the primary consideration is still the patient's desire. However, the physician should beware of situations involving judgments of the value of life. One court ruled that a court order would be required to withhold painful cancer therapy from a mentally retarded man [16]. Similarly, care of seriously ill newborns has attracted much legal attention. Imminently terminal or irreversibly comatose patients, however, generally may be treated based on the judgment of their physicians with input from the family [2, 13, 16].

3. **Psychiatric commitment.** States have specific rules for involuntary treatment of psychiatric patients that usually include a short period of involuntary detention for evaluation and procurement of commitment orders. The hospital's procedures should be in accordance with local laws on the subject, and physicians must know these rules and procedures. Generally, the standard for psychiatric commitment requires some evidence that the patient presents a danger to self or others if not detained.

V. **Release of information**

A. **Confidentiality of medical records.** Patient medical records are confidential. The information regarding treatment should not be disclosed without written authorization from the patient or, if the patient is unable to give consent, from a family member who could give consent to treatment. A valid subpoena will require disclosure.

B. **Release of patient identification and condition.** Disclosure of a patient's identification and general condition is allowed, unless the patient has requested otherwise. The hospital may be liable for breaching an agreement to keep such information about a particular patient confidential.

C. **Release of information to physicians.** Disclosure rules are usually more flexible when a treating physician is disclosing patient information to other treating physicians. If prompt release of information is necessary to protect the patient and facilitate treatment, consent is implied.

D. Federal law requires a specific court order for the release of any record dealing with certain kinds of alcohol and drug abuse and for the release of records concerning venereal disease and birth control in minors. In such cases, the physician should consult with the hospital's administration or attorney.

VI. **Reportable events.** The law requires that these events be reported to some other authority.

A. **Deaths.** All states require that certain deaths be reported to the coroner for investigation, particularly if the death is suspicious or if the treating physician has not had an adequate opportunity to know the cause of death. Frequently, reportable cases include suicides, dead on arrival, miscellaneous violent deaths, deaths from unknown causes without prior medical care, deaths from poisonings and criminal acts, hospital deaths with no available diagnosis, deaths for which the attending physician cannot or will not sign the death certificate, and accidental deaths. Once a death is reported, the coroner may or may not assume jurisdiction of the case.

B. **Certain infectious diseases,** particularly those spread through sexual contact, must be reported to state or federal authorities. The requirements may change from time to time, and physicians should be aware of the hospital's policies in this area, which should accurately reflect local law.

C. **Criminal acts and suicides** may need to be reported to agencies other than the coroner, generally the police. This requirement will depend on state law, which varies.

D. **Child abuse** must be reported in most states, and an increasing number of states require that abuse of adults be reported as well. Violation of these requirements may result in criminal penalties. In addition, medical personnel who do not file a required abuse report may be subject to liability if the abuse is followed by additional injury [7].

E. State law frequently requires reports of suspected food poisoning from commercial establishments in order to enable authorities to investigate and correct the problem.

Situations with Medicolegal Implications

I. **Telephone advice.** It is possible to establish a physician-patient relationship by phone, which creates a full duty to the patient and full exposure to liability for incomplete or inappropriate advice. Consequently, it is not wise to give telephone advice, except to stabilize the patient until help or transportation to the hospital arrives. For similar reasons, emergency department personnel should not offer telephone advice to patients who have left the facility. If it is necessary to give limited advice over the phone, the details should be recorded in the patient's chart (if there is one) and in a log in which all calls are recorded. Only complete records of all such calls can protect against liability from telephone contact.

II. **Child abuse**
A. **Reporting.** As indicated above (see **Medicolegal Issues,** sec. **VI.D**), there may be criminal or civil liability for failure to report child abuse in most states. In contrast, the laws often protect the person reporting abuse from liability for slander, libel, or related actions, as long as the reporting activities are reasonable. The laws encourage involvement of appropriate governmental agencies in potential child abuse situations, leaving the responsibility to follow up in their hands. The physician's critical role is in establishing the diagnosis, documenting the victim's condition at the time of treatment, and involving the appropriate juvenile agency personnel.
B. **Complete documentation** is essential, as the medical record likely will appear in court. A claim of abuse may result in a parent losing custody of the child; alternatively, failure to properly document abuse could result in failure to establish a case and subsequent death or serious injury to the child. Both consequences should be considered when dealing with potential child abuse.

III. **Psychiatric patients** present a collection of unique problems. It is important to remember that a mentally ill patient who can understand his or her condition and the options for treatment is entitled to full consent rights. Failure to consent to psychiatric or other treatment alone does not indicate incompetence rendering that decision invalid.
A. **Involuntary admissions.** All states have procedures governing involuntary admission of patients. Such admissions require some sort of court determination that the patient is a potential danger to self or others. Physicians must know their state laws, as they must be followed exactly to avoid violation of the patient's common law and constitutional rights.
B. **Voluntary admissions** of psychiatric patients present no problem. The patient is admitted voluntarily and is free to leave at will. Psychiatric illness alone does not preclude competence to give consent, so voluntary treatment occurs as a result of valid patient consent. Most states' laws allow hospitals to obtain court permission to "convert" a voluntary admission to an involuntary one when necessary. Once that occurs, the patient must be treated as an involuntary admission.
C. **Physically abusive patients** may be physically or chemically restrained, but not to any greater degree than necessary to protect the patient, other patients, and staff.
D. **Dangerous patients.** Emergency physicians have some latitude in keeping a potentially dangerous patient for evaluation; failure to do so could result in liability if the patient is released and subsequently injures self or others. The law expects physicians to take advantage of the opportunity it provides to evaluate potentially dangerous psychiatric patients through involuntary admissions. However, this law is always balanced against the patient's basic right to leave at will. The two concepts almost always are involved in varying degrees in emergency psychiatric admissions and require astute exercise of physician judgment [16].
E. **Underlying disease.** It is essential to look for underlying physical problems, possibly masked by patient behavior. Failure to do so could result in malpractice liability.

IV. **Intoxicated patients and blood alcohol tests**
A. **Blood alcohol tests.** Several states have laws that create implied consent for blood alcohol tests at the request of arresting police officers for patients suspected of alcohol or drug-related offenses. Medical personnel must know the state law and follow it with careful documentation. If the police follow all the required steps, the hospital will be absolved of liability to the patient for taking the sample without consent, but only for the sample to be used for legal purposes. All samples for routine medical purposes must be obtained with actual or implied patient consent.
B. **Release of information.** Information, including alcohol and drug levels, on patients admitted strictly for medical purposes is confidential and should not be revealed, even to the police, without a valid release, subpoena, or warrant.

V. **Police cases**
A. **Reporting.** Some states may require reports on patients with certain injuries, such as gunshot or stab wounds, or in possession of such illegal items as weapons or drugs. Hospital staff should be familiar with state law, as there could be liability for

improper failure to report or liability to the patient for reporting if there is no requirement.

   B. Patient rights. Unless a special informed consent or disclosure law applies, **patients brought in by the police have the same consent and disclosure rights as other patients.**

   C. Special care is necessary with police cases, as these patients may have latent injuries in addition to the conditions that caused the police to take them to the hospital. For example, an apparently intoxicated person may have an underlying injury or illness.

VI. Weapons

   A. Reporting. Hospital staff may need to report the possession of firearms or other weapons, depending on state law.

   B. Removal of weapons. Patients with weapons or reasonably suspected to have weapons, and who present a danger to the staff or other patients, may be searched, stripped, and restrained (with care and appropriate precautions). The staff may remove potential weapons from the patient's possession. Whether or not they are returned to the patient with the rest of the inventoried possessions depends on state requirements for licensing and reporting possession of firearms, which vary widely.

VII. Alleged rape

   A. Documentation. Since the medical record may be important to later civil or criminal legal action, all facts reported by the patient must be recorded completely and as accurately as possible. In addition, all aspects of the patient's injuries and condition must be documented carefully, using standard medical terminology. In particular, physical findings such as lacerations or bruises must be accurately recorded. Other important observations include the condition of the genitalia and the results of the testing of any samples obtained. Legal terms or conclusions such as "self-defense" and "rape" should not be used. Such legal phrases should appear in the record only when they are quotations from the victim, and then they should be labeled as such.

   B. Rape protocol. If the hospital has an established rape protocol, it should be followed. A patient who is unable to prosecute or pursue civil remedies due to the hospital's failure to follow its own procedures may try to recover from the physician or the hospital.

   C. Chain of custody. It is important to document a chain of custody on any physical items such as the victim's clothing. Giving these articles to the police is the best way to protect the evidence with minimum hospital involvement. If personal items are returned to the patient, that should be documented as well. The hospital should be able to account for the condition and location of such items during the time they are under hospital control. Careful documentation of the handling of laboratory specimens is important as well, including their condition and the identity of any person who transports them.

VIII. Terminally ill patients

   A. No resuscitation policy. It is important to know the hospital's policy and procedures for "do not resuscitate" or "no code" patients and follow them relentlessly. If all the requirements for documentation of a "no code" status have not been met for a terminally ill patient in the emergency department, resuscitation should be initiated.

   B. Decision regarding treatment. The patient has the final decision regarding treatment; unwanted treatment should not be forced on a patient who is competent to understand the decision. All the discussion above of the patient's right to refuse treatment (see **Medicolegal Issues,** sec. **IV**) applies equally to end-stage patients.

   C. It is important for the physician to establish a rapport with family members, especially if a no code decision is possible, since they will be the ones who might file a lawsuit.

IX. Chart documentation. Careful and accurate chart documentation is essential, because staff rarely spend enough time with emergency patients to remember them months or years later. The emergency record should include the patient's complaints, the vital signs, condition of the patient, evaluation (including any tests performed and their results), diagnosis, arrangements for follow-up, and instructions given to the patient or the family.

X. Continuity of care

   A. Follow-up care. For patients to be discharged from the emergency department, there is a duty to take reasonable steps to ensure follow-up care. This process generally involves referring the patient to his or her private physician, another physician, or a specialty clinic. It may be necessary in some cases to actually make the follow-up appointment for the patient. Failure to take such steps may result in liability for "abandonment," a form of malpractice. The patient or a family member should sign an acknowledgment that such instructions for follow-up have been received.

B. **Responsibility regarding admitted patients.** The emergency physician has a responsibility to make sure that the patient receives continuity of care when admitted to the hospital. This may involve consulting with the receiving physician or nurses or writing appropriate admission orders to assure a smooth transition to inpatient status. Once safe transition has occurred, the responsibility of the emergency physician should terminate.

XI. **Disputes regarding patient management.** The emergency physician is responsible for the care given to the patient in the emergency department. If a dispute as to proper treatment develops between the emergency staff and the private physician, the physician who is present and in control is most likely to face legal liability and thus should act accordingly.

Bibliography

1. *Application of the President of Georgetown College,* 331 F.2d 1000 (D.C. Cir.), *cert. denied,* 377 U.S. 978 (1964).
2. *In re Dinnerstein,* 6 Mass. App. Sh. 466, 380 N.E.2d 134 (1978).
3. *Fabian v. Matzko,* 344 A.2d 569 (Pa. Super. 1975).
4. *Hallisey, The Fetal Patient and the Unwilling Mother: A Standard for Judicial Intervention,* 14 Pac. L.J. 1065 (1983).
5. *Hospital Survey and Construction Act of 1944,* 42 U.S.C. §§291 *et seq.* (1944) (Hill-Burton Act).
6. Joint Commission on Accreditation of Hospitals. *Accreditation Manual for Hospitals.* Chicago: JCAH, 1986.
7. *Landeros v. Flood,* 131 Cal. Rptr. 69, 551 P.2d 389 (S. Ct. en banc 1976).
8. *Mercy Medical Center of Oshkosh v. Winnebago County,* 58 Wis. 2d 260, 206 N.W.2d 198, 201 (1973).
9. *Muhlenberg Hospital v. Patterson,* 128 N.J. Super. 498, 320 A.2d 518 (1974).
10. *Nance v. James Archer Smith Hospital,* 329 So. 2d 377 (Fla. App. 1976).
11. *Niles v. City of San Rafael,* 42 Cal. App. 3d 230, 116 Cal. Rptr. 733 (1974).
12. *In re Osborne,* 294 A.2d 372 (D.C. Ct. App. 1972).
13. *In re Quinlan,* 355 A.2d 647 (N.J. 1976).
14. *Robbins v. Jewish Hospital of St. Louis,* 663 S.W.2d 341 (Mo. App. 1983).
15. *Roe v. Wade,* 410 U.S. 113, 93 S. Ct. 705, 35 L. Ed. 2d 147, *reh'g denied,* 410 U.S. 959, 93 S. Ct. 1409, 35 L. Ed. 2d 694 (1973).
16. *Superintendent of Belchertown School v. Saikewicz,* 373 Mass. 728, 370 N.E.2d 417 (1977).
17. *Thomas v. Corso,* 265 Md. 84, 288 A.2d 379, 387–388 (Ct. App. 1972).
18. *Wallace v. Labrenz,* 411 Ill. 618, 104 N.E.2d 769, *cert. denied,* 344 U.S. 824 (1952).
19. *Wilmington General Hospital v. Manlove,* 54 Del. 15, 174 A.2d 135 (1961).

38

Arthrocentesis and Intraarticular Injection

Jeffrey L. Kaine

Arthrocentesis with synovianalysis is a safe and minimally painful procedure with a critical role in the management of patients with undiagnosed arthritis. Synovial fluid usually can be aspirated from inflamed ankles, knees, wrists, elbows, or shoulders. Arthrocentesis of the small joints of the hands and feet, however, is difficult and frequently unsuccessful. Hips generally should be aspirated under fluoroscopic guidance. Joint aspiration should be performed only by experienced physicians.

I. **Indications**
   A. **Diagnostic indications** for arthrocentesis include the diagnosis of infectious arthritis, crystalline arthritis, and intraarticular hemorrhage as well as the determination of the degree of synovial inflammation in any unknown arthritis.
   B. **Therapeutic indications.** Arthrocentesis with intraarticular corticosteroid injection can produce symptomatic relief in any of the synovial-based arthritides. Occasionally, traumatic arthritis and osteoarthritis will benefit from corticosteroid injection. These drugs can also be injected into bursae and tendon sheaths with dramatic improvement. However, intraarticular corticosteroid injection should be viewed only as a palliative procedure. Symptomatic relief may persist for up to 6 months. All other antirheumatic therapeutic modalities can be used concomitantly with intraarticular steroid injections.

II. **Contraindications**
   A. **Contraindications to joint aspiration**
      1. Aspirating through potentially **infected skin** should be avoided whenever possible. However, if septic arthritis is a diagnostic consideration, joint aspiration may be performed with relative safety.
      2. Patients with a **bleeding diathesis** (e.g., anticoagulation, hemophilia, thrombocytopenia) may develop intraarticular hemorrhage following joint aspiration. Reversal of the underlying defect (e.g., by factor VIII infusion or platelet transfusion) should be performed prior to aspiration whenever possible.
      3. Inserting the needle through previously **damaged skin** (e.g., psoriasis, eczema) should be avoided, if possible.
   B. **Contraindications to intraarticular corticosteroid injection**
      1. Intraarticular corticosteroid injections are contraindicated in patients with possible or documented **infectious arthritis.**
      2. In the rare situation in which a patient is allergic to the vehicle, the drug should not be administered.

III. **Procedure**
   A. **Joint aspiration.** General principles of aseptic technique are observed, although gloves and gown are not required.
      1. The skin overlying the joint is cleaned with povidone-iodine and alcohol in routine fashion.
      2. **Anesthesia** is provided with ethyl chloride spray for 10 seconds. Subcutaneous anesthesia with lidocaine is usually unnecessary.
      3. **Aspiration.** The joint is aspirated with an 18- and 20-gauge needle to facilitate removal of viscous fluid.
      4. **Synovianalysis.** Fluid removed is analyzed with a polarizing microscope for crystals and sent for a white blood cell (WBC) count with differential, glucose determination, Gram stain, and culture.

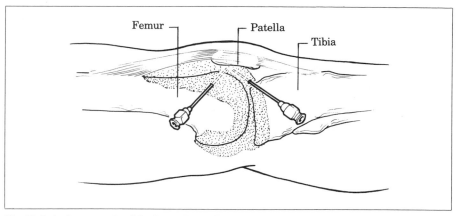

Fig. 38-1. Arthrocentesis of the knee. From the lateral or medial aspect of the knee, an 18-gauge needle is advanced just posteriorly and parallel to the patella into the joint space.

B. Intraarticular injection
1. Multiple microcrystalline **corticosteroid suspensions** are available, although prednisolone tebutate and triamcinolone hexacetonide generally are preferred because of their lower solubility. Both agents are dispensed in individual dose vials in a concentration of 20 mg/ml.
2. **Corticosteroid dosages** vary depending on the joint being injected: ankle, 20 mg; knee, 20–40 mg; wrist, 10–20 mg; and shoulder, 20–40 mg.
3. The drug generally is mixed with 1 ml of lidocaine prior to injection. This mixture provides short-term immediate relief, which assures the physician that the joint space was entered effectively.
4. All joint fluid is aspirated prior to corticosteroid injection.

C. Approach to specific joints
1. The **knee** (Fig. 38-1). Either a medial or lateral approach can be used. With the patient supine and the joint fully extended, an 18-gauge needle is advanced through the skin perpendicular to the medial or lateral aspect of the knee and directed just posteriorly and parallel to the patella into the joint space. Compression of the suprapatellar area may facilitate removal of fluid.
2. The **shoulder** (Fig. 38-2) can be aspirated using either an anterior or posterior approach. For each approach, the arm is held in slight internal rotation, with the elbow flexed across the chest.
   a. Using the **anterior approach,** the glenohumeral joint is injected at a site 1 cm inferior and lateral to the coricoid process; an 18-gauge needle is angled mediodorsally and slightly superiorly.
   b. The **posterior approach,** although slightly more difficult, should be attempted whenever difficulty is encountered with the anterior approach. The needle is inserted at a site 1 cm inferior to the lateral aspect of the acromion and angled ventromedially.
   c. The **subdeltoid bursa** is entered immediately inferior to the most lateral aspect of the scapula.
3. The **wrist** (Fig. 38-3) is entered from its dorsal surface at the most distal aspect of the radius. A 20- or 22-gauge needle is directed perpendicularly to the dorsal wrist surface at a site immediately ulnar to the thumb extensor tendon.
4. The **ankle** (Fig. 38-4) is held in slight plantar flexion.
   a. Using a **medial approach,** a 20-gauge needle is advanced through the skin 1 cm distal and anterior to the medial malleolus and directed posterolaterally.
   b. With the **lateral approach,** the needle is advanced through the skin 1 cm distal and anterior to the lateral malleolus and directed posteromedially.
5. The **elbow** (Fig. 38-5) is entered posterolaterally just lateral to the olecranon process and inferior to the humeral epicondyle. With the arm incompletely extended, an 18- or 20-gauge needle is directed medially and proximally to the head of the radius.

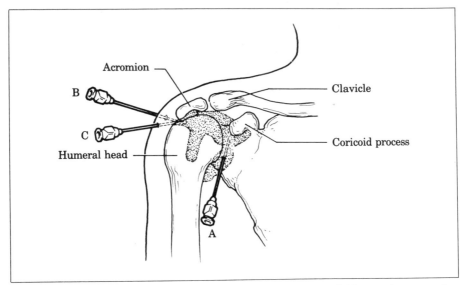

Fig. 38-2. Arthrocentesis of the shoulder showing the (A) anterior and (B) posterior approach and (C) access to the subdeltoid bursa.

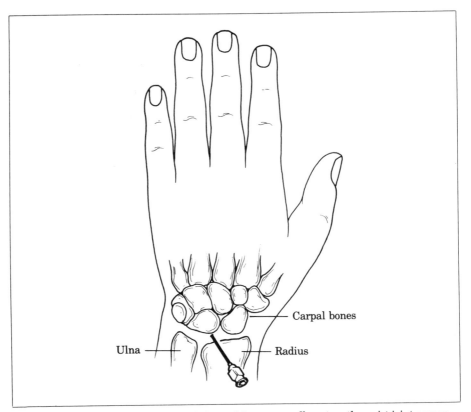

Fig. 38-3. Arthrocentesis of the wrist. A 20- or 22-gauge needle enters the wrist joint perpendicularly to the dorsal surface immediately ulnar to the thumb extensor tendon.

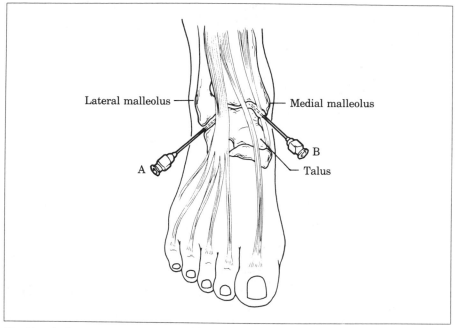

Fig. 38-4. Arthrocentesis of the ankle. A 20-gauge needle enters the joint space from a site 1 cm distal and anterior to the (A) lateral malleolus or (B) medial malleolus.

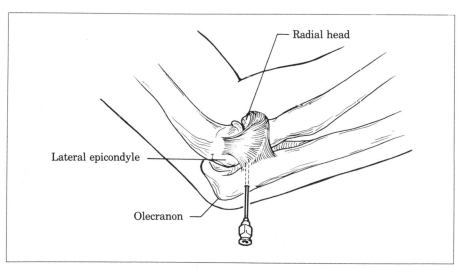

Fig. 38-5. Arthrocentesis of the elbow. The elbow joint is entered with an 18- or 20-gauge needle from a site just lateral to the olecranon process and inferior to the humeral epicondyle.

IV. Complications of joint aspiration or steroid injection are uncommon.
  A. Infection occurs in approximately 0.01% or less of aspirations.
  B. Intraarticular hemorrhage is a rare complication when patients with hemostatic disorders are excluded.
  C. A self-limited **postinjection synovitis** occasionally occurs within 12–48 hours following steroid injection. No specific treatment is warranted; however, patients need to be warned about this potential complication prior to injection. If needed, a mild oral analgesic may be administered.
  D. Since systemic absorption of intraarticular steroids is minimal, **glucose intolerance** in diabetic patients is only very rarely observed.

Autotransfusion

Richard E. Larson

Autotransfusion is defined as the collection and reinfusion of a patient's own blood (autologous) for the purpose of intravascular volume replacement. Although repletion of intravascular volume in a traumatized patient is initiated with crystalloid solutions, administration of blood is usually required if the patient is still in shock after the infusion of 2 liters of crystalloid. Autotransfusion is a relatively uncomplicated procedure that can provide compatable blood immediately to the patient who requires it. Autotransfusion is particularly useful for patients with thoracic trauma where pooled blood within the chest cavity is readily available via tube thoracostomy and is usually not contaminated.

  I. Indications. Autotransfusion is indicated in the presence of an **acute blood loss of 1500 ml or more** into the chest or abdomen from a traumatic or nontraumatic event. Because of the ease of blood retrieval and relatively low risk of contamination, autotransfusion is particularly well suited for blood replacement in the presence of an acute hemothorax. It is particularly useful when homologous blood is unavailable or in short supply (e.g., due to a blood bank shortage or cross-match incompatibility) or when the patient's religious beliefs preclude the use of homologous blood replacement.

  II. Contraindications
  A. Presence of a malignant lesion in the area of traumatic blood pooling and collection.
  B. Pooled blood more than 6 hours old because of the increased risk of bacterial contamination and excessive hemolysis (from the blood having been exposed to the pleura or peritoneum for this length of time).
  C. Contamination of the pooled blood (controversial). It is generally accepted that autotransfusion of potentially contaminated blood (e.g., due to the presence of a concomitant bowel perforation) should be avoided (unless autologous blood is needed to avert a life-threatening situation). Reinfusion of contaminated autologous blood, however, has not been shown to significantly increase morbidity or mortality [31, 56, 66]. It is suggested that if the clinical situation demands the use of contaminated autologous blood because the patient will exsanguinate without it, the patient should receive concomitant IV broad-spectrum antibiotics [31, 56, 66].
  D. Renal insufficiency is a theoretical contraindication to the use of autotransfusion, because the increased levels of plasma-free hemoglobin in autotransfused patients may theoretically precipitate renal failure.

  III. Advantages
  A. Immediate availability of blood.
  B. Identical cross-match compatability of blood.
  C. Risk of transmitting infectious diseases (e.g., hepatitis, acquired immunodeficiency syndrome [AIDS], syphilis) is avoided.
  D. Viable platelets and clotting factors are retained (except for chest blood that is devoid of fibrinogen).
  E. Metabolic alterations of stored blood (e.g., acidosis, hyperkalemia, hypocalcemia, decreased 2,3-diphosphoglyceric acid [2,3-DPG]) are avoided.
  F. Hypothermia associated with transfusion of cold bank blood is avoided.
  G. Lower medical cost. Type and cross-match is not required, and the cost of bank blood is avoided.

  IV. Disadvantages. The following disadvantages are rarely clinically significant.
  A. A coagulopathy secondary to decreased platelets or a low fibrinogen level is possible if the autotransfused blood volume is equal to or greater than half the patient's total blood volume.

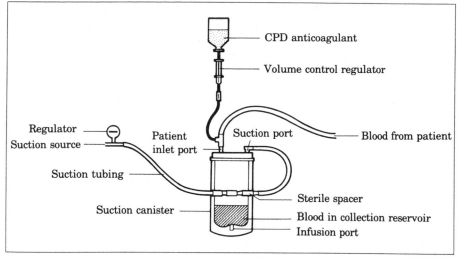

Fig. 38-6. Sorenson autotransfusion system. Blood collected from the patient is mixed with CPD anticoagulant in a ratio of 7:1 and then reinfused.

    B. Red blood cell (RBC) hemolysis may occur with prolonged contact of the pooled blood to serosal surfaces and secondary to mechanical factors (e.g., high suction pressure) during collection and reinfusion.

    C. Elevated plasma-free hemoglobin.

    D. Transient increase in serum creatinine.

    E. Decreased serum hematocrit.

    F. Increased plasma levels of fibrin-split products comparable to that seen with banked blood.

    G. Marginal prolongation of both the prothrombin time (PT) and partial thromboplastin time (PTT) that is self-corrected within 72 hours.

    H. Theoretical risk of sepsis by reinfusing contaminated blood.

    I. Air embolism, usually associated with the automated roller-pump type units.

    J. Microemboli and fat emboli have essentially been eliminated by the use of filters (macropore and micropore) during collection and reinfusion of the patient's blood.

V. The device. Most physicians agree that because the Sorenson autotransfusion system (Fig. 38-6) is easy to use (i.e., does not require a trained technician) and has a relatively low cost (approximately $220 for the initial trauma kit, which contains two complete devices, and about $25 for each additional liner), it is well suited for emergency department use. The apparatus consists of a rigid reusable outer canister and an inner disposable, sterilized plastic bag that holds approximately 1900 ml of blood. The bag serves as a collection, filtering, and reinfusing reservoir. The reservoir contains three ports, two on the top used during collection and one on the bottom used for reinfusion. One top port is connected to controlled suction, and the other is connected to both the patient's source of autologous blood and an anticoagulant source; citrate-phosphate-dextrose (CPD) is the anticoagulant of choice because it is inexpensive, relatively small volumes are required, and it is rapidly metabolized in the liver. The system contains a macropore and micropore filter to remove unwanted microemboli and debris during collection and reinfusion of the patient's blood, respectively.

VI. Procedure

    A. The **source of autologous blood** is tapped (e.g., by tube thoracostomy or insertion of a peritoneal dialysis catheter).

    B. Setup. The appropriate end of the autologous blood drainage system is connected to the patient inlet port on the reservoir bag. The bag is then inserted into the canister and mounted on an IV pole, and the anticoagulant (CPD) source is connected to the patient inlet port via a T connector. The vacuum tubing and regulator are then connected to the suction port, and the vacuum pressure set not to exceed 30 mm Hg.

    C. Collection of blood. The patient's blood is collected in the reservoir bag, and anticoagulant (CPD) is added in a ratio of 1 volume of anticoagulant to 7 volumes of blood.

D. To begin the **autotransfusion,** the tube from the patient's source of blood (e.g., chest tube) is clamped, and the collection bag is removed and replaced with a new one. Any air is removed from the collection bag by squeezing it with care so as not to lose any blood through the open ports. The suction and patient inlet ports are connected to each other, making a closed system. The port on the bottom of the collection bag is then pierced with a micropore filter, and a standard IV blood administration set attached. The blood is then infused via gravity or an in-line blood infusion pump.

E. Massive autotransfusion. Although there is no contraindication to reinfusing a large amount (i.e., > 4000 ml) of autologous blood when blood loss has been extensive, infusing such an amount of autologous blood using CPD anticoagulant may lead to citrate toxicity. To prevent this, it is recommended that after the infusion of 4000 ml of autologous blood, 1 gm of calcium chloride be administered to the patient for each additional 1000 ml of infused autologous blood.

Cricothyrotomy
Robert H. Marcus

Cricothyrotomy involves cannulating the airway through an incision made at the cricothyroid membrane. In general, cricothyrotomy is the surgical procedure of choice for establishing an airway emergently, because at this level there are no vital structures between the skin and airway, the cricoid cartilage prevents inadvertent puncture of the posterior wall of the larynx, and the cricothyroid membrane is usually readily identifiable. Also, cricothyrotomy can be performed without extending the neck in patients with a cervical spine injury. Thus, cricothyrotomy is the fastest, simplest, and safest surgical approach for gaining emergent access to the airway.

I. **Indications. Cricothyrotomy is indicated when rapid access to the airway is required and cannot be achieved by less invasive methods** (e.g., endotracheal intubation, percutaneous transtracheal ventilation). It is particularly useful in patients with upper airway obstruction (e.g., from a foreign body, trauma, edema, or laryngospasm) or in patients with a cervical spine injury in whom nasotracheal intubation is contraindicated or unsuccessful.

II. **Contraindications**
   A. Absolute contraindications
   1. When a less invasive means of establishing an airway can be performed safely.
   2. When obstruction of the airway is distal to the cricothyroid membrane (e.g., fractured or crushed cricoid cartilage, foreign body obstruction at the carina).
   B. Relative contraindications include the following: (1) a coagulopathy, (2) an overlying tumor or hematoma, (3) an age less than 10 years old (because the less prominent small cricothyroid membrane is difficult to identify and cannulate, and the small tracheal diameter at the level of the cricoid cartilage greatly increases the risk of subsequent stenosis), (4) acute laryngeal disease (because of the increased risk of subglottic stenosis), or (5) indistinct landmarks (e.g., from previous surgery, obesity, or swelling).

III. **Procedure**
   A. The neck is hyperextended (unless there is a suspected cervical spine injury) and the anterior aspect of the neck is prepped with a povidone-iodine solution.
   B. Using sterile technique (if time allows), the cricothyroid membrane is identified as an indentation between the prominent thyroid cartilage and cricoid cartilage.
   C. In awake patients, the tissue overlying the cricothyroid membrane is anesthetized with a 1% lidocaine solution.
   D. A 1- to 2-cm horizontal incision is made over the cricothyroid membrane with a scalpel with a No. 15 blade. The incision is extended through the skin, platysma muscle, and cricothyroid membrane.
   E. A hemostat is used to spread the incised cricothyroid membrane while a No. 4–8 tracheostomy tube (or, alternatively, a size 5- or 6-mm cuffed endotracheal tube) is advanced caudally into the trachea.

IV. **Complications** from cricothyrotomy are far less common than from tracheostomy. However, reported complications include damage to the thyroid cartilage or vocal cords, subcutaneous or mediastinal emphysema, hemorrhage, extratracheal tube placement, a pneumothorax, laryngeal edema, laceration of the esophagus or trachea, and a prolonged procedure time with attendant anoxic injury. Delayed complications include infection at the cricothyrotomy site, tracheal erosion, subglottic or tracheal stenosis, a persistent tracheocutaneous fistula, and voice alteration.

Culdocentesis

Diane F. Merritt

Culdocentesis is the procedure whereby intraperitoneal fluid (e.g., transudate, exudate, blood) is aspirated from the rectouterine cul-de-sac (pouch of Douglas, or Douglas' cul-de-sac) by puncture of the posterior vaginal fornix.

I. **Indications** include (1) a suspected ectopic pregnancy, (2) suspected hemoperitoneum (e.g., ruptured corpus luteum, intraabdominal injury), or (3) suspected salpingitis or pelvic inflammatory disease.

II. **Contraindications**
   A. Presence of a pelvic abscess is a relative contraindication to culdocentesis, although this is controversial.
   B. The procedure is difficult if the uterus is retroflexed, and may be technically unfeasible if the uterus is fixed in a retroflexed position.

III. **Procedure** (Fig. 38-7)
   A. The patient is placed in the lithotomy position with the head of the bed slightly elevated, and a bimanual examination is performed to ascertain the position of the uterus and the presence of any masses.
   B. A speculum is placed in the vagina, and an appropriate antiseptic solution (e.g., povidone-iodine) is used to prep the cervix and the posterior fornix of the vagina.
   C. The posterior lip of the cervix is then grasped with a tenaculum and elevated.
   D. An 18-gauge spinal needle with a 10-ml syringe attached is thrust firmly through the midline of the posterior fornix (about 1 cm posterior to the cervix) into the cul-de-sac. As a test for intraperitoneal placement, approximately 5 ml of air is injected; lack of resistance denotes proper positioning of the needle.
   E. Suction is then applied to the syringe, and the return noted. If no fluid is obtained, the procedure may be repeated with the needle repositioned.

IV. **Interpretation of results**
   A. **Diagnostic tap.** If, on aspiration, a substantial amount of free blood is obtained, a hemoperitoneum exists; the presence of clots may indicate very active bleeding. Straw-colored peritoneal fluid indicates proper placement of the needle in the cul-de-sac and no active bleeding at the time of the procedure. Serosanguineous fluid may be spun down to document a low hematocrit and substantiate the diagnosis of no hemoperitoneum. Purulent fluid is diagnostic of infection and should be Gram stained and cultured.

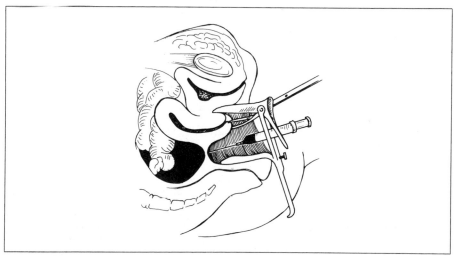

Fig. 38-7. Culdocentesis. An 18-gauge needle attached to a 10-ml syringe is advanced through the midline of the posterior vaginal fornix into the cul-de-sac. (From B. Z. Taber. *Manual of Gynecologic and Obstetric Emergencies* (2nd ed.). Philadelphia: Saunders, 1984. With permission.)

B. Nondiagnostic tap. Obtaining a "dry tap" is nondiagnostic and cannot be presumed to exclude a hemoperitoneum. Obtaining less than 1 ml of blood that clots may indicate a traumatic tap. In these situations, a second attempt is indicated.

V. Complications. Minor bleeding from the tenaculum and puncture sites may be controlled with pressure or cauterization with a silver nitrate stick. Laceration of a pelvic vein (with bleeding) or puncture of bowel (usually without sequelae) may occur.

Endotracheal Intubation

Robert J. Stine

Endotracheal intubation, which may be achieved by the oral or nasal route, is a means to secure a protected airway; ventilate or hyperventilate patients; or clear secretions, blood, or foreign matter from the pulmonary tract.

I. Indications for endotracheal intubation
- **A. Ventilation** of patients with the following:
  1. Cardiac or respiratory arrest.
  2. Respiratory insufficiency.
  3. Significant flail chest.
  4. Upper airway obstruction (e.g., epiglottitis).
  5. Severe shock.
- **B. Hyperventilation** to reduce the intracranial pressure in patients with cerebral edema or an intracranial mass lesion (e.g., patients with anoxic encephalopathy, head injury, or severe cerebrovascular accident).
- **C. Protection of the airway** against aspiration or upper airway obstruction in patients with the following:
  1. Depressed level of consciousness (e.g., drug overdose, head injury).
  2. Absent gag reflex.
  3. Impending upper airway obstruction (e.g., epiglottitis, oral burns).
- **D. Maintenance of a clear pulmonary tract** in patients with the following:
  1. Copious secretions (e.g., pulmonary edema).
  2. Severe hemoptysis.
  3. Aspiration of vomitus or foreign matter.

II. Methods. Nasotracheal intubation is preferred over **orotracheal intubation** in the following situations:
- **A.** Conscious patients.
- **B.** Patients who cannot lie supine.
- **C.** Patients with significant oropharyngeal injuries (e.g., fractured mandible).
- **D.** Patients with suspected cervical spine injury.
- **E.** Inability to gain oral access (e.g., secondary to trismus, oral cavity neoplasm).
- **F.** Need for long-term tracheal intubation.

III. Contraindications. In the emergent situation, there are no absolute contraindications to endotracheal intubation. Relative contraindications are as follows:
- **A. Contraindications to orotracheal intubation**
  1. Suspected cervical spine injury.
  2. Severe mandibular or oral injuries.
- **B. Contraindications to nasotracheal intubation**
  1. Apnea (if blind technique is used).
  2. Severe maxillofacial injuries, in particular, suspected fracture of the cribriform plate.
  3. Bleeding diathesis, including anticoagulation.
  4. Epiglottitis (if blind technique is used).
  5. Foreign body or tumor in the upper airway (if blind technique is used).
  6. Nasal polyps or tumors bilaterally.

IV. Procedure
- **A.** The key to successful tracheal intubation is **proper positioning of the patient's head and neck.** The ideal position is when the axes of the mouth, pharynx, and larynx are aligned [54]. This position, the sniffing position, can be achieved by flexing the neck (by elevating the head on one or two towels) and extending the head at the atlantooccipital joint [54]. However, these maneuvers are contraindicated in the presence of a possible cervical spine injury; in such a situation, the neck must be maintained in a neutral position.

B. The necessary **equipment** is selected and, if time permits, checked to ascertain that it is functioning properly. If orotracheal intubation is to be attempted, the laryngoscope blade can be either curved (MacIntosh blade) or straight (e.g., Miller blade, Flagg blade), depending on personal preference. The curved blade generally is easier to use in visualizing the glottic opening, especially in individuals with a short, thick neck; the straight blade, however, is preferred in infants and small children. Generally, the adult male glottis can accommodate an 8.0- to 9.0-mm cuffed endotracheal tube, and the female glottis a 7.5- to 8.5-mm tube. For children, the outer diameter of the tube should approximate the diameter of the child's little finger, and no cuff is required for children less than 8 years old. If the nasal route is to be used, a 7.0- to 8.0-mm tube generally may be selected for adults. For orotracheal (but not nasotracheal) intubation in adults, the endotracheal tube should be fitted with an inner stylet, which must be recessed 1–2 cm from the end of the tube; the stylet facilitates intubation by maintaining a gentle curve to the distal end of the tube and enabling the operator to better direct the tip of the tube through the glottis.

C. Oxygenation. Prior to attempted intubation and between unsuccessful attempts, the patient must be well oxygenated. Depending on the clinical situation, oxygenation may require ventilation with a mask and bag-valve device or any other means available. During attempted intubation, it is important that ventilation not be interrupted for more than 30 seconds at any one time.

D. Mechanical measures. Prior to attempted intubation, the patient's mouth should be opened widely, any dentures or foreign bodies manually removed, and secretions and any vomitus suctioned.

E. Pharmacologic measures

   1. Topical anesthesia. To facilitate endotracheal intubation in awake patients, the mucosa leading to the trachea should be anesthetized with a topical anesthetic agent (e.g., lidocaine, Cetacaine). If time permits, 4% cocaine, which has the added advantage of shrinking mucosa, may be used to anesthetize the nasal passage.

   2. Depending on the clinical situation, administration of a **sedative** (e.g., diazepam) or a **narcotic analgesic** (e.g., morphine, fentanyl) IV in judicious doses may facilitate intubation in awake patients.

   3. Succinylcholine chloride, a short-acting depolarizing skeletal muscle relaxant (paralyzing agent) generally should not be used as an adjunct to endotracheal intubation. However, in situations where endotracheal intubation is emergently needed but not possible to achieve because of trismus, laryngospasm (not responsive to forced bag ventilation with a mask or application of topical anesthesia), or patient resistance, succinylcholine in a dosage of 1.5 mg/kg IV may facilitate intubation [64]. In addition, in patients with a severe head injury or cerebrovascular accident, succinylcholine may facilitate a difficult intubation without adversely elevating the intracranial pressure [64]. If succinylcholine is used, the **Sellick maneuver** (i.e., application of downward pressure on the cricoid cartilage) should be performed to occlude the esophagus and lessen the chance of aspiration, and an alternate means to establish an airway (e.g., percutaneous transtracheal ventilation, cricothyrotomy) must be readily available. Any resultant bradycardia may be treated with atropine.

   Contraindications to the use of succinylcholine include (1) possible inability to establish an airway; (2) partial airway obstruction (because of the risk of complete obstruction with muscle relaxation); (3) presence of an anatomic disorder involving the head and neck rendering intubation difficult or unlikely, even with muscle relaxation; (4) a penetrating eye injury or glaucoma (because of the increase in intraocular pressure associated with the use of the drug); (5) when any of the following are present for more than a few days: severe trauma, extensive burns, CNS (including spinal cord) injury, or a neuromuscular disorder (because of the risk of severe hyperkalemia from release of potassium from muscle cells); and (6) preexisting hyperkalemia.

F. Intubation

   1. Orotracheal intubation (Fig. 38-8). With the laryngoscope held in the operator's left hand and the patient's mouth opened widely, the blade is inserted into the right side of the mouth. The blade is advanced, elevating and sweeping the tongue to the left, until the epiglottis is visualized. If a curved blade is used, its tip is placed in the vallecula anterior and superior to the epiglottis. If a straight blade is used, it is inserted just beyond the epiglottis. With steady traction (not

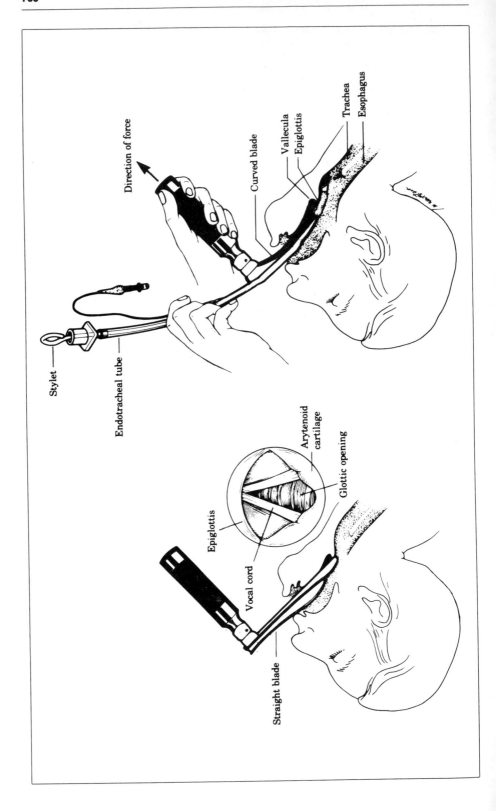

leverage) applied to the handle, the laryngoscope is lifted up and away from the operator at a 45-degree angle to the bed, displacing the base of the tongue and the epiglottis anteriorly and exposing the vocal cords and glottic opening. To avoid damage to the teeth, it is important that they not be used as a fulcrum. External pressure applied to the cricoid cartilage (the Sellick maneuver) by an assistant will facilitate visualization of the glottic opening and, by occluding the upper end of the esophagus, lessen the risk of aspiration. The endotracheal tube, with its distal aspect lubricated and an inner stylet in place, is inserted into the right aspect of the patient's mouth with the operator's right hand and advanced between the vocal cords into the trachea. If the glottis cannot be visualized despite appropriate efforts, the endotracheal tube should be directed in an anterior direction just caudal to the epiglottis. Following insertion of the tube beyond the glottis, the inner stylet is removed and the tube is advanced to its proper position. The cuff is then inflated with 5–10 cc of air, and the patient is ventilated with a bag-valve device as needed.

2. **Nasotracheal intubation.** A well-lubricated endotracheal tube (without a stylet) is inserted into the most patent naris and advanced along the floor of the nose into the oropharynx. With the operator listening to breath sounds at the proximal end of the tube, the tube is slowly advanced until the breath sounds are maximum in intensity, signifying that the distal end of the tube is near the glottic opening. Then during inspiration, the tube is advanced with a single rapid but gentle motion. Inspection and palpation of the patient's neck will aid the operator in placing the tube within the trachea. If the end of the tube impinges on the neck anteriorly, the head needs to be flexed forward [52]; if the tube passes into the esophagus, the head should be hyperextended [52]; or if the end of the tube strikes the neck laterally, the tube should be rotated toward the midline. In addition, the Sellick maneuver generally facilitates intubation. Alternatively, with the aid of a laryngoscope, Magill forceps, and an assistant to advance the tube, the tube may be passed through the glottic opening into the trachea under direct visualization. Following insertion of the tube, the cuff is inflated with 5–10 cc of air, and assisted ventilation is provided as needed.

G. **Tube placement.** Following insertion of the tube, its position must be checked. Signs that the tube has been placed properly within the trachea include air exiting from the tube with exhalation in spontaneous breathing patients, the absence of gurgling sounds indicative of esophageal intubation when the left upper abdomen is auscultated, and the presence of bilateral breath sounds of equal intensity on auscultation of the chest. If the breath sounds are diminished or absent over one hemithorax (almost always the left) suggesting intubation of a mainstem bronchus, the cuff is deflated and the tube withdrawn 1–2 cm at a time until the breath sounds are equal bilaterally. The tube is then taped in place, and, if need be, an oropharyngeal airway is inserted to prevent the patient from biting on the tube. A chest x-ray is then obtained to determine that the distal end of the tube is properly positioned proximal to the carina.

V. **Complications.** In the emergent situation, the complication rate is significant [61]. Common complications include prolonged apnea, failure of tracheal intubation, esophageal intubation, intubation of a mainstem bronchus (almost always the right), aspiration, and injury to the teeth, lips, and oral mucosa. Other complications include hemorrhage (epistaxis with nasotracheal intubation), pharyngeal and retropharyngeal lacerations [68] (which may lead to infection), laryngospasm, laryngeal edema, injury to the vocal cords, arrhythmias, tracheal perforation, pneumothorax, and intracranial intubation (with nasotracheal intubation in the presence of a cribriform plate fracture). Following tracheal intubation, the tube may become dislodged or obstructed.

Fig. 38-8. Endotracheal intubation. With the patient in the sniffing position, a straight blade (left) is advanced to just beyond the epiglottis to lift the epiglottis, or a curved blade (right) is placed so that its tip is in the vallecula anterior and superior to the epiglottis. By applying firm and steady traction to the laryngoscope up and away from the operator at a 45-degree angle, the glottic opening is exposed for intubation by an appropriately sized endotracheal tube with an inner stylet.

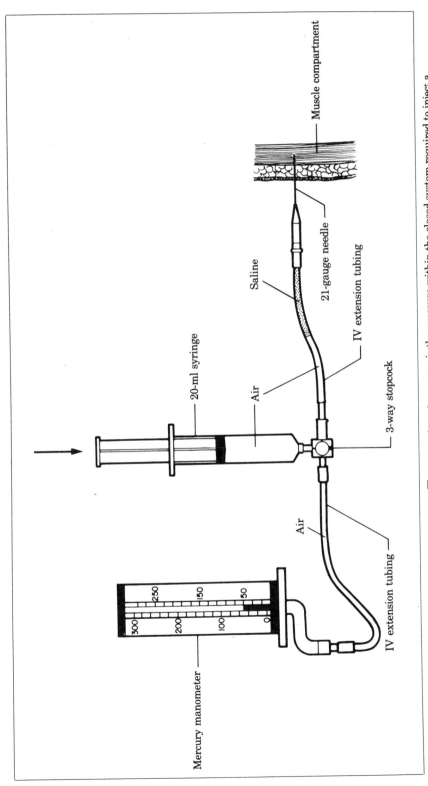

Fig. 38-9. Intracompartment tissue pressure measurement. The compartment pressure is the pressure within the closed system required to inject a small quantity of saline into the tissue compartment. (From T. E. Whitesides, Jr., et al. Tissue pressure measurements as a determinant for the need of fasciotomy. *Clin. Orthop.* 113:43, 1975. With permission.)

Intracompartment Tissue Pressure Measurement

Marc K. Allen

Measurement of tissue pressure within a muscular compartment provides objective data regarding muscle tissue perfusion. An elevated pressure (i.e., > 40 mm Hg) indicates probable compartment hypoperfusion and the need for surgical intervention. A knowledge of anatomic compartments and neurovascular distribution is essential for appropriate use of compartment pressure measurement.

I. **Indications.** Measurement of intracompartmental tissue pressure is indicated in the presence of an extremity injury (e.g., crush injury, closed fracture, snake bite, electrical injury, circumferential burn) with associated signs or symptoms suggestive of a compartment syndrome (e.g., pain out of proportion to the injury, pain on passive stretching, paresthesias without known nerve injury, pallor, pulselessness, paralysis).

II. **Contraindications**
   A. Bleeding diathesis (relative).
   B. A completely open compartment.

III. **Procedure**
   A. The involved extremity is positioned at the level of the heart. The skin overlying the entire compartment is prepped in the usual fashion with an antiseptic solution (e.g., povidone-iodine) and draped, allowing access to multiple sites for pressure sampling.
   B. The sites for pressure testing are anesthetized intradermally with 1% lidocaine. Sites over vessels or nerves should be avoided.
   C. Measurement of intracompartmental pressure is performed with the **equipment** assembled as in Fig. 38-9. Sterile saline is present in the extension set from the patient halfway to the stopcock.
   D. A 21-gauge needle is inserted through an anesthetized site into the muscle compartment.
   E. **Pressure measurement** is performed with the stopcock open to all three ports. Pressure is added to the system via the syringe until the fluid in the extension set begins to move toward the patient (i.e., into the muscle compartment). A pressure reading is taken at this point. Multiple readings are then recorded at different sites within the compartment.

IV. **Interpretation of results.** Intracompartmental pressure readings should be analyzed with regard to the patient's blood pressure. In normotensive patients, a normal tissue pressure is in the 0- to 3-mm Hg range. Above a pressure of 40 mm Hg, a compartment syndrome is rarely in doubt, and surgical intervention is indicated. Patients with elevated pressures less than 40 mm Hg should receive appropriate consultation and repeat measurements within 1 hour. It is important to realize that hypotensive patients are at a higher risk for a compartment syndrome at lower compartmental pressures.

V. **Complications**
   A. Infection.
   B. Hemorrhage.
   C. An early compartment syndrome may be missed because of failure to repeat the study when pressure measurements are equivocal.

Lumbar Puncture

Octavio de Marchena

A **lumbar puncture (LP)** allows examination of the cerebrospinal fluid (CSF) to determine whether infection, blood, or neoplastic cells are present. It also allows measurement of the CSF pressure.

I. **Indications.** An LP is indicated if any of the following is suspected:
   A. **Bacterial or viral meningitis.**
   B. **Encephalitis.**
   C. **Subarachnoid hemorrhage.**
   D. **Carcinomatous meningitis.**
   E. **Pseudotumor cerebri.**

II. **Contraindications**
   A. **Brain herniation or a suspected focal mass** in the brain.
   B. **Cerebellar or other posterior fossa mass.**

    C. Infection at the site of the LP. CSF can still be obtained, however, with a C1–C2 puncture or cisternal puncture.

    D. Bleeding disorder or low platelet count, unless corrected.

    E. Spinal cord compression with block is a relative contraindication.

III. Procedure

    A. Correct positioning is the most important step in doing an LP. The patient should be in the lateral decubitus position with the thoracolumbar spine horizontal. The head is flexed toward the chest, and the legs are flexed toward the head.

    B. Sterile gloves are put on, and a large area of lumbosacral skin is prepped with an antiseptic solution (e.g., povidone-iodine) and draped.

    C. The iliac crest is palpated and a vertical line visualized to the intersection with the spine. A space is then selected between two spinous processes at this level, which is usually at the L4–L5 interspace.

    D. A local anesthetic is injected intradermally.

    E. A 20-gauge spinal needle with a stylet in place and bevel up is introduced perpendicular to the back and directed slightly cephalad. Frequently a soft pop is felt when the needle penetrates the dura.

    F. The stylet is removed, and CSF is returned if the tap was successful. Since most unsuccessful taps result from the operator missing the midline, a change in the angle in a vertical plane is likely to be helpful.

    G. The CSF pressure should be measured with a manometer. Samples should be collected for protein, glucose, cell count and differential, cultures, and serologies.

IV. Complications

    A. The most common complication is a **post-LP headache,** which is a headache produced by a low CSF pressure. The treatment is bed rest and hydration.

    B. The most serious complication is **herniation,** if a mass lesion is present. Immediate management is discontinuing the LP and administering mannitol. Definitive treatment is directed toward correction of the mass lesion.

    C. An epidural or subdural hematoma is a rare complication seen in patients with a bleeding disorder or on an anticoagulant.

MAST Suit

Robert J. Stine

The **MAST (military antishock trousers)** suit has been shown to be a useful and safe device in the management of shock [71]. Studies in humans and dogs have demonstrated the following hemodynamic effects of the MAST suit: (1) elevation of the systolic and diastolic pressures [19, 48, 71], right atrial pressure (central venous pressure [CVP]) [48], and left ventricular end-diastolic pressure [48]; (2) a reflex reduction in heart rate [71]; (3) an increase in peripheral vascular resistance [19, 48]; (4) an increase in carotid blood flow [4, 36]; and (5) variable alterations in stroke volume and cardiac output [19, 48]. Thus, by applying external pressure (up to a maximum of 104 mm Hg) to the lower extremities and abdomen, the MAST suit effects an increase in blood pressure and preferential perfusion of the vital organs in the upper part of the body (i.e., the heart and brain). Initially, it was thought that these hemodynamic effects were due to an autotransfusion of 750–2000 ml of blood from the venous capitance system to the central circulation. It has now been shown, however, that less than 5% of the total blood volume (i.e., < 300 ml) is displaced to the central circulation [5]. It now appears that the hemodynamic effects produced by the MAST suit are due primarily to an increase in peripheral vascular resistance (afterload) secondary to compression of the arterial system beneath the suit [19, 48]. In addition to its hemodynamic actions, the MAST suit has been shown to be effective in tamponading external and internal bleeding from sites underlying the device by reducing the transmural pressure and size of the vascular defect(s) [17, 51]. Also, by applying external pressure to the lower half of the body, the MAST suit effectively immobilizes fractures of the pelvis [17] and femur.

I. Indications

    A. Shock with a systolic pressure below 90 mm Hg. Although the primary indication for use of the MAST suit is hemorrhagic shock, the suit has also been shown to be useful in the management of other forms of shock in which an increase in afterload is not detrimental (e.g., nonhemorrhagic hypovolemia, anaphylaxis, sepsis, neurogenic shock).

    B. Control of suspected hemorrhage arising from below the level of the diaphragm.

The MAST suit has been shown to be useful in arresting intraabdominal hemorrhage [51] and hemorrhage associated with pelvic fractures [17].

C. **Immobilization of suspected fractures** of the pelvis and femur. By acting as an air splint, the MAST suit can stabilize these fractures and thus lessen associated blood loss, soft-tissue injury, and pain.

D. **Cardiac arrest.** Because of its ability to increase blood pressure [4, 36], carotid blood flow [4, 36], and possibly coronary perfusion during cardiopulmonary resuscitation (CPR), the MAST suit may be a useful adjunct in the management of cardiac arrest [38]. However, this use of the MAST suit must be considered experimental, pending clarification by further studies.

II. **Contraindications**

A. **Congestive heart failure, pulmonary edema,** and **cardiogenic shock** are contraindications to the use of the MAST suit. By increasing the afterload, the device will likely be detrimental in such situations.

B. **Gravid uterus.** The abdominal compartment of the suit should not be inflated because of risk of injury to the fetus (unless deemed necessary to save the mother's life).

C. **Evisceration** of abdominal contents is a relative contraindication to use of the abdominal compartment of the suit.

D. The presence of an **impaled object** involving the abdomen is a contraindication to inflation of the abdominal compartment of the suit (unless it is deemed essential to remove the impaled object and inflate the compartment).

E. **Burns.** Because of the possibility of increasing tissue ischemia and thus exacerbating the burn depth, the MAST suit should not be inflated over burns (unless absolutely necessary).

F. In patients with **cardiac tamponade** or a **tension pneumothorax,** the abdominal compartment of the MAST suit generally should not be inflated because of a possible deleterious effect resulting from an increase in intrathoracic pressure further impairing venous return to the heart [50].

G. Although there are theoretical considerations for not using the MAST suit in patients with a head injury or hemorrhage from above the diaphragm because of the risk of increasing the intracranial pressure or enhancing blood loss, the suit has never been shown to be detrimental in such situations. Considering this and that it is essential to achieve adequate perfusion of the heart and brain, these conditions should not be considered a contraindication to the use of the MAST suit.

III. **Procedure**

A. **Application**

1. The MAST suit consists of three compartments, an abdominal and two separate lower extremity chambers. The patient either is placed on the MAST suit, or the lower half of the patient is lifted and the suit placed beneath the patient. The suit is positioned so that the upper aspect of the abdominal section is just below the costal margin.

2. The patient's lower extremities and abdomen are encircled with the respective sections of the device (preferably after removing the patient's clothing); the individual sections are then secured in place with the Velcro fasteners.

3. The separate compartments then are connected to the foot pump, and the stopcocks are opened for inflation.

4. The lower extremity compartments are inflated first; then, if necessary, the abdominal section is inflated. Inflation continues until the systolic pressure reaches 100 mm Hg or the internal pressure of the suit reaches a maximum pressure of 104 mm Hg, at which the Velcro fasteners begin to loosen and the popoff valves are activated. The internal pressure of the suit is then maintained by closing the stopcocks. To minimize complications associated with use of the device, the lowest effective inflation pressure should be used.

B. **Removal.** The MAST suit should not be removed until the intravascular volume has been repleted sufficiently with intravenous fluids to maintain an acceptable blood pressure without the device. Since it may not be known when this endpoint has been reached, deflation of the MAST suit must be performed slowly and cautiously, one compartment at a time, with careful monitoring of the blood pressure, to avoid a precipitous and harmful decline in the blood pressure. If the patient requires surgery, the suit should not be deflated until after the induction of anesthesia. If abdominal surgery is required, the abdominal section is deflated, but the lower extremity sections remain inflated until they can be safely deflated. The deflation procedure is as follows.

1. The abdominal section is deflated first by disconnecting it from the foot pump and opening the stopcock. The leg compartments are then deflated sequentially. Deflation occurs slowly in small decrements with constant monitoring of the blood pressure.
2. If the blood pressure declines by 5 mm Hg, deflation is discontinued until IV fluid repletion returns the blood pressure to the previous level. A more precipitous drop in blood pressure requires reinflation of the compartment.
3. Following deflation, the deflated suit should be left in place (for reinflation if necessary) until it is clear that the suit is no longer needed.

IV. **Complications.** The MAST suit is generally a safe device [71]. It has been employed safely in patients for up to 72 hours [71]. Complications, however, have been reported. They can be minimized by proper use of the suit and use of the lowest effective inflation pressure.

A. The most common serious problem is **hypotension** following premature deflation of the suit. The hypotension may be profound and followed by irreversible shock or cardiac arrest.
B. A **metabolic acidosis** secondary to impaired perfusion of tissues underlying the device commonly occurs, usually becoming manifest following deflation of the suit, but is rarely of serious consequence [71].
C. **Ischemic skin changes** can occur but usually do not require skin grafting [71].
D. Compartment syndrome and vascular thrombosis are rare complications of the use of the MAST suit.
E. Respiratory compromise generally is not a problem unless the suit is improperly applied above the costal margins [71]. Although small decreases in vital capacity and tidal volume can occur following inflation of the abdominal segment of the MAST suit, alveolar ventilation usually is not significantly impaired [53].
F. Renal failure following the use of the MAST suit is likely due to shock rather than to the use of the suit.

Microbiologic Stains

William G. Powderly and
J. William Campbell

Proper staining of clinical specimens facilitates early diagnosis of etiologic agents of infection and initiation of appropriate therapy.

I. **Gram stain** (for identification of bacteria)
A. **Preparation of smear.** A thin film of the material to be examined is placed on a clean glass slide using a sterile loop or swab. The specimen is air-dried and then heat-fixed by passing the slide through a flame several times.
B. **Stain**
1. The slide is flooded with crystal violet for 10 seconds and then rinsed with running water.
2. The slide is then flooded with Gram's iodine for 10 seconds and rinsed.
3. The smear is then decolorized with 95% ethanol until the thinnest parts of the smear are colorless and rinsed with water.
4. The specimen is counterstained, e.g., with Safranin, for 10 seconds and rinsed with water.
5. The slide is then air-dried or blotted dry.
C. **Examination.** The specimen should be examined under low-power magnification for the presence of granulocytes. In a properly prepared smear the nuclei are pink (when Safranin is the counterstain). The oil-immersion lens should be used when examining for bacteria. Gram-positive organisms are stained blue-black. Gram-negative organisms and host cells take up the counterstain, usually red.

II. **Acid-fast stain: Kinyoun method** (for identification of acid-fast bacilli)
A. The **smear** is prepared as for a Gram stain (see sec. I.A).
B. **Stain**
1. The slide is flooded with Kinyoun carbol-fuchsin for 5 minutes and then rinsed with water.
2. The smear is decolorized thoroughly with acid-alcohol until all color disappears from the washing and is then rinsed.
3. The specimen is counterstained with methylene blue for 1 minute and rinsed with water.

    C. Examination. The specimen is examined under an oil-immersion lens. Acid-fast bacilli are stained red.

III. Tzanck preparation (for diagnosis of herpetic infection)

    A. Obtaining the specimen. The lesion (vesicle or pustule) is opened, and its base is scraped vigorously with a scalpel blade. The material obtained is placed onto a glass slide and allowed to air dry.

    B. Stain. Toluidine blue is dropped onto the slide and left for 15 seconds. The slide is then rinsed with water and the specimen covered with a coverslip.

    C. Examination under high magnification reveals multinucleated giant cells in the presence of infection with herpes simplex or varicella-zoster virus.

Nasal Packing

Harlan R. Muntz

I. Indications. If other less invasive techniques for stopping a nose bleed have not been successful, nasal packing is indicated.

II. Contraindications. If acute epistaxis is present, there are no absolute contraindications to nasal packing.

III. Procedure. With the use of a nasal speculum and head light, the nose is observed by anterior rhinoscopy. The ala is opened with the nasal speculum, and the anterior portion of the septum is observed. Any active bleeding or blood clot within the nasal vault is aspirated with a Frasier sucker. Anesthesia of the nasal mucosa plus vasoconstriction may be achieved with 4% cocaine (or lidocaine in combination with a vasoconstrictor) applied by placing a cotton-soaked pledget in the nasal passage. If the bleeding site is identified, it may be cauterized (e.g., with silver nitrate). If cautery is ineffective or unsuccessful or if the point of bleeding is not obviously seen, nasal packing should be performed.

    A. Anterior pack. Three major forms of nasal packing are available: salt pork, absorbable oxycellulose, and gauze packing.

        1. Salt pork is useful in patients with a coagulopathy because of coagulant factors in the pork material. It is usually stored frozen and may be available from the pharmacy. Small portions of this material are broken off and very gently placed with a bayonet forceps in the nose next to the bleeding site.

        2. Oxycellulose is available in a number of forms, e.g., the cotton-type pledget (Oxycel). Small whisps of this cotton are placed firmly next to the area of bleeding with a bayonet forceps, using enough of the material to apply pressure to the bleeding site.

        3. Gauze for packing may be impregnated with an ointment, usually either an antibiotic (but not tetracycline) ointment or petroleum jelly (Vaseline). Packing the nose is done in a layered fashion, beginning at the floor of the nose (Fig. 38-10). The gauze is grasped approximately 3 in. from its end with a bayonet forceps and gently placed on the floor of the nose. Successive layers are then placed superiorly by grasping the material approximately 3 in. from the nasal verge and introducing it in a similar fashion through the anterior nasal vestibule. Because pressure is needed to stop the bleeding, it is important to make sure that as the packing is introduced, it is successively packed toward the floor of the nose. Care must be taken to leave the nasal vestibule relatively free of packing until the end, since it is the only opening to the superior portion of the nasal vault. Finally, the nasal vestibule is packed firmly with the gauze, and a cotton ball placed at the meatus. The layering not only allows greater pressure to be obtained in the packing but also helps prevent the gauze from falling into the posterior pharynx. By far, the most common mistake in packing the nose is to underestimate the extent to which the nose should be packed. Petrolatum gauze for nasal packing is commercially available in a ½-in. width and a length of 72 in. One side of the average female nose should be able to accommodate at least one 72-in. pack, and the male nose more.

    B. Posterior pack. If anterior nasal packing is unable to terminate the nasal bleeding, a posterior nasal pack, which will fill the nasopharynx, is required. There are two commonly used forms of posterior packing.

        1. Lambswool packing (Fig. 38-11) is a ball of tightly knitted wool tied with three heavy black silk strings. A red rubber catheter is placed through the nose (after the anterior nasal packing is removed) and is grasped by a long clamp in the

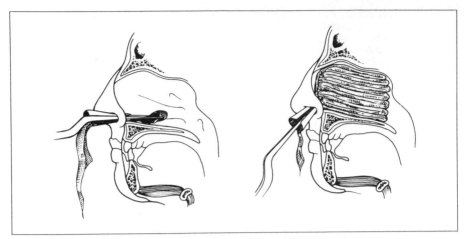

Fig. 38-10. Anterior nasal packing is accomplished by packing successive layers of impregnated gauze from the floor of the nose to the roof.

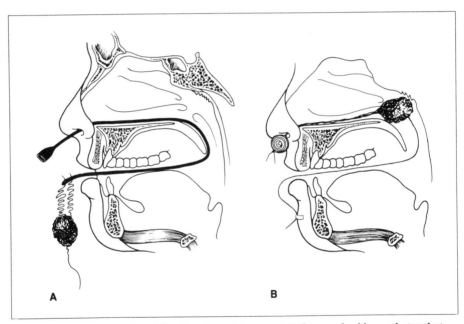

A   **B**

Fig. 38-11. Posterior nasal packing. Lambswool (or gauze) tied to a red rubber catheter that has been passed through the nose and out the mouth (A) is positioned in the nasopharynx (B) by withdrawing the catheter through the nose and held in place by ties to a foam rubber bolster at the nasal verge.

posterior oropharynx and extracted from the mouth. Two of the strings attached to the lambswool pack are then tied to the catheter. By pulling the catheter back through the nose, the pack is introduced gently through the mouth and tucked behind the soft palate to fill the nasopharynx. The two strings are then tied to a foam rubber bolster to help prevent alar necrosis. The third string is allowed to come out of the mouth and is taped on the side of the cheek; it is used to assist removal and avoid aspiration of the pack. An anterior pack is then placed as described in **A.3.**

2. **A balloon-tamponade device** is often effective in controlling bleeding and is more easily placed than the conventional lambswool (or gauze) pack.

    a. A variety of inflatable **double-balloon** devices for providing both a posterior and anterior tamponading effect are commercially available (e.g., Noz-Stop). After the device is lubricated with an anesthetic ointment, it is advanced through the nose until the posterior balloon is within the nasopharynx. The posterior balloon is then inflated with 5–10 ml of saline and the device retracted anteriorly until the posterior balloon is lodged in place. The anterior balloon is then inflated with 10–25 ml of saline.

    b. **A Foley catheter** with a 30-ml balloon may be used (Fig. 38-12). It is passed through the anterior nose (after the anterior nasal packing is removed) until the balloon is within the nasopharynx. Between 5–30 ml of normal saline is then introduced into the balloon to fill the nasopharynx; this will be uncomfortable to the patient. The catheter is then slowly retracted anteriorly until the balloon is wedged into position. While maintaining gentle tension on the catheter to retain the balloon's position, the anterior nasal vault is then packed. After the anterior nasal packing is finally introduced, a piece of foam rubber should be placed over the catheter at the nasal verge to protect the nasal ala. A C-clamp or hemostat is then attached to the catheter to hold it in the proper position.

IV. Complications of anterior nasal packing primarily include rhinitis, sinusitis, and epiphora. Patients with a posterior packing are at significant risk of developing reflex hypoxia and arrhythmias. An otitis media and tissue necrosis may also occur.

Percutaneous Central Venous Catheterization

Robert H. Marcus

Percutaneous central venous catheterization can be achieved via the cephalic or basilic vein in the arm, external or internal jugular vein in the neck, subclavian vein (infra- or supraclavicular approach), or femoral vein. This section will discuss catheterization of the internal jugular vein (central and posterior approach), subclavian vein (infraclavicular approach), and femoral vein.

I. Indications

  A. Access to the venous circulation for the following purposes:

    1. Administration of drugs.

    2. Certain radiographic procedures.

  B. Access to the central circulation for the following purposes:

    1. Monitoring of cardiovascular parameters (e.g., central venous pressure, pulmonary artery occlusive pressure).

    2. Percutaneous pacemaker placement.

    3. Administration of hypertonic or irritating solutions (e.g., hyperalimentation).

    4. Administration of drugs during cardiac arrest in order to decrease their circulation time to the heart and increase their concentration at the heart (controversial indication) [33, 35].

  C. Femoral venipuncture to obtain venous blood samples when peripheral veins are unaccessible.

II. Contraindications

  A. Absolute contraindications include (1) infection over the insertion site, (2) suspected injury or obstruction of the vessel or a drainage vessel proximal to the catheterization site, (3) lack of procedural experience or knowledge of the anatomy, or (4) lack of indication for the procedure.

  B. Relative contraindications include (1) a coagulopathy; (2) a burn overlying the

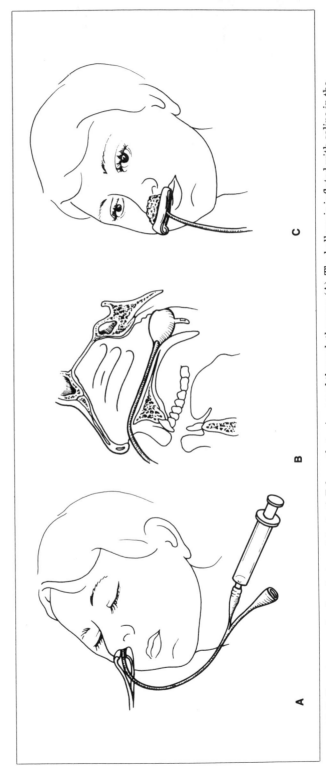

Fig. 38-12. Balloon tamponade of posterior epistaxis. A Foley catheter is passed through the nose (A). The balloon is inflated with saline in the nasopharynx (B) and held in place by a C-clamp at the nasal verge (C).

insertion site; (3) distorted anatomic structures (e.g., from obesity, previous surgery, local deformity, local trauma, or local radiation therapy); (4) an agitated, uncooperative patient; (5) contralateral attempts at subclavian or internal jugular venous catheterization following unsuccessful attempts on the first side (unless there is no hematoma formation and no pneumo- or hemothorax on a chest x-ray); or (6) for subclavian vein catheterization (and, to a lesser extent, internal jugular vein catheterization), any condition that increases the risk of causing a pneumothorax or in which a pneumothorax may precipitate serious pulmonary decompensation (e.g., a contralateral pneumothorax, need for assisted ventilation, borderline pulmonary reserve, presence of chronic obstructive pulmonary disease [COPD]).

III. Procedure

A. Position. For subclavian or internal jugular venous catheterization, the patient is placed in a supine position with the head turned away from the side selected for catheterization. A 15- to 20-degree Trendelenburg position is recommended in order to cause distention of the vein and lessen the chance of an air embolus.

B. Preparation. The area is widely prepped with a povidone-iodine solution. Sterile drapes are then applied around the insertion site, allowing for visualization of anatomic landmarks. For femoral vein catheterization, the groin should be shaved, if time allows. Sterile technique with the use of sterile gloves is important.

C. In awake patients, local **anesthesia** with 1% lidocaine should be infiltrated at the catheterization site.

D. Catheter. A 14-gauge intracatheter (catheter inside a needle) is recommended for percutaneous central venous catheterization in adults. Use of this intracatheter will allow a 16-gauge catheter to be introduced. For placement of the catheter in the superior vena cava, the appropriate catheter insertion length (about 15 cm for subclavian or internal jugular venous catheterization) may be estimated by the distance from the venipuncture site to the manubrial-sternal junction (which overlies the superior vena cava).

E. Venipuncture. An 18- or 20-gauge needle can be used to locate the vein initially. A 6-cm long, 14-gauge intracatheter needle attached to a 5-ml syringe is advanced slowly, maintaining negative pressure on the syringe. If the vein is not entered, negative pressure should be maintained while the needle is slowly withdrawn; the needle is then slowly readvanced in a slightly different direction. When the vein is entered, there will be free flow of venous blood into the syringe. The appearance of a forceful or pulsatile flow of bright red blood indicates arterial puncture; if this occurs, pressure must be applied to the puncture site for at least 10 minutes. The appearance of air bubbles in the syringe may indicate pulmonary penetration; if air is obtained, an occlusive dressing should be applied over the puncture site and a chest x-ray obtained. Specific venipuncture approaches are as follows:

1. Femoral vein venipuncture (Fig. 38-13)

a. The femoral artery is located by its pulsation. If no pulsation is palpable, the artery's position can be estimated as being midway between the anterosuperior iliac spine and the symphysis pubis.

b. The needle is inserted at a 45-degree angle to the skin in a cephalad direction at a site 2–3 cm below the inguinal ligament and 1 cm medial to the femoral artery.

2. Infraclavicular subclavian venipuncture (Fig. 38-14)

a. The needle is inserted at a site 1 cm below the junction of the middle and medial third of the clavicle and directed toward the posterosuperior aspect of the sternal end of the clavicle.

b. The needle should be advanced under the clavicle as parallel to the chest wall as possible in order to minimize the risk of causing a pneumothorax.

c. If an initial attempt at subclavian venipuncture is unsuccessful, the needle should be withdrawn and then redirected in a slightly more cephalad direction. However, occasionally redirecting the needle toward the inferior margin of the suprasternal notch may be necessary.

3. Internal jugular venipuncture (Fig. 38-15). The right side is preferred, since (1) it provides a straighter course to the right atrium, (2) the thoracic duct is avoided, and (3) the dome of the right lung is lower than that of the left lung. Since the internal jugular vein runs through the triangle formed by the two heads of the sternocleidomastoid muscle and the clavicle, an attempt to identify these structures is important; this triangle may be made more prominent by having the patient raise his or her head while the head is turned to one side.

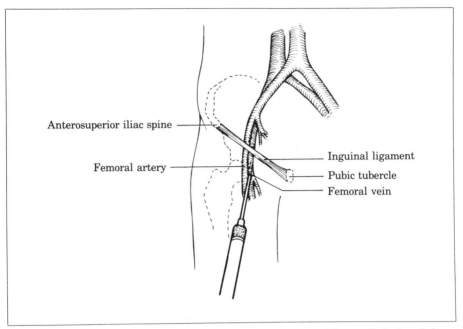

Fig. 38-13. Femoral vein venipuncture. The femoral vein is entered from a site 2–3 cm below the inguinal ligament and 1 cm medial to the femoral artery or, in the absence of a femoral pulse, from a site midway between the anterosuperior iliac spine and symphysis pubis.

> **a. Central approach**
>> **(1)** The needle is inserted at the apex of the sternocleidomastoid-clavicular triangle at a 45-degree angle to the frontal plane and directed at the ipsilateral nipple.
>> **(2)** To lessen the risk of arterial puncture, the carotid artery should be identified and retracted medially with the operator's fingers.
>> **(3)** If cannulation of the vein is unsuccessful, the needle should be withdrawn and then redirected slightly more medially (but without crossing the sagittal plane to avoid puncture of the carotid artery).
>
> **b. Posterior approach**
>> **(1)** The needle is inserted at the junction of the middle and lower third of the lateral border of the sternocleidomastoid muscle.
>> **(2)** The needle is then advanced under the sternocleidomastoid muscle toward the suprasternal notch.

F. Catheterization of the vein. After successful venipuncture, the syringe is removed and the needle hub occluded with a finger in order to avoid an air embolus. If difficulty is encountered in removing the syringe from the needle, a hemostat may be used to grasp the needle and hold the needle in place. The catheter (with the stylet removed) is then introduced through the needle to the appropriate distance, and the needle is withdrawn. If the catheter cannot be threaded into the vein, the catheter and needle should be removed together as a unit; withdrawing the catheter through the needle is contraindicated, since the catheter may be sheared, resulting in a catheter embolus.

G. The catheter is attached to IV tubing (connected to a fluid source), and the needle guard applied (with care not to pinch the catheter with the guard). Venous placement should then be confirmed by noting a return of blood into the tubing when the bag or bottle of fluid is lowered to a level below the patient's chest.

H. The catheter is sutured in place, an antiseptic ointment applied to the puncture site, and a sterile dressing secured in place with tape.

I. Following catheterization of the subclavian or internal jugular vein, a chest x-ray must be obtained to determine catheter placement and assess for a pneumo- or hemothorax.

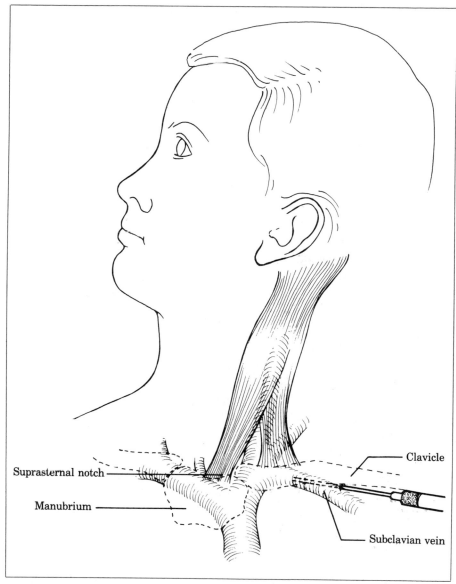

Fig. 38-14. Infraclavicular subclavian venipuncture. From a site 1 cm below the junction of the middle and medial third of the clavicle, a needle is advanced beneath the clavicle and directed toward the posterosuperior aspect of the sternal end of the clavicle.

IV. Complications common to venous catheterization procedures include hematoma formation, local infection, thrombosis, phlebitis, sepsis, pulmonary thromboembolism, air embolism, catheter fragment embolism, injury to an adjacent artery, injury to other adjacent structures (e.g., nerve, lung, thoracic duct), extravasation of IV fluids, and catheter malposition, kinking, or knotting.

A. Femoral vein catheterization is associated with an increased incidence of infection and venous thrombosis (which may extend into the iliac vein or inferior vena cava). Other complications include inadvertent femoral artery cannulation, injury to the femoral nerve, septic arthritis of the hip, penetration of a viscus in an unrecognized femoral hernia, and a psoas abscess.

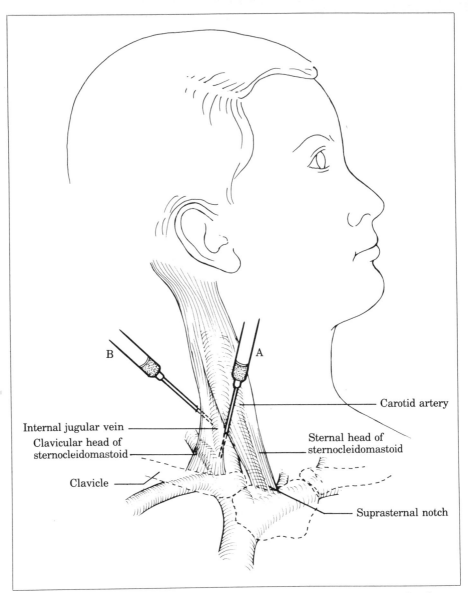

Fig. 38-15. Internal jugular venipuncture. A. Central approach. A needle is inserted at the apex of the sternocleidomastoid-clavicular triangle and directed at a 45-degree angle to the skin toward the ipsilateral nipple. B. Posterior approach. A needle is inserted at the junction of the middle and lower third of the lateral border of the sternocleidomastoid muscle and advanced beneath the muscle toward the suprasternal notch.

B. Subclavian or internal jugular vein catheterization may be complicated by a hemo- or pnemothorax (which is more common with the subclavian approach), extrusion of the catheter out of the vein with infusion of fluids into the pulmonary cavity or mediastinum, cardiac arrhythmias due to intracardiac catheter placement, perforation of the atrium or ventricle leading to cardiac tamponade, thoracic duct injury resulting in a chylothorax (from a left-sided approach), and interruption of CPR in order to perform the catheterization procedure.

  1. Unique complications associated with subclavian vein catheterization include subclavian or internal mammary artery puncture, tracheal penetration (and possible puncture of an endotracheal tube cuff), injury to the brachial plexus or the vagus or phrenic nerve, osteomyelitis of the clavicle, and septic arthritis of the sternoclavicular joint.

2. **Unique complications associated with internal jugular vein catheterization** include carotid artery puncture, stellate ganglion puncture resulting in a Horner's syndrome, and discomfort from decreased neck mobility secondary to securing the catheter to the neck.

Percutaneous Suprapubic Cystostomy

Russell E. Tackett and
Leonard D. Gaum

Percutaneous suprapubic cystostomy is a technique that allows drainage of the bladder when urethral catheterization fails or when a disease state (e.g., prostatitis) contraindicates urethral catheterization. Several suprapubic cystostomy kits are available commercially; all kits employ a trocar-type technique and provide satisfactory bladder drainage.

I. **Indications**
   A. **Urinary retention** and (1) inability to pass a urethral catheter, (2) known urethral stricture disease, or (3) bacterial prostatitis or epididymitis.
   B. **Periurethral abscess.**

II. **Contraindications**
   A. Contracted or decompressed bladder.
   B. Urinary retention secondary to blood clots.
   C. Previous bowel or pelvic surgery, because bowel held to the abdominal wall by adhesions may be encountered during trocar puncture.
   D. Extremely obese patients.
   E. Pelvic fracture, because an extraperitoneal hematoma may be entered during trocar puncture.

III. **Procedure** (Fig. 38-16)
   A. The patient is placed in the supine position, the distended bladder is palpated, and the suprapubic area is shaved, prepped, and draped.
   B. Following local anesthesia with 1% lidocaine, a stab incision is made in the midline two finger breadths above the pubic symphysis and carried down to include the anterior rectus fascia.
   C. The bladder is localized using a 3- to 4-in. spinal needle directed at the coccyx; aspiration of urine into a syringe confirms the correct position.
   D. With the catheter in place over the trocar needle and a syringe attached, the trocar is advanced into the bladder following the same path the spinal needle used to localize the bladder.
   E. When urine is aspirated, the catheter is advanced over the trocar into the bladder, and the trocar is removed.
   F. The catheter is connected to a closed drainage system. The catheter is then sutured to the skin, and a sterile dressing applied.

IV. **Complications**
   A. Hematuria and extravesical bleeding from passage of the trocar.
   B. Bowel penetration, usually secondary to bowel adhesions from prior surgery.
   C. Poor drainage secondary to blockage of the lumen with blood clots, mucus, or bladder mucosa. Irrigation or position adjustment alleviates these problems.

Percutaneous Transtracheal Ventilation

Robert J. Stine

Percutaneous transtracheal ventilation (PTV) is a rapid means of providing emergency ventilatory support on a temporary basis. PTV involves introducing a large-bore IV catheter through the cricothyroid membrane caudally into the trachea, connecting the catheter to a high-pressure oxygen source (i.e., wall or tank oxygen at 50 lb/sq in. [psi]), and ventilating the patient with intermittent 1- to 1.5-second bursts of oxygen

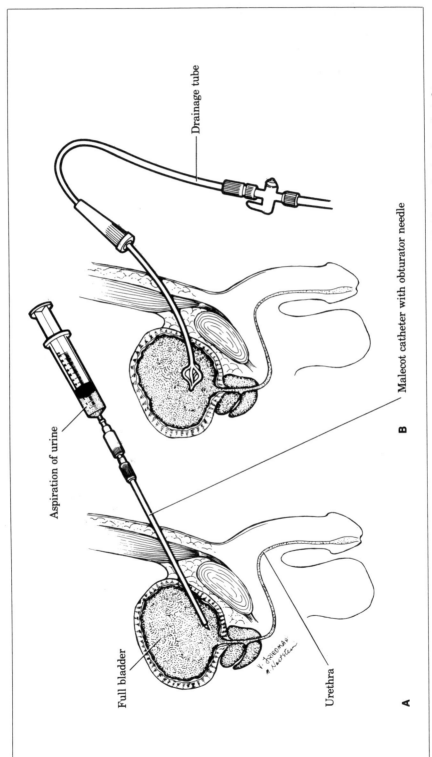

Fig. 38-16. Percutaneous suprapubic catheterization. A. A trocar with an outer catheter is advanced into the bladder, and urine is aspirated to assure proper placement. B. After removal of the trocar, the catheter remains in the bladder and is connected to a closed drainage system.

Drainage tube

Malecot catheter with obturator needle

B

Aspiration of urine

Full bladder

Urethra

A

12–15 times/minute. Even in the presence of upper airway obstruction, which generally is inspiratory and not expiratory, exhalation occurs via the oral cavity by passive recoil of the chest and lungs. In complete upper airway obstruction, however, a second catheter must be inserted through the cricothyroid membrane to act as a vent. When the system is connected to a wall- or tank-oxygen source at 50 psi pressure either directly or via a flow-meter set at the flush position, flow rates of 550 to 850 ml/second can be achieved through a 16- or 14-gauge catheter; thus, the corresponding tidal volumes will be 550 to 1275 ml, depending on the duration of the ventilatory bursts. Unless there is a complete upper airway obstruction, a portion of the insufflated volume escapes through the oral cavity (possibly carrying secretions and foreign bodies with it and clearing the upper airway); yet, adequate ventilation is achieved. Studies of PTV in apneic humans and dogs for up to 30 minutes generally have yielded PaO_2 values in excess of 300 mm Hg and $PaCO_2$ values of about 40 mm Hg [14, 28, 37]. Since PTV does not provide complete control of the airway, a definitive airway should be established as soon as possible. Generally, PTV should not be used for more than 1 hour.

I. **Indications.** PTV is indicated when emergent ventilatory support is required but cannot be achieved by other means (e.g., via a bag-valve-mask device or an endotracheal tube). It is particularly useful when there is upper airway obstruction; it may also be used to achieve ventilation in cardiac or respiratory arrest.

II. **Contraindications.** Considering that PTV is used to establish emergency ventilatory support when other methods have failed, there are no contraindications to its use. Caution, however, is required in the presence of indistinct landmarks (secondary to obesity or soft-tissue swelling), a coagulopathy, or thyromegaly.

III. **Procedure**

A. The neck is hyperextended (unless there is a suspected cervical spine injury), and the anterior aspect of the neck is prepped with a povidone-iodine solution.

B. Using sterile technique, the **cricothyroid membrane** is located between the thyroid and cricoid cartilages by palpation.

C. **Local anesthesia** is obtained by infiltrating the skin and subcutaneous tissue overlying the cricothyroid membrane with 1% lidocaine, if time permits.

D. A 14- or 16-gauge **extracatheter** (catheter over a needle) attached to a syringe is advanced in a caudal direction through the midline of the cricothyroid membrane at an angle of 45 degrees with the skin. The syringe is kept on aspiration (negative pressure); and when air is returned, the catheter is advanced over the needle into the trachea, and the inner needle withdrawn. The intraluminal position of the catheter is confirmed by reaspiration of air, and the catheter is taped in place. The catheter is then connected via a three-way stopcock or Y connector and oxygen tubing to a wall- or tank-oxygen source at 50 psi pressure by direct connection or via a flow meter set at the flush position (Fig. 38-17). To expedite this procedure, the connecting tubing should be set up in advance and readily available.

E. **Ventilation.** The patient is then ventilated with 1- to 1.5-second bursts of 100% oxygen, 12–15 times/minute, by intermittently occluding the open port of the stopcock or Y connector. The ventilatory rate and duration of the inspiratory phase should be adjusted according to the arterial blood gas results. However, the inspiratory phase should not be prolonged beyond 1.5 seconds, as dangerously high airway pressures may result, especially if there is upper airway obstruction.

F. Although uncommon, if there is complete upper airway obstruction, a second 14- or 16-gauge catheter must be inserted through the cricothyroid membrane to act as a **vent** for expiration.

G. A **definitive airway** (e.g., tracheostomy) should be established as soon as possible.

H. An alternate arrangement is as follows [58]. The 14- or 16-gauge catheter, which has been inserted into the trachea through the cricothyroid membrane, is attached to a 3-ml plastic syringe from which the plunger has been removed. A standard 15-mm adapter from an 8-mm endotracheal tube is then fitted into the barrel of the syringe, and a bag-valve device connected to an oxygen source is attached. The patient is then ventilated with the bag-valve device at a rate of 12–15 times/minute.

IV. **Complications.** Although the complication rate of PTV is low, the following problems have been reported: coughing, subcutaneous and mediastinal emphysema (secondary to incorrect catheter placement or leakage of air at the tracheal puncture site), hemorrhage, minor tracheal mucosal damage, hypercapnia, pneumothorax, esophageal perforation, pneumatocyst formation, and kinking of the catheter. Careful attention to proper technique, however, will minimize the incidence of these complications.

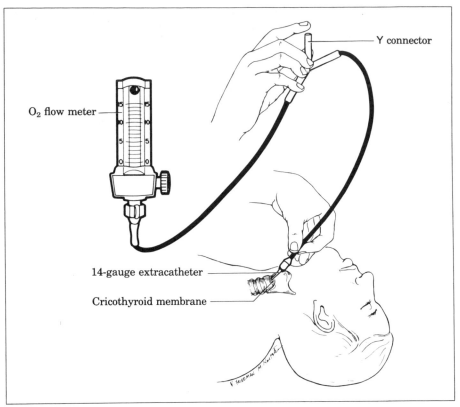

Fig. 38-17. Percutaneous transtracheal ventilation. The patient is ventilated with oxygen via a 14-gauge extracatheter placed in the trachea (through the cricothyroid membrane) by occluding the open port of the Y connector for 1.0–1.5 seconds 12–15 times/minute.

Pericardiocentesis

Bruce D. Lindsay and
Allan S. Jaffe

I. **Indications.** Pericardiocentesis may be performed for diagnostic or therapeutic reasons.
  A. **Therapeutic.** Pericardiocentesis is indicated for relief of decompensated cardiac tamponade (secondary to a traumatic or nontraumatic condition), pending definitive surgical decompression and/or repair.
  B. **Diagnostic.** Pericardiocentesis is indicated in patients with a pericardial effusion thought to be due to a nonviral infectious etiology; otherwise, its diagnostic sensitivity is quite limited.
II. **Contraindications.** There are no absolute contraindications to a therapeutic pericardiocentesis. A diagnostic pericardiocentesis should be avoided in the presence of a coagulopathy (including systemic anticoagulation).
III. **Procedure.** Pericardiocentesis should be performed by experienced personnel using fluoroscopic guidance whenever possible. However, immediate blind pericardiocentesis is mandated for acute pericardial tamponade with hemodynamic collapse. The subxiphoid approach is preferred.
  A. **Position.** The patient's head and thorax should be elevated to a 30-degree angle to increase pooling of pericardial fluid anteriorly and inferiorly.
  B. The skin in the region of the xiphoid process is prepped widely with a povidone-iodine solution and draped. Sterile technique is essential.
  C. **Anesthesia.** In conscious patients, the skin and subcutaneous tissue at the left xiphocostal angle are anesthetized with 1% lidocaine.

   D. A small **skin incision** is made with a No. 11 scalpel blade 1 cm caudal and to the left
   of the xiphoid process.
   E. Electrocardiographic monitoring. The V lead of a properly grounded electrocardiographic machine is attached via an alligator clamp to the hub of a 4- to 8-in. short-
   beveled 16- or 18-gauge needle, and the limb leads are attached to the patient. The
   V lead of the ECG is then monitored.
   F. The **needle** is attached to a 30-ml syringe and advanced toward the right scapula at
   a 30-degree angle to the skin, with continuous aspiration until fluid is obtained. ST-
   segment elevation or premature atrial or ventricular beats indicate epicardial contact, which necessitates withdrawing the needle until the ST-segment elevation or
   arrhythmia resolves.
   G. Aspiration of fluid. Sufficient fluid is withdrawn for diagnostic tests (e.g., Gram
   stain, cultures) or to cause hemodynamic improvement and provide time for definitive surgical therapy. A three-way stopcock can be interposed between the needle
   and syringe to facilitate removal of fluid. A catheter can be advanced into the
   pericardial space for continued drainage, if needed.
   H. A sterile **dressing** is applied to the entry site following termination of the procedure
   or if a drainage catheter is left in place. A follow-up chest x-ray is essential.
IV. Complications include arrhythmias (induced by needle contact with the heart), myocardial injury, pneumothorax, and laceration of a coronary artery.

Peritoneal Lavage

Robert J. Stine

Peritoneal lavage is a rapid, accurate, and sensitive means of assessing whether there
is intraperitoneal injury. Although used primarily in assessment of the abdomen in
trauma victims, peritoneal lavage is also useful in detecting hemorrhage and peritonitis
secondary to nontraumatic conditions. Although this technique is intended primarily
for assessment of blunt abdominal trauma [16], it has also been shown to be of benefit in
assessing whether there is visceral injury in suspected penetrating abdominal trauma
[49, 60, 62, 65]. In addition, peritoneal lavage has been shown to be of value in detecting
whether there is peritoneal penetration in gunshot wounds adjacent to the abdomen
[43]. Peritoneal lavage consistently has been shown to be more accurate than the
physical examination in assessing the abdomen, with an accuracy for blunt and penetrating trauma generally exceeding 98% and 90%, respectively [16, 43, 60, 62, 63, 65].
This technique has its limitations, however, which include (1) inability to reliably
detect retroperitoneal and diaphragmatic injuries [16, 18], (2) a high incidence of false-
negative lavages in patients with diaphragmatic rupture (due to herniation of injured
organ(s) into the thoracic cavity [16, 18], (3) inability to identify the injured organ(s)
and differentiate between trivial and serious injuries, (4) a high incidence of false-
positive lavages in patients with pelvic fractures (due to leakage of an extraperitoneal
hematoma into the peritoneal cavity) [25], and (5) possible inaccuracy in detecting
bowel perforations (due to the 4- to 6-hour delay in mounting a peritoneal leukocyte
count) [45]. Peritoneal lavage can be performed by either the open (minilaparotomy) or
percutaneous (puncture) technique; the former, in which the lavage catheter is inserted
into the peritoneal cavity under direct visualization, is technically more difficult but has
a higher accuracy rate and a lower incidence of complications [44, 49].
 I. Indications. Peritoneal lavage is indicated whenever there is the need for rapid assessment of the abdomen (i.e., the peritoneal cavity) and there is uncertainty regarding its
status. It is particularly useful (1) when the physical examination is unreliable (i.e.,
when the patient has an altered mental status secondary to a head injury or drug
intoxication, a spinal cord injury is present [67], or a communication barrier exists), (2)
when there is unexplained hypotension or blood loss, or (3) when the patient will be lost
to observation for a period of time (e.g., while undergoing general anesthesia for extraabdominal surgery). Although peritoneal lavage is primarily indicated in the evaluation of the trauma victim with equivocal abdominal findings, it is also useful in
determining whether there is a hemoperitoneum or peritonitis secondary to a nontraumatic condition.
 II. Contraindications
   A. Absolute contraindications to peritoneal lavage include the following:
       1. A **predetermined decision** regarding the treatment plan (e.g., because of a
       mandatory indication for an exploratory laparotomy) eliminates the need for
       peritoneal lavage.

   2. If the percutaneous technique is to be used, the procedure is contraindicated
   in the presence of previous abdominal surgery, a gravid uterus, an undecompressed bladder, or massively distended bowel (on a plain film).
   B. Relative contraindications. If the open technique is to be used, previous abdominal
   surgery, a gravid uterus, an undecompressed bladder, and massively distended
   bowel (on a plain film) are relative contraindications to peritoneal lavage.
III. Procedure
   A. If time permits, an upright or left lateral decubitus **abdominal film** is obtained prior
   to the procedure to look for free intraperitoneal air.
   B. A **Foley catheter** is inserted (unless contraindicated) to decompress the bladder,
   and a **nasogastric tube** is passed to decompress the stomach.
   C. The **lavage site** is selected. Normally this site is in the midline of the abdomen at
   an infraumbilical site one-third of the distance from the umbilicus to the symphysis
   pubis. However, in the presence of a major pelvic fracture, a midline supraumbilical
   site should be selected to avoid entering an extraperitoneal hematoma. A supraumbilical site should also be used if there is an advanced pregnancy or a lower abdominal surgical scar. If there is a previous upper and lower midline surgical scar, a left
   or right lower quadrant site may be chosen.
   D. With the patient in the supine position, the lavage site is shaved, prepped with a
   povidone-iodine solution, and draped.
   E. Local anesthesia is obtained by infiltrating the skin and subcutaneous tissue at the
   lavage site with 1% lidocaine with epinephrine.
   F. Either the **open or the percutaneous technique** can be used for inserting the
   lavage (peritoneal dialysis) catheter into the peritoneal space. The open method is
   preferred because of the higher accuracy and lower incidence of complications [44,
   49].
      1. The open (minilaparotomy) technique (Fig. 38-18). With good hemostasis, a 3-
      to 5-cm vertical midline (unless a lower quadrant approach is used) incision
      through the skin and subcutaneous tissue is made and carried down to the linea
      alba. If the rectus muscle is encountered by being off the midline, the muscle is
      retracted laterally. The linea alba or posterior rectus sheath is then incised
      vertically for a distance of 2–4 cm, exposing the peritoneum. After cleaning the
      preperitoneal fat off the underlying peritoneum, the peritoneum is grasped with
      two hemostats, and a 2- to 4-mm incision is made in the peritoneum. A perito-
      neal dialysis catheter without the trocar is then inserted through the incision
      into the peritoneal cavity and directed caudally toward a pelvic gutter. A purse-
      string suture of 2-0 absorbable material is then placed through the peritoneum
      around the catheter to create a watertight seal, and the wound is covered with a
      sterile dressing.
      2. The percutaneous (closed) technique. A small (5-mm) nick is made in the
      skin, and hemostasis is achieved. A peritoneal dialysis catheter with an inner
      trocar in place is then inserted through the skin incision and, with gentle but
      firm pressure and one hand grasping the distal end of the catheter so as to
      prevent too deep a penetration into the peritoneal cavity, advanced in a poste-
      rior and caudal direction at an angle of about 60 degrees with the skin. When
      the catheter passes through the fascia and underlying peritoneum, a "give" or
      "pop" is felt. The catheter is then advanced over the trocar, which is held
      stationary, into the peritoneal cavity and directed toward a pelvic gutter; the
      trocar is then removed.
   G. Aspiration. After placement of the lavage catheter in the peritoneal space, the
   catheter is aspirated with a syringe. If more than 10 ml of blood or if bile or bowel
   contents are obtained, the test is positive, and there is no need to perform a lavage.
   In this situation, the lavage catheter is removed, and the patient is prepared for an
   exploratory laparotomy.
   H. Lavage. If less than 10 ml of blood and no bile or intestinal contents are aspirated,
   lavage is performed.
      1. One liter (15 ml/kg in children) of Ringer's lactate or normal saline solution is
      rapidly instilled into the peritoneal cavity via an IV infusion set and the lavage
      catheter. If the patient's condition permits, he or she should be rolled from side
      to side during the infusion to disperse the lavage fluid within the peritoneal
      space.
      2. When the infusion is nearly complete, the infusion bottle or bag is placed on the
      floor and the lavage fluid collected by gravity siphonage. It is important not to
      allow air to gain access into the infusion (drainage) tubing, as this may negate

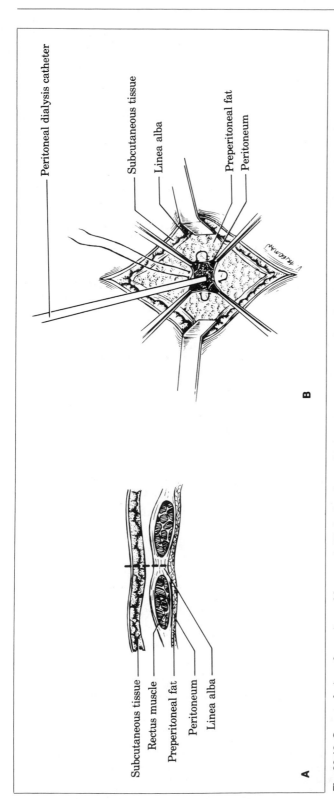

Peritoneal dialysis catheter

Subcutaneous tissue

Linea alba

Preperitoneal fat

Peritoneum

B

Subcutaneous tissue

Rectus muscle

Preperitoneal fat

Peritoneum

Linea alba

A

Fig. 38-18. Open technique for peritoneal lavage. A. Under local anesthesia, a 3- to 5-cm vertical midline incision is carried down through the linea alba with good hemostasis to expose the peritoneum. B. After a 2- to 4-mm incision is made in the peritoneum, a peritoneal dialysis catheter is advanced into a pelvic gutter and secured in place with a purse-string suture.

the siphon effect. A valid test requires retrieval of at least one-third of the instilled volume. If less is returned, the test is nondiagnostic; in such a situation, the lavage catheter should be checked to confirm that it is in the peritoneal space. The catheter should then be gently manipulated, and the patient placed in a slight reverse Trendelenburg position. If sufficient return is still not obtained, an additional 500–1000 ml of lavage fluid may be instilled and collected by siphonage.

I. If the return is grossly bloody, contains bile or intestinal contents, or exits via the Foley catheter or a chest tube, the lavage is positive. Otherwise, aliquots of the lavage return are obtained for erythrocyte and leukocyte counts and a Gram stain. An amylase assay, however, is of low yield and not cost-effective [1].

J. If the lavage is positive, the catheter is removed, the wound packed with sterile gauze, and the patient prepared for surgery. On the other hand, if the lavage is negative, the catheter is removed, the fascia closed with 0-gauge nonabsorbable suture, the skin closed with 3-0 nonabsorbable suture, and the patient admitted for observation.

IV. **Criteria for a positive lavage** (signifying the need for an exploratory laparotomy) include the following [16]:

A. **Aspiration of greater than 10 ml of blood.**

B. **Lavage fluid exits via the Foley catheter or a chest tube.**

C. **Grossly bloody lavage return.**

D. **RBC count greater than 100,000/mm³.** Some authorities use an RBC count greater than 5000/mm³ as indicative of a positive lavage in gunshot wounds to the abdominal region or in stab wounds to the lower chest in which there is the possibility of a diaphragmatic injury [43].

E. **WBC count greater than 500/mm³** [1, 69].

F. **Presence of bile, vegetable matter (gastrointestinal contents), or bacteria.**

G. An elevated amylase level (> 175 units/dl). However, this test is not cost-effective and thus is not recommended [1].

V. **Complications.** The complication rate is low, generally less than 2%, especially when the open technique is used [16, 49]. The most common complication is inadequate return of the lavage fluid due to mechanical problems or extraperitoneal infusion of the fluid. Other complications include bleeding at the lavage site yielding a false-positive result, wound problems (e.g., wound infection, hematoma formation, or incisional hernia), small- or large-bowel perforation, bladder perforation, omental laceration, and vessel laceration.

Regional Anesthesia

Barbel Holtmann,
William B. Strecker, and
V. Leroy Young

I. **Anesthetic agents**

A. **Pharmacologic properties.** Local anesthetics act by stabilizing nerve cell membranes, making the nerve impermeable to sodium in response to partial depolarization. The most frequently used local anesthetics are amides and esters. The chemical composition of the amides is similar to that of the esters, except for the presence of an amide linkage that slows the rate of metabolism and consequently increases the duration of action and risk of toxicity. The maximum dosage and duration of action of the various local anesthetics are given in Table 38-1.

1. **Lidocaine** (Xylocaine) is the most widely used amide anesthetic. Its major advantages are its rapid onset and minimal local irritation. Ninety percent of the drug is metabolized in the liver, and the remainder excreted by the kidneys. Lidocaine has a low incidence of allergic reactions and can be used safely in patients allergic to an ester anesthetic.

2. **Bupivacaine** (Marcaine), an amide derivative, is more potent and nearly 3 times longer-acting than lidocaine. This increased duration of action probably results from increased protein-binding.

3. **Procaine** is the only ester currently in use for local anesthesia in the United States. It causes minimal systemic toxicity, has a large safety margin, and is inexpensive but has a short duration of action.

Table 38-1. Dosage and duration of action of local anesthetics

Anesthetic	Maximum adult dosage	Duration of action
Lidocaine	4.5 mg/kg	1.5–3.0 hr
Bupivacaine	2.5 mg/kg	3–10 hr
Procaine	5.0–8.6 mg/kg	45–90 min

Source: Adapted from P. M. Weeks, *Acute Bone and Joint Injuries of the Hand and Wrist: A Clinical Guide to Management.* St. Louis: Mosby, 1981.

B. Adverse reactions
1. **Local tissue irritation** is uncommon with the currently available agents.
2. **Allergic reactions** including anaphylaxis can occur; however, they are less common with the amide derivatives.
3. **Toxic levels** of circulating local anesthetics can result from inadvertent intravascular injection, rapid injection in a vascular area, or exceeding the recommended maximum dose of a specific anesthetic. Systemic reactions to a toxic drug level primarily involve the central nervous, respiratory, and cardiovascular systems and include nervousness, dizziness, blurred vision, tinnitus, tremor, drowsiness, seizures, unconsciousness, arrhythmias, hypotension, and respiratory or cardiac arrest.

II. Facial anesthesia. Three practical nerve blocks can be performed in this region, since major areas of facial skin sensation are supplied by the terminal branches of the trigeminal nerve that emerge onto the face through foramina that lie in the vertical plane of the pupil when the eye is looking directly forward (Fig. 38-19). These blocks have the advantage of limiting the amount of local anesthetic agent needed to anesthetize the area and are particularly useful in anxious patients, including children. However, they have the disadvantage of not providing immediate analgesia afforded by local infiltration of an anesthetic agent and require a 10- to 15-minute waiting period before the procedure can be started. The preferred method for performing these nerve blocks is to use a 27-gauge needle and a solution of 1% lidocaine with epinephrine 1:200,000.

A. A **supraorbital block** provides analgesia in the distribution of the supraorbital and supratrochlear nerves.
1. **Indications**
   a. Anesthesia for procedures limited to the forehead and frontal scalp back to about the level of a line connecting the two external auditory meati.
   b. Avoidance of local infiltration anesthesia that would distort anatomic landmarks (e.g., forehead wrinkle lines) requiring precise alignment in approximating wound edges.
2. **Contraindications**
   a. Procedures beyond the limits of supraorbital and supratrochlear nerve innervation.
   b. When the vasoconstrictive effect of epinephrine injected directly into the wound (with local infiltration anesthesia) is desirable.
3. **Method**
   a. The lower forehead skin just above the eyebrow is prepped with a povidone-iodine solution.
   b. The supraorbital foramen or notch on the upper margin of the orbit is palpated about 2.5 cm from the midline (or about one finger's breadth from the lateral side of the nose).
   c. A 27-gauge needle is inserted directly over the supraorbital foramen or notch and advanced to the bone.
   d. After aspirating to assure that the injection will not be intravascular, 1–2 ml of a local anesthetic is injected at this point. Without withdrawing the needle from the skin, the needle tip is redirected 1 cm medially, and an additional 1–2 ml of local anesthetic is injected.
   e. The needle is withdrawn, and time is allowed for analgesia to become complete before starting the procedure. If analgesia is incomplete, the nerve block is repeated or augmented with local infiltration anesthesia.
4. **Complications** include (1) incomplete analgesia, (2) hematoma formation at the injection site, (3) a temporary motor nerve block involving the temporal branch

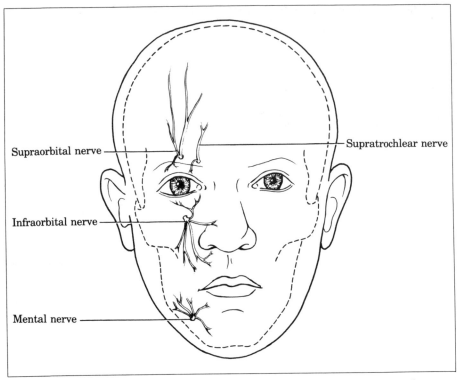

Fig. 38-19. Terminal branches of the trigeminal nerve that can be blocked for regional anesthesia of the face.

of the facial nerve, particularly if the injection is too far lateral, (4) intravascular injection, and (5) nerve injury.

B. Infraorbital nerve block anesthesia can be administered extra- or intraorally; the extraoral approach is preferred for procedures on the external face.

   1. Indications

      a. Anesthesia for procedures limited to the lower eyelid, medial cheek, lateral aspect (but not dorsum) of the lower part of the nose, and upper lip, particularly those areas difficult to inject directly (e.g., thick, lateral nostril skin).

      b. Anesthesia without distortion of anatomic landmarks (e.g., nasolabial crease, lower eyelid margin or wrinkle lines, upper lip vermilion border, alar crease or margin) associated with local infiltration anesthesia.

   2. Contraindications

      a. Procedures beyond the limits of infraorbital nerve innervation.

      b. When the direct vasoconstrictive effect of epinephrine in the wound (with local infiltration anesthesia) is desirable.

   3. Method

      a. Extraoral approach

         (1) The skin of the central cheek below the infraorbital rim is prepped with a povidone-iodine solution.

         (2) A 27-gauge needle is inserted at a point 2.5 cm lateral to the ala nasi. While palpating the infraorbital rim with the other hand, the needle is advanced cephalad at an angle of 45 degrees toward the infraorbital foramen. The foramen, which is difficult to palpate, is approximately 1 cm below the midpoint of the infraorbital rim. The needle tip is advanced until bone is reached or the foramen is entered.

         (3) After aspirating, 2–3 ml of a local anesthetic is injected at this point.

         (4) The needle is withdrawn; and when analgesia is complete, the procedure is started.

      b. For injection via the **intraoral approach,** the needle is passed cephalad through the mucosa above the root of the first premolar, and an anesthetic injected.

4. Complications include (1) incomplete analgesia, (2) a hematoma at the injection site, (3) a temporary motor nerve block involving the zygomatic or buccal branch of the facial nerve, (4) injection into the orbit or globe if the needle tip is advanced too far or misdirected, (5) intravascular injection, and (6) nerve injury.

C. Mental nerve block anesthesia can be administered extra- or intraorally.

   1. Indications

      a. Anesthesia for procedures limited to the lower lip and chin.

      b. Anesthesia without distortion of anatomic landmarks (e.g., lower lip vermilion border, anterior mental crease) associated with local infiltration anesthesia.

   2. Contraindications

      a. Procedures beyond the limits of mental nerve innervation.

      b. When the direct vasoconstrictive effect of epinephrine in the wound (with local infiltration anesthesia) is desirable.

   3. Method

      a. Extraoral approach

         (1) The skin of the lower cheek over the anterior body of the mandible is prepped with a povidone-iodine solution.

         (2) A 27-gauge needle is inserted midway between the upper and lower borders of the mandible at the level of the second premolar (except in edentulous patients in whom the mental foramen is much closer to the upper border and the position of the pupil can be used as a guide for inserting the needle). The needle tip is advanced to the bone or until the foramen is entered.

         (3) After aspirating, 1–2 ml of a local anesthetic is injected at this point.

         (4) The needle is withdrawn; and when analgesia is complete, the procedure can be started.

      b. For injection via the **intraoral approach,** the needle is passed through the mucosa below and slightly anterior to the root of the second premolar, and an anesthetic injected.

   4. Complications include (1) incomplete analgesia, (2) hematoma formation at the injection site, (3) a temporary motor nerve block involving the marginal mandibular branch of the facial nerve, (4) intravascular injection, and (5) nerve injury.

III. Extremity anesthesia

  A. Anesthesia of the hand. Anesthesia for hand injuries and infections can be obtained by digital or regional blocks using common local anesthetic agents. Safe and effective blocks, however, require a detailed knowledge of the innervation of the hand and an understanding of local anesthetic agents and techniques.

   1. Indications

      a. Anesthesia of the involved part in order to conduct a more thorough motor examination or wound exploration.

      b. Anesthesia of the involved part for repair or treatment.

   2. Contraindications

      a. Anesthetics to which the patient has demonstrated hypersensitivity are to be avoided.

      b. Anesthetics containing epinephrine are contraindicated in digital blocks because of the risk of inducing ischemia.

      c. Digital and wrist blocks should be avoided until thorough sensory and motor examinations of the part have been performed.

      d. Local anesthetic agents containing a vasoconstrictor should be avoided in patients having a history of coronary artery disease or arrhythmias.

   3. Anatomy. Innervation of the hand from the distal wrist crease to the ends of the digits is supplied by the median and ulnar nerves and the sensory branch of the radial nerve. The sensory distribution of these nerves is shown in Fig. 23-1. It is important to remember that when total anesthesia of a digit is necessary, both the palmar digital nerves and the dorsal sensory branches must be anesthetized.

   4. Method (Fig. 38-20)

      a. Median nerve block at the wrist. The median nerve at the wrist lies immediately beneath the transverse carpal ligament. It can be anesthetized by

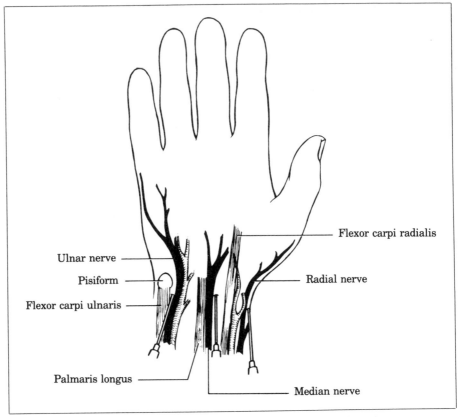

Ulnar nerve

Pisiform

Flexor carpi ulnaris

Palmaris longus

Flexor carpi radialis

Radial nerve

Median nerve

Fig. 38-20. Anatomy and injection sites for performing nerve blocks at the wrist.

inserting a 25- to 27-gauge needle through the distal forearm fascia just radial to the palmaris longus tendon at the proximal wrist crease. If paresthesias are elicited, the needle should be retracted a small distance. Following aspiration to prevent intravascular injection, 5–10 ml of 1% lidocaine is instilled.

b. **Ulnar nerve block at the wrist.** The ulnar nerve can be anesthetized by inserting a needle just beneath the forearm fascia along the radial side of the flexor carpi ulnaris tendon at the proximal wrist crease and instilling 5–10 ml of 1% lidocaine.

c. **Blocks of the dorsal sensory branches of the radial and ulnar nerves.** If anesthesia of the dorsum of the hand is desired, the radial sensory nerve can be blocked by injecting 5–10 ml of 1% lidocaine into the subcutaneous tissue proximal to the anatomic snuff box; this will provide anesthesia on the radial side of the dorsum of the hand. The dorsal sensory branch of the ulnar nerve can be blocked by infiltrating the subcutaneous tissues at the level of the ulnar styloid.

d. **Digital nerve blocks** can be performed by inserting a long 27-gauge needle vertically through the web space into the palm, injecting 5 ml of 1% lidocaine **without epinephrine;** the opposite side of the finger is then anesthetized in a similar manner. To anesthetize the radial aspect of the index finger or ulnar aspect of the little finger, 1–3 ml of 1% lidocaine (without epinephrine) is infiltrated into the corresponding aspect of the finger at the base of the proximal phalanx. For anesthesia of the dorsal aspect of the fingers, lidocaine (without epinephrine) is injected dorsally at the base of the proximal phalanx. In blocking the thumb, a circumferential block may be needed, as the thumb is supplied by multiple branches from the radial and median nerves. In performing digital nerve blocks, local anesthetics containing a vasoconstricting agent must not be used because of the risk of ischemia.

5. **Complications** include allergic or toxic reactions, intravascular injection, distal ischemia, and nerve injury.

B. Anesthesia of the foot

1. **Indications.** Ankle nerve blocks are indicated to anesthetize portions of the foot for repair of lacerations, removal of foreign bodies, or surgical procedures.

2. **Anatomy.** Sensation to the foot is supplied by the posterior tibial nerve, sural nerve, and superficial peroneal nerve. In addition, the anterior tibial nerve supplies sensation to the lateral aspect of the big toe and the medial aspect of the second toe, and the saphenous nerve provides sensation to the anteromedial aspect of the ankle.

   a. The **posterior tibial nerve,** a branch of the sciatic nerve, enters the foot (accompanied by the posterior tibial artery, to which it lies posterior and deep) by passing posterior to the medial malleolus. It then gives off the medial calcaneal branch, which supplies sensation to the inside of the heel, and divides into its terminal branches, the medial and lateral plantar nerves, which provide sensation to the sole of the foot.

   b. The **sural nerve** enters the foot by passing posterior to the lateral malleolus. It supplies sensation to the heel and lateral aspect of the foot, and the posterolateral aspect of the ankle.

   c. The **superficial peroneal nerve** arises from the common peroneal nerve (which originates from the sciatic nerve). It courses down the anterior aspect of the distal leg, entering the foot anteriorly to supply the dorsum of the foot via its subcutaneous branches (except for a small area between the first and second toes that is innervated by the anterior tibial nerve).

   d. The **saphenous nerve** courses distally along with the great saphenous vein, passing anterior and medial to the medial malleolus to supply sensation to the anteromedial aspect of the ankle.

3. **Method**

   a. **Posterior tibial nerve block.** The patient is placed in the prone position, and the posterior tibial artery is palpated. A 23-gauge needle is inserted perpendicular to the skin just anteromedial to the Achilles tendon at the level of the upper border of the medial malleolus and advanced just posterior to the artery until it strikes the tibia. Between 5 and 10 ml of 1% lidocaine is then injected while the needle is slowly withdrawn.

   b. **Sural nerve block.** The patient is placed in the prone position. A 23-gauge needle is inserted just anterolateral to the Achilles tendon at the level of the superior aspect of the lateral malleolus and advanced to a point just posterior to the superior aspect of the lateral malleolus. From 5 to 10 ml of 1% lidocaine is then infiltrated into the subcutaneous tissue just posterior to the distal fibula and extending to the Achilles tendon.

   c. **Superficial peroneal nerve block.** With the patient in the supine position, 5–10 ml of 1% lidocaine is infiltrated subcutaneously (via a 23-gauge needle) along a line extending from the anterior border of the tibia to the anterior aspect of the lateral malleolus.

   d. **Saphenous nerve block.** With the patient in the supine position, 5 ml of 1% lidocaine is infiltrated subcutaneously (via a 23-gauge needle) from the medial aspect of the extensor hallucis longus tendon to the anterior border of the medial malleolus.

   e. **Digital nerve blocks** of the toes can be performed in a similar manner to blocks of the fingers (see **A.4.d**).

C. Bier (IV regional) block

1. **Indications.** The Bier block is useful to anesthetize distal extremities for wound debridement and fracture reduction.

2. **Contraindications.** Anesthesia required for greater than 60–90 minutes and proximal extremity anesthesia are contraindications to the use of this block.

3. **Method.** The limb is first exsanguinated by applying an Esmarch bandage. The upper tourniquet of a double tourniquet is then inflated to about 100 mm Hg above the systolic pressure, and the bandage is removed. An IV bolus of 0.5% lidocaine **without epinephrine** is injected into a distal vein in the extremity. Usually 40–50 ml of a 0.5% solution will be required for an upper-extremity block, and 60–80 ml for a lower-extremity block; however, no more than 5 mg/kg of lidocaine should be used. If the patient experiences tourniquet pain during

the procedure, the lower tourniquet should be inflated and the upper one deflated. This block usually will allow for 60–90 minutes of comfortable anesthesia.

4. The major **complication** is early deflation of the tourniquet (which should be maintained inflated for at least 20 minutes) with release of an IV bolus of lidocaine and resultant toxicity (e.g., arrhythmias, seizures).

D. Axillary nerve block
1. **Indications.** This block is indicated when there is the need for proximal upper-extremity anesthesia, particularly prolonged (i.e., 8–10 hours or more) anesthesia.
2. **Contraindications** include a known allergy to the anesthetic agent.
3. **Method.** The patient is placed supine with the shoulder and elbow at 90 degrees to the body, and the axillary artery is palpated. Using a 1½-in. 25-gauge needle, the needle is advanced until the artery is punctured and then advanced further until no blood can be aspirated. The perivascular region is then infiltrated with 30 ml of 1% lidocaine. The needle is withdrawn through the artery until no blood can be aspirated, and another 10 ml of the anesthetic is infiltrated.
4. **Complications** include a toxic reaction from intravascular injection and obliteration of the radial pulse.

E. Joint block
1. **Indications.** A joint block is indicated to anesthetize joints in order to judge ligamentous integrity.
2. **Contraindications** include an allergy to the anesthetic agent and peripheral joints not amenable to arthrocentesis.
3. **Method.** After aspiration (see **Arthrocentesis and Intraarticular Injection**), 2–5 ml of 1% lidocaine is instilled into the joint. Once anesthesia is achieved, a stress examination can be carried out.
4. **Complications.** Septic arthritis is a rare complication.

F. Hematoma block
1. **Indications.** This block is useful to anesthetize fractures locally, particularly at the wrist, for reduction.
2. **Contraindications.** Open fractures are a contraindication to this procedure.
3. **Method.** Between 2 and 10 ml of lidocaine is injected into the fracture and its hematoma.
4. **Complications.** Compartmental swelling can occur.

Temporary Ventricular Pacemaker Insertion

John A. Boerner and
Michael E. Cain

I. **Indications** for temporary pacing are presented in Chap. 4 (see **Treatment, sec. VIII**). Transthoracic pacemakers are indicated only in life-threatening emergencies, generally in the setting of cardiac arrest; otherwise, transvenous pacemakers should be used.

II. **Contraindications.** Relative contraindications include a marked bleeding diathesis or ventricular irritability due to digitalis toxicity, ongoing myocardial ischemia, or hypothermia.

III. **Method**
A. Transvenous cardiac pacing
1. **Percutaneous entry** into the femoral, subclavian, or internal jugular vein should be accomplished as described under **Percutaneous Central Venous Catheterization.**
2. The pacemaker electrode is passed directly through the needle, which is then withdrawn over the electrode, or through a venous sheath having a sideport for IV solutions. If a balloon-tipped catheter is used, the catheter is advanced 15 cm into the vein and the balloon is then inflated.
3. **Electrode placement**
   a. **Fluoroscopic guidance.** If fluoroscopy is available, the electrode catheter is advanced under fluoroscopic guidance through the tricuspid valve. If a balloon-tipped catheter is used, the balloon is deflated after passing the tricuspid valve. The catheter is then advanced and positioned with the tip against

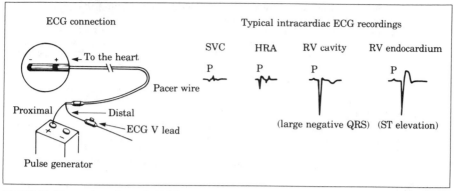

Fig. 38-21. Pacemaker electrode ECG connection and typical intracardiac ECG recordings. The distal jack is connected to the V lead of a grounded ECG machine, and the proximal jack to the positive terminal of the pulse generator. SVC = superior vena cava; HRA = high right atrium.

the right ventricular wall. Greatest stability is achieved with the electrode tip at the apex of the right ventricle (RV).

   b. Electrocardiographic guidance. If fluoroscopy is not available, electrode placement can be guided by monitoring the intracardiac electrocardiogram (ECG) (Fig. 38-21). The distal jack is connected to the chest (V) lead of a grounded ECG machine, and the proximal jack to the positive terminal of the pacemaker box; the ECG machine must be properly grounded to prevent accidental current flow to the heart. The catheter is then advanced with continual monitoring of the V lead. Entry into the RV is signaled by a large negative QRS deflection; if a balloon-tipped catheter is used, the balloon is deflated at this point. The catheter is then advanced an additional 3–5 cm until premature beats or ST elevation indicates contact with the endocardium.

   c. Blind positioning. Although this technique is the least optimal, it may be necessary in acute situations, especially in the presence of asystole. The pacemaker electrode is connected to the pacemaker box (see **4**) immediately after insertion into the vein, the current set at the maximum, the rate set faster than the patient's intrinsic rate, and the pacemaker electrode advanced blindly until ventricular capture is achieved. If the electrode is calibrated, the distance from the internal jugular or subclavian insertion site to the RV apex is usually 30–35 cm.

4. Cardiac pacing. Unless done previously (see **3.c**), the ends of the electrode are connected to the pacemaker box with the distal jack attached to the negative terminal and the proximal jack to the positive terminal, and the pacemaker turned on. The pacing threshold (i.e., the minimum current required for consistent capture) is then established, and the pacemaker is set at twice the threshold current and at an appropriate rate.

5. The electrode catheter is secured to the skin with tape or a suture to prevent accidental displacement, and a chest x-ray is obtained to confirm proper electrode placement.

B. Transthoracic cardiac pacing

   1. Whenever possible, the **subxiphoid approach** should be used. In this technique, the transthoracic needle is inserted in the left subxiphoid space and advanced at a 30-degree angle to the skin toward the sternal notch until free blood return indicates right ventricular puncture. Alternatively, the needle can be placed at the left sternal edge at the fourth intercostal space and directed posteriorly and slightly toward the right; however, this approach is more likely to lacerate the internal mammary or left anterior descending coronary artery.

   2. Electrode placement. The pacing stylet is passed through the needle into the ventricular cavity until the second stylet marker reaches the needle hub; at this point the curve of the pacing stylet has reformed inside the ventricle. The needle is then withdrawn over the pacing stylet, leaving the position of the latter unchanged within the ventricle.

3. **Cardiac pacing.** After connecting the pacing stylet to the pacemaker box, the pacemaker is turned on and set to the maximal current output at a rate faster than the patient's intrinsic rate. The pacing stylet is slowly pulled back until ventricular capture is achieved. The pacemaker is then set at twice the threshold current and at an appropriate rate.

4. The pacing stylet is secured to the skin with tape or a suture, and a chest x-ray is obtained.

IV. Complications

A. A transvenous pacemaker electrode can perforate the right atrium or ventricle, causing pericardial tamponade. More commonly, ventricular perforation is well tolerated and indicated only by an altered QRS morphology (i.e., loss of ventricular capture, an increased threshold, or diaphragmatic pacing). Repositioning the catheter is frequently all that is required.

B. Insertion of a transthoracic pacemaker stylet can lacerate the left internal mammary or left anterior descending coronary artery, especially if the left parasternal approach is used. A hemopericardium with tamponade can occur.

C. **Loss of appropriate sensing and capture** is due most commonly to electrode dislodgment and can be corrected by repositioning the electrode. Other causes include an equipment malfunction or electrolyte imbalance.

D. Phlebitis and thrombosis at the site of transvenous electrode insertion are common; the incidence increases with increased duration of temporary pacing.

E. A pneumothorax can occur during placement of either a transvenous or transthoracic pacemaker.

F. Air embolism can occur with pacemaker placement via the internal jugular or subclavian vein.

G. Accidental delivery of electrical current to the heart via the pacing electrode can result in ventricular fibrillation (VF); proper grounding of equipment, especially the ECG machine, during electrode placement is essential.

Thoracentesis

Daniel P. Schuster

I. **Indications.** A thoracentesis may be performed for either diagnostic purposes or therapeutic reasons (i.e., drainage of a pleural effusion or relief of a pneumothorax in a patient with respiratory compromise). Diagnostic studies (see Chap. 7) should be performed whenever pleural fluid may be exudative in nature.

II. **Contraindications** to a thoracentesis include (1) an uncooperative patient, (2) a bleeding diathesis, or (3) infection at the insertion site.

III. **Procedure**

A. If a pleural effusion is present, the superior extent of the pleural effusion is located by either percussion or sonography.

B. An appropriate **site** is selected for needle puncture (e.g., the sixth or seventh intercostal space in the midscapular or posterior axillary line for removal of fluid, the fifth intercostal space in the midaxillary line for removal of air), and the area is prepped with a povidone-iodine solution and draped.

C. Local **anesthesia** is achieved by infiltrating the skin, subcutaneous tissue, and intercostal space superior to the rib with 1% lidocaine, if time permits.

D. **Needle insertion.** A 14- to 18-gauge catheter-needle combination (extracatheter) attached to a syringe (with a three-way stopcock interposed) is inserted through the intercostal space, following the superior edge of the lower rib (to avoid the intercostal vessels which lie along the inferior edge of each rib). During insertion, negative pressure is maintained on the syringe. The catheter-needle combination is advanced slowly until the pleural space is entered, and pleural fluid (i.e., transudate, exudate, or blood) or air is obtained.

E. **Aspiration of pleural contents**

1. **Diagnostic thoracentesis.** Fluid is aspirated for diagnostic tests (see Chap. 7).

2. If a **therapeutic thoracentesis** is being performed, the catheter is advanced over the needle, the needle removed, and the syringe (with stopcock) reattached. Air or fluid from the pleural space is then aspirated into the syringe and eliminated via the stopcock (in the case of fluid, by way of IV tubing to a drainage bottle). In order to avoid reexpansion pulmonary edema, no more than

1 liter of fluid should be removed at a time, except in the case of a traumatic hemothorax. If such is the case, the pleural space should be drained completely; this may require a tube thoracostomy.

F. Following removal of fluid or air, the catheter is removed, and a sterile dressing is applied to the puncture site. A chest x-ray is then obtained to assess for a pneumothorax, and the patient is carefully observed (with monitoring of the vital signs) for the next few hours.

IV. Complications. The major complications include a pneumothorax (if not already present), bleeding, infection (empyema), and inadvertent intraabdominal organ puncture or laceration (e.g., liver, spleen, gut). Unilateral pulmonary edema can occur if a large volume of air or fluid (i.e., > 1 liter) is rapidly removed (see **Tube Thoracostomy**).

Tube Thoracostomy

Jon F. Moran

Expeditious insertion of a chest tube into one or both pleural cavities can be lifesaving in the setting of a tension pneumothorax, significant hemothorax, or empyema.

I. Indications
  A. Removal of air or fluid from the pleural space
    1. **Traumatic pneumothorax.**
    2. **Spontaneous pneumothorax** exceeding 20%.
    3. **Hemothorax.**
    4. **Empyema.**
    5. Penetrating or severe blunt thoracic trauma (with fractured ribs) without evidence of a pneumothorax in a patient about to undergo positive pressure ventilation. In this situation, a chest tube may be placed prophylactically to avert a possible tension pneumothorax from positive pressure ventilation.
  B. Instillation of a chemotherapeutic agent into the pleural space following removal of a malignant effusion.
II. Contraindications. There are no absolute contraindications to tube thoracostomy. Relative contraindications include a coagulopathy or a skin infection at the insertion site.
III. Procedure. A chest tube is inserted into the portion of the pleural cavity containing air or fluid to be drained, as determined by a chest x-ray if time permits.
  A. The **insertion site** depends on whether the chest tube is being placed to drain primarily air or fluid.
    1. For a **simple spontaneous pneumothorax,** the chest tube generally is inserted into the thorax through the second or third intercostal space in the midclavicular line and directed superiorly. Placing a chest tube in this position avoids any trapped apical cap of air as the lung expands and the two pleural surfaces seal; in addition an anteriorly placed chest tube most directly drains the most frequent area of air leakage. However, such anterior placement requires penetrating the pectoralis muscle, which can be substantial. Alternatively, to avoid placing the tube through this muscle, an entry site in the midaxillary line at the fifth or sixth intercostal space can be used, and the tube directed anterosuperiorly.
    2. When there is any **blood** or **fluid** in the pleural space, the chest tube should be inserted through the fifth or sixth interspace in the midaxillary line and directed posteriorly and superiorly, so that the tube will be posterior to the lung and in the dependent portion of the pleural space when the patient is recumbent. This tube will also effectively drain air from the pleural space, as in a hemopneumothorax.
    3. The insertion site must be individualized when the fluid or air to be drained is loculated.
  B. The chosen insertion site is prepped with an antiseptic solution (e.g., povidone-iodine) and draped with sterile towels.
  C. Local anesthesia. Between 10 and 30 ml of 1% lidocaine (i.e., 100–300 mg) is infiltrated rather widely at the chosen site for chest tube insertion. The periosteum of the rib above and below the chosen interspace, as well as the muscles of the interspace itself, should be generously infiltrated with the anesthetic, if time permits.
  D. Air or fluid is aspirated through the intended site for chest tube penetration to confirm that the chosen entry site communicates with the pleural space and material to be drained.

E. A 2-cm horizontal **incision** is made through the skin and subcutaneous tissue overlying the rib below the selected interspace.

F. A **tunnel** is then made through the deep subcutaneous tissue from the incision site toward the chosen area for penetration of the intercostal muscles by spreading a curved clamp. It is important to remember that the direction (vector) of the tunnel created through the subcutaneous tissue and intercostal muscles will determine the direction that the chest tube will point after it is inserted.

G. **Penetration of the pleural space.** The intercostal muscles are penetrated by passing the curved clamp just over the top of the rib above the skin incision and spreading the jaws of the clamp widely. The pleural space is then entered with the clamp. A common error is to open the curved clamp widely after the tips have penetrated the pleural space; this can lead to damage to the lung. The tract should be sufficiently wide to easily admit an index finger.

H. **Palpation.** Before inserting the tube through the chest wall, a finger should be passed through the tract to confirm that the pleural space has been entered and is free of adherent lung or the dome of the diaphragm.

I. The chosen **chest tube** (e.g., 20F for removal of air, 36F for removal of blood) is grasped with a curved clamp near the tip of the tube, with the tip protruding no more than 1–2 mm from the closed jaws of the curved clamp and the tube resting along the convexity of the curve of the clamp. By holding the tube near the chest wall, an accurate estimation can be made of the length of tube that will need to be inserted in order for the tip to reach the apex of the pleural cavity. Using the curved clamp, the tube is passed through the same tract that was made. Once the tip of the tube is clearly within the pleural space, the curved clamp is released, and the tube threaded into the pleural space without exerting any appreciable force. A rotating motion applied to the tube as it is advanced will encourage it to follow the direction of the tract and not kink on itself. The chest tube is advanced until the final hole is definitely within the pleural space and is connected to an underwater-seal bottle or drainage system. Suction can then be applied at 10–15 cm of water pressure.

J. The skin incision is closed, and the tube secured in place with heavy nonabsorbable sutures. A sterile dressing (including Xeroform or petrolatum gauze) is applied, and the tube is securely taped on the patient's chest wall. A chest x-ray is then obtained to verify both the tube position and adequacy of expansion of the ipsilateral lung.

IV. Complications

A. **Failure to place the tube into the pleural space**
1. **Subcutaneous placement.** It is possible to insert a chest tube into a deep subcutaneous tunnel that never penetrates between the ribs. Such a tube may cause significant bleeding and does not function to drain the pleural space.
2. **Subdiaphragmatic placement.** In the presence of intraabdominal injury or splinting of the chest wall, it is not unusual for the hemidiaphragms to be markedly elevated. In these settings, choosing an insertion site that is too caudal may lead to subdiaphragmatic placement of the chest tube with significant injury to the liver or spleen with hemorrhage.

B. **Damage to underlying lung tissue.** It is important to be certain that the lung underlying the selected site for chest tube insertion is not adherent to the chest wall. Otherwise, the chest tube can be inserted into the substance of the adherent underlying lung, leading to external hemorrhage, a hemothorax, or hemoptysis and simultaneously creating an air leak from the lung.

C. **Injury to vascular structures.** A tube insertion tract passing just under (rather than just over) a rib may damage the intercostal artery, causing significant bleeding either around the tube or into the chest. Injury to the heart or great vessels may occur, especially if a trocar device is used for chest tube insertion.

D. An **empyema** can result if sterile technique is not meticulously followed.

E. **Malfunctioning thoracostomy tube.** A chest tube can become clogged or kinked; in such a situation, air or blood (or other fluid) will collect in the pleural space and may leak around the tube. If one of the tube holes is left outside the pleural space or if a break occurs in the underwater-seal system (e.g., secondary to a hole in the tubing or disconnection of the tubing), an open pneumothorax, subcutaneous emphysema (if the tube hole is in the thoracic wall), or a persistent air leak will occur.

F. **Unilateral pulmonary edema** can occur following rapid lung reexpansion or use of excessive negative pressure, particularly when lung collapse exceeds 72 hours.

Emergency Thoracotomy

Jon F. Moran

Emergency thoracotomy, although rarely indicated, can be lifesaving in certain selected circumstances. The survival rate correlates inversely with the depth of shock on admission to the emergency department and is best for patients with penetrating thoracic injuries and worse for patients with blunt trauma [3, 6]. By definition, this procedure must be carried out rapidly when indicated. The thoracotomy performed must be a relatively simple procedure and versatile enough to be extended to expose practically all intrathoracic structures. An anterolateral thoracotomy can be performed rapidly with very limited equipment and provides wide, easily extendable exposure to the anterior mediastinum and the pleural space (including the hilum of the lung). Most frequently, a left thoracotomy is performed, unless there is penetrating trauma confined to the right hemithorax.

I. **Indications.** Although somewhat controversial, a thoracotomy in the emergency department can be lifesaving in the following situations:

A. **Trauma victims** who are (1) **in extremis** despite appropriate resuscitative efforts and will not tolerate transport to the operating suite or (2) **in cardiac arrest** where the conditions in **1, 2,** or **3** apply are candidates for a thoracotomy in the emergency department [6]. Otherwise, the survival rate approaches 0%, making the procedure not useful.

1. **Penetrating thoracic injuries and signs of life in the field.**
2. **Penetrating abdominal injuries and signs of life in the emergency department.**
3. **Blunt trauma and signs of life in the emergency department.**

B. Patients in **cardiac arrest** of a presumed cardiopulmonary etiology in whom external chest compressions are ineffective (because of an anatomic deformity, severe emphysema, or cardiac tamponade) may benefit from internal chest compressions.

C. Patients with **cardiac tamponade** and a deteriorating hemodynamic status despite pericardiocentesis require an immediate thoracotomy.

II. **Contraindications** to performing a thoracotomy in the emergency department include the following:

A. Trauma victims responding to initial resuscitative efforts with resultant improvement in hemodynamic parameters should be transported to the operating suite for surgery and not undergo a thoracotomy in the emergency department.

B. Trauma victims not satisfying the criteria listed in sec. **I.A** are not candidates for an emergent thoracotomy, because the salvage rate approaches 0% in these patients.

C. Unfamiliarity with the procedure or unavailability of appropriate backup personnel or an operating suite facility is a contraindication to performing a thoracotomy in the emergency department.

III. **Procedure**

A. **Preparation.** The patient must be intubated and receiving positive pressure ventilation. An IV line should be in place for delivery of fluids and drugs. With the patient supine or rolled slightly to one side (with a folded sheet under the scapula and lower posterior ribs of the hemithorax to be entered) and the ipsilateral arm elevated above the head to expose the axilla, the entire anterior chest, upper abdomen, clavicular region, lateral chest, and axilla are prepped with an antiseptic solution (e.g., povidone-iodine). Using sterile towels or sheets, a wide field is then draped, if time permits.

B. The most frequently employed **incision** enters the thorax through the left third or fourth intercostal space. However, if there is penetrating trauma confined to the right hemithorax, a right-sided incision is preferred. The skin, subcutaneous tissue, and chest wall muscles (pectoralis muscle) are incised along the intercostal space with a scalpel (with a No. 10 blade) from the lateral edge of the sternum to the posterior axillary line, passing just beneath the nipple (or in the inframammary crease in women). The incision is carried down through the intercostal muscles, entering the pleural space just along the upper border of the anterior fourth or fifth rib in the anterior axillary line. Dividing the intercostal muscles along the upper border of the rib avoids damage to the intercostal neurovascular bundle. Chest wall bleeding will be minimal in the hypotensive patient. Once the pleural space is entered laterally, a finger or sponge-stick is inserted behind the intercostal muscles to protect the underlying lung and pericardium while dividing the intercostal muscles along the entire length of the incision from laterally to the sternum, using a scalpel or scissors. The internal mammary vessels should be ligated superiorly and inferiorly whenever it is necessary to divide them.

C. Exposure. A small chest retractor is inserted to spread the ribs apart enough to allow inspection of the pericardium and left lung. Further exposure may be obtained by extending the incision across the sternum into the opposite intercostal space. Occasionally, extension of the incision parasternally in the cephalad direction, with division of the costochondral junctions of the upper ribs, can be helpful in gaining increased exposure of the upper mediastinum or the apex of the pleural space.

D. Specific procedures

1. If **relief of a pericardial tamponade** or **open cardiac massage** is indicated, the pericardium is grasped with a forceps or small clamp and incised longitudinally anterior to the phrenic nerve with a scalpel or scissors. Any clotted blood is removed.

2. **Internal cardiac massage,** if needed, is performed by gently compressing the heart in the palm of a hand, with care to avoid pressing the tips of the fingers or thumb into the heart, or by compressing the heart between two hands at a rate of 80–100/minute in adults and in children and at a rate of at least 100/min in infants.

3. **Delivery of fluids and drugs.** For rapid delivery of fluids, sterile IV tubing can be inserted directly into an atrial appendage (preferably the right) of the heart and secured in place with a purse-string suture. Cardiac drugs can be injected directly into the heart via a 22-gauge needle, if necessary.

4. **Defibrillation,** if needed, should be initiated with 5 joules of energy delivered by internal paddles applied to the heart and should not exceed 50 joules/shock.

5. **Management of cardiac wounds**

   a. **Control of cardiac bleeding**

      (1) **Bleeding from a ventricular wound** generally can be controlled by placing a finger over the wound. For larger wounds in which bleeding is difficult to control, a Foley catheter can be passed through the wound into the heart, the balloon inflated, and traction applied to the catheter.

      (2) **Bleeding from an atrial wound** can be controlled by compression of the wound between the thumb and index finger or by application of a vascular clamp.

   b. **Repair of cardiac wounds**

      (1) **Repair of ventricular wounds** can be accomplished with interrupted simple sutures for small wounds or with horizontal mattress sutures for larger wounds or wounds near vessels, using 3-0 Prolene (see **Wound-Closure Techniques**). The sutures should pass down to but not through the endocardium and should be tied just tight enough to stop the bleeding (to avoid tearing the myocardium). Passing the sutures through Teflon pledgets on each side of the wound will help prevent the sutures from cutting through the myocardium. Care must be taken to avoid the coronary arteries when placing sutures.

      (2) **Repair of atrial wounds** generally can be achieved with interrupted sutures of 4-0 Prolene.

6. **Management of injuries** to the hilum or great vessels

   a. **Control of bleeding.** Bleeding can be controlled by application of compression pressure using the thumb and index finger or a vascular clamp.

   b. **Repair** of these injuries generally should be undertaken in the operating suite. Small vascular wounds can be repaired with interrupted simple sutures, and larger wounds with horizontal mattress sutures, using 4-0 Prolene (see **Wound-Closure Techniques**).

7. **Occlusion of the thoracic aorta.** In the presence of severe intraabdominal bleeding or severe hypovolemia, the thoracic aorta can be occluded just above the diaphragm with a vascular clamp (after incising the overlying pleura) in order to retard intraabdominal blood loss and increase perfusion of the heart and brain.

E. Definitive care. If the patient is successfully resuscitated in the emergency department, he or she should be promptly transferred to the operating suite for definitive surgical care.

IV. Limitations. An emergent anterolateral thoracotomy generally does not provide adequate exposure to repair damage to the esophagus or to easily permit the institution of routine cardiopulmonary bypass. However, the esophagus is rarely injured by blunt or penetrating trauma and even more rarely requires emergent thoracotomy. Likewise, cardiopulmonary bypass is rarely needed, since even penetrating cardiac injuries are usually controllable without using bypass.

V. Complications

   A. Damage to the lung. It is possible to damage the lung if the incision through the intercostal muscles penetrates too deep or if the lung is adherent to the anterior chest wall.

   B. Injury to vascular structures. The heart can be damaged if care is not taken in opening the chest or pericardium or in performing internal cardiac massage. The coronary arteries can be injured (e.g., ligated) if care is not taken in repairing cardiac lacerations. The intercostal or internal mammary vessels can be lacerated in opening the chest.

   C. Injury to the phrenic nerve can occur in opening the pericardium.

   D. Infection. Wound infection following emergency thoracotomy is surprisingly uncommon, probably occurring in less than 2% of survivors. Irrigation of the wound prior to closure and use of prophylactic antibiotics will help avoid this complication.

Tonometry

Lawrence A. Gans

The **measurement of intraocular pressure** by tonometry is an integral part of the adult eye examination. The normal range is from 11–21 mm Hg. Pressures over 24 mm Hg occur in less than 0.15% of the normal population and thus require appropriate follow-up evaluation by an ophthalmologist. It is important to realize that the normal range of intraocular pressure is a statistical concept. An abnormal elevation of pressure, however, identifies patients in whom glaucoma may be present or may develop later.

 I. Indications. It is particularly important to measure the intraocular pressure in the following situations: any disturbance in vision, a history or suspicion of glaucoma, a pupillary abnormality, ocular inflammation (but not infection), blunt trauma to the eye, presence of a hyphema, or eye pain.

 II. Contraindications include penetrating trauma to the eye, a ruptured globe, or an uncooperative patient. In addition, use of a tonometer should be avoided on infected eyes.

 III. Method

   A. Shiötz tonometry determines the intraocular pressure by measuring the depth to which a plunger of specific weight indents the cornea. The scale on the tonometer reads the depth of indentation, and the intraocular pressure is determined from a chart which lists pressures corresponding to various combinations of scale readings and plunger weights. For any given plunger weight, the higher the scale reading, the lower the pressure.

   1. A topical anesthetic is instilled.

   2. The patient is positioned so that the head and eyes are pointing straight up. The patient should stare at a point on the ceiling with both eyes so that the eye to be tested assumes an absolutely vertical position.

   3. The tonometer is held by the finger grips and checked by resting the foot plate on the testing surface (a silvery metal dome) in the instrument case. This metal surface cannot be indented by the plunger and thus gives a scale reading of zero with proper calibration.

   4. Holding the eyelids apart (taking care not to press on the globe because this will artificially increase the ocular pressure), the foot plate is gently rested on the cornea and the scale reading noted. Shiötz tonometry is most accurate when the scale reading is between 4 and 6 units. Therefore, the appropriate weight should be added to the plunger so that this optimal range is obtained.

   5. The scale reading and plunger weight (i.e., 5.5 gm, unless supplemental weight is added) are used to determine the intraocular pressure from the tonometer chart.

   B. Applanation tonometry determines the intraocular pressure by measuring the force required to flatten a standard area of the cornea. The tonometer head is a split-image prism through which the examiner observes the tear film around the area of the cornea being flattened. The tonometer is usually mounted on a slit lamp, but portable, hand-held models are also available. Applanation tonometry is more accurate and more easily performed than Shiötz tonometry.

1. A topical anesthetic is instilled.
2. The tear film is stained by touching it with a sterile fluorescein paper strip.
3. The patient is positioned at the slit lamp (or in any comfortable position for a hand-held tonometer).
4. The wide slit beam with the blue filter in place is directed at about a 60-degree angle to illuminate the applanation prism.
5. The patient is instructed to stare at an object so that the eye to be tested assumes a central position between the eyelids.
6. Holding the eyelids apart (taking care not to press on the globe, which will artificially increase the pressure), the prism is gently moved forward until contact is made in the center of the cornea.
7. Under low power, two semicircles are observed through the prism. The prism position is adjusted until the semicircles are of equal size.
8. The knob on the side of the tonometer is turned until the semicircles interlock, with the inner edge of the upper semicircle touching the inner edge of the lower. Variations in the pulse pressure may cause the semicircles to move in and out slightly. If the semicircles are very thick, too much fluorescein is present; and the eye and tonometer should be wiped to reduce the amount of stain. If the semicircles cannot be separated, the whole instrument may be too far forward.
9. The scale on the tonometer knob reveals the grams of force required to flatten the cornea. The area of the prism head is designed so that the intraocular pressure in millimeters of mercury is 10 times the scale reading.

IV. **Complications**
   A. **Minor disturbances in the corneal epithelial surface** occur with Shiötz and applanation tonometry. These minor disturbances may cause slightly blurred vision for several hours. Significant corneal abrasions, however, are uncommon.
   B. **Infectious diseases** can be transmitted to patients by a contaminated tonometer. Care should be taken to wipe the contact surface of any tonometer with a clean dry tissue.

Venous Cutdown

Robert H. Marcus

Venous cutdown can be performed on the basilic, cephalic, or brachial vein in the antecubital fossa; on the cephalic vein in the deltopectoral groove; on the proximal saphenous vein or the saphenous vein at the ankle; or on the external jugular vein. The saphenous vein at the ankle is the preferred cutdown site in the emergency setting, since there are no other important structures in the vicinity and the vein has a constant location. A proximal saphenous vein cutdown is particularly useful for fluid replacement in profoundly hypovolemic patients because of its constant superficial location and large diameter capable of accommodating a large-bore cannula (such as IV extension tubing), but its use should be limited to the initial management of these patients. The basilic vein is the preferred vein for cutdown in the arm.

I. **Indications**
   A. **Access to the venous circulation** for administration of drugs or fluids when other veins are unaccessible (especially in children).
   B. **Placement of a large-bore cannula** for fluid replacement in patients with profound hypovolemia.
   C. **Placement of a central venous catheter or pacemaker electrode** via a peripheral vein.

II. **Contraindications**
   A. **Absolute contraindications** include (1) infection over the cutdown site, (2) phlebitis of the vein to be catheterized, (3) suspected injury or obstruction of the vessel proximal to the catheterization site, (4) lack of procedural experience or knowledge of the anatomy, or (5) lack of indication for the procedure.
   B. **Relative contraindications** include a burn over the cutdown site or significant trauma to an extremity proximal to the proposed cutdown site.

III. **Procedure**
   A. A **tourniquet** may be placed proximal to the cutdown site to distend the vein, when appropriate.
   B. **Sterile technique** should be used. The cutdown site is prepped with a povidone-iodine solution and draped. Sterile gloves should be worn.

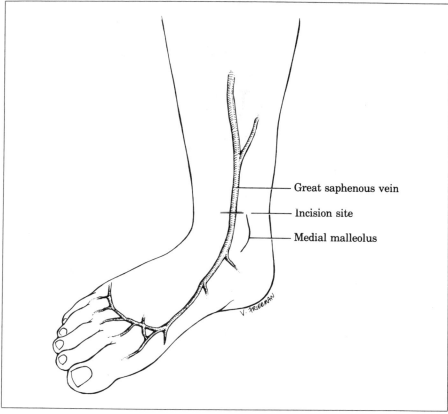

Fig. 38-22. Saphenous vein cutdown at the ankle. A 2.5-cm transverse incision is made just anterior and superior to the medial malleolus.

C. In awake patients, local **anesthesia** should be infiltrated at the cutdown site.
D. A **skin incision** is made with a No. 15 scalpel blade transverse to the axis of the vein. Specific incision (cutdown) sites are as follows:
  1. **Saphenous vein cutdown at the ankle** (Fig. 38-22). With the foot externally rotated to expose the medial malleolus, a 2.5-cm transverse skin incision is made just anterior and superior to the medial malleolus.
  2. **Basilic vein cutdown** (Fig. 38-23). With the arm supinated and extended at the elbow, a 2.5-cm transverse skin incision is centered on the volar surface at a site 2–3 cm superior and lateral to the medial epicondyle of the humerus.
  3. **Proximal saphenous vein cutdown** (Fig. 38-24). With the thigh externally rotated, a 5-cm transverse skin incision is centered about a point 5–6 cm below the junction of the middle and medial third of a line extending from the pubic tubercle to the anterosuperior iliac spine.
E. Vascular access. Blunt dissection through the subcutaneous tissues with a curved hemostat is used to expose the vein. The vein is identified as a thin-walled, blue, pulseless vessel that blanches with pressure. However, in profound shock, the artery may not appear to pulsate, and the vein may appear white. In this setting, the vein can be identified by aspirating (with a small needle) blue, nonpulsatile blood. Once the vein is identified, it is isolated with two 2-0 or 3-0 silk sutures, and the distal suture is tied.
F. Venous catheterization. A small incision is made through the anterior wall of the vein with an iris scissors. A mosquito forceps may then be attached to the cut edge of the vein to provide countertraction during catheterization. A catheter is introduced into the vein and is connected to IV tubing (attached to a fluid source). The

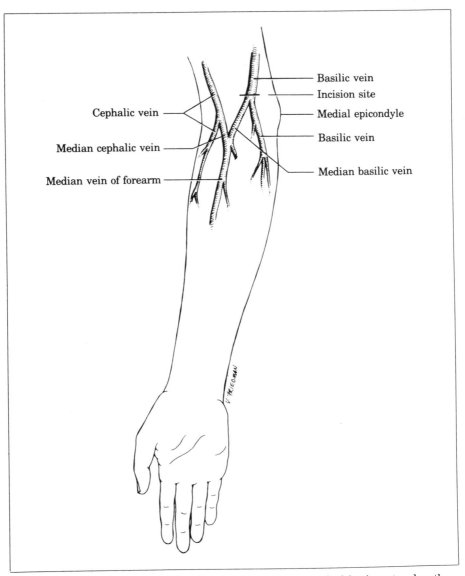

Cephalic vein —

Median cephalic vein —

Median vein of forearm —

Basilic vein

Incision site

Medial epicondyle

Basilic vein

Median basilic vein

Fig. 38-23. Basilic vein cutdown at the elbow. A 2.5-cm transverse incision is centered on the volar surface at a site 2–3 cm superior and lateral to the medial epicondyle of the humerus.

proximal suture is then tied. In patients with profound hypovolemia, sterile IV extension tubing may be cut to form a beveled edge and introduced directly into the vein, if the size of the vein allows.

G. The incision site is sutured closed, the catheter sutured in place, and an antibiotic ointment applied. A sterile dressing is then applied and secured with tape.

IV. Complications include hematoma formation, local infection, thrombosis, phlebitis, sepsis, pulmonary thromboembolism, air embolism, catheter fragment embolism, injury to adjacent structures (e.g., artery, nerve), inadvertent transection of the vein, venospasm, extravasation of IV fluids, and catheter malposition, kinking, or knotting. Also, catheterization of the proximal saphenous vein negates its use as a future vascular substitute.

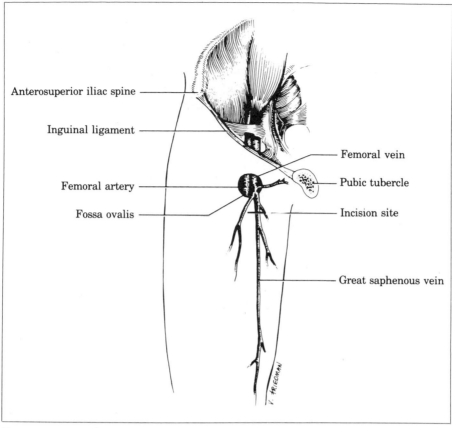

Fig. 38-24. Proximal saphenous vein cutdown. A 5-cm transverse incision is centered at a site 5–6 cm below the junction of the middle and medial third of a line joining the pubic tubercle and anterosuperior iliac spine.

Wound-Closure Techniques

Barbel Holtmann

I. **General principles.** The various steps in wound management leading up to wound repair, characteristics of various suture materials, and factors in scar production are detailed in Chap. 22.

II. **Suture techniques.** In most instances, the following suture techniques can be used on any tissue layer; but for illustrative purposes, descriptions are limited to suture placement in skin.

A. **Interrupted sutures.** Individually placed and tied sutures afford the best control for accurate tissue approximation and precise correction of wound edge malalignment and produce lesser amounts of tissue strangulation because tension can be adjusted individually on each suture. With any of these techniques, the closer the needle enters to the wound edge, the greater its ability to control that edge.

1. **Simple sutures** (Fig. 38-25) are the most commonly used, the easiest to master, and produce the least amount of tissue damage resulting from placement.

   a. **Indications**
      (1) Closure of any tissue layer with little or no tension between the cut edges.
      (2) Skin approximation in most wounds.

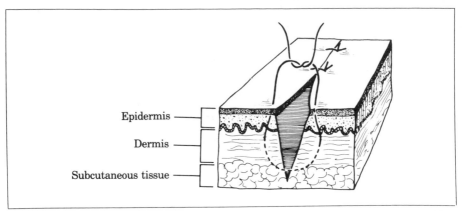

Epidermis

Dermis

Subcutaneous tissue

Fig. 38-25. Interrupted simple skin sutures. To produce eversion of the skin edges, the needle should be placed to form a wider loop in the depths of the wound than at the skin surface.

      (3) Approximation of subcutaneous fat and dermis, when indicated, in wound repair.
  b. Contraindications
      (1) When the tissue layer will be under significant tension.
      (2) When motion during the postoperative period can result in sutures cutting through and pulling out of the tissues with detrimental results (e.g., joint capsule repair).
  c. Method
      (1) The needle enters the skin 1–2 mm from the wound edge on the first side at an angle of 90 degrees or greater, including sufficient subcutaneous tissue in the bite to cause eversion of the raw interface.
      (2) Directly opposite the point of exit on the first side, the needle passes through a comparable amount of subcutaneous tissue on the second side (except when the wound edges are of unequal thickness) and begins to angle back toward the wound edge so that the needle's angle of exit through skin on the second side is the same as its angle of entry on the first side and the same distance from the wound edge.
      (3) The suture ends are tied together across the wound in a secure knot with just enough tension to coapt the wound edges. Both ends are then cut, leaving a tail.
      (4) When wound edges of unequal thickness cannot be equalized by undermining or judicious placement of subcutaneous or dermal sutures, the skin can be aligned by inclusion of less subcutaneous tissue in the suture bite placed in the higher wound margin and inclusion of more subcutaneous tissue in the suture bite on the depressed side (i.e., a more superficial bite on the raised edge and a deeper bite on the depressed edge).
  d. Complications
      (1) Failure of the suture to hold tissues together because of tension, motion, or improper placement.
      (2) Tissue strangulation and necrosis when the suture is tied too tightly.
2. Vertical mattress sutures (Fig. 38-26) provide excellent skin edge eversion and have better holding power in tissue layers closed under tension but damage more tissue when placed and potentially strangulate more tissue.
  a. Indications
      (1) When adequate eversion of skin edges is difficult or impossible to achieve with simple sutures (e.g., skin of hands or feet). These sutures may be used alone or alternating with simple sutures.
      (2) When tension on tissue approximation is significant during wound closure or anticipated to be significant during the postoperative period.
      (3) Skin wounds with troublesome bleeding from dermal edges where hemostasis by other means is difficult to achieve (e.g., scalp wounds).

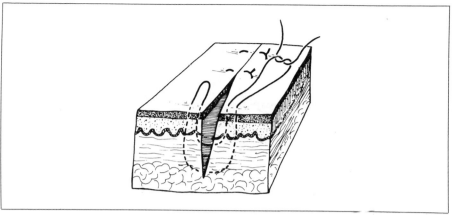

Fig. 38-26. Interrupted vertical mattress sutures.

    (4) In relatively deep wounds where a single-layer closure is preferred (e.g., scalp wounds), vertical mattress sutures can eliminate dead space effectively while providing precise approximation of the skin edges.
  b. Contraindications
    (1) When simple sutures will produce the same result.
    (2) When suture marks are a consideration in the ultimate scar produced (e.g., facial wounds).
    (3) Most skin closures in children, because these sutures are more traumatic to remove than the other types.
  c. Method
    (1) The needle enters the skin 5–10 mm from the wound edge on the first side and includes and exits through the subcutaneous tissue on that side.
    (2) The needle then enters the subcutaneous tissue directly opposite and at the same depth on the second side, exiting the skin on the second side at the same distance from the wound edge as the point of entry on the first side.
    (3) The needle reenters the skin on the second side 1–2 mm from the wound edge (medial to and in the same plane as the point of exit of the first bite) and then passes into and out of the dermis on the second side.
    (4) The needle next enters the dermis on the first side at the same depth and directly opposite the point of exit on the second side and then exits the skin 1–2 mm from the wound edge on the first side, directly medial to the point of entry of the first bite.
    (5) The suture ends are tied together on the same side of the wound. Both ends are then cut, leaving a tail.
    (6) To equalize wound edges of unequal thickness, both bites must be more superficial on the raised edge, and both bites must be deeper on the depressed edge.
  d. Complications
    (1) Difficult and painful suture removal if the skin loops become buried.
    (2) More obvious suture marks.
    (3) A greater chance for tissue strangulation and necrosis, especially when the suture is tied under tension.
3. Horizontal mattress sutures (Fig. 38-27) provide good eversion of the skin edges but are not quite as effective as vertical mattress sutures in obliterating dead space or in providing dermal edge hemostasis.
  a. Indications
    (1) When adequate skin-edge eversion cannot be obtained with simple sutures.
    (2) When tension on tissue approximation is significant.
  b. Contraindications
    (1) When simple sutures will produce the same result.
    (2) When suture marks are a potential problem.

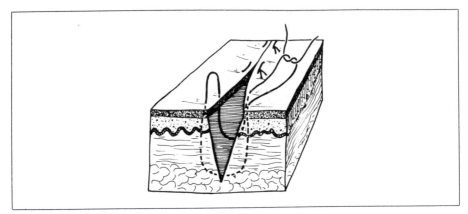

Fig. 38-27. Interrupted horizontal mattress sutures.

(3) Most skin closures in children.

(4) When a single-layer skin closure is expected to obliterate significant dead space in addition to providing precise skin-edge alignment.

c. Method

(1) The needle enters the skin 1–4 mm from the wound edge on the first side and includes and exits through the subcutaneous tissue on that side.

(2) The needle enters the subcutaneous tissue directly opposite and at the same depth on the second side, exiting the skin on the second side at the same distance from the wound edge as the point of entry on the first side.

(3) The needle reenters the skin on the second side at the same distance from the wound edge and 2–5 mm away from the point of exit of the first bite, including the same amount of subcutaneous tissue as the first bite.

(4) The needle then enters the subcutaneous tissue on the first side directly opposite and at the same depth, exiting the skin at the same distance from the wound as the point of entry of the first bite and at a distance from the initial point of entry equal to the distance between the exit and entry points on the second side.

(5) The suture ends are tied together on the same side of the wound. Both ends are then cut, leaving a tail.

(6) To equalize wound edges of unequal thickness, both bites must be more superficial on the raised edge and deeper on the depressed edge.

d. Complications

(1) Difficult suture removal if the skin loops cut through the skin and become buried.

(2) More obvious suture marks.

(3) A greater chance for tissue strangulation and necrosis.

4. Half-buried horizontal mattress sutures (Fig. 38-28) provide excellent skin-edge approximation and are useful in suturing wounds where one edge has potentially decreased vascularity.

a. Indications

(1) Repair of flaplike lacerations.

(2) Suture of the flap tip of triangular wounds (Fig. 38-29).

(3) Wounds at the scalp-skin junction, because the dermal component avoids skin suture marks.

(4) To equalize skin edges in wounds with vertical discrepancies.

b. Contraindications

(1) When simple sutures will produce the same result.

(2) When suture marks are a potential problem.

(3) Most skin closures in children.

(4) When a single-layer skin closure is expected to obliterate dead space in addition to providing precise skin-edge alignment.

c. Method

(1) The needle enters the skin 1–3 mm from the wound edge and perpendicular to it on the first side, penetrating into and out of the dermis.

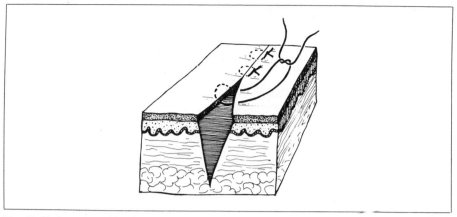

Fig. 38-28. Interrupted half-buried horizontal mattress sutures.

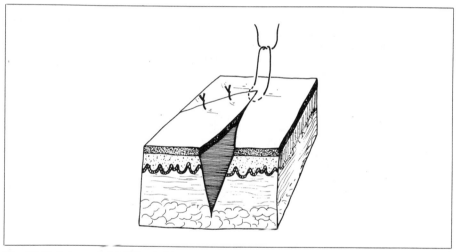

Fig. 38-29. Interrupted half-buried horizontal mattress suture placed in the tip of a triangular flap.

(2) With the needle parallel to the skin surface, it enters the dermis on the second side directly opposite at the same depth as the point of exit on the first side and is looped through the dermis for a distance of 2–5 mm, exiting the dermis on the second side at the same depth as the point of entry.

(3) With the needle perpendicular to the skin, it reenters the dermis on the first side (or enters the third wound edge for triangular flap tips) directly opposite at the same depth as the point of dermal exit of the first bite and exits the skin at the same distance from the wound edge as the point of entry of the first bite.

(4) The suture ends are tied together on the same side of the wound. Both ends are then cut, leaving a tail.

(5) When suturing flaplike lacerations, the dermal component of the suture is placed in the flaplike wound edge.

(6) To equalize wound margins of unequal thickness, the buried (dermal) portion of the suture passes through the raised wound edge. The suture enters and exits the skin and is tied on the depressed edge.

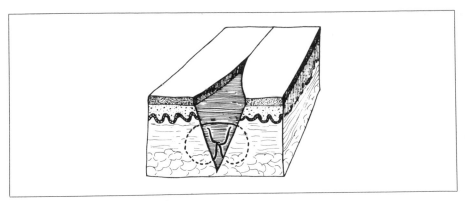

Fig. 38-30. Interrupted subcuticular sutures.

   d. Complications
      (1) Difficult suture removal if the skin loop becomes buried.
      (2) Potentially more significant suture marks.
      (3) Necrosis of the flap edge or tip if the dermal bite is too large or if the suture is tied with too much tension.
5. Subcuticular sutures (Fig. 38-30) are completely buried simple sutures placed beneath the epidermis. They are excellent for coapting skin margins but have the disadvantage of creating a foreign body reaction close to the skin surface. The skin coaptation they produce is usually reinforced with another technique of skin approximation (e.g., simple sutures or skin tapes).
   a. Indications
      (1) Any wound where a gap exists between the skin edges and buried sutures are not contraindicated.
      (2) To reduce tension on skin sutures.
      (3) When skin approximation with tapes is planned.
   b. Contraindications
      (1) Wounds in which the skin margins fall together, with or without closure of deeper layers.
      (2) Wounds in which buried suture material is likely to be detrimental (e.g., animal bites or other wounds with a high likelihood of becoming infected).
   c. Method
      (1) Perpendicular to the wound margin, the needle enters the base of the dermis (or includes variable amounts of subcutaneous fat if obliteration of dead space is indicated) along the raw interface on the first side.
      (2) The needle then passes vertically and more superficially through the dermis, exiting the dermis on the first side just beneath the epidermis (without passing through the epidermis at any point along the suture bite).
      (3) The needle enters the superficial dermis on the second side directly opposite and at the same depth as the point of exit on the first side.
      (4) The needle then passes vertically through the dermis to a deeper level on the second side and exits the second side directly opposite and at the same depth as the point of entry on the first side.
      (5) The suture is tied securely. Both ends are then cut directly on the knot to prevent the suture ends from sticking out between the skin edges.
      (6) In areas where the dermis is thin, it may be necessary to orient subcuticular sutures horizontally in the dermis, making them completely intradermal in location, with the points of entry and exit at the same depth on both sides of the wound.
      (7) To equalize wound margins of unequal thickness, the bites must be more superficial on the raised edge and deeper on the depressed edge.
   d. Complications
      (1) Foreign body reaction close to the skin surface.

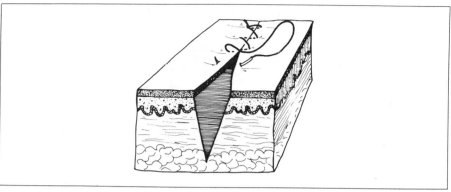

Fig. 38-31. Continuous simple over-and-over sutures (baseball stitch).

       (2) Early and late extrusion of sutures through the skin edges, with or without localized suture abscesses.

       (3) Failure of the sutures to maintain coaptation of the skin edges.

B. Continuous (running) sutures. Continuous sutures enter the wound at one point (usually one end), pass back and forth from one wound edge to the other, and exit the wound at some distant point (usually the other end). Continuous sutures take less time to insert than interrupted sutures, but longitudinal and vertical wound-edge malalignments are considerably harder to correct with continuous sutures. It is difficult or impossible to control tension on individual suture bites; therefore, the potential for tissue strangulation and necrosis is greater with sutures placed using a continuous technique.

  1. Simple over-and-over sutures (Fig. 38-31) represent the most common continuous technique used for repair of deep-tissue layers. They may also be used for skin closure in some instances.

    a. Indications

       (1) Closure of wounds when decreased operative time is desirable.

       (2) Skin closure in wounds without longitudinal or vertical discrepancies.

       (3) Skin closure when suture marks are inconsequential (e.g., scalp wounds).

       (4) Closure of deep-tissue layers in a wound (e.g., muscle fascia).

    b. Contraindications

       (1) Wounds requiring realignment of longitudinal or vertical marginal discrepancies (e.g., most skin closures).

       (2) Wound margins with decreased vascularity of one or both edges.

       (3) Wounds requiring obliteration of dead space plus precise skin alignment, using only a single-layer skin closure.

       (4) Wounds with a high likelihood of becoming infected.

    c. Method

       (1) At one end of the wound, the needle enters the skin at an angle of 90 degrees or greater 1–3 mm from the edge on the first side, including sufficient subcutaneous tissue in the bite to cause eversion of the raw interface.

       (2) Directly opposite the point of exit on the first side, the needle passes through a comparable amount of subcutaneous tissue on the second side (except when the wound edges are of unequal thickness) and then begins to angle back toward the wound edge so that the needle's exit through the skin on the second side is the same distance from the wound edge as its entry on the first side and at the same angle.

       (3) Most of the suture is pulled through the wound, the suture is tied in a secure knot, and only the end of the suture without the needle is cut, leaving a tail.

       (4) The needle reenters the skin on the first side at the same distance from the wound edge as the first bite, passing through the same thickness of subcutaneous tissue as the first bite at a 45-degree angle and several millimeters away from the tied first stitch.

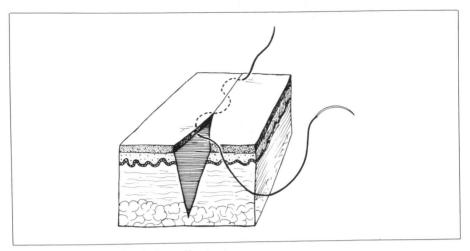

Fig. 38-32. Running subcuticular pull-out suture.

(5) The needle passes through a comparable amount of subcutaneous tissue directly opposite on the second side and then exits the skin at the same distance from the wound edge as on the first side.

(6) The entire length of the suture is pulled through the wound, and mild tension is held on it as successive sutures are placed.

(7) The needle then reenters the skin on the first side at a 45-degree angle and several millimeters away from the last skin suture loop, maintaining the same distance from the wound edge as before.

(8) The above steps are repeated until the other end of the wound is reached (or until termination of the continuous suture is desired).

(9) A knot is tied between the remaining suture end attached to the needle and the last skin suture loop, which is left long enough to permit an instrument tie. All suture ends are then cut, leaving a tail.

(10) To equalize wound margins of unequal thickness (not very precise using this technique), suture bites must be more superficial on the raised edge and deeper on the depressed edge.

d. **Complications**

(1) A greater chance for suture-mark scars to occur.

(2) Depressed scars from failure to adequately evert the skin edges.

(3) Puckering of the wound margins from imprecise suture placement.

2. **Subcuticular (intradermal) sutures** (Fig. 38-32) are excellent for producing precise skin-edge approximation. They may be left in place longer than other sutures, because the risk of leaving suture marks has been virtually eliminated. They may also be left in place permanently (with buried knots at both ends), but the pull-out technique is preferred. Prolene of 3-0, 4-0, or 5-0 caliber (depending on the wound location) is the suture material of choice for the pull-out technique, because its tensile strength and smoothness make it the suture least likely to break when it is removed.

a. **Indications**

(1) Skin closure under tension (so the sutures can be left in place for 2–3 weeks).

(2) Skin closure in children (because of the ease of removal).

b. **Contraindications**

(1) Wounds with a high likelihood of becoming infected (e.g., animal-bite lacerations).

(2) Wounds in which the skin closure must correct longitudinal and major vertical discrepancies of the margins.

(3) Wounds in which the skin closure must also obliterate dead space between underlying tissue layers.

(4) Triangular or stellate wounds.

(5) Short wounds.

    c. Method (pull-out technique)

        (1) The needle penetrates the skin vertically 2–5 mm distal to the corner of one end of the wound, passes through dermis only, and exits from the dermis 2–3 mm from the corner on the first side.

        (2) The needle passes horizontally for a distance of 2–5 mm through dermis only on the second side, entering 1–2 mm proximal (closer to the wound corner just entered) to the exit point on the first side, and entering and exiting at the same depth on the second side as the exit point on the first side.

        (3) The needle then passes horizontally through the dermis on alternating sides of the wound for 2- to 5-mm distances each time, keeping the entry and exit sites at the same depth and backing up the entry point of each bite 1–2 mm to prevent the entry and exit sites from being directly opposite each other.

        (4) The gliding ability of the suture must be checked frequently. If gliding decreases significantly, the suture should be brought through the skin at that point. The same suture (leaving a redundant loop) may be used to continue the running subcuticular suture, or a new suture may be started. In either case, the needle should enter the skin directly opposite the point of exit of the previous suture, and the running subcuticular suture is continued as described in the preceding steps. If gliding of the suture ceases completely, the suture (and needle) must be backed out until gliding returns. **A running subcuticular suture that does not glide at the time of wound closure will not glide at the time of suture removal.**

        (5) When the opposite wound corner is reached, the needle passes vertically from the dermis through the skin 2–5 mm distal to the corner.

        (6) The suture ends may be taped to the skin under moderate tension, with the tails long enough (e.g., several centimeters) to prevent retraction beneath the skin; tied together in a large, fairly loose loop; or individually knotted on the skin surface.

        (7) The skin approximation is frequently reinforced with tapes or interrupted simple sutures.

        (8) To equalize skin edges with minor vertical discrepancies using this technique, the dermal bites must be more superficial on the raised edge and deeper on the depressed edge.

    d. Complications

        (1) Failure to maintain skin coaptation with loss of tension on the suture.

        (2) Failure to coapt skin edges adequately due to improper suture placement.

        (3) Breakage of suture material during suture removal.

  3. Other continuous suture techniques include vertical, horizontal, and half-buried horizontal mattress and simple running locked (blanket stitch) sutures. All produce significant amounts of tissue strangulation and necrosis. Therefore, their use is rarely, if ever, indicated.

III. Suture care. Most skin sutures should be covered with a firm bandage of appropriate size for approximately 24 hours to absorb minor amounts of blood or drainage. After removal of the bandage, suture-line care should begin. This care consists of cleaning sutures one or more times/day with diluted hydrogen peroxide, using a cotton-tipped applicator to remove dry crusts. A thin layer of a topical antibiotic ointment (e.g., Polysporin) should then be applied to the suture line. Bandages should be reapplied only if necessary to prevent contamination or repeated trauma to the area. Although it is wise to admonish patients to keep sutures dry (because the water's wicking effect can introduce bacteria along suture tracts), this is often impractical and sometimes ill-advised (e.g., the bacterial population of unwashed hair can multiply rapidly). It is better to instruct patients to keep sutures as clean as possible (regardless of the method) and dry them carefully if they do get wet.

IV. Suture removal. Sutures removed at or before 7 days leave no appreciable permanent skin marks. Sutures left in the skin 14 days or longer leave significant skin suture marks. Sutures tied under tension constrict the skin and cause necrosis, which in turn causes scarring and deformity. To avoid additional scarring from suture marks, these factors must be considered in determining the length of time skin sutures should be left in place, although tension should have been considered at the time of wound closure and appropriate action taken (e.g., reduction of tension on skin sutures with judiciously placed buried sutures or use of a pull-out running subcuticular suture for skin closure). For practical purposes, skin suture removal is chiefly dependent on the wound location.

A. Eyelid sutures are removed within 5 days to prevent epithelialization of suture tracts and formation of small inclusion cysts (milia).

B. Facial sutures are removed at 5–7 days.

C. Scalp, neck, and **trunk** sutures are removed at 7–10 days.

D. Extremity sutures are removed at 10–14 days.

E. Running subcuticular pull-out sutures can be left in place 2–3 weeks and can alter the time of suture removal in any of the above areas.

V. Nonsuture techniques of skin closure. Microporous surgical adhesive tape (Steri-Strip) or stainless-steel skin staples or clips are occasionally indicated for skin closure in emergency department procedures.

A. Tapes are available as ¼-in. to ½-in. wide sterile strips. They are placed across the wound edges perpendicular to the longitudinal axis of the wound, with or without the use of skin glue (e.g., Benzoin). Their advantages include easier application and removal than sutures, little or no skin reaction, no possibility of suture marks (although blistering under tapes may result in minor skin scars), the ability to be left in place for long periods of time under dressings or casts, and the ability to be applied without an anesthetic. Their disadvantages include failure to produce eversion of skin edges; failure to correct malalignment of skin edges; failure to adhere to oily or moist skin, hirsute areas, or areas of constant motion (e.g., lips, neck); and failure to stay in place reliably (e.g., they usually come loose when bathing or with any wound bleeding or drainage and are easily removed prematurely by children or uncooperative patients). They are used most frequently to reinforce skin approximation after skin suture removal or when running subcuticular sutures are used.

B. Skin staples and clips are loaded in a magazine and inserted with an applicator that makes application fairly rapid. They are made of stainless steel and therefore produce minimal skin reaction. They are removed with a special clip remover or the point of a small hemostat, either of which spreads the points of the clip and lifts it from the skin. Use of skin clips requires an assistant who must hold the skin edges with forceps to evert them. Despite this, inversion, rather than eversion, of skin edges frequently occurs, resulting in a wider, depressed skin scar. Patients frequently find them unaesthetic. They are rarely indicated for skin closure in emergency department procedures.

Bibliography

1. Alyono, D., and Perry, J. F. Value of quantitative cell count and amylase activity of peritoneal lavage fluid. *J. Trauma* 21:345, 1981.
2. Anderson, J. E. *Grant's Atlas of Anatomy* (7th ed.). Baltimore: Williams & Wilkins, 1978.
3. Baker, C. C., Thomas, A. N., and Trunkey, D. D. The role of emergency room thoracotomy in trauma. *J. Trauma* 20:848, 1980.
4. Bircher, N., Safar, P., and Stewart, R. A comparison of standard, "MAST" augmented, and open-chest CPR in dogs. *Crit. Care Med.* 8:147, 1980.
5. Bivins, H. G., et al. Blood volume displacement with inflation of antishock trousers. *Ann. Emerg. Med.* 11:409, 1982.
6. Bodai, B. I., et al. Emergency thoracotomy in the management of trauma. A review. *J.A.M.A.* 249:1891, 1983.
7. Converse, J. M. Introduction to Plastic Surgery. In J. M. Converse (ed.), *Reconstructive Plastic Surgery* (2nd ed.). Philadelphia: Saunders, 1977.
8. Cordell, W. H., Nugent, S. K., and Ehrenwerth, J. Using neuromuscular blocking agents to facilitate tracheal intubation. *Emerg. Med. Reports* 5:141, 1984.
9. Crikelair, G. F. Skin suture marks. *Am. J. Surg.* 96:631, 1958.
10. Crikelair, G. F., Ju, D. M. C., and Cosman, B. Scars and Keloids. In J. M. Converse (ed.), *Reconstructive Plastic Surgery* (2nd ed.). Philadelphia: Saunders, 1977.
11. Dannewitz, S. R., Lilja, G. P., and Ruiz, E. Effect of pneumatic trousers on intracranial pressure in hypovolemic dogs with an intracranial mass. *Ann. Emerg. Med.* 10:176, 1981.
12. Davidson, S. J. Correct use of autotransfusion in the emergency patient. *E.R. Reports* 2:73, 1981.
13. Dronon, S. C., et al. Proximal saphenous vein cutdown. *Ann. Emerg. Med.* 10:328, 1981.

14. Dunlap, L. B. A modified, simple device for the emergency administration of percutaneous transtracheal ventilation *J.A.C.E.P.* 7:42, 1978.
15. DuPriest, R. W., Jr., et al. A technique for open diagnostic peritoneal lavage. *Surg. Gynecol. Obstet.* 147:241, 1978.
16. Fischer, R. P., et al. Diagnostic peritoneal lavage. Fourteen years and 2,586 patients later. *Am. J. Surg.* 136:701, 1978.
17. Flint, L. M., et al. Definitive control of bleeding from severe pelvic fractures. *Ann. Surg.* 189:709, 1979.
18. Freeman, T., and Fischer, R. P. The inadequacy of peritoneal lavage in diagnosing acute diaphragmatic rupture. *J. Trauma* 16:538, 1976.
19. Gaffney, F. A., et al. Hemodynamic effects of medical anti-shock trousers (MAST garment). *J. Trauma* 21:931, 1981.
20. Gatter, R. A. *A Practical Handbook of Joint Fluid Analysis.* Philadelphia: Lea & Febiger, 1984.
21. Grabb, W. C. Basic Techniques of Plastic Surgery. In W. C. Grabb and J. W. Smith (eds.), *Plastic Surgery* (3rd ed.). Boston: Little, Brown, 1979.
22. Gray, R. G., and Gottlieb, N. L. Corticosteroid injections in RA: How to get the best results. *J. Musculo. Med.* 1:48, 1984.
23. Grossman, J. A. *Minor Injuries and Disorders: Surgical and Medical Care.* Philadelphia: Lippincott, 1984.
24. Hollinshead, W. H. *Anatomy for Surgeons: Volume 1. The Head and Neck* (2nd ed.). New York: Hoeber Medical Division, Harper and Row, 1968.
25. Hubbard, S. G., et al. Diagnostic errors with peritoneal lavage in patients with pelvic fractures. *Arch. Surg.* 114:844, 1979.
26. Iserson, K. V. Blind nasotracheal intubation. *Ann. Emerg. Med.* 10:468, 1981.
27. Jacobs, H. B. Emergency percutaneous transtracheal catheter and ventilator. *J. Trauma* 12:50, 1972.
28. Jacobs, H. B., Smyth, N. P., and Witorsch, P. Transtracheal catheter ventilation: Clinical experience in 36 patients. *Chest* 65:36, 1974.
29. Jacobs, L. M., and Hsieh, J. W. A clinical review of autotransfusion and its role in trauma. *J.A.M.A.* 251:3283, 1984.
30. Kaback, K. R., Sanders, A. B., and Meislin, H. W. MAST suit update. *J.A.M.A* 252:2598, 1984.
31. Klebinoff, G., Phillips, J., and Evans, W. Use of a disposable autotransfusion unit under varying conditions of contamination. *Am. J. Surg.* 120:351, 1970.
32. Knopp, R. Venous cutdowns in the emergency department. *J.A.C.E.P.* 7:439, 1978.
33. Knopp, R., and Dailey, R. H. Central venous cannulation and pressure monitoring. *J.A.C.E.P.* 6:358, 1977.
34. Kress, T. D., and Balasubramanian, S. Cricothyroidotomy. *Ann. Emerg. Med.* 11:197, 1982.
35. Kuhn, G. J., et al. Peripheral or central circulation times during CPR: A pilot study. *Ann. Emerg. Med.* 10:417, 1981.
36. Lee, H. R., et al. MAST augmentation of external cardiac compression: Role of changing intrapleural pressure. *Ann. Emerg. Med.* 10:560, 1981.
37. Levinson, M. M., et al. Emergency percutaneous transtracheal ventilation (PTV). *J.A.C.E.P.* 8:396, 1979.
38. Mahoney, B. D., and Mirick, M. J. Efficacy of pneumatic trousers in refractory prehospital cardiopulmonary arrest. *Ann. Emerg. Med.* 12:8, 1983.
39. Matsen, F. A., III. *Compartmental Syndromes.* New York: Grune & Stratton, 1980.
40. McCabe, J. B., Niemann, J. T., and Wasserberger, J. New concepts concerning pneumatic antishock trousers. *Emerg. Med. Reports* 5:85, 1984.
41. McGill, J., et al. Cricothyrotomy in the emergency department. *Ann. Emerg. Med.* 11:361, 1982.
42. McIntyre, K. M., and Lewis, A. J. *Textbook of Advanced Cardiac Life Support.* Dallas: American Heart Association, 1983.
43. Moore, E. E., et al. Mandatory laparotomy for gunshot wounds penetrating the abdomen. *Am. J. Surg.* 140:847, 1980.
44. Moore, J. B., et al. Diagnostic peritoneal lavage for abdominal trauma: Superiority of the open technique at the infraumbilical ring. *J. Trauma* 21:570, 1981.
45. Mueller, G. L., Burney, R. E., and Mackenzie, J. R. Sequential peritoneal lavage and early diagnosis of colon perforation. *Ann. Emerg. Med.* 10:131, 1981.
46. Murphy, T. M. Nerve Blocks. In R. D. Miller (ed.), *Anesthesia.* New York: Churchill Livingstone, 1981.

47. Natanson, C., Shelhamer, J. H., and Parrillo, J. E. Intubation of the trachea in the critical care setting. *J.A.M.A.* 253:1160, 1985.
48. Nieman, J. T., et al. Hemodynamic effects of pneumatic external counterpressure in canine hemorrhagic shock. *Ann. Emerg. Med.* 12:661, 1983.
49. Pachter, H. L., and Hofstetter, S. R. Open and percutaneous paracentesis and lavage for abdominal trauma. *Arch. Surg.* 116:318, 1981.
50. Palafox, B. A., et al. ICP changes following application of the MAST suit. *J. Trauma* 21:55, 1981.
51. Pelligra, R., and Sandberg, E. C. Control of intractable abdominal bleeding by external pressure. *J.A.M.A.* 241:708, 1979.
52. Pointer, J. Utilizing nasotracheal intubation to full potential. *E.R. Reports* 3:143, 1982.
53. Ransom, K., and McSwain, N. E. Respiratory function following application of MAST trousers. *J.A.C.E.P.* 7:15, 1978.
54. Salem, M. R., Mathrubhutham, M., and Bennett, E. J. Current concepts. Difficult intubation. *N. Engl. J. Med.* 295:879, 1976.
55. Simon, R. R., and Brenner, B. E. *Procedures and Techniques in Emergency Medicine.* Baltimore: Williams and Wilkins, 1982.
56. Smith, R. N., Yaw, P. B., and Glover, J. L. Autotransfusion of contaminated intraperitoneal blood: An experimental study. *J. Trauma* 18:341, 1978.
57. Spoerel, W. E., Narayanan, P. S., and Singh, N. P. Transtracheal ventilation. *Br. J. Anaesth.* 43:932, 1971.
58. Stinson, T. W. A simple connector for transtracheal ventilation. *Anesthesiology* 47:232, 1977.
59. Swanson, R. S., et al. Emergency intravenous access through the femoral vein. *Ann. Emerg. Med.* 13:244, 1984.
60. Talbert, J., Gruenberg, J. C., and Brown, R. S. Peritoneal lavage in penetrating thoracic trauma. *J. Trauma* 20:979, 1980.
61. Taryle, D. A., et al. Emergency room intubations—complications and survival. *Chest* 75:541, 1979.
62. Thal, E. R. Evaluation of peritoneal lavage and local exploration in lower chest and abdominal stab wounds. *J. Trauma* 17:642, 1977.
63. Thal, E. R., May, R. A., and Bessinger, D. Peritoneal lavage. Its unreliability in gunshot wounds of the lower chest and abdomen. *Arch. Surg.* 115:430, 1980.
64. Thompson, J. D., Fish, S., and Ruiz, E. Succinylcholine for endotracheal intubation. *Ann. Emerg. Med.* 11:526, 1982.
65. Thompson, J. S., et al. The evolution of abdominal stab wound management. *J. Trauma* 20:478, 1980.
66. Thurer, R. L., and Hauer, J. M. Autotransfusion and blood conservation. *Curr. Probl. Surg.* 19:98, 1982.
67. Tibbs, P. A., et al. Diagnosis of acute abdominal injuries in patients with spinal shock: Value of diagnostic peritoneal lavage. *J. Trauma* 20:55, 1980.
68. Tintinalli, J. E., and Claffey, J. Complications of nasotracheal intubation. *Ann. Emerg. Med.* 10:142, 1981.
69. Vij, D., et al. The importance of the WBC count in peritoneal lavage. *J.A.M.A.* 249:636, 1983.
70. Walt, A. J. (ed.). *Early Care of the Injured Patient* (3rd ed.). Philadelphia: Saunders, 1982.
71. Wayne, M. A., and Macdonald, S. C. Clinical evaluation of the antishock trouser: Retrospective analysis of five years of experience. *Ann. Emerg. Med.* 12:342, 1983.
72. Weeks, P. M. *Acute Bone and Joint Injuries of the Hand and Wrist. A Clinical Guide to Management.* St. Louis: Mosby, 1981.
73. Westreich, M. Preventing complications of subclavian vein catheterization. *J.A.C.E.P.* 7:368, 1978.
74. Whitesides, T. E., Jr., et al. Tissue pressure measurements as a determinant for the need of fasciotomy. *Clin. Orthop.* 113:43, 1975.
75. Young, G. P., and Purcell, T. B. Emergency autotransfusion. *Ann. Emerg. Med.* 12:180, 1983.

Appendixes

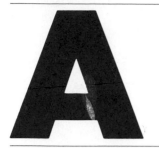

Nomogram for Estimation of Surface Area

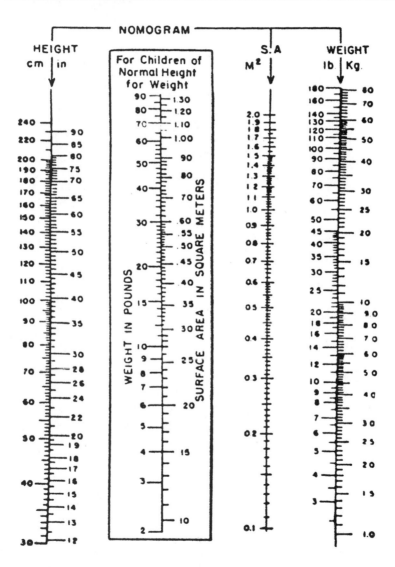

Appendix A. Nomogram for estimation of surface area (SA). The surface area is determined by the intersection of the surface area column and a straight line connecting the patient's height and weight. Alternatively, for children of normal height and weight, the surface area can be estimated from the patient's weight alone. (Nomogram modified from data of E. Boyd by C. D. West. From R. E. Behrman and V. C. Vaughan III (eds.), *Nelson Textbook of Pediatrics* (12th ed.). Philadelphia: Saunders, 1983. Pg. 1814. With permission.)

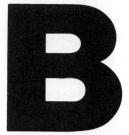

Infusion Rates in Adults of Select Cardiovascular Medications

Table B-1. Dopamine hydrochloride (Intropin) (800 mg/500 ml = 1600 µg/ml)

Dosage (µg/kg/min)	Body weight												
	88 / 40	99 / 45	110 / 50	121 / 55	132 / 60	143 / 65	154 / 70	165 / 75	176 / 80	187 / 85	198 / 90	209 / 95	220 / 100 lb / kg
1.0	2	2	2	2	2	2	3	3	3	3	3	4	4
2.5	4	4	5	5	6	6	7	7	8	8	8	9	9
5.0	8	8	9	10	11	12	13	14	15	16	17	18	19
7.5	11	13	14	15	17	18	20	21	23	24	25	27	28
10.0	15	17	19	21	23	24	26	28	30	32	34	36	38
15.0	23	25	28	31	34	37	39	42	45	48	51	53	56
20.0	30	34	38	41	45	49	52	56	60	64	68	71	75
25.0	38	42	47	52	56	61	66	70	75	80	84	89	94
30.0	45	51	56	62	67	73	78	84	90	96	101	107	113
35.0	53	59	66	72	79	85	92	98	105	112	118	125	131
40.0	60	68	75	83	90	98	105	113	120	128	135	143	150
45.0	68	76	84	93	101	110	118	127	135	143	152	160	169
50.0	75	84	94	103	113	122	131	141	150	159	169	178	188

Infusion rate: microdrops/min = ml/hr (60 microdrops/ml)

Table B-2. Dobutamine hydrochloride (Dobutrex) (250 mg/250 ml = 1000 µg/ml)

Dosage (µg/kg/min)	Body weight												
lb	88	99	110	121	132	143	154	165	176	187	198	209	220
kg	40	45	50	55	60	65	70	75	80	85	90	95	100
1.0	2	3	3	3	4	4	4	5	5	5	5	6	6
2.5	6	7	8	8	9	10	11	11	12	13	14	14	15
5.0	12	14	15	17	18	20	21	23	24	26	27	29	30
7.5	18	20	23	25	27	29	32	34	36	38	41	43	45
10.0	24	27	30	33	36	39	42	45	48	51	54	57	60
12.5	30	34	38	41	45	49	53	56	60	64	68	71	75
15.0	36	41	45	50	54	59	63	68	72	77	81	86	90
20.0	48	54	60	66	72	78	84	90	96	102	108	114	120
30.0	72	81	90	99	108	117	126	135	144	153	162	171	180
40.0	96	108	120	132	144	156	168	180	192	204	216	228	240

Infusion rate:
microdrops/min = ml/hr
(60 microdrops/ml)

Table B-3. Sodium nitroprusside (Nipride) (50 mg/250 ml = 200 µg/ml)

Dosage (µg/kg/min)	Body weight												
lb	88	99	110	121	132	143	154	165	176	187	198	209	220
kg	40	45	50	55	60	65	70	75	80	85	90	95	100
0.5	6	7	8	8	9	10	11	11	12	13	14	14	15
1.0	12	14	15	17	18	20	21	23	24	26	27	29	30
2.0	24	27	30	33	36	39	42	45	48	51	54	57	60
3.0	36	41	45	50	54	59	63	68	72	77	81	86	90
4.0	48	54	60	66	72	78	84	90	96	102	108	114	120
5.0	60	68	75	83	90	98	105	113	120	128	135	143	150
6.0	72	81	90	99	108	117	126	135	144	153	162	171	180
7.0	84	95	105	116	126	137	147	158	168	179	189	200	210
8.0	96	108	120	132	144	156	168	180	192	204	216	228	240
9.0	108	122	135	149	162	176	189	203	216	230	243	257	270
10.0	120	135	150	165	180	195	210	225	240	255	270	285	300

Infusion rate:
microdrops/min = ml/hr
(60 microdrops/ml)

Table B-4. Nitroglycerin (Tridil) (25 mg/250 ml = 50 mg/500 ml = 100 μg/ml)

Dosage (μg/min)	Infusion rate microdrops/min = ml/hr (60 microdrops/ml)
5	3
10	6
20	12
30	18
40	24
50	30
60	36
70	42
80	48
90	54
100	60
110	66
120	72
130	78
140	84
150	90
160	96
170	102
180	108
190	114
200	120

Table B-5. Isoproterenol (Isuprel) (2 mg/250 ml = 8 μg/ml)

Dosage (μg/min)	Infusion rate microdrops/min = ml/hr (60 microdrops/ml)
1	8
2	15
4	30
6	45
8	60
10	75
12	90
16	120
20	150

Table B-6. Norepinephrine (Levophed) (4 mg/250 ml = 16 μg/ml)

Dosage (μg/min)	Infusion rate microdrops/min = ml/hr (60 microdrops/ml)
1	4
2	8
4	15
6	23
8	30
10	38
12	45
16	60
20	75
24	90
28	105

Table B-7. Lidocaine (2 gm/500 ml = 4 mg/ml)

Dosage (mg/min)	Infusion rate microdrops/min = ml/hr (60 microdrops/ml)
1	15
2	30
3	45
4	60

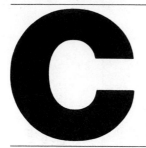

Infusion Rates in Children of Select Cardiovascular Medications

Table C-1. Epinephrine or isoproterenol (Isuprel), or norepinephrine (Levophed) (2 mg/100 ml = 20 μg/ml)

Infusion rate: microdrops/min = ml/hr (60 microdrops/ml)

Dosage (μg/kg/min)	Body weight															
lb	4	9	11	13	18	22	26	31	33	35	40	44	55	66	77	88
kg	2	4	5	6	8	10	12	14	15	16	18	20	25	30	35	40
0.1	1	1	2	2	2	3	4	4	5	5	5	6	8	9	11	12
0.2	1	2	3	4	5	6	7	8	9	10	11	12	15	18	21	24
0.4	2	5	6	7	10	12	14	17	18	19	22	24	30	36	42	48
0.5	3	6	8	9	12	15	18	21	23	24	27	30	38	45	53	60
0.6	4	7	9	11	14	18	22	25	27	29	32	36	45	54	63	72
0.8	5	10	12	14	19	24	29	34	36	38	43	48	60	72	84	96
1.0	6	12	15	18	24	30	36	42	45	48	54	60	75	90	105	120

Table C-2. Dopamine hydrochloride (Intropin) (40 mg/100 ml = 400 μg/ml)

Infusion rate: microdrops/min = ml/hr (60 microdrops/ml)

Dosage (μg/kg/min)	Body weight															
lb	4	9	11	13	18	22	26	31	33	35	40	44	55	66	77	88
kg	2	4	5	6	8	10	12	14	15	16	18	20	25	30	35	40
2.0	1	1	2	2	2	3	4	4	5	5	5	6	8	9	11	12
5.0	2	3	4	5	6	8	9	11	11	12	14	15	19	23	26	30
7.5	2	5	6	7	9	11	14	16	17	18	20	23	28	34	39	45
10.0	3	6	8	9	12	15	18	21	23	24	27	30	38	45	53	60
12.5	4	8	9	11	15	19	23	26	28	30	34	38	47	56	66	75
15.0	5	9	11	14	18	23	27	32	34	36	41	45	56	68	79	90
17.5	5	11	13	16	21	26	32	37	39	46	47	53	66	79	92	105
20.0	6	12	15	18	24	30	36	42	45	48	54	60	75	90	105	120

Table C-3. Dobutamine hydrochloride (Dobutrex) (250 mg/500 ml = 500 µg/ml)

Dosage (µg/kg/min)	lb / kg																
	4 / 2	9 / 4	11 / 5	13 / 6	18 / 8	22 / 10	26 / 12	31 / 14	33 / 15	35 / 16	40 / 18	44 / 20	55 / 25	66 / 30	77 / 35	88 / 40
2.5	1	1	2	2	2	3	4	4	5	5	5	6	8	9	11	12
5.0	1	2	3	4	5	6	7	8	9	10	11	12	15	18	21	24
7.5	2	4	5	5	7	9	11	13	14	14	16	18	23	27	32	36
10.0	2	5	6	7	10	12	14	17	18	19	22	24	30	36	42	48
12.5	3	6	8	9	12	15	18	21	23	24	27	30	38	45	53	60
15.0	4	7	9	11	14	18	22	25	27	29	32	36	45	54	63	72
20.0	5	10	12	14	19	24	29	34	36	38	43	48	60	72	84	96

Body weight

Infusion rate:
microdrops/min = ml/hr
(60 microdrops/ml)

Table C-4. Lidocaine (100 mg/100 ml = 1000 µg/ml)

Dosage (µg/kg/min)	lb / kg																
	4 / 2	9 / 4	11 / 5	13 / 6	18 / 8	22 / 10	26 / 12	31 / 14	33 / 15	35 / 16	40 / 18	44 / 20	55 / 25	66 / 30	77 / 35	88 / 40
20	2	5	6	7	10	12	14	17	18	19	22	24	26	36	42	48
30	4	7	9	11	14	18	22	25	27	29	32	36	40	54	63	72
40	5	10	12	14	19	24	29	34	36	38	43	48	53	72	84	96
50	6	12	15	18	24	30	36	42	45	48	54	60	66	90	105	120

Body weight

Infusion rate:
microdrops/min = ml/hr
(60 microdrops/ml)

Index

Index